Mucocutaneous Manifestations of

VIRAL DISEASES

Compliments of

3M Pharmaceuticals

Mucocutaneous Manifestations of
VIRAL DISEASES

edited by

Stephen K. Tyring

*University of Texas Medical Branch
Galveston, and
University of Texas Medical Branch
Center for Clinical Studies
Houston, Texas, USA*

Associate Editor

Angela Yen-Moore

*University of Texas Southwestern Medical Center
Dallas, Texas, USA*

MARCEL DEKKER, INC.   NEW YORK · BASEL

ISBN: 0-8247-0450-9

This book is printed on acid-free paper.

Headquarters
Marcel Dekker, Inc.
270 Madison Avenue, New York, NY 10016
tel: 212-696-9000; fax: 212-685-4540

Eastern Hemisphere Distribution
Marcel Dekker AG
Hutgasse 4, Postfach 812, CH-4001 Basel, Switzerland
tel: 41-61-261-8482; fax: 41-61-261-8896

World Wide Web
http://www.dekker.com

The publisher offers discounts on this book when ordered in bulk quantities. For more information, write to Special Sales/Professional Marketing at the headquarters address above.

PRINTED IN THE UNITED STATES OF AMERICA

Preface

The skin is the window of the body. Many viral diseases express themselves through changes in skin appearance, eruptions on the skin, swelling, and so forth. Often the skin becomes a warning of internal manifestations signaling the physician to look beyond the window for other impacts. The contributors to *Mucocutaneous Manifestations of Viral Diseases* interact on a regular basis with other dermatologists and virologists, or combinations thereof. The book is an outgrowth of those daily consultations and discussions with other colleagues in various fields of medicine. As family practitioners are increasingly being called upon to provide the diagnosis and treatment of a wider variety of illnesses (those previously referred to a specialist), a quick reference is needed. This book not only helps distinguish the cutaneous manifestations of one virus from another, but also helps differentiate viral diseases from other infectious and noninfectious diseases. It is intended for internists, dermatologists, pediatricians, and family practitioners worldwide.

The goal of this book is to enhance the expertise of physicians in the diagnosis, treatment, and pathogenesis of viral diseases that express their presence in the skin and its affiliated membranes. No other text currently addresses the issues of the skin manifestations of viral diseases. Photographs to aid diagnoses are usually black and white and of limited use to the physician. Many color atlases only encompass one or a few viral diseases, leaving the practitioner with a desire for more detail and/or a better explanation of possible mimics of the diseases.

The contributing authors and I have provided a text that serves as a central resource for each of the viral diseases described. It should be of interest to physicians worldwide as we have included many diseases previously known only in third-world, developing countries. Given the global aspects of international transportation, social exchange, and political boundaries, it is entirely feasible that one or more of these rarer viral diseases could present itself at any physician's office in the world. Animal vectors and reservoirs are often immigrants on baggage or agricultural products. Each chapter includes, as appropriate, a timeline of infection and progress of the disease, numerous quality color illustrations of characteristic epidermal and cellular manifestations, a means to reference the differential diagnosis of viral diseases from other infectious or noninfectious diseases, a brief taxonomy and history of the disease, incidence among gender and age groups by geographical region, pathogenesis, clinical manifestations, dermatopathology, laboratory findings, differential diagnosis, and treatment/prophylaxis. To the extent possible, we have used tabular information for quick reference by the physician.

Mucocutaneous Manifestations of Viral Diseases is unique in that it covers the field of viral diseases having mucocutaneous manifestations and offers the quality color photographs associated with an atlas. The book also serves as a bibliography for physicians wishing to broaden their knowledge of the primary literature. I envision the physician using the color photographs in considering possible diagnoses. The differential diagnosis section helps the physician narrow the search for the virus causing the epidermal insult. The text would then provide suggestions as to which laboratory tests might be useful to confirm diagnosis. Finally, it outlines the appropriate treatment, including specific types of antiviral drugs and vaccines.

In summary, it is hoped that the book will fill a void in the medical literature and provide a valuable resource to a variety of practicing physicians worldwide.

ACKNOWLEDGMENTS

Publication of this book would not have been possible without the combined efforts of many individuals. Therefore, I wish to thank the contributors for writing, rewriting, and updating their manuscripts. Likewise, I wish to thank my colleagues on six continents for contributing quality photographs of the clinical manifestations of viral diseases. I deeply appreciate the efforts of the following individuals in their extremely valuable roles:

Charlene Hoff for typing and retyping the manuscripts;
Linda Roberts for helping to coordinate the efforts of many individuals;
Tricia J. Brown, M.D., for assuring the scientific integrity of the text;
Nancy Bell, Ph.D., for all aspects of the editing and production process; and
Angela Yen-Moore, M.D., for proofreading the entire text and helping to rewrite chapters for consistency and clinical accuracy.

Most of all, I wish to thank my wife, Patricia Lee, M.D., for her support, encouragement, and dedication throughout the long journey that led to the publication of *Mucocutaneous Manifestations of Viral Diseases*.

Stephen K. Tyring

Contents

Preface   *iii*
Contributors   *vii*

1. Cutaneous Virology   1
   Stephen K. Tyring

2. Cutaneous Resistance to Viral Infections   25
   Omeed M. Memar, Pedram Geraminejad,
   Istvan Arany, and Stephen K. Tyring

3. Poxviruses   39
   Dayna G. Diven

4. Herpes Simplex Virus   69
   Richard J. Whitley and John W. Gnann, Jr.

5. Varicella-Zoster Virus (Herpes 3)   119
   Monica McCrary, Tricia J. Brown, and
   Stephen K. Tyring

6. Epstein-Barr Virus   145
   Dennis M. Walling, Angela Yen-Moore, and
   S. David Hudnall

7. Cytomegalovirus   173
   Istvan Boldogh, Janak A. Patel, Stephen K.
   Tyring, and Tasnee Chonmaitree

8. Human Herpesvirus 6   197
   Samuel A. Shube, Andrea M. Dominey, and
   Tricia J. Brown

9. Human Herpesvirus 7   213
   Tricia J. Brown and Angela Yen-Moore

10. Human Herpesvirus 8   219
    Tricia J. Brown, Angela Yen-Moore,
    and Stephen K. Tyring

11. Herpes B Virus   235
    Paul Rockley and Stephen K. Tyring

12. Human Papillomaviruses   247
    Claire P. Mansur

13. Parvovirus B19   295
    Karen Wiss and Tricia J. Brown

14. Cutaneous Manifestations of HIV Infection   307
    Clay J. Cockerell and Philip R. Cohen

15. Colorado Tick Fever   397
    Michael R. Weir and Tracey E. Weir

16. Measles   403
    Vera Y. Soong and Tricia J. Brown

17. Marburg and Ebola Hemorrhagic Fevers   421
    Michael R. Weir and Tracey E. Weir

18. Bunyaviridae and Arenaviridae   429
    Michael R. Weir and Tracey E. Weir

19. Cutaneous Manifestations of Enterovirus
     Infections   455
     Wesley King Galen

20. Flaviviridae   473
     Michael R. Weir and Tracey E. Weir

21. Togaviridae   503
     Michael R. Weir and Tracey E. Weir

22. Rubella (German Measles)   519
     *Lourdes Tamayo, Edith Garcia-Gonzalez,
     and Tricia J. Brown*

23. Hepatitis Viruses   529
     *A. Michele Hill, Catherine C. Newman,
     Tricia J. Brown, and Sharon S. Raimer*

Index   *551*

Contributors

Istvan Arany, Ph.D.   Department of Internal Medicine, University of Arkansas School of Medicine, Little Rock, Arkansas, USA

Istvan Boldogh, D.M.&B., Ph.D.   Department of Microbiology and Immunology, University of Texas Medical Branch, Galveston, Texas, USA

Tricia J. Brown, M.D.   Department of Dermatology, University of Oklahoma Health Sciences Center, Oklahoma City, Oklahoma, USA

Tasnee Chonmaitree, M.D.   Departments of Pediatrics and Pathology, University of Texas Medical Branch, Galveston, Texas, USA

Clay J. Cockerell, M.D.   Departmant of Dermatology, University of Texas Southwestern Medical Center, Dallas, Texas, USA

Philip R. Cohen, M.D.   Department of Dermatology, University of Texas—Houston Medical School, Houston, Texas, USA

Dayna G. Diven, M.D.   Department of Dermatology, University of Texas Medical Branch, Galveston, Texas, USA

Andrea M. Dominey, M.D.   Rockwood Clinic, Spokane, Washington, USA

Wesley King Galen, M.D.   Clinical Faculty, Tulane University, New Orleans, and Louisiana State University School of Medicine, New Orleans, Louisiana, USA

Edith Garcia-Gonzalez, M.D.   Department of Dermatology, Instituto Nacional de Perinatología, Mexico City, Mexico

Pedram Geraminejad, M.D.   Department of Dermatology, University of Illinois at Chicago School of Medicine, Chicago, Illinois, USA

John W. Gnann, Jr., M.D.   Departments of Medicine and Microbiology, University of Alabama at Birmingham School of Medicine, Birmingham, Alabama, USA

A. Michelle Hill, M.D.   Division of Dermatology, Department of Medicine, Kansas University School of Medicine, Kansas City, Kansas, USA

S. David Hudnall, M.D.   Department of Pathology, University of Texas Medical Branch, Galveston, Texas, USA

Claire P. Mansur, M.D.   Department of Dermatology, Tufts University, Boston, and New England Medical Center, Boston, Massachusetts, USA

Monica McCrary, M.D.   Department of Dermatology, Medical College of Georgia, Augusta, Georgia, USA

Omeed M. Memar, M.D., Ph.D.   Academic Dermatology & Skin Care Institute, Chicago, Illinois, USA

Catherine C. Newman, M.D. Department of Dermatology, University of Texas Medical Branch, Galveston, Texas, USA

Janak A. Patel, M.D. Department of Pediatrics, University of Texas Medical Branch, Galveston, Texas, USA

Sharon S. Raimer, M.D. Departments of Dermatology and Pediatrics, University of Texas Medical Branch, Galveston, Texas, USA

Paul Rockley, M.D. Private Practice, Cosmetic, Laser, and Classic Dermatology, North Miami Beach, Florida, USA

Samuel A. Shube, M.D. Department of Radiology, Boca Raton Community Hospital, Boca Raton, Florida, USA

Vera Y. Soong, M.D. Department of Dermatology, University of Alabama at Birmingham School of Medicine, Birmingham, Alabama, USA

Lourdes Tamayo, M.D. Department of Dermatology, Instituto Nacional de Pediatría, Mexico City, Mexico

Stephen K. Tyring, M.D., Ph.D. Departments of Dermatology, Microbiology/Immunology, and Internal Medicine, University of Texas Medical Branch, Galveston, and University of Texas Medical Branch Center for Clinical Studies, Houston, Texas, USA

Dennis M. Walling, M.D. Department of Internal Medicine, University of Texas Medical Branch, Galveston, Texas, USA

Michael R. Weir, M.D. Department of Pediatrics, Scott and White Clinic and Memorial Hospital, Temple, Texas, USA

Tracey E. Weir, M.D. Department of Emergency Medicine, Brackenridge Hospital, Austin, Texas, USA

Richard J. Whitley, M.D. Departments of Pediatrics, Microbiology, and Medicine, University of Alabama at Birmingham School of Medicine, Birmingham, Alabama, USA

Karen Wiss, M.D. Department of Dermatology, University of Massachusetts Medical School, Worcester, Massachusetts, USA

Angela Yen-Moore, M.D. Department of Dermatology, University of Texas Southwestern Medical Center, Dallas, Texas, USA

1

Cutaneous Virology

Stephen K. Tyring

*University of Texas Medical Branch, Galveston, Texas, USA,
and University of Texas Medical Branch Center for Clinical Studies, Houston, Texas, USA*

Viral diseases may produce mucocutaneous manifestations either as the result of viral replication in the epidermis or as a secondary effect of viral replication elsewhere in the body. Most primary epidermal viral replications result from three groups of viruses: human papillomaviruses (HPV), herpesviruses, and poxviruses. Secondary skin lesions are produced by virus families such as retroviruses, paramyxoviruses, togaviruses, parvoviruses, and picornaviruses. Rhabdoviruses, rotavirus, reoviruses, and the like rarely induce skin lesions and are beyond the scope of this book. Likewise, the mucocutaneous manifestations, if any, of subviral agents, such as viroids and prions, have not been well described and are not discussed further.

A number of cutaneous diseases appear to be viral exanthemas, but no virus has been proved to be the etiologic agent in some of these diseases. For example, pityriasis rosea (PR) is an acute, self-limiting cutaneous eruption with a distinctive course. The initial lesion, the herald patch, is followed after 1 to 2 weeks by a generalized secondary rash that typically lasts about 6 weeks (Fig. 1–1). Like most viral infections, PR shows seasonal variability with an increased incidence in autumn and winter and a decreased incidence in summer. A preceding upper respiratory infection is often noted with PR, as are clusters of cases in time and space. Most recently, PR was hypothesized to be due to infection with human herpesvirus type 7 (HHV-7), but controlled studies have failed to support this hypothesis.

Likewise, asymmetrical periflexural exanthem of childhood (APEC) or unilateral laterothoracic exanthem (ULE)

is suspected to be of viral etiology. It presents in children 6 months to 5 years of age in winter and spring. The rash is unilateral on the trunk, often in the axillae or large flexures of the limbs (Figs. 1–2 and 1–3). It spreads centrifugally and to the contralateral side over 2 to 4 weeks and resolves in 6 weeks. Red, 3-mm papules appear first, followed by a scarlatiniform or eczematous rash. There are no constitutional symptoms, but an enlarged lymph node is usually observed at the primary site. Viruses that are suspected, but not proved to be of etiologic significance, include parainfluenza 2 or 3 and adenoviruses.

Conversely, several new viral diseases or viral diseases in new geographic areas have been described recently. These diseases include West Nile, Nipah, and Rift Valley fever viruses. When cutaneous manifestations of such viruses are reported, the description in the general medical literature rarely is more specific than "rash" or "skin rash." More specific descriptions in the dermatology literature might aid in the more rapid diagnosis of these diseases.

CLINICAL MANIFESTATIONS

Viral infections can result in a wide spectrum of skin lesions. HPV infection frequently results in verrucous papules, but the range of presentations includes erythematous macules in epidermodysplasia verruciformis, smooth papules in bowenoid papulosis, and fungating Buschke-Lowenstein tumors. The primary lesions in herpes simplex virus (HSV), varicella-zoster virus (VZV), and many cox-

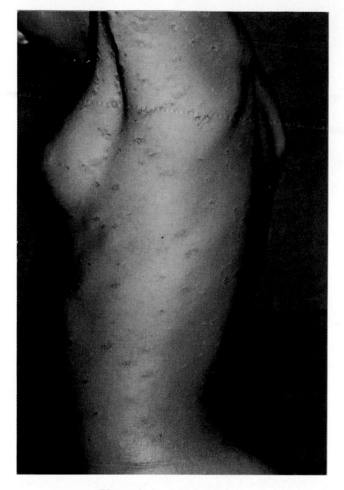

Figure 1–1. Pityriasis rosea.

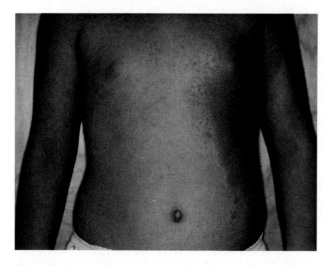

Figure 1–2. Asymmetrical periflexural exanthem of childhood (unilateral laterothoracic exanthem). (Courtesy of Karen Wiss, M.D., Dermatology Division, University of Massachusetts, Worcester, MA.)

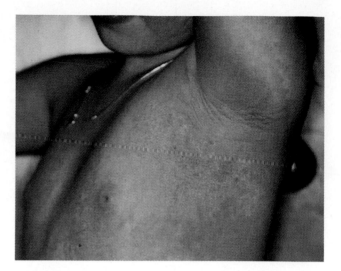

Figure 1–3. Asymmetrical periflexural exanthem of childhood (unilateral laterothoracic exanthem). (Courtesy of Karen Wiss, M.D., Dermatology Division, University of Massachusetts, Worcester, MA.)

sackievirus infections are vesicles. Erythema and papules often precede the vesicles, which are followed by pustules, crusts, or shallow ulcers. Cytomegalovirus (CMV) infections of the skin and mucous membranes, as well as HSV, VZV, or coxsackievirus infections of mucous membranes, can present as ulcers without other stages. Measles and rubella can be associated with both macules and papules. Epstein-Barr virus (EBV), human HHV-6, and parvovirus B19 infections may result in macules that coalesce into larger erythematous patches. A spectrum of nonspecific skin lesions, such as erythema multiforme, urticaria, and petechiae, may be viral or nonviral in etiology.

Mucocutaneous manifestations of viral diseases can range from very specific (e.g., dermatomal vesicles of herpes zoster) to very general (e.g., urticaria); thus, the differential diagnosis must take the total clinical presentation of the patient into consideration (Table 1–1). Some skin changes may be highly suggestive of a specific viral disease, such as the verrucous papules seen with papillomavirus infection or smooth umbilicated papules resulting from poxvirus infection. Further diagnostic tests often may not be needed for these conditions. A differential diagnosis, including both viral and nonviral etiologies, may be suggested by vesicles induced by HSV-1 or HSV-2 or VZV, or they may be diagnostic. The diagnosis may not be obvious when any of these three viruses produce mucous membrane lesions and further diagnostic procedures may be required. Less frequent skin manifestations may be produced by other herpesviruses such as EBV, CMV, and HHV-6. These infections are most accurately diagnosed only when the systemic manifestations of the viral infection

Table 1–1. Viral Exanthems

Type of rash	Associated virus
Macular/ maculopapular	Rubella
	Echovirus (especially 9,16)
	Coxsackievirus (especially A5, A9, A16, B5)
	Epstein-Barr virus (infectious mononucleosis)
	Human herpesvirus 6 (roseola)
	Rubeola
	Arboviruses (dengue fever)
	Parvovirus B19 (erythema infectiosum)
	Hepatitis B and C
	Human immunodeficiency virus 1
Papular	Human papillomaviruses
	Orf
	Human herpesvirus 8 (Kaposi's sarcoma)
	Milker's nodule
	Molluscum contagiosum
	Human immunodeficiency virus 1
Patches	Epstein-Barr virus (oral hairy leukoplakia)
Petechial/ purpuric	Coxsackieviruses A5, A9
	Hemorrhagic fever viruses
	Congenital rubella
	Congenital cytomegalovirus
	Echovirus 9
	Epstein-Barr virus
Urticarial	Human immunodeficiency virus 1
	Hepatitis B
	Coxsackieviruses A5, A9
	Epstein-Barr virus
Vesicular/ vesiculopustular	Varicella-zoster
	Vaccinia
	Variola
	Herpes simplex virus types 1 and 2
	Coxsackievirus (hand, foot, and mouth disease) (Herpangina)
	Vesicular stomatitis
	Echovirus

are simultaneously considered. The cutaneous manifestations would indicate the need to evaluate systemic signs and symptoms and to institute appropriate diagnostic tests in other diseases in which viral replication is not in the epidermis.

PATHOPHYSIOLOGY

Three different routes are used by viruses to infect the skin: direct inoculation, local spread from an internal focus, and/ or systemic infection. Papillomaviruses, most poxviruses (except smallpox), and primary HSV infect the skin by direct inoculation. The skin in primary VZV is infected from systemic infection, and recurrent VZV (shingles) or recurrent HSV reaches the skin from an internal focus.

Skin lesions may be the direct effect of virus replication in infected cells, or the skin lesions may be the result of the host response to the virus. Alternatively, an interaction of viral replication and the host response may produce the lesions. Viruses that replicate in the epidermis, for example, are generally directly responsible for the lesions. Skin lesions of rubella and measles, on the other hand, are thought to be at least partly due to the cell-mediated immune response to the virus.

DIAGNOSIS

Confirmation of suspected viral diseases is usually via one of five general methods of laboratory diagnosis: viral cultures, microscopic examination of infected tissue, detection of viral antigens, detection of viral DNA or RNA, or serology. The preferred method of diagnosis is viral culture when a good culture system is available. A positive culture can be obtained in 1 or 2 days when HSV-1 or HSV-2 is responsible for the lesion. Generally, however, high rates of positivity are seen only when lesions are in the vesicular stage, whereas later stages of healing are less likely to be positive. Even when fresh vesicular fluid is used to inoculate the appropriate cell culture, positive cultures are more difficult to obtain from VZV.

Papillomaviruses and many other common viral diseases of the skin do not have available culture systems. Microscopic examination of biopsy material can reveal changes consistent with a viral family in such cases, but it is usually not helpful in identifying the specific virus responsible. Histological changes induced by HPV in benign warts, for example, have similar microscopic appearances. Similar microscopic changes are induced by HSV-1 and HSV-2, as well as by VZV, but are distinctive from changes associated with other herpesviruses. The Tzanck smear is a procedure more rapid than microscopic examination of biopsy tissue to detect changes associated with HSV-1 and HSV-2 and VZV. A smear containing cells scraped from the base of a vesicle is prepared on a glass slide and stained (e.g., with Wright's or Giemsa stain). Multinucleated giant cells will help to confirm that one of the three viruses is responsible for the vesicle, but they cannot specify which virus. Molluscum contagiosum (MC) is another viral infection that can be diagnosed directly from smears from a skin lesion. Intracytoplasmic inclusion bodies (Table 1–2) will help to distinguish papules associated with MC from skin lesions of *Cryptococcus neoformans,* which can appear very similar in human immunodeficiency virus (HIV)–infected patients.

Rapid diagnostic tests for viral antigens are widely available. Fluorescent antibody detection of HSV-1 and HSV-2, as well as VZV, is frequently used in the detection of viral infections of the skin. The three viruses can be distinguished by this technique (in contrast to the Tzanck smear). HPV capsid antigens are sometimes detected by immunoperoxidase techniques, but this technique can be associated with false-negative results with oncogenic HPV types in which viral DNA may be present without capsid antigens. Viral antigens also may be detected by radioimmunoassay or enzyme-linked immunosorbent assay (ELISA). Viral particles or viral antigens can also be detected by labor-intensive techniques such as electron microscopy or immunoelectron microscopy.

Viruses for which no effective culture system (or serologic assay) is available can be identified by the use of assays to detect viral nucleic acid. HPV is an example, but any virus should be detectable with these methodologies if sufficient knowledge is available regarding the viral genome in order to design specific probes and primers. In situ hybridization is the most widely available technique for detection of viral nucleic acids. Detection of the viral nucleic acid and histological localization of the virus to specific cells is possible with this technique. Southern hybridization (considered the "gold standard") is a more sensitive technique for viral nucleic acid detection and is the basis for greater than 100 HPV types described thus far. The polymerase chain reaction (PCR) is the most sensitive technique for viral nucleic acid detection. A range of viruses within a particular family (i.e., using consensus primers) can be detected, or primers used in PCR can be designed to be specific for a particular virus (i.e., type-specific primers). In situ PCR that combines the sensitivity of PCR with specific histological localization of the virus is even more sophisticated. The Hybrid Capture Assay II is a molecular technique with sensitivity similar to that of PCR that has recently become available commercially.

Serology provides a fifth technique for diagnosis by using the detection of antibodies elicited by the viral infection. A recent infection is indicated by a fourfold rise in serum antibodies to a specific virus between acute and convalescent sera (usually 4 weeks). A true primary herpetic infection (which would be associated with high levels of immunoglobulin [Ig] M) can be distinguished from a first-episode nonprimary infection or a recurrence (i.e., high levels of IgG) by serology. Antibodies to viruses can be detected by a variety of techniques. The responsible virus determines, at least partly, the usefulness of a particular technique. ELISA is considered a screening test for antibodies against HIV, for example. Confirmation with Western blotting must be completed before a definitive diagnosis can be made owing to the possibility of a false-positive test. Specificity between HSV-1 and HSV-2 antibodies is not adequate with the currently available ELISAs, but de-

Table 1–2. Viral Inclusion Bodies in Human Diseases

Virus	Location	Eponym
Adenovirus	Nucleus	
Cytomegalovirus	Nucleus, cytoplasm	"Owl's eye"
Herpes simplex (types 1 and 2)	Nucleus	Cowdry type A, Lipschütz body
Measles	Cytoplasm	
Molluscum contagiosum	Cytoplasm	Henderson-Paterson body
Papillomaviruses[a]	Nucleus, cytoplasm	
Rabies	Cytoplasm	Negri body
Varicella	Nucleus	Cowdry type A
Variola, vaccinia	Cytoplasm	Guarnieri body

[a] Keratohyaline granules.

tection of antibodies against HSV can be made accurately with this test. Antibodies to HSV-1 can be distinguished with sensitivity and specificity from those to HSV-2 using the Western blot.

DIFFERENTIAL DIAGNOSIS

A spectrum of nonviral and viral conditions must be considered in the differential diagnosis of various types of viral exanthemata. HSV-1, HSV-2, VZV, poxviruses, hand-foot-mouth viruses, as well as other coxsackieviruses, may produce vesicles. During the process of healing, most vesicles develop into pustules. Nonviral entities such as bullous impetigo, insect bite reactions, drug eruptions, contact dermatitis, and gonococcemia must be included in the differential diagnosis of vesiculopustules. Rubella, EBV infections (i.e., infectious mononucleosis), HHV-6 infection (i.e., roseola), as well as a variety of coxsackieviruses (A and B), and echovirus infections, may produce macules. Drug eruptions and bacterial infections (e.g., scarlet fever, Rocky Mountain spotted fever, erysipelas) are possible nonviral etiologies of macules. Measles, echovirus infections, and human parvovirus B19 infections (i.e., erythema infectiosum) may result in macules presenting with papules. Any of the macular or papular nonviral conditions noted previously, as well as erythema multiforme, which is commonly of viral etiology (i.e., HSV), may produce maculopapular lesions, or they may be associated with nonviral infections or with drug eruptions. A spectrum of poxvirus and HPV infections, as well as in the Gianotti-Crosti syndrome, which may be a manifestation of hepatitis B or a variety of other viral infections, may manifest as papules. Bacterial infections (e.g., Bartonella, Mycobacterium), fungal infections (e.g., cryptococcus), and noninfectious conditions (e.g., seborrheic keratoses, basal cell carcinomas) may also be papules. Poxvirus infections (e.g., orf, milker's nodules), HPV (e.g., squamous cell carcinomas associated with HPV-16), or herpes virus 8 (e.g., Kaposi's sarcoma), mycobacterial and Bartonella infections (e.g., bacillary angiomatosis), and noninfectious tumors (e.g., basal cell carcinomas, squamous cell carcinoma, melanoma, pyogenic granuloma) may be nodular. Allergic reactions, including drug eruptions, as well as hepatitis B or coxsackie A9 virus infections, are usually associated with urticaria. Dengue fever and other hemorrhagic fevers (e.g., Lassa fever) may result in petechiae, but this finding may occur in nonviral conditions producing thrombocytopenia. Viral infections such as HSV-1, HSV-2, VZV, CMV, and hand-foot-mouth disease commonly cause ulcerations of the mucous membranes. Immunocompromised persons sometimes suffer oral or anogenital ulcers owing to CMV,

or such ulcers may involve a coinfection of CMV and HSV. Nonviral ulcers such as aphthous stomatitis must be distinguished from oral ulcers of viral etiology. Stasis dermatitis or other causes of decreased circulation may cause cutaneous ulcers.

DNA VIRUSES

Poxviruses

Poxviruses are large DNA viruses that are members of the family poxviridae; those of clinical significance include smallpox, vaccinia, molluscum contagiosum, orf, and milker's nodules (Table 1–3). The only one of these viruses with significant mortality, smallpox, has been eradicated via worldwide vaccination programs that resulted in the last patient with epidemic smallpox being treated in 1977 [1].

Smallpox

Although smallpox replicates in the epidermis, it is spread not only via direct skin contact and fomites but also by respiratory transmission. Patients experience 3 days of apprehension, preceding development of skin lesions; this is followed by sudden prostrating fever, severe headache, back pain, and vomiting. Tense, deep-seated papules and vesicles are preceded by erythematous macules. Pustules follow the vesicles, then crusts, and finally scar formation. All lesions are in the same stage of development, with the rash appearing in a centrifugal distribution. The hemorrhagic form of smallpox results in almost 100% mortality even before development of skin lesions, although the overall mortality rate with smallpox is approximately 25%.

Vaccinia

Vaccination against the vaccinia virus is no longer routinely used because smallpox has been eradicated (Tables 1–4 and 1–5). Although use of the vaccinia virus to immunize against smallpox was one of the greatest success stories in medical history, use of this live virus occasionally led to complications in susceptible individuals such as bacterial superinfection, abnormal viral replication, or altered reactivity [2].

Molluscum Contagiosum

The most prevalent poxvirus is MC; the incubation period of MC is 2 to 7 weeks. MC presents as 3- to 6-mm skin-colored papules with a central umbilication. Although two different strains of MC (I and II) have been identified (based on restriction endonuclease digestion patterns), both strains produce similar clinical pictures. MC often follows one of two patterns of clinical presentation in immunocompetent individuals: widespread papules on the trunk and

Table 1–3.   Taxonomy of Human Viruses

Family DNA viruses	Subfamily, genus	Type species or example	Morphology	Envelope	Chapter
dsDNA viruses					
Poxviridae			Ovoid	+	3
	Chordopoxvirinae				
	Orthopoxvirus	Vaccinia virus, variola			
	Parapoxvirus	Orf virus			
	Molluscipoxvirus	Molluscum contagiosum virus			
	Yatapoxvirus	Yaba monkey tumor virus			
Herpesviridae			Icosahedral	+	
	Alphaherpesvirinae				
	Simplexvirus	Human herpesviruses (HSV) 1 and 2			4
		Cercopithecine herpesvirus 1 (herpesvirus B)			11
	Varicellovirus	Human herpesvirus 3 (VZV)			5
	Betaherpesvirinae				
	Cytomegalovirus	Human herpesvirus 5 (CMV)			7
	Roseolovirus	Human herpesvirus 6 and 7[a]			8, 9
	Gammaherpesvirinae				
	Lymphocryptovirus	Human herpesvirus 4 (EBV)			6
	Rhadinovirus	(HHV-8)			10
Adenoviridae	*Mastadenovirus*	Human adenoviruses	Icosahedral	–	
			Icosahedral	–	
Papovaviridae	Polyomavirus	JC virus			
	Papillomavirus	Human papillomaviruses			
ssDNA viruses					12
Parvoviridae			Icosahedral	–	
	Parvovirinae				
	Erythrovirus	B19 virus			
	Dependovirus	Adeno-associated virus 2[a]			13
DNA and RNA reverse transcribing viruses					
Hepadnaviridae	*Orthohepadnavirus*	Hepatitis B virus	Icosahedral	–	23
Retroviridae			Spherical	+	
	"BLV-HTLV retroviruses"	HTLV-I and II			1
	Lentivirus	Human immunodeficiency virus			14
	Spumavirus	Human spumavirus[a]			
RNA viruses					
DsRNA viruses					
Reoviridae			Icosahedral	–	
	Orthoreovirus	Reovirus 3[a]			
	Orbivirus	Kemerovo viruses			
	Rotavirus	Human rotaviruses			
	Coltivirus	Colorado tick fever virus			15
DNA viruses					
Negative-stranded					
ssRNA viruses			Spherical	+	
Paramyxoviridae					
	Paramyxovirinae				
	Paramyxovirus	Human parainfluenza viruses			
	Morbillivirus	Measles virus			
	Rubulavirus	Mumps virus			16

(*continued*)

Table 1–3. *(continued)*

Family DNA viruses	Subfamily, genus	Type species or example	Morphology	Envelope	Chapter
	Pneumoniavirinae				
	Pneumovirus	Human respiratory syncytial virus			
Rhabdoviridae			Bacilliform	+	
	Vesiculovirus	Vesicular stomatitis virus			
	Lyssavirus	Rabies virus			
Filoviridae	Filovirus	Ebola virus	Bacilliform	+	17
Orthomyxoviridae			Spherical	+	
	Influenzavirus A, B	Influenza A virus			
	Influenzavirus C	Influenza C virus			
Bunyaviridae			Amorphic	+	
	Bunyavirus	Bunyamwera virus, LaCrosse virus			18
	Hantavirus	Hantaan virus, Sin Nombre virus			18
	Nairovirus	Crimean-Congo hemorrhagic fever virus			
	Phlebovirus	Rift Valley fever virus			
Arenaviridae	Arenavirus	Lymphocytic choriomeningitis virus	Spherical	+	
Positive-stranded ssRNA virus					
Picornaviridae			Icosahedral		
	Enterovirus	Polioviruses, Coxsackieviruses, Echovirus		–	19
	Rhinovirus	Human rhinoviruses			
	Hepatovirus	Hepatitis A virus		–	23
Caliciviridae	Calicivirus	Hepatitis E virus	Icosahedral		
		Norwalk virus			
Astroviridae	Astrovirus	Human astrovirus 1	Icosahedral	–	
Coronaviridae	Coronavirus	Human coronavirus	Pleomorphic	+	
Flaviridae	Flavivirus	Yellow fever virus, Dengue	Spherical	+	20
	"Hepatitis C–like viruses"	Hepatitis C virus			23
Togaviridae	Alphavirus	Western equine encephalitis virus	Spherical		21
	Rubivirus	Rubella virus		+	22
Subviral agents: satellites, viroids, and agents of spongiform encephalopathies					
Satellites (single-stranded RNA)	*Deltavirus*	Hepatitis delta (D) virus	Spherical	–	
Prion protein agents		Creutzfeld-Jakob agent	?	–	

a Human virus with no recognized human disease.

Table 1–4. Timeline of Virus Vaccine Development[a]

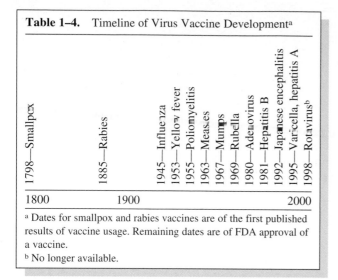

1800	1900	2000

a Dates for smallpox and rabies vaccines are of the first published results of vaccine usage. Remaining dates are of FDA approval of a vaccine.
b No longer available.

face of children transmitted by direct skin-to-skin (nonsexual) contact and genital papules in adults spread by sexual contact. In either case, it is unusual to see more than 20 lesions per patient [3]. In immunocompromised persons, especially those who are HIV positive, MC can present with thousands of papules and be a major source of morbidity; prevalence rates in this population range from 9% to 18% [4].

Orf

Contagious ecthyma, orf, is a less common poxvirus that is transmitted from sheep, goats, and the like to the hands of humans. The cutaneous presentation of orf is usually nodules averaging 1.6 cm in diameter associated with regional lymphadenopathy, lymphangitis, and fever. Orf lesions spontaneously progress through six stages, resulting in healing in about 35 days [5].

Milker's Nodules

A paravaccinia virus causes milker's nodules, which is similar to orf except that lesions result from manual contact with teats of infected cows, and milker's nodules have an incubation period of 4 to 7 days. The nodules heal in 4 to 6 weeks after progressing through six clinical stages similar to orf [6].

Primary viremia follows local multiplication in the respiratory mucosa and regional lymphoid tissue after contact with smallpox via the respiratory route. A secondary viremia is associated with the initiation of the prodrome after spread throughout the reticuloendothelial system. Thrombocytopenia accompanies development of skin lesions, which, in hemorrhagic forms of smallpox, can become severe and result in disseminated intravascular coag-

ulation with decreases in accelerator globulin, prothrombin, and proconvertion, ending with extensive hemorrhage and death.

Regional lymphadenopathy sometimes accompanies a local reaction to vaccinia replication in the epithelium. The host immune response limits systemic manifestations except in cases of depressed immunity or in diseases with inadequate epithelial barriers. Generalized vaccinia can result, but it is rarely a lethal disease like smallpox. Viral replication in MC, orf, and milker's nodules is generally limited to the epidermis, but dermal changes are also seen in milker's nodules.

Pathology. Lesional biopsy of smallpox reveals cytoplasmic eosinophilic inclusion bodies (Guarieri's bodies) along with papules, vesicles, or pustules. Electron microscopy or fluorescent antibody staining can identify smallpox, or the virus can be isolated with appropriate tissue culture systems. A history of vaccination along with the clinical presentation is usually sufficient for diagnosis of vaccinia, but diagnostic tools similar to those used for smallpox may be used to detect this virus.

A hypertrophied and hyperplastic epidermis overlying a normal-appearing basal layer characterizes MC histologically. Multiple Feulgen-positive intracytoplasmic inclusion bodies (Henderson Paterson bodies or molluscum bodies) are seen in the enlarged epidermal cells.

Laboratory Findings. Laboratory findings with orf and milker's nodules, as with MC, are generally limited to histology. The histopathology varies with the clinical stage in the case of the latter two diseases. In the early stages, both intracytoplasmic and intranuclear inclusions may be observed.

Management. The only effective management of smallpox proved to be prevention via vaccination. Management of symptoms and prevention of bacterial superinfection were paramount for patients with smallpox or disseminated vaccinia. Thiosemicarbezone and antivariola or antivaccinia sera had limited effectiveness (Table 1–6). Liquid nitrogen, curetting, imiquimod, or cidofovir can be used to treat MC. In immunocompromised persons, recurrences are common. Excision and cautery can remove lesions of orf or milker's nodules, but this is usually not necessary because spontaneous resolution can be expected in approximately 6 weeks.

Human Papillomaviruses

HPVs are nonenveloped, double-stranded DNA viruses that belong to the family Papovaviridae. Regional tropism (i.e., whether they produce genitomucosal lesions, nongenital lesions in the general population, or lesions associated

Table 1–5. Virus Vaccines: Recommendations for Administration[a]

Vaccine	Target population	Route	Dosage	Comments
MMR(measles, mumps, rubella)	Children	SC	2 doses at 12–15 mo and 4–6 yrs	Also available: Measles and rubella (live):MRVAX II® Measles (live attenuated): ATTENUVAX® Mumps (live): MUMPSVAX Rubella (live): MERUVAX Rubella + Mumps (live): BIAVAX II
Varicella-zoster Varivax®	Children and susceptible adults	SC	Ages 12 mo–12 yr: 1 dose ≥ 13 yr: 2 doses (4–8 wks apart in susceptible persons	
Influenza Fluzone® Fluvirin® Fluogen® Flushield®	Persons ≥ 65 yrs, residents of chronic care facilities, those with chronic cardiopulmonary diseases, or those who may transmit the virus to high-risk persons.	IM	6 mo–8 yr: 1 or 2 doses of split virus only, at least 1 mo apart 9–12 yr: 1 dose of split virus only > 12 yr: 1 dose of whole or split virus	Vaccinate from September to November
Hepatitis A	Children and susceptible adults	IM	2 doses: Havrix®—>2 yr: 0 mo & 6–12 mo Vaqta®—2–17 yr: 0 mo & 6–18 mo >17 yr: 0 mo & 6 mo	Havrix® now available in combination with Engerix-B® as Twinrix®
Hepatitis B Recombivax HB® Engerix B® Comvax® (with haemophilus influenza type B Vaccine)	Children and susceptible adults	IM	3 doses: Infants: birth to 2 mo, 1–4 mo & 6–18 mo Children and adolescents: mo 0, 2, & 4 Adults: mo 0,1, & 6	Infants with HbsAG-positive mothers receive 1st dose within 12 hr of birth. 2nd dose at 1 mo, and 3rd dose at 6 mo Engerix-B® now available in combination with Havrix® as Twinrix®.
Rabies RABIE-VAX®	Persons at risk of rabies exposure or those recently exposed.		Pre-exposure: 3 doses on days 0,7, & 21 or 28	
		IM	Human diploid cell rabies vaccine (HDCV): Imovax®	
		IM	PCEC: RabAvert™	Previously vaccinated persons require only 2 doses after rabies exposure, on days 0 & 3.
		ID	Rabies Vaccine Absorbed HDCV: Imovax® Rabies ID Postexposure: 5 doses on days 9,3,7,14, & 28	
		IM	HDCV	
		IM	Rabies Vaccine Absorbed	
		IM	PCEC	

(continued)

Table 1–5. (*continued*)

Vaccine	Target population	Route	Dosage	Comments

Poliomyelitis
  Poliovax®
  IPOL®
  Orimune® (live, oral)
	Children	SC	Sequential series: 4 doses
			2 mo: IPV
			4 mo: IPV
			6–18 mo: IPV
			4–6 yr: IPV
				Routine vaccination should always use IPV (completely inactivated poliovirus vaccine). All IPV doses are indicated for immunosuppressed patients or contacts. All OPV dosing is accepted in certain circumstances only.

Yellow fever YF-VAX®	Persons traveling to endemic countries (parts of Africa and South America)	SC	1 dose	Booster given every 10 yr for recertification for travel into endemic countries.
Japanese encephalitis JE-VAX®	Persons traveling to certain parts of Asia	SC	3 doses, on days 0, 7, & 30	
Adenovirus (types 4 and 7)	Military	Oral	1 dose	

IM = intramuscular; SC = subcutaneous; ID = intradermal;
HDCV = human diploid cell vaccine; PCEC = purified chick embryo cell culture vaccine.
[a] Vaccinia vaccine for prevention of smallpox not generally available (or recommended) and when available, limited to certain military forces.

Table 1–6. Immunoglobulins (IG): Indications for Administration [a]

Immunoglobulin	Generic/trade name	Approved indication
Intramuscular IG	BAYGAM	Exposure to measles or hepatitis A in susceptible persons; varicella (if VZIG unavailable); rubella
Hepatitis B-IG	BAYHEPB, NABI-HB, HYPER HEP	Hepatitis B exposure in susceptible persons
Human rabies IG	BAYRAB, IMOGAM-Rabies, HYPERAB	Rabies exposure in previously unvaccinated persons
Varicella-zoster IG	VZIG	Susceptible persons exposed to varicella who have a high risk for complications (e.g., immunocompromised patients and neonates)
Respiratory syncytial virus IG	Respigam® (Palivizumab) Synagis®	Prophylaxis in high-risk infants (e.g., those with bronchopulmonary dysplasia or prematurity)
Cytomegalovirus	Cytogam	CMV prophylaxis in seronegative transplant recipients of a kidney from a CMV-positive donor

[a] Vaccinia immune globulin generally not available and, when available, limited to certain military forces.

with epidermodyplasia verruciformis [EV]) can be used to categorize HPV. Location of the lesions, quantity of HPV in the lesion, degree and nature of the contact, and immune status of the exposed individual determine the transmission of HPV. Genital (venereal) warts, condyloma acuminatum, are the most prevalent clinical form of viral genitomucosal lesions; the incidence of these warts has risen sixfold during the past three decades. Classification of HPVs also may be according to their malignant potential. More than 99% of condyloma acuminatum are clinically benign and are due to HPV-6 or HPV-11. HPV types 31, 33, and 35 have intermediate malignant potential. In contrast, HPV-16 and HPV-18 have high malignant potential; over 90% of cervical and other anogenital cancers contain DNA from one of the latter two types [7–9]. Orogenital sex can transmit these HPV types to other mucous membranes, resulting in oral condyloma acuminatum, or HPV may be transmitted nonsexually such as during vaginal delivery [10]. HPV from vaginal warts in the latter case may be transmitted to the oral or respiratory tract of the infant and present as respiratory (laryngeal) papillomas [11]. As a result of HPV acquired during vaginal delivery, anogenital warts may also develop in infants within a few months of birth. Although sexual abuse can produce anogenital warts in children, a significant proportion of such warts results from incidental spread from cutaneous warts [12]. Oral warts not of genital origin can be seen in focal epithelial hyperplasia, which contains such unique HPV types as 13 or 32, and they present most commonly in certain ethnic groups [13]. In the general population, cutaneous warts are very common and can present as verruca vulgaris (HPV-2), plantar warts (HPV-1), or verruca plana (HPV-3). These verrucous papules rarely lead to major medical problems but can be annoying and difficult to eradicate.

Conversely, cutaneous warts in EV can lead to major morbidity and mortality [14]. EV was the first model of cutaneous viral oncogenesis in humans and is a rare condition that can occur sporadically or in an autosomal recessive manner. During childhood, disseminated warty papules and erythematous macules develop in EV patients. Approximately one third of these patients will develop cutaneous carcinomas in adulthood. EV is associated with at least 17 HPV types. HPV-3 and HPV-10 are also found in flat warts in the general population, but most types are unique to EV. Malignant transformation in EV is mostly associated with HPV-5 and HPV-8. Oncogenic HPV in EV appears to be necessary but not sufficient for malignant transformation, which is analogous to the situation with HPV-16 and HPV-18 in anogenital cancers in the general population. In both cases, cofactors appear to be necessary. Cofactors, including cigarette smoking, other transactivating viruses, genetics, and diet, may be important in anogen-

ital malignancies, but the individual role of each cofactor is not clear [15]. The most important cofactor in EV is ultraviolet irradiation, which is illustrated by the fact that the highest incidence of carcinomas in EV patients is in areas of greatest sunlight exposure [16].

HPV DNA replication, RNA transcription, and late protein production are coordinated by the state of differentiation of the epithelial cell following infection of the basal layer of the epidermis. Early (E) proteins direct viral replication. Late (L) proteins, L1 and L2, are viral capsids, which are synthesized and assembled into virions in the nuclei of the granular layer [17]. Verruca are produced in approximately 2 to 9 months, but HPV DNA can remain in a latent state in normal-appearing skin or mucous membranes for much longer periods of time. Therefore, in some cases, the incubation time from infection to lesion development may be years.

Because newer warts tend to have more virions than do older verrucae, the copy number of HPV DNA varies according to the age of the lesions. Plantar warts usually have more virions than do condyloma acuminatum, and benign warts have more virions than do dysplastic or neoplastic HPV-related lesions.

Pathology. If the lesion is assumed to be HPV related and benign, often no laboratory tests are carried out. The following general patterns may be observed in tissues from biopsies of verrucae: acanthosis, papillomatosis, hyperkeratosis, parakeratosis, and prominent and often thrombosed dermal capillary vessels. Often such features as koilocytes, large keratinocytes with an eccentric, pyknotic nucleus surrounded by a perinuclear halo, are observed. A biopsy sometimes is taken to determine if the lesion is dysplastic or neoplastic. Such biopsies would most likely be taken in the anogenital region in the general population. Dysplastic or neoplastic lesions are most frequent on the cervix and would be detectable via cytopathology taken with the Papanicolaou smear.

Laboratory Findings. Immunohistochemical staining for HPV capsid antigens for more specific detection of HPV can be done. This method may give false-negative results with such lesions because dysplastic or neoplastic lesions contain few, if any, capsid antigens. The only specific method of diagnosing HPV is via DNA detection methods because HPV cannot be readily grown in tissue culture nor is serology routinely useful. Over 100 HPV types are recognized based on Southern hybridization [18]. A new HPV genotype is designated if the virus differs more than 10% in nucleotide sequence in the "late gene" L1 open reading frame from previously identified HPV types. Although in situ hybridization and Hybrid Capture Assay II have become widely available, detection of specific HPV types is more frequently a research tool than a routine laboratory procedure. Hybrid Capture Assay II and PCR, however, are by far the most sensitive methods of detecting HPV DNA [19].

Management.   Treatment for most benign verrucae includes surgery, cryotherapy, or topical chemotherapy. The objective in each case is to eradicate the lesion and allow the immune system to hold latent HPV in surrounding (normal-appearing) tissue in check so as to prevent recurrences. Simple excision, electrodesiccation, and removal with a CO_2 laser are all types of surgical therapy. Liquid nitrogen for destruction of the lesion is a form of cryotherapy. Podophyllin resin, purified podophyllotoxin, 5-fluorouracil, retinoic acid, cantharidin, salicylic acid, lactic acid, bichloroacetic acid, and trichloroacetic acid are options for topical chemotherapy [20–22]. The size and location of the wart, as well as the history of previous therapies, are determinants in selection of the most appropriate therapy.

Interferon (IFN-α) for treatment of condyloma acuminatum was the first antiviral therapy approved for HPV (Table 1–7) [23]. Although IFN-α is effective in eradicating 50% to 70% of genital warts, its most effective use is in combination therapy [24]. IFN-α given subcutaneously following laser excision of condyloma acuminatum, for example, markedly reduces the recurrence rate. Surgery is used for therapy of HPV-related malignant lesions; and, if metastases are present, chemotherapy is usually included. Antisense oligonucleotides and cidofovir (a broad-spectrum agent active against a variety of DNA viruses) are new treatments for HPV-related lesions currently under study [25,26]. An immunomodulatory agent demonstrated to be very effective for condyloma acuminatum is imiquimod [27]. The patient applies imiquimod topically, and it produces minimal local inflammation and no systemic side effects. The mode of action of imiquimod is via induction of endogenous IFN-α as well as a wide variety of other cytokines. Recurrence rates following clearance of lesions with imiquimod are very low. Controlled trials are cur-

rently being conducted with recombinant HPV protein vaccines for the prophylaxis and therapy of HPV-associated lesions.

Human Herpesviruses

The family herpesviridae is composed of double-stranded DNA viruses and is divided into three subfamilies: alphaherpesviruses (HSV-1, HSV-2, VZV, and B virus); betaherpesviruses (CMV, HHV-6, HHV-7), and gammaherpesviruses (EBV, HHV-8). Primary VZV reaches the skin as a result of a secondary viremia but primary HSV infects the skin via direct inoculation. The skin is infected by local spread from an internal focus (i.e., the nerve) in recurrent HSV and VZV. Viral replication at nonepithelial sites can result in the infrequent skin lesions secondary to EBV or CMV. Although HHV-6 infection frequently produces an exanthem, viral replication is occurring in the peripheral blood mononuclear cells (especially T cells). Although no specific disease has yet been linked to HHV-7 infection, PR has been suggested. HHV-8 has been identified in both the endothelial cells of Kaposi's sarcoma and the epithelial cells of squamous cell carcinomas of organ transplant patients, but its role in the etiology of the latter tumor is not clear. Herpesvirus simiae, an animal herpes virus (B virus), can also cause human disease, most significantly a fatal encephalomyelitis. The virus can be recovered from vesicular skin lesions at the point of inoculation as well as from vesicles possibly arising from reactivation of latent B virus infection.

Herpes Simplex Viruses 1 and 2

Although most known for causing cold sores and genital herpes, respectively, HSV-1 and HSV-2 cause several other mucocutaneous infections, such as gingivostomatitis, herpes gladiatorum, eczema herpeticum, herpes whitlow, neonatal herpes, lumbosacral herpes, herpetic keratoconjunctivitis, and herpes encephalitis. Erythema multiforme is usually caused by HSV. These viruses typically cause a primary mucocutaneous infection followed by a latent infection when the virus remains dormant in the neuronal ganglia. Viral reactivation and movement down the nerve to produce active mucocutaneous infections is seen with recurrent disease.

Three to 14 days following sexual exposure to an infected partner, primary genital herpes may occur. In most transmissions, the source partner may be shedding HSV asymptomatically. Widespread genital vesicles and ulcers, edema, pain, inguinal lymphadenopathy, discharge, dysuria, malaise, fever, photophobia, and occasionally aseptic meningitis can be seen during the primary episode. The severity of these signs and symptoms usually is greater in

Table 1–7. FDA-approved Anti-HPV Agents (i.e., FDA Approval for Condyloma Acuminatum Only)

Generic name	Trade name
Interferon-α	Roferon A,
	Intron A
	Alferon
Imiquimod	Aldara[a]

[a] Approved as an immune response modifier because the antiviral activity is indirect.

women than in men; 3 to 4 weeks are often required for complete healing. Viral shedding lasts up to approximately 10 days in men and 14 days in women [28].

The first recognized episode of genital HSV, however, is often not truly primary. This first clinical manifestation of a virus that has remained latent in the infected nerve for an extended period of time (i.e., months or even years) would be considered a first episode, nonprimary outbreak. In such case, signs and symptoms are usually less severe than in true primary genital HSV and may require only 2 to 3 weeks for complete healing. The pre-existence of sufficient levels of IgG to attenuate the disease is the major reason for the decreased severity of first episode, nonprimary genital herpes.

An increasing proportion (e.g., 30%) of first-episode genital herpes is due to HSV-1, which is often attributable to orogenital contact. Outbreaks of genital herpes due to HSV-1, however, are usually less severe than those due to HSV-2.

Whereas at least 45 million individuals in the United States are estimated to be seropositive for HSV-2, approximately 11 million persons have recognized recurrent genital herpes [29–31]. Approximately one half of seropositive persons who deny a history of genital herpes can be taught to recognize signs and symptoms of the disease, according to one study [30]. Another investigation demonstrated that the majority of persons seropositive for HSV-2 via Western blotting shed the virus asymptomatically at least occasionally [31]. Virus traveling down the sensory nerve first causes prodromal sensations of pruritus or tingling followed shortly by the formation of vesicles. This is the result of reactivation of HSV, which lies dormant in neuronal ganglia. A variety of factors, such as emotional or physical stress (e.g., menstrual periods) or mild trauma (e.g., sexual intercourse), may trigger recurrences. HSV recurrent episodes are usually less severe than initial outbreaks and often heal in 7 to 10 days without therapy. Genital herpes due to HSV-2 recurs more frequently than HSV-1–associated disease. Women suffer 20% fewer recurrences of genital herpes than do men, a factor that may contribute to the higher rate of herpes transmission from men to women than from women to men. HSV recurrences in immunocompromised patients may be chronic and result in large ulcerations if not treated.

HSV-1 is associated with greater than 90% of orolabial herpes, which is usually acquired early in life [32,33]. Primary HSV-1 infection may present as acute gingivostomatitis with a peak incidence between the ages of 1 and 5 years. Five to 10 days after exposure to HSV, primary gingivostomatitis often presents with sore throat, regional lymphadenopathy, fever, and widespread painful ulcerations of the oral cavity and lips.

Up to 90% of adults in various seroepidemiologic surveys have serologic evidence of HSV-1 infection [33]. Recurrent herpes labialis, however, is seen in 20% to 40% of the population. The majority of orolabial herpes infections remain asymptomatic, analogous to the situation with genital herpes. In certain susceptible individuals, not only stress and trauma but also exposure to sufficient ultraviolet light can induce recurrent episodes of herpes labialis. Erythema and vesicle formation are preceded by a few hours of prodromal symptoms of pruritus, tingling, and pain. Formation of vesicles usually occurs on the vermilion border of the lip but occasionally may be seen around the lips. Such lesions contain culturable HSV for approximately 4 days. During the next 10 days vesicles ulcerate, crust, and usually undergo complete healing.

Varicella–Zoster Virus

The presentation of VZV can be as primary varicella (chickenpox) or as the recurrent form, herpes zoster (shingles) [34]. Children usually develop primary varicella, which presents with the simultaneous onset of rash, low-grade fever, and malaise. The exanthem is often preceded by up to 3 days of prodromal symptoms in older children and adults, including headache, myalgia, anorexia, nausea, and vomiting. The face and trunk first develop lesions, which appear as erythematous macules and rapidly progress over the next 12 to 14 hours to papules, vesicles, pustules, and crusts. Most skin lesions are seen on the trunk and on proximal extremities. Pruritus is the most prevalent symptom. Varicella is characterized by the simultaneous presence of lesions in all stages of development in the same anatomic region owing to the rapid evolution of successive crops of lesions. Shallow, painful ulcers develop from rapid erosion of vesicles, which appear on mucous membranes. Scarring, which may be due to bacterial secondary infection, is the most common cutaneous complication of varicella in immunocompetent persons. Significant morbidity and occasional mortality can result from such complications as central nervous system (CNS) involvement, varicella pneumonia, or varicella hepatitis in adults and in immunocompromised individuals. A 2% risk of congenital malformations is associated with maternal varicella if infection occurs during the first 20 weeks of pregnancy.

VZV persists in sensory ganglia and reactivates, usually after many years, in 20% of immunocompetent persons and in 20% to 50% of immunocompromised patients. This reactivation causes a transient viremia and spreads down the sensory nerve, producing radiculoneuritis [35]. Vesicles appear along the distribution of the sensory nerve after a few days (to weeks) of pain. Fever, regional lymphadenopathy, malaise, and occasionally a flu-like syndrome can be associated with pain. It is not unusual for a few lesions to appear in neighboring dermatomes although vesicles generally occur only along one dermatome. The areas usually affected most severely by primary varicella are those same anatomic regions (i.e., face and trunk) that have the greatest predilection for zoster. Pustules result after a few days when the vesicles are infiltrated by leukocytes. Pustules begin to dry after 1 to 2 weeks, resulting in crusts that are usually lost by 1 month after the appearance of the first vesicle.

Cutaneous complications are rare, although scarring can occur, particularly in darker-skinned individuals [36]. Postherpetic neuralgia, which can be defined as any pain remaining after full cutaneous healing, is the most prevalent complication. The pain can be extremely severe, can be treatment resistant, and can last months to years. Disseminated herpes zoster, defined as more than 20 vesicles outside the primary and adjacent dermatomes, is rare in normal hosts; but severely immunocompromised patients have a risk of dissemination approaching 40%. Cutaneous dissemination can herald significant morbidity and mortality, because it may be a marker of visceral involvement (i.e., liver, lungs, CNS).

Vision impairment or blindness with involvement of the ophthalmic branch of the trigeminal nerve is another complication of herpes zoster, not uncommonly seen in normal hosts [37]. Involvement of the facial and auditory nerves can result in the Ramsey-Hunt syndrome. CNS involvement or motor paralysis less commonly can result from herpes zoster [38,39].

Cytomegalovirus

The seroprevalence for CMV increases with age, such that most adolescents are seropositive and nearly 100% of older individuals are CMV seropositive. In immunocompetent persons, primary infection is asymptomatic and usually subclinical. In most normal hosts, the virus remains latent. However, it can produce clinical symptoms in neonates and in immunocompromised persons, but skin involvement is rare. During pregnancy, primary CMV infection results in intrauterine infection in 55% of fetuses. If infection occurs during the first trimester, sequelae are most severe [40]. Infection with CMV is the major infectious cause of mental retardation and deafness in the United States and is the most common congenital viral infection. CMV can produce purpuric macules and papules due to persistent dermal hematopoiesis, like other causes of the TORCH syndrome (i.e., toxoplasmosis, other [syphilis/bacterial sepsis], rubella, CMV, HSV), resulting in the clinical picture termed *blueberry-muffin baby* [41]. A variety of skin lesions from vesicles to verrucous plaques have been reported in association with immunocompromised patients.

The most prevalent cutaneous manifestation of CMV is ulceration, especially in the perianal area [42,43].

Epstein-Barr Virus

In immunocompetent individuals, the most prevalent clinical manifestation of EBV infection is infectious mononucleosis [44]. In infectious mononucleosis, the incubation period of EBV is 30 to 50 days, followed by a prodrome characterized by malaise, headache, and fatigue, followed by fever, sore throat, and cervical adenopathy. Small petechiae are observed at the border of the hard and soft palate in approximately one third of patients. Cutaneous manifestations of infectious mononucleosis, such as macules or papules and, less commonly, erythema, vesicles, petechiae, or purpura, occur in 3% to 16% of patients [45]. These lesions are more common on the trunk and upper arms, last 1 to 7 days, and present during the first week of illness. A high percentage of patients develop erythematous macules and papules over the trunk and extremities after approximately 1 week if ampicillin or certain other penicillins are given to a person with infectious mononucleosis [46]. After about 1 week, these lesions are followed by desquamation.

The epithelial cells of oral hairy leukoplakia, an oral lesion closely associated with HIV infection, also contain EBV DNA [47,48]. In addition, B-cell lymphomas of immunocompromised individuals often produce mucocutaneous lesions and contain EBV DNA. Symmetrical, nonpruritic, lichenoid papules of the face, limbs, and buttocks, known as the Gianotti-Crosti syndrome, have also been associated with primary EBV infection [49].

Human Herpesvirus Type 6

HHV-6 is presently recognized as the cause of exanthem subitum (roseola infantum), which was also termed *sixth disease* long before HHV-6 was isolated (Table 1–8) [50]. Exanthem subitum usually occurs after an incubation period of 5 to 15 days, in infants from 6 months to 2 years of age, with high fever lasting 3 to 5 days. The infant may

Table 1–8. The Classic Childhood Exanthems (Named in Early 1900s)

First disease	Rubeola (measles)
Second disease	Scarlet fever
Third disease	Rubella
Fourth disease	Filatov-Dukes (staphylococcus scalded skin syndrome?)
Fifth disease	Erythema infectiosum
Sixth disease	Exanthem subitum (roseola infantum)

not appear in distress despite the high fever, but can have such signs as palpebral edema, inflammation of the pharynx, and lesions of the soft palate. A macular to papular eruption appears on the trunk and neck as the fever resolves. Manifestations of the disease, including the rash, usually fade in 1 to 2 days without treatment [51–53].

Human Herpesvirus Type 7

HHV-7 has been associated with certain cases of roseola infantum as well as with PR, but it is not presently recognized as the etiological factor in any disease.

Human Herpesvirus Type 8

HHV-8 has been detected both in Kaposi's sarcoma from HIV-infected persons and classic (HIV-negative) Kaposi's sarcoma and was termed *Kaposi's sarcoma-related herpesvirus* [54–57]. The same viral sequences have been reported from squamous cell carcinomas and other epithelial lesions from patients with organ transplants [58]. The role of HHV-8 in epithelial tumors is unknown, but this virus is considered necessary, but not sufficient, to cause Kaposi's sarcoma. Cofactors for development of this tumor are under study.

B Virus (Herpesvirus Simiae)

Many nonhuman herpesviruses exist, but B virus is of particular importance owing to the high mortality rate from encephalomyelitis in humans infected with this simian herpesvirus [59]. Humans become infected with this virus following a bite or scratch from a macaque monkey. Fever, lymphangitis, lymphadenopathy, gastrointestinal symptoms, and myalgia follow development of erythema, induration, and vesicles at the inoculation site. Rapid progression to the neurological signs and symptoms of encephalomyelitis follow these symptoms [60,61]. The prognosis is very poor with B virus infection.

Pathology. Ballooning degeneration and cell fusion are seen with HSV-1, HSV-2, and VZV infections, resulting in multinucleated giant cells. The uninfected stratum corneum is elevated to form a vesicle by degeneration of epithelial cells and influx of edema fluid. Infiltration of leukocytes forms pustules. Both intranuclear and intracytoplasmic inclusions may be seen in cells infected with CMV. Intranuclear inclusions in HSV- or VZV-infected cells are similar to those observed in cytomegalic cells, but the CMV intranuclear inclusions are larger, surrounded by a clear halo, and resemble "owls' eyes." Viral infection of the vascular endothelium and subsequent destruction of blood vessels cause cutaneous ulcerations in CMV.

It is not certain whether EBV enters epithelial cells by interaction with a specific receptor or by fusion of the epithelial cell with an infected lymphocyte. It is not completely understood how EBV produces rash in infectious

mononucleosis (with or without ampicillin) or in oral hairy leukoplakia.

It is not fully known how HHV-6 produces an exanthem. The presence of HHV-8 sequences has been documented in endothelial cells of Kaposi's sarcoma as well as in epithelial cells of squamous cell carcinomas by in situ hybridization, but HHV-8 is not firmly established as the cause of epithelial tumors. Ballooning degeneration, multinucleated cells, vesicle formation, and necrosis are seen in cutaneous lesions with B virus infection.

Laboratory Findings. The most definitive method of demonstrating a herpesvirus as the probable cause of a vesicle is viral culture. In 1 to 2 days, both HSV-1 and HSV-2 grow readily. VZV has a much lower recovery rate than HSV and requires 7 to 10 days to produce a cytopathic effect. Culturable virus is much less likely to be found in pustules than in vesicles, virus can only rarely be cultured from crusts. HSV or VZV can be grown in either fibroblast or epithelial (amnion) cell cultures, but CMV grows only in fibroblast cultures. EBV or HHV-6 grows in lymphocytes; growth of HHV-8 in the laboratory has been reported recently.

Multinucleated giant cells of HSV and VZV will be revealed by scraping of the base of a vesicle and subsequent staining (Tzanck smear). The Tzanck smear can differentiate HSV- or VZV-associated changes from those associated with nonviral etiologies similar to a skin biopsy or electron microscopy, but it cannot distinguish among HSV-1, HSV-2, and VZV. Differentiation of skin lesions associated with each of these three viruses can, however, be accomplished using direct fluorescent antigen staining.

Diagnosis of infection with herpesviruses is possible via serologic tests. ELISA testing is used to detect antibodies to HSV-1 or HSV-2, but cross-reactivity confounds differentiation of the two viruses. Western blotting provides differentiation of antibodies with high sensitivity and specificity. True primary genital herpes can be differentiated from first episode, nonprimary genital herpes by the predominance of IgM in the former and IgG in the latter presentation. A fourfold or greater increase in the antibody titer to VZV between acute and convalescent titers can retrospectively diagnose herpes zoster.

Any of the eight human herpesviruses can be detected via PCR. Whereas this technique is the most sensitive, it is also associated with a significant incidence of false positivity if proper controls are not used.

Management. Thirteen antiviral drugs are FDA approved for therapy of herpesvirus infections (Table 1–9) [62]. Ophthalmic preparations of trifluridine and vidarabine are used for treatment of HSV- and VZV-associated keratitis and keratoconjunctivitis. Topical, oral, and intra-

Table 1–9. FDA-approved Anti-herpesvirus Agents

Human herpes virus	Generic name	Trade name
Herpes simplex virus 1 & 2 and/or herpes zoster virus	Acyclovir	Zovirax
	Valacyclovir	Valtrex
	Famciclovir	Famvir
	Foscarnet (acyclovir-resistant HSV and VZV)	Foscavir
	Penciclovir (topical only)	Denavir
	Trifluridine (optical only)	Viroptic
	Vidarabine (optical only)	Vira A
	n-Docosanol (topical only)	Abreva[a]
Cytomegalovirus	Ganciclovir	Cytovene, Vitrasert
	Valganciclovir	Valcyte
	Foscarnet	Foscavir
	Cidofovir	Vistide
	Fomivirsen (intravitreal only)	Vitrasene
Human herpesvirus-8 (AIDS-related Kaposi's sarcoma)	Interferon-α	Roferon-A Intron-A

[a] Over the counter, has antiviral activity, but not specifically approved as an antiviral drug.

venous formulations of acyclovir are available. Topical acyclovir has very low efficacy but continues to be used for therapy of HSV infections. Oral, genital, and other HSV infections are treated with oral acyclovir [63]. Primary varicella and herpes zoster require a fourfold higher dose of acyclovir [64,65]. Frequent dosing and low (i.e., 15–20%) bioavailability limit the efficacy of oral acyclovir. Therefore, the intravenous preparation is favored in immunocompromised patients with HSV or VZV infections, especially with disseminated disease. Acyclovir is not only very effective in suppressing signs and symptoms of genital herpes but also was recently demonstrated to reduce asymptomatic viral shedding of HSV-2 by 95% [66–68].

Two additional drugs, famciclovir [69] and valacyclovir [70], were approved for treatment of herpes zoster to overcome the limitations of oral acyclovir. More convenient dosing and greater bioavailability after oral dosing are provided by famciclovir and valacyclovir than with acyclovir. These newer drugs are also approved for treatment, and suppression of genital herpes. Penciclovir, a metabolite of famciclovir, and n-docosanal are approved in topical formulations for the therapy of herpes labialis. Fomivirsen is an antisense compound directed against CMV and is given via intraocular injection. Fomivirsen, valganciclovir, cidofovir, foscarnet, and ganciclovir are approved for treatment of CMV infections. The latter three drugs are administered intravenously and are associated with markedly higher rates of toxicities than are the three antiviral agents approved for systemic therapy of HSV and VZV infections.

Ganciclovir in the oral and ocular implant forms is approved for CMV prophylaxis in immunocompromised patients; valganciclovir is approved for induction and maintenance therapy of CMV retinitis; foscarnet is also approved for therapy of acyclovir-resistant HSV infections.

VZV is the only herpesvirus for which a vaccine is currently available for prophylaxis (Table 1–5) [71]. Approval for this live, attenuated viral vaccine (Oka strain) came in 1995; the vaccine produces a 95% seroconversion rate. Studies are ongoing with recombinant glycoprotein vaccines for the prophylaxis (and possible therapy) of HSV infections [72].

Parvoviruses

The only parvovirus known to infect humans is parvovirus B19, which is the cause of erythema infectiosum (fifth disease) (Table 1–8) [73]. Erythema infectiosum presents most commonly in children and often occurs in epidemics in late winter and early spring [74]. This syndrome begins with nonspecific symptoms approximately 4 to 14 days after exposure to parvovirus B19, which is transmitted primarily by the respiratory route. Erythematous, confluent, edematous plaques appear on the cheeks after about 2 days of low-grade fever, headache, and coryza. A ''slapped'' appearance of the cheeks is accompanied by continuation of the previously mentioned symptoms and the appearance of cough, conjunctivitis, pharyngitis, malaise, myalgias, nausea, diarrhea, and occasional arthralgias. The facial rash fades after 1 to 4 days concomitant with the appearance of erythematous macules and papules with a reticulated pattern on the extensor surfaces of the extremities, neck, and trunk. The rash usually lasts for 1 to 2 weeks but can persist for months and can be pruritic. Because parvovirus B19 is usually not found in respiratory secretions or in the serum after appearance of cutaneous manifestations, patients with erythema infectiosum appear to be infectious only before appearance of the rash.

Acute arthropathy without rash is often associated with primary parvovirus B19 infection in adults [75]. Transient aplastic crisis in patients with chronic hemolytic anemias, parvovirus-related chronic anemia in immunocompromised patients, and nonimmune fetal hydrops are other clinical presentations of parvovirus B19 infection potentially much more serious than erythema infectiosum but uncommonly accompanied by rash.

Pathology. Although the rash appears 17 to 18 days following infection, viremia appears 6 to 14 days after a susceptible patient contracts parvovirus B19 via the respiratory route. The pathogenesis of erythema infectiosum is not understood and may relate to immune complex formation, but the systemic manifestations of parvovirus B19 infection involve viral lysis of erythroid precursor cells. There are no diagnostic histologic changes in the skin of these patients.

Laboratory Findings. Complete blood counts and serum chemistries are usually normal in erythema infectiosum. Recent infection is indicated by detection of serum IgM directed to parvovirus B19 via radioimmunoassay (RIA) or ELISA. After 1 month, serum levels of IgM start to decline but are still detectable for 6 months after infection. One week following infection, parvovirus B19–specific IgG can be detected and persists for years. Less readily available tests exist for detection of the virus such as RIA, immunoelectrophoresis, ELISA, dot blot hybridization, and PCR. Human erythroid progenitor cells can be used to culture the virus.

Management. Treatment of erythema infectiosum is aimed at relief of symptoms because no antiviral therapy exists for parvovirus B19. Development of a vaccine appears feasible because one infection with the virus produces lifelong immunity.

RNA VIRUSES

Enteroviruses

Enteroviruses, such as coxsackieviruses, are small RNA viruses belonging to a subgroup of the family Picornaviridae. The two most distinctive clinical syndromes are hand-foot-mouth disease (HFMD) and herpangina, although a variety of enteroviruses, particularly coxsackieviruses, cause mucocutaneous manifestations. Most epidemic cases of HFMD are associated with coxsackievirus A16, but HFMD may be associated with coxsackieviruses A4–7, A9, A10, B2, and B5. Coxsackieviruses A2, A4, A5, A6, A8, and A10 cause herpangina.

Hand-Foot-Mouth Disease

Persons in their preteen to early teen years are most susceptible to HFMD [76]. HFMD is spread via oral or fecal-oral routes. A prodrome characterized by low fever, malaise, and abdominal or respiratory symptoms develops after an incubation period of 3 to 6 days; this prodrome precedes the mucocutaneous lesions by 12 to 24 hours. Most common on the hard palate, tongue, and buccal mucosa, oral lesions begin as macules that rapidly progress to vesicles and then to shallow, yellow-to-gray ulcers with an erythematous halo. Concomitant with or soon after the oral lesions, cutaneous vesicles appear and are most prevalent on the hands and feet. Cutaneous and oral lesions are usually tender or painful. In 5 to 10 days, both types of lesions resolve without treatment.

Herpangina

Herpangina is caused by viruses spread via routes similar to those causing HFMD. Children from 1 to 7 years of age are most commonly seen with herpangina, which begins abruptly with fever, sore throat, dysphagia, and malaise [77]. Appearing on the posterior palate, uvula, and tonsils are small gray-white vesicles surrounded by erythema. The vesicles usually ulcerate. Within 4 to 5 days, systemic symptoms usually resolve, and the ulcers heal spontaneously within 1 week.

Pathology. Viral infection of the buccal mucosa extends to regional lymph nodes in HFMD or herpangina. A viremia carries the virus to mucocutaneous sites approximately 48 hours later, resulting in intraepidermal vesicles containing neutrophils, mononuclear cells, and proteinaceous eosinophilic material. A perivascular polymorphous infiltrate composed of lymphocytes and neutrophils is observed in the edematous subvesicular dermis.

Laboratory Findings. A mild leukocytosis (i.e., 10,000 to 15,000/mm^3) may be seen in both HFMD and herpangina. The responsible virus may be recovered using tissue culture techniques or type-specific serology can identify the responsible coxsackievirus.

Management. Because no vaccine or antiviral drug is available for HFMD or herpangina, management is symptomatic.

Paramyxoviruses

Paramyxoviruses (paramyxoviridae), such as measles, are enveloped, single-stranded RNA viruses.

Measles

Measles (rubeola) is seen primarily in winter and spring and is most prevalent in children 5 to 10 years of age. An incubation period of 10 to 11 days precedes a prodromal phase. The prodrome is characterized by high fever, cough, coryza, conjunctivitis, malaise, and Koplik's spots on the buccal mucosa, which persist 3 to 4 days. Developing first behind the ears and over the forehead, an erythematous macular and papular rash then spreads to the face, neck, trunk, and extremities within 3 days. The fever, cough, and conjunctivitis are most severe when the lesions reach confluence over the face and upper back. Two to 3 days after the appearance of the rash, the Koplik's spots disappear. The rash fades within 5 or 6 days, sometimes with fine desquamation. Encephalitis and purpura are uncommon complications. Subacute sclerosing panencephalitis is a rare, but usually fatal, complication of measles. Persons previously given killed measles virus vaccine who are subsequently exposed to wild-type measles or to live attenuated measles virus vaccine can develop atypical measles [78].

Pathology.   Respiratory secretions spread the measles virus throughout the prodrome until 4 days after initiation of the rash. The appearance of skin lesions concomitant with detectable serum antibody suggests that virus-antibody complexes may initiate the damage, although the rash may be partly due to viral damage to epithelial and vascular endothelial cells. Likewise, immune complexes may cause the complications of encephalitis and thrombocytopenic purpura. Hyaline necrosis of epithelial cells, formation of a serum exudate around superficial dermal vessels, proliferation of endothelial cells followed by a leukocytic infiltrate of the dermis, and lymphocytic cuffing of vessels are seen in biopsies of the measles exanthem.

Laboratory Findings.   In measles, routine laboratory tests are usually unremarkable, but specific tests can include viral culture or detection of viral antigens in secretions. Measles infection is confirmed more commonly via serology using ELISA, complement fixation, neutralization, or hemagglutination inhibition tests.

Management.   Treatment is supportive therapy because no approved antiviral drug exists for measles. The live attenuated measles vaccine for prevention is effective (Table 1–5). If serum immunoglobulin is administered within 6 days of exposure to the virus, passive immunity may modify or prevent measles (Table 1–6).

Togaviruses

Togaviruses (togaviridae), such as rubella, are enveloped, single-stranded RNA viruses.

Rubella

Between 14 and 21 days following exposure to the virus, the prodrome of rubella (German measles, 3-day measles) develops and becomes more prominent with the increasing age of the patient. Low-grade fever, headache, conjunctivitis, cough, sore throat, and marked lymphadenopathy can be observed during the prodrome; arthritis can be seen in adults. An erythematous macular to papular rash appears first on the face and then on the neck, trunk, and extremities 1 to 4 days after initiation of the prodrome. The rash clears with fine desquamation after 2 to 3 days. Rubella is most common during spring months. Intrauterine infection produces congenital malformations in 50% of infected neonates, but the sequelae of rubella are rare in children and adults. The teratogenic findings, which can affect a wide variety of organ systems, especially the heart, eyes, auditory system, bone, and CNS, are most severe if the infection is early during pregnancy. The characteristic cutaneous findings of the TORCH syndrome, petechiae and ecchymoses, are produced by infection of the bone marrow [79,80].

Pathology.   The virus can be recovered from the pharynx from 7 days before the rash until almost 2 weeks after the rash and is spread via the respiratory route. The initial measurable antibody response appears simultaneously with the rash, suggesting that the exanthem may be due to the inflammatory effects of antibody-virus complexes rather than direct viral infection of the vascular endothelium. Only nonspecific acute and chronic inflammatory changes are seen in skin biopsies of the rubella rash.

Laboratory Findings.   The peripheral blood may contain increased numbers of atypical lymphocytes and plasma cells, but they are not diagnostic. Hemagglutination inhibition, RIA, ELISA, and the like are serological tests to detect rubella antibodies. Viral RNA can be found with PCR, or the virus may be cultured. Direct immunofluorescence may detect viral antigen.

Management.   Because no antiviral drug is approved for rubella, treatment is symptomatic. A live attenuated vaccine that is administered along with the mumps and measles vaccines (i.e., MMR) is used for prevention (Table 1–5).

Retroviruses

Retroviruses (retroviridae) such as HIV contain a central core surrounding two identical copies of the single-stranded viral RNA genome. An envelope formed by budding from the cell membrane covers the core. HIV, like other retroviruses, contains an RNA-dependent DNA polymerase (i.e., reverse transcriptase), which allows viral RNA to be converted into a proviral DNA sequence.

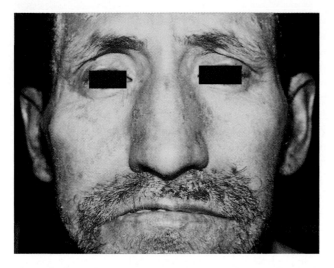

Figure 1–4. Infective dermatitis of the upper lip associated with HTLV-1. (Courtesy of Francisco Bravo Puccio, M.D., Instituto Dermatologico, Lima, Peru.)

Human Immunodeficiency Virus

The most important retrovirus medically, epidemiologically, and in terms of cutaneous manifestations is human T-cell leukemia virus type III (HTLV-III), more commonly known as HIV-1. Other retroviruses, however, such as HTLV-I and HTLV-II can have cutaneous manifestations, particularly owing to the association of HTLV-I and adult T-cell lymphoma/leukemia and infective dermatitis (Figs. 1–4 and 1–5) [81].

The signs and symptoms that lead to suspicion and sero-

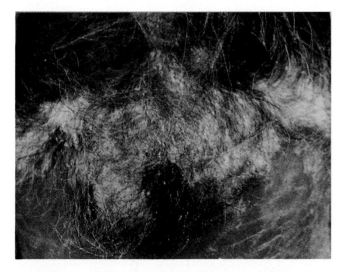

Figure 1–5. Infective dermatitis of the scalp associated with HTLV-1. (Courtesy of Francisco Bravo Puccio, M.D., Instituto Dermatologico, Lima, Peru.)

logic testing for HIV in individuals at high risk are often due to the mucocutaneous manifestations of HIV infection. Progression from asymptomatic HIV infection to full-blown acquired immunodeficiency syndrome (AIDS) may be reflected in a variety of mucocutaneous manifestations [82,83]. Sexual contact with an infected person, significant exposure to infected blood or blood products (including intravenous drug abuse), or perinatal exposure are the primary routes of transmission of HIV.

The incubation period in many persons infected with HIV may be 10 or more years before appearance of signs or symptoms. Primary HIV infection occasionally is manifested by fever and mild systemic symptoms that may be accompanied by a papulosquamous exanthem that is similar to those seen with a variety of other viral diseases. Within 2 weeks, the exanthem and symptoms generally resolve spontaneously [84].

Over 90% of patients will develop secondary mucocutaneous manifestations of their infection as the disease progresses from asymptomatic HIV infection through advanced AIDS [85,86]. Infectious, neoplastic, or noninfectious/nonneoplastic signs may be observed. Herpesviruses, poxviruses (i.e., MC), and papillomaviruses are examples of opportunistic viral infections commonly presenting clinically in HIV-positive individuals. Not only are relatively common organisms such as *Staphylococcus aureus, Streptococcus, Pseudomonas aeruginosa,* and *Treponema pallidum* responsible for opportunistic bacterial infections, but multiple species of Mycobacterium and unique infections, such as with *Bartonella quintana* and *B. henselae* (which cause bacillary angiomatosis), also have mucocutaneous manifestations. A variety of species of tinea as well as systemic fungi, including *Candida* sp., *Cryptococcus neoformans,* and *Histoplasma capsulatum,* produce mycotic infections. Kaposi's sarcoma is the most common neoplasm in HIV-positive patients and is associated with HHV-8. Inflammatory diseases (e.g., psoriasis and Reiter's disease), vascular diseases, hypersensitivities to drugs, insect bites, and ultraviolet light, pruritus, xerosis, ichthyosis, and seborrheic dermatitis are all common nonneoplastic/noninfectious mucocutaneous findings.

Pathology. The virus infects CD4+ T lymphocytes by attaching to the CD4 molecule. HIV also infects monocytes and macrophages, which help to spread the virus to susceptible cells in the brain, lymph node, skin, lung, and gastrointestinal tract. Disease is produced by HIV killing CD4+ cells, by syncytia formation, and by induction of certain cytokines that may play a direct role in induction of malignancy, neurological disease, and other clinical manifestations. Several weeks are usually required after infection for detectable antibody formation to HIV, in some cases seroconversion may follow infection by more than 1 year. The exanthem associated with primary HIV infection usually demonstrates nonspecific changes such as a superficial perivascular and perifollicular mononuclear cell infiltrate predominantly composed of CD4+ cells.

Laboratory Findings. Marked leukopenia, anemia, and thrombocytopenia may be found with progression of disease, as well as an elevated erythrocyte sedimentation rate and lymphocytic cerebral spinal fluid pleocytosis. Marked declines in CD3+ cells, CD4+ cells, and a reversed CD4/CD8 cell ratio accompanies disease progression. Seropositivity to the virus using ELISA with confirmation by Western blotting documents HIV infection. Isolation of virus from the blood or demonstration of HIV p24 antigenemia demonstrates the presence of HIV.

Management. Six synthetic nucleoside analogues, zidovudine, zalcitabine, didanosine, stavudine, lamivudine, and abacavir, are approved for therapy of HIV infection (Table 1–10). All six drugs work by inhibition of HIV reverse transcription [87–91]. Three nonnucleoside analogues, nevirapine, delaviridine, and efavirenz, are also approved. The first nucleotide analogue, tenofovir, was approved most recently (October 2001). Protease inhibitors are approved for treatment of HIV. Saquinavir was the first of these agents approved (December 1995). Other available protease inhibitors include ritonavir, indinavir, nelfinavir, amprenavir, and lopinavir. Combinations of antiviral drugs from different classes appear to produce greater efficacy than higher doses of individual agents, thereby reducing both adverse events and viral resistance. Such combinations usually include at least one protease inhibitor and two drugs from the other classes, although combinations of nucleoside and nonnucleoside analogues recently have been demonstrated to be effective. Together these agents form "highly active antiretroviral therapy" (HAART). HAART has produced marked reductions in morbidity and mortality of AIDS patients since 1996. Clinical trials are ongoing with a variety of other antiretroviral drugs, including integrase inhibitors and fusion inhibitors, as are prophylactic and therapeutic HIV vaccines. Management of HIV-positive patients also requires treatment and prophylaxis of a variety of opportunistic infections and neoplasms in addition to using drugs aimed at the responsible retrovirus [92].

MISCELLANEOUS VIRUSES

Hepatitis B, hepatitis C, several hemorrhagic fever viruses, and a variety of other viral diseases have occasional cutaneous manifestations, but pathogenesis and histology of the rash in these diseases are often not well understood, or the eruption may not be specific for a particular viral infection (Table 1–11). Therefore, the rash of these viral infections may be of less diagnostic or prognostic significance as

Table 1–10. FDA-approved Anti-retroviral Agents

Category of drug	Generic name	Trade name
Nucleoside analogues	Zidovudine	Retrovir
	Didanosine	Videx
	Zalcitibine	Hivid
	Stavudine	Zerit
	Lamivudine	Epivir
	Zidovudine + Lamivudine	Combivir
	Abacavir	Ziagen
	Abacavir + lamivudine + zidovudine	Trizivir
Non-nucleoside analogues	Nevirapine	Viramune
	Delaviridine	Rescriptor
	Efavirenz	Sustiva
Nucleotide analogue	Tenofovir	Viread
Protease inhibitors	Saquinavir (hard gel)	Invirase
	Saquinavir (soft gel)	Fortovase
	Ritonavir	Norvir
	Indinavir	Crixivan
	Nelfinavir	Viracept
	Amprenavir	Agenerase
	Lopinavir + ritonavir	Kaletra

Table 1–11. FDA-approved Anti-hepatitis Agents

Hepatitis virus	Generic name	Trade name
Hepatitis B virus	Interferon-α	Intron A
	Lamivudine	Epivir-HBV
Hepatitis C virus	Interferon-α	Roferon-A, Intron A, Infergen
	Interferon-α + ribavirin	Rebetron
	Peginterferon Alfa-2b + ribavirin	Peg-Intron + Rebetol

in the previously discussed viral diseases. Although these viruses are covered by individual chapters in this text, viruses having no (or very rare) mucocutaneous manifestations, such as rhinoviruses, influenza, respiratory syncytial virus, and rabies, are not discussed further (Table 1–12).

Recognition of characteristic mucocutaneous manifestations, however, of a variety of viral diseases either directly helps to determine the etiologic agent or assists the clinician in deciding which additional diagnostic tests to order. Proper management of the patient can be initiated from the results of such tests.

An important concept in the control of viral diseases is that antiviral drugs are generally virostatic, not virocidal. Therefore, prevention of viral infections takes on an even greater level of importance. Such control includes good public health measures such as sanitation, hand washing (and the use of disposable examination gloves), safe sex (abstinence, condoms), control of mosquitoes (and other vectors), testing of blood products, and single use of needles. Otherwise, the single most effective medical intervention is the use of vaccines. The prototype of a successful vaccine campaign was the eradication of smallpox. Recently, the only known stocks of smallpox virus, maintained by the governments of the United States and Russia, were to be destroyed. That plan has now been put on hold. Because widespread vaccination of the general public stopped around 1980, the majority of the world's population has no immunity to smallpox. Therefore, smallpox is considered to be a leading pathogen that could be used for bioterrorism.

Generally, the FDA-approved vaccines are several orders of magnitude safer, in terms of morbidity and mortality, than the diseases that they are designed to prevent. One vaccine, however, was recently removed from the market due to safety issues. Rotashield® was a live, oral tetravalent, rotavirus vaccine that was associated with several cases of intussusception and is considered to be causal [93]. Most associations between vaccines and adverse events are not, however, demonstrated to be causal. For example, the MMR vaccine was reported very recently not to have a causal relationship to autism [94,95]. Likewise, a causal relationship between the hepatitis B vaccine and a variety of autoimmune diseases has been disproved. This vaccine does not increase the risk of multiple sclerosis [96] nor does it cause a relapse of pre-existing multiple sclerosis (97). Nevertheless, suspected relationships between vaccines and adverse events need to be reported to the "Vaccine Adverse Event Reporting System" (1–800–822–7967) so that the excellent safety record of vaccines can be maintained.

It is anticipated that the future will bring safe and effective vaccines for a variety of viral diseases, for example, HIV, hepatitis C, HSV, and HPV. Although no vaccine is available for the therapy of a viral disease, our concept of vaccines is now being expanded by ongoing clinical trials of therapeutic vaccines, for example, for HIV, HSV, and HPV.

Table 1–12. FDA-approved Anti-influenza Agents

Generic name	Trade name	Indication
Amantadine	Symmetrel	Influenza A
Ramantadine	Flumadine	Influenza A
Oseltamivir	Tamiflu	Influenza A and B
Zanamivir	Relenza	Influenza A and B

REFERENCES

1. JG Bremen, I Arita. The confirmation and maintenance of smallpox eradication. N Engl J Med 303:1263–1273, 1980.
2. S Sussman, M Grossman. Complications of smallpox vaccination. Effects of vaccinia immune globulin therapy. J Pediatr 67:1168–1173, 1965.
3. CD Porter, NW Blahi, LC Archard, MF Muhlemann, N Rusedale, JJ Cream. Molluscum contagiosum virus types

in genital and non-genital lesions. Br J Dermatol 120:37–41, 1989.

4. DS Goodman, ED Teplitz, A Wishner, RS Klein, PG Burk, E Hershenbaum. Prevalence of cutaneous disease in patients with acquired immunodeficiency syndrome (AIDS) or AIDS-related complex. J Am Acad Dermatol 17:210–220, 1987

5. UW Leavell Jr, MJ McNamara, R Muelleng, WM Talbert, RC Ruches, J Dalton. Orf: report of 19 human cases with clinical and pathological observations. JAMA 203: 657–664, 1968.

6. AE Friedman-Kien, WP Rowe, WG Bonfield. Milker's nodules: isolation of a poxvirus from a human case. Science 140:1335–1339, 1963.

7. K Syrjanen, S Syrjanen. Papillomavirus Infections in Human Pathology. New York: J Wiley & Sons, 2000, pp. 117–142.

8. MW Cobb. Human papillomavirus infection. J Am Acad Dermatol 22:547–566, 1990.

9. DR Brown, KH Fife. Human papillomavirus infections of the genital tract. Med Clin North Am 74:1455–1485, 1990.

10. SM Syrjanen. Human papillomavirus infections in the oral cavity. In: K Syrjanen et al. eds. Papillomaviruses and Human Disease. Berlin: Springer, 1987, p. 104.

11. P Mounts, KV Shah. Respiratory papillomatosis: etiological relation to genital tract papillomaviruses. Prog Med Virol 29:90–114, 1984.

12. S Obalek, S Jablonska, M Favre, L Walczak, G Orth. Condyloma acuminata in children: frequent association with human papillomaviruses responsible for cutaneous warts. J Am Acad Dermatol 23:205–213, 1990.

13. H Pfister, I Hettich, U Runne, L Gissman, GN Chilf. Characterization of human papillomavirus type 13 from focal epithelial hyperplasia Heck lesions. J Virol 47:363–366, 1983.

14. S Jablonska, G Orth. Epidermodysplasia verruciformis. Clin Dermatol 3:83–96, 1985.

15. H zur Hausen. Human papillomaviruses in the pathogenesis of ano-genital cancer. Virology 184:9–13, 1991.

16. S Jablonska, J. Dubrowski, K Jukubowicz. Epidermodysplasia verruciformis as a model in studies on the role of papovavirus in oncogenesis. Cancer Res 32:583–589, 1972.

17. BA Werness, K Munger, PM Howley. Role of the human papillomavirus oncoproteins in transformation and carcinogenic progression. In: JT DeVita, ed. Important Advances in Oncology. Philadelphia: Lippincott-Raven, 1991, p. 3.

18. E De Villiers. Heterogeneity of the human papillomavirus group. J Virol 63:4898–4903, 1989.

19. PL Rady, R Chin, I Arany, TK Hughes, SK Tyring. Direct sequencing of consensus primer generated PCR fragments of human papillomaviruses. J Virol Methods 43:335–350, 1993.

20. KR Beutner, MA Conant, AE Friedman-Kien, M Illeman, NN Artman, RA Thisted, et al. Patient-applied podofilox for treatment of genital warts. Lancet 1:831–834, 1989.

21. DK Goette. Topical chemotherapy with 5-fluorouracil. J Am Acad Dermatol 4:633–649, 1981.

22. WS Sawchuk, PJ Weber, DR Lowy, LM Dzubow. Infectious papillomavirus in the vapor of warts treated with carbon dioxide laser or electrocoagulation: detection and protection. J Am Acad Dermatol 21:41–49, 1989.

23. RC Reichman, D Oakes, W Bonnez, D. Brown, HR Mattison, A Bailey-Farchione, MH Stoler, LM Demeter, SK Tyring, et al. Treatment of condyloma acuminatum with three different interferon-α preparations administered parenterally: a double-blind, placebo-controlled trial. J Infect Dis 162:1270–1276, 1990.

24. R Reid, MD Greenberg, DJ Pizzuti, KH Omoto, LH Rutledge, W Soo. Superficial laser vulvectomy. V. Surgical debulking is enhanced by adjuvant systemic interferon. Am J Obstet Gynecol 166:815–820, 1992.

25. LM Cowsert, MC Fox, G Zon, C Mirabelli. In vitro evaluation of phosphorothioate oligonucleotides targeted to the E2 mRNA of papillomavirus: potential treatment for genital warts. Antimicrob Agents Chemother 37:171–177, 1993.

26. E Van Cutsem, R Snoeck, M Van Ranst, P Fiten, G Opdenakker, K Geboes, J Janssens, P Rutgeerts, G Vantrappen, E de Clercq, et al. Successful treatment of a squamous papilloma of the hypopharynxesophagus by local injections of (S)-1-(3-Hydroxy-2-phosphonylmethoxypropyl) cytosine. J Med Virol 45:230–235, 1995.

27. L Edwards, A Ferenczy, L Eron, D Baker, ML Owens, TL Fox, AJ Hougham, KA Schmitt. Self-administered topical 5% imiquimod cream for external anogenital warts. Arch Dermatol 134(1):25–30, 1998.

28. L Corey, HG Adams, ZA Brown, KK Holmes. Genital herpes simplex virus infections: clinical manifestations, course and complications. Ann Intern Med 98:958–972, 1983.

29. AJ Nahmias, FK Lee, S Beckman-Nahmias. Sero-epidemiological and sociological patterns of herpes simplex virus infection in the world. Scand J Infect Dis 69(suppl): S19–S36, 1990.

30. RE Johnson, AI Nahmias, LS Maydei, FK Lee, CA Brooks, CB Snowden. A seroepidemiologic study of the prevalence of herpes simplex virus type 2 infection in the United States. N Engl J Med 321:7–12, 1989.

31. JJ Gibson, CA Harnung, GR Alexander, FK Lee, WA Potts, AJ Nahmias. A cross-sectional study of herpes simplex virus types 1 and 2 in college students: occurrence and determinants of infection. J Infect Dis 162:306–312, 1990.

32. JA Embil, RG Stephens, FR Manuel. Prevalence of recurrent herpes labialis and aphthous ulcers among young adults in six continents. Can Med Assoc J 113:627–630, 1975.

33. C Bader, CS Crumpacker, LE Schnipper, B Ransil, JE Clark, K Arndt, IM Freedberg. The natural history of recurrent facial-oral infection with herpes simplex virus. J Infect Dis 138:897–905, 1978.

34. J Cohen, S Straus. Varicella-zoster virus. In: BN Fields, DM Knipe, PM Howley, eds. Virology. 3rd ed. New York: Lippincott-Raven, 1996, pp 2525–2585.

35. KD Croen, SE Straus. Varicella-zoster virus latency. Annu Rev Microbiol 45:265–282, 1991.

36. RE Hope-Simpson. Postherpetic neuralgia. J R Col Gen Prac 25:571–575, 1975.

37. SP Harding, JR Lipton, JC Wells. Natural history of herpes zoster ophthalmicus: predictors of postherpetic neuralgia and ocular involvement. Br J Ophthalmol 71:353–358, 1987.

38. FC Rose, EM Brett, J Burston. Zoster encephalomyelitis. Arch Neurol 11:155–172, 1964.

39. D Kendall. Motor complications of herpes zoster. BMJ 1: 616–618, 1957.

40. CA Alford, S Stagno, RF Pass, WJ Britt. Congenital and perinatal cytomegalovirus infections. Rev Infect Dis 12: S745–S753, 1990.

41. TORCH syndrome and TORCH screening (editorial). Lancet 335:1559–1561, 1990.

42. TD Horn, AF Hood. Cytomegalovirus is predictably present in perineal ulcers from immunocompromised patients. Arch Dermatol 126:642–644, 1990.

43. JL Lesher. Cytomegalovirus and the skin. J Am Acad Dermatol 18:1333–1338, 1988.

44. JC Niederman, RW McCallum, G Henle, W Henle. Infectious mononucleosis: clinical manifestations in relation to EB virus antibodies. JAMA 203:205–209, 1968.

45. JT McCarthy, RJ Hoagland. Cutaneous manifestations of infectious mononucleosis. JAMA 187:153–154, 1964.

46. BM Petel. Skin rash with infectious mononucleosis and ampicillin. Pediatrics 40:910–911, 1967.

47. D Greenspan, JS Greenspan, M Conant, V Petersen, S Silverman, Y de Souza. Oral ''hairy'' leukoplakia in male homosexuals: evidence of association with both papillomavirus and a herpes-group virus. Lancet 2:831–834, 1984.

48. D Greenspan, JS Greenspan, NG Hearst, LZ Pan, MA Conant. Oral hairy leukoplakia: human immunodeficiency virus strains and risk for development of AIDS. J Infect Dis 155: 475–481, 1987.

49. L Lowe, AA Herbert, M Duvic. Gianotti-Crosti syndrome associated with Epstein-Barr virus infection. J Am Acad Dermatol 20:336–338, 1989.

50. K Yamanashi, T Okuno, K Shiraki, M Takahashi, T Kondo, Y Asano, T Kurata. Identification of human herpesvirus-6 as a causal agent for exanthem subitum. Lancet 1: 1065–1067, 1988.

51. C Lopez. Human herpesvirus 6 and 7: molecular biology and clinical aspects. In: B Roizman, RJ Whitley C Lopez, eds. The Human Herpesviruses. New York: Lippincott-Raven, 1993, p. 309.

52. MT Caserta, CB Hall. Human herpesvirus-6. Annu Rev Med 44:377–383, 1993.

53. Y Asano, T Yoshikawa, S Suga, I Kobayashi, T Nakashima, T Yazaki, Y Kajita, T Ozaki. Clinical features of infants with primary human herpesvirus 6 infection (exanthem subitum, roseola infantum). Pediatrics 93:104–108, 1994.

54. Y Chang, F Cesarman, MS Pessin, F Lee, J Culpepper, DM Knowles, PS Moore. Identification of herpesvirus-like DNA sequences in AIDS-associated Kaposi's sarcoma. Science 266:1865–1869, 1994.

55. YQ Huang, JJ Li, MH Kaplan, B Poiesz, E Katabira, WC Zhang, D Feiner, AE Friedman-Kien. Human herpesvirus like nucleic acid in various forms of Kaposi's sarcoma. Lancet 345:759–761, 1995.

56. N Dupin, M Grandadam, V Calvez, I Gorin, JT Aubin, S Harvard, et al: Herpesvirus-like DNA sequences in patients with Mediterranean Kaposi's sarcoma. Lancet 345: 761–762, 1995.

57. PL Rady, A Yen, RW Martin 3rd, I Nedelcu, TK Hughes, SK Tyring. Herpesvirus-like DNA sequences in classic Kaposi's sarcomas. J Med Virol 47:179–183, 1995.

58. PL Rady, A Yen, JL Rollefson, I Orengo, S Bruce, TK Hughes, SK Tyring. Herpesvirus-like DNA sequences in non–Kaposi's sarcoma skin lesions of transplant patients. Lancet 345:1339–1340, 1995.

59. RJ Whitley. The biology of B virus (cercopithecine virus). In: B Roizman, RJ Whitley, C Lopez, eds. The Human Herpesviruses. New York: Lippincott-Raven, 1993, p. 317.

60. PM Benson, SL Malane, R Banks, CB Hicks, J Hilliard. B virus (herpesvirus simiae) and human infection. Arch Dermatol 125:1247–1248, 1989.

61. GP Holmes, JK Hilliard, KC Klontz, AH Rupert, CM Schindler, E Parrish, DG Griffin, GS Ward, ND Bernstein, TW Bean, et al. B virus (herpesvirus simiae) infection in humans: epidemiologic investigation of a cluster. Ann Intern Med 112:833–839, 1990.

62. E DeClerq. Antivirals for the treatment of herpesvirus infections. J Antimicrob Chemother 32(suppl A):121–123, 1993.

63. RC Reichman, GJ Badger, GJ Mertz, L Corey, DD Richman, JD Conner, D Redfield, MC Savoia, MN Oxman, Y Bryson, et al. Treatment of recurrent genital herpes simplex infections with oral acyclovir. JAMA 251:2103–2107, 1984.

64. JC Huff, JL Drucker, A Clemmer, OL Laskin, JD Connor, YJ Bryson, HH Balfour. Effect of oral acyclovir on pain resolution in herpes zoster: a reanalysis. J Med Virol (suppl 1):93–96, 1993.

65. HH Balfour Jr, JM Kelly, CS Suarez, RC Heussner, JA Englund, DD Crane, PV McGuirt, AF Clemmer, DM Aeppli. Acyclovir treatment of varicella in otherwise healthy children. J Pediatr 116:633–639, 1990.

66. LH Goldberg, R Kaufman, TO Kurtz, MA Conant, LJ Eron, RL Batenhorst, GS Boone. Long-term suppression of recurrent genital herpes with acyclovir. A 5-year benchmark. Acyclovir Study Group. Arch Dermatol 129:582–587, 1993.

67. A Wald, J Zeh, G Barnum, LG Davis, L Corey. Suppression of subclinical shedding of herpes simplex virus type 2 with acyclovir. Ann Intern Med 124:8–15, 1996.

68. A Wald, L Corey, R Cone, A Hobson, G Davis, J Zehl. Frequent genital herpes simplex virus 2 shedding in immunocompetent women. Effect of acyclovir treatment. J Clin Invest 99:1092–1097, 1997.

69. S Tyring, RA Barbarash, J Nahlik, A Cunningham, J Marley, M Heng, T Jones, T Rea, R Boon, R Saltzman. Famciclovir for the treatment of acute herpes zoster: effects on

acute disease and postherpetic neuralgia. A randomized, double-blind, placebo-controlled trial. Collaborative Famciclovir Herpes Zoster Study Group. Ann Intern Med 123: 89–96, 1995.

70. KR Beutner, DJ Friedman, C Forszpaniak, PL Anderson, MJ Wood. Valaciclovir compared with acyclovir for improved therapy for herpes zoster in immunocompetent adults. Antimicrob Agents Chemother 39:1546–1553, 1995.

71. B Watson, R Gupta, T Randall, S Starr. Persistence of cell-mediated and humoral immune responses in healthy children immunized with live attenuated varicella vaccine. J Infect Dis 169:197–199, 1994.

72. RJ Whitley, B Meignier. Herpes simplex vaccines. Biotechnology 20:223–254, 1992.

73. T Chorba, LJ Anderson. Erythema infectiosum (Fifth disease). Clin Dermatol 7:65–74, 1989.

74. J Thurn. Human parvovirus B-19: historical and clinical review. Rev Infect Dis 10:1005–1011, 1988.

75. ML Keeler. Human parvovirus B-19; not just a pediatric problem. J Emerg Med 10:39–44, 1992.

76. I Thomas, CK Janniger. Hand, foot, and mouth disease. Cutis 52:265–266, 1993.

77. T Nakayama, T Urano, M Osano, Y Hayashi, S Sekine, T Ando, S Makinom. Outbreak of herpangina associated with coxsackievirus B3 infection. Pediatr Infect Dis J 8:495–498, 1989.

78. JD Cherry. Contemporary infectious exanthems. Clin Infect Dis 16:199–205, 1993.

79. C Bialecki, HM Feder Jr, JM Grant-Kels. The six classic childhood exanthems: a review and update. J Am Acad Dermatol 21:891–903, 1989.

80. JD Cherry. Rubella. In: RD Feigin, Cherry JD, eds. Textbook of Pediatric Infectious Diseases. 3rd ed. Philadelphia: WB Saunders, 1992, p. 1792.

81. HL Chan, I-J Su, T-T Kuo, YZ Kuan, MJ Chen, LY Shih, T Eimoto, Y Maeda, M Kikuchi, M Takeshita. Cutaneous manifestations of adult T cell leukemia/lymphoma. J Am Acad Dermatol 13:213–219, 1985.

82. H Libman, RA Witzburg. HIV Infection: A Clinical Manual. 2nd ed. Boston: Little, Brown, 1993.

83. TG Berger. Dermatologic manifestations of HIV infection. In: PT Cohen, MA Sande, PA Volberding, eds. The AIDS Knowledge Base: A Textbook of HIV Disease from the University of California, San Francisco, and the San Francisco General Hospital. Waltham, MA: The Medical Publishing Group, 1990, p. 531.

84. RA Johnson, JS Dover. Cutaneous manifestations of human immunodeficiency virus disease. In: TB Fitzpatrick, AZ Eisen, K Wolff et al, eds. Dermatology in General Medicine. 4th ed. New York: McGraw-Hill, 1993, p. 2637.

85. MJ Zalla, WP Su, AF Fransway. Dermatologic manifesta-
tions of human immunodeficiency virus infection. Mayo Clin Proc 67:1089–1108, 1992.

86. MH Kaplan, N Sadick, NS McNutt, M Meltzer, MG Sarngadharan, S Pahwa. Dermatologic findings and manifestations of acquired immunodeficiency syndrome (AIDS). J Am Acad Dermatol 16:485–506, 1987.

87. PA Volberding, SW Lagakos, MA Koch, C Pettinelli, MW Meyers, DK Booth, HH Balfour Jr, RC Reichman, JA Bartlett, MS Hirsch, et al. Zidovudine in asymptomatic human immunodeficiency virus infection. A controlled trial in persons with fewer than 500 CD4-positive cells per cubic millimeter. N Engl J Med 322:941–949, 1990.

88. EM Connor, RS Sperling, R Gelber, P Kiselev, G Scott, MJ O'Sullivan, R VanDyke, M Bey, W Shearer, RL Jacobson, et al. Reduction of maternal-infant transmission of human immunodeficiency virus type 1 with zidovudine treatment. N Engl J Med 331(18):1173–1180, 1994.

89. KM Butler, RN Husson, FM Balis, P Brauwers, J Eddy, D el-Amin, J Gress, M Hawkins, P Jarosinski, H Moss, et al. Dideoxyinosine in children with symptomatic human immunodeficiency virus infection. N Engl J Med 324: 137–144, 1991.

90. TC Meng, MA Fischl, AH Booth, SA Spector, D Bennett, Y Bassiakos, SH Lai, B Wright, DD Richman. Combination therapy with zidovudine and dideoxycytidine in patients with advanced human immunodeficiency virus infection. Ann Intern Med 116:13–20, 1992.

91. DA Cooper, PO Pehrson, C Pederson, M Moroni, E Oksenhendler, W Rozenbaum, N Clumeck, V Faber, W Stille, B Hirschel, et al. The efficacy and safety of zidovudine alone or as cotherapy with acyclovir for the treatment of patients with AIDS and AIDS-related complex: a double-blind, randomized trial. AIDS 7:197–207, 1993.

92. TG Berger. Treatment of bacterial, fungal, and parasitic infections in the HIV-infected host. Semin Dermatol 12: 296–300, 1993.

93. TY Murphy, PM Gargiullo, MS Massoudi, DB Nelson, AO Jumaan, CA Okoro, CA Okoro, LR Zanardi, S Setia, E Fair, CW LeBaron, M Wharton, JR Livingood. Intussusception among infants given an oral rotavirus vaccine. N Engl J Med 344:564–572, 2001.

94. L Dales, SJ Hammer, NJ Smith. Time trends in autism and in MMR immunization coverage in California. JAMA 285: 1183–1185, 2001.

95. JA Kaye, M del Mar Melero-Montes, H Jick. Mumps, measles and rubella vaccine and the incidence of autism recorded by general practitioners: a time trend analysis. Br Med J 322:460–463, 2001.

96. A Ascherio, SM Zhang, MA Hernan, MJ Olek, PM Caplan, K Brodoviczl. Hepatitis B vaccine and the risk of multiple sclerosis. N Engl J Med 344:327–332, 2001.

97. C Confavreux, S Suissa, P Saddier, V Bourdes, S Vukusic. Vaccinations and the risk of relapse in multiple sclerosis. N Engl J Med 344:319–326, 2001.

2

Cutaneous Resistance to Viral Infections

Omeed M. Memar
Academic Dermatology & Skin Care Institute, Chicago, Illinois, USA

Pedram Geraminejad
University of Illinois at Chicago School of Medicine, Chicago, Illinois, USA

Istvan Arany
University of Arkansas School of Medicine, Little Rock, Arkansas, USA

Stephen K. Tyring
*University of Texas Medical Branch, Galveston, Texas, USA,
and University of Texas Medical Branch Center for Clinical Studies, Houston, Texas, USA*

The skin permits primary immune sensitization, retains immunological memory and houses immunocytes, and can be preferentially affected by T-cell malignancies. Based on this information, Streilein proposed a specific relationship between the immune system and the integument, similar to that existing in gut-associated lymphoid tissue [1]. He then advanced the concept of skin-associated lymphoid tissue (SALT) [2]. SALT is composed of (1) keratinocytes, which can phagocytize, release many cytokines, and even express major histocompatibility complex (MHC) class II antigens upon incubation with interferon (IFN-γ); (2) epidermal Langerhans' cells, dendritic cells that have surface expression of MHC class II, CD1, CD3, and CD4 molecules and are the predominant scavenger antigen-presenting cells of the epidermis; (3) skin tropic T cells, which in the epidermis include mainly "inactive" memory T cells of predominantly CD8 + phenotype, although CD4 + and CD4 −, CD8 −, and $\gamma\delta$ + T cells are also present; and (4) skin endothelial cells, which direct cellular traffic in and out of the skin. The epidermis contains the basic elements needed for an immune response (T cells, antigen-presenting cells, and cytokines). The epidermis, in conjunction with its anatomical structure, serves as a primary line of defense against infections. Therefore, we will review the components of SALT and their interactions with viruses having cutaneous manifestations.

LANGERHANS' CELLS

Langerhans' cells are the professional antigen-presenting cells of the epidermis. They capture exogenous antigens and process them into peptides for presentation to CD4 + T cells in the context of MHC class II. Todate, two predominant methods of antigen capture have been described in Langerhans' cells: one is micropinocytosis, and the other involves a mannose receptor–mediated mechanism. Additionally, when they are infected with a virus such as human immunodeficiency virus (HIV), Langerhans' cells present viral peptides to CD8 + T cells in the context of a different MHC class (class I).

Skin biopsies from 7 of 40 HIV-positive individuals reacted with anti–HIV-1 core protein in an indirect immunofluorescence assay [3]. The only cells infected with HIV that could be detected were Langerhans' cells, although Heng and coworkers have shown that keratinocytes, which do not express CD4, can be coinfected with HSV-1 and HIV in vivo [4]. Berger et al. demonstrated that Langerhans' cells could be infected with HIV in vitro and that Langerhans' cells from HIV-positive individuals could infect mononuclear phagocytes from HIV-negative individuals [5]. Cimarelli et al. quantified the proviral DNA in Langerhans' cells and found that this value correlated with the frequency of peripheral blood CD4 + T cells infected with HIV in acquired immune deficiency syndrome (AIDS) patients [6]. Two important questions arise: How are the Langerhans' cells infected? How do they contribute to the pathology associated with AIDS?

HIV is the causative agent of AIDS. HIV is a retrovirus that can incorporate into cellular DNA through reverse transcriptase. Infection leads to a progressive weakening of cell-mediated immune function and a progressive decline in the numbers of peripheral blood CD4 + cells. The effect on the humoral immune system is the induction of hypergammaglobulinemia, which enables diagnosis but is not sufficient to eliminate HIV infection. HIV has a particular tropism for activated CD4 + cells [7]. Phagocytes containing the proviral form of HIV have been isolated from AIDS patients [8].

Langerhans' cells normally reside in the epidermis. When they are activated, these cells migrate to the draining lymph nodes and come in contact with T cells. By using the HIV animal model of simian immunodeficiency virus (SIV) and rhesus macaques, it was shown that dendritic cells of the lamina propria are the first to be infected with intravaginal inoculation of virus [9]. Four rhesus macaques were inoculated intravaginally and then killed 2, 5, 7, and 9 days later. The animal killed at 2 days postinoculation showed productive infection only in the dendritic cells of the lamina propria. Conversely, no infection could be detected by polymerase chain reaction in the epithelial layer, including in Langerhans' cells. Interestingly, SIV-infected cells in the lamina propria were found only immediately beneath the single columnar epithelium of the endocervix. However, other investigators have shown that up to 40% of infected cells of the vaginal tract in rhesus macaques with chronic SIV infection are intraepithelial Langerhans' cells [10]. Miller and Hu were the first to provide in vivo evidence that Langerhans' cells of the genital tract are infected with SIV. These same investigators claim that the dendritic cells of the epithelial layer are the first to be infected with SIV during vaginal inoculation [10].

Some studies agree that dendritic cells are the first to be infected during vaginal inoculation of virus, but the how and where of occurrence are unclear. Also unclear is whether the site of first infection is the dendritic cells of the dermis or the Langerhans' cells of the epithelial layer. Blauvelt et al. propose that productive infection of dendritic cells by HIV-1 and the cells' ability to capture virus

are mediated through separate pathways [11]. Although productive infection is dependent on the CD4 ligand and coreceptor stimulation, HIV capture and transmission can take place independently of these factors. Epithelial Langerhans' cells capture viruses and deliver them to the draining lymph nodes. During activation by T cells in the cytokine-rich lymph nodes, Langerhans' cells may subsequently become productively infected. Recirculation of these cells to the epithelial layer may explain the 40% composition of infected cells in the vagina [10]. Another possibility is that some Langerhans' cells carrying virus migrate to the dermis and infect dermal CD4 + and dendritic cells. This idea is supported by evidence from other laboratories using a hybrid murine/human in vitro model [12]. Murine dendritic cells that are known to be nonpermissive to HIV infection were incubated with HIV and then cocultured with human T lymphocytes. Transfer of virus to T cells was observed. Previously described mechanisms of antigen capture by Langerhans' cells include micropinocytosis and mannose receptor–mediated uptake [11]. However, it is unknown whether HIV antigens are taken up by one of these or by another as yet unknown method.

Consistent with this viral transfer model is the recent discovery of a new lectin, designated DC-SIGN. DC-SIGN binds ICAM-3 and HIV and maintains them on the cell surface for days in a native conformation conducive to infection. Langerhans' cells are not known to express DC-SIGN; once in the dermis, however, dendritic cells express this lectin. Since epidermal, i.e., DC-SIGN-negative dendritic cells, are more selective for M-tropic HIV-1, the Langerhans' cells most likely transmit M-tropic HIV to the dermal dendritic cells, which become DC-SIGN-positive to facilitate HIV transmission [13,14].

Alternatively, seeding of Langerhans' cells may occur by direct inoculation and productive infection. This is particularly plausible in coinfection scenarios where, for example, a herpetic lesion has compromised the cornified layer of the epidermis. The lesion attracts and activates CD4 + cells. This leaves Langerhans' cells and other cells in the epidermis and possibly the dermis vulnerable to primary infection. This idea is supported by the finding in the rhesus macaques model that the only DC-SIGN-positive cells of the lamina propria that were infected were those directly beneath the single columnar epithelium [9]. This epithelial barrier is easier to penetrate than that of squamous epithelium. Additionally, the epithelium of the vagina is not as tight and impenetrable as that of the skin. It is moist, and fluid is continually passing through the intercellular spaces. These epithelial cells are connected by discontinuous patches of desmosomes, the weakest form of intercellular junction [9].

A significant reduction of epidermal Langerhans' cells in HIV-positive individuals has been demonstrated [15].

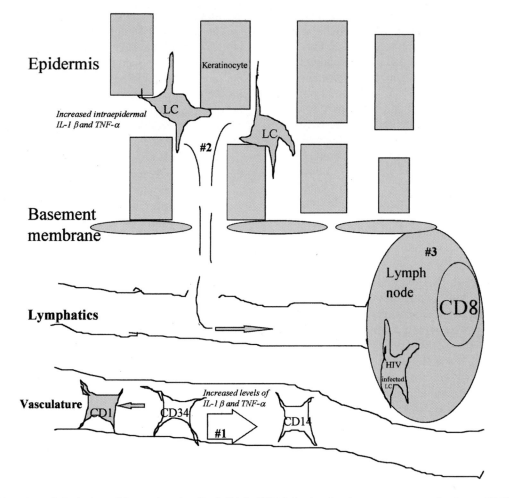

Figure 2–1. Intradermal depletion of Langerhans' cells (LCs) in HIV infection by three separate mechanisms: (1) IL-1β and TNF-α influence precursors of CD34 LCs to differentiate toward CD14 dermal dendritic cells rather than toward CD1 LCs, (2) LCs migrate toward the draining lymph nodes, (3) cytotoxic lymphocytes within lymph nodes destroy HIV-infected LCs.

HIV infection can result in a milieu in which levels of various cytokines, especially interleukin-1β (IL-1β) and tumor necrosis factor-α (TNF-α), are chronically elevated [16] (Fig. 2–1). These cytokines are essential and powerful stimulators of Langerhans' cell migration out of the epidermis [17,18]. Cytokine stimulus may partly explain the reduction of epidermal Langerhans' cells in HIV infection. Langerhans' cells originate from CD34 + marrow-derived cells that can differentiate along two primary pathways. One pathway leads to the formation of a group of cells most known for their expression of CD1 that become the Langerhans' cells of the epidermis [19]. The alternative pathway leads to the dendritic cells of the dermis, noted for expression of CD14. Whereas the CD1 + cells of the epidermis promote cell-mediated immunity (CMI), the CD14 + cells of the dermis tend to initiate a humoral response [19]. When the hypergammaglobulinemia and defi-

ciency of CMI in HIV infection are considered, speculation is that direct or indirect cytokine manipulation by HIV results in a preference for the CD14 + pathway. This might be a second factor in the depletion of epidermal Langerhans' cells. Last, HIV infection has definite cytopathic effects on Langerhans' cells. After migrating to lymph nodes and activating T cells, dendritic cells do not leave the lymph nodes in the efferent lymphatics. In vitro studies have shown that HIV-infected dendritic cells could serve as targets of cytotoxic lymphocytes (CTL) [20]. In one study as many as 50% of the dendritic cells were lysed after 3 days of HIV exposure, which was then followed by exposure to activated cytotoxic lymphocytes.

Cytokines strongly influence HIV-infected Langerhans' cells. Leonard and coworkers created a transgenic mouse with the HIV long terminal repeat (LTR) that contains all known HIV transcriptional response elements, linked to a reporter gene [21]. Langerhans' cells from the mouse skin had a higher reporter gene activity when compared with other cells of the monocyte/macrophage lineage. This indicates that HIV provirus is easily induced in Langerhans' cells. The transgenic mouse macrophages treated with a variety of cytokines (colony-stimulating factor-1, granulocyte-monocyte colony-stimulating factor (GM-CSF), IL-1α, and IL-2) had much higher reporter gene activity than macrophages incubated in the absence of these cytokines. The results indicate that these cytokines are involved in modulating SALT, and it would be important to elucidate their role in human skin from HIV-positive patients.

In healthy skin, IL-1 is constitutively made by keratinocytes, whereas Langerhans' cells make IL-1 upon activation and depend on it for their proper maturation [22]. IL-1 upregulates IL-2 and IL-2 receptor production by T cells, a process necessary for an antigen-specific immune response. Stage of disease, by Centers for Disease Control classification, has been correlated with epidermal Langerhans' cell numbers. Subsequently, Dreno et al. have shown a relationship between intraepidermal levels of IL-1 in normal skin of HIV-positive patients and the stage of their disease [23]. All stage II patients had high levels of intraepidermal IL-1. Significant decreases in IL-1 were seen in stage III patients and even lower or in some cases undetectable levels in stage IV^c and stage IV^d patients. It is likely that the paucity of intraepidermal Langerhans' cells in these later stages is directly responsible for the lower levels of IL-1. The subsequent lower levels of IL-2 leave the epidermis devoid of T cells, vulnerable to infections, at risk for development of neoplasms, and anergic to recall antigens.

In addition to decreased numbers of epidermal Langerhans' cells, symptom-free HIV-positive individuals have reduced intraepidermal CD4 + cell counts. After IL-2 injection, however, local accumulation of T cells, monocytes, and Langerhans' cells occurs [24]. Although epidermal infiltration of CD4 + cells is normally reduced in HIV-positive patients, IL-2 induces a CD4 + infiltrative response equivalent to that seen in HIV-negative individuals and results in enhanced recall response to antigens [4]. Therefore, inoculation of IL-2, which is usually made by T cells in response to IL-1, converts a relatively sterile epidermis in HIV patients into an antigen-responsive milieu.

A great majority of T cells in the human epidermis have αβ T-cell receptors. Some of these T cells lack the coreceptors CD4 and CD16, and their function in the epidermis is unknown. In humans, epidermal γδ + cells are not dendritic and are involved in many diseases. CD1, which is expressed on Langerhans' cells, can act as an antigen-presenting molecule for γδ + T cells [25]. γδ + cells, through non-MHC-restricted cytolytic activity, contribute greatly to immune surveillance against malignancies and viral infections [26]. In HIV infection, local γδ subtype ratios of bronchial-associated lymphoid tissue (BALT) are altered relative to HIV-negative individuals [27]. Hermier et al. observed higher γδ + cells in the blood of relatively healthy HIV-positive patients than in symptomatic HIV-positive patients [28]. HIV-positive patients with oral candidiasis had even lower blood γδ T cell counts than did other HIV-positive patients. Numerous infectious, neoplastic, and idiopathic cutaneous manifestations in HIV patients, along with the known effects of HIV on γδ + cells in other lymphoid tissues, would suggest that γδ + cells are functionally affected in the skin of HIV-positive patients. Unfortunately, it is not known whether γδ counts increase or decrease in the epidermis of HIV-positive individuals. Indirect immunofluorescence assays of punch biopsies of skin using pan-γδ antibodies should be a simple and direct method of answering this question.

A decrease in intraepidermal Langerhans' cells is a common phenomenon of viral infections. However, some viruses have adapted other mechanisms of influencing Langerhans' cells. Mature dendritic cells release the cytokines necessary for T-cell activation and to ward off herpes simplex virus (HSV) infections [29,30]. Salio et al. showed that infected dendritic cells are unable to upregulate costimulatory molecules, do not produce cytokines, and do not acquire responsiveness to those chemokines required for migration to secondary lymphoid organs [31]. To compare infected and uninfected dendritic cells, a recombinant replication defective HSV1 encodes a green fluorescent protein. Normally dendritic cells are the primary producers of IFN-α. It may be that the disregulation of dendritic cells by HSV, as described above, allows the virus to evade the immune system [32].

KERATINOCYTES

Keratinocytes are squamous epithelial cells that take part in SALT by the production of cytokines, presentation of endogenous viral antigens in the context of MHC class I to CD8 + T cells, and expression of MHC class II when stimulated with interferon. Human papilloma virus (HPV) is a DNA virus that can directly infect keratinocytes (Fig. 2–2). HPV gains entry into the epidermis through a break in the skin and remains in the basal layer. It replicates just below the granular layer and gives rise to a slow-growing lesion. There are over 100 different recognized HPV genotypes [33]. HPV is categorized by regional tropism and the potential for malignant transformation. For example, HPV 6 and 11 are tropic for the genital skin and mucous membranes, giving rise to condyloma acuminatum, which has a low probability of undergoing malignant transformation.

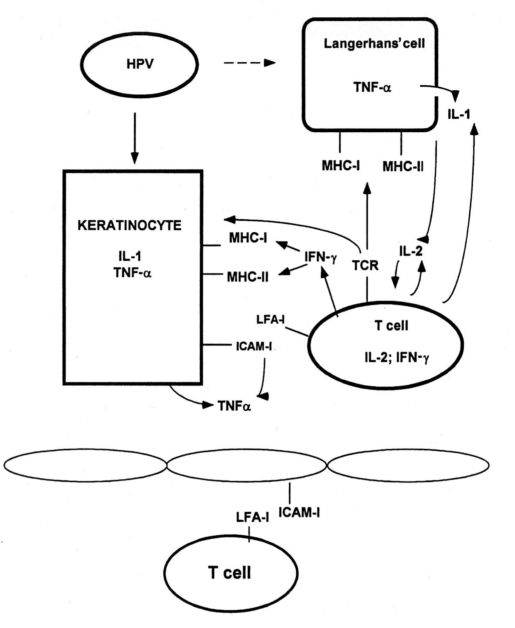

Figure 2–2. Necessary immune mechanisms for effective HPV clearance, including MHC II presentation of HPV antigens to CD4 cells by Langerhans' cells with costimulation by B7 and stabilization by ICAM-1. MHC I and II, IL-1, TNF-α, IL-2, ICAM-1, IFN-γ and costimulatory molecules, are commonly deficient in chronic HPV infections. (Leukocyte functional antigen = LFA.)

Epidermodysplasia verruciformis is characterized by persistent disseminated wartlike skin lesions associated with HPV 5 and 8. One third of patients with these lesions later experience malignant transformation of the HPV-infected lesions.

Recently, the active role of SALT in HPV infections has been further elucidated. Generally, regressing flat wart lesions are accompanied by CD4+ and CD8+ cellular infiltrates, a reduction in epidermal Langerhans' cells, an increase in dermal Langerhans' cells, and the appearance of human leukocyte antigen (HLA)-DR+ cells in the dermis. In general cutaneous viral infections lead to a reduction in the number of epidermal Langerhans' cells [34]. Furthermore, lesions positive for HPV viral antigens are more likely to have reduced Langerhans' and HLA-DR+ cell counts in the epidermis [35]. Keratinocytes are known to express HLA-DR but not HLA-DQ in HPV infections. Therefore, staining for HLA-DR in the lesion reveals its expression on keratinocytes but not on Langerhans' cells. Viac et al. observed HLA-DR + keratinocytes only in condyloma acuminatum and laryngeal papillomas and not in plantar and hand warts [36]. HLA-DR expression directly correlated with the intraepithelial upregulation of intercellular adhesion molecule-1 (ICAM-1) and lymphocyte function-associated antigen-1 (LFA-1) [36]. ICAM-1 is expressed on keratinocytes in condyloma but not in flat warts. LFA-1, the natural ligand for ICAM-1, is expressed on lymphocytes and directs lymphocytes to the epidermis. Normally, ICAM-1 is expressed at low levels on dermal endothelial cells, not in the epidermis. Upregulation of ICAM-1 and other adhesion molecules leads to lymphocytic infiltration. This, along with upregulation of HLA-DR in the epidermis, could facilitate antigen presentation to infiltrating CD4 + T cells and lead to clearance of infection [37,38].

We have addressed the role of HPV pathology in skin by identifying HPV gene products and immunological and cellular responses in patients. We probed for TNF-α and TGF-β1 levels in HPV 6- and 11-induced condylomas and found a dramatic reduction in their levels when compared with those in normal skin [39]. Majewski et al. found increased expression of TNF-α and TGF-β1 in epidermodysplasia verruciformis lesions [40]. The disparity of TNF-α and TGF-β1 levels between epidermodysplasia verruciformis and condyloma lesions might indicate part of the underlying defect in epidermodysplasia verruciformis patients. There may be a lack of proper T-cell repertoire [41] necessary to mount a regulatory or effector function, a cytokine receptor defect [42], or active neutralization of the cytokines by HPV products [43]. The viral oncoprotein/cellular protein interactions are well established in "high-risk" HPV types, but very little is known concerning lesions caused by "low-risk" HPV types. mRNAs of the early papilloma virus proteins E2, E5, E6, and E7, as well as the late L1 protein, can be detected by reverse transcriptase-polymerase chain reaction (RT-PCR) [39] in low-risk HPV-containing condylomas. Especially important is the high abundance of E7 and E6 messages since they can inhibit pRb and p53, respectively, two well-known tumor suppressor genes. Also important is E2, which regulates expression of HPV genes. The L1 gene encodes the major capsid protein and plays a critical antigenic role in cellular immunity. Viral oncoproteins, such as high-risk E6 and E7, interact with cellular regulatory proteins (e.g., p53, pRb, E2F) by displacing them in specific cellular pathways. Low-risk E6 and E7 proteins probably are not capable of binding cellular proteins, or at least bind with lower affinity, but they are still able to transregulate certain host genes like their high-risk counterparts [44,45].

In condyloma lesions, there are decreased levels of growth-inhibitory genes (TGF-β1 and p53). Also present are increased mRNA levels of hyperphosphorylated (inactive) retinoblastoma tumor suppressor gene product (pRB), reduced levels of p53 tumor suppressor gene product, increased levels of cdc2-kinase, and increased levels of c-*myc* [39]. Although HPV 6 and 11 are low risk for malignant progression, the condyloma lesional milieu is conducive to proliferation, i.e., a slow-growing lesion. Elevated cdc2-kinase levels lead to elevated cdc2 protein levels, presumably allowing for higher kinase activity. Elevated cdc2 protein most probably leads to hyperphosphorylation and inactivation of pRB. The underphosphorylated (i.e., active) pRB has strong transcriptional regulatory functions and can upregulate TGF-β1 as well as other growth control factors [46]. Underphosphorylated pRB also binds and inhibits the transcription factors for the enzymes of DNA replication. With reduced active pRB, the TGF-β1 levels would drop and the transcription factors necessary to produce the enzymes of DNA replication would be upregulated, leading to unregulated hyperproliferation of cells and subsequent growth of lesions.

The above data demonstrate an increase in proliferation but a decrease in differentiation and growth suppressive signals by the presence of low risk types of HPVs. Since experimental data suggest a negative effect of HPVs on cytokine/lymphokine secretion in vitro, these changes may be attributable to the expression of viral genes [47]. The downregulation of TGF-β, TNF-α, and IFN-β is particularly interesting because these cytokines and others (such as GMC-SF and IL-1s) have the capacity to influence MHC class I and class II expression, and potentially antigen presentation [48,49].

Condylomas have very low levels of MHC class I and II mRNAs compared with those in uninfected skin [50]. This significant decrease of MHC mRNA, a marker for Langerhans' cells, suggests a decline of these cells [51]. Quantitative and morphological changes of cutaneous Langerhans' cells have been observed in condylomas. Because HLA-DR is expressed chiefly by Langerhans' cells and keratinocytes of condylomas, the reduced numbers of Langerhans' cells must cause the net reduction. Diminished levels of IL-1α and IL-1β further affect the ability of epidermal cells to present antigens, thus influencing dendritic Langerhans' cells. This lack of Langerhans' cells probably hampers keratinocyte presentation of antigen and leads to a decrease in the immunological surveillance process.

The very low levels of IL-2 mRNAs in condylomas further suggest a significant decrease in numbers of lymphocytes [52]. Indeed, CD4 and CD8 mRNA levels are significantly lower in infected skin than in uninfected skin. Tay et al. detected a lower helper-suppressor T-cell ratio in condyloma acuminatum compared to that in normal tissue [53]. Other data indicate that CD8 mRNA exceeds CD4 mRNA levels in infected skin and are in agreement with these findings [39]. This depletion of intraepithelial lymphocytes, together with the depletion of Langerhans' cells, the selective depletion of CD4+ cells, and the change in the ratio of CD4+ and CD8+ subsets, supports the suggestion that there is a local intraepithelial immune deficiency associated with HPV infection. This might facilitate a prolonged HPV infection and expression of other long-term effects, such as malignancy.

Suppression of class I MHC expression (e.g., HLA-B7) in HPV-infected cells may be virally mediated [54]. Given the extent to which MHC class I levels can be affected by indirect means, such as availability of stimulatory or inhibitory cytokines, care must be taken in assigning modulations of surface class I levels to direct virus intervention. On the other hand, in vitro experiments clearly demonstrate that the presence of HPV may contribute to the loss of responsiveness of infected cells to potent MHC-inducing cytokines [47].

The presence of HPV can influence MHC gene expression directly or indirectly. A direct influence might be elicited through the expression of E7 or E5 early genes, which seem to interact with the antigen processing system in in vivo studies [55]. Indirect effects of E7 or other HPV early gene products may be exerted through different cytokines (e.g., TGF-β, TNF-α, IL-1) or oncogenes (c-*myc*), which then can influence MHC class I or II synthesis [56]. Another direct effect of HPV gene products on MHC levels and antigen presentation might relate to a high abundance of early viral genes (especially E7). This differential expression can have multiple effects, leading to immunological hyporesponsiveness. First, in vitro experiments demonstrate that the HPV E7 proteins are masked in the infected cell nuclei, probably as a result of complex formation with cellular proteins. The consequence of this masking might be an inappropriate immune recognition, which could be the case in nonresponder tumors [57]. Second, keratinocytes, which lack costimulatory molecules, might render E7-specific T cells anergic through peripheral tolerance [58].

Upon an active immune response, HPV-infected keratinocytes release TNF-α, which is toxic to HPV replication. Patients with more advanced cervical carcinoma in situ were found to have lower levels of TNF-α in affected areas, whereas in areas of normal epidermis, there was constitutively expressed TNF-α from keratinocytes. Another consistent finding in cervical carcinoma was the lack of expression of any adhesion or costimulatory molecules by epithelial Langerhans' cells [59]. The lack of TNF-α, a known stimulator of Langerhans' cells, may have been responsible. TNF-α also normally upregulates the expression of ICAM-1 on keratinocytes, which attracts T cells. Therefore, ICAM-1 levels may also be inappropriately low. This, in combination with the decreased numbers of Langerhans'

cells in the epidermis, may be contributory to the progression of the carcinoma. Keratinocytes, however, were found to have increased expression of HLA DR, CD 54, and CD 58, thus increasing their antigen-presenting capacity [59]. This increased expression may be futile in light of the depressed activity of Langerhans' cells secondary to decreased TNF-α and other Langerhans' cell–activating cytokines.

The deficiency in TNF-α, with subsequent downregulation of ICAM-1 and T cells, results in decreased levels of IFN-γ. Therefore MHC class II is not upregulated and antigen presentation is not facilitated (see Fig. 2–2). Elevations of TGF-β1, IFN-β, and underphosphorylated (active) pRB and reduced levels of cdc2-kinase and c-*myc* follow intralesional IFN treatment of HPV-infected sites [60], indicating a more complicated role of IFN action. The IFN causes an initial immune modulatory effect and stimulates the immune system to overtake the infection. Thus, the cytokine and anti-oncogene responses reflect a normal status.

Despite the wealth of knowledge regarding the virulence and oncogenic factors of HPV, some individuals continue to be more susceptible to these factors than others. The successful clearance of HPV from the epidermis is dependent on an intact immune system. Among immunosuppressed transplant patients, 77% eventually develop viral warts [36]. Some recent investigations found a correlation between HLA type and HPV susceptibility and immunity [61–66]. Although a critical role for HLA antigens is likely, the results vary among investigators, and the data at this point are preliminary. One study has shown strong cytotoxic T lymphocyte responses following T-cell exposure to dendritic cells pulsed with recombinant E7 protein [67]. This may indicate that effective antigen presentation may be the area of deficiency in those with chronic HPV infection.

T CELLS

T cells are important regulatory and effector components in SALT. Herpes simplex virus (HSV) exemplifies the role of T cells in SALT, as T cells are necessary to prevent reactivation of HSV infection. Skin-homing lymphocytes express a sialyl Lewis a- and x- closely related antigen called cutaneous lymphocyte–associated antigen (CLA) [68]. CLA is a selectin ligand that is expressed on transition of T cells from the naive to the memory status in the presence of IL-12 and TGF-β and binds E-selectin of the endothelium [69]. Therefore, for memory T cells to traffic to skin, they normally express CLA.

HSV1 and 2 are DNA viruses with extensive cutaneous manifestations, including interactions with SALT. This leads to modulation of immunocyte subsets and the epidermal upregulation of IL-1β, TNF-α, and IL-6 [70]. HSV types 1 and 2 cause a primary infection and then retire to their respective neuronal ganglia to asymptomatically shed viral particles. In immunocompetent individuals, HSV remains in a latent phase, with only mild or subclinical reactivations. In immunocompromised patients, reactivation is more common and severe. One important question is the role of SALT in preventing HSV reactivation.

Overcoming a cutaneous HSV infection requires intact antigen presentation and both CD4+ and CD8+ T cells [71–73]. In most viral infections, including HSV, CD8+ cytotoxic lymphocytes (CTL) are major effector cells, but in HSV, CD4+ cells are involved in both immune modulation and direct cell killing. Jennings et al. reported the requirement of CD4+ T cells in mounting a primary CTL response to HSV infection and identified a similar requirement for the presence of CD4+ cells in a secondary CTL response [74]. Williams and coworkers demonstrated that although the epidermis is the primary site of inoculation and subsequent HSV infection, Langerhans' cells failed to invoke a HSV-specific proliferation of T cells from naive animals [75]. This suggests that epidermal Langerhans' cells may not invoke the primary T-cell response against HSV. Instead, they acquire this ability only after maturation in an extra-epidermal site where there is sufficient cytokine stimulation. This lag in time might allow the HSV viral infection to enter the protective dorsal ganglia. Also, Langerhans' cells actively invoke a secondary T-cell proliferative response to HSV, abrogated by anti-MHC class II antibodies and complement [75]. Therefore, both the primary and secondary (i.e., memory) CD4+ T cell responses to HSV require HSV presentation in the context of MHC class II.

The CD4+ Th cells have been categorized into two major subsets, Th1 and Th2 [76]. The Th1 cells mainly secrete IL-2, IFN-γ, and TNF, whereas Th2 cells mainly secrete IL-4, IL-5, and IL-10. Interestingly, the cytokine activity of each Th subset downregulates the activity of the other subset. Th1 cells are generally efficient in controlling viral and intracellular pathogens, whereas Th2 cells better control bacterial and parasitic infections by augmenting humoral immunity. The presence of Th1 and Th2 differences in skin and their involvement in cutaneous disease have been demonstrated [77]. Not surprisingly, the data support an obvious role for Th1 cells. Administration to mice of HSV-2 plasmid vaccines encoding the gD protein, as well as the Th1 cytokines IL-1, IL-12, IL-15 and IL-18, resulted in immunity to subsequent challenge with HSV-2. However, mice inoculated with plasmids encoding the same HSV-2 gD protein but with Th2 cytokines IL-4 and IL-10 had increased morbidity and mortality [30]. If the Th2 cytokines downregulate the Th1 response, decreased

cellular immunity, the primary defense against cutaneous herpes infection, is experienced. Other vaccine-based studies have shown that vaccination with HSV-2 DNA plasmid vaccines favors a Th1 response, whereas induction of immunity with recombinant protein gD induces a Th2 response. Although both were protective against lethal challenge, only the plasmid DNA vaccine induced a response that was protective against subsequent herpetic lesions and HSV-induced morbidity [78]. While cell-mediated immunity (CMI) is most relevant to cutaneous manifestations, the humoral response offers protection from HSV encephalitis and HSV-induced mortality [29,78].

Eta-1, or osteopontin, a newly described cytokine, further supports the role of CMI in HSV-1 infection. Eta-1 is a necessary component of CMI [79]. Without this cytokine, IFN-γ and IL-12 do not increase appropriately, and IL-10 levels rise inappropriately. Eta-1 -/- mice infected with HSV-1 were unable to mount a delayed type hypersensitivity (DTH) reaction when further inoculated in the foot pad with HSV-1. Eta-1 +/+, HSV-1 infected mice displayed a strong DTH response in the foot pad when inoculated with HSV-1. Use of the antibody against Eta-1 results in similar findings. Although this study does not deny a role for Th2 and the humoral response in protection against HSV, it emphasizes the overwhelming significance of CMI.

ENDOTHELIAL CELLS

In many respects the endothelium is the gatekeeper of the skin, only allowing certain cells and components through. Adhesion molecules expressed by endothelial cells play a significant role in leukocyte entry into the skin. E-selectin, P-selectin, ELAM-1, ICAM-1, ICAM-2, and VCAM-1 are the predominant adhesion molecules of endothelial cells used for interaction with leukocytes. The first part of this interaction involves the slowing of blood flow and the margination of cells toward the periphery of the vasculature near the endothelium. Selectins mediate the next step, known as rolling, which consists of loose and transient associations between the white cells and the endothelium. This is followed by the firm and stable adhesions formed by integrins such as ICAM-1, ICAM-2, and VCAM-1. This, in turn, leads to diapedesis, mediated in part by ICAM-1 [80]. During this process endothelial cells are an important element in the eradication of pathogens. However, certain pathogens show tropism for endothelial cells and can infect them. Cytomegalovirus (CMV) is a virus well documented

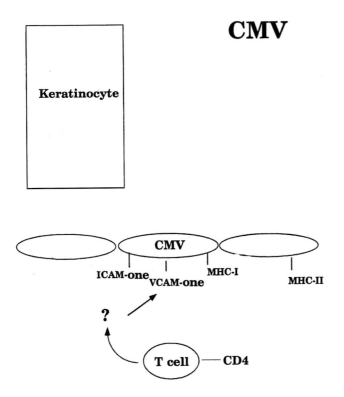

Figure 2–3. Cytomegalovirus (CMV) is disseminated to healthy tissue through endothelial infection. (1) CMV causes endothelial upregulation of vascular adhesion molecules by a paracrine mechanism; (2) transendothelial migration by white cells results in infection from adjacent endothelial cells; (3) infected white cells disseminate CMV into healthy tissue.

to have endothelial involvement (Fig. 2–3). Although CMV has numerous mucocutaneous manifestations, especially in immunocompromised patients, the majority of research on endothelial involvement of CMV has been carried out on extracutaneous tissues.

CMV infection of endothelial cells directly affects transendothelial migration of white cells and further dissemination of the CMV virus. Studies with human umbilical vein endothelial cells (HUVEC) have shown that CMV infection upregulates endothelial expression of E-selectin, ELAM-1, ICAM-1, and VCAM-1 [81,82]. ELAM-1 and ICAM-1 caused increased adhesion of polymorphonuclear (PMN) cells and T lymphocytes, whereas VCAM-1 resulted in increased adhesion of monocytes and T lymphocytes to endothelial cells [81]. IL-1β may mediate the increased expression of these endothelial surface antigens. CMV infection of endothelial cells results in increased secretion of IL-1β, which affects adjacent noninfected endothelial cells by a paracrine route. Significantly, studies have shown that certain white cells, such as neutrophils, can

become infected during transmigration across infected endothelial cells and subsequently disperse this infection to other cells [83,84]. This can tremendously increase the dissemination of the virus and the inflammatory response throughout the body.

Endothelial cells also express MHC class I and II antigens, subsequent to IFN-γ [85]. In the past few years a host of other escape mechanisms for CMV have been proposed, and many of these involve the influence of CMV on MHC class I and II expression by the endothelium. In one study it was shown that CMV disrupts the signal transduction pathway that normally results in expression of IFN-α [86]. Specifically, CMV decreases the expression of Janus Kinus 1 and p48, important signal transducers involved in the expression of IFN-α. Decreased IFN-α, a key antiviral cytokine, secondarily results in MHC-I, IFN regulatory factor-1, MxA, and 2′, 5-oligoadenylate synthetase gene expression in fibroblasts and endothelial cells infected with CMV. Similarly, another group showed that CMV-infected arterial and venous endothelial cells are refractory to upregulation of MHC-II by IFN-γ [87]. CMV has the ability to interrupt signal transduction of the JAK/STAT pathway, which is induced by IFN-γ and normally upregulates MHC-II [88]. The combination of these two findings results in decreased expression of both class I and II antigens by the endothelium. The result is an impaired ability to induce an immune response and clear CMV infection. Only with a competent immune system can important molecules be sufficiently upregulated, allowing for effective antigen presentation and immunoresponsiveness.

HIV infection also affects the endothelial component of SALT. HIV-infected cells release many different cytokines, with TNF-α being the most common [89]. TNF-α contributes to endothelial leakiness by (1) induction of cytokine release, (2) expression of adhesion molecules, and (3) direct enhancement of endothelial permeability. Furthermore, the HIV-derived transactivator (tat) protein, which is secreted into extravascular tissue, directly stimulates endothelial cells to express E-selectin, ICAM-1, VCAM-1, and ELAM-1 [90–92]. The molecules are necessary for endothelial trapping of leukocytes in the vasculature. IL-6 synthesis, enhanced by tat, increases endothelial permeability, which facilitates leukocyte passage out of the vasculature [93]. This aids in the dissemination of infected cells into virus-free tissue. This may also be deleterious to epithelial homing of leukocytes and contribute to epidermal depletion of Langerhans' cells.

Interactions between the HIV tat protein and the endothelium may be responsible for the highly aggressive behavior of AIDS malignancies. As mentioned earlier, increased expression of VCAM-1, ICAM-1, ELAM-1, and alpha v beta 3 integrin as well as other vascular adhesion molecules is thought to be a direct consequence of the tat protein. These proteins increase cellular motility and transendothelial migration. It has been shown that the tat protein increases the motility of cells from the AIDS-related Burkitt's lymphoma cell lines and AIDS primary effusion lymphoma cell lines. Tat not only enhances the migration of lymphoma cells but also increases their adhesion to endothelial cells. This study gives one explanation for the malignant behavior of non-Hodgkins lymphoma in patients with AIDS. Interestingly, antibodies against VCAM-1 inhibited this increased motility. Other actions of tat have also been studied and described.

Human herpesvirus 8 (HHV8), discovered by Chang in 1994, is the causative agent of Kaposi's sarcoma. However, the increased incidence of Kaposi's sarcoma in AIDS patients may be partially related to the HIV tat protein. One mechanism by which the tat protein has been shown to act is by mobilization of b-fibroblast growth factor (b-FGF) [91]. Heparin sulfate proteoglycans normally provide binding sites for b-FGF. Tat competes for these sites and increases the concentration of free b-FGF (well-known angiogenic factor). The tat protein b-FGH and HHV8 may act synergistically in the development of KS [93].

CONCLUSION

SALT is composed of keratinocytes, Langerhans' cells, skin tropic T cells, and lymphatic endothelial cells of the skin. The epidermis, which is involved in many viral infections, contains all of the components needed for an effective immune response: antigen presenting Langerhans' cells, T cells, and cytokines from leukocytes and keratinocytes. There have been some recent advances in the study of the cutaneous immunology involved in infections with the human immunodeficiency, human papilloma, and herpes simplex viruses and cytomegalovirus (Fig. 2–4). In general, viral diseases with cutaneous manifestations lead to a decline in epidermal Langerhans' cells numbers, which is probably a reflection of the Langerhans' cells emigration out of the epidermis and into regional lymph nodes. These events lead to the activation of Langerhans' cells and antigen presentation to T cells. In HSV, there is subsequent T-cell infiltration of the epidermis, consisting of CD4+ cells that have both immune modulatory action and direct cytotoxic action. In HIV, in which there is a systemic depletion of CD4+ cells, the epidermis is left with reduced numbers of T cells. Intradermal injection of IL-2, however,

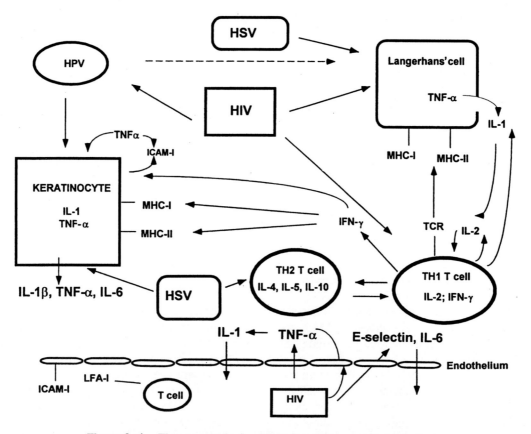

Figure 2–4.   The presumed role of SALT in cutaneous viral infections.

leads to an epidermal cellular infiltration in HIV-positive individuals. In HPV-induced condyloma acumination intralesional IFN increases Langerhans' cells, CD4 +, and CD8 + cells in the skin, as well as TGF-β1, TNF-α, pRB, and p53. Therefore, viral infections involving the epidermal immune system have certain similar characteristics, whereas other parameters are unique to the infecting virus. The immune system resident in the epidermis is significantly affected by infections with CMV, HIV, HPV, and HSV. SALT is able to eradicate a cutaneous viral infection and retain memory of the infection to ward off future infections. In certain instances, SALT does the opposite and enhances the pathology of a cutaneous viral infection. One common feature in HIV, HPV, and HSV infections is reduction in epidermal Langerhans' cell counts, but this does not indicate a common mechanism. For example, HIV is known to infect Langerhans' cells and have cytopathic effects, although this has not been shown for HPV or HSV. Possibly, viral infections of the epidermis require the presence of Langerhans' cells only in extra-epidermal sites (e.g., lymph nodes), where antigen processing takes place. All these viruses affect epidermal T-cell counts and subset proportions differently and may indicate the differential cytokine levels or patterns of expression that might exist in different viral infections. Although much has been learned about cutaneous viral immunology during the past few years, further studies are needed to enhance our understanding of the role of SALT in viral infections.

REFERENCES

1. JW Streilein. Lymphocyte traffic, T-cell malignancies and the skin. J Invest Dermatol 71:167–171, 1978.
2. JW Streilein. Skin-associated lymphoid tissues (SALT): the next generation. In: JD Bos, (ed). Skin Immune System (SIS). Boca Raton, FL: CRC Press, 1990, pp 25–48.
3. E Tschachler, V Groh, K Popovic, et al. Epidermal Langerhans cells—a target for HTLV-III/LAV infection. J Invest Dermatol 88:233–237, 1987.
4. MCY Heng, SY Heng, SG Allen. Co-infection and synergy of human immunodeficiency virus-1 and herpes simplexvirus-1. Lancet 343:255–258, 1994.
5. R Berger, S Gartner, K Rappersberger, et al. Isolation of human immunodeficiency virus type 1 from human epidermis: virus replication and transmission studies. J Invest Dermatol 99:271–277, 1992.
6. A Cimarelli, G Zambruno, A Marconi, et al. Quantitation by competitive PCR of HIV-1 proviral DNA in epidermal Langerhans cells of HIV-infected patients. J Acquir Immune Defic Syndr 7:230–235, 1994.
7. D Kiatzinann, F Barre-Sinoussi, MR Nugeyre, et al. Selective tropism of lymphadenopathy associated virus (LAV) for helper-inducer T lymphocytes. Science 225:59–63, 1984.
8. DD Ho, TR Rota, MS Hirsch. Infection of monocyte/macrophages by human T lymphotropic virus type III. J Clin Invest 77:1712–1715, 1986.
9. A Spira, P Marx, B Patterson, J Mahoney, R Koup, et al. Cellular targets of infection and route of viral dissemination after an intravaginal inoculation of simian immunodeficiency virus into rhesus macaques. J Exp Med 183: 215–225, 1996.
10. C Miller, J Hu. T cell-tropic simian immunodeficiency virus (SIV) and simian-human immunodeficiency viruses are readily transmitted by vaginal inoculation of rhesus macaques, and Langerhans' cells of the female genital tract are infected with SIV. J Infect Dis 179(suppl 3):S413–S417, 1999.
11. A Blauvelt, H Asada, W Saville, V Klaus-Kovtun, D Altman et al. Productive infection of dendritic cells by HIV-1 and their ability to capture virus are mediated through separate pathways. J Clin Invest 100:2043–2053, 1997.
12. C Masurier, N Guettari, C Pioche, R Lacave, B Salomon, et al. The role of dendritic cells in the transport of HIV to lymph nodes analysed in mouse. Adv Exp Med Biol 417: 411–414, 1997.
13. TBH Geijtenbeek, DS Kwon, R Torensma, SJ van Vilet, GCF van Duijnhoven, et al. DC-Sign, a dendritic cell–specific HIV-1-binding protein that enhances trans-infection of T cells. Cell 1000:587–597, 2000.
14. TBH Geijtenbeek, R Torensma, SJ van Vliet, GCF van Duijnhoven, GJ Adema, et al. Identification of DC-SIGN, a novel dendritic cell-specific ICAM-3 receptor that supports primary immune responses. Cell 100:575–585, 2000.
15. DV Belsito, MR Sanchez, RL Baer, F Valentine, GJ Thorbecke. Reduced Langerhans' cell la antigen and ATPase activity in patients with the acquired immunodeficiency syndrome. N Engl J Med 810:1279–1282, 1984.
16. K Lore, A Sonnerborg, J Olsson, B Patterson, T Fehniger, et al. HIV-1 exposed dendritic cells show increased proinflammatory cyokine production but reduced IL-1ra following lipopolysaccaride stimulation. AIDS 13: 2013–2021, 1999.
17. M Cumberbatch, R Dearman, I Kimber. Stimulation of Langerhans cell migration in mice by tumour necrosis factor α and interleukin 1β. Adv Exp Med Biol 417:121–124, 1997.
18. M Cumberbatch, R Dearman, I Kimber. Langerhans cells require signals from both tumour necrosis factor α and interleukin 1β for migration. Adv Exp Med Biol 417: 125–128, 1997.
19. C Caux, C Massacrier, B Vanbervliet, B Dubois, B Saint-Vis, et al. CD34 + hematopoietic progenitors from human cord blood differentiate along two independent dendritic cell pathways in response to GM-CSF + TNFα. Adv Exp Med Biol 417:21–25, 1997.
20. S Knight, B Askonas, S Macatonia. Dendritic cells as targets for cytotoxic T lymphocytes. Adv Exp Med Biol 417: 389–394, 1997.
21. J Leonard, JS Khillan, BE Gendelman, et al. The human

immunodeficiency virus long terminal repeat is preferentially expressed in Langerhans cells in transgenic mice. AIDS Res Hum Retroviruses 5:421–430, 1989.

22. C Heufler, F Koch, G Schuler. Granulocyte/macrophage colony stimulating factor and interleukin 1 mediate the maturation of murine epidermal Langerhans cells into potent immunostimulatory dendritic cells. J Exp Med 167: 700–705, 1988.

23. B Dreno, B Milpied, IL Dutartre, P Litoux. Epidermal interleukin 1 in normal skin of patients with HIV infection. Br J Dermatol 123:487–492, 1990.

24. H Muller, S Weier, G Kojouharoff, et al. Distribution and infection of Langerhans cells in the skin of HIV-infected healthy subjects and AIDS patients. Res Virol 144:59–67, 1993.

25. S Procelli, MB Brenner, JL Greenstein, et al. Recognition of cluster of differentiation I antigens by human CD4- CD8- cytolytic T lymphocytes. Nature 341:447–450, 1989.

26. D Kabelitz. Function and specificity of human gamma/delta-positive T cells. Crit Rev Immunol 11:281–303, 1992.

27. C Agostini, R Zambello, L Trentin, et al. Gamma delta T cell receptor subsets in the lung of patients with HIV-I infection. Cell Immunol 153:194–205, 1994.

28. F Hermier, E Comby, A Delaunay, et al. Decreased blood TCR gamma delta + lymphocytes in AIDS and p24-antigenemic HIV-1-infected patients. Clin Immunol Immunopathol 9:248–250, 1993.

29. JI Sin, M Bagarazzi, C Pachuk, DB Wiener. DNA priming-protein boosting enhances both antigen-specific antibody and Th-1-type cellular immune responses in a murine herpes simplex virus-2 gD vaccine model. DNA Cell Biol 18: 771–778, 1999.

30. JI Sin, JJ Kim, JD Boyer, RB Ciccarelli, TJ Higgins, DB Weiner. In vivo modulation of vaccine-induced immune responses toward a Th1 phenotype increases potency and vaccine effectiveness in a herpes simplex virus type 2 mouse model. J Virol 73:501–509, 1999.

31. M Salio, M Cella, M Suter, A Lanzavecchia. Inhibition of dendritic cell maturation by herpes simplex virus. Eur J Immunol 29:3245–3253, 1999.

32. ML Eloranta, GV Alm. Splenic marginal metallophilic macrophages and marginal zone macrophages are the major interferon-alpha/beta producers in mice upon intravenous challenge with herpes simplex virus. Scand J Immunol 49: 391–394, 1999.

33. S Tyring. Human papillomavirus infections: epidemiology, pathogenesis, and host immune response. J Am Acad Dermatol 43:S18–S26, 2000.

34. M Drijkoningen, C De Wolf-Peeters, H Degreef, V Desmet. Epidermal Langerhans cells, dermal dendritic cells, and keratinocytes in viral lesions of skin and mucous membranes: an immunohistochemical study. Arch Dermatol Res 280: 220–227, 1988.

35. Y Charsonnet, J Viac, J Thivolet. Langerhans cells in human warts. Br J Dermatol 115:669–675, 1986.

36. J Viac, C Soler, Y Chardonnet, S Euvrard, D Schmitt. Expression of immune associated surface antigens of keratinocytes in human papillomavirus-derived lesions. Immunobiology 188:392–402, 1993.

37. IH Frazer, R Thomas, J Zhou, GR Leggat, L Dunn, N McMillan et al. Potential strategies utilized by papillomavirus to evade host immunity. Immunol Rev 168:131–142, 1999.

38. FM Brodsky, L Lem, A Solache, EM Bennett. Human pathogen subversion of antigen presentation. Immunol Rev 168:199–215, 1999.

39. I Arany, P Rady, SK Tyring. Alterations in cytokine/antioncogene expression in skin lesions caused by ''low risk'' types of human papillomaviruses. Viral Immunol 6: 255–265, 1993.

40. S Majewski, N Hunzelmann, R Nischt, et al. TGF beta-1 and TNF alpha expression in the epidermis of patients with epidermodysplasia verruciformis. J Invest Dermatol 97: 862–867, 1991.

41. KD Cooper, EJ Androphy, D Lowy, SI Katz. Antigen presentation and T-cell activation in epidermodysplasia verruciformis. J Invest Dermatol 94:769–776, 1990.

42. A Kimchi, X-F Wang, RA Weinberg, S Cheifetz, J Massague. Absence of TGF-beta receptors and growth inhibitory responses in retinoblastoma cells. Science 240: 196–199, 1988.

43. JA Pietenpol, RW Stein, E Moran, et al. TGF beta-1 inhibition of c-*myc* transcription and growth in keratincytes is abrogated by viral transforming proteins with pRB binding domains. Cell 61:777–785, 1990.

44. K Munger, WC Phelps. The human papillomavirus E7 protein as a transforming and transactivating factor. Biochem Biophys Acta 1155:111–123, 1993.

45. CP Mansur, EJ Androphy. Cellular transformation by papillomavirus oncoproteins. Biochem Biophys Acta 1155: 323–345, 1993.

46. S-J Kim, H-D Lee, PD Robbins, K Busain, MB Spom, AB Roberts. Regulation of transforming growth factor beta I gene expression by the product of the retinoblastoma-susceptibility gene. Proc Natl Acad Sci USA 88:3052–3056, 1991.

47. CD Woodworth, S Simpson. Comparative lymphokine secretion by cultured normal human cervical keratinocytes, papillomavirus-immortalized, and carcinoma cell lines. Am J Pathol 142:1544–1555, 1993.

48. S Grabbe, S Bruvers, RD Granstein. Interleukin I alpha but not transforming growth factor beta inhibits tumor antigen presentation by epidermal antigen-presenting cells J Invest Dermatol 102:67–73, 1994.

49. J Viac, L Guerin-Reverchon, Y Chardonnet, A Bremond. Langerhans cells and epithelial cell modification in cervical intraepithelial neoplasia. Correlation with human papillomavirus infection. Immunobiology 180:328–338, 1993.

50. OM Memar, I Arany, SK Tyring. Skin-associated lymphoid tissue in human immunodeficiency virus-1, human papillomavirus, and herpes simplex virus infections. J Invest Dermatol 105:99S–104S, 1995.

51. AE Morelli, C Sananes, G Di Paola, A Paredes, L Fainbom. Relationship between types of human papillomavirus and Langerhans cells in cervical condyloma and intraepithelial neoplasia. Am J Clin Pathol 99:200–206, 1993.

52. H Matsue, PD Cruz Jr, PR Bergstresser, A Takashima. Cytokine expression by epidermal cell subpopulations. J Invest Dermatol 99:42S–45S, 1992.

53. SK Tay, D Jenkins, P Maddox, A Singer. Lymphocyte phenotypes in cervical intraepithelial neoplasia and human papillomavirus infection. Br J Obstet Gynecol 94:16–21, 1987.

54. FV Cromme, CJ Meijer, PJ Snijders, et al. Analysis of MHC class I and II expression in relation to presence of HPV genotypes in premalignant and malignant cervical lesions. Br J Cancer 67:1372–1380, 1993.

55. G Fadden, K Kane. How DNA viruses perturb functional MHC expression to alter immune recognition. Adv Cancer Res 63:117–209, 1994.

56. DJ Maudsley. Role of oncogenes in the regulation of MHC antigen expression. Biochem Soc Trans 19:291–196, 1991.

57. T Kanda, S Zamma, S Watanbe, SA Furuno, K Yoshiiki. Two immunodominant regions of the human papillomavirus type 16 E7 protein and masked in the nuclei of monkey COS-1 cells. Virology 182:723–731, 1991.

58. V Bal, A McIndoe, G Denton, et al. Antigen presentation by keratinocytes induces tolerance in human T-cells. Eur J Immunol 20:1893–1897, 1990.

59. F Mota, N Rayment, S Chong, A Singer, B Chain. The antigen-presenting environment in normal and human papillomavirus (HPV)-related premalignant cervical epithelium. Clin Exp Immunol 116:33–40, 1999.

60. I Arany, P Rady, SK Tyring. Interferon treatment enhances the expression of underphosphorylated (biologically-active) retinoblastoma protein in human papillomavirus-infected cells through the inhibitory TGF beta-1/IFN beta cytokine pathway. Antiviral Res 23:131–141, 1994.

61. SN Tabrizi, CK Fairley, S Chen, AJ Borg, P Baghurst, et al. Epidemiological characteristics of women with high grade CIN who do and do not have human papillomavirus. Br J Obstet Gynecol 106:252–257, 1999.

62. EJ Krul, RF Schipper, GM Schreuder, GJ Fleuren, et al. HLA and susceptibility to cervical neoplasia. Hum Immunol 60:337–342, 1999.

63. L Aaltonen, J Partanen, E Auvinen, H Rihkanen, A Vaheri. HLA-DQ alleles and human papillomavirus DNA in adult-onset laryngeal papillomatosis. J Infect Dis 179:682–685, 1999.

64. TD de Gruijl, HJ Bontkes, JM Walboomers, P Coursaget, MJ Stukart, C Dupuy, et al. Immune responses against human papillomavirus (HPV) type 16 virus-like particles in a cohort study of women with cervical intraepithelial neoplasia. I. Differential T-helper and IgG responses in relation to HPV infection and disease outcome. J Gen Virol 80(Pt 2):339–408, 1999.

65. L Montoya, I Saiz, G Rey, F Vela, N Clerici-Larradet. Cervical carcinoma: human papillomavirus infection and HLA-associated risk factors in the Spanish population. Eur J Immunogenet 25:329–337, 1998.

66. A Helland, AO Olsen, K Gjoen, HE Akselsen, T Sauer, P Magnus, et al. An increased risk of cervical intra-epithelial neoplasia grade II-III among human papillomavirus positive patients with the HLA-DQA1*0102-DQB1*0602 haplotypes: a population-based case-control study of Norwegian women. Int J Cancer 76:19–24, 1998.

67. AD Santin, PL Hermonat, A Ravaggi, M Chiriva-Internati, D Zhan, et al. The induction of human papillomavirus-specific CD4(+) and CD8(+) lymphocytes by E7-pulsed autologous dendritic cells in patients with human papillomavirus type 16- and 18- positive cervical cancer. J Virol 73:5402–5410, 1999.

68. EL Berg, T Yoshino, LS Rott, MK Robinson, RA Warnock, TK Kishimoto et al. The cutaneous lymphocyte antigen is a skin lymphocyte homing receptor for the vascular lectin endothelial cell-leukocyte adhesion molecule 1. J Exp Med 174:1461–1466, 1991.

69. LJ Picker, JR Treer, B Ferguson-Darnell, PA Collins, BR Bergstresser, LW Terstappen. Control of lymphocyte recirculation in man. II. Differential regulation of the cutaneous lymphocyte-associated antigen, a tissue-selective homing receptor for skin-homing T cells. J Immunol 150:1122–1136, 1993.

70. E Sprecher, Y Becker. Detection of IL1-beta, TNF-alpha, and IL-6 gene transcription by the polymerase chain reaction in keratinocytes, Langerhans cells and peritoneal exudate cells during infection with herpes simplex virus-1. Arch Dermatol 126:253–269, 1992.

71. EL Howes, W Taylor, NA Mitchison, E Simpson. MHC matching shows that at least two T cells subsets determine resistance to HSV. Nature 277:67–68, 1979.

72. RK Johnson, D Lancki, AI Sperling, et al. A murine CD4-, CD8- T cell receptor-gamma delta T cell lymphocyte clone specific for herpes simplex glycoprotein I. J Immunol 148:983–988, 1992.

73. AL Cunningham, JR Noble. Role of keratinocytes in human recurrent herpetic lesions. J Clin Invest 83:490–496, 1989.

74. SR Jennings, RH Bonneau, RH Smith, RM Wolcott, R Chervenak. CD4-positive T lymphocytes are required for the generation of the primary but not the secondary CD-positive cytolytic T lymphocyte response to herpes simplex virus in C57 Bl/6 mice. Cell Immunol 133:234–252, 1991.

75. NA Williams, TJ Hill, DC Hooper. Murine epidermal antigen-presenting cells in primary and secondary T-cell proliferative responses to herpes simplex virus in vitro. Immunology 72:34–39, 1991.

76. Mosmann TR, Cherwinski H, Bound MW, Giedlin MA, Coffman RL. Two types of murine T cell clone I. Definition according to profiles of lymphokine activities and secreted proteins. J Immunology 136:2348–2357, 1986.

77. G Saed, DP Fiverson, Y Naidu, BJ Nickoloff. Mycosis fungoides exhibits a Th1-type cell-mediated cytokine profile whereas Sezary syndrome expresses Th2-type T cells. J Invest Dermatol 103:29–33, 1994.

78. JI Sin, V Ayyavoo, J Boyer, J Kim, RB Ciccarelli, DB Weiner. Protective immune correlates can segregate by vac-

cine type in a murine herpes model system. Int Immunol 11:1763–1773, 1999.

79. S Ashkar, G Weber, V Panoutsakopoulou, M Sanchirico, M Jansson, S Zawaideh, et al. Eta-1 (osteopontin): an early component of type-1 (cell mediated) immunity. Science 287:860–864, 2000.

80. TA Springer. Traffic signals for lymphocyte recirculation and leukocyte emigration: the multistep paradigm. Cell 76: 301–314, 1994.

81. S Shahgasempour, SB Woodroffe, HM Garnett. Alterations in the expression of ELAM-1, ICAM-1 and VCAM-1 after in vitro infection of endothelial cells with a clinical isolate of human cytomegalovirus. Microbiol Immunol 41:121–129, 1997.

82. TJ Dengler, MJ Raftery, M Werle, R Zimmermann, G Schonrich. Cytomegalovirus infection of vascular cells induces expression of pro-inflammatory adhesion molecules by paracrine action of secreted interleukin-1 beta. Transplantation 69:1160–1168, 2000.

83. JE Grundy, KM Lawson, LP MacCormac, JM Fletcher, KL Yong. Cytomegalovirus-infected endothelial cells recruit neutrophils by the secretion of C-X-C chemokines and transmit virus by direct neutrophil-endothelial cell contact and during neutrophil transendothelial migration. J Infect Dis 177:1465–1474, 1998.

84. JL Craigen, KL Yong, NJ Jordan, LP MacCormac, J Westwick, et al. Human cytomegalovirus infection up-regulates interleukin-8 gene expression and stimulates neutrophil transendothelial migration. Immunology 92:138–145, 1997.

85. JS Pober, T Collins, MA Gimbrone, P Libby, CS Reiss. Inducible expression of class II major histocompatibility complex antigens and the immunogenicity of vascular endothelium. Transplantation 41:141–146, 1986.

86. DM Miller, Y Zhang, BM Rahill, WJ Waldman, DD Sedmak. Human cytomegalovirus inhibits IFN-alpha-stimulated antiviral and immunoregulatory responses by blocking multiple levels of IFN-alpha signal transduction. J Immunol 162:6107–6113, 1999.

87. DA Knight, WJ Waldman, DD Sedmak. Human cytomegalovirus does not induce human leukocyte antigen class II expression on arterial endothelial cells. Transplantation 63: 1366–1369, 1997.

88. DM Miller, BM Rahill, JM Boss, MD Lairmore, JE Durbin, et al. Human cytomegalovirus inhibits major histocompatibility complex class II expression by disruption of the Jak/Stat pathway. J Exp Med 187:675–683, 1998.

89. ZF Rosenberg, AS Fauci. Immunopathogenic mechanisms of HIV infection: cytokine induction of HIV expression. Immunol Today 11:176–180, 1990.

90. RG Chirivi, G Taraboletti, MR Bani, L Barra, G Piccinini, M Giacca et al. Human immunodeficiency virus-1 (HIV-1)-Tat protein promotes migration of acquired immunodeficiency syndrome-related lymphoma cells and enhances their adhesion to endothelial cells. Blood 94:1747–1754, 1999.

91. G Barillari, C Sgadari, V Fiorelli, F Samaniego, S Colombini, V Manzari, et al. The Tat protein of human immunodeficiency virus type-1 promotes vascular cell growth and locomotion by engaging the alpha5beta1 and alphavbeta3 integrins and by mobilizing sequestered basic fibroblast growth factor. Blood 94:663–672, 1999.

92. S Dhawan, RK Puri, A Kumar, H Duplan, JM Masson, BB Aggarwal. Human immunodeficiency virus-1-tat protein induces the cell surface expression of endothelial leukocyte adhesion molecule-1, vascular cell adhesion molecule-1, and intercellular adhesion molecule-1 in human endothelial cells. Blood 90:1535–1544, 1997.

93. G Barillari, C Sgadari, C Palladino, R Gendelman, A Caputo, CB Morris, et al. The inflammatory cytokines synergize with the HIV-1 Tat protein to promote angiogenesis and Kaposi's sarcoma via induction of basic fibroblast growth factor and alpha v beta3 integrin. J Immunol 163: 1929–1935, 1999.

3

Poxviruses

Dayna G. Diven
University of Texas Medical Branch, Galveston, Texas, USA

INTRODUCTION TO POXVIRIDAE

The poxvirus family affects both humans and animals (Fig. 3–1). The poxviruses are the largest of all animal viruses and are easily visualized on light microscopy. When seen under the electron microscope, the poxviruses are brick-shaped or oval 200–400 nm structures (Fig. 3–2). The nucleosome contains double-stranded DNA, surrounded by a membrane. The outer surface of the lipoprotein bilayer has randomly arranged surface tubules, which give the virion its characteristic textured appearance. The lipid composition of the membrane is different from that of the host cell membrane [1]. The nucleoprotein core, lateral bodies, and membrane constitute an infectious collective unit, and the virus may acquire an envelope as well.

Dermatologists are interested in the epitheliotropic aspects of poxviruses. There are a large number of poxvirus species, as outlined in Table 3–1.

Replication occurs autonomously in the cytoplasm of cells. After uncoating, the virion produces early enzymes and early virion proteins and late enzymes and late virion proteins [1]. These replication "factories" are independent of the host nucleus and are discernible on light microscopy as basophilic staining B-type inclusion bodies. The genome undergoes spontaneous recombination.

The toxic effect of poxviruses on cells causes cell round-

Portions of this chapter were published in the *Journal of the American Academy of Dermatology* 44:1–14, 2000. Used with permission.

ing and clumping, degeneration of cell architecture, and the production of cytoplasmic vacuoles. Different poxviruses are capable of producing a localized, self-limited infection by inoculation to the skin (e.g., ORF) or a fulminant systemic disease (e.g., variola). The same virus can affect different species differently. Other poxviruses cause localized cell proliferation, for example, molluscum contagiosum virus.

Poxviruses that are not known to infect humans (such as camelpox and sheep and goat lumpy skin disease complex) are capable of producing great economic hardship in communities that are dependent on the affected animal species [2]. Our review includes only those poxviruses that infect humans.

ORTHOPOXVIRUSES

Smallpox

Definition

An infection caused by the variola virus that only affects humans.

History

The history of the rise and fall of the smallpox virus is both fascinating and unique. The saga includes centuries of death and disfigurement followed by scientific triumph, although the future of the fate of the virus is undecided. For generations the interaction of smallpox and humans has been characterized by unparalleled persistence and diffusion [3]. Smallpox is thought to have originated in Africa

TAXONOMY OF VIRUSES

Poxviridae family
Chordopoxvirinae subfamily
Orthopoxvirus genus (vaccinia, cowpox, variola, monkeypox)
Parapoxvirus genus (orf, bovine papular stomatitis, pseudocowpox)
Yatapoxvirus genus (tanapox)
Molluscipoxvirus genus (molluscum contagiosum)

WORLDWIDE GEOGRAPHICAL INCIDENCE

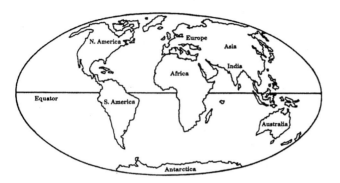

Figure 3–1. Taxonomy and incidence of poxviruses.

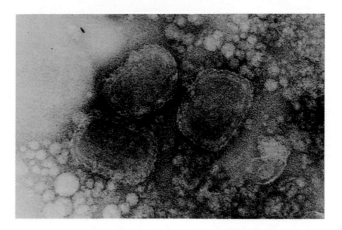

Figure 3–2. Poxvirus (vaccinia) brick-shaped to oval virus particles with electron-dense DNA core and visible outer membrane are seen in the vacuolated keratinocyte cytoplasm ($\times$ 20, 160). (Photograph courtesy of Harvey Blank, M.D., Department of Dermatology, University of Miami School of Medicine, Miami, FL.)

Table 3–1. Hosts and Portal of Entry for Selected Poxvirus Species

Genus	Species	Hosts	Portal of Entry (for Humans)
Orthopoxvirus	Vaccinia virus	Humans	Skin
	Cowpox virus	Humans, cats, cattle	Skin
	Variola virus	Rodents, humans	Respiratory tract
	Monkeypox virus	Humans, monkeys, rodents	Skin
Parapoxvirus	Orf virus	Goats, sheep, camels, humans	Skin
	Bovine papular stomatitis virus	Cattle, humans	Skin
	Pseudocowpox virus	Cattle, humans	Skin
	Red deer poxvirus	Red deer	
Avipoxvirus	FowlPox virus	Birds	
Capripoxvirus	Sheep-Pox virus	Sheep, goats, cattle	
Leporipoxvirus	Myxoma virus	Squirrels, rodents, rabbits	
Suipoxvirus	Swinepox virus	Swine	
Molluscipoxvirus	Molluscum contagiosum virus	Humans (chimpanzees)	Skin
Yatapoxvirus	Tanapox virus	Humans, monkeys	Mosquitoes suspected
	Yabapox	Humans, monkeys	Skin

* Adapted from Buller and Palumbo [1], 1991, Tables 1 and 3, p. 82 and 98.

and then to have spread to India and China thousands of years before Christ. The first recorded smallpox epidemic was in 1350 B.C., during the Egyptian-Hittite war [3]. It began to affect Europe between the 5th and 7th centuries. Smallpox occurred in the West Indies in 1507 and followed the Spanish conquest into the new world [4]. The immunity of the Spanish troops and the susceptibility of the peoples of Mexico and Peru to smallpox may have been a factor in the outcome of that conquest. During the 17th and 18th centuries, epidemics occurred in the North American colonies [4]. At one time smallpox was endemic throughout the world except in Australia and on certain islands [4]. Large-scale epidemics caused millions of deaths in Europe and Mexico [3]. In the 1700s, the observation that survivors of smallpox were immune to further outbreaks led to the practice of variolation in China, India, and Turkey. Variolation was the deliberate inoculation of an uninfected person with the smallpox virus by contact with the pustular maker as a prophylaxis against a more severe form of smallpox. Lady Mary Wortley Montague, herself a smallpox survivor, is credited with advancing the smallpox variolation in England [5,6]. Late in the 18th century, Edward Jenner, acting on reports of smallpox immunity in milkmaids who had developed cowpox, developed the smallpox vaccine. The Council of the Royal Society rejected his idea as it was ''in variance with established knowledge'' and ''incredible.'' Jenner self-financed the publication, and the vaccine was used for nearly 200 years (see Section on Vaccinia) [3].

The decline of smallpox during the 20th century is linked to a rise in smallpox vaccination (see section on Vaccinia). In the latter half of the 20th century, other countries, especially in Africa and Asia, continued to suffer major disease outbreaks whereas most of North America, Western Europe, Australia, and New Zealand were free of the disease. In 1967, the World Health Organization (WHO) set forth with a worldwide campaign to eradicate smallpox. By 1976, only Ethiopia and surrounding areas were still affected by the disease. On May 8, 1980, the World Health Assembly declared the world free of smallpox [6]. The spread of smallpox evolved over thousands of years, the global spread occurred for hundreds of years, and its eradication was sealed 13 years after the WHO program was begun (Fig. 3–3).

Incidence
In the United States, the last outbreak of smallpox occurred in Texas in 1949 (eight cases one death) [7]. The last endemic case of smallpox occurred in Somalia in October of 1977 [7]. A laboratory-associated outbreak occurred at a university in England in 1978 [7,8]. The infected person worked on a floor above the laboratory and died 1 month after infection [8]. By 1984, all countries had ceased vacci-

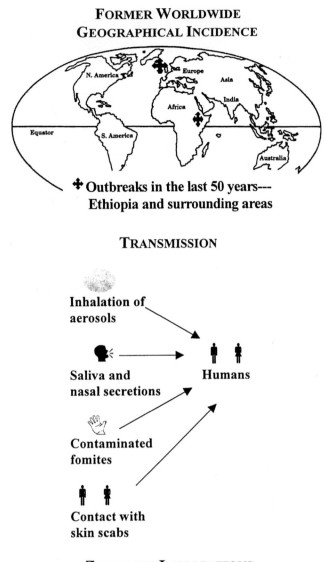

Figure 3–3. Incidence and transmission of smallpox.

nating the general population, nor did they require travelers to certify vaccination [9]. Routine vaccination in the United States continued until 1971. The vaccine was given sporadically after this until in 1983 vaccine producers were urged to reserve the vaccine for military personnel only [10]. In 1986, it was recommended that military personnel no longer be vaccinated [11]. Smallpox vaccination was officially discontinued in U.S. military recruits (except for special units) in 1990. At the time of this writing, most of the population of unvaccinated people is under 30 years of age. The WHO has investigated rumors of smallpox, all

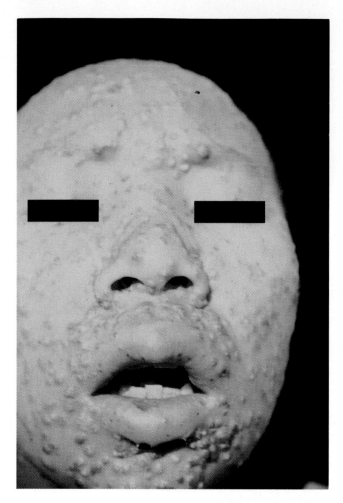

develop from inhalation of aerosolized virus, contact with saliva or nasal secretions, contact with the skin scabs, or through contaminated fomites, such as bedding [13]. No significant subclinical carrier state exists [4] (Fig. 3–4). Population density and immunity affect the extent of spread. Eradication was obtainable because there are no known animal reservoirs for smallpox. Infected people are contagious from the onset of illness until the last crusts of the lesions are gone, although infectivity is greatest in the earlier stages of disease. The rate of infectivity for susceptible contacts is 30% [14]. Generally, environmental conditions do not affect the virility of the virus.

Clinical Manifestations

The incubation period is 12–13 days (Table 3–2). The initial lesions on the palms and soles feel firm like "BB shots" when palpated [4]. The development of fever is followed by an exanthem of deep, firm multiloculated vesicles in a centrifugal and extensor distribution.

Figure 3–4. Smallpox in a Chinese soldier. (Photograph courtesy of Harvey Blank, M.D., Department of Dermatology, University of Miami School of Medicine, Miami, FL.)

of which turned out to be misdiagnosed varicella or other skin diseases. Two known high-security laboratories in Atlanta and Moscow contain the virus. However, some believe that whole virus is no longer needed to make the vaccine because the variola virus gene pool has been cloned in bacterial plasmids [9,11,12]. After 1986, it was no longer considered necessary to maintain global reserves of smallpox vaccine. In the year 2000, however, fears of biological warfare led to renewal of vaccine production for use by the military. In this posteradication era, it still remains a possibility that unsanctioned laboratories are storing variola viruses; therefore physicians should familiarize themselves with the signs and symptoms of this infection (see section on Future Considerations).

Pathogenesis/Epidemiology

The spread of smallpox usually occurs through intimate contact via the respiratory tract [1]. However, infection can

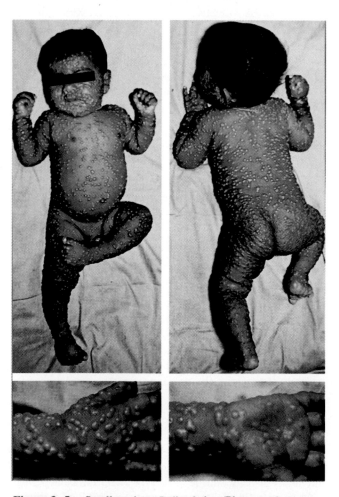

Figure 3–5. Smallpox in an Indian baby. (Photograph courtesy of the World Health Organization, Geneva, Switzerland.)

Table 3–2. Clinical Manifestations of Smallpox Infection

Time After Exposure	Clinical Manifestations	Laboratory Analyses	Other Notes
12–13 days	Prodrome of fever, malaise and backache—lasts 3–4 days ↓ Exanthem appears and quickly evolves:	Silver impregnation or fluorescent antibody stain of skin lesion smears;* electron microscopy; chick embryo or tissue culture (reserved for specialized laboratories); fourfold increase in antibody titer	Portal of entry—respiratory tract Infectivity is maximal during the first week of rash Initial eruption on palms of hands and soles of feet; distribution is centrifugal and on extensor surfaces
14–16 days	↓ macules ↓ papules ↓ Vesicles		All lesions are in a similar stage at any one time
19–20 days	↓ Pustules		Overall mortality rate is 30%
25–27 days	↓ Crusts (see Fig. 3–5), new epithelial formation		Scarring may occur; corneal infections may result in blindness Scarring may be severe

* A negative smear does not exclude disease.

There are four clinical types of smallpox: ordinary, modified (by previous vaccination), flat, and hemorrhagic, with the latter two having the highest fatality rates [5]. Variola major, the severe form of infection, could cause pulmonary edema from heart failure, leading to death. Variola minor (alastrim) resulted in few fatalities. There is no identifiable difference in the virus among these variants [4], although the epidemiology suggests that subspecies of the virus produce either variola minor or variola major. The case mortality rate in adults varied between 20% and 60%. Survivors often had disfiguring scars. Corneal infection frequently resulted in blindness. See Table 3–3 for differential diagnosis.

Table 3–3. Differential Diagnoses of Smallpox

Varicella (chickenpox): Small delicate vesicles, concentrated on trunk, face, and flexor extremities, with rare deep scarring. Lesions are generally in various states of development

Syphilis: Resembles early smallpox but does not progress as smallpox does

Monkeypox: Has a greater tendency to produce both lymphadenopathy and skin lesions in "crops"

Dermatopathology

Ballooning degeneration and cytoplasmic inclusion bodies (Guarnieri bodies) within keratinocytes are seen. Reticular degeneration and dermal hemorrhage ensue, with massive polymorphonuclear cell infiltrates. This is followed by crusting and new epithelial formation [15].

Laboratory Findings

Laboratory confirmation may be obtained from silver impregnation or florescent antibody staining of smears taken from skin lesions [4]. Electron microscopy can also be used to identify the virus. A negative smear does not exclude the disease. A laboratory designed to handle the virus uses chick embryo or tissue culture for identification. A fourfold or greater rise in antibody titer is also diagnostic.

Treatment/Prophylaxis

If the diagnosis of smallpox is considered, immediate isolation of the patient is in order, after which the Centers for Disease Control (CDC) should be contacted. All patient contacts should be identified. No antiviral treatment for smallpox exists. Supportive care and treatment of bacterial infections are necessary (Table 3–4).

Smallpox vaccination may be indicated for the following groups: laboratory persons who handle variola or monkeypox viruses or the staff of surveillance teams who study

Table 3–4. Symptomatic Treatment of Smallpox

Secondary Symptoms	Treatment
Fever	Antipyretics
Secondary bacterial infection of open lesions	Systemic antibiotics
Pulmonary edema	Morphine, oxygen, intravenous loop diuretics, afterload reduction, inotropic support, aminophylline

monkeypox virus in Africa [9]. Opinions vary as to whether or not laboratory workers who handle other orthopoxviruses that infect humans (e.g., cowpox and vaccinia viruses) should undergo vaccination.

Future Considerations

There is a debate regarding whether all stocks of the variola virus should be destroyed. Opponents of destruction argue that more scientific inquiry requiring the whole virus could be done to identify the virulence segment of the genome [16–19]. Opponents also believe that variola's unique host specificity makes it valuable for future research and that completely destroying the virus would set a bad precedent. Additionally, they argue that specimens collected during epidemics could still be in existence and that similar viruses such as monkeypox could mutate [16–19].

Those who want the virus destroyed argue that the genomes of reference strains have been cloned and sequenced. Also, monkeypox virus DNA is easier to study than variola in that it is similar to variola, has an animal host, and requires less stringent laboratory precautions [12].

The smallpox virus is a potentially dangerous agent of biological terrorism [12] because a large proportion of the world's population is not immune to smallpox, no effective treatment exists, and the secondary attack rate is 25%–40% with a case fatality rate of 30%. It has been proposed that plans to protect against biological warfare, including the large-scale production of vaccine, should be delineated now [12].

In mid-1999, the World Health Assembly recommended a delay in the destruction of known smallpox reserves. The WHO was directed to appoint a new group of experts to establish what research, if any, had to be carried out to reach a global consensus on the timing for the destruction of existing variola virus stocks. This action permits further research into antiviral agents, improved vaccines, genetic structure analysis, and pathogenesis of smallpox.

Conclusion

For centuries smallpox terrorized the civilized world and affected millions of people [3]. Worldwide eradication of this virus is a unique event in history. The efforts of WHO and strategies in this matter are outlined in other publications [7,20]. Controversy still exists regarding the fate of the remaining stores of virus [18–20].

Vaccinia

Definition

An orthopoxvirus that affects a wide range of vertebrate hosts.

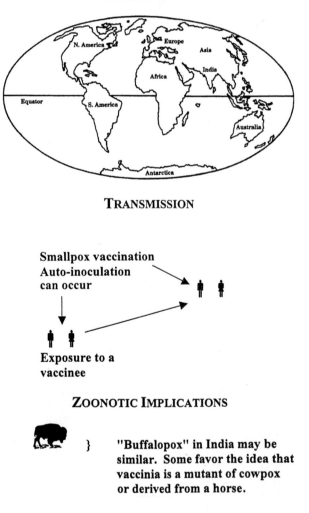

Figure 3–6. Incidence and transmission of vaccinia.

History

Vaccinia virus is the poxvirus that has been best studied. Edward Jenner first used vaccinia in 1796 [2]. It was then used for nearly 200 years as a vaccine for smallpox. The virus was originally thought to be isolated from infected cows and later horses [21–23]. However, it is now considered to be a laboratory virus with no natural reservoir [2].

Incidence

Infection with vaccinia virus occurs only in laboratory workers (Fig. 3–6). The vaccine strain is considered to be a relatively safe virus because it does not cause serious disease in immunocompetent humans or animals [24].

Pathogenesis

As with smallpox vaccination, the vaccinia virus is introduced into the outer layers of the skin. A localized infection occurs owing to the host immune response. Regional lymphadenopathy and systemic symptoms may sometimes occur in healthy individuals. Persons with eczema or immunosuppression may develop more severe cases, as will be discussed later. When the area of vaccination contacts other areas of the body or unvaccinated individuals, accidental inoculation may also occur.

Clinical Manifestations

A papule occurs 2 to 3 days after vaccination with a bifurcated needle multiple puncture technique (Table 3–5). The appearance of a pustule at day 7 confirms successful vacci

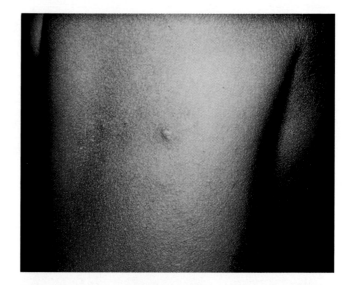

Figure 3–7. Vaccinia vesicopustule—a sign of successful vaccination. (Photograph courtesy of Harvey Blank, M.D., Department of Dermatology, University of Miami School of Medicine, Miami, FL.)

nation (Figs. 3–7, 3–8). In the past, vaccination scars were used with considerable accuracy to assess the vaccination status of the individual or of populations [25]. Table 3–6 contains the differential diagnosis.

Complications of Vaccination

Recovery from generalized vaccinia as a result of viremia is expected [22]. Autoinoculation or inoculation of another

Table 3–5. Clinical Manifestations of Vaccinia

Time After Exposure	Clinical Manifestations	Laboratory Analyses	Other Notes
2–3 days	Papule appears ↓ (loculated and umbilicated) jennerian vesicle ↓	Laboratory analysis is usually not indicated since the source of infection is known	Lesion formation confirms successful vaccination Generalized vaccinia can occur at 6–9 days. Reaction may be more severe (see Figs. 3–9, 3–10, 3–11)
10 days	Pustule with surrounding erythema and induration (Fig. 3–7) ↓		Inoculation into eczema may occur. Infants and the elderly are at risk of spread, as are those with immune deficits
12–13 days	Maximum erythema; lymphadenopathy; fever and malaise ↓		
22–24 days	Scab falls off		Pitted scar remains as evidence of vaccination (Fig. 3–8)

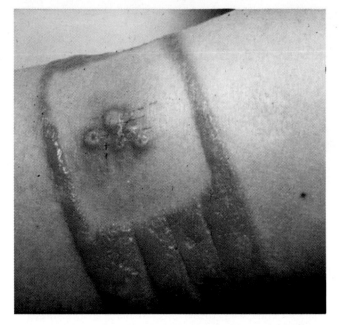

Figure 3–8. Vaccination site with contact dermatitis from tape.

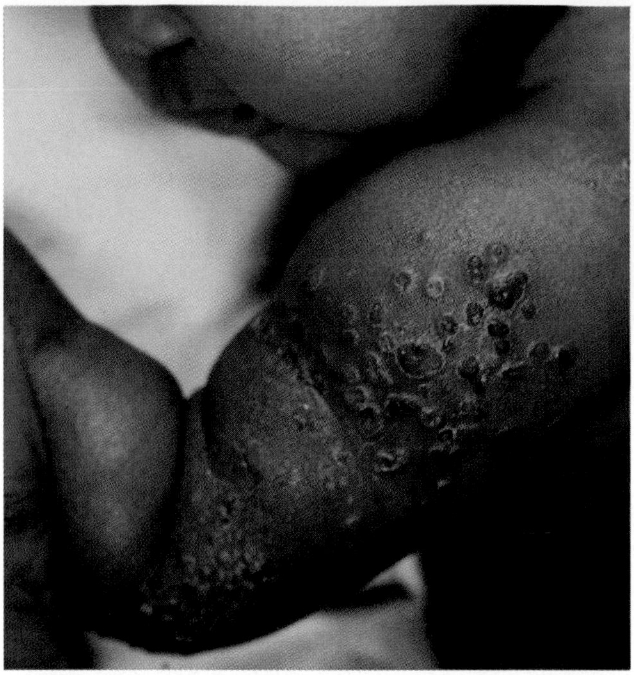

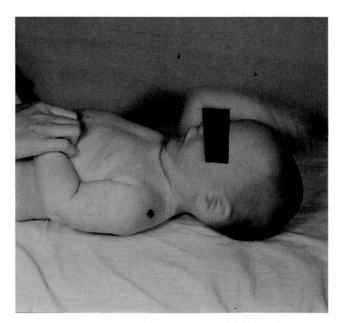

Figure 3–9. Local dissemination of vaccinia from vaccine site.

person from the vaccination site is possible. As the vaccinia virus was not attenuated, it did at times cause serious complications. ''Eczema vaccinatum'' or extensive lesions in eczematous patients or eczematous family contacts of vaccinees was an occasional but serious problem (Figs. 3–9 to 3–15). Mortality was about 5% [20]. Encephalopathy in infants and postvaccinial encephalitis in elderly persons are other possible complications. Thymic aplasia, thymic dysplasia, acquired immune defects, and other impaired cell-mediated immunities contribute to progressive vaccinia, which is a very serious disease. Those with partial immune deficiencies have a better recovery rate if they are administered vaccinia immune globulin [25]. A 1997 report describes an immunocompromised patient who was inadvertently given a vaccinia melanoma oncolysate vaccination, which led to progressive vaccinia [26]. Baxby summarizes the opinions regarding vaccination and acquired immunodeficiency syndrome (AIDS) [2]. Because vaccinia virus is handled by laboratory personnel, a practical guide for such personnel was published in 1993 [27].

Table 3–6. Differential Diagnoses of Vaccinia

Smallpox: Similar to generalized vaccinia but history of exposure to vaccinia via research or vaccination would differentiate

Figure 3–10. ''Vaccinial roseola,'' a transient erythematous eruption following vaccination. (Photograph courtesy of Harvey Blank, M.D., Department of Dermatology, University of Miami School of Medicine, Miami, FL.)

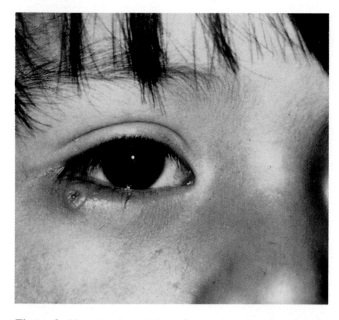

Figure 3–11. Autoinoculation of vaccinia to the lower eyelid produced a pustule. (Photograph courtesy of Roberto Arenas, M.D., Mexico City, Mexico.)

Future Applications

Genetically engineered recombinant viruses may be used as immunogenic vectors. One of the most promising seems to be vaccinia virus, because the large genome allows for large or multiple foreign gene insertion to create recombinant vaccinia virus. Its broad host range, including humans, laboratory animals, and common tissue culture cells, al-

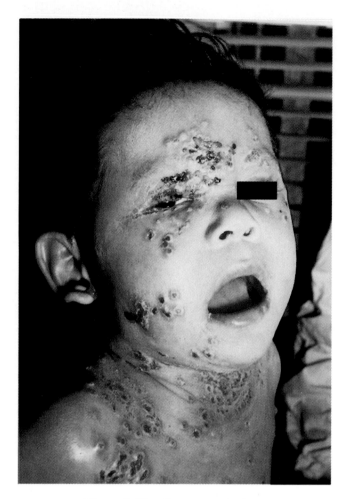

Figure 3–13. Eczema vaccinatum.

lows for many potential applications [28,29]. Because vaccinia virus replicates in the cytoplasm, problems with host cell DNA integration and nuclear transcription errors do not occur [24].

Recombinant vaccinia virus strains that express influenza hemagglutinin, hepatitis B surface antigen, and *Plasmodium falciparum* antigens have been produced [24]. An oral wild-life rabies vaccine has been developed [30]. Potential laboratory applications include the insertion of virtually any coding sequence for a protein into the vaccinia virus genome, but its clinical use depends upon improving the safety of live vaccines and achieving high immune responses to recombinant protein [30,31]. Mass production of vaccinia may be needed for use as a vaccine for smallpox virus in case of acts of warfare or terrorism [12].

Conclusion

The incidence of vaccinia decreased when routine smallpox vaccination with vaccinia was discontinued. In the fu-

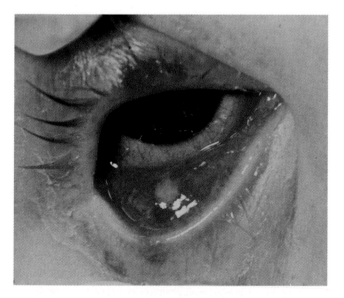

Figure 3–12. Conjunctival autoinoculation of vaccinia.

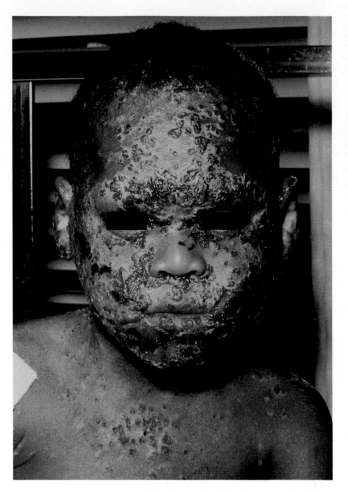

Figure 3–14.   Eczema vaccinatum.

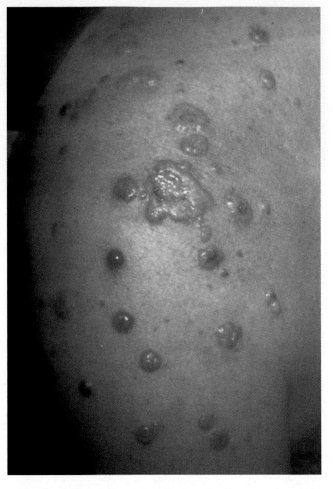

Figure 3–15.   Early vesicopustules of eczema vaccinatum.

ture, the incidence of vaccinia may increase if immuno-compromised individuals are vaccinated with vaccinia-based vaccines.

Monkeypox

Definition

Monkeypox is an orthopoxvirus that occasionally infects humans and that has been monitored closely in the post–smallpox eradication era.

History

Human monkeypox infection was identified in 1970. Travelers to and residents of western and central Africa (mostly Zaire, now referred to as the Democratic Republic of the Congo) are most likely to be infected. Squirrels and monkeys in the rain forests of this area are the identified reservoirs (Fig. 3–16). Smallpox vaccination protects against monkeypox or lessens the severity of disease. Unvacci-

nated children are mostly affected, and deaths have occurred [2,6]. Preliminary DNA studies indicate only minor genetic variation among animal strains collected from 1970 through 1979 [32]. In 1986, the committee on orthopoxvirus infections identified human monkeypox as a nonsignificant worldwide health problem because of its low incidence in humans and their belief that interhuman transmission did not occur [10]. Since that time, human-to-human transmission has accounted for most of the identified cases occurring in 1996 and 1997 [32]. The WHO in collaboration with the CDC, investigated two outbreaks of 92 and 419 suspected cases [33]. The secondary attack rate of 9% was lower than that for smallpox and case mortality rates were much lower [12]. Table 3–7 presents clinical manifestations and Table 3–8 provides differential diagnoses.

Pathogenesis/Epidemiology

Monkeypox virus has two different forms of transmission. Primary transmission occurs after skinning or handling

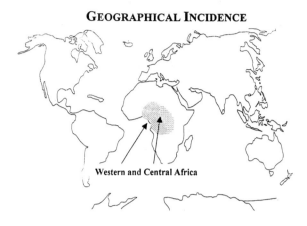

GEOGRAPHICAL INCIDENCE

Western and Central Africa

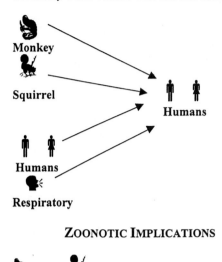

TRANSMISSION

Primary:Skinning or handling of wild animals; consumption of incompletely cooked wild monkey meat.
Secondary:Close contact with infected humans.

Monkey

Squirrel

Humans

Humans

Respiratory

ZOONOTIC IMPLICATIONS

Monkey Squirrel } Near tropical rainforest areas of West and Central Africa

Figure 3–16. Incidence and transmission of monkeypox.

Table 3–7. Clinical Manifestations of Monkeypox

Time after Exposure	Clinical Manifestations	Laboratory Analyses	Other Notes
1 day 2–10 days	Local inflammation ↓ Febrile response, with lymphadenopathy lasting 1–3 days, particularly in submandibular, cervical, and inguinal locations ↓	Isolation of virus from vesicular fluid or scabs (PCR) or hemagglutination	Transmission from animals was the most common form until 1996, when human-to-human transmission became more prominent
11 days	Severe headache, backache, and malaise ↓ Papule ↓ Vesicle ↓		Infection is most common in children and the unvaccinated Mucous membrane involvement is common Monkeypox is a milder illness in those who received the vaccinia vaccine for smallpox
Up to 4 weeks	Pustule ↓ Crust		Severe generalized infection has approximately 10% mortality

Table 3–8. Differential Diagnoses of Monkeypox

Smallpox: Clinically similar to smallpox, but monkeypox has a greater tendency to produce both lymphadenopathy and skin lesions that occur in "crops"
Varicella: Scabs and vesicles are not simultaneously present in monkeypox as they are in varicella

wild animals or consuming incompletely cooked wild monkey meat. Acquisition of the virus is probably from small lesions on the skin or mucous membrane of the animal. The second transmission form involves close contact with infected humans, such as sharing a bed. Viral spread resembles that of smallpox. In 282 cases of monkeypox, 50% of cases involved children 4 years of age or younger, and an additional 40% occurred in children from 4 to 14 years old [34]. The case fatality rate is generally 10% [35].

Conclusion

Monkeypox produces a clinical disease in humans that is indistinguishable from smallpox, except for the more pronounced enlargement of cervical and sometimes inguinal lymph nodes and a tendency for lesions to occur in crops. The incidence of this viral disease is increasing in frequency. Those without smallpox vaccinations have increased susceptibility to monkeypox and increased severity of the illness.

Cowpox

Definition

An orthopoxvirus that infects cats, cows, possibly rodents, and occasionally humans (Fig. 3–17)

History

Cowpox is thought to be the original isolate used by Edward Jenner in the 18th century for development of his vaccine. This signaled the beginning of the age of vaccination [36].

Incidence

Cowpox now appears to occur primarily in Europe and the former USSR [22,37]. Rare outbreaks in cattle are of unknown origin. Infection in humans is relatively rare but can be severe.

Pathogenesis

Cowpox virus is transmitted to humans through contact with infected animals [38,39]. Typically, a broken area of skin, such as a minor abrasion, comes in contact with ulcers or lesions on an infected animal.

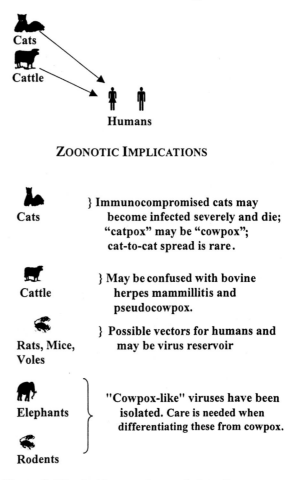

GEOGRAPHICAL INCIDENCE

← Europe and former USSR

TRANSMISSION
Contact with infected animals through broken skin.

Cats
Cattle
→ Humans

ZOONOTIC IMPLICATIONS

Cats   } Immunocompromised cats may become infected severely and die; "catpox" may be "cowpox"; cat-to-cat spread is rare.

Cattle   } May be confused with bovine herpes mammillitis and pseudocowpox.

Rats, Mice, Voles   } Possible vectors for humans and may be virus reservoir

Elephants
Rodents   } "Cowpox-like" viruses have been isolated. Care is needed when differentiating these from cowpox.

Figure 3–17. Incidence and transmission of cowpox.

Clinical Manifestations

Infected humans, after a week-long incubation period, develop a painful papule or papules that quickly become vesicles (Table 3–9). Umbilicated pustules, which may become hemorrhagic, develop with surrounding edema and ery-

Table 3–9. Clinical Manifestations of Cowpox

Time after Exposure	Clinical Manifestations	Laboratory Analyses	Other Notes
7 days	Painful papule(s); most patients have only 1 lesion ↓	Electron microscopy of skin lesions to view virions [39,45]; screen samples to determine epidemiology by DNA restriction endonuclease analysis of viral isolates; tissue culture of virions	Agent may be from exposure to domestic cats [2, 37, 38]. Most common in July-October [37] and in young girls. Infection in humans rare but severe
11–12 days	Vesicles ↓ Umbilicated pustules with surrounding edema and erythema ↓ Crust, eschar, or ulcer ↓	Serum samples for antibody detection are useful later in the course of the disease [37]	Pustules are usually hemorrhagic. Lesions most commonly on hands or face [22, 37] Lymphadenitis and general flu-like symptoms are common The draining lymph node may become enlarged and swollen. One third of patients are hospitalized. Severe cases may take as long as 12 weeks to heal
6–8 weeks	Cutaneous healing of lesions begins (with probable scarring)	Orthopoxvirus antibodies in paired sera may be used but are not definitive [43]	Atopic patients (e.g., on corticosteroids) may have lesions that resemble those of smallpox

thema; those transform into a crust, eschar, or ulcer (Figs. 3–18, 3–19). Lymphadenopathy is common, and fever or influenza-like illness may occur. Severe and rarely fatal infection has been reported in atopic patients. In one fatal case, an 18-year-old eczematous patient on corticosteroids for asthma developed a smallpox-like eruption [37,40]. Recently a boy was infected with a cowpox virus after a suspected rat bite [41].

Dermatopathology

The histological appearance of cowpox is similar to that of vaccinia but with less necrosis and more hemorrhage [22]. Cytoplasmic inclusions are larger than the Guarnieri bodies of vaccinia and smallpox [42].

Diagnosis

Painful orflike lesions in a human with a history of exposure to cats should raise the possibility of cowpox infection. Differential diagnoses are shown in Table 3–10.

Treatment/Prophylaxis

No known treatment for cowpox exists; healing is spontaneous. In a severe case, homologous vaccinia antiserum was given [40]. The prediction has been that orthopoxvirus infections (variola and vaccinia) would provide protection against cowpox infection [36]. This may not be true because infection has occurred in a recently vaccinated adult [38].

Conclusion

Cowpox infection usually affects humans by contact with an infected cat or other animal [40–45]. The infection is usually localized but can be severe. Geographical locations of infections thus far are limited to Europe and the former USSR. The virus appears to have low infectivity for humans [37].

PARAPOXVIRUS INFECTIONS

Orf

Definition

Orf is a parapoxvirus that infects sheep, goats, and humans. It is also referred to as ecthyma contagiosum, scabby mouth, sore mouth, contagious pustular dermatosis, and infectious pustular dermatitis (see section on Pseudocowpox/Milker's Nodules) (Fig. 3–20 and 3–21).

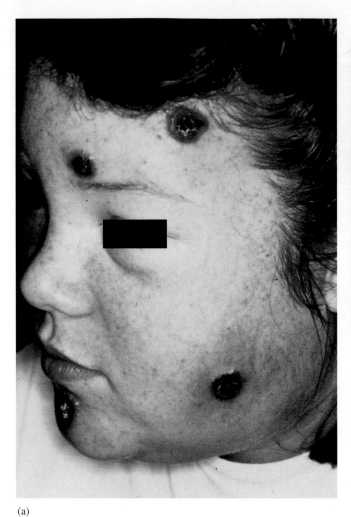

(a)

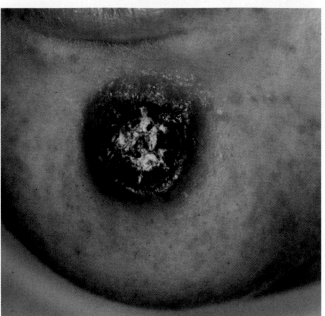

(b)

Figure 3–18. (a) Facial appearance of cowpox, showing marked left-sided swelling and periorbital edema and four crusted lesions. (b) Close view of crusted lesion on the chin. (Photographs from Lewis-Jones et al., Br J Dermatol 129:625–627, 1993, used with permission, and courtesy of M. S. Lewis-Jones, M.D., Department of Dermatology, Ninewells Hospital and Medical School, Dundee, Scotland.)

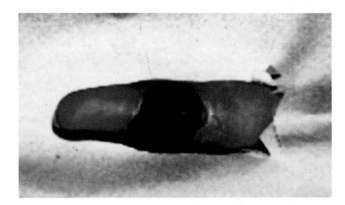

Figure 3–19. Eschar of the finger resulting from cowpox. (Photograph from Vestey et al., Int J Dermatol 30:696–698, 1991, used with permission, and courtesy of James Vestey, M.D., Department of Dermatology, University of Edinburgh, Edinburgh, Scotland.)

Table 3–10. Differential Diagnoses of Cowpox

Vaccinia: Has more necrosis and less hemorrhage; has smaller cytoplasmic inclusions (Guarnieri bodies)
Smallpox: Multiple lesions with more generalized spread
Orf/Milker's nodules: More granulomatous lesions, which are not usually painful
Anthrax: Relatively painless and progresses more rapidly to an eschar in 5–6 days
Herpesvirus infection: Usually not hemorrhagic or as erythematous as cow pox. Lesions are more superficial than in cowpox. Patients often have a history of recurrent lesions

WORLDWIDE GEOGRAPHICAL INCIDENCE

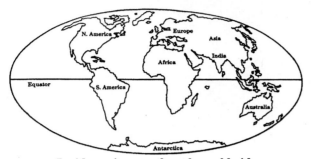

Incidence is rare, though worldwide

TRANSMISSION

Contaminated fomites, such as knives and barbed wire. Virus remains infective for years at room temperature.

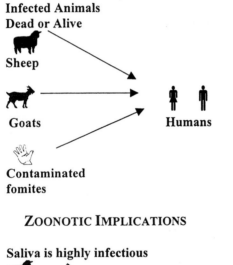

ZOONOTIC IMPLICATIONS

Saliva is highly infectious

Sheep Goats **} Vesicopapular eruption on gums, lips, nose, or groin**

Figure 3–20. Incidence and transmission of orf.

History

In 1937, George Peterkin reported the occurrence of orf in humans from contagious pustular dermatitis of sheep [46,47]. The word orf is derived from the Anglo-Saxon name for cattle [48]. In 1520 Pope Leo X referred to Martin Luther, the founder of the Reformation, as a "scabby sheep" infecting "the flock," obviously a reference to orf. [48].

Incidence

The economic impact of this parapoxvirus is important; infected lambs may fail to grow properly and lesions can become secondarily infected [49]. Although the infection is relatively trivial in humans, the disease has a worldwide distribution. One author stated that apparently only "whites" have been infected [50]. However, Figure 3–22 shows an affected Hispanic male who was a sheepherder.

Pathogenesis

Transmission to humans occurs from infected lesions on animals or from fomites, such as wire fencing, barn doors, feeding troughs, or shears [49]. The virus remains infective on fomites for years at room temperature. It is able to survive heating and drying but is sensitive to ether [49]. The saliva of the infected animal is highly infectious. Person-to-person transmission under natural conditions has not been demonstrated, although a nurse who changed the dressing of an infected patient contracted the disease [51].

Clinical Manifestations

Orf is characterized by six stages lasting approximately 6 days each. These sequential stages are described in Table 3–11 and are illustrated in Figures 3–21 to 3–25. Secondary bacterial infection is rare but can occur during disease progression (Table 3–11). Possible secondary complications include (1) lymphadenopathy and lymphangitis [50]; (2) fever [48]; (3) erythema multiforme and vesicular eruption [52,53]; and (4) secondary spread of lesions to face and hands associated with active atopic dermatitis [54]. A "giant orf" lesion measuring 6 cm failed to regress in a patient with chronic lymphocytic leukemia [55]. Fortunately, in one study orf virus contracted during late pregnancy showed no effects on the infant or placenta [56]. No underlying predisposition for infection has been found.

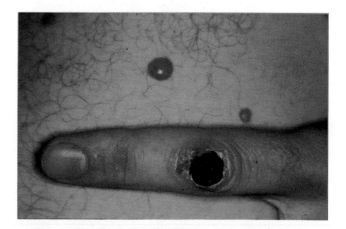

Figure 3–21. Acute stages in orf infection.

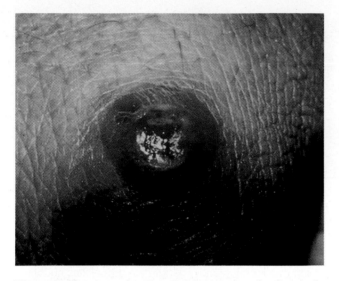

Figure 3–22. Acute weeping nodule stage in orf on hand of a Mexican shepherd.

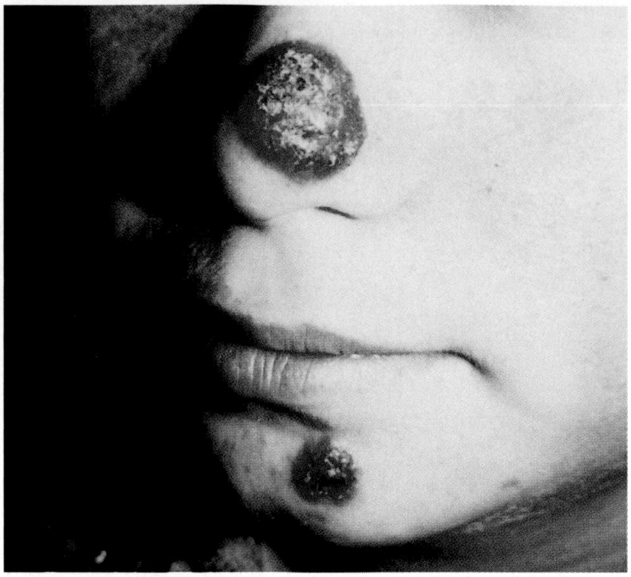

Typically, lesions of orf undergo spontaneous resolution, passing through the six stages over a period of 35 to 36 days.

Dermatopathology

Routine histopathologic studies can be helpful in the diagnosis. Cells in the upper third of the epidermis are vacuolated and have intracytoplasmic inclusions. In the weeping

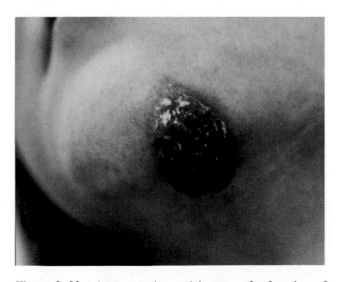

Figure 3–23. Acute weeping nodule stage of orf on jaw of woman who rested her chin on the head of her pet sheep. (Photograph courtesy of Dearl Dodson, M.D., Department of Dermatology, University of Texas Medical Branch at Galveston, Galveston, TX.)

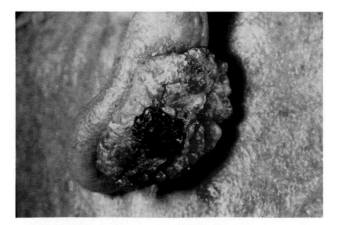

Figure 3–24. Early regenerative dry stage of orf.

and regenerative stages, the following signs are seen: multilocular vesicles [48]; lymphohistiocytic dermal infiltrates with plasma cells; reticular degeneration of the epidermis; and dilated hair follicles. Papillomatous and regressive stages of orf have finger-like downward projections that produce acanthosis and papillomatosis. Electron microscopic examination of lesional skin shows the characteristic brick-shaped viral particles 200–380 nm long. Intranuclear inclusions are occasionally seen [57].

Laboratory Findings

The immune response of humans to the orf virus has been studied in a series of patients [58], although this method

Figure 3–25. Papillomatous stage of orf.

Table 3–11. Clinical Manifestations of Orf

Time After Exposure	Clinical Manifestations	Laboratory Analyses	Other Notes
3–7 days	One to four papules on hand (typically only one lesion); begins as a red maculopapular lesion ↓ Vesicle ↓	Can confirm by histologic study, viral culture, increase in serologic titers, or complement fixation Electron microscopy of lesional skin shows brick-shaped viral particles (200–380 nm in length) (Fig. 3–2); intranuclear inclusions are occasionally seen	Systemic symptoms are rare but may include lymphadenopathy and lymphangitis, fever, rigors, drenching sweats, malaise, and urticaria
10–14 days	Target lesion with red center, white middle ring, and red halo ↓		
14–21 days	Acute weeping stage (Figs. 3–22, 3–23) ↓		Lesions are relatively painless
21–28 days	Regenerative dry stage with black dots (Fig. 3–24) ↓		
28–35 days	Papillomatous stage (Fig. 3–25) ↓		Typically no scarring occurs
35 days	Regressive stage with dry crust and eventual shedding of the scab (Fig. 3–21)		

is not commonly employed for clinical diagnosis. Soon after infection, subjects developed a vigorous lymphoproliferative immune response including peripheral blood mononuclear cells. Western blot analysis and enzyme-linked immunosorbent-assay (ELISA) demonstrate a rise in orf virus antibody levels as early as 2 weeks after infection. With serial sampling, the majority of patients have a fourfold or greater rise in orf virus antibody titers.

Diagnosis

The diagnosis of orf infection can be made by patient history and physical examination. If necessary, this may be confirmed by using cell culture, complement fixation, fluorescent antibody testing, or by biopsy of a lesion for examination by routine histologic study or electron microscopy [57]. See Table 3–12 for differential diagnoses.

Treatment

There is no specific antiviral treatment for orf. Lesions resolve spontaneously. A live vaccine is available for animals [59]. Antibiotics are warranted only if secondary infection is present. Isolation of infected animals helps limit the spread of disease. Infection confers lasting immunity in humans.

Conclusion

Orf is a self-limited viral infection of humans. Cross-immunity for variola or other orthopoxviruses (vaccinia or cowpox) does not result from infection [58,60].

Table 3–12. Differential Diagnoses of Orf

Milker's nodules: Clinically identical; source of infection is cattle
Cowpox: Early lesions of cowpox are similar
Anthrax: More hemorrhagic and lesions progresses more rapidly to an eschar
Tularemia: Typically, tularemia has systemic symptoms, with high fever, headache, malaise, and myalgias. The skin ulcer is more chancrelike
Tuberculosis (primary inoculated): Most lesions occur in children. A painless shallow ulcer develops and heals poorly
Mycobacterial infection (atypical): Lesions often last 1 to 2 years before healing
Syphilitic chancre: Lesions typically occur on the genitalia rather than on the hand
Sporotrichosis: Begins as a single necrotic nodule, but multiple nodules arise in a linear fashion along the lymphatics
Pyogenic granuloma: Juicy red papule that bleeds easily, often with an epidermal collarette at the base
Keratoacanthoma: Appears as a dome-shaped papule or plaque with a central crater filled with keratin
Giant molluscum contagiosum: Lesions do not weep or become necrotic and often appear in clusters

Pseudocowpox-Bovine Papular Stomatitis Virus-Milker's Nodules

Definition

Pseudocowpox or paravaccinia is a parapoxvirus that infects the teats of cattle (Fig. 3–26). In humans it is called

FORMERLY WORLDWIDE GEOGRAPHICAL
INCIDENCE

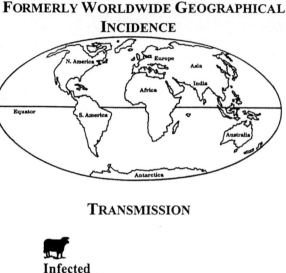

TRANSMISSION

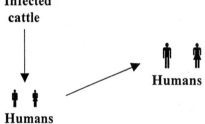

ZOONOTIC IMPLICATIONS

Cattle   }**Teats that are infected have observable lesions similar to those on humans; bovine papular stomatitis is characterized by papules in the oral cavity or muzzle.**

Reindeer, muskox, red deer   } **Reported to have other parapoxvirus infections.**

Figure 3–26. Incidence and transmission of pseudocowpox.

milker's nodules, milker's node, or paravaccinia. The DNA of ovine (orf) and bovine (pseudocowpox, paravaccinia) and papular stomatitis strains is distinct [61,62]. Others, however, consider these differences to be too slight to separate orf and milker's nodules into different species [2].

Infection in the bovine mouth is called bovine papular stomatitis. The viruses responsible for pseudocowpox and bovine papular stomatitis are designated as separate species by most investigators [61,62]; however, some contend that only one virus may be involved [63].

History

Jenner grouped milker's nodules or pseudocowpox under the heading of "spurious cowpox" because it did not immunize against smallpox [64]. In 1957, Wheeler and Cawley suspected a viral etiology for milker's nodules and its relationship to vaccinia [64]. In 1963, Friedman-Kien et al. isolated a poxvirus from a case of milker's nodule [65].

Incidence

New milkers (young people, vacation milkers or persons who have switched jobs) have been infected worldwide [64]. Veterinary students who have contact with the mouths of cows during feeding or endotracheal tube placement are susceptible to bovine papular stomatitis [66].

Pathogenesis

The pseudocoxpox virus is transmitted to humans through contact with infected lesions on cows. Infection of human wounds from contaminated fomites occurs rarely, and human-to-human spread has not been reported.

Clinical Manifestations

Pseudocowpox infection of the teats of cattle produces observable lesions similar to those produced in humans (Table 3–13). Bovine papular stomatitis, a mild disease, is difficult to diagnose because papules in the oral cavity and muzzle area are difficult to see. When humans are infected with either pseudocowpox or bovine papular stomatitis virus, the lesions are identical to those of orf (see Orf section) (Figs. 3–27, 3–28). Milker's nodules associated with burn wounds have been reported in which the source of inoculation was assumed to be contaminated water or grass (Fig. 3–29)[67]. See Table 3–14 for differential diagnoses.

Dermatopathology
See section on Orf.

Laboratory Findings, Differential Diagnosis, and Treatment
See section on Orf.

Conclusion

Paravaccinia viruses affect cattle causing oral or cutaneous teat infections. When either type of infection is transmitted

Table 3–13. Clinical Manifestations of Pseudocowpox/Paravaccinia (Milker's Nodules)

Time After Exposure	Clinical Manifestations	Laboratory Analysis	Other Notes
5–7 days	Papular stage with hemispherical, extremely vascular papule(s); Generally only one lesion but can be up to four ↓	Electron microscopy; viral culture; complement fixation; routine histopathology	Usually infects new or recent milkers, veterinary students
12–14 days	Target stage—large purple nodule up to 2 cm in diameter with a red center surrounded by a white ring and a red halo ↓ Weeping and erosion ↓		Infection generally induces long-lasting immunity Lesions are painless but may have pruritus. No frank ulceration occurs
19–21 days	Firm, crusted nodule ↓		Occasionally there is mild swelling of draining lymph nodes
26–28 days	Regressive stage; granulation tissue is absorbed and the crust		
4–6 weeks	sloughs off		

to humans, the result is a self-limited disease identical to orf.

OTHER PARAPOXVIRUS INFECTIONS

Cutaneous infections can occur in humans from contact with a reindeer or a musk ox with a parapoxvirus infection [44,68]. Mercer, in 1997, stated that the parapoxvirus of red deer in New Zealand (PNVZ) had not yet infected humans [69]. Tentative members of the genus are camel contagious ecthyma, chamois contagious ecthyma, and sealpox viruses [62].

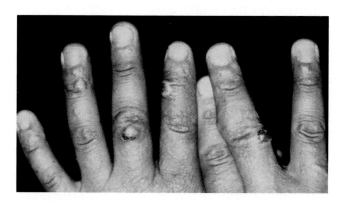

Figure 3–27. Milker's nodules of the hands. (Photograph courtesy of Roberto Arenas, M.D., Mexico City, Mexico.)

Tanapox

Definition

This "unclassified" poxvirus affecting humans and monkeys [70] is usually placed in the genus *Yatapox* [1,71] (Fig. 3–30).

History

The virus was first isolated in 1962 after causing epidemics in 1957 and 1962 near the Tana river valley in Kenya

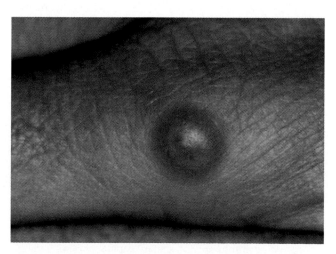

Figure 3–28. This milker's nodule was identical to the nodules of orf.

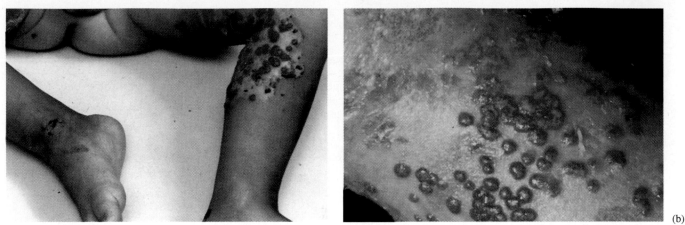

(a)   (b)

Figure 3–29.   (a) Milker's nodules within a burn scar. (b) Closer view of milker's nodules. (Photographs from Schuler et al., JAAD, 334–339, 1982, used with permission, and courtesy of Klaus Wolff, M.D., Department of Dermatology, University of Vienna School of Medicine, Vienna, Austria.)

[70,72]. Now Central Africa, including Zaire, is affected [45].

Incidence

All age groups are affected, apparently only in tropical Africa (Zaire and Kenya) [70,73]. Most cases have occurred in individuals who worked or played close to the river [70]. The incidence of tanapox infection has a seasonal variation, with an increased frequency during the 5-month period from November to March [70].

Pathogenesis

The mode of transmission of tanapox is not completely known. Direct contact transmission occurs when animal handlers are scratched by monkeys. However, many individuals have acquired the disease with no known exposure to monkeys or their carcasses. Mosquitoes have been suspected as vectors of infection from monkeys to humans [45,70,72,73]. Most infected patients can recall repeated

GEOGRAPHICAL INCIDENCE

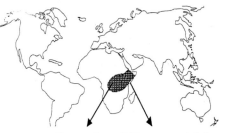

Central and Eastern Africa

TRANSMISSION

Mosquitoes suspected as vectors of infection from monkeys to humans.

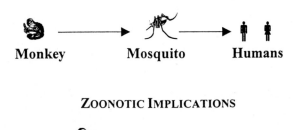

Monkey   Mosquito   Humans

ZOONOTIC IMPLICATIONS

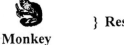

                        } **Reservoir of infection**
Monkey

Figure 3–30.   Incidence and transmission of tanapox.

Table 3–14.   Differential Diagnoses of Pseudocowpox/Bovine Papular Stomatitis Virus/Milker's Nodules

Orf: Lesions are identical but source of infection is sheep
Bovine papular stomatitis: Similar to milker's nodules, but bovine papular stomatitis rarely occurs
Anthrax: Lesions are hemorrhagic and progress to an eschar more rapidly
Herpetic whitlow: Characterized as more vesicular, not as nodular and elevated, and more painful
Pyogenic granuloma: Vascular papule, often with collarette of epidermis at the base

Table 3–15. Clinical Manifestations of Tanapox

Time Since Exposure	Clinical Manifestations	Laboratory Analysis	Other
3–5 days	Short febrile illness, at times with headache, backache, and lymphadenopathy, lasting 3–4 days ↓	Electron microscopy of skin samples or necrotic tissue	Incubation and clinical features not fully known
Commonly appear during febrile stage	1–10 skin lesions, about 1.5 cm in diameter, usually on exposed body parts, especially the torso [66]. The face is often spared. Most patients have only 1 lesion ↓		Generally a benign illness Human-to-human spread is extremely rare Lesions consist of pruritic, indurated, and sometimes umbilicated papules that become necrotic and are surrounded by edematous skin; lymphadenopathy is common Scarring occurs
Rapid growth	Pruritic papule with induration ↓ Papule becomes poxlike with little or no fluid but with a significant amount of necrotic tissue ↓ Raised nodule, often firm and deep-seated ↓		High probability of lifelong immunity
Slow process of healing 6 weeks	Frequent ulceration, with a base of soft necrotic tissue and slightly raised border; pain and pruritus ↓ Complete healing		

bites from blood-sucking insects prior to developing the disease, and most lesions have occurred on exposed body parts [70]. In addition, the seasonal increase in tanapox disease corresponds with a similar increase in blood-sucking insects, such as mosquitoes.

Clinical Manifestations

Lymphadenopathy is common [70] (see Tables 3–15 and 3–16).

Treatment/Prophylaxis

This is usually a benign illness that heals within 6 weeks. Smallpox vaccination does not protect an individual from tanapox infection [70].

Table 3–16. Differential Diagnoses of Tanapox

Monkeypox: Rapidly develops into vesicles and pustules, with no ulceration. Lesions are smaller (≤5 mm) than those of tanapox

Tropical ulcers: Tropical ulcers are characterized by larger lesions than occur in tanapox. Most have a foulsmelling, grey-green membranous covering and purulent discharge

Conclusion

Tanapox is generally a mild disease with a limited geographic distribution. Further studies of the natural history of viruses such as tanapox could provide clues about the human immune system and, perhaps, a better understanding of viral evolution [74].

Molluscum Contagiosum

Organism

Molluscum contagiosum is a virus of the Molluscipox virus genus that produces multiple umbilicated skin lesions. Only humans are known to be affected, except for one report each of molluscum contagiosum occurring in chimpanzees and a horse [75,76](Fig. 3–31).

History

In 1817 Bateman described the lesions characteristic of this infection and assigned its name [77]. In 1841 Henderson and Paterson described the intracytoplasmic inclusion bodies now known by their names or as "molluscum bod-

GEOGRAPHICAL INCIDENCE

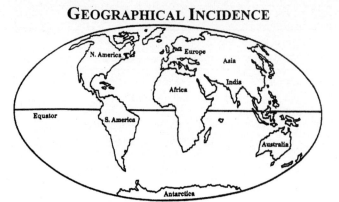

Incidence more prevalent in tropical areas

TRANSMISSION

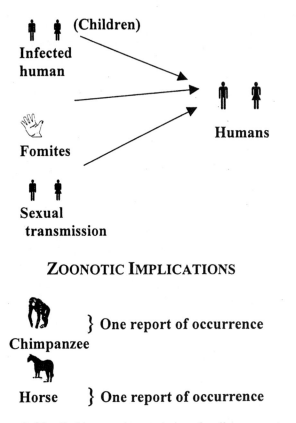

Figure 3–31. Incidence and transmission of molluscum contagiosum.

Incidence

Molluscum contagiosum virus (MCV) has a worldwide distribution but is more prevalent in tropical areas. It mainly affects children, sexually active adults, and individuals with impaired cellular immunity. Its incidence in the United States has been increasing since the 1960s, mainly as a sexually transmitted disease [82]. Those most commonly affected in 1966–1983 were 15- to 29-year olds [82]. The subtypes of molluscum contagiosum virus, MCV I and MCV II, occur in both genital and nongenital lesions. Patients usually have either MCV I or MCV II. In one study, patients under 15 years of age had only MCV I [83]. MCV I is more prevalent than MCV II, except in HIV-infected individuals [84]. Less than 5% of children in the United States are believed to be infected with molluscum virus; however, infected children without clinical manifestations may go undiagnosed [83]. In one study, the incidence of molluscum contagiosum was found to be twice as high in children who went to swimming pools than children who did not [85]. Some authors refer to the type II variants as MCV III [86]; others designate a type IV rarely [87].

Pathogenesis

Transmission of this virus is primarily through direct skin contact with an infected individual. Sexual transmission also occurs. Fomites have been suggested to be another source of infection, with molluscum contagiosum reportedly acquired from bath towels, tattoos, and in beauty parlors and Turkish baths [88].

The virus has not been grown reproducibly in cell cultures, which has hindered studies of infection and immune detection. The pathogenesis of skin lesions involves hyperplasia and hypertrophy of the keratinocytes [89]. Free virus cores have been found in all layers of the epidermis. "Viral factories" are located in the malpighian and granular cell layers [89]. The molluscum bodies contain large numbers of maturing virions. These are contained intracellularly in a collagen- and lipid-rich saclike structure that is thought to deter immunological recognition by the host [90]. Rupture and discharge of the infectious virus-packed cells occurs in the crater of the lesion. MCV induces a benign tumor instead of the usual necrotic "pox" lesion associated with other poxviruses.

Clinical Manifestations

Any cutaneous surface may be involved but favored sites include the axillae, the antecubital and popliteal fossae, and the crural folds (Fig. 3–32) [91,92]. Autoinoculation is common. Rarely, molluscum contagiosum lesions occur

ies" [78]. In the first decade of the 20th century, Juliusberg showed transmissibility of these lesions by a filterable agent [79], and Lipshutz granules within the molluscum bodies were described [80]. Inoculation experiments have not been reliable [81].

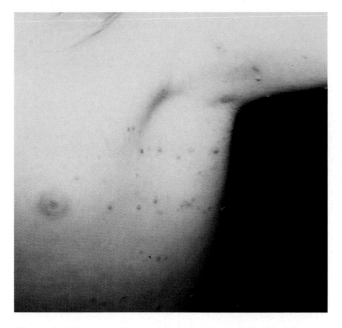

Figure 3–32. Umbilicated shiny papules of molluscum contagiosum acquired by casual contact in a child.

in the mouth [93] or conjunctivae [94,95]. Table 13–17 outlines the progression of the infection. The lesions produced by MCV I and II are clinically indistinguishable. Molluscum contagiosum in adults is often acquired sexually and affects the groin, genital area, thighs, and lower abdomen (Fig. 3–33). Children usually acquire molluscum nonsexually. They may have genital lesions, but this is in addition to lesions in extragenital areas. Patients with atopic dermatitis can have a disseminated eruption (Fig. 3–34). Eruptions in immunocompromised adults are very resistant to treatment [96–98]. Potential differential diagnoses are shown in Table 3–18.

Molluscum dermatitis, or an eczematous reaction around a molluscum papule, occurs occasionally. Resolution of the papule is presumably as a result of the host immune response to viral antigens [99,100]. Occasionally, molluscum lesions can become inflamed and resemble a pyoderma [100,101]. Molluscum contagiosum can infect the conjunctiva [94,95] or be the cause of unilateral chronic conjunctivitis when the lesion is on the eyelid [102]. Molluscum contagiosum in patients with HIV infection is often widespread. Treatment is resistant and frequently involves

Table 3–17. Clinical Manifestations of Molluscum Contagiosum (MCV)

Time Since Exposure	Clinical Manifestations	Laboratory Analysis	Other
1 week to several months	Small, firm, umbilicated papule with smooth, wavy, or pearly surface (1 mm to 1 cm in diameter) (Fig. 3–35) Span of individual papule is 2 months	Virus does not grow reproducibly in cell cultures Use of PCR to detect MCV in skin lesions	10–20 lesions are most common; autoinoculation (Koebner's reaction) may occur. MCV produces benign tumors rather than the usual necrotic pox lesion
Months to years	Spontaneous resolution Remission	Histologic examination—cells of lesions demonstrate inclusion bodies	Immunocompromised hosts show widespread eruption, especially on the face (Fig. 3–26)
Subsequent months to years	Relapse and reappearance of lesion	Electron microscopy shows characteristic poxvirus structure (Fig. 3–2) Polyclonal antibody recognizes MCV in fixed tissue In situ hybridization for MCV DNA	Solitary lesion can resemble a furuncle or a pyogenic granuloma MCV can infect the conjunctiva or cause unilateral chronic conjunctivitis when the eyelid is involved

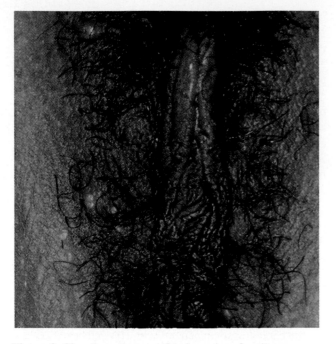

Figure 3–33. Sexually transmitted papules of molluscum contagiosum of the right labia majora.

Table 3–18. Differential Diagnoses of Molluscum Contagiosum

Herpes simplex virus: HSV lesions are vesicular and often are accompained by burning pain. Lesions progress and heal more rapidly

Verruca vulgaris: Hyperkeratotic and verrucous without central umbilication of MC

Syringoma or other adnexal tumors: Usually occurs as dermal papules that do not resolve

Pyodermas: Pyoderma is crusty or purulent and may spread

Papular granuloma annulare: Diffuse papules, usually widespread

Condyloma acuminata: Verrucous papules and plaques in genital region

Cutaneous cryptococcosis: May be found in immunocompromised hosts (requires biopsy)

Histoplasmosis: May be found in immunocompromised hosts (requires biopsy)

Keratoacanthoma: May be confused with a single molluscum lesion and require biopsy confirmation

Epidermal inclusion cyst: A dermal cyst, often with overlying pore

Basal cell carcinoma: May be confused with a single molluscum lesion and require biopsy confirmation

Neurilemmoma: Firm nodule usually located along nerve trunks

Pyogenic granuloma: May be confused with a single molluscum lesion and require biopsy for confirmation. It is usually more vascular in appearance

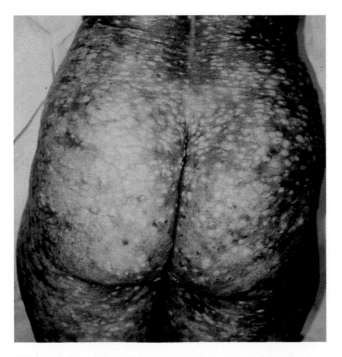

Figure 3–34. Disseminated molluscum contagiosum in a patient with atopic dermatitis.

the face, which is an unusual location for MCV in HIV-seronegative persons (Figs. 3–35 to 3–39).

Dermatopathology

Histologically, molluscum contagiosum exhibits intraepidermal lobules with central cellular and viral debris (Fig. 3–40). In the basal layer, enlarged basophilic nuclei and mitotic figures are seen. Progressing upward, the cells show cytoplasmic vacuolization and then eosinophilic globules. The nucleus becomes compressed at the periphery of the cell and at the level of the granular cell layer and the molluscum bodies lose their internal structural markings. Undisrupted lesions show an absence of inflammation, but dermal changes can include an infiltrate that is lymphohistiocytic, neutrophilic, or granulomatous. The granulomatous form has been found in solitary lesions [92].

Laboratory Findings

Antibody to MCV by indirect immunofluorescence has been found in 69% of patients with visible lesions [103].

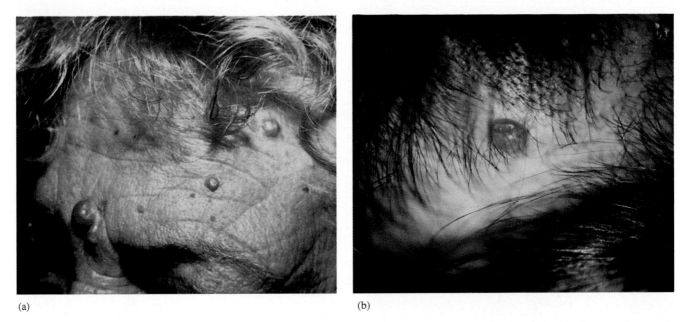

(a)   (b)

Figure 3–35. (a) Large molluscum contagiosum lesions in a patient with AIDS. (b) The umbilication is seen in this close-up photograph of another AIDS patient.

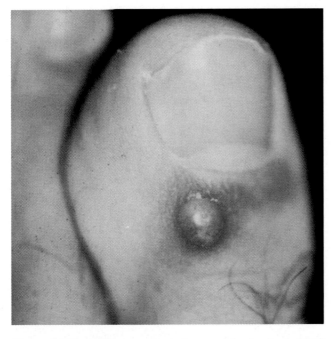

Figure 3–36. Molluscum contagiosum of the toe in an AIDS patient. (Photograph courtesy of Mario Marini, M.D., Department of Dermatology, University of Buenos Aires School of Medicine, Buenos Aires, Argentina.)

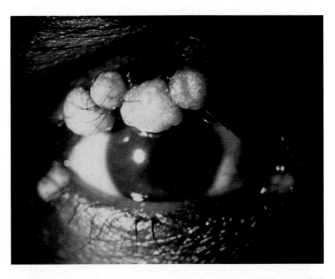

Figure 3–37. Molluscum contagiosum of the eyelid in an AIDS patient. (Photograph courtesy of J. K. Maniar, M.D., Department of Dermatovenereology and AIDS Medicine, G.T. Hospital, Grant Medical College, Mumbai, India.)

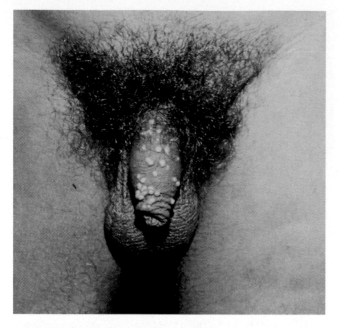

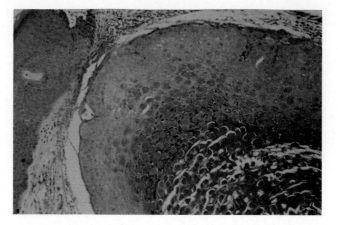

Figure 3–40. Molluscum contagiosum. Intraepidermal lobule containing cellular and viral debris. Large eosinopilic globules within keratinocytes are termed "molluscum bodies" (H & E × 100).

Figure 3–38. Molluscum contagiosum of the penis in an AIDS patient. (Photograph courtesy of J. K. Maniar, M.D., Department of Dermatovenereology and AIDS Medicine, G.T. Hospital, Grant Medical College, Mumbai, India.)

Polymerase chain reaction (PCR) can detect MCV in skin lesions [104,105]. Currently, there is no in vitro or animal model for MCV. MCV can undergo an abortive infection in some cell lines, which can cause confusion with herpes simplex virus by laboratories [106]. Two sets of investigators have infected human skin with molluscum contagiosum and grafted it onto athymic mice, although there was no continued viral replication [107,108].

Diagnosis

The diagnosis of molluscum contagiosum is a clinical one. When necessary, histological examination of a curetted or biopsied lesion is diagnostic. The curetted material can be crushed on a slide and left unstained or stained with the Wright's, Giemsa, Gram, or Papanicolaou stains to demonstrate the inclusion bodies. Electron microscopy shows characteristic poxvirus structures. Penneys and coworkers

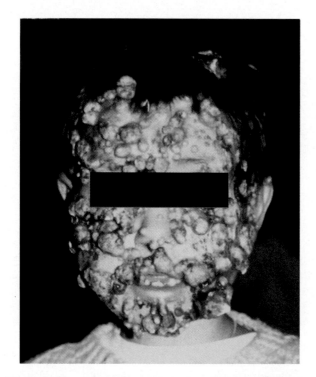

Figure 3–39. Molluscum contagiosum of the face of a 13-year-old girl with AIDS in Romania. (Photograph courtesy of Mark Klein, M.D., Department of Pediatrics, Baylor College of Medicine, Houston, TX.)

Table 3–19. Treatment of Molluscum Contagiosum

Symptoms	Treatment
Shiny umbilicated papules seen in children and young adults	Can be handled with "benign neglect," but many destructive methods are available. Antiretroviral therapy has benefited the cause of facial molluscum in the immunocompromised patient
	Immunotherapy: imiquimod
	Antiviral therapy: cidofovir

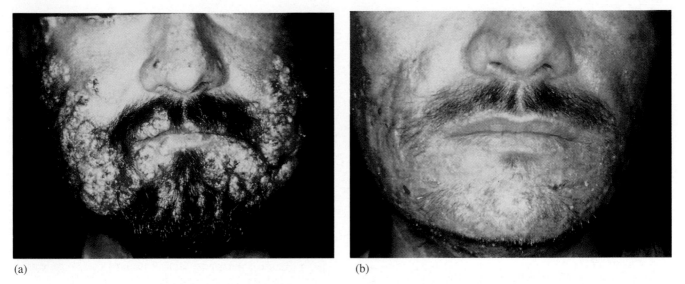

(a)   (b)

Figure 3–41. Molluscum contagiosum of the face of an AIDS patient before (a) and after (b) cidofovir therapy. (Photographs from Meadows et al., Arch Dermatol 133:987–990, 1997, used with permission, and courtesy of Kappa Meadows, M.D., Department of Dermatology, University of Utah School of Medicine, Salt Lake City, UT.)

generated a polyclonal antibody that recognizes molluscum contagiosum in fixed tissue using immunohistochemical methods [109]. In situ hybridization for MCV DNA has been used [110].

Treatment/Prophylaxis

Molluscum contagiosum may be left untreated, as most papules will eventually resolve. Many patients seek medical attention to rid themselves of the papules; in these cases many methods have been used (Table 3–19), including curettage, liquid nitrogen, cantharidin, podophyllin, podophyllotoxin, salicylic acid/lactic acid, phenol, tincture of iodine, tretinoin cream or gel, silver nitrate, trichloroacetic acid, oral cimetidine, repeated application and removal of tape (tape stripping), squeezing with blunt forceps, or diathermy. Recently reported treatments include use of the carbon dioxide or pulsed-dye laser or topical photodynamic therapy [111,112]. Lesions, clinically undetectable at the time of examination, may appear later and necessitate multiple treatments.

Treatment of the facial molluscum lesions on those with AIDS poses a great challenge. Partial success has been achieved using photodynamic therapy with 5-aminolevulinic acid [111], antiretroviral therapy [113,114], cidofovir given intravenously or topically [115–117] (Fig. 3–41), or imiquimod [118].

Conclusion

MCV causes a benign cutaneous infection in humans with normal immunological responses. It differs from other pox-

viruses in that it does not cause a "poxlike" vesicular lesion but rather causes spontaneously regressing tumors of the skin. Many local treatments are at least temporarily effective, except in the immunocompromised host, whose infection is difficult to eradicate but who may respond to antiviral or immunomodulatory therapy.

REFERENCES

1. RML Buller, GJ Palumbo. Poxvirus pathogenesis. Microbiol Rev 55:80–122, 1991.
2. D Baxby. Human poxvirus infection after the eradication of smallpox. Epidemiol Infect 100:321–334, 1988.
3. N Barquet, P Domingo. Smallpox: the triumph over the most terrible of the ministers of death. Ann Intern Med 127:635–642, 1997.
4. AS Klainer. Smallpox. Clin Dermatol 7:19–22, 1989.
5. J Rathbone. Lady Mary Wortley Montague's contribution to the eradication of smallpox. Lancet 347:1566, 1996.
6. World Health Organization: The global eradication of smallpox. Final report of the Global Commission for the Certification of Smallpox Eradication. Geneva, Switzerland: World Health Organization, 1980.
7. A Deria, Z Jezek, K Markvart, P Carrasco, J Weisfeld. The world's last endemic case of smallpox: surveillance and containment measures. Bull World Health Organ 58:279–283, 1980.
8. Centers for Disease Control. Laboratory associated smallpox—England/Smallpox follow-up. MMWR 27:319–320, 346, 1978.

9. Z Jezek, LN Khodakevich, JF Wickett. Smallpox and its post eradication surveillance. Bull World Health Organ 65:425–434, 1987.

10. F Fenner, DA Henderson, I Arita, et al. Smallpox and its eradication. Geneva, Switzerland: World Health Organization, 1988.

11. Committee on orthopoxvirus infections: report of the fourth meeting. Wkly Epidemiol Rec 61:289–293, 1986.

12. JG Breman, DA Henderson. Poxvirus dilemmas—monkeypox, smallpox, and biologic terrorism. N Engl J Med 339:556–559, 1998.

13. AW Downie, G Meiklejohn, L St. Vincent, AR Rao, BV Sundara Babu, CH Kempe. The recovery of smallpox virus from patients and their environment in a smallpox hospital. Bull World Health Organ 33:615–622, 1965.

14. WH Foege, JD Millar, DA Henderson. Smallpox eradication in West and Central Africa. Bull World Health Organ 52:209–222, 1975.

15. F Fenner, R Wittek, KR Dumbell. The Orthopoxviruses. San Diego, CA: Academic Press, 1989, p. 107.

16. WK Joklik, B Moss, BN Fields, DH Bishop, LS Sandakhchiev. Why the smallpox virus stocks should not be destroyed. Science 262:1225–1226, 1993.

17. B Roizman, W Joklik, B Fields, B Moss. The destruction of smallpox virus stocks in national repositories: a grave mistake and a bad precedent. Infect Agents Dis 3:215–217, 1994.

18. W Joklik. The remaining smallpox virus stocks are too valuable to be destroyed. Scientist 10:11, 1996.

19. BW Mahy, JW Almond, KI Berns, RM Chanock, DK Lvov, RF Pettersson, HG Schatzmayr, F Fenner. The remaining stocks of smallpox virus should be destroyed. Science 262:1223–1224, 1993.

20. DA Henderson. Principles and lessons from the smallpox eradication programme. Bull World Health Organ 65:535–546, 1987.

21. D Baxby, RM Gaskell, CJ Gaskell, M Bennett. Ecology of orthopox viruses and use of recombinant vaccinia vaccines. Lancet 2:850–851, 1986.

22. AS Highet, J Kurst. Viral infections. In: RH Champion, ed. Textbook of Dermatology, 5th ed. Oxford: Blackwell Scientific Publications, 1992, pp. 872–873.

23. CE Taylor. Did vaccinia virus come from a horse? Equine Vet J 25:8–10, 1993.

24. DE Hruby. Present and future applications of vaccinia virus as a vector. Vet Parasitol 29:281–292, 1988.

25. F Fenner, R Wittek, KR Dumbell. The Orthopoxviruses. San Diego, CA: Academic Press, 1989, p 152.

26. AM Kesson, JK Ferguson, WD Rawlinson, AL Cunningham. Progressive vaccinia treated with ribavirin and vaccinia immune globulin. Clin Infect Dis 25:911–914, 1997.

27. NR Williams, BM Cooper. Counseling of workers handling vaccinia virus. Occup Med (Lond) 43:125–127, 1993.

28. CS Chung, JC Hsiao, YS Chang, YS Chang. A27L protein mediates vaccinia virus interaction with cell surface heparan sulfate. J Virol 72:1577–1585, 1998.

29. WB Minich, M Behr, U Loos. Expression of a functional tagged human thyrotropin receptor in HeLa cells using recombinant vaccinia virus. Exp Clin Endocrinol Diabetes 105:282–290, 1997.

30. B Moss. Genetically engineered poxviruses for recombinant gene expression, vaccination, and safety. Proc Natl Acad Sci USA 93:11341–11348, 1996.

31. B Moss. Vaccinia virus: a tool for research and vaccine development. Science 252:1662–1667, 1991.

32. Centers for Disease Control and Prevention. Human monkeypox—Kasai Oriental, Zaire, 1996–1997. MMWR 46:304–307, 1997.

33. Centers for Disease Control and Prevention. Human monkeypox—Kasai Oriental, Democratic Republic of Congo, February 1996–October 1997. MMWR 46:1168–1171, 1997.

34. Z Jezek, M Szczeniowski, KM Paluku, M Mutombo. Human monkeypox: clinical features of 282 patients. J Infect Dis 156:293–298, 1987.

35. Z Jezek, B Grab, M Szczeniowski, KM Paluku, M Mutombo. Clinico-epidemiological features of monkeypox patients with an animal or human source of infection. Bull World Health Organ 66:459–464, 1988.

36. JP Vestey, DL Yirrel, M Norval. What is human catpox/cowpox infection? Int J Dermatol 30:696–698, 1991.

37. D Baxby, M Bennett. Cowpox: a reevaluation of the risks of human cowpox based on new epidemiological information. Arch Virol 13:1–12, 1997.

38. D Baxby, M Bennett, B Getty. Human cowpox 1969–93: a review based on 54 cases. Br J Dermatol 131:598–607, 1994.

39. E Willemse, HF Egberink. Transmission of cowpox virus infection from domestic cat to man. Lancet 1:1515, 1985.

40. AM Eis-Hubinger, A Gerritzen, KE Schneweis, B Pfeiff, H Pullmann, A Mayr, CP Czerny. Fatal cowpox-like virus infection transmitted by cat [letter]. Lancet 336:880, 1990.

41. BH Postma, RJA Diepersloot, GJCM Niessen, RP Droog. Cowpox-virus-like infection associated with rat bite. Lancet 337:733–734, 1991.

42. J Nagington, A Rook, AS Highet. Virus and related infections. In: A Rook, ed. Textbook of Dermatology, 4th ed. Oxford: Blackwell Scientific Publications, 1986, pp 657–723.

43. JP Vestey, DL Yirrel, RD Aldridge. Cowpox/catpox infection. Br J Dermatol 124:74–78, 1991.

44. F Fenner, R Wittek, KR Dumbell. The Orthopoxviruses. San Diego, CA: Academic Press Inc, 1989, pp 186.

45. D Baxby, M Bennett. Poxvirus zoonoses. J Med Microbiol 46:17–20, 28–33, 1997.

46. IE Newsom, F Cross. Sore mouth in sheep transmissible to man. J Am Vet Med Assoc 84:790–802, 1934.

47. AG Peterkin. Occurrence in humans of contagious pustular dermatitis of sheep (''orf''). Br J Dermatol 49:492–497, 1937.

48. RH Bainton. Here I Stand. The Life of Martin Luther. New York: Abingdon-Cokesbury Press, 1950.

49. UW Leavell Jr, MJ McNamara, R Muelling, WM Talbert, RC Rucker, AJ Dalton. Orf: report of 19 human cases with clinical and pathological observations. JAMA 203: 657–664, 1968.

50. UW Leavell Jr, RJ Jacob. Orf. In: IM Freedberg, AZ Eisen, K Wolff et al., eds. Fitzpatrick's Dermatology in General Medicine, 5th ed. New York: McGraw-Hill, 1999, pp 2474–2478.

51. HO Wespahl. Human to human transmission of orf. Cutis 11:202–205, 1973.

52. MF Ferrando, C Leaute-Labreze, H Fleury, A Taieb. Orf and erythema multiforme in a child [letter]. Pediatr Dermatol 14:154–155, 1997.

53. K Bassioukas, A Orfanidou, CH Stergiopoulou, J Hatzis. Orf. Clinical and epidemiologic study. Australas J Dermatol 34:119–123, 1993.

54. A Dupre, B Christol, JL Bonafe, J Lassere. Orf and atopic dermatitis. Br J Dermatol 105:103–104, 1981.

55. S Hunskaar. Giant orf in a patient with chronic lymphocytic leukaemia. Br J Dermatol 114:631–634, 1986.

56. WJ Watson, MW Meyer, DL Madison. Orf virus infection in pregnancy. Sou Dakota J Med 46:423–424, 1993.

57. B Mendez, JW Burnett. Orf. Cutis 44:286–287, 1989.

58. DL Yirrell, JP Vestey, M Norval. Immune responses of patients to orf virus infection. Br J Dermatol 130:438–443, 1994.

59. RA Fox. Orf vaccine supplies. Vet Recl 20:624, 1987.

60. AJ Robinson, AA Mercer. Orf virus and vaccinia virus do not cross-protect sheep. Arch Virol 101:255–259, 1988.

61. U Gassman, R Wyler, R Witter. Analysis of poxvirus genomes. Arch Virol 83:17–31, 1985.

62. E Paoletti. Poxvirus recombinant vaccines. Ann NY Acad Sci 590:309–325, 1990.

63. CR Rossi, GK Kiesel, MH Jong. A paravaccinia virus isolated from cattle. Cornell Vet 67:72–90, 1977.

64. CE Wheeler, EP Cawley. The etiology of milker's nodules. Arch Dermatol 75:249–259, 1957.

65. AE Friedman-Kien, WP Rowe, WG Banfield. Milker's nodules: isolation of a poxvirus from a human case. Science 140:1335–1336, 1963.

66. KF Bowman, RT Barbery, LJ Swango, PR Schnurrenberger. Cutaneous form of bovine papular stomatitis in man. JAMA 246:2813–2818, 1981.

67. G Schuler, H Honigsmann, K Wolff. The syndrome of milker's nodules in burn injury. J Am Acad Dermatol 6: 334–339, 1982.

68. ES Falk. Parapoxvirus infections with reindeer and musk ox associated with unusual human infections. Br J Dermatol 99:647–654, 1978.

69. A Mercer, S Fleming, A Robinson, P Nettelton, H Reid. Molecular genetic analysis of parapoxviruses pathogenic for humans. Arch Virol Suppl 13:25–34, 1997.

70. Z Jezek, I Arita, M Szczeniowski, KM Paluku, K Ruti, JH Nakano. Human tanapox in Zaire: clinical and epidemiological observations on cases confirmed by laboratory studies. Bull World Health Organ 63:1027–1035, 1985.

71. JC Knight, FJ Novembre, DR Brown, CS Goldsmith, JJ Esposito. Studies on tanapox virus. Virology 172: 116–124, 1989.

72. AW Downie, CH Taylor-Robinson, AE Caunt, GS Nelson, PE Manson-Bahr, TC Matthews. Tanapox: a new disease caused by a pox virus. Br Med J 1:363–368, 1971.

73. JS Axford, AW Downie. Tanapox. A serological survey of the lower Tana River Valley. J Hygiene 83:273–276, 1979.

74. F Fenner. Adventures with poxviruses of vertebrates. FEMS Microbiol Rev 24:123–133, 2000.

75. JD Douglas, KN Tanner, JR Prine, DC Van Riper, SK Derwelis. Molluscum contagiosum in chimpanzees. J Am Vet Med Assoc 151:901–904, 1967.

76. IB Van Resburg, MG Collett, N Ronen, T Gerdes. Molluscum contagiosum in a horse. J S Afr Vet Assoc 62: 72–74, 1991.

77. F Bateman. Molluscum contagiosum. In: WB Shelley, JT Crissey, eds. Classics in Dermatology. Springfield, IL: Charles C Thomas, 1953, p 20.

78. ST Brown, JF Nalley, SJ Kraus. Molluscum contagiosum. Sex Transm Dis 8:227–234, 1981.

79. M Juliusberg. Zur Kenntnis des virus des molluscum contagiosum. Dtsch Med Wochenschr 31:1598–1599, 1905.

80. B Lipshutz. Weitere beitrage zur Kenntnis des molluscum contagiosum. Arch Derm Syph 287–396, 1911.

81. H Goldschmidt, AM Kligman. Experimental inoculation of humans with ectodermotrophic viruses. J Invest Dermatol 31:175–182, 1958.

82. TM Becker, JH Blout, J Douglas, FM Judson. Trends in molluscum contagiosum in the United States, 1966–1983. Sex Transm Dis 13:88–92, 1986.

83. CD Porter, NW Blake, LC Archard, MF Muhlemann, N Rosedale, JJ Cream. Molluscum contagiosum virus types in genital and non-genital lesions. Br J Dermatol 120: 37–41, 1989.

84. H Yamashita, T Uemura, M Kawashima. Molecular epidemiologic analysis of Japanese patients with molluscum contagiosum. Int J Dermatol 35:99–105, 1996.

85. K Niizeki, O Kano, Y Kondo. An epidemic study of molluscum contagiosum. Dermatologica 169:197–198, 1984.

86. J Scholz, A Rosen-Wolff, J Bugert, H Reisner, MI White, G Darai, R Postlethwaite. Epidemiology of molluscum contagiosum using genetic analysis of the viral DNA. J Med Virol 27:87–90, 1989.

87. J Nakamura, Y Muraki, M Yamada, Y Hatano, S Nii. Analysis of MCV genomes isolated in Japan. J Med Virol 46: 339–348, 1995.

88. R Postlethwaite. Molluscum contagiosum. Arch Environ Health 21:432–452, 1970.

89. SA Billstein, VJ Mattaliana. The "nuisance" sexually transmitted diseases: molluscum contagiosum, scabies, and crab lice. Med Clin North Am 74:1487–1505, 1990.

90. JJ Bugert, G Darai. Recent advances in molluscum contagiosum virus research. Arch Virol Suppl 13:35–47, 1997.

91. TG Hawley. The natural history of molluscum contagiosum in Fijiian children. J Hyg (Camb) 68:631–632, 1970.

92. TR Funt. Solitary molluscum contagiosum—clinical histological study of nine cases. Cutis 3:339–344, 1967.

93. SB Whitaker, SE Wiegand, SD Budnick. Intraoral molluscum contagiosum. Oral Surg Oral Med Oral Pathol. 72:334–336, 1991.

94. S Vannas, K Lapinleimu. Molluscum contagiosum of the skin, caruncle, and conjunctiva. Acta Ophthalmol 45:314–321, 1967.

95. HJ Ingraham, DB Schoenleber. Epibulbar molluscum contagiosum. Am J Ophthalmol 125:394–396, 1998.

96. DW Cotton, C Cooper, DF Barrett, BJ Leppard. Severe atypical molluscum contagiosum infection in an immunocompromised host. Br J Dermatol 116:871–876, 1987.

97. M Katzman, JT Carey, CA Elmets, GH Jacobs, MM Lederman. Molluscum contagiosum and the acquired immunodeficiency syndrome: clinical and immunological details of two cases. Br J Dermatol 116:131–138, 1987.

98. JJ Schwartz, PL Myskowski. Molluscum contagiosum in patients with HIV infection; a review of 27 patients. J Am Acad Dermatol 27:583–588, 1992.

99. HF Kipping. Molluscum dermatitis. Arch Dermatol 103:106–107, 1971.

100. F Brandrup, P Asschenfeld. Molluscum contagiosum-induced comedo and secondary abscess formation. Pediatr Dermatol 6:118–121, 1989.

101. H Takematsu, H Tagamitt. Proinflammatory properties of molluscum bodies. Arch Dermatol Res 287:102–106, 1994.

102. BJ Curtin, FH Theodure. Ocular molluscum contagiosum. Am J Ophthalmol 39:302–307, 1955.

103. PV Shirodaria, RS Matthews. Observations on the antibody responses in molluscum contagiosum. Br J Dermatol 96:29–34, 1977.

104. A Nunez, JM Funes, M Agromayor, M Moratilla, AJ Varas, JL Lopez-Estebaranz, M Esteban, A Martin-Gallardo. Detection and typing of molluscum contagiosum virus in skin lesions by using a simple lysis method and polymerase chain reaction. J Med Virol 50:342–349, 1996.

105. CH Thompson. Identification and typing of molluscum contagiosum virus in clinical specimens by polymerase chain reaction. J Med Virol 53:205–211, 1997.

106. JL Hovenden, TE Bushell. Molluscum contagiosum: possible culture misdiagnosis as herpes simplex [letter]. Genitourin Med 67:270, 1991.

107. RM Buller, J Burnett, W Chen, J Kreider. Replication of molluscum contagiosum virus. Virology 213:655–659, 1995.

108. KH Fife, M Whitfield, H Faust, MP Goheen, J Bryan, DR Brown. Growth of a molluscum contagiosum virus in a human foreskin xenograft model. Virology 226:95–101, 1996.

109. NJ Penneys, S Matsuo, R Mogollon. The identification of molluscum infection of immunohistochemical means. J Cutan Pathol 13:97–101, 1986.

110. CH Thompson, IM Biggs, RT DeZwart-Steffe. Detection of molluscum contagiosum virus DNA by in-situ hybridization. Pathology 22:181–186, 1990.

111. Z Smetana, Z Malik, A Orenstein, E Mendelson, E Ben-Hur. Treatment of viral infections with 5-aminolevulinic acid and light. Lasers Surg Med 21:351–358, 1997.

112. PS Hughs. Treatment of molluscum contagiosum with the 585 nm pulsed dye laser. Dermatol Surg 24:229–230, 1998.

113. MA Hurni, L Bohlen, H Furrer, LR Braathen. Complete regression of giant molluscum contagiosum lesions in an HIV-infected patient following combined antiretroviral therapy with saquinavir, zidovudine and lamivudine. AIDS 11:1784–1785, 1997.

114. CB Hicks, SA Myers, J Giner. Resolution of intractable molluscum contagiosum in a human immunodeficiency virus-infected patient after institution of antiretroviral therapy with ritonovir. Clin Infect Dis 24:1023–1025, 1997.

115. KP Meadows, SK Tyring, AT Pavia, TM Rallis. Resolution of recalitrant molluscum contagiosum virus lesions in human immunodeficiency virus-infected patients treated with cidofovir. Arch Dermatol 133:987–990, 1997.

116. EG Davies, A Thrasher, K Lacey, J Harper. Topical cidofovir for severe molluscum contagiosum. Lancet 353:2042, 1999.

117. J Toro, LV Wood, NK Patel, ML Turner. Topical cidofovir. Arch Dermatol 136:983–985, 2000.

118. R Buckley, K Smith. Topical imiquimod therapy for chronic giant molluscum contagiosum in a patient with advanced human immunodeficiency virus 1 disease. Arch Dermatol 135:1167–1169, 1999.

4

Herpes Simplex Virus

Richard J. Whitley and John W. Gnann, Jr.
University of Alabama at Birmingham School of Medicine, Birmingham, Alabama, USA

Mucocutaneous lesions are by far the most common manifestation of herpes simplex virus (HSV) infection. Genital herpes infection is one of the most important and common sexually transmitted diseases throughout the world. Our knowledge of HSV infections has increased dramatically since the initial historical descriptions of the clinical manifestations and histopathology of HSV lesions. Advances in our understanding of the natural history and pathogenesis of HSV infections have been paralleled by the development of both sensitive and specific tests that distinguish HSV-1 from HSV-2 infections and antiviral drugs that are selective inhibitors of viral replication. Type-specific serological markers of infection have allowed for a detailed evaluation of the epidemiology of infection. Establishing the unequivocal value of antiviral therapy has permitted clinicians to alter the spectrum of human disease and has implications for long-range control of HSV infections. The current level of biomedical knowledge sets the stage for application of the tools of molecular biology to the evaluation of human HSV disease, the evaluation of genetically engineered vaccines, and the development of antiviral therapeutics designed to be effective against newly identified virus-specific molecular targets [1–3]. These are practical future goals that should be achievable. This chapter summarizes the current status of our knowledge of the epide-

miology, clinical manifestations, and treatment of HSV infections (Fig. 4–1).

HISTORY

Herpes simplex virus infections of humans have been recognized since ancient times [4,5]. Records of human HSV infections began with descriptions of cutaneous spreading lesions thought to be of herpetic etiology, particularly in the writings of Hippocrates, as reviewed by Nahmias and Dowdle [4]. Scholars of Greek civilization define the word ''herpes'' as ''to creep or crawl,'' in reference to the spreading nature of the skin lesions [5,6]. The Roman scholar Herodotus associated mouth ulcers and lip vesicles with fever and defined this association as ''herpes febralis'' [7]. Later descriptions were predicated on Galen's deduction that the appearance of such lesions was an attempt by the body to rid itself of evil humors and perhaps led to the name of ''herpes excretins'' [5]. However, some of these original descriptions of skin lesions bear little resemblance to later reports from the 19th and 20th centuries of HSV infections [7].

It was not until the 18th century that Astruc, physician to the King of France, drew the appropriate correlation between herpetic lesions and genital infection [8]. By the early 19th century, the vesicular nature of lesions associated with herpetic infections was well characterized. However, it was not until 1893 that Vidal specifically recognized human-to-human transmission of HSV infections [5].

Work performed and reported by the author was supported by Contract N0-1-AI-65306 from the Division of Virology of the National Institute of Allergy and Infectious Diseases, a grant from the Division of Research Resources (RR-032) from the National Institutes of Health, and a grant from the state of Alabama.

GEOGRAPHICAL INCIDENCE

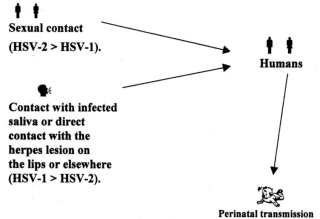

TAXONOMY

Herpesviridae family
Alphaherpesvirinae subfamily

TRANSMISSION

Sexual contact
(HSV-2 > HSV-1).

Contact with infected
saliva or direct
contact with the
herpes lesion on
the lips or elsewhere
(HSV-1 > HSV-2).

Humans

Perinatal transmission

ZOONOTIC IMPLICATIONS

None

Figure 4–1. Incidence and transmission of HSV.

Observations at the beginning of the 20th century advanced our knowledge of HSV infections beyond simple descriptions. First, histopathological studies identified the multinucleated giant cells associated with herpesvirus infections [9]. Second, the infectivity of HSV was recognized by Lowenstein in 1919, whereby virus retrieved from the lesions of humans with HSV keratitis or the vesicles of HSV labialis produced lesions on the rabbit cornea [10]. Furthermore, vesicle fluid from patients with herpes zoster failed to reproduce similar dendritic lesions in the rabbit eye model. In fact, these observations were originally made during earlier investigations by Gruter, who performed vir-

tually identical experiments around 1910 but did not report them until much later [11].

Investigations reported between 1920 and the early 1960s focused on the biological manifestations of infections caused by HSV as well as the natural history of human disease. Studies performed over these decades have been summarized in several reviews [12–15]. In the early 1930s, Andrews and Carmichael defined the presence of neutralizing antibodies to HSV in the serum of previously infected adults [16]. Subsequently, some of these patients developed recurrent labial lesions, although less severe than those associated with the initial episode. This observation led to the recognition of a unique biological property of HSV, namely, the ability of these viruses to recur in the presence of humoral immunity, a characteristic known as reactivation of latent infection. By the late 1930s, infants with severe stomatitis who shed a virus thought to be HSV subsequently developed neutralizing antibodies during the convalescent period [17,18]. Later in life, some of these children had apparent recurrent lesions of the lip, as had been reported for adults.

The medical literature of the 1940s and 1950s was replete with articles describing specific disease entities such as primary and recurrent infections of mucous membranes, (e.g., gingivostomatitis, herpes labialis, and genital HSV infections), the skin manifestations of herpetic whitlow or eczema herpeticum [19], keratoconjunctivitis [20], neonatal HSV infection, visceral HSV infections of the immunocompromised host, and herpes simplex encephalitis (HSE) [21]. Furthermore, the clinical spectrum of HSV infection was expanded to include Kaposi's varicella-like eruption and recurrent infections of the immunocompromised host.

Antigenic differences between HSV types were first suggested by Lipschitz [22] on clinical grounds over 80 years ago and by others from laboratory observations [23,24], but it was not until 1968 that these differences between HSV type 1 and HSV type 2 were demonstrated by Nahmias and Dowdle [4]. These two investigators demonstrated that HSV type 1 was more frequently associated with nongenital infection, whereas, HSV type 2 was associated with genital disease. This observation was seminal for many of the clinical, serological, immunological, and epidemiological studies that have followed during the ensuing 30 years.

Several other critical advances over the past decade have aided our understanding of the natural history and pathogenesis of HSV infections. First, unequivocally successful antiviral therapy was established for herpes simplex encephalitis [25] and, subsequently, for genital HSV infections [25–29] and HSV infections in the immunocompromised host [30,31], as reviewed [32]. Second, differences between strains of HSV were demonstrated by restriction endonuclease analyses of viral DNA. This technology has become an important tool for molecular epidemiological studies [33]. Third, the utilization of type-specific antigens has advanced our understanding of the epidemiology of infection [34]. Fourth, the elucidation of the molecular events of viral replication and the resultant gene products will aid in the development of vaccines and further antiviral drugs. A principal goal of these efforts is to define the biological properties of these gene products, a task that is in very early stages of accomplishment. Fifth, the engineering of HSV and the expression of specific genes will provide technology for new vaccines [35]. Finally, the still controversial observation of a latency-associated transcript and a gene contributing to neurovirulence may lead to clues regarding the molecular pathogenesis of infection [36,37]. Many of these advances have been previously summarized [13,38].

INCIDENCE

Herpes simplex viruses are distributed worldwide and have been reported in both developed and underdeveloped societies, including remote Brazilian tribes [39]. Animal vectors for human HSV infections have not been described, and humans remain the sole reservoir. Virus is transmitted from infected to susceptible individuals during close personal contact. There is no seasonal variation in the incidence of infection. Because infection is rarely fatal and because these viruses become latent, it is estimated that over one third of the world's population has recurrent HSV infections and is capable of transmitting HSV during episodes of productive infection. As has been well appreciated, many individuals are exposed to HSV but do not develop evidence of clinical disease. For children less than 10 years of age, antibodies directed to HSV are invariably of the HSV-1 type. Primary HSV-1 infections usually occur in young children and are most often asymptomatic. Cross-sectional seroprevalence studies in developing countries have shown that seroconversion is influenced by age (occurring early in life) and socioeconomic status.

Predictably, middle-class individuals of industrialized societies acquire antibodies to HSV significantly later in life. Utilizing type-specific serological assays, seroprevalence studies indicate that by the age of 5, over 35% of black children versus 18% of Caucasian children have been infected with HSV-1. Through adolescence, blacks had an approximately twofold higher prevalence of antibodies to HSV-1 as compared with their Caucasian counterparts. Females had a slightly higher prevalence of HSV-1 antibodies than males. By the age of 40, both blacks and Caucasians

had a high prevalence of antibodies. Similar analyses performed worldwide in individuals 20 to 40 years of age have detected antibody prevalence in excess of 95% in Spain, Italy, Rwanda, Zaire, Senegal, China, Taiwan, Haiti, Jamaica, and Costa Rica [40–42].

Recurrent herpes labialis is indicative of the reservoir of HSV infection in a community. A positive history of recurrent herpes labialis was prevalent in 38% of 1800 University of Pennsylvania students [43,44]. Among several studies, recurrence has a frequency that is approximately 33% [45–47]. Even though there are no clinical symptoms, asymptomatic excretion (viral shedding) following recurrence is approximately 1% in normal children [48,49] and ranges from 1–5% in normal adults [50–54].

Because infections with HSV-2 are usually acquired through sexual contact, antibodies to this virus are rarely found before the age of onset of sexual activity [55–64]. Most genital HSV infections are caused by HSV-2, but an ever-increasing incidence is attributable to HSV-1 [55–58]. The incidence of primary genital HSV infection has been conservatively estimated to be 500,000 to 1,000,000 individuals per year in the United States. Predicated upon newer serological methods for detection of prior HSV-2 infection, the prevalence of infection is probably over 40 to 60 million individuals in the United States [65].

Women are reported to have higher rates of infection than men, particularly prostitutes and those with multiple sex partners. The appearance of type-specific HSV-2 antibodies can be positively correlated with the onset of sexual activity [66–68], although crowded living conditions may indirectly contribute to antibody prevalence [69]. Historically, if HSV-2 antibodies are sought in healthy women, there is a wide discrepancy in prevalence, ranging from 10–21% in Americans to 77% in Ugandans [70,71]. As many as 50–60% of women of lower socioeconomic status in the United States and elsewhere develop antibodies to HSV-2 by adulthood [72]. Overall, 35% of middle class women receiving care through an Atlanta Health Maintenance Organization were seropositive for HSV-2 [73]. The seroprevalence of HSV-2 increases from 6.9% at 15 to 29 years of age to 23.4% by the age of 60. Importantly, if the populations were analyzed according to race, these percentages were 4.6% and 19.7% for Caucasians and 21.8% and 64.7% for blacks, respectively. Factors found to influence acquisition of HSV type 2 include sex (in women more than men) [74]; race (in blacks more than whites); marital status (divorced more than single or married); and place of residence (city more than suburb). In addition, the number of sexual partners has been reported to influence acquisition of infection [75–77]. The estimated risk of a susceptible female for contracting genital HSV from an infected male is 80% following a single sexual contact [75,76]. In most studies the existence of HSV-1 antibodies appears to reduce the risk of acquisition of HSV-2, especially in women [78]. Nevertheless, seropositivity for both HSV-1 and HSV-2 is relatively common. The colonization and reactivation of the two HSV types in the same anatomical region, however, appears to be rare, but it has been documented in the genital area [79]. Use of condoms also appears to reduce the risk of acquisition of HSV-2, although it appears to be highly protective for women but less so for men [80]. The risk of HSV-2 acquisition in discordant couples decreases over time, possibly reflecting heterogeneity in susceptibility, decline in infectiousness of the source partner, or changes in sexual behavior. Susceptibility appears to be partly genetically determined and associated with human leukocyte antigen (HLA) expression. Lekstrom-Himes et al. [81] showed associations of HLA-B27 and -Cw2 with symptomatic disease, indicating that immunological factors linked to the major histocompatibility complex (MHC) influence the risk of HSV-2 infection and disease expression. Because HSV-2 infection causes ulcerative disease, its occurrence correlates with acquisition of both HIV-1 (human immunodeficiency virus) and HTLV-1 (human T-cell lymphotropic virus), resulting in at least twofold increased risk [42,82–84]. The reader is referred to more detailed reviews [85–87].

The seroprevalence of HSV-2 has increased by 32% in the last two decades [71]. Considering that public health promotion of safe sex and condom use has increased during this time, factors responsible for the elevated rate of HSV-2 may be difficult to ascertain. One factor, however, may be the public's lack of recognition that most HSV-2 transmission is associated with asymptomatic or subclinical viral shedding.

Having sex while lesions are present is likely to increase the risk of transmission of HSV-2, but most couples avoid sex during outbreaks because (1) they want to avoid transmitting HSV-2, and (2) genital lesions decrease the pleasure of sex. Recurrent genital infection is the largest reservoir of HSV-2. Recurrent HSV-2 infection can be either symptomatic or asymptomatic, as with HSV-1; however, recurrence is usually associated with a shorter duration of viral shedding and fewer lesions. The frequency of recurrences varies somewhat between males and females, with calculations of 2.7 and 1.9 recurrences per 100 patient days, respectively [55]. Overall, several studies have implicated a frequency of recurrence as high as 90% in individuals with a symptomatic primary infection [68,69,88]. The type of genital infection, HSV-1 versus HSV-2, appears predictive of the frequency of recurrence [59]. Herpes simplex type 1 infections recur less frequently in the genital area (i.e., an average of once per year) than those caused by HSV-2 (i.e., an average of four times per year). Of further

importance, when polymerase chain reaction is utilized to detect viral DNA, shedding can be detected up to 15–18% of days in women and is usually asymptomatic.

One prospective study demonstrated that over 50% of women with serological evidence of HSV-2 infection but without evidence of disease on initial history were found to actually have symptomatic disease after being taught to distinguish symptoms of herpes infection from those of other genitourinary infections [89]. This finding was recently confirmed both in men and in women by Wald et al. [90]. They reported that rates of subclinical viral shedding were similar among subjects with previously unrecognized genital herpes and those with recognized infection; rates of subclinical shedding among women approximated those in men. Even those seropositive individuals who had no recognizable (even after education about herpes) clinical signs or symptoms of genital herpes were found to shed HSV-2 asymptomatically.

PATHOGENESIS

For infection to occur, the virus must come in contact with mucosal surfaces or abraded skin. Therefore, intimate personal contact of a susceptible person with another person excreting HSV is necessary for transmission of HSV. Viral replication occurs at the site of infection. An intact viron or the capsid travels to the dorsal root ganglia via retrograde axonal flow [91]. This mechanism has been demonstrated in animal models [92]. Replication of the virus is necessary for disease occurrence, including life-threatening nervous system infections. These occur during primary infection and will spread beyond the dorsal root ganglia. This may cause disseminated neonatal HSV infection with multiorgan involvement, multiorgan disease of pregnancy, and, infrequently, dissemination in patients who are markedly immunocompromised (e.g., organ transplant recipients). Normally the virus replicates on the mucosal surfaces, travels to the dorsal root ganglia, and undergoes a host-virus interaction that causes latency. If an appropriate stimulus occurs later, the virus will begin replicating, and viral infection will appear as skin vesicles or mucosal ulcers. If the host immune system is not capable of limiting replication to mucosal surfaces, widespread organ involvement occurs.

Contaminated saliva or direct contact with infected secretions (labial vesicular fluid) is the route of infection with HSV-1. The oropharyngeal mucosa hosts the viral replication, with latency occurring in the cells of the trigeminal ganglia. Sexual transmission is usually the cause of HSV-2. The virus replicates in the dermis or mucosal surfaces of the genitalia and latency later occurs in the sacral sensory ganglia.

Operative definitions of the nature of the host's infection are of relevance whether examining the pathogenesis of human or animal HSV infection. For individuals susceptible to HSV infections, namely, those without pre-existing antibodies, first infection with either HSV-1 or HSV-2 is defined as ''primary infection.'' The epidemiology and clinical characteristics of primary infection are distinctly different from those associated with recurrent infection. After latency is established, a recurrence of HSV is known as ''reactivated'' or ''recurrent infection.'' This form of infection results in recurrent vesicular skin lesions such as HSV labialis or recurrent HSV genitalis. An individual with pre-existing antibodies to only one type of HSV (type 1 or type 2) can experience a first infection with the other virus type. Under such circumstances, the infection is known as a nonprimary initial infection rather than a primary one. An example of a nonprimary initial infection would be in an individual who has pre-existing HSV-1 antibodies acquired after HSV gingivostomatitis who then acquires a genital HSV-2 infection. Reinfection with a different strain of either HSV type can occur but is rare. This circumstance is defined as ''exogenous reinfection.''

Latency allows HSV to persist in an apparently inactive state for varying periods of time, and then be reactivated by the proper stimulus [93–98]. The molecular basis of latency has been reviewed extensively [95–97]. The biological phenomenon of latency has been recognized since the beginning of this century [98–105]. In 1905, Cushing noted that patients treated for trigeminal neuralgia by sectioning a branch of the trigeminal nerve developed herpetic lesions along the areas innervated by the sectioned branch [106], as noted subsequently by others [107–111] Similarly, surgery of the lower back with manipulation of the sacral ganglia may result in reactivation of genital HSV infections [112,113].

Viral replication can be induced by axonal injury. The sectioning of a peripheral nerve results in the appearance of virus within the ganglia 3 to 5 days after the surgical manipulation [114]. Not surprisingly, if an attempt is made to excise the lesions induced by HSV, vesicles will still recur adjacent to the site of excision [114,115]. Figure 4–2 illustrates a patient with recurrent genital HSV infection in whom a surgeon attempted to excise the virus. Recurrences appear in the presence of both cell-mediated and humoral immunity. Virus can be isolated from patients during interim periods (those times between recurrences) at or near the usual site of recurrent lesions. Recurrences are spontaneous, but there have been associations with physical or emotional stress, fever, exposure to ultraviolet light, tissue damage, and immune suppression [104,116–121]. Latent virus has been retrieved from the trigeminal, sacral, and vagal ganglia of humans [93,99,100,122].

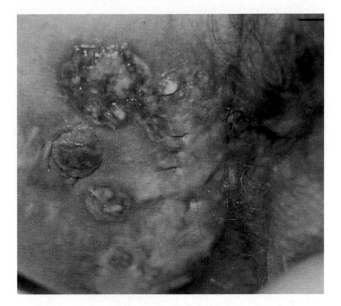

Figure 4–2.   Genital HSV (type 2) infection in immunocompromised host. Note that the physician attempted surgical excision of lesions.

Clinical evidence, reported as early as 1968, has suggested that lesions could also be caused by exogenous reinfection [4]. Unequivocal demonstration of exogenous reinfection became possible only after the development of the technique of restriction endonuclease analysis of viral DNA [123]. Analyses of numerous HSV-1 and HSV-2 isolates from a variety of clinical situations and widely divergent geographical areas demonstrated that epidemiologically unrelated strains yielded distinct HSV DNA fragment patterns. In contrast, HSV DNA derived from the same individual obtained years apart or from epidemiologically related sources (such as mothers and their newborns, monogamous sexual partners, or following short and long passages in vitro) had identical cleavage patterns after restriction endonuclease digestion. When this technique was applied to HSV genital isolates, analyses of endonuclease digestion patterns of HSV DNA fragments revealed that isolates from the same patients or their respective sexual partners could be either the same or different [33,124]. Stated differently, a given patient might have nonidentical isolates obtained from lesions at adjacent sites. This finding indicates that an individual can be infected with multiple different strains. Similar findings will likely become apparent for orolabial HSV-1 infections when properly studied. The frequency of this occurrence has been evaluated in two reasonably large studies and appears to be extremely uncommon in the immunocompetent host [125,126]. In women, infection with HSV-2 is associated with a persistent cervical mucosal cellular immune response, thus preventing reinfection [127].

Reinfection with the same strain of HSV can occur by autoinoculation at a distant site. Thus, HSV-1 can be mechanically transmitted from one site to either an adjacent site or a distal one. These instances have been reported in cases of mouth-to-genital transmission via scratching [128] or intentional inoculation of vesicle fluid to "bolster immunity" [129–132]. This event is most likely to occur during or soon after a primary episode of herpes. During recurrent episodes of herpes, systemic immunity prevents most cases of autoinoculation.

CLINICAL MANIFESTATIONS OF HERPES LABIALIS

Great variability exists in the clinical symptoms of primary HSV-1 infections (Table 4–1). Manifestations of infection can range from a total absence of symptoms to combinations of fever, sore throat, ulcerative and vesicular lesions, gingivostomatitis, edema, localized lymphadenopathy, anorexia, and malaise. Asymptomatic infection is the rule rather than the exception. Mucosal and skin surfaces are the usual sites of primary or initial infection. The mouth and lips are clearly the most common sites of HSV-1 infections. The most common manifestation of oropharyngeal infection is gingivostomatitis. Primary infection in young adults has also been associated with pharyngitis and a mononucleosis-like syndrome [50]. Under such circumstances, ulcerative tonsilar lesions on an erythematous base with associated submandibular lymphadenopathy are common [50].

Symptomatic disease in children is characterized by involvement of the buccal and gingival mucosa, as shown in Figure 4–3. It is not at all uncommon for children with symptomatic primary infection to be unable to swallow

Table 4–1. Clinical Manifestations of Herpes Labialis

Time After Exposure	Clinical Manifestations	Laboratory Analyses	Other Notes
2–12 days, average of 4 days	Onset of fever, soreness of mouth and throat, and development of painful vesicles on the lips, anterior tongue or hard palate, gingiva, or buccal mucosa. The lesions are typically on an erythematous base	Viral culture (specific) Tzanck smear (not specific)	Fever may range between 101°F and 104° F
18–25 days	↓ Progression to ulcerations ↓ Resolution of symptoms and lesions, usually within 2–3 weeks ↓	Direct fluorescent antigen (specific) Type-specific serology	Submandibular lymphadenopathy is commonly associated with primary HSV gingivostomatitis but rarely with recurrent infections
Time varies greatly	↓ Prodrome of burning pain, tingling, or itching for several hours or days prior to recurrence ↓ One or more papules arise in the localized area ↓ Lesions evolve into vesicles. With healing, the vesicular fluid may become pustular with the recruitment of more inflammatory cells ↓ Ulceration of each vesicle typically occurs		Precipitating factors, such as stress, sunlight, local trauma, or infection may precede the onset of recurrences
Within 7-9 days of onset of recurrent lesions	Lesions crust and resolve. Scarring uncommon but has been noted in patients with frequently recurrent lesions		Frequency of recurrences varies among individuals

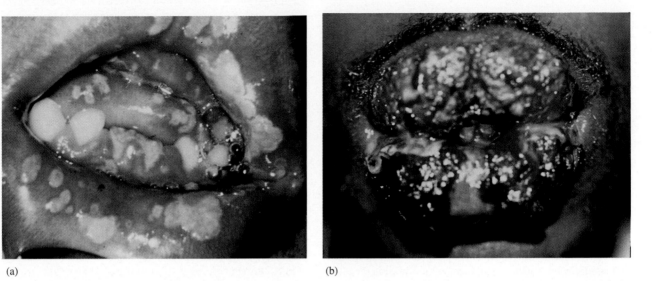

(a)   (b)

Figure 4–3. (a) An example of primary gingivostomatitis secondary to HSV type 1 in a child. (b) Such manifestations of primary infections are rarely seen in adults.

liquids because of the significant edema and ulcerations of the oropharyngeal membranes and the associated pain.

With recurrent episodes, vesicles appear most commonly at the vermillion border of the lip and persist in most patients for 48 hours or less, as shown in Figure 4–4. Vesicles generally number from three to five. The total area of involvement is usually less than 100 mm², and

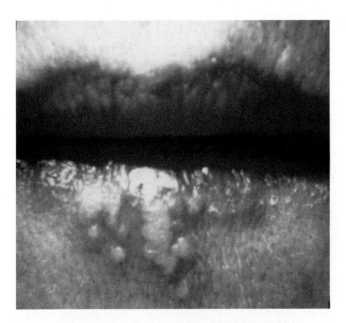

Figure 4–4. Herpes simplex labialis (type 1).

lesions progress to the pustular or ulcerative and crusting stage within 72 to 96 hours. Pain is most severe at the outset and resolves quickly over 96 to 120 hours (Table 4–2) [133–135].

CLINICAL MANIFESTATIONS OF HERPES GENITALIS

The most severe clinical disease is encountered with primary genital herpetic infection (Table 4–3). There are both similarities and differences in the clinical symptoms of men and women with genital herpes [55,136]. Primary infection is associated with larger quantities of virus replicating in the genital tract ($>10^6$ viral particles per 0.2 ml of inoculum) and a period of viral excretion that may persist for an average of 3 weeks. Systemic complications in the male are relatively uncommon; however, aseptic meningitis can appear. Furthermore, paresthesias and dysesthesias can result as a consequence of genital herpetic infection.

In women with primary infection, lesions usually appear on the vulva bilaterally as shown in Figure 4–5A, but occasional vesicles can be observed as far away as the plantar surface of the foot (Fig. 4–5B). The cervix is invariably involved, as shown in Figure 4–6. Lesions usually are excruciatingly painful, associated with inguinal adenopathy and dysuria, and may involve the vulva, perineum, buttocks, cervix, and/or vagina. A urinary retention syndrome may be encountered in 10–15% of women patients, and

Table 4–2. Differential Diagnosis of Herpes Labialis

Herpangina: Herpes infection typically affects the anterior portion of the mouth, while enteroviral infection involves the posterior oropharynx and may have an associated eruption on the distal extremities (hand-foot-and-mouth disease)

Aphthous stomatitis: This condition typically presents as a solitary ulcer, usually on the buccal mucosa, with no associated vesicles

Stevens-Johnson syndrome: While this condition affects the mucosal surfaces, it is also characteristically associated with erythema multiforme skin lesions

Epstein-Barr virus–induced mononucleosis: Diffuse hyperemia and hyperplasia of oropharyngeal lymphoid tissue; gelatinous greyish-white exudative tonsillitis; small petechiae at the border of the hard and soft palates

Oral candidiasis: A white coating containing yeast is seen on the tongue, buccal mucosa, and pharynx

penis or the penile shaft, as shown in Figure 4–7. The total number of lesions can vary significantly from six to ten to many more. Recurrent outbreaks are usually unilateral and involve fewer vesicles (Fig. 4–8). Extragenital lesions can occur on the thigh, buttocks, and perineum (Table 4–4) (Fig. 4–9).

As reviewed, the severity of primary infection and frequency of complications are statistically higher in women than in men for unknown reasons [55]. Systemic complaints are more common in women, occurring in >70% of all cases. The most common complications include aseptic meningitis (approximately 10%) and extragenital lesions (approximately 20%). Complications following primary genital herpetic infection also include sacral radiculomyelitis, which can lead to urinary retention, neuralgia, and meningoencephalitis [137–141]. Primary perianal and anal HSV-2 infections, as well as associated proctitis, are common in male homosexuals, as shown in Figure 4–10 [142,143]. As with HSV-1, many primary HSV-2 infections are subclinical, involving the mouth or the uterine cervix [61,62,144].

Nonprimary but initial genital infection (i.e., occurring in an individual with pre-existing heterologous antibody) is less severe symptomatically and heals more quickly than primary infection. The number of lesions, severity of pain, and likelihood of complications are significantly de-

as many as 25% of women develop a clinical picture of aseptic meningitis.

In males, primary genital HSV infections are most often associated with vesicular lesions superimposed on an erythematous base, usually appearing bilaterally on the glans

Table 4–3. Clinical Manifestations of Herpes Genitalis

Time After Exposure	Clinical Manifestations	Laboratory Analyses	Other Notes
2–12 days, average of 4 days	Onset of painful grouped vesicles or papules (either painful or painless) that become vesicles, typically with an erythematous base ↓	Viral culture (specific) Tzanck smear (not specific)	Associated signs and symptoms include fever, malaise, dysuria, polyuria, headache, and tender inguinal lymphadenopathy. Other symptoms may include urethral and vaginal discharge, vulvar irritation, and scrotal, vulvar, or perianal fissures
	Lesions become ulcerated ↓	Direct fluorescent (antigen (specific)	
18–25 days	Resolution of symptoms and lesions, typically after 2–3 weeks ↓		
Time course varies greatly	↓	Type-specific serology	Precipitating factors, such as stress, sunlight, local trauma, or infection may precede onset of recurrences. Recurrent genital herpetic infection in both men and women is characterized by a prodrome and localized irritation.
	Recurrent papules or vesicles appear in the localized area, progressing to ulcerations ↓		
	Crusting and resolution of lesions, typically after 7–10 days. Scarring is uncommon but has been noted in patients with frequently recurrent lesions		With healing, the vesicular fluid becomes pustular with recruitment of more inflammatory cells

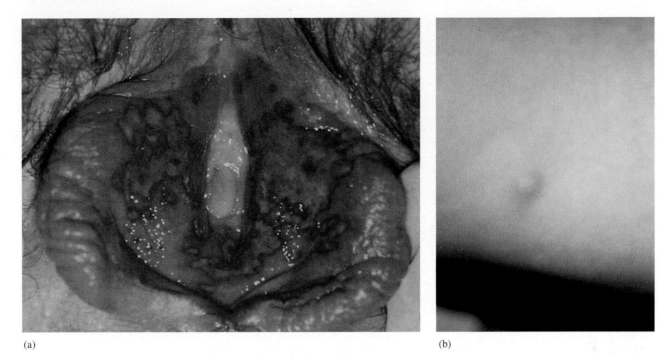

(a)
(b)

Figure 4–5. (a) Primary genital herpes in a female (type 2). (b) Occasionally vesicles can be observed as far away as the plantar surface of the foot.

creased. The mildest form of genital herpetic infection is that associated with recurrent disease. With recurrent genital herpetic infection, a limited number of vesicles, usually three to five, appear on the shaft of the penis of the male or simply as a vulvar irritation in the female [145]. Neuro-

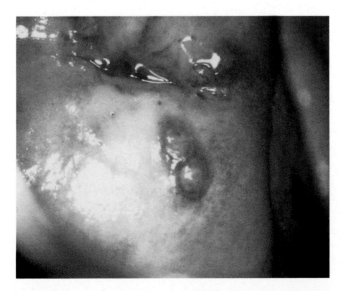

Figure 4–6. Recurrent cervical lesions secondary to HSV (type 2).

logical or systemic complications are uncommon with recurrent disease. Virus is shed for only 2 to 5 days (average of 3) and at lower concentrations (approximately $10^2–10^3$ per 0.2 ml of inoculum in tissue culture systems) in women with recurrent genital infection. Events of healing in the presence of an asymptomatic infection are not well defined. The major problem with genital HSV infection is the frequency of recurrences, which varies from one individual to the next. The severity of primary infection correlates directly with the frequency of recurrences; the more severe the primary infection, the more likely and frequent the recurrences. It is estimated that one third of patients with recurrences have in excess of eight or nine per year, one third of patients have less than three per year, and the remaining one third of patients between four to seven [55]. Obviously, with recurrences, either symptomatic or asymptomatic, the patient can transmit infection to sexual partners.

A particularly serious but fortunately uncommon problem encountered with HSV infections during pregnancy is that of widely disseminated disease in women. As first reported by Flewett et al. [146] in 1969, infection was demonstrated to involve multiple visceral sites in addition to cutaneous dissemination. In a limited number of cases, dissemination after primary oropharyngeal or genital infection led to severe manifestations of disease such as necrotizing hepatitis with or without thrombocytopenia, leukopenia,

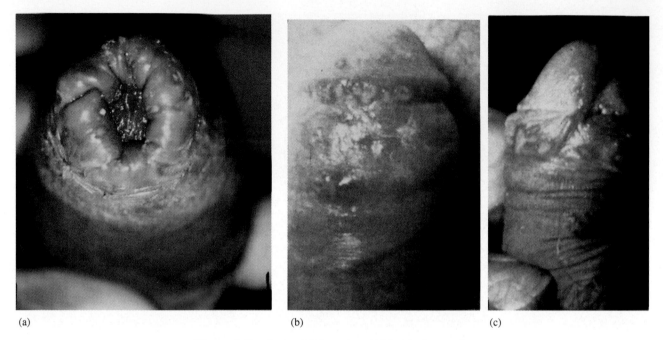

(a)   (b)   (c)

Figure 4–7.   (a, b, c) Primary genital herpes in a male.

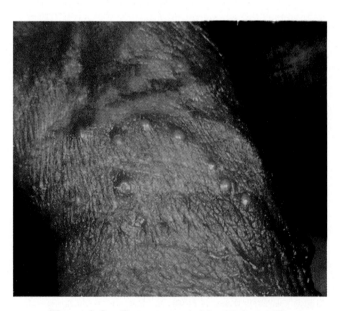

Figure 4–8.   Recurrent genital herpes in a male.

Table 4–4.   Differential Diagnosis of Herpes Genitalis

Syphilis: Chancre, usually not painful, not preceded by vesicles or pustules, and not recurrent

Chancroid: Ulcers are usually tender and multiple; the base is usually covered by a yellowish-grey exudate over granulation tissue; not recurrent

Granuloma inguinale: Nodular ulcerovegetative, hypertrophic, and cicatricial varieties

Lymphogranuloma venereum: Painless erosion in minority of patients, followed by secondary inguinal lymphadenopathy with "groove sign"

Behçet's disease: Genital and/or oral aphthosis, can be recurrent and may be associated with any of the following: synovitis, posterior uveitis, cutaneous pustular vasculitis

Crohn's disease: Sinuses and fistules may develop around the anus and vulva but are deeper than ulcers of herpes and are not associated with vesicles

Candidiasis: Associated with white discharge and occasionally with superficial erosions but not often with discrete ulcers

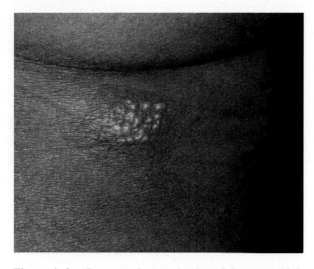

Figure 4–9. Recurrent herpes simplex of the upper thigh.

disseminated intravascular coagulopathy, and encephalitis. Although only a small number of patients have suffered from disseminated infection, the mortality rate among these pregnant women is reported to be higher than 50%. Fetal deaths occurred in more than 50% of cases, although fetal mortality did not necessarily correlate with the death of the mother. Surviving fetuses were delivered by cesarean section either during the acute illness or at term, and none showed evidence of neonatal HSV infection. The cumulative experience, then, suggests that factors associated with pregnancy may place both mother and fetus (for those succumbing) at increased risk for severe infection, possibly because of altered cell-mediated immunity [147–152].

MISCELLANEOUS CUTANEOUS HSV INFECTIONS

Skin infections caused by HSV may sometimes manifest in a variety of ways, such as eczema herpeticum, also known as Kaposi's varicelliform eruption, as illustrated in Fig. 4–11 [153–155]. This variant of HSV infection is most commonly seen in individuals with atopic dermatitis, but it may also develop in patients with thermal burns,

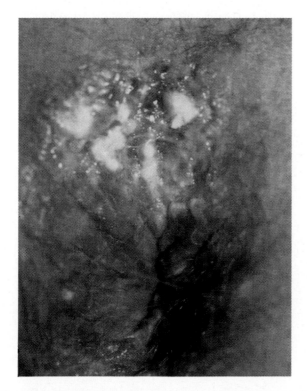

Figure 4–10. Perianal HSV-2 lesions in an HIV-infected individual.

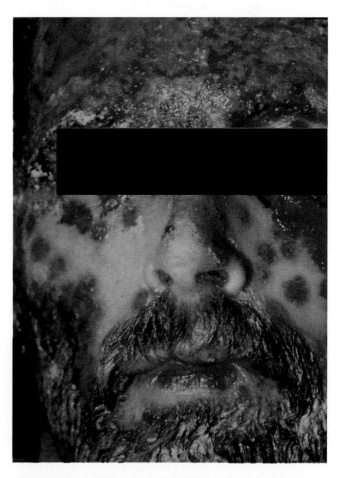

Figure 4–11. HSV type 1 lesions in a patient with eczema herpeticum.

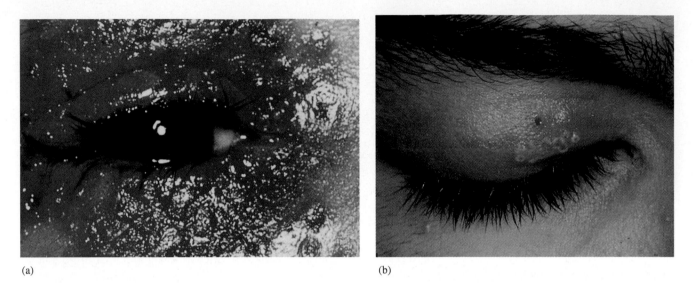

(a)   (b)

Figure 4–12. Periocular HSV type 1 lesions in (a) a patient with eczema herpeticum, and (b) in an immunocompetent person.

pemphigus, mycosis fungoides, keratosis follicularis, or congenital ichthyosiform erythroderma. Infants and children are most often affected, although this condition may occur in a patient of any age. With eczema herpeticum, the extent of involvement is usually disseminated [156], although lesions can also be localized, resembling those of herpes zoster with a dermatomal distribution. Internal organs may occasionally be involved with infection. Examples of periocular herpes simplex in an immunocompetent patient and in a patient with Kaposi's varicelliform erup-

tion appear in Figure 4–12. Another variant of HSV infection is the involvement of recurrent HSV lesions with erythema multiforme, as depicted in Figure 4–13. HSV is actually the most common identifiable etiological agent of erythema multiforme [157].

HSV infections of the digits, known as herpetic whitlow, were especially common among dental and medical personnel [158] before the routine use of examination gloves, with an estimated occurrence rate of 2.4 cases per 100,000 population per year. An increasing incidence of

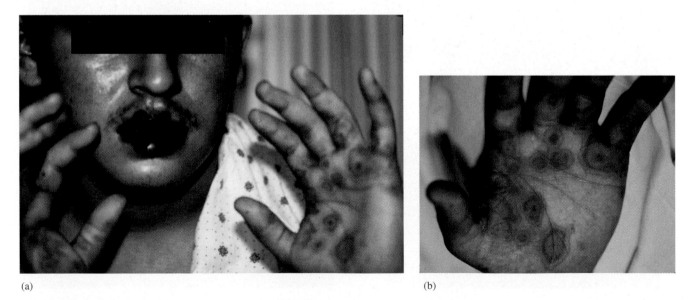

(a)   (b)

Figure 4–13. HSV type 1 lesions associated with erythema multiforme. (a) Recurrent herpes labialis with erythema multiforme of the palms. (b) Target lesions of erythema multiforme of the palms.

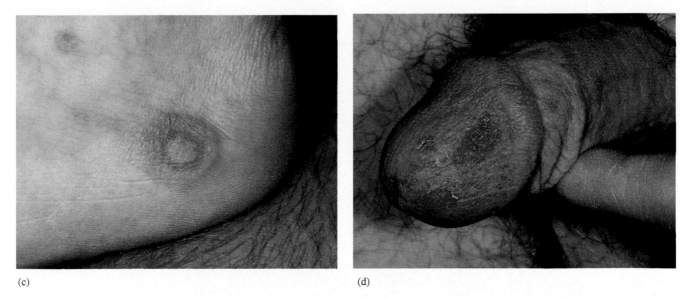

(c)   (d)

Figure 4–13. (*Continued.*) (c) Target lesions of erythema multiforme of the heel. (d) Patch of erythema multiforme of the head of the penis associated with herpes labialis.

HSV-2 whitlow has been recognized in the community [159] as a result of digital-genital contact. An example of herpetic whitlow appears in Figure 4–14 and can be followed by cutaneous HSV infection of the hand and secondary lymphadenitis (Fig. 4–15). Toxic epidermal necrolysis can occur in association with recurrent HSV infection, as displayed in Figure 4–16. Additional common presentations of HSV infections include HSV infection of the face, ear, neck, arm, and nipple (Figure 4–17) and HSV folliculitis (Fig. 4–18).

Overall, studies performed in dermatology clinics identify about 2% of men and 1.5% of women with herpetic

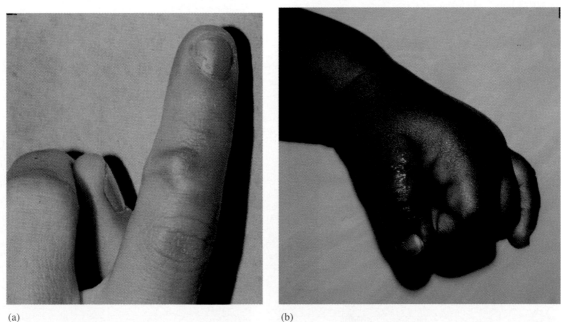

(a)   (b)

Figure 4–14. (a,b) HSV type 1: herpes whitlow.

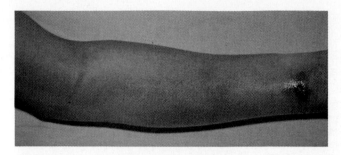

Figure 4–15. Cutaneous HSV lesions with secondary lymphangitis.

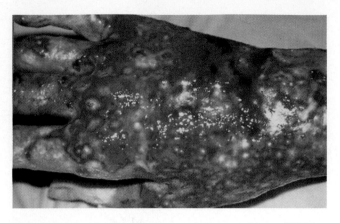

Figure 4–16. Toxic epidermonecrolysis secondary to HSV infection.

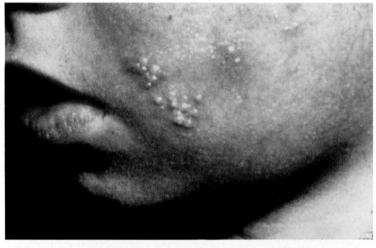

(a)

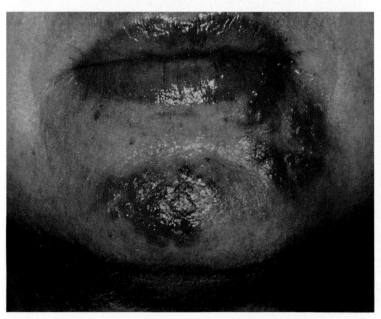

(b)

Figure 4–17. HSV infection of the (a, b) face; (c) ear.

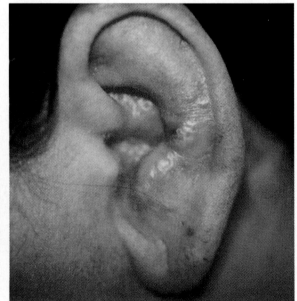

(c)

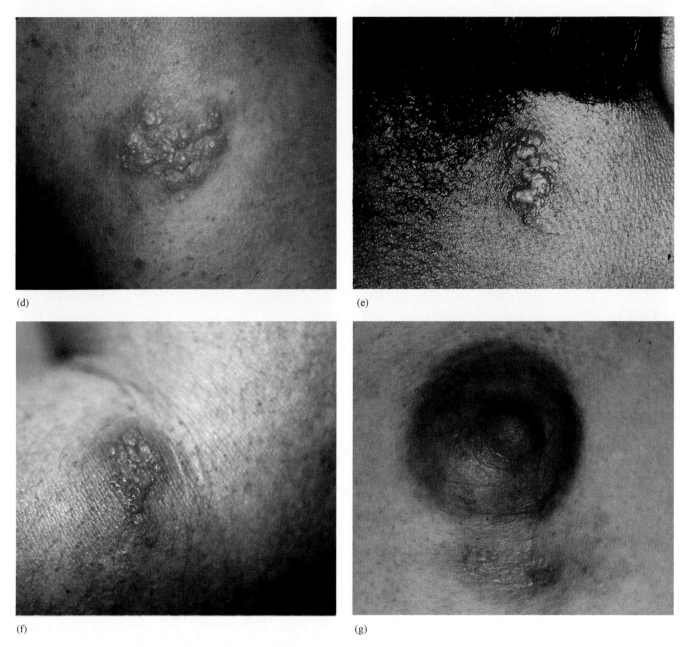

(d)

(e)

(f)

(g)

Figure 4–17. (*Continued.*) (d, e) Neck; (f) arm; and (g) nipple.

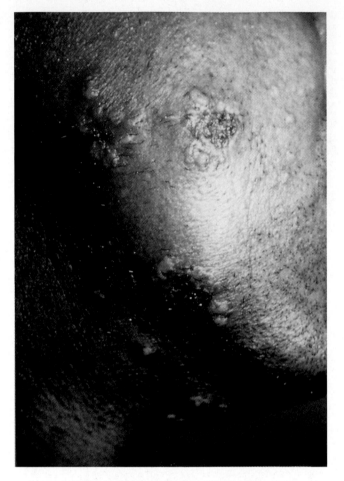

Figure 4–18. HSV facial folliculitis.

unilateral or bilateral conjunctivitis (which can be follicular in nature), followed soon after by preauricular adenopathy. Herpes simplex virus infection of the eye also causes photophobia, tearing, eyelid edema, and chemosis with the pathognomonic finding of branching dendritic lesions, as shown in Figure 4–19. Less commonly, advanced disease can result in a geographical ulcer of the cornea, as shown in Figure 4–20. As disease advances, uveitis can be a complication, as shown in Figure 4–21. Healing of the cornea can take as long as 1 month, even with appropriate antiviral therapy.

Recurrent HSV infections of the eye are common and are usually unilateral. Characteristically, either dendritic ulcerations or stromal involvement appears. Visual acuity

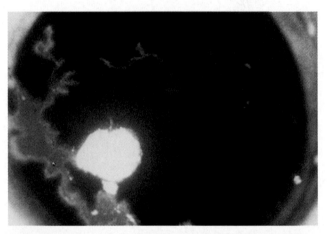

(a)

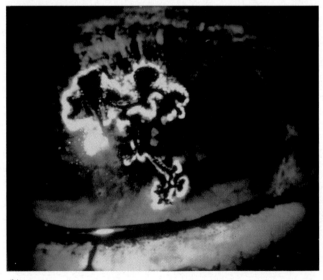

(b)

Figure 4–19. (a, b) Dendritic lesions secondary to herpes simplex (type 1) keratoconjunctivitis.

skin infections [160]. In addition to individuals with atopic disease, patients with skin abrasions or burns appear particularly susceptible to HSV-1 or HSV-2 infections, and some may develop disseminated infection [161]. Disseminated cutaneous HSV infections have also been reported among wrestlers and are referred to as herpes gladitorium [162], as previously summarized [163]. Other skin disorders associated with extensive cutaneous HSV lesions include Darier's disease and Sézary's syndrome [164,165].

HERPES SIMPLEX KERATOCONJUNCTIVITIS

Viral infections of the eye occurring beyond the newborn age are usually caused by HSV-1 [166–168]. Approximately 300,000 cases of HSV infections of the eye are diagnosed yearly. These infections are second only to trauma as a cause of corneal blindness in the United States. Primary herpetic keratoconjunctivitis may result in either

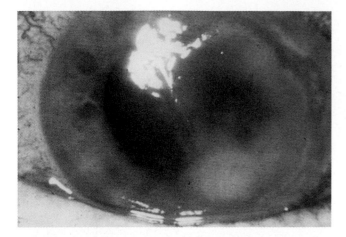

Figure 4–20. Geographical ulcer as a complication of herpes simplex keratoconjunctivitis.

is decreased in the presence of the ulcers, and with progressive stromal involvement, opacification of the cornea may occur. Repeated individual attacks may last for weeks or even months following appropriate antiviral therapy. Progressive disease can result in visual loss and even rupture of the globe.

HERPES SIMPLEX VIRUS INFECTIONS IN THE IMMUNOCOMPROMISED HOST

Patients compromised by immunosuppressive therapy, underlying disease, or malnutrition are at increased risk for severe HSV infections. Renal and cardiac transplant recipients are at particular risk for increased frequency and severity of HSV infection [159,169,170]. An example of cuta-

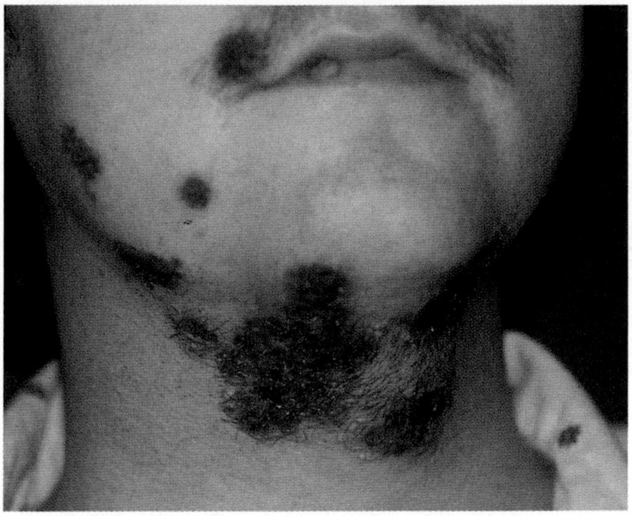

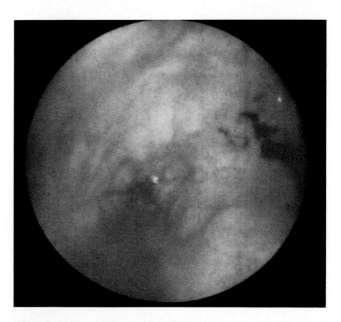

Figure 4–22. Disseminated facial HSV (type 1) infection in an organ transplant recipient.

neous dissemination following shaving in a renal transplant recipient is shown in Figure 4–22. The virus was probably autoinoculated to multiple skin sites by the razor blade, although this remains speculative. In organ transplant recipients, the presence and quantity of antibodies to HSV before transplantation predict the individuals at greatest risk for recurrence. These patients may develop progressive disease involving the respiratory tract, esophagus (Fig. 4–23), or even the gastrointestinal tract [171,172]. The se-

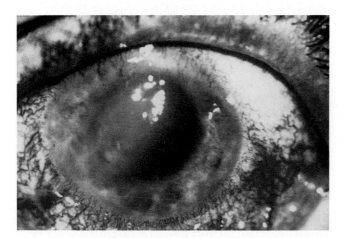

Figure 4–21. HSV uveitis.

Figure 4–23. HSV esophagitis in an immunocompromised host.

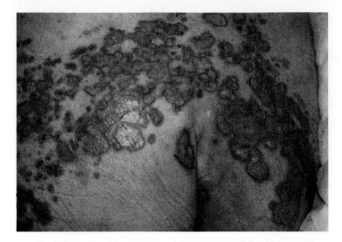

Figure 4–24. Disseminated sacral HSV (type 2) infection in an immunocompromised host.

vere nature of progressive disease in these patients appears to be directly related to the degree of immunosuppressive therapy employed [173]. Reactivation of latent HSV infections can occur at multiple sites, and healing in these patients with severe progressive disease occurs over an average of 6 weeks [174]. An example of progressive cutaneous dissemination of HSV-2 at sacral sites appears in Figure 4–24.

Since the first reports of the acquired immunodeficiency

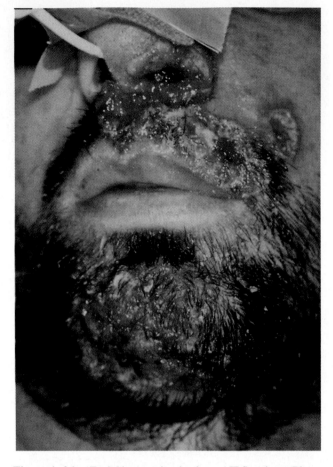

Figure 4–26. Facial herpes simplex in an AIDS patient. (Photograph courtesy of Jeffery Callen, M.D., Department of Dermatology, University of Louisville, Louisville, KY.)

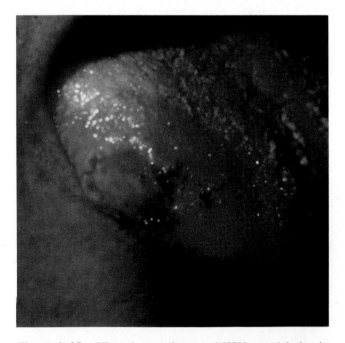

Figure 4–25. Ulcerative oropharyngeal HSV type 1 lesion in an HIV-infected individual.

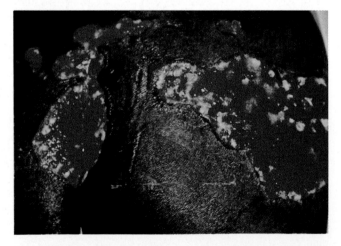

Figure 4–27. Aggressive herpes simplex of the buttocks in an AIDS patient. (Photograph courtesy of Margaret Muldrow, M.D., Aurora, CO.)

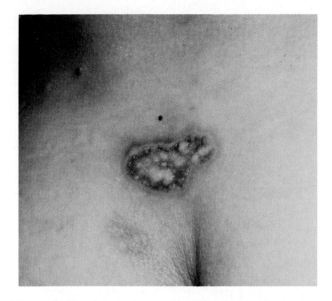

Figure 4–28. Sacral ulcer resulting from herpes simplex in an AIDS patient.

syndrome (AIDS), the severity of HSV clinical disease in these severely immunocompromised hosts has become apparent [175]. An example of intraoral HSV-1 in an AIDS patient appears in Figure 4–25. AIDS patients may develop very severe herpes simplex infections of the face (Fig. 4–26) or anogenital area (Fig. 4–27). A sacral ulcer resulting from herpes simplex in an AIDS patient is seen in Figure 4–28. Exophytic, verrucous herpetic lesions have also been reported in AIDS patients (Fig. 4–29). Disseminated herpes simplex is also seen in patients with thermal burns (Fig. 4–30). Extensive herpetic disease in the cancer patient has been reported and has become an important target for antiviral therapy (Fig. 4–31).

NEONATAL HSV INFECTIONS

Although centers caring for infants with neonatal HSV infections have observed fluctuations in disease incidence, the estimated rate of occurrence is approximately one in 2000 to one in 5000 deliveries [176,177]. At least four factors appear to have the greatest effect on disease transmission. First, the type of maternal genital infection at delivery influences the duration and quantity of virus excreted and the time to total healing. Primary infection is most severe, whereas initial and recurrent maternal genital infections are less so [55,136]. For example, the incidence of neonatal herpes in babies born to women with primary or initial genital HSV infection was 33% as compared with 3% in those born to women with recurrent infections [178]. Second, transplacental maternal neutralizing and antibody-dependent cellular cytotoxicity (ADCC) antibodies appear to have an ameliorative effect on the acquisition of infection by babies exposed to the virus [179–181]. Third, the duration of ruptured membranes is an important indicator of risk for acquisition of neonatal infection. Women

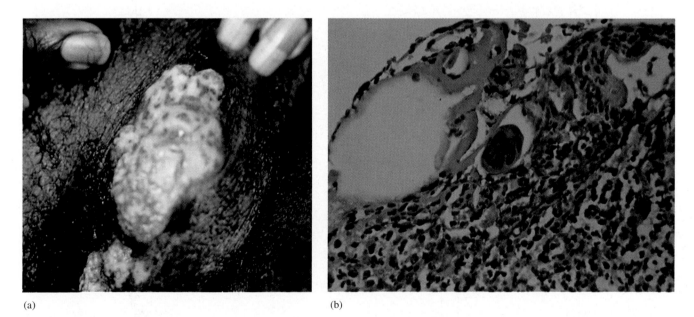

(a)   (b)

Figure 4–29. (a,b) Exophytic, verrucous lesions of herpes simplex of the scrotum in an AIDS patient as confirmed by culture and histological examination.

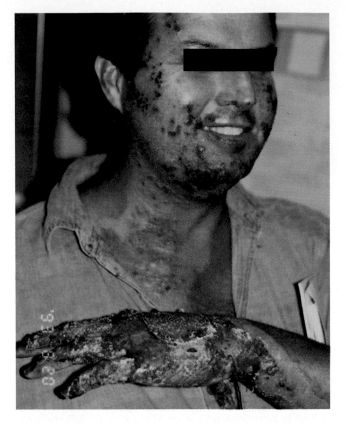

Figure 4–30. Disseminated herpes simplex in a patient with thermal burns.

with active genital lesions at the time of onset of labor usually have their infants delivered by cesarean section. Infection of the newborn has occurred in spite of delivery by cesarean section [182]. Fourth, fetal scalp monitors can create a site of inoculation of virus [183,184]. HSV infection of the newborn can be acquired at one of three times: in utero, intrapartum, or postnatally. The mother is the most common source of infection for the first two of these routes of transmission of infection to the newborn. Although intrapartum transmission accounts for 75–80% of all cases, the other two routes must be considered in a child with suspected disease for both public health and prognostic purposes.

The clinical presentation of infants with neonatal HSV infection is a direct reflection of the site and extent of viral replication. Neonatal HSV infection is almost invariably symptomatic and frequently lethal. Congenital intrauterine infection usually is identified within the first 48 hours following birth. Infants infected intrapartum or postnatally with HSV infection can be divided into three categories, namely, those with: (1) disease localized to the skin, eye, and/or mouth; (2) encephalitis with or without skin, eye, and/or mouth involvement; and (3) disseminated infection that involves multiple organs, including central nervous system, lung, liver, adrenals, skin, eye, and/or mouth [185].

Intrauterine infection is characterized by the triad of skin vesicles or skin scarring, eye disease, and the far more severe manifestations of microcephaly or hydranencephaly [186]. Often chorioretinitis, alone or in combination with

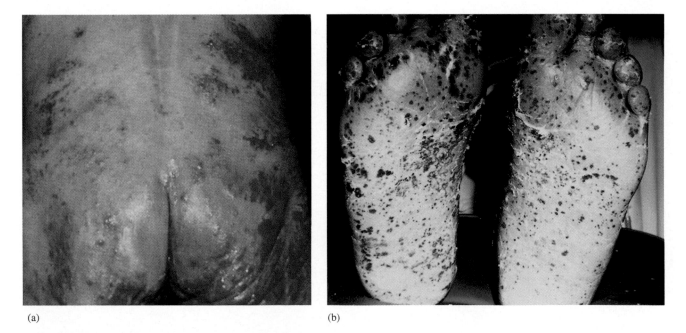

(a)

(b)

Figure 4–31. (a, b) Disseminated herpes simplex in patients with cutaneous T-cell lymphoma. (Photographs courtesy of Margretta A. O'Reilly, M.D., University of Utah, Salt Lake City, UT.)

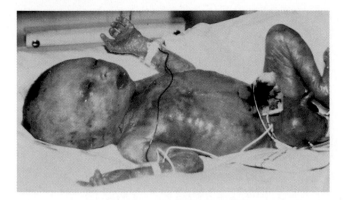

Figure 4–32. Intrauterine HSV infection (newborn).

other eye findings such as keratoconjunctivitis, is a component of the clinical presentation [187]. An example of a child with bullous skin lesions secondary to intrauterine infection appears in Figure 4–32.

Infants with the worst prognosis for both morbidity and mortality are those with disseminated infection. Children with disseminated infection usually are seen at tertiary care centers for therapy between 9 and 11 days of life. The principal organs involved following disseminated infection are the liver and adrenals. However, infection can involve multiple other organs, including the larynx, trachea, lungs, esophagus, stomach, lower gastrointestinal tract, spleen, kidneys, pancreas, and heart. Constitutional signs and symptoms include irritability, seizures, respiratory distress, jaundice, bleeding diatheses, shock, and frequently the characteristic vesicular exanthem often considered pathognomonic for infection. Encephalitis appears to be a common component of this form of infection, occurring in about 60–75% of children with disseminated infection. The vesicular rash, as described below, is particularly important in the diagnosis of HSV infection. However, over 20% of children with disseminated infection do not develop skin vesicles during the course of their illness [182]. Mortality in the absence of therapy exceeds 80%.

Infection of the central nervous system, alone or in combination with disseminated disease, is manifested by the findings indicative of encephalitis in the newborn. Brain infection can occur either as a component of multiorgan disseminated infection or as encephalitis alone with or without skin, eye, and mouth involvement. Nearly one third of all infants with neonatal HSV infection have only the encephalitic component of disease. Clinical manifestations of encephalitis (alone or in association with disseminated disease) include seizures (both focal and generalized), lethargy, irritability, tremors, poor feeding, temperature instability, bulging fontanelle, and pyramidal tract signs. Whereas babies with disseminated infection often have

skin vesicles in association with brain infection, the same is not true for those with encephalitis alone. This latter group of children have skin vesicles at any time in the disease course in only about 60% of cases [182,188,189]. Cultures of cerebrospinal fluid yield virus in 25–40% of all cases. Anticipated findings on cerebrospinal fluid examination include pleocytosis and proteinosis (as high as 500–1000 mg/dl). Death occurs in 50% of babies with localized central nervous system disease who are not treated and is usually related to brain stem involvement. With rare exceptions, survivors are left with neurological impairment [185].

Infection localized to the skin, eyes and/or mouth is associated with lower mortality, but it is not without significant morbidity. When infection is localized to the skin, the presence of discrete vesicles remains the hallmark of disease, as illustrated in Figure 4–33. Clusters of vesicles often appear initially on the presenting part of the body that was in direct contact with the virus during birth, such as the scalp (Fig. 4–34). With time, the rash can progress to involve other areas of the body as well. Vesicles occur in 90% of children with skin, eye, or mouth infection, usually 1 to 2 mm in diameter. They can progress to larger bullous lesions more than 1 cm in diameter. These larger lesions and their progression are illustrated in Figure 4–35. Although discrete vesicles on various parts of the body are usually encountered, crops and clusters of vesicles have also been described. Infections involving the eye may man-

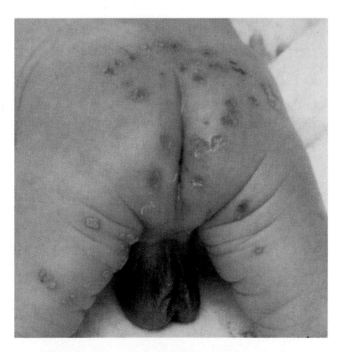

Figure 4–33. Cutaneous HSV lesions in a newborn.

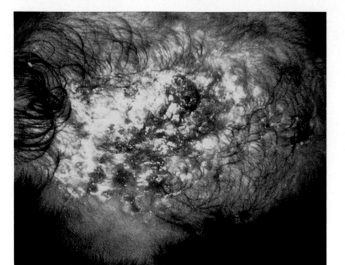

Figure 4–34. Scalp lesions caused by HSV infection in a newborn.

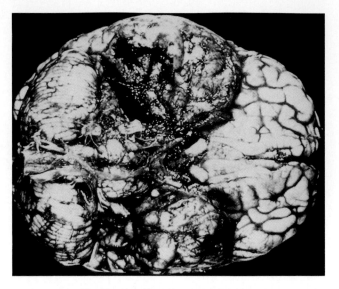

Figure 4–36. Herpes simplex encephalitis.

HERPES SIMPLEX ENCEPHALITIS

ifest as keratoconjunctivitis in newborns or later as chorioretinitis. Children with disease localized to the skin, eyes, or mouth generally are identified at about 10 to 11 days of life. Those infants with skin lesions invariably suffer from recurrences over the first 6 months (and longer) of life, regardless of whether therapy was administered or not. Although death is not associated with disease localized to the skin, eyes, and/or mouth, approximately 30% of these children eventually develop evidence of neurological impairment [185]. The reader is referred to more thorough reviews of neonatal HSV infection for more detailed descriptions of the disease and its management [185].

Herpes simplex encephalitis (HSE) is one of the most devastating of all HSV infections (Fig. 4–36). It is considered the most common cause of sporadic, fatal encephalitis in the United States [190]. The incidence of severe hemorrhagic focal encephalitis is approximately one in 200,000 individuals per year, for a national annualized rate of approximately 1250 cases.

The actual incidence of HSE remains unknown, as no national reporting system exists for any HSV infection, even for life-threatening diseases such as HSE. The manifestations of HSE in the older child and adult reflect the areas of pathology in the brain. Figure 4–37 indicates the

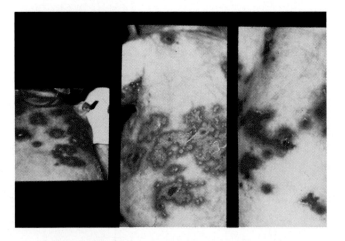

Figure 4–35. Evolution of cutaneous HSV lesions.

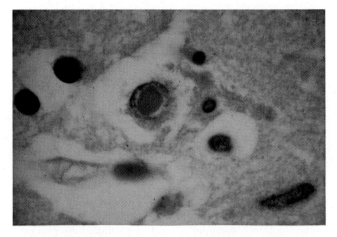

Figure 4–37. Cowdry type A intranuclear inclusion.

classic Cowdry type A intranuclear inclusion evident on brain biopsy from a patient with HSE. The most common findings include a focal encephalitis associated with fever, altered consciousness, bizarre behavior, disordered mentation, and localized neurological findings. These clinical signs and symptoms can often be correlated with localized temporal lobe disease, as demonstrated by neurodiagnostic procedures [25]. There is no characteristic set of findings pathognomonic for HSE; however, a progressively deteriorating level of consciousness, fever, an abnormal cerebrospinal fluid formula, and focal neurological findings in the absence of other causes should make this disease highly suspect. Other diagnostic evaluations should be initiated immediately, since other treatable diseases may mimic HSE [191]. Mortality in untreated patients is in excess of 70%, and only 2.5% of all patients recover full neurological function. Factors that influence outcome include age, level of consciousness (Glasgow Coma Score) at the outset of therapy, and disease duration.

In addition to encephalitis with cortical disease, HSV can involve virtually any anatomical areas of the nervous system. HSV has been associated with meningitis, myelitis, radiculitis, and other syndromes. The relationships between HSV infections of the brain and chronic degenerative disease, psychiatric disorders, or Bell's palsy require further definition [192–194].

DIAGNOSIS

The appropriate utilization of laboratory techniques is essential if a diagnosis of HSV infection is to be established, as reviewed [195]. Virus isolation remains the definitive diagnostic method. If skin lesions are present, a scraping of skin vesicles should be made and transferred in appropriate virus transport media to a diagnostic virology laboratory. Clinical specimens should be expeditiously shipped and processed for inoculation into cell culture systems that are appropriate for the demonstration of the cytopathic effects characteristic of HSV replication, as illustrated in Figure 4–38. In addition to skin vesicles, other sites from which virus may be isolated include the cerebrospinal fluid, stool, urine, throat, nasopharynx, and conjunctivae. It may also be useful in infants with evidence of hepatitis or other gastrointestinal abnormalities to obtain duodenal aspirates for HSV isolation. The virological results of cultures from these anatomical sites should be used in conjunction with clinical findings to define the extent of disease in the newborn and immunocompromised host. Typing of an HSV isolate may be done by one of several techniques, but they may not all be routinely available. Since treatment outcome does not appear related to the virus type, typing is only of

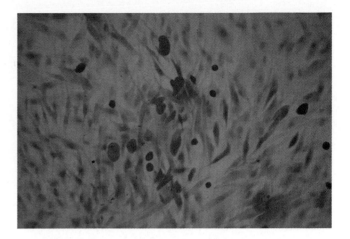

Figure 4–38. Cytopathic effect of HSV in cell culture.

epidemiological and pathogenetic importance and, therefore, is not routinely necessary.

Every effort should be made to confirm infection by viral isolation. In industrialized countries, such efforts are both reasonable and appropriate. In the absence of diagnostic virology facilities, cytological examination of cells from the maternal cervix or the infant's skin, mouth, conjunctivae, or corneal lesions may be useful in making a presumptive diagnosis of HSV infection. These methods have a sensitivity of only approximately 60–70% and, therefore, should not be the sole diagnostic determinant of infection in the newborn [72]. Alternative methods, such as a direct fluorescent antigen (DFA) assay, have a higher sensitivity and specificity in adults with genital herpes [196] (Fig. 4–39). Cellular material obtained by scraping the periphery

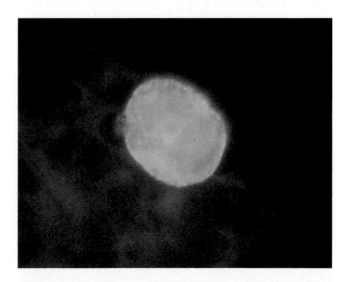

Figure 4–39. Positive direct fluorescence antigen assay for HSV-2.

of the base of lesions should be smeared on a glass slide and promptly fixed in cold ethanol. The slide can be stained according to the methods of Papanicolaou, Giemsa, or Wright before examination by a trained cytologist. Tzanck smears (Fig. 4–40) probably will not demonstrate the presence of intranuclear inclusions but typically reveal multinucleated giant cells from the majority of early herpetic lesions. The presence of intranuclear inclusions and multinucleated giant cells are indicative but not diagnostic of HSV infection. It is important to recognize that the Tzanck smear cannot differentiate HSV from other human herpesviruses, such as varicella zoster virus. Even electron microscopic assays are continuing to be developed [197]. Figure 4–41 illustrates a classic electron micrograph of HSV.

Polymerase chain reaction (PCR) is another method employed in the diagnosis of HSV in certain situations. It can be used to detect HSV in routine skin biopsy specimens. Currently, PCR amplification of HSV DNA in cerebrospinal fluid is the diagnostic method of choice for infections of the brain, whether in the newborn or adult [198–200].

Therapeutic decisions cannot await the results of serological studies. The inability of most commercially available serological assays to distinguish between antibodies to HSV-1 or HSV-2, as well as between transplacentally acquired maternal and endogenously produced immunoglobulin G, makes the assessment of the neonate's serological status difficult during acute infection. Serial antibody assessment may be useful if a mother without a prior history of HSV infection has a primary infection late in gestation and transfers very little or no antibody to the fetus. The most commonly used tests for measurement of HSV antibodies are complement fixation, passive hemagglutination, neutralization, immunofluorescence, and the enzyme-

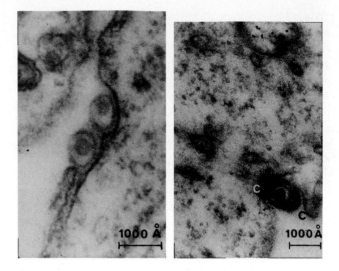

Figure 4–41. Electron micrograph of HSV at time of absorption and penetration.

linked immunosorbent assay (ELISA) Western blot assay is available for the diagnosis of HSV infection only in research laboratories, but it has high sensitivity and specificity in differentiating between HSV-1 and HSV-2 [201].

There are two types of commercial HSV serological assays. One type uses whole virus lysates of prototype strains of HSV-1 and HSV-2 to measure antibodies. Although immunoglobulin G and immunoglobulin M antibodies to such prototype strains are reported by commercial laboratories, e.g., titers to HSV-1 and HSV-2, these titers mostly measure antibodies to type-common antigens and hence are not reliable in defining whether the person has antibodies to HSV-1 only, HSV-2 only, or both HSV-1 and HSV-2. They are only reliable for defining whether a person is seronegative or seropositive for HSV-1 or HSV-2.

The second test employs the predominantly type-specific response to glycoprotein G-2 for HSV-2 and to glycoproteins G-1 and C-1 for HSV-1. Therefore, a type-specific serological HSV-2 test must be based on detection of antibodies to glycoprotein G-2. Recently, assays that recognize antibodies to glycoprotein G-2 for HSV-2 infection and G-1 for HSV-1 infection have been licensed. Four of these novel type-specific serological assays are currently approved by the Federal Drug Administration (FDA). Others are under development. All four FDA-approved tests have been compared with the University of Washington Western blot assay, which has been extensively evaluated and shown to be type-specific. The sensitivity and specificity of these tests vary, depending on the test and the setting. In general, the sensitivity and specificity have been greater

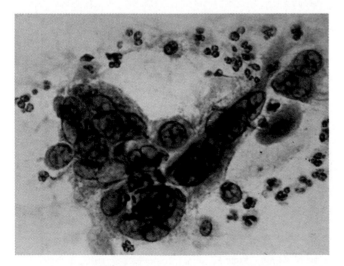

Figure 4–40. Tzanck smear.

for detection of antibodies to HSV-2 than to HSV-1. The cost of the tests varies as well.

The performance and unique characteristics of these tests are as follows:

- A recently approved, easy and rapid point-of-care assay for the detection of specific HSV-2 antibodies is expected to streamline the diagnosis and treatment for many patients with suspected genital herpes [202]. This POCKit HSV-2 test is a membrane-based immunoassay using a native glycoprotein of G-2 as antigen. This in-office diagnostic test is extremely accurate when compared with the Western blot assay, with a sensitivity of 92–97.7% and a specificity of 94–100% [203,204]. The test takes approximately 6 to 10 minutes to provide results.

- Meridian Premier Type-Specific HSV-1 or HSV-2 gG ELISA detects HSV-1 or HSV-2 antibodies, respectively. This is a laboratory-based test performed on patient's serum. This test appears to provide negative results for a long time after initial infection.

- Microbiology Reference Laboratory (MRL) Diagnostics has two types of test formats for detection of type-specific serologies: ELISA and immunoblot. Both employ recombinant glycoprotein G-1 for HSV-1 antibody detection and G-2 for HSV-2 antibody detection. Both tests are performed on sera and are laboratory-based. Both are more sensitive for HSV-1 and HSV-2 than the respective Meridian Premier ELISAs.

Standard neurodiagnostic procedures used in the evaluation of patients with suspected HSE include cerebrospinal fluid examination, electroencephalogram, and one or more scanning procedures such as technetium, computed tomography (Fig. 4–42), or magnetic resonance imaging. For the diagnosis of HSE, characteristic abnormalities of the cerebrospinal fluid include pleocytosis (usually mononuclear cells) and elevated protein levels. Red blood cells are found in most (but not all) cerebrospinal fluid samples obtained from patients with HSE. Upon examination of serial cerebrospinal fluid, protein concentration and cell counts virtually always increase dramatically. This observation is helpful in distinguishing HSV infection of the central nervous system from other viral infections. The electroencephalogram generally localizes spike and slow wave activity to the temporal lobe. A burst suppression pattern is considered characteristic. Early after onset, imaging may reveal only evidence of edema. As the disease progresses, this finding is followed by evidence of temporal lobe hemorrhage and midline shift in the cortical structures.

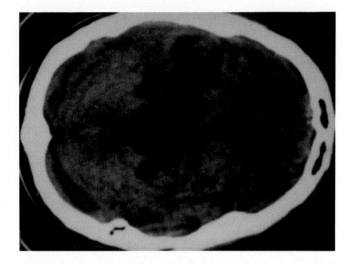

Figure 4–42. Computed tomographic scan from patient with herpes simplex encephalitis.

PATHOLOGY

The pathological changes induced by the replication of HSV are similar for both primary and recurrent infection but vary in the extent of cytopathology. The histopathological characteristics of a skin lesion induced by HSV are shown in Figure 4–43. These changes represent a combination of virus-mediated cellular death and an associated inflammatory response. Changes induced by viral infection of skin include ballooning of infected cells and the appear-

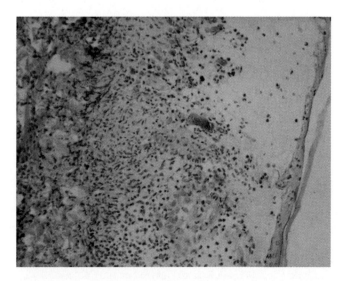

Figure 4–43. Histopathological findings of cutaneous HSV infection with multinucleated giant cells and lymphocytic infiltration.

ance of chromatin within the nuclei, followed by degeneration of the cellular nuclei, generally within parabasal and intermediate cells of the epithelium. Multinucleated giant cells form as cells lose intact plasma membranes, as demonstrated by a Tzanck smear obtained by scraping cutaneous lesions (Fig. 4–40). With cell lysis, clear fluid containing large quantities of virus accumulates between the epidermis and the dermal layer and forms a vesicle. The vesicular fluid also contains cell debris, inflammatory cells, and multinucleated giant cells. In deeper dermal structures there is an intense inflammatory response, usually in the corneum of the skin, more so in primary infection than with recurrent infection.

Vascular changes that have been reported in the area of infection include perivascular cuffing and areas of hemorrhagic necrosis, as shown in Figure 4–44, which is a hematoxylin and eosin stained section of brain tissue from a patient with HSE. These histopathological findings become particularly prominent when organs other than skin are involved, as is encountered with HSE or disseminated neonatal HSV infection. In such cases, widespread areas of hemorrhagic necrosis, mirroring the area of infection, become prominent. When the brain is involved, oligodendrocytic involvement and gliosis are common as well as astrocytosis, but these changes develop late in the disease course. Local lymphatics can show evidence of infection with intrusion of inflammatory cells, since the lymphatic channels allow for the drainage of infected fluid from the area of viral replication. The intensity of the inflammatory response is significantly less with recurrent disease. As host defenses are mounted, an influx of mononuclear cells can be detected in infected tissue.

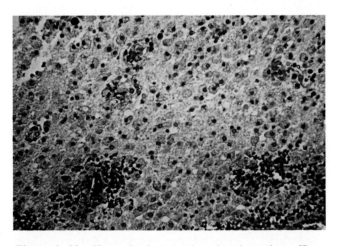

Figure 4–44. Hemorrhagic necrosis and perivascular cuffing.

TREATMENT

Compared to the remarkable progress made in the treatment of bacterial infections over the past four decades, only a few antiviral drugs of proven clinical value are available for a limited number of indications. Acyclovir, the prototype drug, has proved its value since its development in 1974 and introduction to medical treatment in 1983. Acyclovir has served as a model for the development of many subsequent and possibly future antiviral therapies.

Viruses are obligate intracellular parasites that utilize many biochemical pathways of the infected host cell. Historically, it has been difficult to achieve clinically useful antiviral activity without also adversely affecting normal host cell metabolism and causing toxic effects in uninfected cells. As will be noted below, acyclovir is selectively activated by the thymidine kinase of HSV and, therefore, has a selectivity of its mechanism of action. Early diagnosis of viral infection is crucial for effective antiviral therapy because by the time symptoms appear, several cycles of viral multiplication usually have occurred and replication is waning. Precise diagnosis is exceedingly difficult for many viral infections because of the lack of specificity of many viral syndromes, e.g., coryza and cough for rhinovirus infection, pneumonitis attributed to cytomegalovirus (CMV), or the encephalopathy associated with HSE. As a consequence, effective antiviral therapy is dependent on rapid, sensitive, specific, and practical means of diagnosing viral disease. Nevertheless, there are some viral infections, such as herpes zoster or genital herpes, for which clinical diagnosis is relatively straightforward. Since many of the disease syndromes caused by viruses are common, relatively benign, and self-limiting, the therapeutic index (or ratio of efficacy to toxicity) must be extremely high in order for therapy to be acceptable. The exceptions to this rule are infections that are associated with high morbidity such as HSE or CMV chorioretinitis.

Fortunately, the explosion of research in molecular biology is helping several of these problems. It has been possible to identify enzymes unique to viral replication and, therefore, clearly distinguish between virus and host cell functions. Unique events in viral replication are sites that serve as ideal targets for antiviral agents; examples include the thymidine kinase (TK), protease, or unique protein kinases of HSV. Second, several early, sensitive, and specific diagnostic methods for viral illnesses have been made possible by advances in biotechnology, e.g., the use of monoclonal antibodies, DNA hybridization techniques, and PCR, which has the sensitivity of detecting one viral genome per tissue sample.

As with all infectious diseases, the efficacy of antiviral

therapy is often dependent on host defenses, and this principle is of paramount importance when considering the value of antiviral agents such as acyclovir. The special risk of immunocompromised patients for the development of symptomatic herpesvirus infections deserves special note. The ability of all herpesviruses to become latent results in an extremely high incidence of reactivated infection in this patient group. In renal transplant recipients, for example, reactivation rates are 40–70% for latent HSV infections, 80–100% for CMV infections, and 5–35% for varicella zoster virus infections within one year, as summarized [205]. Not only is the incidence of reactivation high, but these infections are often much more severe in the immunocompromised population, e.g., varicella in children with leukemia, mucocutaneous HSV infections in organ transplant recipients, and CMV infection in bone marrow transplant recipients and AIDS patients.

The documented value of therapy for herpesvirus infections has provided the foundation from which other antiviral drugs have evolved. Following the discovery of idoxuridine in the mid-1950s and its successful demonstration as a topical therapeutic agent for HSV keratoconjunctivitis, other herpesvirus infections have subsequently become targets for experimental antiviral therapy and, ultimately, have become amenable to treatment. After licensing of the topical formulation of idoxuridine (Stoxil) for HSV infections of the eye, it was another decade before significant advances were achieved in therapy of other herpesvirus infections, as summarized [32]. Vidarabine (Vira-A), the first compound licensed for systemic use as an antiviral agent, was approved for the treatment of HSE in 1978. Vidarabine was originally synthesized in the early 1960s as a potential anticancer agent but was found to have antiviral activity against HSV and vaccinia viruses in cell culture [206,207]. Subsequently, acyclovir, a second-generation antiviral agent, was shown to be activated selectively by HSV TK. The resultant hope that acyclovir would be more effective and less toxic than vidarabine has been borne out in clinical trials, and this drug has become the foundation of treatment for HSV infection.

Acyclovir

As a selective inhibitor of herpesvirus replication, acyclovir (ACV) represents one of the most important advances in antiviral therapy and to this day serves as the prototype for future antiviral drug development. ACV was synthesized in 1974 by Drs. Lilia Beauchamp and Howard Schaffer of Burroughs Wellcome Company as a part of a program designed to produce anticancer drugs. These compounds were screened both for inhibition of cell replication and for antiviral activity [3]. ACV, 9-([2-hydroxye-

thoxy]methyl) guanine, demonstrated significant antiviral activity against herpesviruses, especially HSV and varicella zoster virus [2]. After extensive preclinical studies revealed an extremely favorable toxicity profile, ACV was started in clinical trials for a number of herpesvirus infections [208,209].

The first reports of clinical efficacy of ACV began to appear in both the European and United States medical literature almost two decades ago. In the intervening decade, it has become the most widely prescribed and clinically effective antiviral drug available to date, and active research on new indications is ongoing. The indications as well as limitations of ACV therapy are summarized in Table 4–5 [210].

ACV is a synthetic acyclic purine nucleoside analogue that is a selective inhibitor of HSV types 1 and 2 and varicella zoster virus replication [2,3]. It is converted by virus-encoded TK to its monophosphate derivative, an event that does not occur to any significant extent in uninfected cells [211]. Subsequent di- and tri-phosphorylation are catalyzed by cellular enzymes, resulting in ACV-triphosphate concentrations 40 to 100 times higher in HSV-infected cells than in uninfected cells. ACV triphosphate inhibits viral DNA synthesis by competing with deoxyguanosine triphosphate as a substrate for viral DNA polymerase [212]. Because ACV triphosphate lacks the $3'$ hydroxyl group required for DNA chain elongation, viral DNA synthesis is terminated. Viral DNA polymerase is tightly associated with the terminated DNA chain and is functionally inactivated [213]. Also, the viral polymerase has greater affinity for ACV triphosphate than does cellular DNA polymerase, resulting in little incorporation of ACV into cellular DNA [214]. In vitro, ACV is most active against HSV-1 (average IC (inhibitory concentration) 50—0.04 μg/ml), HSV-2 (0.10 μg/ml), and varicella zoster virus (0.50 μg/ml). Epstein-Barr virus (EBV) requires higher ACV concentrations for inhibition [215], and cytomegalovirus (CMV), which lacks a virus-specific TK, is resistant. These observations indicated that ACV was the first truly specific inhibitor of HSV replication, making it a second-generation antiviral therapeutic.

ACV was originally released in topical and intravenous preparations and subsequently became the first orally administered therapeutic for herpesvirus infections. Absorption of ACV after oral administration is slow and incomplete, with oral bioavailability of about 15–30% [216]. After multidose oral administration of 200 mg or 800 mg of ACV, the mean steady-state peak levels are about 0.57 and 1.57 μg/ml, respectively [217]. Much higher plasma ACV levels can be achieved with intravenous administration. Steady-state peak ACV concentrations following intravenous doses of 5 mg/kg or 10 mg/kg every 8 hours

Table 4–5.   Treatment of Herpesvirus Infections

Symptom	Treatment
Herpes labialis:	Topical application of 1% penciclovir cream every 2 hours while awake for 4 days. (Mucous membrane application is not recommended)
	Topical application of 10% docosanol cream five times daily
	Acyclovir is often used off label for oral treatment of herpes labialis, at 400 mg 5 times daily for 5 days
	Famciclovir is often used off label for oral treatment of herpes labialis, at 125 mg twice daily for 5 days, although a recent study showed that high dosages are more optimal (500 mg three times daily for 5 days)
	Valacyclovir is often used off label for oral treatment of herpes labialis, at 500 mg twice daily for 5 days, but current studies suggest higher doses may be more efficacious
	For chronic suppression, if needed (off label): Acyclovir, 400 mg twice daily, or famciclovir, 250 mg twice daily, or valacyclovir, 500 mg once daily
Herpes genitalis:	Acyclovir, 200 mg five times daily (or 400 mg tid for 10 days initial infection) or 5 days (recurrent attacks). Intravenous acyclovir may be given for severe primary infections, at 5 mg/kg over 1 hour every 8 hours for 7 days, followed by oral therapy. Daily suppressive therapy may be given to prevent frequent attacks, at 400 mg twice daily
	Valacyclovir, 1 g twice daily for 10 days for initial episodes, and 500 mg twice daily for 6 days for recurrent attacks. For chronic suppressive therapy, 1 g daily is given for patients with 10 or more recurrences per year, and 500 mg once daily is given for those with less frequent outbreaks
	Famciclovir, 250 mg tid for 10 days for initial episodes, and 125 mg twice daily for 5 days for recurrent outbreaks only. For continuous suppressive therapy, 250 mg twice daily is given
Other cutaneous HSV infections (i.e., herpetic whitlow):	Although no controlled studies have evaluated acyclovir for therapy of HSV infections in other cutaneous areas, if disease is severe and recurrent, it would seem prudent to prescribe oral acyclovir (or valacyclovir or famciclovir) initially at dosages utilized to treat primary genital HSV infections. If suppressive therapy is planned those dosages utilized for frequently recurrent genital HSV infection would seem appropriate
Mucocutaneous HSV infections in immunocompromised patients:	Intravenous acyclovir infusion at 5 mg/kg over 1 hour, given every 8 hours for 7 days. For children less than 12 years of age, the dosage is 250 mg/m^2 at the same schedule
	For limited disease, topical application of acyclovir 5% ointment every 3 hours (six times daily) for 7 days
Recurrent orolabial or genital HSV infections in HIV-infected patients:	Famciclovir, 500 mg twice daily for 7 days. This same dosage is also used off label on a daily basis for chronic suppression of recurrent episodes in HIV-infected persons
	Valacyclovir, 500 mg to 1000 mg bid, can also be used off label for episodic therapy (e.g., 7 days) or on a daily basis for chronic suppression in these patients
Herpes simplex keratoconjunctivitis:	Trifluridine 1% ophthalmic solution for primary keratoconjunctivitis and recurrent epithelial keratitis due to HSV, given as one drop in the affected eye(s) every 2 hours while awake (maximum of 9 drops per day). This is continued until re-epithelialization of the corneal ulcer occurs, followed by one drop every 4 hours while awake for 7 more days
	Vidarabine 3% ophthalmic ointment applied in the lower conjunctival sac five times daily at 3-hour intervals. This is continued until complete re-epithelialization of the ulcer occurs, followed by twice daily application for 7 additional days
	Topical acyclovir for HSV ocular infections is effective but probably not superior to trifluridine [280–282] and is no longer recommended
Herpes simplex encephalitis:	Intravenous acyclovir infusion at 10 mg/kg over 1 hour, given every 8 hours for 14 days. For children ages 6 months to 12 years of age, the dosage is adjusted to 500 mg/m^2
Neonatal herpes simplex infection:	Intravenous acyclovir infusion at 20 mg/kg over 1 hour, given every 8 hours for skin, eye, mouth (SEM) disease for 14–21 days (encephalitis or multiorgan disease)
Neonatal HSV:	Intravenous acyclovir infusion at 10 mg/kg every 8 hours for 10 to 14 days
Acyclovir-resistant HSV infections:	Intravenous foscarnet infusion at 40 mg/kg over 1 hour either every 8 or 12 hours, for 2–3 weeks or until all lesions are healed
	Cidofovir 1% cream or gel may be compounded as an alternative therapy

are about 9.9 and 20.0 pg/ml, respectively [218]. ACV penetrates well into most body tissues, including the brain. Its terminal plasma half-life is 2 to 3 hours in adults with normal renal function. ACV is minimally metabolized and about 85% is excreted unchanged in the urine via renal tubular secretion and glomerular filtration. Dosage adjustment is required in patients with impairedrenal function. For patients with severe renal failure (creatinine clearance < 10 ml/min), the dose of oral ACV should be reduced to 200 mg every 12 hours. The drug is readily removed by hemodialysis but not by peritoneal dialysis.

Both primary and initial genital HSV infections can be treated with topical, oral, or intravenous ACV. Topical application of ACV reduces the duration of viral shedding and the time to complete lesion crusting but is less effective than oral or intravenous therapy [27,29]. Intravenous ACV is the most effective treatment for first-episode genital herpes and results in a significant reduction in the median duration of viral shedding, pain, and time to complete healing (8 versus 14 days on average) [28,219]. Since intravenous ACV therapy usually requires hospitalization, it should be reserved for patients with severe local disease or systemic complications (e.g. meningitis, urinary retention, transverse myelitis). Oral therapy is nearly as effective as intravenous ACV for first-episode genital herpes [26,220] and has become the standard treatment. Unfortunately, neither intravenous nor oral ACV treatment of acute HSV infection alters the frequency of subsequent recurrences [26,219].

As previously described, recurrent genital herpes is less severe and resolves more rapidly than primary or initial infection, offering a shorter time interval for successful antiviral chemotherapy. Topically-applied ACV reduces the duration of virus shedding but has no significant effect on the clinical symptoms [152,221]. Orally-administered ACV shortens the duration of virus shedding and time to healing (6 versus 7 days) when initiated early (within 24 hours of onset), but the duration of pain and itching and the time to subsequent recurrence are not affected [222–224]. While the effects of oral ACV therapy indicate statistically significant benefit, clinical improvement perceived by the patient is limited, suggesting that episodic treatment is not indicated in most patients with recurrent genital herpes.

Oral ACV administration is dramatically effective for suppression of frequently recurring genital herpes [224–227]. Daily administration of ACV reduces the frequency of recurrences by up to 80%, and 25–30% of patients have no further recurrences while taking ACV (see Table 4–5). Successful suppression for up to 10 years has been reported with no evidence of significant adverse effects [226–228]. Titration of ACV (400 mg twice daily or 200 mg two to five times daily) may be required to establish the minimum ACV dose that is most effective and economical. Treatment may be interrupted at 12-month intervals to reassess the need for continued suppression [229]. Emergence of ACV-resistant HSV appears to be an infrequent occurrence in immunologically normal individuals [230]. These data taken in sum indicate the first effective approach to the reduction in the frequency of reactivation of genital HSV infections. Although suppressive antiviral therapy is generally recommended for patients with frequent (e.g., ≥6 per year) recurrences of genital herpes, a variety of additional reasons are emerging to support antiviral suppression (Table 4–6).

Although an early study did not demonstrate a decrease in the rate of asymptomatic viral shedding with ACV compared with placebo [231], a subsequent investigation showed a 95% reduction in subclinical shedding with ACV (defined as viral shedding on days without genital lesions) [232]. These differences may be attributable to different daily doses of ACV (600 mg versus 800 mg), differing definitions of asymptomatic versus subclinical shedding, or other variations in study design. Although the reductions in the latter study [232] were not a total elimination of shedding (19% of women in the study still had subclinical shedding), the study does indicate that suppressive ACV decreases subclinical shedding. Another investigation of daily samples of genital secretions from HSV-2 infected women found that those taking ACV 400 mg twice a day had an 80% reduction in the frequency of HSV DNA detection, which was reversible upon discontinuation of ACV [233]. While it is logical that such reductions would have a positive impact on transmission rates, thus far no studies have been completed to confirm this relationship.

The use of ACV for primary HSV gingivostomatitis has only been minimally studied, with the need for further clinical evaluation [234]. However, many children and adults have received therapy in an attempt to avoid hospitalization for rehydration. Thus, therapy, to a great extent, has been designed for those with more severe courses of

Table 4–6. Reasons to Consider Suppression versus Episodic Therapy with Acyclovir, Valacyclovir or Famciclovir

Immunocompromised patient?
Frequency of outbreaks?
Time since first outbreak?
Severity of outbreaks?
Presence of prodromes?
Gender of partner?
If susceptible partner is female, is she pregnant?

reactivation. Despite early suggestions that topical therapy with 5% ACV was effective for HSV-1 orolabial infections [235], subsequent studies showed no clinical benefit in immunocompetent persons [236–238], probably because of poor penetration of drug to the site of viral replication. Current data do not support the use of topical ACV treatment for herpes labialis in otherwise healthy patients.

Orally-administered ACV (at a dose of 200 mg five times daily for 5 days) reduces the time to loss of crust by approximately one day (7 versus 8 days) but does not alter the duration of pain or time to complete healing [239]. If the dose is increased to 400 mg five times daily for 5 days, treatment started during prodrome or erythema stages reduces the mean duration of pain by 36% and time to loss of crusts by 27% [240]. Thus, oral ACV has modest clinical benefit only if initiated very early after recurrence and cannot be recommended for routine therapy of herpes labialis. It may be of value in the small group of individuals whose recurrence is associated with protracted clinical illness.

Oral ACV can alter the severity of sun-induced reactivation of labial herpes. Administration of 200 mg of ACV five times daily to skiers resulted in a similar frequency of HSV reactivation for treatment and placebo recipients, but significantly fewer lesions formed on days 5 to 7 among ACV recipients [241]. Short-term prophylactic ACV administration may benefit some patients with recurrent herpes labialis who anticipate high-risk activity (e.g., intense sunlight exposure). Intermittent ACV administration does not alter the frequency of subsequent recurrences. Although it is not FDA-approved for this purpose, chronic suppression with oral ACV for herpes labialis has been shown to result in 53% reduction in the number of clinical recurrences [242].

Remarkable clinical benefit from the treatment of immunocompromised persons with intravenous ACV was documented in placebo-controlled trials [243]. In the early 1980s, when these data were first presented, they provided real hope for the advancement of antiviral therapy. ACV recipients had a significantly shorter duration of viral shedding and experienced accelerated lesion healing (Fig. 4–45) [244]. Oral ACV therapy is also very effective for these conditions [245]. Both formulations are used to treat HSV infections in the immunocompromised host, according to the area of the hospital in which care is provided (inpatient versus ambulatory). Although the topical application of ACV in polyethylene glycol has been shown to be useful [174], its use should be discouraged in favor of oral therapy.

ACV prophylaxis of HSV infections is of significant clinical value in severely immunocompromised patients, especially those undergoing induction chemotherapy or transplantation. Intravenous or oral ACV administration reduces the incidence of symptomatic HSV infection from about 70% to 5–20% [31,246–248]. Parenthetically, these

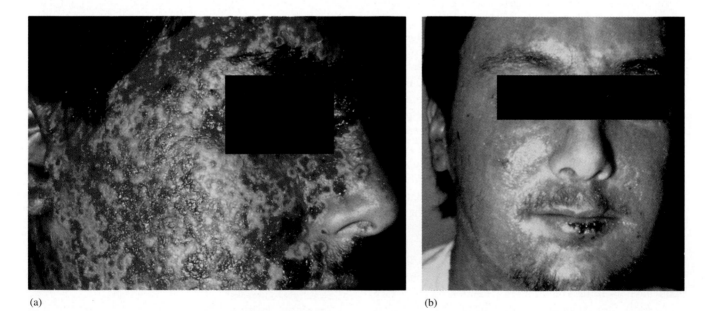

(a)   (b)

Figure 4–45. (a) Eczema herpeticum in a patient with atopic dermatitis before therapy. (b) Same patient following 7 days of intravenous aciclovir therapy.

clinical studies were among the first to establish both the efficacy and safety of this drug in controlled clinical trials. A sequential regimen of intravenous ACV followed by oral ACV for 3 to 6 months can virtually eliminate symptomatic HSV infections in transplant recipients (i.e., while the drug is being taken) [249]. A variety of oral dosing regimens, ranging from 200 mg three times daily to 800 mg twice daily, have been used successfully. Among bone marrow transplant recipients, ACV-resistant HSV isolates have been identified more frequently following therapeutic ACV administration than during prophylaxis [250]. ACV has become a therapeutic mainstay for physicians treating and suppressing herpesvirus infections in immunocompromised patients, including those with AIDS.

For the treatment of neonatal HSV infections, ACV has been shown to be as effective as vidarabine treatment [251]. No infant whose disease was localized to the skin, eyes, or mouth has died, whereas 18% and 55% of babies with CNS or disseminated infection have died. For babies with HSV localized to the skin, eyes, and mouth, it was found that 90% and 98% of vidarabine and ACV recipients, respectively, were developing normally 2 years after infection. For infants surviving encephalitis, 50% and 43% of vidarabine and ACV recipients were developing normally. For survivors of disseminated infection, 62% and 57% of vidarabine and ACV recipients were developing normally. Thus, unlike therapy of HSE in older patients, there were no significant differences in either morbidity or mortality between ACV and vidarabine treatments in infants. Clearance of virus in babies who received ACV was slower than from studies of immunocompromised adults, implying a requirement for host defense as well. To improve outcome, if therapy is to be employed, it must prevent progression of infection to the central nervous system or disseminated disease. However, ideally, prevention of neonatal HSV infection either by immunization of the at-risk mother or by immunoprophylaxis and therapy of the newborn delivered to the mother with an asymptomatic primary infection would be far more desirable. Both of these later approaches are purely hypothetical at this time and will require many studies before acceptance. The safety and ease of administration of ACV prompts its recommendation as the treatment of choice for neonatal HSV infections. Long-term oral suppressive therapy may be of value and warrants further study [252].

For the treatment of HSV encephalitis, intravenous ACV therapy has been shown to reduce mortality at 3 months to 19%, as compared with approximately 50% among vidarabine recipients [253]. Over time, mortality directly attributable to HSE increases to approximately 30% overall. Furthermore, 38% of ACV recipients returned to normal function. Patients with a Glasgow Coma Score of less than 6, individuals over 30 years of age, and those with encephalitis (any clinical sign or symptom) lasting longer than 4 days had a significantly poorer outcome. For the most favorable outcome, therapy must be instituted before semicoma or coma develops. These data stress the need for improved therapeutic regimens for HSE. Because of the safety of ACV therapy, as noted below, ACV is often used empirically and in the absence of definitive diagnostic efforts. The recent application of PCR to the evaluation of cerebrospinal fluid from patients with suspect HSE should be useful, as discussed above. Brain biopsy should be reserved for those patients for whom the diagnosis is still unclear and who are experiencing progressive neurological deterioration in spite of ACV therapy [254].

The spectrum of HSV infections continues to expand. Case reports have described the successful use of ACV in the treatment of other HSV infections such as hepatitis, pulmonary infections, herpetic esophagitis, and proctitis [255–257].

ACV therapy is associated with very few adverse effects. Renal dysfunction induced by ACV has been reported but appears to be very uncommon and is usually reversible [258,259]. Creatinine level elevations have been noted in patients given high doses of ACV by rapid intravenous infusion and have been attributed to crystallization of drug in the renal tubules and collecting ducts, resulting in a transient nephropathy [260]. The risk of nephrotoxicity can be minimized by administering ACV by slow infusion over 1 hour and ensuring adequate hydration. Oral ACV therapy, even at doses of 800 mg five times daily, has not been associated with renal dysfunction [261]. A few reports have linked intravenous ACV use to central nervous system disturbances, including agitation, hallucinations, disorientation, tremors, and myoclonus [262,263].

An ''Acyclovir in Pregnancy Registry'' has gathered data on prenatal ACV exposures. Although no significant risk to the mother or fetus has been documented, the total number of monitored pregnancies remains too small to detect any low-frequency events [264]. From the outcomes of this registry, ACV has not been associated with an increased risk of birth defects [265]. Since ACV crosses the placenta and can concentrate in amniotic fluid, there is valid concern about the potential for fetal nephrotoxicity, although none has been observed [266].

ACV has been evaluated in several studies for the suppression of recurrent genital herpes in order to prevent transmission of HSV to the neonate and to eliminate the need for cesarean section. A significant reduction in herpes recurrences and in cesarean sections was demonstrated in one study of 46 pregnant women with first-episode genital herpes treated with ACV three times a day versus placebo [267]. Whereas 9 of 25 women in the placebo group had a cesarean delivery as a result of herpes infection, women who received ACV had vaginal deliveries. Other studies [268,269] have demonstrated similar results. No adverse reactions to ACV were seen in mothers or infants in any of these trials.

Valacyclovir

Valacyclovir is a prodrug of ACV with greatly improved oral bioavailability, which is three to five times that of ACV [270]. Because valacyclovir is quickly metabolized to form ACV and L-valine after absorption, its mechanism of action, its efficacy, and its safety profile are all identical to those of ACV. Many different clinical studies have shown valacyclovir to be well tolerated and as effective as ACV for the treatment of first-episode genital herpes [271], recurrent genital herpes [272], and chronic suppression of genital herpes [273].

One large study for first-episode genital herpes comparing oral valacyclovir 1000 mg twice a day versus ACV 200 mg five times daily for 10 days showed the two therapies to be equally effective, with no differences in the duration of viral shedding, pain, other symptoms, or lesion healing [271]. Side effects and tolerability profiles of ACV, valacyclovir, and placebo were all similar.

Two large multicenter studies comparing valacyclovir, 500 mg twice a day and 1000 mg twice a day with ACV, 200 mg five times daily for 5 days, showed no significant difference between the two in terms of the speed of lesion healing, duration of pain, duration of viral shedding, number of aborted episodes, or safety profiles [272,274]. Another investigation found that valacyclovir, 500 mg twice daily and 1000 mg twice daily, to be equally effective [275]. Therefore, the lower dose was approved by the FDA and is widely used. Recently, valacyclovir, 500 mg twice a day for 3 days, was found to be as effective for episodic treatment of recurrent genital herpes as was 500 mg twice a day for 5 days [276].

Valacyclovir is also very effective for the suppression of recurrent genital herpes; valacyclovir, 500 mg daily, was demonstrated to prolong the time to first recurrence [277]. Recently a study of multiple doses of valacyclovir found that all doses (250 mg twice daily and 250 mg, 500 mg, 1000 mg once daily) decreased recurrence rates [273]. Furthermore, the investigation found that patients with a history of fewer than 10 recurrences per year were effectively managed with valacyclovir 500 mg once daily, whereas

doses of valacyclovir 250 mg twice daily, valacyclovir 1000 mg once daily, or ACV 400 mg twice daily were more effective for those persons suffering 10 or more recurrences annually. Therefore the FDA recommends 1 g daily dosing for those patients with 10 or more recurrences annually and 500 mg once daily dosing for those with fewer than 10 recurrences annually.

Current studies are investigating valacyclovir for the treatment of herpes labialis, but no data are available. Data from an initial 4-month trial of valacyclovir for suppression of recurrent herpes labialis suggested 500 mg daily was safe and effective for this purpose (278). Laser resurfacing frequently leads to outbreaks of orofacial herpes. One study reported that valacyclovir was safe and effective prophylaxis against such recurrences.

In addition, valacyclovir has been studied for the treatment and suppression of recurrent anogenital herpes in HIV-seropositive persons. In one investigation valacyclovir, 1000 mg twice daily, was equally safe and effective as ACV, 200 mg five times daily, for treatment of recurrent genital herpes in HIV-positive persons (279). In a 1-year study in HIV-seropositive subjects, valacyclovir, 500 mg twice daily, was equally safe but more effective than valacyclovir, 1000 mg once daily, or ACV, 400 mg twice daily, in preventing or delaying recurrences of HSV (280).

Famciclovir

Famciclovir is the oral prodrug of penciclovir, a drug that is available only topically because of its extremely poor oral bioavailability. Like ACV, penciclovir and famciclovir are acyclic guanosine analogues that competitively inhibit viral DNA polymerase after phosphorylation by viral TK and cellular kinases. However, they are not obligate DNA-chain terminators, as is ACV [281]. Famciclovir has been shown to be well tolerated and significantly effective for the treatment of recurrent genital herpes [282]. After the treatment of first-episode genital herpes, famciclovir delayed the time to first recurrence in one clinical trial [283]. This drug has also been shown to be effective for chronic suppression of recurrent genital herpes [284,285]. Famciclovir, 250 mg three times a day for 10 days, was safe and equally effective as ACV, 200 mg five times daily, for the therapy of first-episode genital herpes [283]. For recurrent genital herpes, famciclovir, 125 mg, 250 mg, or 500 mg twice daily for 5 days, initiated by patients within 6 hours of the onset of symptoms, was demonstrated to speed lesion healing, decrease the duration of viral shedding, decrease the duration of lesion edema, vesicles, ulcers and crusts, and increase the likelihood that viral shedding would be aborted [282]. Unlike oral ACV trials, famciclovir also was found to reduce the duration of all lesional symptoms, including pain, tenderness, and burning. Although no direct comparisons of ACV and famciclovir antiviral efficacies for recurrent genital herpes have been published, famciclovir twice daily is at least as effective as ACV five times daily. The 125 mg twice daily dosing has been FDA approved for therapy of recurrent genital herpes.

Famciclovir, 125 mg twice daily, 250 mg twice daily, or 250 mg three times daily, were all safe and effective in delaying initial recurrences of genital herpes and increasing the percentage of patients free of recurrences throughout the duration of suppressive therapy compared to placebo (90% versus 48%) [285,286]. The 250 mg twice daily dose of famciclovir is FDA approved for suppression of recurrent genital herpes.

Famciclovir has been investigated for the treatment of herpes labialis in two small trials. In a dose-ranging study, famciclovir, 500 mg three times daily for 5 days, decreased lesion size and time of lesion healing when given 48 hours after ultraviolet radiation–induced herpes labialis modeling early episodic intervention [287]. In a second study, Spruance et al. [288] used the same dose and schedule of famciclovir, but half of the patients also used topical fluocinonide 0.05% gel three times daily for 5 days, while the other half used a control (vehicle) gel. Patients using combination therapy experienced markedly reduced median maximum lesion size, and the number of patients who suffered pain was reduced by approximately one half compared with the control group (59% versus 100%). Adverse events were minimal in both groups. Famciclovir is not FDA-approved for therapy of herpes labialis, nor have any studies been reported using famciclovir for daily suppression of herpes labialis. Famciclovir, 125 mg twice daily, or 250 mg twice daily, begun 1 to 2 days before laser resurfacing and continued for 5 days after surgery, significantly reduced postsurgical orofacial herpes outbreaks compared to placebo [289]. The metabolite of famciclovir, penciclovir, is FDA-approved for episodic therapy of herpes labialis. Topical 1% penciclovir cream applied every 2 hours (when patient is awake) for 4 days decreases the duration of lesion healing, pain, and viral shedding [290].

Famciclovir has been demonstrated to be safe and effective for the episodic treatment of recurrent HSV infection in HIV-positive patients [291]. In a double-blind study of daily suppressive therapy in HIV-positive patients with a mean CD4 count of 384, famciclovir, 500 mg twice daily, effectively decreased the number of days with symptoms, reduced symptomatic and asymptomatic viral shedding,

and decreased the frequency, duration, and severity of breakthrough reactivations [292].

Foscarnet

Foscarnet is the only FDA-approved drug indicated for the treatment of ACV-resistant HSV infections in immunocompromised patients. All of the aforementioned antiviral agents are acyclic nucleoside analogues that rely on the viral TK for initial phosphorylation. Foscarnet, on the other hand, is a pyrophosphate analogue that does not require this viral enzyme and is effective against TK-negative viral strains [293]. Foscarnet works by competitively blocking the pyrophosphate binding site of the virus-specific DNA polymerase, preventing further primer-template extension for replication of virus [294,295].

The role of foscarnet in the treatment of HSV is significantly limited by its many adverse effects and the need for intravenous administration because of its extremely poor oral absorption. Renal impairment is the major dose-limiting toxicity of foscarnet, which requires adequate hydration and frequent monitoring of the serum creatinine levels. Other adverse effects frequently seen include electrolyte imbalances, nausea and vomiting, diarrhea, headache, fever, anemia, and central nervous system disturbances. Foscarnet can also induce penile ulceration in some patients [296–301]. This complication is a contact dermatitis caused by local accumulation of foscarnet in the urine, which can be prevented by proper hygiene and adequate hydration.

Cidofovir

Cidofovir is an acyclic nucleotide analogue that is phosphorylated in cells to the active metabolite cidofovir diphosphate (independently of viral TK). In a multicenter phase I–II dose escalation study for the treatment of recurrent genital herpes in otherwise healthy persons, cidofovir gel at various strengths decreased the median time to negative virus cultures in a dose-dependent fashion. Cidofovir use was associated with a nonstatistically significant reduction in complete healing. Application site reactions were observed at all doses of cidofovir, but the 1% gel reaction was not different from the vehicle gel [302]. Intravenous cidofovir is effective for treatment of ACV-resistant herpes in immunocompromised hosts but is associated with nephrotoxicity and neuropenia [303]. A placebo-controlled clinical trial using 0.3% or 1% cidofovir gel for ACV-resistant herpes produced accelerated lesion healing and a reduced duration of pain and HSV shedding in AIDS patients [304]. Therefore 1% cidofovir gel (or cream) appears to offer the alternative to intravenous foscarnet with the best therapeutic index. Although not FDA-approved for the treatment of ACV-resistant herpes, topical cidofovir is recommended by the Centers for Disease Control as a ''user friendly'' alternative to foscarnet. Since it is available only in the intravenous form (for CMV infection), cidofovir must be compounded into a topical preparation.

Docosanol

Recently, docosanol 10% cream became the first over-the-counter product approved by the FDA as therapy for herpes labialis. Docosanol (behenyl alcohol, a saturated 22-carbon aliphatic alcohol) inhibits fusion between the plasma membrane and the viral envelope, blocking viral entry and subsequent replication. In clinical trials, docosanol 10% cream significantly reduced the healing time of patients' herpes labialis episodes when compared with placebo times. Docosanol-treated patients also experienced significant reductions in the duration of related symptoms [305]. Application of docosanol cream is recommended five times daily during episodes of herpes labialis. It has not been evaluated in trials versus topical penciclovir or topical ACV. Since in vitro studies demonstrated that n-docosanol can enhance the antiviral activity of nucleoside analogues against replication of herpesviruses, clinical trials of such combination therapy are being planned.

Resiquimod

Resiquimod is a topically active immune response modifier that induces cytokines including, IFN-α (interferon) and IL-2 (interleukin). In a phase II, double-blind, dose-ranging study, patients with a history of at least six recurrences of genital herpes in the preceding year were randomized to receive resiquimod gel or a matching vehicle [306]. Various dosing schedules were evaluated. After treatment of one episode of genital herpes, the time to the next recurrence was 169 days with resiquimod patients compared with 57 days with vehicle patients ($p < 0.01$). All resiquimod regimens in the study appeared to delay the recurrence of genital herpes, possibly via enhancement of herpes-specific cellular immunity. Phase III studies with the 0.01% gel have been initiated.

OTHER (EXPERIMENTAL) THERAPIES FOR HERPES SIMPLEX INFECTIONS

A large number of other interventions have been studied for the therapy of herpes simplex infections, including foscarnet cream [307], edoxudine [308], alpha-interferon gel [240], laser [309], tetracaine [310], and ascorbic acid [242,311–315].

VIRAL RESISTANCE

Herpes simplex virus resistance to ACV can develop through mutations in the viral gene encoding TK via generation of TK-deficient mutants or the selection of mutants possessing a TK that are unable to phosphorylate ACV [316–319]. ACV-resistant herpes simplex virus infections were first described in 1982 [320]. Resistant viral strains generally develop in immunosuppressed patients who have had episodic (in contrast to suppressive) ACV therapy [321]. The rates of ACV-resistant HSV in immunosuppressed patients depend on the extent of exposure and currently vary from 2–10.9% in this patient population [243,322–324]. Clinical isolates resistant to ACV are almost uniformly deficient in TK, although DNA polymerase mutants have also been recovered from HSV-infected patients [325]. Drug resistance was considered rare and resistant isolates were thought to be less pathogenic [250] until a series of ACV-resistant HSV isolates from patients with AIDS were characterized [326]. These resistant mutants were deficient in TK but remained sensitive to vidarabine and foscarnet, drugs that do not require viral TK for activation [327,328]. ACV-resistant HSV isolates have been identified as the cause of pneumonia [329], encephalitis [330], esophagitis [325], mucocutaneous infections [331–333], and disseminated disease [334], almost always occurring in immunocompromised patients. ACV-resistant HSV has been reported in at least one immunocompetent patient, although this is extremely rare [335]. HSV strains resistant to foscarnet [336] or both foscarnet and acyclovir [337–339] have arisen more recently, particularly in AIDS patients. In general, such infections can be treated with cidofovir.

PREVENTION

Over the past several years, significant attention has been directed toward the prevention of HSV disease, particularly since antiviral treatment cannot prevent the development of latency and lifelong infection. Vaccines have been under development and evaluation for both the treatment and prevention of HSV infection. Three different types of HSV vaccines are currently in clinical trials, including an adjuvant subunit vaccine, a DNA vaccine, and a replication-incompetent viral mutant vaccine, also known as a disabled infectious single cycle (DISC) vaccine. The construction

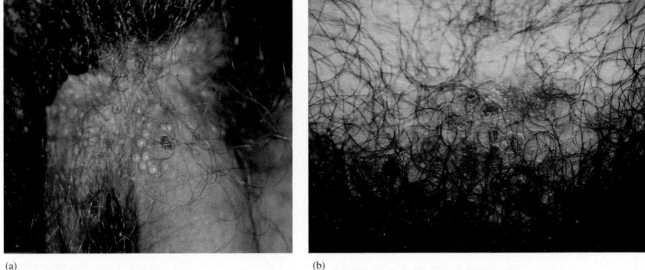

(a)   (b)

Figure 4–46. Primary herpes simplex in men who gave histories of always using condoms during sexual intercourse. (a) vesicles at the base of the penis; (b) suprapubic erosions.

and utilization of these vaccines is discussed in detail in greater depth elsewhere [340–346].

Two randomized, double-blind, placebo-controlled multicenter trials of a recombinant subunit vaccine containing two major HSV-2 surface glycoproteins (g-B2 and g-D2) demonstrated that the vaccine induced high levels of HSV-2–specific neutralizing antibodies. Follow-up of vaccine recipients, however, revealed that vaccination had no significant influence on acquisition rates of HSV-2 or on the duration of clinical first genital HSV-2 episodes or subsequent frequency of reactivation [347].

In contrast, a prophylactic HSV-2 vaccine containing recombinant glycoprotein D2 (g-D2) and a novel adjuvant SBAS4 (containing deacetylated monophosphoryl lipid A) was recently demonstrated to be effective in preventing genital herpes in HSV $1-/2-$ females but not in males or in HSV $1+/2-$ females [78].

Currently available viral vaccines are designed for the prevention of disease. The potential of a therapeutic herpes vaccine has been evaluated [348]. Studies are currently ongoing with the DISC vaccine to evaluate its safety and efficacy in the therapy of recurrent genital herpes.

An important and currently available method of prevention of genital HSV is the use of barrier protection with condoms during sexual exposure [349,350]. As expected, protection only occurs over the specific area covered by the condom, and transmission of virus to and from uncovered skin can still take place (Fig. 4–46). In addition, subclinical viral shedding can occur at any time without apparent lesions [351–353]; therefore condoms can only reduce HSV transmission if used each and every time.

CONCLUSION

Tremendous progress has been made in our understanding of the molecular biology, natural history, and therapy of HSV infections; however, it is apparent that a great deal remains to be learned. Confusion still originates from many diseases that produce vesicles or ulcers and, thus, mimic the lesions of herpes simplex (Fig. 4–47) as well as several nonviral diseases that include the word ''herpes'' (Fig. 4–48). Understanding of the molecular pathogenesis of these infections and prevention of resultant disease with molecularly derived vaccines remain critical goals for future research efforts. The development of antiviral therapy has accelerated the development of our knowledge of HSV infections. The synthesis of ACV was a true milestone in the development of selective and specific inhibitors of viral replication. ACV is the drug of choice for a wide range of infections caused by HSV as well as by other herpesviruses. However, even as the indications for ACV therapy continue to expand, the appearance of isolates resistant to ACV underscores the necessity for continued development of new agents with alternative mechanisms of action. The newer antiviral drugs, including penciclovir, famciclovir, and valacyclovir, have generally been shown to be as effective as ACV but have not been able to further reduce mor-

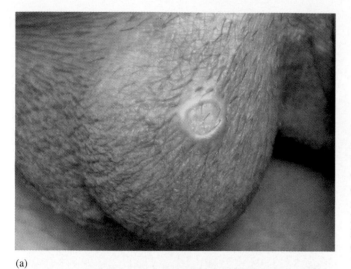

(a)

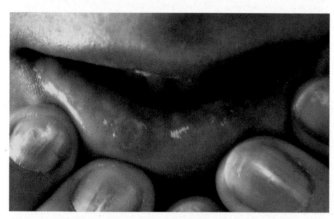

Figure 4–47. Diseases with vesicles or ulcers that may mimic the lesions of herpes simplex. Behcet's disease produces ulcers of the (a) scrotum, (b) lip, and (c) tongue. Primary syphilis may produce ulcers (chancres) of the (d) lips, and (e) *Staphylococcus aureus* can produce bullous impetigo of the inguinal folds. (f) Tularemia may present as vesicles. (Fig. 4–47a–c courtesy of Meltem Onder, M.D., Department of Dermatology, Gazi University School of Medicine, Ankara, Turkey; Fig. 4–47f courtesy of Margretta A. O'Reilly, M.D., University of Utah, Salt Lake City, UT.)

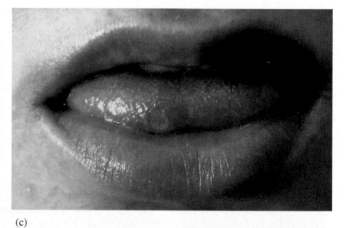

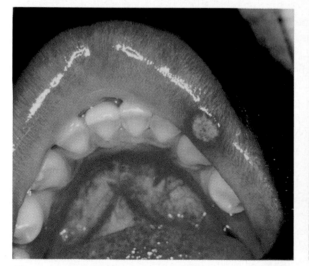

(b)

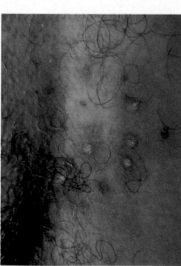

(c)

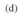

(d)

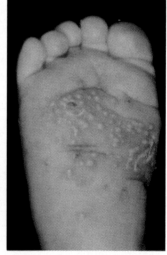

(e)

(f)

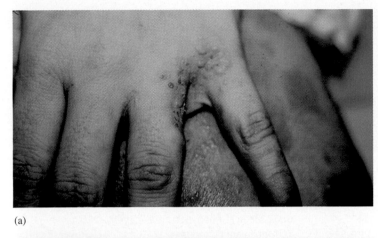

(a)

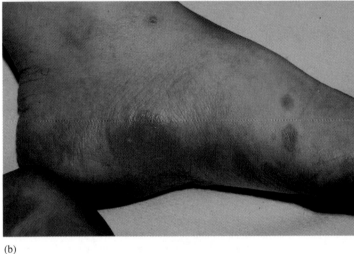

(b)

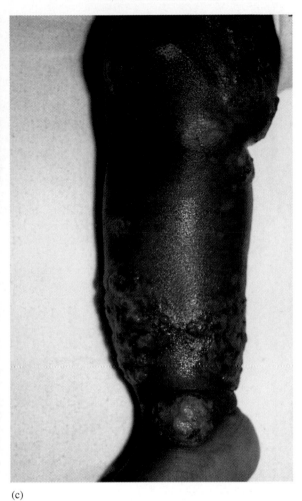

(c)

Figure 4–48. Nonviral diseases sometimes include the word ''herpes'' in their name, such as the following autoimmune diseases: (a, b) ''herpes'' gestationis and (c) dermatitis herpetiformis.

tality and morbidity of serious HSV disease or prevent the establishment of latency and subsequent recurrences. It is hoped that future antiviral drugs and vaccines will be able to overcome these hurdles to the control of herpesvirus infection.

REFERENCES

1. LA Koutsky, CE Stevens, KK Holmes, RL Ashley, NB Kiviat, CW Critchlow, L Corey. Underdiagnosis of genital herpes by current clinical and viral-isolation procedure. N Engl J Med 326:1533–1539, 1992.

2. GB Elion, PA Furman, JA Fyfe, P de Miranda, L Beauchamp, HJ Schaeffer. Selectivity of action of an antiherpetic agent, 9-(2-hydroxyethoxymethyl) guanine. Proc Natl Acad Sci USA 74:5716–5720, 1977.

3. HJ Schaeffer L, Beauchamp, P de Miranda, GB Elion, DJ Baver, P Collins. 9-(2-Hydroxyethoxymethyl) guanine activity against viruses of the herpes group. Nature 272: 583–585, 1978.

4. AJ Nahmias, WR Dowdle. Antigenic and biologic differences in herpesvirus hominis. Prog Med Virol 10: 110–159, 1968.

5. P Wildy. Herpes: history and classification. In: AS Kaplan, ed. The Herpesviruses. New York: Academic Press, 1973, p 1.

6. TS Beswick. The origin and the use of the word herpes. Med Hist 6:214–232, 1962.

7. C Mettler. History of Medicine. New York: McGraw-Hill, 1947, p 356.

8. DC Hutfield. History of herpes genitalis. Br J Vener Dis 42:263–268, 1966.

9. PG Unna. The Histopathology of the Diseases of the Skin. New York: Macmillan, 1886.

10. Lowenstein. Aetiologische untersuchungen uber den fieberhaften, herpes. Munch Med Wochenschr 66:769, 1919.

11. W Gruter. Experimentelle und Klinische untersuchungen uber den sogenannten herpes cornea. Ber Dtsch Ophthalmol Ges 42:162, 1920.

12. R Doerr. Sitzungsberichte der: tesellschaft der schweizerischen. Klin Monatsbl Augenheilkd 65:04, 1920.

13. RJ Whitley. Herpes simplex viruses. In: BN Fields, DM Knipe, PM Howley et al, eds. Field's Virology. New York: Raven Press, 1996, pp 2297–2342.

14. WE Rawls. The Herpesviruses. New York: Academic Press, 1973, pp 291–325.

15. AJ Nahmias, AM Visintine. Herpes simplex. In: JS Remington, JO Kline, eds. Infectious Diseases of the Fetus and Newborn Infant. Philadelphia: W B Saunders, 1976, pp 156–190.

16. CH Andrews, EA Carmichael. A note on the presence of antibodies to herpes virus in post-encephalitic and other human sera. Lancet 1:857–858, 1930.

17. K Dodd, IM Johnston, GJ Buddingh. Herpetic stomatitis. J Pediatr 12:95, 1938.

18. FM Burnet, SW Williams. Herpes simplex: New point of view. Med J Aust 1:637, 1939.

19. S Seidenberg. Zur aetiologic der pustulosis vacciniformis acuta. Schweiz Z Pathol Bakteriol 4:398, 1941.

20. E Gallardo. Primary herpes simplex keratitis: clinical and experimental study. Arch Ophthalmol 30:217–220, 1943.

21. MG Smith, EH Lennette, HR Reames. Isolation of the virus of herpes simplex and the demonstration of intranuclear inclusions in a case of acute encephalitis. Am J Pathol 17:55–68, 1941.

22. B Lipschitz. Untersuchugen uber die atiologic der krankheiten der herpesgruppe (herpes zoster, genitalis and febrilis). Arch Dermatol Res 136:428, 1921.

23. G Plummer. Serological comparison of the herpes viruses. Br J Exp Pathol 45:135–141, 1964.

24. KE Schneweis, AJ Nahmias. Antigens of herpes simplex virus types 1 and 2—immunodiffusion and inhibition passive hemagglutination studies. Z Immunitaetsforsch Exp Klin Immunol 141:471–487, 1971.

25. RJ Whitley, SJ Soong, R Dolin, GJ Galasso, LT Ch'ien, CA Alford. Adenine arabinoside therapy of biopsy-proved herpes simplex encephalitis. National Institute of Allergy and Infectious Diseases Collaborative Antiviral Study. N Engl J Med 297:289–294, 1977.

26. YJ Bryson, M Dillon, M Lovett, G Acuna, S Taylor, JD Cherry, BL Johnson, E Wiesmeier, W Growdon, T Creagh-Kirk, R Keeney. Treatment of first episodes of genital herpes simplex virus infection with oral acyclovir. N Engl J Med 308:916–921, 1983.

27. L Corey, AJ Nahmias, ME Guinan, CW Critchlow, K Holmes. A trial of topical acyclovir in genital herpes simplex virus infections. N Engl J Med 306:1313–1319, 1982.

28. L Corey, KH Fife, JK Benedetti, CA Winter. Intravenous acyclovir for treatment of primary genital herpes. Ann Intern Med 98:914–921, 1983.

29. L Corey, J Benedetti, C Critchlow, G Mertz, J Douglas, K Fife, A Fahnlander, ML Remington, C Winter, J Dragavon. Treatment of primary first episode genital herpes simplex virus infections with acyclovir: results of topical, intravenous, and oral therapy. J Antimicrob Chemother 12:79–88, 1983.

30. JD Meyers, N Flournoy, ED Thomas. Infection with herpes simplex virus and cell-mediated immunity after marrow transplant. J Infect Dis 142:338–346, 1980.

31. R Saral, WH Burns, OL Laskin, GW Santos, AS Leitman. Acyclovir prophylaxis of herpes simplex virus infections. N Engl J Med 305:63–67, 1981.

32. RJ Whitley. Approaches to therapy of viral infections. In: L Barness, ed. Advances in Pediatrics. Chicago: Year Book Medical Publishers, 1987, pp 89–110.

33. TG Buchman, B Roizman, G Adams, BH Stover. Restriction endonuclease fingerprinting of herpes simplex DNA: a novel epidemiological tool applied to a nosocomial outbreak. J Infect Dis 138:488–498, 1978.

34. B Roizman, B Norrild, C Chan, L Pereira. Identification and preliminary mapping with monoclonal antibodies of a herpes simplex virus 2 glycoprotein lacking a known type 1 counterpart. Virology 133:242–247, 1984.

35. B Roizman, FJ Jenkins. Genetic engineering of novel genomes of large DNA viruses. Science 229:1208–1214, 1985.

36. JG Stevens, EK Wagner, GB Devi-Rao, ML Cook, LT Feldman. RNA complementary to a herpesvirus alpha gene mRNA is prominent in latently infected neurons. Science 235:1056–1059, 1987.

37. J Chou, E Kern, RJ Whitley, B Roizman. Mapping of neurovirulence to protein 31.5 encoded by a diploid herpes simplex virus I gene non-essential for growth in cell culture. Science 250:1262–1266, 1990.

38. B Roizman, AE Sears. Herpes simplex viruses and their replication. In: BN Fields, DM Knipe, PM Howley, et al., eds. Field's Virology, 3rd ed. New York: Raven Press, 1996, pp 2231–2295.

39. FL Black. Infectious diseases in primitive societies. Science 187:515–518, 1975.

40. RE Johnson, AJ Nahmias, LS Magder, FK Lee, C Brooks, C Snowden. A seroepidemiologic survey of the prevalence of herpes simplex virus type 2 infection in the United States. N Engl J Med 321:7–12, 1989.

41. AJ Nahmias, C Brooks, R Johnson, et al. Distribution of antibodies to herpes simplex viruses (1 and 2) in the United States as measured by a new antibody type-specific assay. England: Leeds, 1986.

42. AJ Nahmias, FK Lee, S Bechman-Nahmias. Sero-epidemiological and sociological patterns of herpes simplex virus infection in the world. Scand J Infect Dis 69:19–36, 1990.

43. II Ship, AL Morris, RT Durocher, LW Burket. Recurrent aphthous ulcerations and recurrent herpes labialis in a professional school student population. I. Experience. Oral Surg Oral Med Oral Pathol 13:1191–1202, 1960.

44. II Ship, AL Morris, RT Durocher, LW Burket. Recurrent aphthous ulcerations in a professional school student population. IV. Twelve-month study of natural disease patterns. Oral Surg Oral Med Oral Pathol 14:30–39, 1961.

45. E Friedman, AH Katcher, VJ Brightman. Incidence of recurrent herpes labialis and upper respiratory infection: a prospective study of the influence of biologic, social, and psychologic predictors. Oral Surg Oral Med Oral Pathol 43:873–878, 1977.

46. II Ship, VJ Brightman, LL Laster. The patient with recurrent aphthous ulcers and the patient with recurrent herpes labialis: a study of two population samples. J Am Dent Assoc 75:645–654, 1967.

47. II Ship, MF Miller, C Ram. A retrospective study of recurrent herpes labialis (RHL) in a professional population, 1958–1971. Oral Surg Oral Med Oral Pathol 44:723–730, 1977.

48. RE Haynes, P Azimi, H Cramblett. Fatal herpes hominis (herpes simplex virus) infections in children. Clinical, pathological, and virologic characteristics. JAMA 206: 312–319, 1968.

49. L Hellgren. The prevalence of some skin disease and joint disease in total populations in different areas of Sweden. Proc Dermatol Sci 155:162, 1962.

50. WP Glezen, GW Fernald, JA Lohr. Acute respiratory disease of university students with special references to the etiologic role of herpesvirus hominis. Am J Epidemiol 101: 111–121, 1975.

51. KM Lindgren, RG Douglas Jr, RB Couch. Significance of herpesvirus hominis in respiratory secretions of man. N Engl J Med 278:517–523, 1968.

52. LI Hatherley, K Hayes, I Jack. Herpesvirus in an obstetric hospital. II. Asymptomatic virus excretion in staff members. Med J Aust 2:273–275, 1980.

53. LI Hatherley, K Hayes, EM Hennessy, I Jack. Herpesvirus in an obstetric hospital. I: Herpetic eruptions. Med J Aust 2:205–208, 1980.

54. PJ Sheridan, EC Hermann Jr. Intraoral lesions of adults associated with herpes simplex virus. Oral Surg Oral Med Oral Pathol 32:390–397, 1971.

55. L Corey, H Adams, A Brown, K Holmes. Genital herpes simplex virus infections: Clinical manifestations, course and complications. Ann Intern Med 98:958–972, 1983.

56. JE Kalinyak, G Fleagle, JJ Docherty. Incidence and distribution of herpes simplex virus types 1 and 2 from genital lesions in college women. J Med Virol 1:175–181, 1977.

57. IW Smith, JR Peutherer, DH Robertson. Virological studies in genital herpes [letter]. Lancet 2:1089–1090, 1976.

58. S Wolontis, S Jeansson. Correlation of herpes simplex virus types 1 and 2 with clinical features of infection. J Infect Dis 135:28–33, 1977.

59. WC Reeves, L Corey, HG Adams, LA Vontver, KK Holmes. Risk of recurrence after first episodes of genital herpes: relation to HSV type and antibody response. N Engl J Med 305:315–319, 1981.

60. SL Deardourff, FA Deture, DM Drylie, Y Centifanto, HW Kaufman. Association between herpes hominis type-2 and the male genitourinary tract. J Urol 112:126–127, 1974.

61. WE Josey, AJ Nahmias, ZM Naib, PM Utley, WJ McKenzie, MT Coleman. Genital herpes simplex infection in the female. Am J Obstet Gynecol 96:493–501, 1966.

62. JJ Gibson, CA Hornung, GR Alexander, FK Lee, WA Potts, AJ Nahmias. A cross-sectional study of herpes simplex virus types 1 and 2 in college students: occurrence and determinants of infection. J Infect Dis 162:306–312, 1990.

63. WE Josey, AJ Nahmias, ZM Naib. The epidemiology of type-2 (genital) herpes simplex virus infections. Obstet Gynecol Surv 27:295–302, 1972.

64. JD Parker, JE Banatvala. Herpes genitalis: clinical and virological studies. Br J Vener Dis 43:212–216, 1967.

65. LS Magder, AJ Nahmias, RE Johnson, FK Lee, C Brooks, C Snowden. The prevalence and distribution of herpes simplex virus type 1 and 2 antibodies in the United States population. N Engl J Med 321:7–12, 1989.

66. AJ Nahmias, WE Josey, ZM Naib, CF Luce, B Guest. Antibodies to herpesvirus hominis types 1 and 2 in humans. II. Women with cervical cancer. Am J Epidemiol 91:547–552, 1970.

67. WE Rawls, WA Tompkins, JL Melnick. The association of herpesvirus type 2 and carcinoma of the uterine cervix. Am J Epidemiol 89:547–554, 1969.

68. E Adam, RH Kaufman, RR Mirkovic, JL Melnick. Persistence of virus shedding in asymptomatic women after recovery from herpes genitalis. Obstet Gynecol 54:171–173, 1979.

69. WB Becker. The epidemiology of herpesvirus infection in three racial communities in Cape Town. S Afr Med J 40: 109–111, 1966.

70. WE Rawls, E Adam, JL Melnick. Geographical variation in the association of antibodies to herpesvirus type 2 and carcinoma of the cervix. In: PM Biggs, G deThé, LN Payne, eds. Oncogenesis and Herpesviruses. Lyon, France: International Agency for Research on Cancer, 1972, pp 424–427.

71. DT Fleming, GM McQuillan, RE Johnson, AJ Nahmias, SO Aral, FK Lee, ME St Louis. Herpes simplex virus type 2 in the United States, 1976 to 1994. N Engl J Med 337: 1105–1111, 1997.

72. AJ Nahmias, B Roizman. Infection with herpes simplex viruses 1 and 2. N Engl J Med 289:667–674, 1973.

73. FK Lee, RM Coleman, L Pereira, PD Bailey, M Tatsuno, AJ Nahmias. Detection of herpes simplex virus type 2-specific antibody with glycoprotein G. J Clin Microbiol 22:641–644, 1985.

74. GJ Mertz, J Benedetti, R Ashley, SA Selke, L Corey. Risk factors for the sexual transmission of genital herpes. Ann Intern Med 116:197–202, 1992.

75. WE Rawls, HL Gardner. Herpes genitalis: venereal aspects. Clin Obstet Gynecol 15:913–918, 1972.

76. WE Rawls, HL Gardner, RW Flanders, SP Lowry, RH Kaufman, JL Melnick. Genital herpes in two social groups. Am J Obstet Gynecol 110:682–689, 1971.

77. WE Rawls, CH Garfield, P Seth, E Adam. Serological and epidemiological considerations of the role of herpes simplex virus type 2 in cervical cancer. Cancer Res 36: 829–835, 1976.

78. SL Spruance, and the SmithKline Beecham (SB) Herpes Vaccine Efficacy Study Group. Gender-specific efficacy of a prophylactic SBAS4-adjuvanted gD2 subunit vaccine against genital herpes disease (GHD): results of two clinical efficacy trials. Program and Abstracts of the 40th Interscience Conference on Antimicrobial Agents and Chemotherapy, Toronto, Canada, September 2000.

79. G. Sucato, A Wald, E Wababayashi, J Vieira, L Corey. Evidence of latency and reactivation of both herpes simplex virus (HSV)-1 and HSV-2 in the genital region. J Infect Dis 177:1069–1072, 1998.

80. A Wald, A Langenberg, K Link, et al. Declining risk of herpes simplex virus type-2 (HSV-2) acquisition over time in discordant couples. Program and Abstracts of the 39th Interscience Conference on Antimicrobial Agents and Chemotherapy, San Francisco, CA, September, 1999.

81. JA Lekstrom-Himes, P Hohman, T Warren, A Wald, JM Nam, T Simonis, L Corey, SE Straus. Association of major histocompatibility complex determinants with the development of symptomatic and asymptomatic genital herpes simplex type 2 infections. J Infect Dis 179:1077–1085, 1999.

82. FK Keet, F Lee, F van Griensven, J Lange, AJ Nahmias, R Coutinho. Herpes simplex virus type 2 and other genital ulcerative infections as a risk factor for HIV acquisition. Genitourin Med 66:330–333, 1990.

83. SD Holmberg, JA Stewart, AR Gerber, RH Byers, FK Lee, PM O'Malley, AJ Nahmias. Prior herpes simple xirus type 2 infection as a risk factor for HIV infection. JAMA 259: 1048–1050, 1988.

84. E Hook, R Cannon, AJ Nahmias, FF Lee, CH Campbell Jr, D Glasser, TC Quinn. Herpes simplex virus infection as a risk factor for human immunodeficiency virus infection in heterosexuals. J Infect Dis 165:251–255, 1992.

85. WE Stamm, HH Handsfield, AM Rompalo, RL Ashley, PL Roberts, L Corey. The association between genital ulcer disease and acquisition of HIV infection in homosexual men. JAMA 260:1429–1433, 1988.

86. T Schacker, AJ Ryncarz, J Goddard, K Diem, M Shaughnessy, L Corey. Frequent recovery of HIV-1 from genital herpes simplex virus lesions in HIV-1 infected men. JAMA 280:61–66, 1998.

87. JL Severson, SK Tyring. Relation between herpes simplex viruses and human immunodeficiency virus infections. Arch Dermatol 135:1393–1397, 1999.

88. J Benedetti, L Corey, R Ashley. Recurrent rates in genital herpes after symptomatic first-episode infection. Ann Intern Med 121:847–854, 1994.

89. A Langenberg, J Benedetti, J Jenkins, R Ashley, C Winter, L Corey. Development of clinically recognizable genital lesions among women previously identified as having "asymptomatic" HSV-2 infection. Ann Intern Med 110: 882–887, 1989.

90. A Wald, J Zeh, S Selke, T Warren, AJ Ryncarz, R Ashley, JN Krieger, L Corey. Reactivation of genital herpes simplex virus type 2 infection in asymptomatic seropositive persons. N Engl J Med 342:844–850, 2000.

91. ML Cook, JG Stevens. Pathogenesis of herpetic neuritis and ganglionitis in mice: evidence of intra-axonal transport of infection. Infect Immun 7:272–288, 1973.

92. TJ Hill. Herpes simplex virus latency. In: B Roizman, ed. The Herpesviruses. New York: Plenum Publishing, 1985, pp 175–240.

93. JR Baringer. The biology of herpes simplex virus infection in humans. Surv Ophthalmol 21:171–174, 1976.

94. JS Pagano. Diseases and mechanisms of persistent DNA virus infection: latency and cellular transformation. J Infect Dis 132:209–223, 1975.

95. B Roizman. An inquiry into the mechanisms of recurrent herpes infections in man. In: M Pollard, ed. Perspectives in Virology IV. New York: Harper and Row Publishers, 1968, p 283.

96. B Roizman, A Sears. An inquiry into mechanisms of herpes simplex virus latency. Annu Rev Microbiol 41: 543–571, 1987.

97. JC Stevens. Latent herpes simplex virus and the nervous system. Curr Top Microbiol Immunol 70:31–50, 1975.

98. M Terni. Infection due to herpes simplex virus, recurrent disease and the problem of latency. G Mal Infett Parassit 23:433–467, 1971.

99. JR Baringer, P Swoveland. Recovery of herpes simplex virus from human trigeminal ganglions. N Engl J Med 288:648–650, 1973.

100. FO Bastian, AS Rabson, CL Yee. Herpesvirus hominis: isolation from human trigeminal ganglion. Science 178: 306–307, 1972.

101. TJ Hill. Mechanisms involved in recurrent herpes simplex. In: A Nahmias, WR Dowdle, R Schinazi, eds. The Human Herpesvirus: An Interdisciplinary Perspective. Amsterdam: Elsevier/North-Holland, 1981, p 241.

102. AB Nesburn, ML Cook, JG Stevens. Latent herpes simplex virus. Isolation from rabbit trigeminal ganglia between episodes of recurrent ocular infection. Arch Ophthalmol 88: 412–417, 1972.

103. JG Stevens, ML Cook. Latent herpes simplex virus in spinal ganglia of mice. Science 173:843–845, 1971.

104. JG Stevens, ML Cook. Latent herpes simplex virus in sensory ganglia. Perspect Virol 8:171, 1974.

105. KG Warren, SM Brown, A Wrobelwska, D Gilden, H Koprowski, Subak-Sharpe. Isolation of latent herpes simplex virus from the superior cervical and vagus ganglions of human beings. N Engl J Med 298:1068–1069, 1978.

106. H Cushing. Surgical aspects of major neuralgia of trigeminal nerve: report of 20 cases of operation upon the casserian ganglion with anatomic and physiologic notes on the consequences of its removal. JAMA 44:1002, 1905.

107. EW Goodpasture. Herpetic infections with special reference to involvement of the nervous system. Medicine 72: 125–132, 1993.

108. CA Carton, ED Kilbourne. Activation of latent herpes simplex by trigeminal sensory-root section. N Engl J Med 246:172–176, 1952.

109. GJ Pazin, M Ho, PJ Jannetta. Reactivation of herpes simplex after the trigeminal nerve root decompression. J Infect Dis 138:405–409, 1978.

110. GJ Pazin, JA Armstrong, MT Lam, GC Tarr, PJ Jannetta, M Ho. Prevention of reactivated herpes simplex infection by human leukocyte interferon after operation on the trigeminal route. N Engl J Med 301:225–230, 1979.

111. SA Ellison, CA Carlton, HM Rose. Studies of recurrent herpes simplex infections following section of the trigeminal nerve. J Infect Dis 105:161–167, 1959.

112. HW Haverkos, GJ Pazin, M Ho, PB Nelson. Reactivation of type 2 herpes simplex virus by thoracolumbar neurosurgery. Ann Intern Med 101:503–504, 1984.

113. MW Nabors, CK Francis, AI Kobrine. Reactivation of herpesvirus in neurosurgical patients. Neurosurgery 19:599–603, 1986.

114. MA Walz, RW Price, AL Norkins. Latent ganglionic infection with herpes simplex virus types 1 and 2: viral reactivation in vivo after neurectomy. Science 184:1185–1187, 1974.

115. S Kbrick, GW Gooding. Pathogenesis of infection with herpes simplex virus with special reference to nervous tissue. NINDB Monograph Vol II, 1965, p 143.

116. AL Segal, AH Katcher, VJ Brightman, MF Miller. Recurrent herpes labialis, recurrent aphthous ulcers and the menstrual cycles. J Dent Res 53:797–803, 1974.

117. MS Greenberg, VJ Brightman, II Ship. Clinical and laboratory differentiation of recurrent intraoral herpes simplex virus infections following fever. J Dent Res 48:385–391, 1969.

118. MS Greenberg, H Friedman, SG Cohen, SH Oh, L Laster, S Starr. A comparative study of herpes simplex infections in renal transplant and leukemic patients. J Infect Dis 156:280–287, 1987.

119. FM Keddie, RB Rees Jr, NN Epstein. Herpes simplex following artificial fever therapy. JAMA 117:1327–1330, 1941.

120. SL Warren, CM Carpenter, RA Boak. Symptomatic herpes, a sequela of artificially induced fever. J Exp Med 71:155–167, 1940.

121. F Cohen, ME Kemeny, KA Kearney, LS Zegans, JM Neuhaus, MA Conant. Persistent stress as a predictor of genital herpes recurrence. Arch Intern Med 159:2430–2436, 1999.

122. JR Baringer. Recovery of herpes simplex virus from human sacral ganglions. N Engl J Med 291:828–830, 1974.

123. GS Hayward, N Frenkel, B Roizman. Anatomy of herpes simplex virus DNA: strain difference and heterogenicity in the locations of restriction endonuclease cleavage sites. Proc Natl Acad Sci USA 72:1768–1772, 1975.

124. TG Buchman, B Roizman, AJ Nahmias. Demonstration of exogenous genital reinfection with herpes simplex virus type-2 by restriction endonuclease fingerprinting of viral DNA. J Infect Dis 140:295–304, 1979.

125. AD Lakeman, AJ Nahmias, RJ Whitley. Analysis of DNA from recurrent genital herpes simplex virus isolates by restriction endonuclease digestion. J Sex Transm Dis 13:61–66, 1986.

126. Schmidt OW, Fife KH, L Corey. Reinfection is an uncommon occurrence in patients with symptomatic recurrent genital herpes. J Infect Dis 149:645–646, 1984.

127. DM Koelle, M Schomogyi, L Corey. Antigen-specific T cells localize to the uterine cervix in women with genital herpes simplex virus type 2 infection. J Infect Dis 182:662–670, 2000.

128. AJ Nahmias, C Alford, S Korones. Infection of the newborn with herpes virus hominis. Adv Pediatr 17:185–226, 1970.

129. H Blank, HG Haines. Experimental human reinfection with herpes simplex virus. J Invest Dermatol 61:223–225, 1973.

130. L Goldman. Reactions of autoinoculation for recurrent herpes simplex. Arch Dermatol 84:1025–1026, 1961.

131. MP Lazar. Vaccination for recurrent herpes simplex infection: initiation of a new disease site following the use of unmodified material containing the live virus. Arch Dermatol 73:70–71, 1956.

132. P Teissier, P Castinel, J Reilly. L'herpes experimental humain: L'inoculabilité du virus herpetique. J Physiol Pathol Gen 24:271, 1926.

133. SK Young, NH Rowe, RA Buchanan. A clinical study for the control of facial mucocutaneous herpes virus infections. I. Characterization of natural history in a professional school population. Oral Surg Oral Med Oral Pathol 41:498–507, 1976.

134. SL Spruance, CS Crumpacker. Topical 5% acyclovir in polyethylene glycol for herpes simplex labialis: antiviral effect without clinical benefit. Am J Med 73:315–319, 1982.

135. SL Spruance, CS Crumpacker, LE Schnipper, ER Kern, S Marlowe, KA Arndt, JC Overall Jr. Early, patient-initiated treatment of herpes labialis with topical 10% acyclovir. Antimicrob Agents Chemother 25:553–555, 1984.

136. L Corey. The diagnosis and treatment of genital herpes. JAMA 248:1041–1049, 1982.

137. LR Caplan, FJ Kleeman, S Berg. Urinary retention probably secondary to herpes genitalis. N Engl J Med 297:920–921, 1977.

138. JE Hervon Jr. Herpes simplex virus type 2 meningitis. Obstet Gynecol 49:622–624, 1977.

139. DR Hinthorn, LH Baker, DA Romig, C Liu. Recurrent conjugal neuralgia caused by herpesvirus hominis type 2. JAMA 236:587–588, 1976.

140. B Skoldenberg, S Jeansson, S Wolontis. Herpes simplex virus type 2 and acute aseptic meningitis: clinical features of cases with isolation of herpes simplex virus from cerebrospinal fluids. Scand J Infect Dis 7:227–232, 1975.

141. Terni M, Carcialanza D, Cassai E, Kieff E. Aseptic meningitis in association with herpes progenitalis. N Engl J Med 285:503–504, 1971.

142. SE Goodell, TC Quinn, E Mkritchian, MD Schuffler, KK Holmes, L Corey. Herpes simplex virus proctitis in homosexual men. Clinical, sigmoidoscopic, and histopathological features. N Engl J Med 308:868–871, 1983.

143. E Jacobs. Anal infections caused by herpes simplex virus. Dis Colon Rectum 19:151–157, 1976.

144. Yen SS, Reagan JW, MS Rosenthal. Herpes simplex infection in the female genital tract. Obstet Gynecol 25:479–492, 1965.

145. HG Adams, EA Benson, Alexander ER, LA Vontver, MA Remington, KK Holmes. Genital herpetic infection in men and women: clinical course and effect of topical application of adenine arabinoside. J Infect Dis 133:151–159, 1976.

146. TH Flewett, RGF Parker, WM Philip. Acute hepatitis due to herpes simplex virus in an adult. J Clin Pathol 22:60–66, 1969.

147. OM Petrucco, RF Seamark, K Holmes, IJ Forbes, RG Symons. Changes in lymphocyte function during pregnancy. Br J Obstet Gynecol 83:245–260, 1976.

148. YH Thong, RW Steele, MM Vincent, SA Hensen, JA Bellanti. Impaired in vitro cell-mediated immunity to rubella virus during pregnancy. N Engl J Med 289:604–606, 1973.

149. L Corey, A Wald. Genital herpes. In: KK Holmes, PA Mardh, PF Sparling, eds. Sexually Transmitted Diseases, 3rd ed. New York: McGraw Hill, 1999, pp 285–312.

150. AGM Langenberg, L Corey, RL Ashley, WP Leong, SE Straus. A prospective study of new infections with herpes simplex virus type 1 and type 2. Chiron HSV Vaccine Study Group. N Engl J Med 341:1432–1438, 1999.

151. LA Vontver, DE Hickok, Z Brown, L Reid, L Corey. Recurrent genital herpes simplex virus infection in pregnancy: infant outcome and frequency of asymptomatic recurrences. Am J Obstet Gynecol 143:75–84, 1982.

152. JP Luby, JW Gnann Jr, WJ Alexander, VA Hatcher, AE Friedman-Kien, RJ Klein, H Keyserling, A Nahmias, J Mills, J Schachter, et al. A collaborative study of patient-initiated treatment of recurrent genital herpes with topical acyclovir or placebo. J Infect Dis 150:1–6, 1984.

153. RC Pugh, JA Dudgeon, M Bodian. Kaposi's varicelliform eruption (eczema herpeticum) with typical and atypical visceral necrosis. J Pathol Bacteriol 69:67–80, 1955.

154. GT Terezhalmy, MT Tyler, GR Ross. Eczema herpeticum: Atopic dermatitis complicated by primary herpetic gingivostomatitis. Oral Surg Oral Med Oral Pathol 48:513–516, 1979.

155. CEJ Wheeler, DC Abele. Eczema herpeticum, primary and recurrent. Arch Dermatol 93:162–173, 1966.

156. I Ruchman, AL Welsh, K Dodd. Kaposi's varicelliform eruption: isolation of the virus of herpes simplex from the cutaneous lesions of three adults and one infant. Arch Dermatol Syphilol 56:846–863, 1947.

157. JC Huff. Acyclovir for recurrent erythema multiforme caused by herpes simplex. J Am Acad Dermatol 18:197–199, 1998.

158. FE Rosato, EF Rosato, SA Plotkin. Herpetic-paronychia: an occupational hazard of medical personnel. N Engl J Med 283:804–805, 1970.

159. SA Muller, EC Hermann Jr, RK Winkelmann. Herpes simplex infections in hematologic malignancies. Am J Med 52:102–104, 1972.

160. U Eilard, L Hellgren. Herpesvirus infection in burned patients. Dermatology 130:101, 1965.

161. FD Foley, KA Greenwald, G Nash, BA Pruitt. Herpesvirus infection in burned patients. N Engl J Med 282:652–656, 1970.

162. B Selling, S Kibrick. An outbreak of herpes simplex among wrestlers (herpes gladiatorum). N Engl J Med 270:979–982, 1964.

163. EA Belongia, JL Goodman, EJ Holland, CW Andres, SR Homann, RL Mahanti, MW Mizener, A Erice, MT Osterholm. An outbreak of herpes gladiatorum at a high-school wrestling camp. N Engl J Med 325:906–910, 1991.

164. PG Hazen, RB Eppes. Eczema herpeticum caused by herpesvirus type 2. A case in a patient with Darier's disease. Arch Dermatol 113:1085–1086, 1977.

165. JF Hitselberger, RE Burns. Darier's disease: report of a case complicated by Kaposi's varicelliform eruption. Arch Dermatol 83:425–429, 1961.

166. PS Binder. Herpes simplex keratitis. Surv Ophthalmol 21:313–331, 1977.

167. HB Ostler. Herpes simplex: the primary infection. Surv Ophthalmol 21:91–99, 1976.

168. TF Scott. Epidemiology of herpetic infections. Am J Ophthalmol 43:134, 1957.

169. WS Logan, JP Tindal, ML Elson. Chronic cutaneous herpes simplex. Arch Dermatol 103:606–614, 1971.

170. RJ Whitley, S Spruance, FG Hayden, J Overall, CA Alford Jr, JM Gwaltney Jr, SJ Soong. Vidarabine therapy for mucocutaneous herpes simplex virus infections in the immunocompromised host. J Infect Dis 149:1–8, 1984.

171. B Korsager, ES Spencer, CH Mordhorst, HK Andersen. Herpesvirus hominis infections in renal transplant recipients. Scand J Infect Dis 7:11–19, 1975.

172. JZ Montgomerie, MC Croxson, DM Becroft, PB Doak, JD North. Herpes simplex virus infection after renal transplantation. Lancet 2:867–871, 1969.

173. KH Rand, LE Rasmussen, RB Pollard, AM Arvin, TC Merigan. Cellular immunity and herpes virus infections in cardiac transplant patients. N Engl J Med 296:1372–1377, 1977.

174. RJ Whitley, M Levin, N Barton, BJ Hershey, G Davis, RE Keeney, J Whelchel, AG Diethelm, P Kartus, SJ Soong. Infections caused by herpes simplex virus in the immunocompromised host: natural history and topical acyclovir therapy. J Infect Dis 150:323–329, 1984.

175. SL Mann, JD Meyers, KL Holmes, L Corey. Prevalence and incidence of herpesvirus infections among homosexually active men. J Infect Dis 149:1026–1027, 1984.

176. AJ Nahmias, HL Keyserling, CM Kerrick. Herpes simplex. In: JS Remington, JO Klein, eds. Infectious Diseases of the Fetus and Newborn Infant. Philadelphia: WB Saunders, 1983, p 638.

177. AJ Nahmias, HL Keyserling, FK Lee. Herpes simplex viruses 1 and 2. In: AS Evans, ed. Viral Infections of Humans: Epidemiology and Control. New York: Plenum, 1989, pp 393–417.

178. JZ Sullivan-Bolyai, Fife KH, RF Jacobs, Z Miller, L Corey. Disseminated neonatal herpes simplex virus type 1 from a maternal breast lesion. Pediatrics 71:455–457, 1983.

179. AS Yeager, AM Arvin, LJ Urbani, JA Kemp III. Relationship of antibody to outcome in neonatal herpes simplex infections. Infect Immun 29:532–538, 1980.

180. CG Prober, WM Sullender, LL Yasukawa. Low risk of herpes simplex virus infections in neonates exposed to the virus at the time of vaginal delivery to mothers with recurrent genital herpes simplex virus infections. N Engl J Med 316:240–244, 1987.

181. S Kohl. The neonatal human's immune response to herpes simplex virus infection: a critical review. Pediatr Infect Dis J 8:67–74, 1989.

182. RJ Whitley, L Corey, A Arvin, FD Lakeman, CV Sumaya, PF Wright, LM Dunkle, RW Steele, SJ Soong, AJ Nahmias, et al. Changing presentation of neonatal herpes simplex virus infection. J Infect Dis 158:109–116, 1988.

183. LS Parvey, LT Ch'ien. Neonatal herpes simplex virus infection introduced by fetal-monitor scalp electrodes. Pediatrics 65:1150–1153, 1980.

184. AL Florman, AA Gershon, RP Blackett, AJ Nahmias. Intrauterine infection with herpes simplex virus: resultant congenital malformation. JAMA 225:129–132, 1973.

185. RJ Whitley. Herpes simplex virus infections. In: JS Remington, JO Klein, eds. Infectious Diseases of the Fetus and Newborn Infant. Philadelphia: WB Saunders, 1989, pp 282–305.

186. C Hutto, A Arvin, R Jacobs, R Steele, S Stagno, R Lyrene, L Willett, D Powell, R Andersen, J Werthammer, et al. Intrauterine herpes simplex virus infections. J Pediatr 110: 97–101, 1987.

187. S Baldwin, RJ Whitley. Intrauterine herpes simplex virus infection. Teratology 39:1–10, 1989.

188. AM Arvin, AS Yeager, FW Bruhn, M Grossman. Neonatal herpes simplex infection in the absence of mucocutaneous lesions. J Pediatr 100:715–721, 1982.

189. J Sullivan-Bolyai, H Hull, C Wilson, L Corey. Presentation of neonatal herpes simplex virus infections: implications for a change in therapeutic surgery. Pediatr Infect Dis 5: 309–314, 1986.

190. LC Olson, EL Buescher, MS Artenstein. Herpesvirus infections of the human central nervous system. N Engl J Med 277:1271–1277, 1967.

191. DW Barnes, RJ Whitley. CNS diseases associated with varicella zoster virus and herpes simplex virus infections: pathogenesis and current therapy. Neurol Clin 4:265–283, 1986.

192. JF Cleobury, GRB Skinner, MD Thoules. Association between psychopathic disorder and serum antibody to herpes simplex virus (type 1). BMJ 1:438–439, 1971.

193. VS Constantine, RD Francis, LF Montes. Association of recurrent herpes simplex with neuralgia. JAMA 205: 181–183, 1968.

194. DP McCormick. Herpes simplex virus as a cause of Bell's palsy. Lancet 1:937–939, 1972.

195. L Corey. Laboratory diagnosis of herpes simplex virus infections. Principles guiding the development of rapid diagnostic tests. Diagn Microbiol Infect Dis 4(3 Suppl): 111S–119S, 1986.

196. WE Lafferty, S Krofft, M Remington, R Giddings, C Winter, A Cent, L Corey. Diagnosis of herpes simplex virus by direct immunofluorescence and viral isolation from samples of external genital lesions in a high-prevalence population. J Clin Microbiol 25:323–326, 1987.

197. FK Lee, AJ Nahmias, DG Nahmias, JS McDougal. Demonstration of virus particles within immune complexes by electron microscopy. J Virol Methods 7:167, 1983.

198. A Rowley, F Lakeman, R Whitley, S Wolinsky. Diagnosis of herpes simplex encephalitis by DNA amplification of cerebrospinal fluid cells. Lancet 335:440–441, 1990.

199. E Puchhammer-Stockl, T Popow-Kraupp, FX Heinz, CW Mandl, C Kunz. Establishment of PCR for the early diagnosis of herpes simplex encephalitis. J Med Virol 32: 77–82, 1990.

200. MC Bach, SP Bagwell, NP Knapp, KM Davis, PS Hedstrom. 9-(1,3-Dihydroxy-2-propoxymethyl) guanine for cytomegalovirus infections in patients with the acquired immunodeficiency syndrome. Ann Intern Med 103:381–382, 1985.

201. RL Ashley, J Militoni, F Lee, A Nahmias, L Corey. Comparison of Western blot (immunoblot) and glycoprotein G-specific immunodot enzyme assay for detecting antibodies to herpes simplex virus types 1 and 2 in human sera. J Clin Microbiol 26:662–667, 1988.

202. RL Ashley, M Eagleton, N Pfeiffer. Ability of a rapid serology test to detect seroconversion to herpes simplex virus type 2 glycoprotein G soon after infection. J Clin Microbiol 37:1632–1633, 1999.

203. TD Ly, JE Malkin, JM Bohbot. Performance of a rapid screening test POCkit™ HSV2 rapid test. Int J STD AIDS 10:68–70, 1999.

204. RL Ashley, M Eagleton. Evaluation of a novel point of care test for antibodies to herpes simplex virus type 2. Sex Transm Infect 74:228–238, 1998.

205. RJ Whitley, S Goldsmith, J Gnann. Herpesviruses in the immunocompromised host. In: NJ Dimmock, PD Griffiths, CR Madeley, eds. Control of Virus Diseases. England: Cambridge University Press, 1990, pp 315–339.

206. J DeRudder, F Andreeff, M Privat de Garilhe. Action inhibitrice de la 9-D-xylofuranosyl-adenine sur la multiplication du virus de l'herpes en culture cellulaire. C R Acad Sci Hebd Seances Acad Sci D 264:677–680, 1967.

207. FA Miller, GJ Dixon, J Ehrlich, BJ Sloan, IW McLean Jr. Antiviral activity of 9-b-D-arabinofuranosyladenine (ara-A). I. Cell culture studies. Antimicrob Agents Chemother 8:136–147, 1968.

208. JW Gnann Jr, NH Barton, RJ Whitley. Acyclovir: mechanism of action, pharmacokinetics, safety and clinical applications. Pharmacotherapy 3:275–283, 1983.

209. DI Dorsky, CS Crumpacker. Drugs five years later: acyclovir. Ann Intern Med 107:859–874, 1987.

210. R Whitley, J Gnann. Acyclovir: a decade later. N Engl J Med 327:782–789, 1992.

211. JA Fyfe, PM Keller, PA Furman, RA Miller, GB Elion. Thymidine kinase from herpes simplex virus phosphorylates the new antiviral compound, 9-(2-hydroxyethoxymethyl)guanine. J Biol Chem 253:8721–8727, 1978.

212. D Derse, YC Chang, PA Furman, GB Elion. Inhibition of purified human and herpes simplex virus-induced DNA polymerase by 9-(2-hydroxyethoxymethyl)guanine [acyclovir] triphosphate: effect on primer-template function. J Biol Chem 256:11447–11451, 1981.

213. PA Furman, MH St Clair, T Spector. Acyclovir triphosphate is a suicide inactivator of the herpes simplex virus DNA polymerase. J Biol Chem 259:9575–9579, 1984.

214. PA Furman, PA St Clair, JA Fyfe, JL Rideout, PM Keller, GB Elion. Inhibition of herpes simplex virus induced DNA polymerase activity and viral DNA replication of 9-(2-hydroxyethoxymethyl)guanine and its triphosphate. J Virol 32:72–77, 1979.

215. AK Datta, BM Colby, JE Shaw, JS Pagano. Acyclovir inhibition of Epstein-Barr virus replication. Proc Natl Acad Sci USA 77:5163–5166, 1980.

216. P DeMiranda, MR Blum. Pharmacokinetics of acyclovir after intravenous and oral administration. J Antimicrob Chemother 12:29–37, 1983.

217. OL Laskin. Acyclovir: pharmacology and clinical experience. Arch Intern Med 144:1–6, 1984.

218. RJ Whitley, MR Blum, N Barton, P DeMiranda. Pharmacokinetics in acyclovir in humans following intravenous administration: a model for the development of parenteral antivirals. Am J Med 73:165–171, 1982.

219. JE Peacock, LG Kaplowitz, PF Sparling, DT Durack, JW Gnann, RJ Whitley. Intravenous acyclovir therapy of first episodes of genital herpes: a multicenter double-blind, placebo-controlled trial. Am J Med 85:301–306, 1988.

220. GJ Mertz, CW Critchlow, J Benedetti, RC Reichman, R Dolin, J Connor, DC Redfield, MC Savoia, DD Richman, DL Tyrrell, et al. Double-blind placebo-controlled trial of oral acyclovir in first-episode genital herpes simplex virus infection. JAMA 252:1147–1151, 1984.

221. RC Reichman, GJ Badger, ME Guinan, AJ Nahmias, RE Keeney, LG Davis, T Ashikaga, R Dolin. Topically administered acyclovir in the treatment of recurrent herpes simplex genitalis: a controlled trial. J Infect Dis 147:336–340, 1983.

222. RC Reichman, GJ Badger, GJ Mertz, L Corey, DD Richman, JD Connor, D Redfield, MC Savoia, MN Oxman, Y Bryson, et al. Treatment of recurrent genital herpes simplex infection with oral acyclovir. Controlled trial. JAMA 251:2103–2107, 1984.

223. AE Nilsen, T Aasen, AM Halsos. Efficacy of oral acyclovir in the treatment of initial and recurrent genital herpes. Lancet 2:571–573, 1982.

224. JM Douglas, C Critchlow, J Benedetti, GJ Mertz, JD Connor, MA Hintz, A Fahnlander, M Remington, C Winter, L Corey. Double-blind study of oral acyclovir for suppression of recurrences of genital herpes simplex virus infection. N Engl J Med 310:1551–1556, 1984.

225. SE Straus, HE Takiff, M Seidlin, S Bachrach. Suppression of frequently recurring genital herpes: placebo-controlled double-blind trial of oral acyclovir. N Engl J Med 310:1545–1550, 1984.

226. GJ Mertz, CC Jones, J Mills, Lemon SM. Long-term acyclovir suppression of frequently recurring genital herpes simplex virus infection. JAMA 260:201–206, 1988.

227. LG Kaplowitz, D Baker, L Gelb, J Blythe, R Hale, P Frost, C Crumpacker, S Rabinovich, JE Peacock Jr, J Herndon, et al. Prolonged continuous acyclovir treatment of normal adults with frequently recurring genital herpes simplex virus infections. JAMA 265:747–751, 1991.

228. KF Chopra, PC Lee, SK Tyring. Herpes simplex. Clin Dermatol 3(Unit 14–1):1–22, 1998.

229. SE Straus, KD Croen, MH Sawyer, AG Freifeld, JM Felser, JK Dale, HA Smith, C Hallahan, SN Lehrman. Acyclovir suppression of frequently recurring genital herpes. Efficacy and diminishing need during successive years of treatment. JAMA 260:2227–2230, 1988.

230. S Nusinoff-Lehrman, JM Douglas, L Corey, DW Barry. Recurrent genital herpes and suppressive oral acyclovir therapy. Ann Intern Med 104:786–790, 1986.

231. SE Straus, M Siedin, HE Takiff, JF Rooney, JM Felser, HA Smith, P Roane, F Johnson, C Hallahan, JM Ostrove, et al. Effect of oral acyclovir treatment on symptomatic and asymptomatic shedding in recurrent genital herpes. Sex Transm Dis 16:107–113, 1989.

232. A Wald, J Zeh, G Barnum, LG Davis, L Corey. Suppression of subclinical shedding of herpes simplex virus type 2 with acyclovir. Ann Intern Med 124:8–15, 1996.

233. A Wald, L Corey, R Cone, A Hobson, G Davis, J Zeh. Frequent genital herpes simplex 2 shedding in immunocompetent women. Effect of acyclovir treatment. J Clin Invest 99:1092–1097, 1997.

234. J Amir, L Harel, Z Smetana, I Varsano. Treatment of herpes simplex gingivostomatitis with aciclovir in children: a randomised double blind placebo controlled study. BMJ 314:1800–1803, 1997.

235. PA Fiddian, JM Yeo, R Stubblings, D Dean. Successful treatment of herpes labialis with topical acyclovir. BMJ 286:1699–1701, 1983.

236. SL Spruance, LE Schnipper, JC Overall, ER Kern, B Wester, J Modlin. Treatment of herpes simplex labialis with topical acyclovir in polyethylene glycol. J Infect Dis 146:85–90, 1982.

237. M Shaw, M King, JM Best, JE Banatvala, JR Gibson, MR Klaber. Failure of acyclovir cream in treatment of recurrent herpes labialis. BMJ 291:7–9, 1985.

238. JR Gibson, MR Klaber, SG Harvey, A Tosti, D Jones, JM Yeo. Prophylaxis against herpes labialis with acyclovir cream. A placebo controlled study. Dermatologica 172: 104–107, 1986.

239. GW Raborn, WT McGaw, M Grace, LD Tyrrell, SM Samuels. Oral acyclovir and herpes labialis: a randomized, double-blind, placebo-controlled study. J Am Dent Assoc 115: 38–42, 1987.

240. SL Spruance, JC Stewart, NH Rowe, MB McKeough, G Wenerstrom, DJ Freeman. Treatment of recurrent herpes simplex labialis with oral acyclovir. J Infect Dis 161: 185–190, 1990.

241. SL Spruance, ML Hamill, WS Hoge, G Davis, J Mills. Acyclovir prevents reactivation of herpes simplex labialis in skiers. JAMA 260:1597–1599, 1988.

242. JF Rooney, SE Straus, ML Mannix, CR Wohlenberg, DW Alling, JA Dumois, AL Notkins. Oral acyclovir to suppress frequently recurrent herpes labialis. A double-blind, placebo-controlled trial. Ann Intern Med 118:268–272, 1993.

243. JC Wade, B Newton, C McLaren, N Flournoy, RE Keeney, JD Meyers. Intravenous acyclovir to treat mucocutaneous herpes simplex virus infection after marrow transplantation: double-blind trial. Ann Intern Med 96:265–269, 1982.

244. JD Meyers, JC Wade, CD Mitchell, R Saral, PS Lietman, DT Durack, MJ Levin, AC Segreti, HH Balfour Jr. Multicenter collaborative trial of intravenous acyclovir for treatment of mucocutaneous herpes simplex virus infection in the immunocompromised host. Am J Med 73:229–235, 1982.

245. DH Shepp, BA Newton, PS Dandliker, N Flornoy, JD Meyers. Oral acyclovir therapy for mucocutaneous herpes simplex virus infections in immunocompromised marrow transplant recipients. Ann Intern Med 102:783–785, 1985.

246. JC Wade, B Newton, N Flournoy, JD Meyers. Oral acyclovir for prevention of herpes simplex virus reactivation after marrow transplantation. Ann Intern Med 100: 823–828, 1984.

247. IM Hann, HG Prentice, HA Blacklock, MG Ross, D Brigden, AE Rosling, C Burke, DH Crawford, W Brumfitt, AV Hoffbrand. Acyclovir prophylaxis against herpes virus infections in severely immunocompromised patients: randomised double-blind trial. BMJ 287:384–388, 1983.

248. R Saral, RF Ambinder, WH Burns. Acyclovir prophylaxis against simplex virus infection in patients with leukemia. Ann Intern Med 99:773–776, 1983.

249. DH Shepp, PS Dandliker, N Flournoy, JD Meyers. Sequential intravenous and twice-daily oral acyclovir for extended prophylaxis of herpes simplex virus infection in marrow transplant patients. Transplantation 43:654–658, 1987.

250. JC Wade, C McLaren, JD Meyers. Frequency and significance of acyclovir-resistant herpes simplex virus isolated from marrow transplant patients receiving multiple courses of treatment with acyclovir. J Infect Dis 148:1077–1082, 1983.

251. RJ Whitley, A Arvin, C Prober, S Burchett, L Corey, D Powell, S Plotkin, S Starr, C Alford, J Connor, et al. A controlled trial comparing vidarabine with acyclovir in neonatal herpes simplex virus infection. N Engl J Med 324:444–449, 1991.

252. LT Gutman, CM Wilfert, S Eppes. Herpes simplex virus encephalitis in children: analysis of cerebrospinal fluid and progressive neurodevelopmental deterioration. J Infect Dis 154:415–421, 1986.

253. RJ Whitley, CA Alford Jr, MS Hirsch, RT Schooley, JP Luby, FY Aoki, D Hanley, AJ Nahmias, SJ Soong. Vidarabine versus acyclovir therapy in herpes simplex encephalitis. N Engl J Med 314:144–149, 1986.

254. RJ Whitley, JW Gnann. The epidemiology and clinical manifestations of herpes simplex virus infections. In: B Roizman, RJ Whitley, C Lopez, eds. The human herpes viruses. New York: Raven Press, 1993, pp 69–105.

255. MK Sherry, AS Klainer, M Wolff, H Gerhard. Herpetic tracheobronchitis. Ann Intern Med 109:229–232, 1988.

256. M Niimura, T Nishikawa. Treatment of eczema herpeticum with oral acyclovir. Am J Med 85:49–52, 1988.

257. OL Laskin. Acyclovir and suppression of frequently recurring herpetic whitlow. Ann Intern Med 102:494–495, 1985.

258. DM Speigal, K Lau. Acute renal failure and coma secondary to acyclovir therapy. JAMA 155:1882–1883, 1986.

259. MG Bianchetti, C Roduit, OH Oetliker. Acyclovir induced renal failure: course and risk factors. Pediatr Nephrol 5: 238–239, 1991.

260. D Brigden, AE Rosling, NC Woods. Renal function after acyclovir intravenous injection. Am J Med 73:182–185, 1982.

261. JC Huff, B Bean, HH Balfour, OL Laskin, JD Connor, L Corey, YJ Bryson, P McGuirt. Therapy of herpes zoster with oral acyclovir. Am J Med 85:84–89, 1988.

262. JC Wade, JD Meyers. Neurologic symptoms associated with parenteral acyclovir treatment after bone marrow transplantation. Ann Intern Med 98:921–925, 1983.

263. SMZ Cohen, JA Minkove, WJ Zebley, JH Mulholland. Severe but reversible neurotoxicity from acyclovir. Ann Intern Med 100:920, 1984.

264. EB Andrews, HH Tilson, BA Hurn, JF Cordero. Acyclovir in Pregnancy Registry. An observational epidemiological approach. Am J Med 85:123–128, 1988.

265. Pregnancy outcomes following systemic prenatal acyclovir exposure—June 1, 1984–June 30, 1993. Arch Dermatol 130;153–154, 1994.

266. LM Frenkel, ZA Brown, YJ Bryson, L Corey, JD Unadkat, PA Hensleigh, AM Arvin, CG Prober, JD Connor. Pharmacokinetics of acyclovir in the term human pregnancy and neonate. Am J Obstet Gynecol 164:569–576, 1991.

267. LL Scott, PJ Sanchez, GL Jackson, F Zeray, GD Wendel Jr. Acyclovir suppression to prevent cesarean delivery after first-episode genital herpes. Obstet Gynecol 87: 69–73, 1996.

268. P Brocklehurst, G Kinghorn, O Carney, K Helsen, E Ross,

E Ellis, R Shen, F Cowan, A Mindel. A randomized placebo controlled trial of suppressive acyclovir in late pregnancy in women with recurrent genital herpes infection. Br J Obstet Gynecol 105:275–280, 1998.

269. B Stray-Pedersen. Acyclovir in late pregnancy to prevent neonatal herpes simplex. Lancet 336:756, 1990.

270. J Soul Lawton, E Seaber, N On, R Wootton, P Rolan, J Posner. Absolute bioavailability and metabolic disposition of valaciclovir, the L-valyl ester of acyclovir, following oral administration to humans. Antimicrob Agents Chemother 39:2759–2764, 1995.

271. KH Fife, RA Barbarash, T Rudolph, B Degregario, R Roth. Valaciclovir versus acyclovir in the treatment of first-episode genital herpes infection. Results of an international, multicenter, double-blind, randomized clinical trial. Sex Transm Dis 24:481–486, 1997.

272. SK Tyring, JM Douglas Jr, C Lawrence, SL Spruance, J Esmann. A randomized, placebo-controlled comparison of oral valacyclovir and acyclovir in immunocompetent patients with recurrent genital herpes infections. Arch Dermatol 134:185–191, 1998.

273. M Reitano, S Tyring, W Lang, C Thoming, AM Worm, S Borelli, LO Chambers, JM Robinson, L Corey. Valacyclovir for the suppression of recurrent genital herpes simplex virus infection: a large-scale dose range-finding study. J Infect Dis 178:603–610, 1998.

274. NJ Bodsworth, RJ Crooks, S Berell, G Vejlsgaard, J Paavonen, AM Worm, N Uexkull, J Esmann, A Strand, AJ Ingamells, A Gibb. Valaciclovir versus Acyclovir in patient-initiated treatment of recurrent genital herpes: A randomized, double-blind trial. Genitourin Med 73:110–160, 1997.

275. SL Spruance, SK Tyring, B DeGregoria, C Miller, K Beutner. A large-scale, placebo-controlled, dose-ranging trial of peroral valaciclovir for episodic treatment of recurrent herpes genitalis. Arch Intern Med 156:1729–1735, 1996.

276. P Leone, S Trottier, J Miller, International Valaciclovir Study Group. A comparison of oral valaciclovir 500 mg twice daily for three or five days in the treatment of recurrent genital herpes. International Congress of Infectious Diseases, Boston, MA, May 15–18, 1998.

277. R Patel, NJ Bodsworth, P Woolley, B Peters, G Vejlsgaard, S Saari, A Gibb, J Robinson. Valaciclovir for the suppression of recurrent genital HSV infection: a placebo-controlled study of once daily therapy. Genitourin Med 73: 105–109, 1997.

278. D Baker. Valaciclovir for the suppression of herpes labialis. Program and abstracts of the 40th Interscience Conference on Antimicrobial Agents and Chemotherapy, Toronto, Canada, September, 2000.

279. T Schacker and the International Valaciclovir HSV Study Group. Valaciclovir as acute treatment for recurrent anogenital herpes in immunocompromised (HIV positive) individuals. 13th Meeting of the International Society for Sexually Transmitted Diseases Research, July 11–14, 1999. Denver, CO, Abstract 365.

280. MA Conant, T Schacker, RL Murphy, J Gold, LT Crutchfield, RJ Crooks. Valaciclovir versus aciclovir for herpes simplex virus infection in HIV-infected individuals—two double-blind controlled trials. Int J Std AIDS 13:12–21, 2002.

281. DL Earnshaw, TH Bacon, SJ Darlison, K Edmonds, RM Perkins, RA Vere Hodge. Mode of antiviral action of penciclovir in MRC-5 cells infected with herpes simplex virus type 1 (HSV-1), HSV-2, and varicella-zoster virus. Antimicrob Agents Chemother 36:2747–2757, 1992.

282. SL Sacks, F Aoki, F Diaz-Mitoma, J Sellors, SD Shafran. Patient-initiated, twice-daily oral famciclovir for early recurrent genital herpes. A randomized, double-blind multicenter trial. JAMA 276:44–49, 1996.

283. M Loveless, W Harris, S Sacks. Treatment of first episode genital herpes with famciclovir. Presented before the American Society for Microbiology, 35th ICAAC Meeting, San Francisco, CA. September 1995, Session 8, Abstract 412.

284. SL Sacks, A Hughes, B Rennie, R Boon. Famciclovir (FCV) for suppression of asymptomatic (Asx) and symptomatic (Sx) recurrent genital herpes (RGN) shedding: a randomized double-blind, double dummy, parallel-group, placebo-controlled trial [abstract]. Presented at the 37th Interscience Conference on Antimicrobial Agents and Chemotherapy September 28–October 1, 1997, Toronto, Ontario.

285. F Diaz-Mitoma, RG Sibbald, SD Shafran, R Boon, RL Saltzman. Oral famciclovir for the suppression of recurrent genital herpes: a randomized controlled trial. JAMA 280: 887–892, 1998.

286. GJ Mertz, MO Loveless, MJ Levin, SJ Kraus, SL Fowler, D Goade, SK Tyring. Oral famciclovir for suppression of recurrent genital herpes simplex virus infection in women. A multicenter, double-blind, placebo-controlled trial. Arch Intern Med 157:343–349, 1997.

287. SL Spruance, NH Rowe, GW Raborn, EA Thibodeau, JA D'Ambrosio, DI Bernstein. Peroral famciclovir in the treatment of experimental ultraviolet radiation-induced herpes simplex labialis: a double-blind, dose-ranging, placebo-controlled, multicenter trial. J Infect Dis 179: 303–310, 1999.

288. SL Spruance, MB McKeough. Combination treatment with famciclovir and a topical corticosteroid gel versus famciclovir alone for experimental ultraviolet radiation-induced herpes simplex labialis: A pilot study. J Infect Dis 181:1906–1910, 2000.

289. SH Wall, SJ Ramey, F Wall. Famciclovir as antiviral prophylaxis in laser resurfacing procedures. Plast Reconstr Surg 104:1103–1108, 1999.

290. SL Spruance, TL Rea, C Thoming, R Tucker, R Saltzman, R Boon. Penciclovir cream for the treatment of herpes simplex labialis. A randomized, multicenter, double-blind, placebo-controlled trial. JAMA 277:1374–1379, 1997.

291. G Frechette, B Ramanawski. Efficacy and safety of famciclovir for the treatment of HSV infection in HIV + patients. Presented at the Sixth Annual Canadian Conference

on HIV/AIDS Research, May 22–25, 1997, Oral Presentation 301, Ottawa, Ontario.

292. T Schacker, HL Hu, DM Koelle, J Zeh, R Saltzman, R Boon, M Shaughnessy, G Barnum, L Corey. Famciclovir for the suppression of symptomatic and asymptomatic herpes simplex virus reactivation in HIV-infected persons. A double-blind, placebo-controlled trial. Ann Intern Med 128:21–28, 1998.

293. CS Crumpacker. Mechanism of action of foscarnet against viral polymerases. Am J Med 92(suppl 2A):3S–7S, 1992.

294. FA Pereira. Herpes simplex: evolving concepts. J Am Acad Dermatol 35:503–520, 1996.

295. B Oberg. Antiviral effects of phosphonoformate (PFA, foscarnet sodium). Pharmacol Ther 40:213–285, 1989.

296. TA Schiff, AB Bodian, MR Buchness. Foscarnet-induced penile ulceration. Int J Dermatol 32:526–527, 1993.

297. AS Gross, RH Dretler. Foscarnet-induced penile ulcer in an uncircumcised patient with AIDS [letter]. Clin Infect Dis 17:1076–1077, 1993.

298. LM Evans, ME Grossman. Foscarnet-induced penile ulcer. J Am Acad Dermatol 27:124–126, 1992.

299. JW Van Der Pijl, PH Frissen, P Reiss, HJ Hulsebosch, JG Van Den Tweel, JM Lange, SA Danner. Foscarnet and penile ulceration [letter]. Lancet 335:286, 1990.

300. E Fitzgerald, HM Goldman, WG Miller, SM Purcell. A penile ulceration in a patient with the acquired immunodeficiency syndrome. Foscarnet-induced penile ulceration. Arch Dermatol 131:1449–1452, 1995.

301. G Moyle, S Barton, BG Gazzard. Penile ulceration with foscarnet therapy [letter]. AIDS 7:140–141, 1993.

302. SL Sacks, SD Shafran, F Diaz-Mitoma, S Trottier, RG Sibbald, A Hughes, S Safrin, J Rudy, B McGuire, HS Jaffe. A multicenter, phase I/II dose escalation study of single-dose cidofovir gel for treatment of recurrent genital herpes. Antimicrob Agents Chemother 42:2996–2999, 1998.

303. CM Martinez, DB Luks-Golger. Cidofovir in ACV-resistant herpes infections. Ann Pharmacother 31:1519–1521, 1997.

304. J Lalezari, T Schacker, J Feinberg, J Gathe, S Lee, T Cheung, F Kramer, H Kessler, L Corey, WL Drew, J Boggs, B McGuire, HS Jaffe, S Safrin. A randomized, double-blind, placebo-controlled trial of cidofovir gel for the treatment of acyclovir-unresponsive mucocutaneous herpes simplex virus infection in patients with AIDS. J Infect Dis 176:892–898, 1997.

305. L Habbema. *N*-docosanol 10% cream in the treatment of recurrent herpes labialis: A randomized double-blind, placebo-controlled study. ACTA Derm Venereol (Stockh) 76: 479–481, 1996.

306. SL Spruance, S Tyring, M Smith, T Meng. Application of a topical immune response modifier, resiquimod gel, to modify the recurrence rate of recurrent genital herpes: A pilot study. J Infect Dis 184:196–200, 2001.

307. SL Sacks, J Portony, D Lawee, W Schlech 3rd, FY Aoki, DL Tyrrell, M Poisson, C Bright, J Kaluski, and the Canadian Cooperative Study Group. Clinical course of recurrent genital herpes and treatment with foscarnet cream: results of a Canadian multicenter trial. J Infect Dis 155:178–186, 1987.

308. SL Sacks, LD Tyrrell, D Lawee, W Schlech 3rd, MJ Gill, FY Aoki, AY Martel, J Singer. Randomized double-blind, placebo-controlled, clinic-initiated, Canadian multicenter trial of topical edoxudine 3.0% cream in the treatment of recurrent genital herpes. J Infect Dis 164:665–672, 1991.

309. TM Rallis, SL Spruance. Low-intensity laser therapy for recurrent herpes labialis. J Invest Dermatol 115:131–132, 2000.

310. LH Kaminester, RJ Pariser, DM Pariser, JS Weiss, JS Shavin, L Landsman, HG Haines, DW Osborne. A double-blind, placebo-controlled study of topical tetracaine in the treatment of herpes labialis. J Am Acad Dermatol 41: 996–1001, 1999.

311. T Hovi, A Hirvimies, M Stenvik, E Vuola, R Pippuri. Topical treatment of recurrent mucocutaneous herpes with ascorbic acid-containing solution. Antiviral Res 27: 263–270, 1995.

312. R Boon, JJ Goodman, J Martinez, GL Marks, M Gamble, C Welch. Penciclovir cream for the treatment of sunlight-induced herpes simplex labialis: a randomized, double-blind, placebo-controlled trial. Clin Ther 22:76–90, 2000.

313. G Hovding. A comparison between acyclovir and trifluro-thymidine ophthalmic ointment in the treatment of epithelial dendritic keratitis: a double-blind, randomized parallel group trial. Acta Ophthalmol 67:51–54, 1989.

314. PR Laibson, D Pavan-Langston, WR Yeakley, J Lass. Acyclovir and vidarabine for the treatment of herpes simplex keratitis. Am J Med 73:281–285, 1982.

315. LM Collum, P Logan, IB Hillary, T Ravenscroft. Acyclovir in herpes keratitis. Am J Med 73:290–293, 1982.

316. WH Burns, R Saral, GW Santos, OL Laskin, PS Lietman, C McLaren, DW Barry. Isolation and characterization of resistant herpes simplex virus after acyclovir therapy. Lancet 1:421–423, 1982.

317. SM Swetter, EL Hill, ER Kern, DM Koelle, CM Posavad, W Lawrence, S Safrin. Chronic vulvar ulceration in an immunocompetent woman due to acyclovir-resistant, thymidine kinase-deficient herpes simplex virus. J Infect Dis 177:543–550, 1998.

318. CS Crumpacker, LE Schnipper, SI Marlowe, PN Kowalsky, BJ Herskey, MJ Levin. Resistance to antiviral drugs of herpes simplex virus isolated from a patient treated with acyclovir. N Engl J Med 306:343–346, 1982.

319. JC Pottage Jr, HA Kessler. Herpes simplex virus resistance to acyclovir: clinical relevance. Infect Agents Dis 4: 115–124, 1995.

320. CD Sibrack, LT Gutman, CM Wilfert, C McLaren, MH St Clair, PM Keller, DW Barry. Pathogenicity of acyclovir-resistant herpes simplex virus type 1 from an immunodeficient child. J Infect Dis 146:673–682, 1982.

321. EL Hill, GA Hunter, MN Ellis. In vitro and in vivo characterization of herpes simplex virus clinical isolates re-

covered from patients infected with human immunodeficiency virus. Antimicrob Agents Chemother 35: 2322–2328, 1991.

322. J Christophers, J Clayton, J Craske, R Ward, P Collins, M Trowbridge, G Darby. Survey of resistance of herpes simplex virus to acyclovir in northwest England. Antimicrob Agents Chemother 42:868–872, 1998.

323. JA Englund, ME Zimmerman, EM Swierkosz, JL Goodman, DR Scholl, HH Balfour Jr. Herpes simplex resistance to acyclovir: a study in a tertiary care centre. Ann Intern Med 112:416–422, 1990.

324. P Reusser. Virostatika-Resistenz bei Herpesviren: Mechanismen, Haufigkeit und klinische Bedeutung. Schweiz Med Wochenschr 124;152–158, 1994.

325. SL Sacks, RJ Wanklin, DE Reece, KA Hicks, KL Tyler, DM Coen. Progressive esophagitis from acyclovir-resistant herpes simplex. Clinical roles for DNA polymerase mutants and viral heterogeneity. Ann Intern Med 111: 893–899, 1989.

326. KS Erlich, J Mills, P Chatis, GJ Mertz, DF Busch, SE Follansbee, RM Grant, CS Crumpacker. Acyclovir-resistant herpes simplex virus infections in patients with the acquired immunodeficiency syndrome. N Engl J Med 320: 293–296, 1989.

327. S Safrin, C Crumpacker, P Chatis, R Davis, R Hafner, J Rush, HA Kessler, B Landry, J Mills. A controlled trial comparing foscarnet with vidarabine for acyclovir-resistant mucocutaneous herpes simplex in the acquired immunodeficiency syndrome. N Engl J Med 325:551–555, 1991.

328. KS Erlich, MA Jacobson, JE Koehler. Foscarnet therapy for severe acyclovir-resistant herpes simplex virus type-2 infections in patients with the acquired immunodeficiency syndrome (AIDS). Ann Intern Med 110:710–713, 1989.

329. P Ljungman, MN Ellis, RC Hackman, DH Shepp, JD Meyers. Acyclovir-resistant herpes simplex virus causing pneumonia after marrow transplantation. J Infect Dis 162: 711–715, 1990.

330. A Gateley, RM Gander, PC Jonson, S Kit, H Otsuka, S Kohl. Herpes simplex virus type 2 meningoencephalitis resistant to acyclovir in a patient with AIDS. J Infect Dis 161:711–715, 1990.

331. J Triebwasser, R Harris, RE Bryant, ER Rhoades. Varicella pneumonia in adults: report of seven cases and review of the literature. Medicine 46:409–420, 1967.

332. GL Marks, PE Nolen, KS Erlich, MN Ellis. Mucocutaneous dissemination of acyclovir-resistant herpes simplex virus in a patient with AIDS. Rev Infect Dis 11:474–476, 1989.

333. LF Verdonck, JJ Cornelissen, J Smit, J Lepoutre, GC de Gast, AW Dekker, M Rozenberg-Arska. Successful foscarnet therapy for acyclovir-resistant mucocutaneous infection with herpes simplex virus in a recipient of allogeneic BMT. Bone Marrow Transplant 11:177–179, 1993.

334. TJ Jones, R Paul. Disseminated acyclovir-resistant herpes simplex virus type 2 treated successfully with foscarnet [letter]. J Infect Dis 171:508–509, 1995.

335. RG Kost, EL Hill, M Tigges, SE Straus. Brief report: recurrent acyclovir-resistant genital herpes in an immunocompetent patient. N Engl J Med 329:1777–1182, 1993.

336. S Safrin, S Kemmerly, B Plotkin, T Smith, N Weissbach, D De Veranez, LD Phan, D Cohn. Foscarnet-resistant herpes simplex virus infection in patients with AIDS. J Infect Dis 169:193–196, 1994.

337. CJ Birch, DP Tyssen, G Tachedjian, R Doherty, K Hayes, A Mijch, CR Lucas. Clinical effects and in vitro studies of trifluorothymidine combined with interferon-alpha for treatment of drug-resistant and -sensitive herpes simplex virus infection. J Infect Dis 166:108–112, 1992.

338. E Pelosi, KA Hicks, SL Sacks, DM Coen. Heterogeneity of a herpes simplex virus clinical isolate exhibiting resistance to acyclovir and foscarnet. Adv Exp Med Biol 312: 151–158, 1992.

339. R Snoeck, G Andrei, M Gérard, A Hedderman, J Balzarini, C Sadzot-Delvaux, G Tricot, N Clumeck, E De Clercq. Successful treatment of progressive mucocutaneous infection due to acyclovir- and foscarnet-resistant herpes simplex virus with (S)-1-(3-hydroxy-2-phosphonylmethoxypropyl)cytosine (HPMPC). Clin Infect Dis 18:570–578, 1994.

340. RJ Whitley, B Meignier. Herpes simplex vaccines. In: RW Ellis, ed. Vaccines: New Approaches to Immunological Problems. Boston: Butterworth Publishers, 1991, p 254.

341. RL Burke. Current status of HSV vaccine development. In: B Roizman, JR Whitley, C Lopez, eds. The Human Herpesviruses. New York: Raven Press, 1993, pp 367–379.

342. LR Stanberry, AL Cunningham, A Mindel, LL Scott, SL Spruance, FY Aoki, CJ Lacey. Prospects for control of herpes simplex virus disease through immunization. Clin Infect Dis 30:549–566, 2000.

343. PR Krause, SE Straus. Herpesvirus vaccines. Development, controversies, and applications. Infect Dis Clin North Am 13:61–81, 1999.

344. LR Stanberry. Control of STDs—the role of prophylactic vaccines against herpes simplex virus. Sex Transm Infect 74:391–394, 1998.

345. DI Bernstein, LR Stanberry. Herpes simplex virus vaccines. Vaccine 17:1681–1689, 1999.

346. LR Stanberry. Herpes. Vaccines for HSV. Dermatol Clin 16:811–816, 1998.

347. L Corey, AGM Langenberg, R Ashley, RE Sekulovich, AE Izu, JM Douglas Jr, HH Handsfield, T Warren, L Marr, S Tyring, R DiCarlo, AA Adimora, P Leone, CL Dekker, RL Burke, WP Leong, SE Straus. Recombinant glycoprotein vaccine for the prevention of genital HSV-2 infection: Two randomized controlled trials. JAMA 282:331–340, 1999.

348. SE Straus, L Corey, RL Burke, B Savarese, G Barnum, PR Krause, RG Kost, JL Meier, R Sekulovich, SF Adair, et al. Placebo-controlled trial of vaccination with recombinant glycoprotein D of herpes simplex virus type 2 for immunotherapy of genital herpes. Lancet 343:1460–1463, 1994.

349. MA Conant, DW Spicer, CD Smith. Herpes simplex virus transmission: condom studies. Sex Transm Dis 11:94–95, 1984.

350. H Ward, S Day, J Weber. Risky business: health and safety in the sex industry over a 9 year period. Sex Transm Infect 75:340–343, 1999.

351. A Wald, J Zeh, S Selke, RL Ashley, L Corey. Virologic characteristics of subclinical and symptomatic genital herpes infections. N Engl J Med 333:770–775, 1995.

352. MR Krone, A Wald, SR Tabet, M Paradise, L Corey, CL Celum. Herpes simplex virus type 2 shedding in human immunodeficiency virus-negative men who have sex with men: frequency, patterns, and risk factors. Clin Infect Dis 30:261–267, 2000.

353. A Wald, AGM Langenberg, K Link, A Izu, R Ashley, T Warren, S Tyring, JM Douglas, Jr, L. Corey. Effects of condoms on reducing the transmission of herpes simplex virus type-2 from men to women. JAMA 285:3100–3106, 2001.

5

Varicella-Zoster Virus (Herpes 3)

Monica McCrary
Medical College of Georgia, Augusta, Georgia, USA

Tricia J. Brown
University of Oklahoma Health Sciences Center, Oklahoma City, Oklahoma, USA

Stephen K. Tyring
University of Texas Medical Branch, Galveston, Texas, USA,
and University of Texas Medical Branch Center for Clinical Studies, Houston Texas, USA

Varicella-zoster virus (VZV) is a unique virus, occurring worldwide (Fig. 5–1), that causes two different clinical syndromes: chickenpox (varicella) and shingles (herpes zoster). Primary infection with varicella is typically a self-limited disease of childhood characterized by a pruritic rash. Herpes zoster, predominantly a disease affecting adults, is caused by reactivation of the latent virus. The associated pain during and after zoster infection may lead to significant impairment in affected persons. Varicella and zoster in immunocompromised individuals can often be severe and cause significant illnesses.

HISTORY

Up to the nineteenth century, varicella was frequently confused with smallpox infection. In 1767, Heberden first clearly distinguished the two illnesses [1]. However, in 1892 in his book on clinical medicine, Osler still saw the need to emphasize the distinction between the two diseases [2]. The origin of the name chickenpox is not completely known although it may come from the French word "chiche-pois" used to describe the "chick-pea" size varicella vesicles [3]. Alternatively, the word may have been derived from the Old English word "gican," which means "to itch" [4].

Since ancient times, herpes zoster has been recognized as a separate clinical disease [5]. The origin of the word herpes is derived from the Greek word meaning "to creep." Zoster is derived from the Greek and Latin words meaning "girdle" or "belt" [6].

The association between the varicella and zoster diseases was first postulated by von Bokay in 1888, who noted that varicella often developed in susceptible children following exposure to a patient with herpes zoster infection [7]. Kundratiz (1922) and Bruusgarrd (1932) were then able to show that the same agent was the cause of both diseases by successfully inoculating children with vesicle fluid from patients with zoster [8]. These experiments produced localized varicella lesions at the site of inoculation in some recipients and a generalized varicella-like exanthem in others. The etiology of varicella and herpes zoster was proved later to be identical by Weller, et al., through isolation and propagation of the viruses in vitro [9,10].

INCIDENCE

Infection with varicella occurs worldwide. The virus is more transmittable in temperate climates than in tropical environments. This phenomenon results in unique epide-

GEOGRAPHICAL INCIDENCE

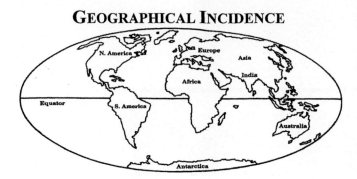

TAXONOMY

Alphaherpesviridae

TRANSMISSION

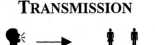

Respiratory   **Humans**
secretions

ZOONOTIC IMPLICATIONS

None

Humans are the only reservoir

Figure 5–1. Incidence and transmission of varicella-zoster virus (herpes 3).

miologic differences among regions [11]. In temperate climates varicella is typically a disease of childhood, whereas in tropical regions the infection more commonly occurs in susceptible adults.

Herpes zoster infection primarily affects adults older than 50 years of age but may occur at any age. Persons with a history of primary varicella infection have a 20% lifetime chance of later developing herpes zoster infection. The incidence and duration of zoster infection increases significantly with age [12]. The annual incidence from ages 20 to 50 years is 2.5 per 1000 persons and increases to 5 per 1000 persons for ages 51 to 79. This incidence doubles again for persons older than 80 years of age (10 per 1000). Zoster infection rarely occurs in childhood, but it is more

frequent in children who had primary varicella infection in the first year of life. As many as 35% of bone marrow transplantation recipients develop zoster within one year after transplantation [13].

PATHOGENESIS

Varicella disease is one of the most contagious infections; 80 to 90% of susceptible household contacts develop clinical infection after exposure to the infected individual [14]. The varicella-zoster virus is transmitted by respiratory droplets from the nasopharynx or by contact with infected skin lesions. Patients with varicella are infectious from 2 days prior to and 5 days after the onset of the rash. Dry crusted scabs are not infectious. Patients with zoster are infectious from the skin lesions and sometimes from the nasopharynx. Susceptible contacts of these patients may develop primary varicella infection. There is no evidence that herpes zoster illness can be acquired directly from contact with patients with varicella or zoster infection [12,15,16].

After exposure to the virus, primary varicella initially colonizes the conjunctiva or the mucosa of the upper respiratory tract. The first cycle of viral replication occurs in the regional lymph nodes 2–4 days after exposure, followed by primary viremia that develops 4–6 days after exposure. After the viremia, a second cycle of viral replication occurs in the liver, spleen, and other organs. A secondary viremia then develops, seeding the entire body with viral particles. These virions progressively invade the capillary endothelial cells, the capillaries, and the epidermis 14–16 days following exposure [17].

During the course of primary varicella infection, the virus travels from the skin and mucosal lesions into the sensory nerve endings. The varicella-zoster virus then spreads centripetally along nerve fibers to establish a permanent latent state in the dorsal ganglion cells. The exact pathogenesis and reactivation of herpes zoster disease is not completely understood. A decline in virus-specific, cell-mediated immunity, particularly a decrease in T-cell proliferation, to the varicella-zoster virus antigen may be part of the process [18]. Decreased cell-mediated immunity is typically seen in elderly persons or those with immunocompromised conditions, such as human immunodeficiency virus (HIV) infection or organ transplantation or treatment with chemotherapy, radiotherapy [19], or long-term corticosteroids [20]. In the first year following transplantation, 20 to 40% of bone marrow transplant recipients develop herpes zoster [17,21–23]. Similarly, 20 to 50% of patients with Hodgkin's disease develop herpes zoster [24–31], usually within 1 month of induction chemotherapy or 7 months of radiotherapy [32]. Herpes zoster disease also may be the first sign of infection with HIV [33,34]. This patient population may present with atypical or recurrent varicella disease [35–41].

After reactivation of the varicella-zoster virus, the virus undergoes an initial replication cycle in the affected sensory ganglion, which produces active ganglionitis. Severe neuralgia results from the inflammatory response and the neuronal necrosis that occurs. As the virus spreads down the sensory nerve, the pain intensifies and produces radiculoneuritis.

CLINICAL MANIFESTATIONS OF VARICELLA

Primary varicella is usually a mild and self-limited disease in immunocompetent children (Figs. 5–2 to 5–9). Signifi-

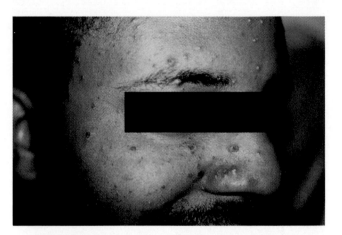

Figure 5–3. Primary varicella in an adult.

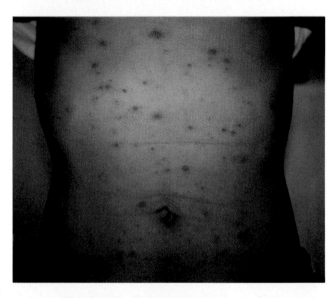

Figure 5–4. Primary varicella in an adult.

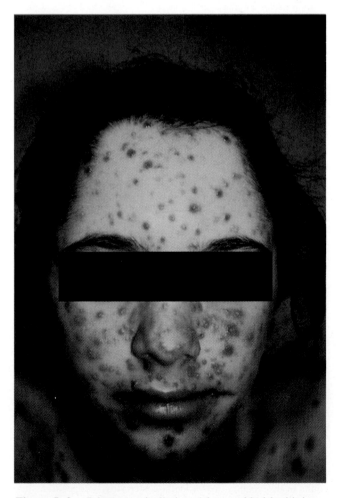

Figure 5–2. Primary varicella in a 16-year-old girl with juvenile rheumatoid arthritis.

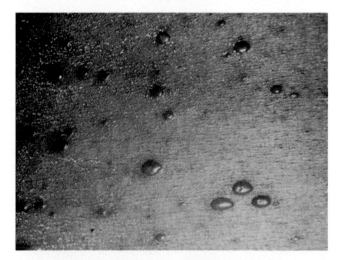

Figure 5–5. Vesicles of primary varicella.

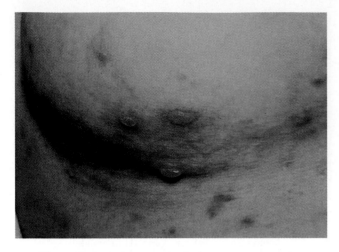

Figure 5–6. Primary varicella in a pregnant woman.

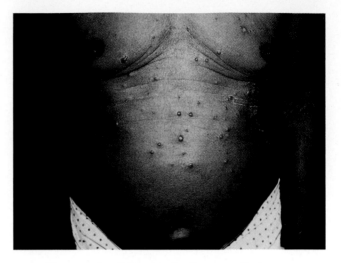

Figure 5–8. Primary varicella in an elderly man.

cant morbidity may sometimes occur, with 11,000 hospitalizations each year in the United States due to complications of varicella infection in children who are often otherwise healthy. Susceptible adults typically develop more frequent complications, more profuse skin lesions, and more prominent constitutional symptoms, such as prolonged fever (Tables 5–1 and 5–2).

Primary varicella infection may result in multiple complications. The most common complication is bacterial superinfection, usually caused by staphylococcus or streptococcus. The superinfection may manifest as cellulitis, impetigo, erysipelas, furuncles, or bullous lesions resulting from the bacterial production of staphylococcal exfoliative toxin [42] (Fig. 5–10). Bacterial infection frequently results in scarring but rarely leads to septicemia [43]. Central nervous system complications occur in less than 1 in 1000 cases and may include Reye's syndrome, acute cerebellar ataxia, encephalitis, meningoencephalitis, polyradiculitis, myelitis, and Guillain-Barré syndrome [44]. Reye's syndrome is rare since aspirin is no longer recommended for

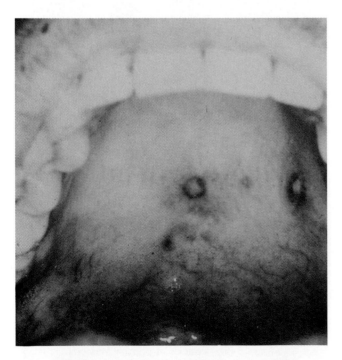

Figure 5–7. Oral vesicles of primary varicella.

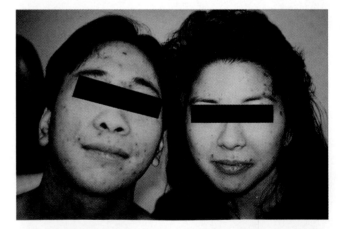

Figure 5–9. Husband and wife with primary varicella. Since both persons were born in the United States and over 90% of adults in this country are varicella-zoster virus seropositive, this is an unusual situation. In this case, the wife acquired primary varicella during her hospital employment. Her husband developed vesicles of primary varicella approximately 2 weeks later.

Table 5–1. Clinical Manifestations of Varicella

Time After Exposure	Clinical Manifestations	Laboratory Analysis	Other Notes
14–15 days	Occasional prodrome symptoms lasting 2–3 days: low-grade fever, chills, headache malaise, backache, anorexia, myalgia, nausea, or vomiting ↓	Tzanck smear of lesion scraping but does not differentiate from varicella or herpes simplex.	Older children and adults may have prodrome symptoms. Younger children usually have an abrupt onset of rash with mild fever and malaise.
16–17 days	Rash with crops of small red macules, beginning on the face and scalp, and spreading rapidly to the trunk. Relative sparing of the distal upper and lower extremities. ↓	Viral culture, serology, and direct immunofluorescense.	Pruritus typically occurs with the rash.
16–17 days	Rash progresses over 12–14 hours to 1–3 mm papules, vesicles, and then pustules. ↓		Vesicles are classically described as "dew drops on a rose petal" (clear serous fluid surrounded by a small red halo). Most children have 250–500 lesions, mostly vesicular.
17–19 days	Crust formation ↓		
23–27 days	Healing		Scarring is rare in uncomplicated cases.

children with varicella or other infections. Varicella pneumonia can be a complication in adults (Fig. 5–11). In a study of otherwise healthy military recruits with varicella, radiographic evidence of pneumonia was found in 16%, but only 4% of subjects had clinical evidence of pulmonary

Table 5–2. Differential Diagnoses of Varicella

Smallpox: Historically, smallpox has been an important differential diagnosis, but no longer occurs.
Herpes simplex virus: Disseminated disease may sometimes mimic varicella, but herpes simplex typically has a predominance of localized vesicle clusters at the primary site of infection.
Hand-foot-and-mouth disease: Lesions are more prominent on the mucous membranes of the mouth and on the distal extremities with hand-foot-and-mouth disease.
Insect bites: Insect bites typically occur on the extremities and have an underlying wheal.
Drug eruption: Fever does not occur; simultaneous appearance of multiple types of lesions is rare.
Scabies: More chronic development of the lesions, which tend to appear in body folds and often have a linear distribution.
Contact dermatitis: Pustules do not tend to form and fever does not occur; lesions are less likely on the trunk than on the extremities.

involvement [45]. This complication usually develops within 6 days after the onset of rash. The mortality rate for adults with varicella pneumonia is high, with death occurring in 10% of immunocompetent and 30% of immunocompromised individuals [45]. Other complications of varicella that rarely occur include myocarditis, glomerulonephritis, pancreatitis, hepatitis, appendicitis, orchitis, arthritis, Henoch-Schönlein vasculitis, optic neuritis, keratitis, iritis [46] and varicella gangrenosum (Fig. 5–12) [47].

Varicella infection during pregnancy may produce a wide array of fetal complications, ranging from asymptomatic latency to severe congenital defects [48]. Congenital developmental malformations most commonly occur when maternal infection occurs in the first trimester. These defects may include hypoplastic limbs, cortical atrophy, cicatricial skin lesions, ocular abnormalities, psychomotor re-

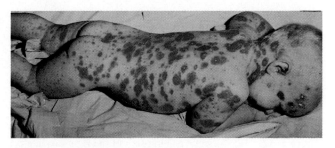

Figure 5–10. Bullous varicella from *Staphlococcus aureus* secondary infection.

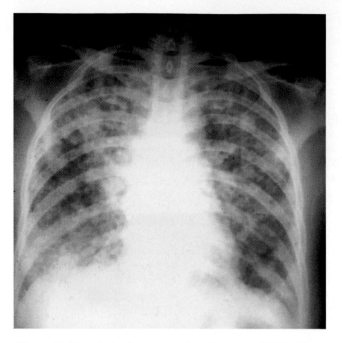

Figure 5–11. Varicella pneumonia. (Courtesy of Siri Chiewchanvit, M.D., Chiang Mai, Thailand.)

Table 5–3. Complications of Varicella

Bacterial superinfection of lungs, bones, or skin, rarely with
    septicemia
Scarring from skin lesions
Pneumonia
Neurologic complications
        Transient cerebellar ataxia
        Aseptic meningitis
        Transverse myelitis
        Reye's syndrome
        Meningoencephalitis
        Guillain-Barré syndrome
Neutropenia
Thrombocytopenia
Renal complications
    Glomerulonephritis
    Nephrotic syndrome
Hemolytic-uremic syndrome
Optic neuritis, keratitis, or iritis
Arthritis
Myocarditis
Pericarditis
Pancreatitis
Orchitis
Vasculitis

tardation, and low birth weight. The absolute risk of embryopathy after primary maternal VZV infection in the first 20 weeks of pregnancy is about 2% [49]. Maternal varicella infection that occurs after the first 20 weeks of pregnancy is associated with a much lower risk of congenital malformation. The risk of congenital problems after maternal herpes zoster infection at any time during pregnancy is much less than with primary VZV infection. The exposure of a pregnant women without a history of chickenpox to a person with a clinically active VZV infection is always of concern. It should be noted, however, that about 85% of adults who report that they have not had

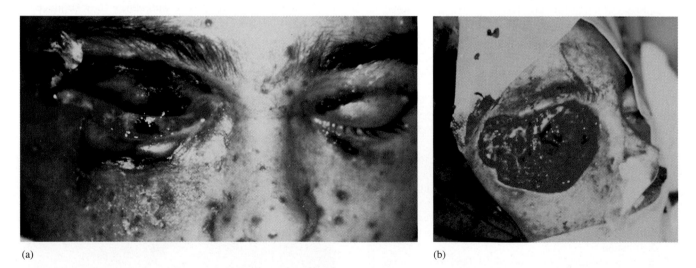

(a)   (b)

Figure 5–12. (a) Varicella gangreosum of the right eye in a previously healthy man with untreated primary varicella. (b) Enucleation of the necrosed right eye. (From Ref. 47. Used with permission.)

chickenpox are actually seropositive for antibodies to VZV [49].

Varicella infection can be associated with significant morbidity and mortality in immunocompromised adults or children. The lack of immunity in these populations allows for continued virus replication and dissemination, leading to persistent viremia; prolonged fever; a more extensive rash (often with hemorrhagic and/or purpuric lesions); and involvement of other organs of the body such as the lungs, liver, or central nervous system [50,51]. Table 5–3 highlights potential complications of varicella.

CLINICAL MANIFESTATIONS OF ZOSTER

A prodrome of intense pain in the involved dermatome precedes the zoster rash in more than 90% of patients. Because the pain is present before cutaneous manifestations, it often leads to a wide array of misdiagnoses, such as myocardial infarction, pleurisy, cholecystitis, peptic ulcer, appendicitis, ovarian cyst, prolapsed intervertebral disk, thrombophlebitis, or renal colic. The pain may be constant or intermittent and may be accompanied by pruritus, tingling, tenderness, or hyperesthesia. Rarely, a patient with dermatomal pain and serologic or virologic evidence of zoster infection never develops cutaneous manifestations of herpes zoster. This condition is known as zoster sine herpete (zoster without rash) [52,53]. This diagnosis is occasionally suspected but rarely confirmed. Laboratory confirmation is, however, possible with paired serology (i.e., acute and chronic) or with the polymerase chain reaction (i.e., to detect VZV DNA). In addition, patients with shin-

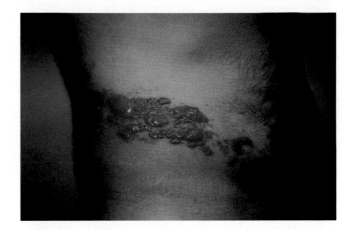

Figure 5–14. Herpes zoster in a thoracic dermatome in an adult.

gles may rarely have skin changes that are zosteriform (e.g., livedo reticularis) but never develop the classic lesions (Fig. 5–13).

The rash of herpes zoster is commonly localized to the skin area innervated by a single sensory ganglion (dermatome) and does not typically cross the midline of the body (Figs. 5–14 to 5–24). However, bilateral zoster has been observed in both immunocompetent (Fig. 5–25) and in immunocompromised persons (Fig. 5–26). The dermatomal rash usually occurs at the site that was most severely affected during primary varicella infection [14]. Any dermatome can be affected, but the most common regions of involvement include the ophthalmic (V1) and midthoracic to upper lumbar (T3-L2) dermatomes [12,54,55].

Herpes zoster in immunocompetent children or young

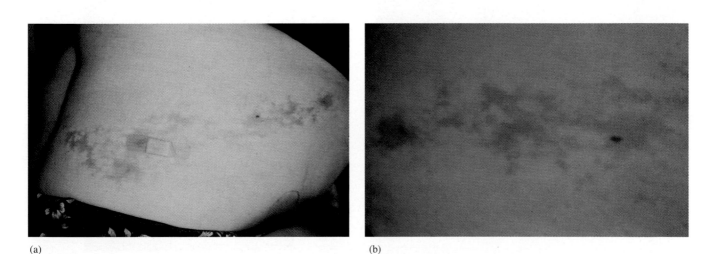

(a)   (b)

Figure 5–13.   (a, b) Livedo reticularis as the only cutaneous manifestation of serologically confirmed herpes zoster.

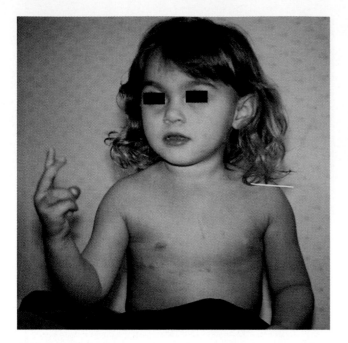

Figure 5–15. Herpes zoster in a thoracic dermatome in a child.

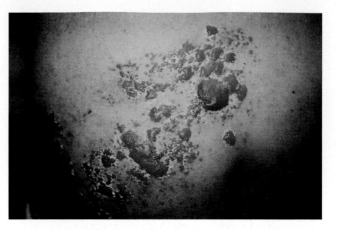

Figure 5–17. Herpes zoster in a sacral dermatome.

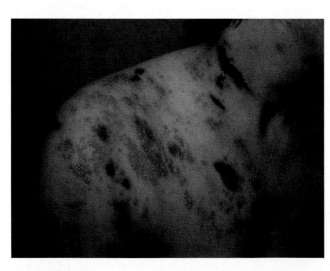

Figure 5–16. Herpes zoster in cervical dermatome.

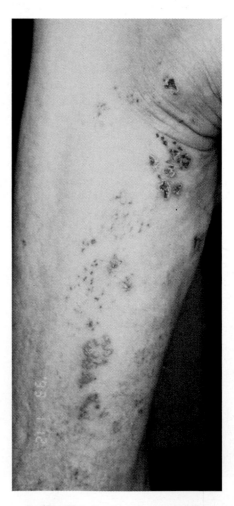

Figure 5–18. Herpes zoster in a sacral dermatome.

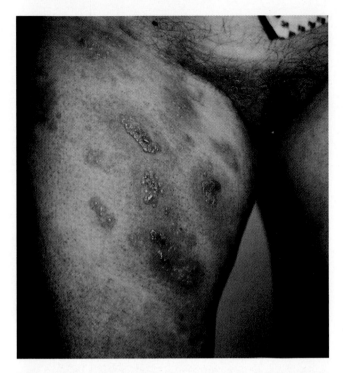

Figure 5–19. Herpes zoster in a lumbar/sacral dermatome in an adult.

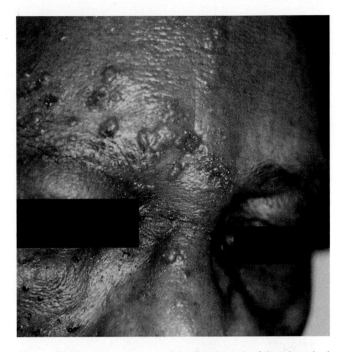

Figure 5–21. Herpes zoster of the first branch of the trigeminal nerve. Vesicles on the nose are termed *Hutchinson's sign.*

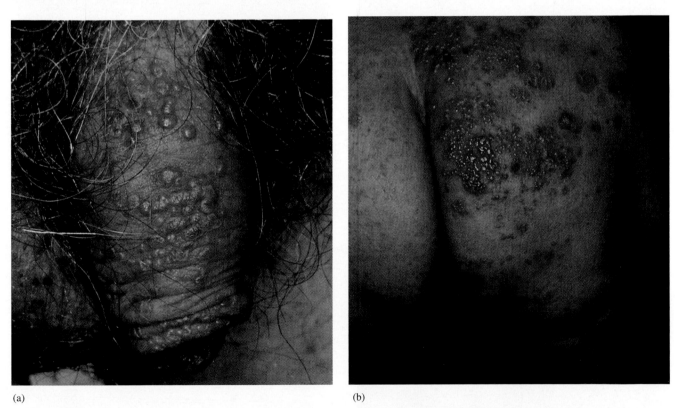

(a)

(b)

Figure 5–20. Herpes zoster in a sacral dermatome in a man. (a) The patient was referred for the treatment of primary genital herpes as the referring physician only observed the penile vesicles. (b) The patient, however, also had vesicles of the right buttock, which confirmed the diagnosis of sacral herpes zoster.

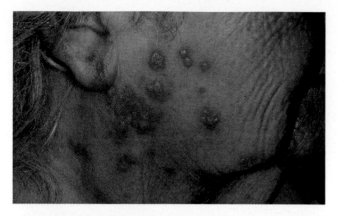

Figure 5–22. Herpes zoster of a cervical dermatome (C3).

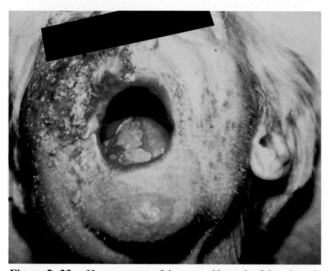

Figure 5–23. Herpes zoster of the second branch of the trigeminal nerve.

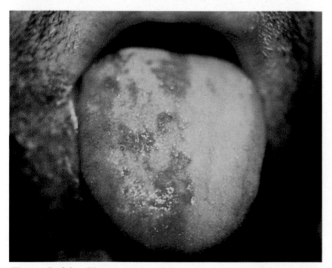

Figure 5–24. Herpes zoster of the second branch of the trigeminal nerve.

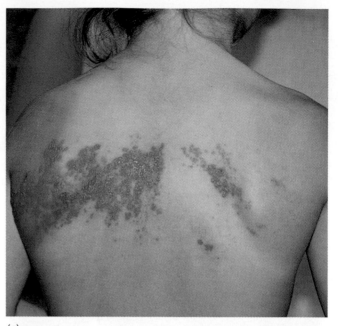

(a)

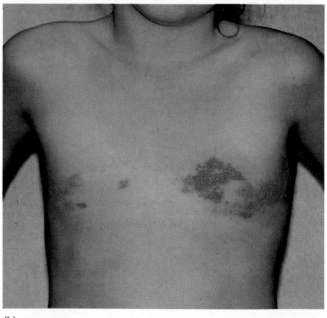

(b)

Figure 5–25. (a, b) Bilateral herpes zoster in an otherwise healthy girl. (Courtesy of Stan Gilbert, M.D., Bellingham, WA.)

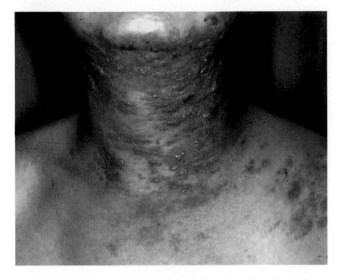

Figure 5–26. Bilateral herpes zoster in an AIDS patient. (Courtesy of Siri Chiewchanvit, M.D., Chiang Mai, Thailand.)

adults tends to evolve rapidly, with few complications, and resolution of the neuralgia as the lesion crusts fall off. In immunocompromised and elderly individuals, the pain and rash of zoster are usually more severe and complications occur more frequently (Fig. 5–27). Postherpetic neuralgia is a common complication, but it has varying definitions in the medical community. It is most commonly referred to as pain that persists after a certain time period or after all crusts have fallen off. This complication occurs in 10 to 15% of zoster cases [56,57], but it infrequently affects

persons under 40 years of age. On the other hand, more than one third of affected individuals 60 years or older develop postherpetic neuralgia [55–57]. The pain of postherpetic neuralgia typically remits or lessens significantly within 1 to 6 months, although the duration is variable [58]. After crusting of the lesions, other abnormal sensations may occur in patients, such as pruritus, paresthesia, dysesthesia, or anesthesia (Table 5–4). The differential diagnoses of herpes zoster are presented in Table 5–5.

Complications from herpes zoster are summarized in Table 5–6. Scarring with hypopigmentation or hyperpigmentation is occasionally seen, especially if the patient did not receive appropriate antiviral therapy (Figs. 5–28 and 5–29). The ophthalmic division of the trigeminal nerve (V1) is involved in 7% of zoster cases and is associated with a high complication rate [45]. Of these cases, 20 to 70% develop associated ocular disease [57], particularly those cases involving the nasociliary division of the ophthalmic nerve. The Hutchinson's sign indicates nasociliary branch involvement and presents as vesicles on the side and top of the nose [59] (see Fig. 5–21). Ocular complications may include scleritis, acute epithelial keratitis, uveitis, cicatricial lid retraction, oculomotor palsies, paralytic ptosis, glaucoma, chorioretinitis, optic neuritis, or panophthalmitis (due to secondary bacterial infection). All of these complications have the potential to produce visual impairment or blindness. Corneal sensation is frequently impaired with ophthalmic zoster and may result in corneal ulceration

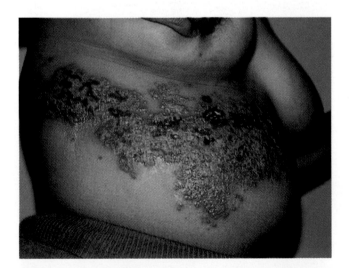

Figure 5–27. Herpes zoster in a pregnant woman with AIDS (Courtesy of Edith Garcia-Gonzalez, M.D., Mexico City, Mexico.)

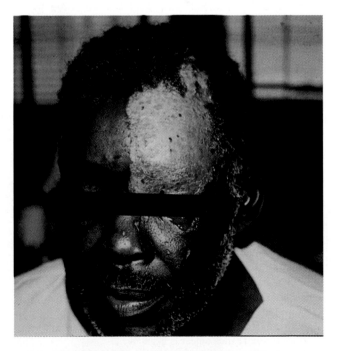

Figure 5–28. Scarring from herpes zoster.

Table 5–4. Clinical Manifestations of Herpes Zoster

Time After Initial Symptoms	Clinical Manifestations	Laboratory Analysis	Other Notes
	Reactivation of the virus may occur up to several decades after initial varicella infection ↓	Tzanck smear of lesion scraping, but does not differentiate from varicella or herpes simplex.	5% of patients (particularly children) will have fever, malaise or headache during the prodrome period. Pain is not normally significant in children.
0 days	Prodrome of localized pain ↓	Viral culture, serology, and direct immunofluorescense.	
3–7 days or more	Unilateral dermatomal rash with erythematous macules and papules ↓		Regional lymphadenopathy is usually present.
4–8 days	Vesicles ↓		Skin lesions resemble varicella but are more confluent.
6–10 days	Pustules ↓		
10–14 days	Crusts ↓		
2 wk, up to 4–6 wk	Complete healing		Scarring may occur with healing, particularly in dark-skinned individuals. Localized hypersensitivity or post herpetic neuralgia may persist for months or years after healing.

or neurotrophic keratitis. Postherpetic neuralgia is also more commonly associated with ophthalmic zoster [60].

Herpes zoster less commonly involves the second and third divisions of the trigeminal nerve or other cranial nerves [61–64]. Involvement of these nerves may result in lesions of the mouth, pharynx, larynx, or ears. The Ramsey-Hunt syndrome is due to involvement of the facial or auditory nerves and consists of ipsilateral facial palsy, in addition to zoster lesions of the external ear, tympanic membrane, or anterior two thirds of the tongue. Involvement of these nerves may also result in tinnitus, vertigo, otalgia, loss of taste, or deafness [61] (Fig. 5–30).

Table 5–5. Differential Diagnoses of Herpes Zoster

Herpes simplex virus: Herpes simplex virus may occasionally simulate zoster, but it is associated with recurrent symptoms and lesions at the same site.
Localized contact dermatitis: Dermatitis is not typically associated with pain, and Tzanck smear is negative.
Localized bacterial skin infection (e.g., bullous impetigo): Tzanck smear is negative.

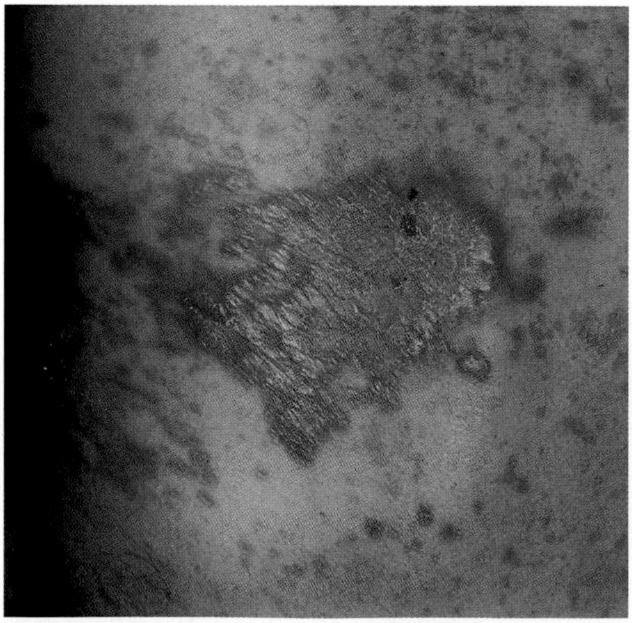

Figure 5–29. Scarring from herpes zoster.

Table 5–6. Complication of Herpes Zoster

Bacterial superinfection
Cutaneous dissemination of lesions
Scarring of skin lesions
Arthritis
Ocular complications
   Cicatricial lid retraction
   Optic neuritis
   Acute epithelial keratitis
   Scleritis
   Uveitis
   Glaucoma
   Oculomotor palsies
   Chorioretinitis
   Panophthalmitis
   Visual impairment
   Paralytic ptosis
   Blindness
Neurologic complications
   Postherpetic neuralgia
   Peripheral nerve palsies
   Sensory loss
   Granulomatous angiitis
   Transverse myelitis
   Cranial nerve palsies
   Deafness
   Meningoencephalitis
   Motor paralysis
Visceral complications
   Pneumonitis
   Hepatitis
   Pericarditis
   Gastritis
   Esophagitis

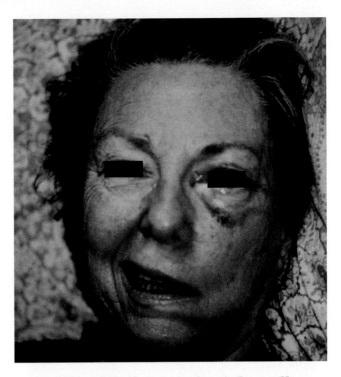

Figure 5–30. Facial palsy resulting from the Ramsey-Hunt syndrome. The suborbital hematoma on the left side was the result of a fall secondary to vertigo (also a manifestation of the Ramsey-Hunt syndrome).

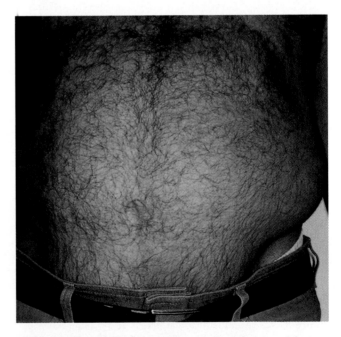

Figure 5–31. Unilateral abdominal distention secondary to motor nerve involvement with herpes zoster. (From Ref 74. Used with permission.)

Other nervous system complications rarely occur with herpes zoster disease. Meningoencephalitis and myelitis have been reported in 0.2 to 0.5% of patients. These conditions are associated with fever, headache, photophobia, meningeal irritation, vomiting, altered mentation, or nerve palsies [44,65–69]. Herpes zoster may involve the vagus nerve or its ganglia, resulting in dysphagia, nausea, vomiting, gastric upset, or cardiac irregularities. Other patients may develop motor paralysis resulting from direct extension of the virus from the sensory ganglion to the anterior horn cells. This complication occurs in 1 to 5% of all zoster cases [70–73] and usually develops in the first 2 to 3 weeks after rash onset. The muscles associated with the involved dermatome are typically affected, and the prognosis for recovery is generally good (Fig. 5–31) [74]. Although mild motor paralysis of the trunk often goes unnoticed, in zoster the incidence of motor deficiencies resulting from herpes zoster of the facial nerve or extremities is 10 to 20% [44].

Granulomatous cerebral angiitis is a delayed central nervous system complication of zoster, developing weeks to months after the zoster rash. This condition predominantly occurs in the elderly and results in signs and symptoms that resemble those of a cerebrovascular hemorrhage or thrombosis [75]. Patients may present with symptoms of transient ischemic attacks, stroke-in-evolution, or isolated or multiple cerebral infarctions. The most frequent central nervous system finding is asymptomatic cerebrospinal fluid abnormalities, such as elevated levels of protein and lymphocytes. The mortality rate with this complication is 15%, and autopsy examination reveals vascular inflammation with thrombosis and microinfarcts [76].

Herpes zoster has a high rate of dissemination (up to 40%) in immunosuppressed individuals, while this complication is rare in immunocompetent persons [45]. In immunocompetent patients, 17 to 35% may have a few vesicles

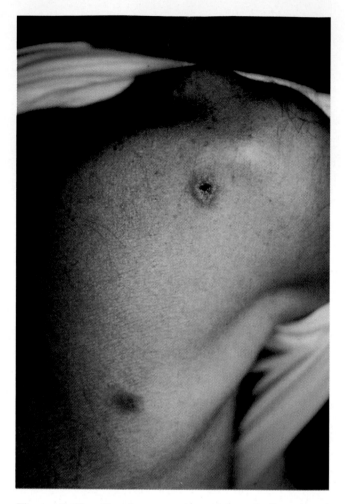

Figure 5–33. Chronic verrucous nodules of disseminated herpes zoster in an AIDS patient.

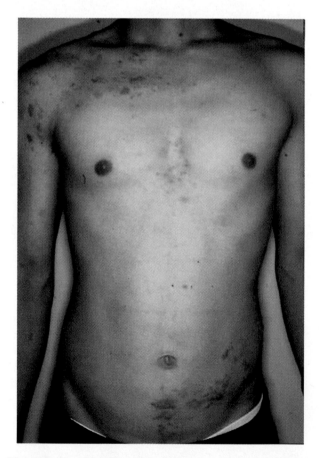

Figure 5–32. Multidermatomal herpes zoster in an AIDS patient. (Courtesy of Siri Chiewchanvit, M.D., Chiang Mai, Thailand.)

located remotely from the primary dermatomal eruption, likely due to hematogenous spread of the virus. Cutaneous dissemination is defined as more than 20 vesicles outside the area of the primary and adjacent dermatomes. This is followed by visceral dissemination (i.e., into lungs, liver, or brain) in 10% of immunosuppressed patients. HIV-infected patients with zoster have been observed to have an increased rate of neurologic complications (e.g., aseptic meningitis, radiculitis, and myelitis) [77] and ophthalmic complications (particularly progressive outer retinal necrosis) [77–79]. Other manifestations of herpes zoster in immunocompromised patients include: (1) multidermatomal zoster (Fig. 5–32), (2) chronic verrucous nodules (Fig. 5–33), and (3) one very unusual case of postherpetic hyperhidrosis (Fig. 5–34) [80].

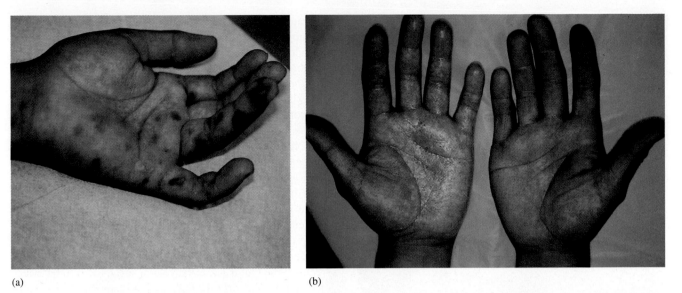

(a)   (b)

Figure 5–34.   Hyperhidrosis following herpes zoster in an AIDS patient. (a) Hemorrhagic vesicles of herpes zoster in cervical dermatome (i.e., C8). (b) Marked sweating in the same dermatome 2 months later.

DERMATOPATHOLOGY

The Tzanck smear is often the initial test of choice, performed by scraping the base of an early lesion and staining it with hematoxylin-and-eosin, Papanicolaou, Giemsa, Wright's, or toluidine blue stains. A smear of varicella or zoster lesions will have multinucleated giant cells and epithelial cells that contain acidophilic intranuclear inclusions. However, herpes simplex infections also have identical findings, and these two infections cannot be differentiated by using a Tzanck smear. The same is true of histopathologic findings from lesion biopsies. Varicella, zoster, and herpes simplex have findings of ballooning degeneration, intranuclear inclusion bodies, and multinucleated giant cells. The multinucleated cells are created by the fusion of adjacent infected cells [81]. This process allows direct cell-to-cell spread of the virus and protects the virus from extracellular neutralization by host antibodies [82].

LABORATORY FINDINGS

Most straightforward cases of varicella and herpes zoster are diagnosed based on history and clinical findings [69,83,84]. Varicella zoster virus can be differentiated from herpes simplex virus by several laboratory tests, such as viral culture, serology, direct immunofluorescence, and molecular techniques. Isolation of the virus by culture is

the most specific test, but it is not always sensitive since the varicella zoster virus is extremely labile [85–87]. Serologic testing for the virus (e.g., complement fixation) is limited by possible cross-reactivity with herpes simplex virus but a retrospective diagnosis of varicella zoster infection can be made [88]. Direct immunofluorescence of cellular material from skin lesions is currently the most useful diagnostic test for varicella zoster infection (Fig. 5–35). Molecular techniques with high sensitivity, such as dot-blot hybridization and polymerase chain reaction, have been used more recently to detect the virus in skin lesions, peripheral blood mononuclear cells, and other tissues of infected patients [86,89,90]. These tests may become the preferred diagnostic methods in the future.

TREATMENT OF VARICELLA

Immunocompetent children with varicella have typically been treated symptomatically, since varicella infection in this population is usually benign and self-limited. With the development of antiviral drugs, acyclovir has been shown to decrease the duration and severity of varicella in this population if begun within 24 hours of the rash onset [91], although some benefits are still seen if acyclovir is initiated between 24 to 72 hours after rash onset (Table 5–7). Acyclovir has been approved for the treatment of varicella in children 2 years of age and older, as well as adults. Several factors have forestalled the wide acceptance of this

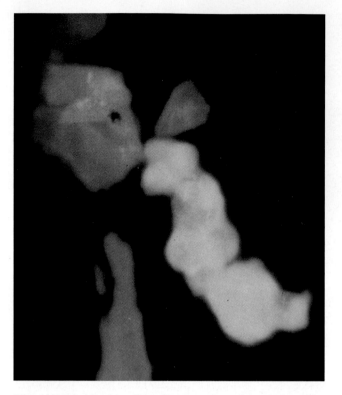

Figure 5–35. Positive direct fluorescence antigen (DFA) staining for VZV.

Table 5–7. Treatment of Varicella

Symptom	Treatment
Fever	Antipyretics (although aspirin should be avoided in children, due to its association with Reye's syndrome [105, 106])
Pruritus	Oral antihistamines, calamine lotion, and tepid baths with baking soda (1/4 cup per bath). Trimming of nails to discourage scratching.

Systemic Antiviral Treatment

Otherwise healthy children: oral acyclovir (20 mg/kg) 4 times a day for 5 days

Immunocompetent adults (and children over 40 kg): oral acyclovir 800 mg 5 times a day for 7 days ; valacyclovir 1 g tid or famciclovir 500 tid for 7 days are commonly used but not specifically FDA approved for primary varicella in adults.

Immunocompromised persons: intravenous acyclovir: 10mg/kg (500 mg/m²) every 8 h for 7–10 days

therapy for children: the high cost of treatment, the delay in rapid institution of therapy, and the concern of possible development of acyclovir resistance. However, with this treatment the child can resume school or play activities 1 to 2 days earlier, which is considered cost effective in working families, because it allows the caretaker to return to work sooner than if no antiviral therapy were used. Because of the increased risk of severe varicella infection and complications in adults, systemic antiviral treatment is clearly indicated in this population. In a clinical study, oral acyclovir significantly reduced the extent of disease and duration of signs and symptoms [92]. Antiviral treatment of varicella is mandatory in immunocompromised patients [93,94]. Intravenous acyclovir continues to be the drug of choice in this population. Although not FDA approved for primary varicella and not studied in controlled trials, famciclovir and valacyclovir are known to be effective against the virus through herpes zoster studies. Vidarabine and interferon alpha also have proved to be effective in the treatment of varicella in immunocompromised persons, but significant toxicity with these drugs have limited their use [95–96].

PREVENTION OF VARICELLA

Because the available treatment for varicella is not optimal, more emphasis remains on prevention of the infection. For immunocompromised patients who have had recent substantial exposure to varicella, varicella-zoster immune globulin (VZIG) is available. This prophylaxis is indicated also for several other exposure situations, such as susceptible pregnant women and neonates whose mothers became infected shortly before delivery. VZIG should be given within 96 hours of varicella exposure, and the duration of protection lasts at least 3 weeks [97]. Unfortunately, one third to one half of individuals still develop clinical infection after VZIG administration [98].

The live attenuated varicella-zoster vaccine (Oka strain) has been shown to be highly efficacious with a 96% seroconversion rate in healthy children [99]. Studies indicate that the vaccine is 71 to 91% effective in preventing all disease and 95% to 100% effective in preventing severe disease. The vaccine is also extremely safe, with only mild side effects such as fever, slight varicelliform rash, and pain at the injection site [100–102]. From 1 to 4% of immunized children develop this mild varicella-like syndrome. Some pregnant women have inadvertently received the vaccine, but no congenital varicella syndromes are known to have resulted from these vaccinations. Moreover, the incidence of zoster in vaccinated children is less than that seen in naturally-infected children [103]. The decreased incidence of zoster after vaccination also holds true for children with leukemia [104]. A clinical study of vaccine efficacy in a

Table 5–8. Prophylaxis of Varicella

Varicella-zoster immune globulin (VZIG)	125 U/10 kg (up to 625 U) within 96 h of exposure for immunosuppressed patients with substantial varicella exposure.
Live attenuated varicella vaccine (Oka strain)	Routine vaccination at 12–18 mo of age. Susceptible persons ages 12 mo to 12 yr require one vaccine dose, while ages 13 and above require 2 doses, 4–8 wk apart.

child-care center showed that 14% of vaccinated children versus 88% of unvaccinated children developed the infection after exposure [105]. The vaccinated children who did become infected had less severe disease with fewer lesions and less days of absence from school than their unvaccinated counterparts. In another clinical trial, the vaccine was 100% efficacious in preventing varicella [106] (Table 5–8). Most states now require children to receive the varicella vaccine in order to attend school (or documentation of previous wild-type chickenpox infection). However, national vaccination coverage for one dose of varicella vaccine among children in the United States ages 19 to 35 months was only 59% in 1999 [107].

There were approximately 4 million cases of chickenpox annually in the United States before the VZV vaccine was licensed in 1995. Each year about 100 persons died of primary varicella, 50% children and 50% adults. In addition, there were approximately 11,000 hospitalizations annually from complications of varicella, such as secondary bacterial infections [107–109]. Therefore, universal coverage with the VZV vaccine has immense potential benefits on reduced morbidity and mortality. Furthermore, an estimated annual societal savings of $384 million would result from the otherwise lost income of parents staying home with sick children, physician office visits, and hospitalizations, as well as the lifetime income of those persons dying of varicella [110]. This estimate, however, does not include the potential reduction in morbidity due to a reduced incidence and severity of herpes zoster later in life. Much remains to be learned about the VZV vaccine, including the question of persistence of immunity. More than 20 years after the first use of the vaccine in Japan, however, there is little evidence that the protection imparted by the vaccine may wane as the individual ages.

TREATMENT OF ZOSTER

Several antiviral agents are used for the treatment of herpes zoster, although no medication has been shown to com-

pletely prevent the development of postherpetic neuralgia (PHN). However, early therapy with antiviral agents has demonstrated reduction in the duration of PHN. Topical idoxuridine was the first agent to be evaluated for the treatment of herpes zoster. Its use has not been recommended because of the high potential for toxicity and the lack of effect on PHN [111,112]. Vidarabine is a systemic antiviral agent given intravenously, which has been shown to decrease the duration of viral shedding, time to cessation of pain and new vesicle formation, healing time, cutaneous dissemination, and complications [49,113]. However, this agent was found later to be no more effective than acyclovir [114], and the significant side effects and difficulty of administration with vidarabine has limited its use (Table 5–9).

Both oral and intravenous acyclovir have a role in the treatment of herpes zoster. Studies have shown that intravenous acyclovir given to immunocompromised and immunocompetent patients with herpes zoster reduced acute pain and the time to cutaneous healing [115–118]. Intravenous administration is indicated for the treatment of significant complications in immunocompetent patients and the treatment of zoster in immunocompromised individuals. The oral form of acyclovir is indicated for therapy in immunocompetent patients and has been shown to lead to accelerated rash healing and reduction in acute pain [119–124]. However, acyclovir has not been shown to reduce the incidence of PHN [115–117]. Adverse effects with acyclovir are rare and include headache, nausea, diarrhea, and renal toxicity. Central nervous system toxicity is also rare and may result in disorientation, delirium, tremor, seizures, or slurred speech [125]. Treatment of PHN is outlined in Table 5–10.

Valacyclovir, the orally administered prodrug of acyclovir, is effective in decreasing the appearance of new zoster lesions, time to crusting, and time to 50% healing [126]. Compared with acyclovir, valacyclovir reduced the

Table 5–9. Treatment of Zoster

Symptoms	Treatment
Local pain and pruritus	Analgesics, oral antipruritics, calamine lotion, cool compresses
	Systemic Antiviral Treatment
Immunocompetent patients (oral therapy):	
acyclovir 800 mg 5 times daily for 7 days	
valacyclovir 1 g tid for 7 days	
famciclovir 500 mg tid for 7 days	
Immunocompromised patients: intravenous acyclovir: 10 mg/kg (500 mg/m²) every 8 h for 7 days	

Table 5–10. Treatment of Postherpetic Neuralgia

Symptom	Treatment
Non-narcotic analgesics	Frequently not effective
Narcotic analgesics	Temporary benefit
Capsaicin cream	Applied topically every 4 h for pain relief, but usually with local burning sensation.
Topical lidocaine gel or patch	For topical pain relief (patch is FDA approved)
Tricyclic antidepressants (amitriptyline, maprotiline, and desipramine)	Doses needed are much less than that used for depression treatment
Anticonvulsants	Especially gabapentin
Sympathetic nerve blockade	Some reports of success
Steroids	Intrathecal methylprednisolone appears effective
Transcutaneous electrical stimulation	Some reports of success

median duration of pain from 60 days to 40 days. In addition, only 19% of patients taking valacyclovir had continued pain at 6 months as compared with 26% of acyclovir recipients [127]. Valacyclovir has a similar side effect profile but with no reports of nephropathy or neurotoxicity [128].

Famciclovir, the prodrug of penciclovir, has been shown to be at least equal to acyclovir in promoting cutaneous healing and reducing the duration of acute pain [129]. In addition, famciclovir has been found to decrease the duration of PHN among elderly patients when compared with placebo [130]. As with all of the antiviral agents, treatment should be initiated as soon as possible after the zoster rash onset, preferably within 72 hours. It has been reported recently, however, that patients may also benefit if antiviral therapy is started after 72 hours of rash onset, but the upper limit of time for initiation of antiviral therapy has not been established [131].

In controlled studies famciclovir has been demonstrated to be equally safe, convenient, and effective as valacyclovir in reducing the duration of PHN in immunocompetent patients over 50 years of age [132]. Famciclovir has also been shown to be equally safe and effective but more convenient than acyclovir for the therapy of herpes zoster in immunocompromised patients [133], as well as for the treatment of ophthalmic zoster in immunocompetent patients [134].

Many practitioners have tried corticosteroids to decrease inflammation and thus decrease the progression of the nerve damage which leads to PHN. This treatment has been used both alone and in combination with antiviral agents. Some clinical trials have shown a reduction in persistent pain [135] or accelerated healing [136]. However, a more definitive study demonstrated no long-term benefit when corticosteroids were added to the acyclovir regimen [137]. The combination treatment led to more rapid rash resolution and a decrease in acute pain, but no effects on PHN were seen. In addition, adverse effects were more frequent with the addition of corticosteroids. A second study revealed no difference in pain at 6 months when comparing a combination of acyclovir and prednisone with acyclovir alone, prednisone alone, and double placebo [138]. In a small study of patients with Bell's palsy, a combination of prednisone plus acyclovir was more effective than prednisone monotherapy for those who presented with zoster sine herpete and also had VZV DNA in their saliva [139].

TREATMENT OF POSTHERPETIC NEURALGIA

No single antiviral agent has been consistently effective in the treatment of PHN. However, the duration and severity of this complication can generally be reduced by early treatment of herpes zoster with the appropriate antiviral agents. The majority of clinical trials have studied and recommended treatment within 72 hours of the first vesicle onset. However, patients frequently present after the 72 hour window of treatment. It appears reasonable to initiate treatment after 72 hours in specific situations if the lesions are not completely crusted and the individual is older than 50 years of age, immunocompromised, and/or has trigeminal zoster [131].

Several other modalities have been employed in the treatment of PHN, such as analgesics, narcotics, tricyclic antidepressants, capsaicin, biofeedback, nerve blocks, and cutaneous stimulation. Systemic analgesics and narcotics are not usually effective against PHN, and long-term narcotic use may lead to drug dependency. However, these agents may be useful for the short-term treatment of acute pain with herpes zoster (Table 5–10).

Tricyclic antidepressants have shown considerable efficacy in the treatment of PHN although the mechanism of action appears to be independent of the antidepressant effects. Some experts recommend the initiation of amitriptyline therapy as soon as possible for all patients with zoster older than 60 years [140]. This medication is typically begun at low doses (10–25 mg) and gradually increased to doses of 50–75 mg over 2–3 weeks. Maprotiline and desipramine are also effective, and desipramine may be more preferable with its lower anticholinergic and sedative effects [141,142]. Antipsychotics (chlorprothixene, flu-phenazine, and haloperidol) have also been tried for the treatment of PHN, often in combination with antidepressants. However, a placebo-controlled study of chlorprothixene demonstrated only marginal efficacy [143].

In a randomized, controlled, multi-center trial gabapentin was studied for the therapy of PHN in persons whose pain had been present for more than 3 months after healing of a herpes zoster rash [144]. This agent was found to be effective in the treatment of pain and sleep interference associated with PHN. In this study, patients received a 4-week titration period to a maximum dosage of 3600 mg/d of gabapentin or matching placebo. Treatment was maintained for another 4 weeks at the maximum tolerated dose. Using an intent to treat analysis, persons receiving gabapentin had a statistically significant reduction in average daily pain scores from 6.3 to 4.2 points compared with placebo recipients whose change was from 6.5 to 6.0 points ($P<.001$).

Changes in pain and sleep interference as well as secondary measures of pain showed improvement with gabapentin ($P<.001$). In this study the following adverse events were observed more frequently in gabapentin recipients than in those persons receiving placebo: somnolence, dizziness, ataxia, peripheral edema, and infection. Study withdrawals, however, were comparable in the two groups. The literature reveals that, while a decrease in PHN severity has been reported with a variety of therapies, there is no clear expectation of what that reduction might be if such therapies were used acutely in combination with an antiviral drug.

Topical treatments also have been beneficial in the treatment of PHN. Capsaicin cream acts by enhancing the release or inhibiting the reaccumulation of substance P from cell bodies and nerve terminals. In a clinical trial, nearly 80% of patients treated with capsaicin experienced some pain relief [145]. However, some patients cannot tolerate the burning sensation associated with capsaicin treatment. Some authors recommend pretreatment with topical anesthetics (lidocaine) to alleviate this problem [146]. Patients should be cautioned against applying capsaicin to any unhealed skin lesions. Topical lidocaine is available in several forms, such as cream, gel, and a patch. In fact, the topical lidocaine patch is the only therapy with an FDA-approved indication for PHN [147–149].

Other local treatments such as EMLA cream, injection of bupivacaine, cryoanalgesia, and sympathetic nerve blockade have led to pain relief in some patients [150–154]. Transcutaneous electrical stimulation has also been tried with some success for the treatment of PHN [155].

Steroids have been used in various preparations, doses,

and schedules for the treatment of PHN, but generally with limited success. Recently, however, Kotani et al. [156] demonstrated that intrathecal administration of methyl-prednisolone with lidocaine produced excellent or good pain relief at 4 weeks and at 1 and 2 years in over 90% of persons who had suffered intractable PHN for at least 1 year. In contrast, relief was reported in only 6% of those who received only lidocaine and 4% of those who received no treatment. Moreover, allodynia was reduced by more than 70% in the methylprednisolone-lidocaine group and less than 25% in the lidocaine-only group. Importantly, no serious adverse events were observed in any of the patients.

PREVENTION OF POSTHERPETIC NEURALGIA BY PROPHYLAXIS OF HERPES ZOSTER

Because the development of herpes zoster has been linked to a decrease in cell-mediated immunity, studies are underway to evaluate the prophylactic effect of the live attenuated varicella-zoster vaccine for this disease. Studies thus far have shown an increase in immunity against the virus in elderly recipients of the vaccine [157,158], although results from one study demonstrated enhanced immunity which lasted only 1 year [159]. In addition, 10 to 15% of vaccinees failed to develop enhanced immunity regardless of dose [159]. Further studies with improved vaccines may show more promising results.

CONCLUSION

Although primary varicella is generally considered a mild, self-limited disease of children, the increased population of immunosuppressed patients will likely lead to an overall increase in morbidity from this illness. The potential morbidity of herpes zoster, particularly in the elderly and immunosuppressed persons, can also be quite devastating. Considering that 20% of otherwise healthy individuals and approximately 50% of markedly immunocompromised persons will eventually develop herpes zoster, the clinician's level of suspicion for this condition should remain high. This fact is especially important as initiation of antiviral therapy early in the course of the disease can reduce or eliminate complications. Therefore, it is important to differentiate herpes zoster from the many other conditions that may have zosteriform cutaneous presentations (Figs. 5–36 to 5–41) [160]. It is expected that the epidemiology and incidence of both of these diseases will be changing with widespread vaccination against the VZV. Although the available treatment for these illnesses has advanced dramatically in recent years, there is a continued need for

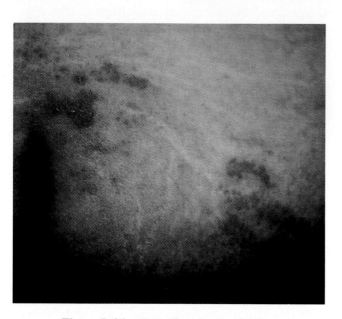

Figure 5–36. Zosteriform herpes simplex.

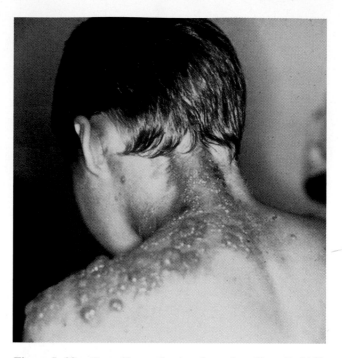

Figure 5–38. Zosteriform echovirus 6 eruption. (From Ref 160. Used with permission.)

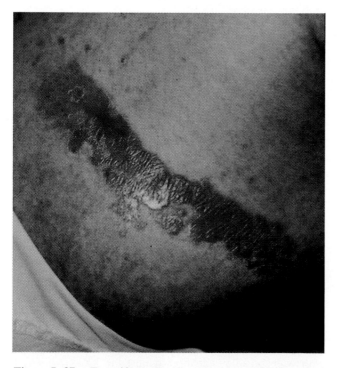

Figure 5–37. Zosteriform allergic contact dermatitis to surgical tape.

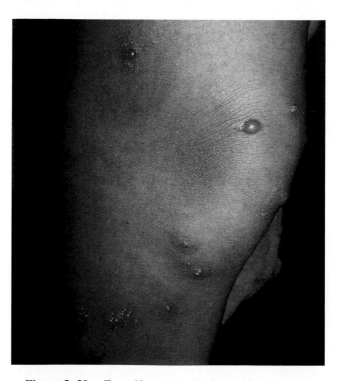

Figure 5–39. Zosteriform vesicular insect bite reactions.

more effective medications, particularly for postherpetic neuralgia.

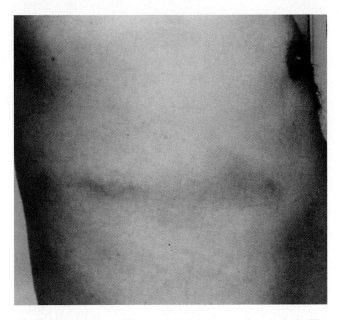

Figure 5-40. Zosteriform eruption due to gnathostomiasis. The patient became infected with the responsible organism, *Gnathostoma spinigerum,* by eating ceviche (raw fish). (Courtesy of Francisco Bravo, M.D., Universidad Peruana Cayetano Heredia, Lima, Peru.)

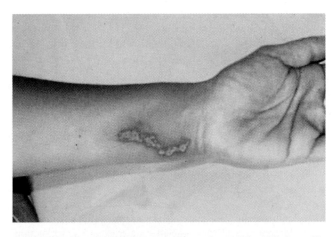

Figure 5-41. Zosteriform paederus dermatitis ("latigazo"). The pustules resulted from contact of the skin with an insect, which is a member of the order Coleoptera, the paederus. (Courtesy of Francisco Bravo, M.D., Universidad Peruana Cayetano Heredia, Lima, Peru.)

REFERENCES

1. JE Gordon. Chickenpox: an epidemiological review. Am J Med Sci 244:362–389, 1962.
2. W Osler. The Principles and Practice of Medicine. New York:Appleton, 1892, pp 65.
3. C Grose, TI Ng. Intracellular synthesis of varicella-zoster virus. J Infect Dis 166(Suppl 1):S7–S12, 1992.
4. Scott- JH Wilson. Why "chicken" pox? Lancet 1:1152, 1978.
5. MN Oxman, R Alani. Varicella and herpes zoster. In: TB Fitzpatrick, AZ Eisen, K Wolff, IM Freedberg, KF Austen, eds. Dermatology in General Medicine, 4th ed. New York: McGraw-Hill, 1993, pp 2543–2572.
6. AA Gershon, SJ Silverstein. Varicella-zoster virus. In: DD Richman, RJ Whitley, FG Hayden, eds. Clinical Virology. New York:Churchill Livingstone, 1997, pp 421–444.
7. J von Bokay. Uber den atiologischen Zusammenhang der Varizellan mit gewissen Fallen von Herpes Zoster. Wien Zlin Wochenschr 22:1323–1326, 1909.
8. E Bruusgaard. The mutual relation between zoster and varicella. Br J Dermatol Syphilol 44:1–24, 1932.
9. TH Weller, HM Witton. The etiologic agents of varicella and herpes zoster: serologic studies with the viruses as propagated in vitro. J Exp Med 108:869–890, 1958.
10. TH Weller, HM Witton, EJ Bell. The etiologic agents of varicella and herpes zoster: isolation, propagation, and cultural characteristics in vitro. J Exp Med 108:843–868, 1958.
11. H Kjersem, S Jepsen. Varicella among immigrants from the tropics, a health problem. Scand J Soc Med 18: 171–174, 1990.
12. DH Gilden, AN Dueland, R Cohrs, JR Martin, BK Kleinschmidt-DeMasters, R Mahalingam. Preherpetic neuralgia. Neurology 41:1215–1218, 1991.
13. RM Locksley, N Flournoy, KM Sullivan, JD Meyers. Infection with varicella-zoster virus after bone marrow transplantation. J Infect Dis 152:1172–1181, 1985.
14. AH Ross, E Lencher, G Reitman. Modification of chickenpox in family contacts by administration of gamma globulin. N Engl J Med 267:369–376, 1962.
15. HE Seiler. A study of herpes zoster particularly in its relationship to chickenpox. J Hyg (Camb) 47:253–262, 1949.
16. SE Straus. Shingles: sorrows, salves, and solutions. JAMA 269:1836–1839, 1993.
17. C Grose. Variation on a theme by Fenner: the pathogenesis of chickenpox. Pediatrics 68:735–737, 1981.
18. AM Arvin. Cell-mediated immunity to varicella-zoster virus. J Infect Dis 166(Suppl 1):S35–S41, 1992.
19. JC Ruckdeschel, SC Schimpff, AC Smyth, MR Mardiney Jr. Herpes zoster and impaired cell-associated immunity to the varicella zoster virus in patients with Hodgkin's disease. Am J Med 62:77–85, 1977.

20. AM Arvin. Immune responses to varicella-zoster virus. Infect Dis Clin North Am 10:529–570, 1996.

21. P Ljungman, B Lonnqvist, G Gahrton, O Ringden, VA Sundqvist, B Wahren. Clinical and subclinical reactivations of varicella-zoster in immunocompromised patients. J Infect Dis 153:840–847, 1986.

22. JD Meyers, N Flournoy, ED Thomas. Cell-mediated immunity to varicella-zoster virus after allogenic marrow transplant. J Infect Dis 141:479–487, 1980.

23. CS Han, W Miller, R Huake, D Weisdorf. Varicella zoster infection after bone marrow transplantation: incidence, risk factors and complications. Bone Marrow Transplant 13:277–283, 1994.

24. R Dolin, RC Reichman, MH Mazur, RJ Whitley. Herpes zoster-varicella infection in immunosuppressed patients. Ann Intern Med 89:375–388, 1978.

25. BE Juel-Hensen, FO MacCallum. Herpes simplex, varicella and zoster. Philadelphia:JB Lippincott, 1972, pp 72–77.

26. JE Sokal, D Firat. Varicella-zoster infection in Hodgkin's disease. Am J Med 39:452–463, 1965.

27. S Schimpff, A Serpick, B Stoler, B Rumack, H Mellin, JM Joseph, J Block. Varicella-zoster infection in patients with cancer. Ann Intern Med 76:241–254, 1972.

28. S Feldman, WT Hughes, HY Kim. Herpes zoster in children with cancer. Am J Dis Child 126:178–184, 1973.

29. DR Goffinet, EJ Glatstein, TC Merigan. Herpes zoster-varicella and lymphoma. Ann Intern Med 76:235–240, 1972.

30. R Goodman, N Jaffe, R Filler. Herpes zoster in children with stage I-III Hodgkin's disease. Radiology 118:429–431, 1976.

31. F Reboul, SS Donaldson, HS Kaplan. Herpes zoster and varicella infections in children with Hodgkin's disease: an analysis of contributing factors. Cancer 41:95–99, 1978.

32. JJ Rusthoven, P Ahlgren, T Elhakim, P Pinfold, J Reid, L Stewart, R Feld. Varicella-zoster infection in adult cancer patients: a population study. Arch Intern Med 148:1561–1566, 1988.

33. R Colebunders, JM Mann, H Francis, K Bila, L Izaley, M Ilwaya, N Kakonde, TC Quinn, JW Curran, P Piot. Herpes zoster in African patients: a clinical predictor of human immunodeficiency virus infections. J Infect Dis 157:314–318, 1988.

34. AE Friedman-Kien, FL Lafleur, E Gendler, NP Hennessey, R Montagna, S Halbert, P Rubinstein, K Krasinski, E Zang, B Poiesz. Herpes zoster: a possible early clinical sign for development of acquired immunodeficiency syndrome in high-risk individuals. J Am Acad Dermatol 14:1023–1028, 1986.

35. MA Jacobson, TG Berger, S Fikrig, P Becherer, JW Moohr, SC Stanat, KK Biron. Acyclovir-resistant varicella zoster infection after chronic oral acyclovir therapy in patients with the acquired immunodeficiency syndrome (AIDS). Ann Intern Med 112:187–191, 1990.

36. PR Cohen, VP Beltrani, ME Grossman. Disseminated herpes zoster in patients with human immunodeficiency virus infection. Am J Med 84:1076–1080, 1988.

37. CC Linnemann Jr, KK Biron, WG Hoppenjans, AM Solinger. Emergence of acyclovir-resistant varicella zoster virus in an AIDS patient on prolonged acyclovir therapy. AIDS 4:577–579, 1990.

38. PE LeBoit, M Limova, TS Yen, JM Palefsky, CR White Jr, TG Berger. Chronic verrucous varicella-zoster virus infection in patients with the acquired immunodeficiency syndrome (AIDS): histologic and molecular biologic findings. Am J Dermatopathol 14:1–5, 1992.

39. IH Gilson, JH Barnett, MA Conant, OL Laskin, J Williams, PG Jones. Disseminated ecthymatous herpes varicella-zoster infection in patients with acquired immunodeficiency syndrome. J Am Acad Dermatol 20:637–642, 1989.

40. WB Hoppenjans, MR Bibler, RL Orme, AM Solinger. Prolonged cutaneous herpes zoster in acquired immunodeficiency syndrome. Arch Dermatol 126:1048–1050, 1990.

41. E Alessi, M Cusini, R Zerboni, S Cavicchini, C Uberti-Foppa, M Galli. Unusual varicella zoster virus infection in patients with the acquired immunodeficiency syndrome [letter]. Arch Dermatol 124:1011–1013, 1988.

42. ME Melish. Bullous varicella: its association with the staphylococcal scalded-skin syndrome. J Pediatr 83:1019–1021, 1973.

43. JG Bullowa, SM Wishik. Complications of varicella: I. Their occurrence among 2,534 patients. Am J Dis Child 49:923–926, 1935.

44. RR McKendall, HL Klawans. Nervous system complications of varicella-zoster virus. In: PJ Vinken, GW Bruyn, eds. Handbook of Clinical Neurology, Vol 34. Amsterdam: Elsevier, 1978, pp 161.

45. DM Weber, JA Pellecchia. Varicella pneumonia: study of prevalence in adult men. JAMA 257:843–848, 1965.

46. RJ Whitley. Varicella-zoster virus infections. In: GJ Galasso, RJ Whitley, TC Merigan, eds. Antiviral Agents and Viral Diseases of Man. New York: Raven Press, 1990, pp 235.

47. WO Thomas, JA Parker, B Weston, C Evankovich. Periorbital varicella gangrenosa necessitating orbital exenteration in a previously healthy adult. South Med J 89:723–725, 1996.

48. SG Paryani, AM Arvin. Intrauterine infection with varicella-zoster virus after maternal varicella. N Engl J Med 314:1542–1546, 1986.

49. AL Pastuszak, M Levy, B Schick, C Zuber, M Feldkamp, J Gladstone, F Bar-Levy, E Jackson, A Donnenfeld, W Meschino, et al. Outcome after maternal varicella infection in the first 20 weeks of pregnancy. N Engl J Med 330:901–905, 1994.

50. RJ Whitley, SJ Soong, R Dolin, R Betts, C Linnemann Jr, CA Alford Jr. Early vidarabine therapy to control the complication of herpes zoster in immunosuppressed patients. N Engl J Med 307:971–975, 1982.

51. MG Myers. Viremia caused by varicella-zoster: association with malignant progressive varicella. J Infect Dis 140:229, 1979.

52. GW Lewis. Zoster sine herpete. Br Med J 2:418–421, 1958.

53. HG Easton. Zoster sine herpete causing acute trigeminal neuralgia. Lancet 2:1065–1066, 1970.

54. H Head, AW Campbell. The pathology of herpes zoster and its bearing on sensory localization. Brain 23:353, 1900.

55. CF Burgoon, JS Burgoon, GD Baldridge. The natural history of herpes zoster. JAMA 164:265–269, 1957.

56. RE Hope-Simpson. Postherpetic neuralgia. J R Coll Gen Pract 25:571–575, 1975.

57. MW Ragozzino, LJ Melton 3d, LT Kurland, CP Chu, HO Perry. Population-based study of herpes zoster and its sequelae. Medicine (Baltimore) 61:310–316, 1982.

58. RE Hope-Simpson. The nature of herpes zoster: a long-term study and a new hypothesis. Proc R Soc Med 58: 9–20, 1965.

59. JJ Kanski. Clinical ophthalmology, 2nd ed. London:Butterworth-Heineman, 1989, pp 101.

60. TJ Liesegang. Diagnosis and therapy of herpes zoster ophthalmicus. Ophthalmology 98:1216–1229, 1991.

61. D Denny-Brown, RD Adams, PJ Fitzgerald. Pathologic features of herpes zoster: a note on ''geniculate herpes.'' Arch Neurol Psychiatr 51:216–231, 1944.

62. J Clark. Herpes zoster of right glossopharyngeal nerve. Lancet 1:38–39, 1979.

63. M Mesolella, B Testa, C Mesolella, A Giuliano, G Testa. Herpes du larynx. A propos de trois cas [Abstract]. Ann Otolaryngol Chir Cervicofac 110:337–340, 1993.

64. E Tidwell, B Hutson, N Burkhart, JL Gutmann, CD Ellis. Herpes zoster of the trigeminal nerve third branch: a case report and review of the literature. Int Endod J 32:61–66, 1999.

65. WR McCormick, RL Rodnitzky, SS Schochet Jr, AP McKee. Varicella zoster encephalomyelitis. Arch Neurol 21:559–570, 1969.

66. E Gold, FC Robbins. Isolation of herpes zoster virus from spinal fluid of a patient. Virology 6:293, 1958.

67. E Appelbaum, SI Kreps, A Sunshine. Herpes zoster encephalitis. Am J Med 32:25–31, 1962.

68. FH Norris Jr, R Leonards, PR Calanchini, CD Calder. Herpes zoster meningoencephalitis. J Infect Dis 122: 335–338, 1970.

69. J Jemsek, SB Greenberg, L Taber, D Harvey, A Gershon, RB Couch. Hereps zoster-associated encephalitis: clinicopathologic report of 12 cases and review of the literature. Medicine 62:81–97, 1983.

70. AB Christie. Chickenpox (varicella); herpes zoster. In: Infectious Diseases: Epidemiology and Clinical Practice, 3rd ed. Edinburgh:Churchill-Livingstone, 1980, pp 262, 278.

71. BE Juel-Hensen, FO MacCallum. Herpes Simplex, Varicella, and Zoster. Philadelphia:JB Lippincott, 1972, pp 78–85.

72. BD Grant, CR Rowe. Motor paralysis of the extremities in herpes zoster. J Bone Joint Surg (Am) 43A:885–896, 1961.

73. JE Thomas, FM Howard. Segmented zoster paresis: a disease profile. Neurology 22:459–466, 1972.

74. KD Vincent, LS Davis. Unilateral abdominal distention following herpes zoster outbreak. Arch Dermatol 134: 1168–1169, 1998.

75. MF Yoong, PC Blumbergs, JB North. Primary (granulomatous) angiitis of the central nervous system with multiple aneurysms of spinal arteries. J Neurosurg 79:603–607, 1993.

76. DC Hilt, D Buchholz, A Krumholz, H Weiss, JS Wolinsky. Herpes zoster ophthalmicus and delayed contralateral hemiparesis caused by cerebral angiitis: diagnosis and management approaches. Ann Neurol 14:543–553, 1983.

77. MJ Glesby, RD Moore, RE Chaisson. Clinical spectrum of herpes zoster in adults infected with human immunodeficiency virus. Clin Infect Dis 21:370–375, 1995.

78. DJ Forster, PV Dugel, GT Frangieh, PE Liggett, NA Rao. Rapidly progressive outer retinal necrosis in the acquired immunodeficiency syndrome. Am J Ophthalmol 110: 341–348, 1990.

79. TP Sellitti, AJ Huang, J Schiffman, JL Davis. Association of herpes zoster ophthalmicus with acquired immunodeficiency syndrome and acute retinal necrosis. Am J Ophthalmol 116:297–301, 1993.

80. KF Chopra, T Evans, J Severeson, SK Tyring. Acute varicella zoster with postherpetic hyperhidrosis as the initial presentation of HIV infection. J Am Acad Dermatol 41: 119–121, 1999.

81. HN Johnson. Visceral lesions associated with varicella. Arch Pathol 30:292–307, 1940.

82. MN Oxman, R Alani. Varicella and herpes zoster. In: TB Fitzpatrick, AZ Eisen, K Wolff, IM Freedberg, KF Austen, eds. Dermatology in General Medicine, 4th ed. New York: McGraw-Hill, 1993, pp 2543–2572.

83. C Wesselhoeft. The differential diagnosis of chickenpox and smallpox. N Engl J Med 230:15–19, 1944.

84. AA Gershon. Varicella zoster virus. In: RD Feigin, JD Cherry, eds. Textbook of Pediatric Infectious Diseases, 4th ed. Philadelphia: WB Saunders, 1998, pp 1769–1777.

85. M Takahashi. Herpesviridae: varicella zoster virus. In: EM Lennette, P Halonen, FA Murphy, eds. Laboratory Diagnosis of Infectious Diseases: Principles and Practice. Vol 2: Viral Rickettsial, and Chlamydial Diseases. New York: Springer-Verlag, 1988, pp 261–275.

86. NJ Schmidt, D Gallo, V Delvin, JD Woodie, RW Emmons. Direct immunofluorescence staining for detection of herpes simplex and varicella zoster virus antigen in vesicular lesions and certain tissue specimens. J Clin Microbiol 12:651–655, 1980.

87. CM Koropchak, G Graham, J Palmer, M Winsberg, SF Ting, M Wallace, CG Prober, AM Arvin. Investigation of varicella-zoster infection by polymerase chain reaction in the immunocompetent host with acute varicella. J Infect Dis 163:1016–1022, 1991.

88. TH Weller. Varicella and herpes zoster. In: EH Lennette, NJ Schmidt, eds. Diagnostic Procedures for Viral, Rickett-

sial, and Chlamydial Infections, 5th ed. Washington DC: American Public Health Association, 1979, pp 375–388.

89. DH Gilden, AR Hayward, J Krupp, M Hunter-Laszlo, JC Huff, A Vafai. Varicella-zoster virus infection of human mononuclear cells. Virus Res 7:117–129, 1987.

90. GT Nahass, BA Goldstein, WY Zhu, U Serfling, NS Penneys, CL Leonardi. Comparison of Tzanck smear, viral culture, and DNA diagnostic methods in detection of herpes simplex and varicella-zoster infection. JAMA 268: 2541–2544, 1992.

91. LM Dunkel, AM Arvin, RJ Whitley, MK Farrell, RJ Sokol, RJ Rothbaum, FJ Suchy, WF Balistreri. A controlled trial of acyclovir for chickenpox in normal children. N Engl J Med 309:133–139, 1983.

92. MR Wallace, WA Bowler, NB Murray, SK Brodine, EC Oldfield 3d. Treatment of adult varicella with oral acyclovir. A randomized, placebo-controlled trial. Ann Intern Med 117:358–363, 1992.

93. CG Prober, LE Kirk, RE Keeney. Acyclovir therapy of chickenpox in immunosuppressed children: a collaborative study. J Pediatr 101:622–625, 1982.

94. G Nyerges, Z Meszner, E Gyarmati, Kerpel-Fronius. Acyclovir prevents dissemination of varicella in immunocompromised children. J Infect Dis 157:309–313, 1988.

95. RJ Whitley, M Hilty, R Haynes, Y Bryson, JD Connor, SJ Soong, CA Alford. Vidarabine therapy of varicella in immunosuppressed patients. J Pediatr 101:125–131, 1982.

96. AM Arvin, JH Kushner, S Feldman, RL Baehner, D Hammond, TC Merigan. Human leukocyte interferon in the treatment of varicella in children with cancer. N Engl J Med 306:761–765, 1982.

97. Centers for Disease Control and Prevention. Prevention of varicella: recommendations of the Advisory Committee on Immunization Practices (ACIP). MMWR 45(No. RR-11): 1–36, 1996.

98. Centers for Disease Control and Prevention. Varicella-zoster immune globulin for the prevention of chickenpox. MMWR 33:84–90, 95–99, 1984.

99. CJ White, BJ Kuter, CS Hildebrand, KL Isganitis, H Matthews, WJ Miller, PJ Provost, RW Ellis, RJ Gerety, GB Calandra. Varicella vaccine (VARIVAX) in healthy children and adolescents: results from clinical trials, 1987 to 1989. Pediatrics 87:604–610, 1991.

100. AA Gershon. Viral vaccines of the future. Pediatr Clin North Am 37:689–707, 1990.

101. AA Gershon. Live attenuated varicella vaccine. Annu Rev Med 38:41–50, 1987.

102. RP Wise, ME Salive, MN Braun, GT Mootrey, JF Seward, LG Rider, PR Krause. Postlicensure safety surveillance for varicella vaccine. JAMA 284:1271–1279, 2000.

103. HA Guess, DD Broughton, JL Melton 3d, LT Kurland. Epidemiology of herpes zoster in children and adolescents: a population-based study. Pediatrics 76:512–517, 1985.

104. I Hardy, AA Gershon, SP Steinberg, P LaRussa. The incidence of zoster after immunization with live attenuated varicella vaccine. N Engl J Med 325:1545–1550, 1991.

105. HS Izurieta, PM Strebel, PA Blake. Post licensure effectiveness of varicella vaccine during an outbreak in a child care center. JAMA 278:1495–1499, 1997.

106. M Takahachi. Current status and prospects of live varicella vaccine. Vaccine 10:1007–1014, 1992.

107. CDC. National, state, and urban area vaccination coverage levels among children aged 19–35 months—United States, 1999. MMWR 49:585–589, 2000.

108. PK Lichtenstein, JE Heubi, CC Daugherty, MK Farrell, RJ Sokol, RJ Rothbaum. Grade I Reye's syndrome: a frequent cause of vomiting and liver dysfunction after varicella and upper-respiratory-tract infection. N Engl J Med 309: 133–139 1983.

109. VA Fulginiti, PA Brunell, JD Cherry, WL Ector, AA Gershon, SP Gotoff. Aspirin and Reye syndrome. Pediatrics 69:810–812, 1982.

110. TA Lieu, SL Cochi, SB Black, ME Halloran, HR Shinefield, SJ Holmes, M Wharton, AE Washington. Cost effectiveness of a routine varicella vaccination program for US children. JAMA 271:375–381, 1994.

111. KE Wildenhoff, J Ipsen, V Esmann, J Ingemann-Jensen, JH Poulsen. Treatment of herpes zoster with idoxuridine ointment including a multivariate analysis of signs and symptoms. Scand J Infect Dis 11:1–9, 1979.

112. KE Wildenhoff, V Esmann, J Ipsen, H Harving, NA Peterslund, H Schonheyder. Treatment of trigeminal and thoracic zoster with idoxuridine. Scand J Infect Dis 13: 257–262, 1981.

113. RJ Whitley, LT Chien, R Dolin, GJ Galasso, CA Alford Jr. Adenosine arabinoside therapy of herpes zoster in the immunosuppressed. N Engl J Med 294:1193–1199, 1976.

114. RJ Whitley, JW Gnann Jr, D Hinthorn, C Liu, RB Pollard, F Hayden, GJ Mertz, M Oxman, SJ Soong. Disseminated herpes zoster in the immunocompromised host: a comparative trial of acyclovir and vidarabine. J Infect Dis 165: 450–455, 1992.

115. NA Peterslund, J Ipsen, H Schonheyder, K Seyer-Hansen, V Esmann, H Juhl. Acyclovir in herpes zoster. Lancet 2: 827–830, 1981.

116. B Bean, C Braun, HH Balfour Jr. Acyclovir therapy for acute herpes zoster. Lancet 2:118–121, 1982.

117. PJ van den Broek, JW van der Meer, JD Mulder, J Versteeg, H Mattie. Limited value to acyclovir in the treatment of uncomplicated herpes zoster: a placebo-controlled study. Infection 12:338–341, 1984.

118. J McGill, DR MacDonald, C Fall, GD McKendrick, A Copplestone. Intravenous acyclovir in acute herpes zoster infection. J Infect 6:157–161, 1983.

119. JC Huff, B Bean, HH Balfour Jr, OL Laskin, JD Connor, L Corey, YJ Bryson, P McGuirt. Therapy of herpes zoster with oral acyclovir. Am J Med 85(Suppl 2A):84–87, 1988.

120. MJ Wood, PH Ogan, MW McKendrick, CD Care, JI McGill, EM Webb. Efficacy of oral acyclovir in the treatment of acute herpes zoster. Am J Med 85(Suppl 2A): 79–83, 1988.

121. P Morton, AN Thomson. Oral acyclovir in the treatment

of herpes zoster in general practice. N Z Med J 102:93–95, 1989.

122. SP Harding, SM Porter. Oral acyclovir in herpes zoster ophthalmicus. Curr Eye Res 10:177–182, 1991.

123. JC Huff, JL Drucker, A Clemmer, OL Laskin, JD Connor, YJ Bryson, HH Balfour Jr. Efficacy of oral acyclovir on pain resolution in herpes zoster: a reanalysis. J Med Virol suppl 1:93–96, 1993.

124. RT Crooks, DA Jones, AP Fiddian. Zoster-associated chronic pain: an overview of clinical trials with acyclovir. Scand J Infect Dis 80(Suppl):62–68, 1991.

125. JJ Sasadeusz, SL Sachs. Systemic antivirals in herpesvirus infections. Dermatol Ther 11:171–185, 1993.

126. KR Beutner, DJ Friedman, C Forszpaniak, PL Andersen, MJ Wood. Valaciclovir compared with acyclovir for improved therapy for herpes zoster in immunocompetent adults. Antimicrob Agents Chemother 39:1546–1553, 1995.

127. K Beutner. Antivirals in the treatment of pain. J Geriatr Dermatol 6(Suppl 2):23A–28A, 1994.

128. MA Jacobson, J Gallant, LH Wang, D Coakley, S Weller, D Gary, L Squires, ML Smiley, MR Blum, J Feinberg. Phase-1 trial of valaciclovir, the L-valyl ester of acyclovir, in patients with advanced human immunodeficiency disease. Antimicrob Agents Chemother 38:1534–1540, 1994.

129. H Degreef, Famciclovir Herpes Zoster Clinical Study Group. Famciclovir, a new oral antiherpes drug: results of the first controlled clinical study demonstrating its efficacy and safety in the treatment of uncomplicated herpes zoster in immunocompetent patients. Int J Antimicrob Agents 4: 241–246, 1994.

130. S Tyring, RA Barbarash, JE Nahlik, A Cunningham, J Marley, M Heng, T Jones, T Rea, R Boon, R Saltzman. Famciclovir for the treatment of acute herpes zoster: effects on acute disease and postherpetic neuralgia. Ann Intern Med 123:89–96, 1995.

131. I Decroix, H Partsch, R Gonzalez, H Mobacken, CL Goh, L Walsh, S Shukla, B Naisbett. Factors influencing pain outcome in herpes zoster: an observational study with valaciclovir. J Eur Acad Dermatol Venereol 14:23–33, 2000.

132. SK Tyring, KR Beutner, BA Tucker, WC Anderson, RJ Crooks. Antiviral therapy for herpes zoster: a randomized, controlled, clinical trial of valacyclovir and famciclovir therapy in immunocompetent patients 50 years and older. Arch Fam Med 9:863–869, 2000.

133. SK Tyring, R Belanger, W Bezwoda, P Ljungman, R Boon, RL Saltzman. A randomized, double-blind trial of famciclovir versus acyclovir for the treatment of localized dermatomal herpes zoster in immunocompromised patients. Cancer Invest 19:13–22, 2001.

134. SK Tyring, M Engst, C Corriveau, N Robillard, S Trottier, S Van Slycken, RA Crann, LA Locke, R Saltzman, AG Palestine. Famciclovir for ophthalmic zoster: a randomised, aciclovir-controlled study. Br J Ophthalmol 85: 576–581, 2001.

135. WH Eaglstein, R Katy, JA Brown. The effects of early

corticosteroid therapy on the skin eruption and pain of herpes zoster. JAMA 211:1681–1683, 1970.

136. B Post, JT Philbrick. Do corticosteroids prevent postherpetic neuralgia? A review of the evidence. J Am Acad Dermatol 18:605–610, 1988.

137. MJ Wood, RW Johnson, MW McKendrick, J Taylor, BK Mandal, J Crooks. A randomized trial of acyclovir for 7 days or 21 days with and without prenisolone for treatment of acute herpes zoster. N Engl J Med 330:896–900, 1994.

138. RJ Whitley, H Weiss, JW Gnann, S Tyring, GJ Mertz, PG Pappas, CJ Schleupner, F Hayden, J Wolf, SJ Soong. Acyclovir with and without prednisone for the treatment of herpes zoster. Ann Intern Med 125:376–383, 1996.

139. Y Furuta. Early diagnosis of zoster sine herpete and antiviral therapy for the treatment of facial palsy. Neurology 55:708–710, 2000.

140. D Bowsher. The management of postherpetic neuralgia. Postgrad Med J 73:623–629, 1996.

141. CP Watson, M Chipman, K Reed, RJ Evans, N Birkett. Amitriptyline versus maprotiline in postherpetic neuralgia: a randomized, double-blind, crossover trial. Pain 48: 29–36, 1992.

142. R Kishore-Kumar, MB Max, SC Schafer, AM Gaughan, B Smoller, RH Gracely, R Dubner. Desipramine relieves postherpetic neuralgia. Clin Pharmacol Ther 47:305–312, 1990.

143. PW Nathan. Chlorprothixen (Tractan) in post-herpetic neuralgia and other severe chronic pain. Pain 5:367–371, 1978.

144. M Rowbotham, N Harden, B Stacey, MS Bernstein, L Magnus-Miller for the Gabapentin Postherpetic Neuralgia group. Gabapentin for the treatment of postherpetic neuralgia. JAMA 280:1837–1842, 1998.

145. JE Bernstein, NJ Korman, DR Bickers, MV Dahl, LE Millikan. Topical capsaicin treatment of chronic postherpetic neuralgia. J Am Acad Dermatol 21:265–270, 1989.

146. CP Watson, RJ Evans, VR Watt. Postherpetic neuralgia and topical capsaicin. Pain 33:333–340, 1988.

147. MC Rowbotham, PS Davies, C Verkempinck, BS Galer. Lidocaine patch: Double-blind controlled study of a new treatment method for post-herpetic neuralgia. Pain 65: 39–44, 1996.

148. MC Rowbotham, HL Rields. Topical lidocaine reduces pain in post-herpetic neuralgia. Pain 38:297–301, 1989.

149. J Kissin, J McDanal, AV Xavier. Topical lidocaine for relief of superficial pain in postherpetic neuralgia. Neurology 39:1132–1133, 1989.

150. R Tenicela, D Lovasik, W Eaglstein. Treatment of herpes zoster with sympathetic blocks. Clin J Pain 1:63–67, 1985.

151. H Suzuki, S Ogawa, H Nakagawa, T Kanayama, K Tai, H Saitoh, Y Ohshima. Cryocautery of sensitized skin areas for the relief of pain due to postherpetic neuralgia. Pain 9:355–362, 1980.

152. A Colding. The effect of sympathetic blocks on herpes zoster. Acta Anaesthesiol Scand 13:133–141, 1969.

153. A Colding. Treatment of pain: organization of a pain clinic;

treatment of acute herpes zoster. Proc R Soc Med 66: 541–543, 1973.

154. PJ Stow, CJ Glynn, B Minor. EMLA cream in the treatment of post-herpetic neuralgia: efficacy and pharmacokinetic profile. 39:301–305, 1989.

155. PW Nathan, PD Wall. Treatment of post-herpetic neuralgia by prolonged electric stimulation. Br Med J 3:645–647, 1974.

156. N Kotani, T Kushikata, H Hashimoto, F Kimura, M Muraoka, M Yodono, M Asai, A Matsuki. Intrathecal methylprednisolone for intractable postherptic neuralgia. N Engl J Med 343:1514–1519, 2000.

157. A Hayward, E Villaneuba, M Cosyns, M Levin. Varicella-zoster virus (VZV) specific cytotoxicity after immunization of nonimmune adults with OKA strain attenuated VZV vaccine. J Infect Dis 166:260–264, 1992.

158. L Zerboni, S Nader, K Aoki, AM Arvin. Analysis of the persistence of humoral and cellular immunity in children and adults immunized with varicella vaccine. J Infect Dis 177:1701–1704, 1998.

159. MJ Levin, M Murray, GO Zerbe, CJ White, AR Hayward. Immune responses of elderly persons 4 years after receiving a live attenuated varicella vaccine. J Infect Dis 170: 522–526, 1994.

160. RH Mead 3rd, TW Chang. Zoster-like eruption due to echovirus 6. Am J Dis Child 133:283–284, 1979.

6

Epstein-Barr Virus

Dennis M. Walling and S. David Hudnall
University of Texas Medical Branch, Galveston, Texas, USA

Angela Yen-Moore
University of Texas Southwestern Medical Center, Dallas, Texas, USA

The Epstein-Barr virus (EBV) is a human herpesvirus of the gamma subfamily that is related to the lymphocryptoviruses of the old world primates [1]. EBV consists of a 170 to 180-kb double-stranded DNA genome that encodes 80 to 100 genes. EBV isolates can be classified on the basis of levels of genome complexity. There are two distinct types of EBV, similar to the difference between herpes simplex virus 1 and 2. Within each EBV type, distinct strains can be identified based on nucleotide substitution patterns within specific genes. Viral variants are created through genetic recombination within or between different types and strains. The infectious particle of EBV consists of linear viral DNA packaged within a hexagonal protein nucleocapsid and surrounded by a lipid envelope.

EBV routinely infects human mucosal epithelial cells and B lymphocytes and is capable of infecting other cell types under certain conditions [1]. As with all human herpesviruses, EBV infection persists for the life of the host. The state of EBV infection may be productive or latent. In productive infection, the viral genome is repeatedly replicated by viral DNA polymerase. This high level of replication ultimately results in the production and release of infectious virions from the host cell. In the latent state of infection, no infectious virions are produced. Each latent viral genome within a host cell is replicated only once by the host cell DNA polymerase as the cell divides. Over the life of the host, EBV may transit between latent and productive infection many times.

HISTORY

In 1964, an African Burkitt's lymphoma was found to contain a herpesvirus that was subsequently named Epstein-Barr virus after its two discoverers [2]. In 1968, an association was made between EBV and the previously described infectious mononucleosis syndrome [3]. Since that time, EBV has been associated with a variety of different diseases and syndromes that can be classified by the infected cell type and the predominant state of viral infection (Table 6–1). Worldwide (Fig. 6–1), the most common and clinically important EBV-associated diseases include the infectious mononucleosis syndrome, Hodgkin's lymphoma, African Burkitt's lymphoma, and nasopharyngeal carcinoma. In the United States, the infectious mononucleosis syndrome, Hodgkin's lymphoma, and the lymphoproliferative diseases of immunocompromised patients account for most of the EBV-associated morbidity and mortality. EBV is

Table 6–1. Epstein-Barr Virus (EBV)–Associated Diseases and Syndromes

I. EBV in lymphocytes
  A. Latent Infection
    1. Infectious mononucleosis
    2. African Burkitt's lymphoma
    3. Hodgkin's lymphoma
    4. Lymphoproliferative diseases of immunocompromised patients
      a) Polyclonal nonmalignant lymphoproliferations
      b) Monoclonal malignant lymphomas of various histologic types
    5. T-cell lymphomas
      a) Angioimmunoblastic lymphadenopathy type
      b) Nodal T-cell immunoblastic lymphoma
      c) Peripheral T-cell lymphoma with hemophagocytosis
    6. Kikuchi's histiocytic necrotizing lymphadenitis
II. EBV in smooth muscle cells
  A. Latent infection
    1. Leiomyomas of immunocompromised patients
    2. Leiomyosarcomas of immunocompromised patients
III. EBV in epithelial cells
  A. Latent infection
    1. Lymphoepithelial carcinoma
      a) Nasopharynx
      b) Salivary glands
      c) Gastric mucosa
      d) Thymus
      e) Lung
    2. Squamous cell carcinoma of the oropharynx
  B. Productive infection
    1. Oral hairy leukoplakia

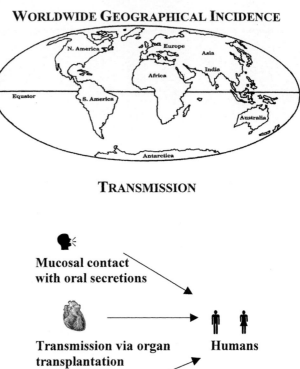

TAXONOMY

Herpesviridae (Human herpes virus 4)

WORLDWIDE GEOGRAPHICAL INCIDENCE

TRANSMISSION

Mucosal contact with oral secretions

Transmission via organ transplantation

Humans

Blood transfusion or congenital exposure

ZOONOTIC IMPLICATIONS
None

Figure 6–1. Incidence and transmission of Epstein-Barr virus (EBV; human herpes virus 4.)

now recognized as an oncogenic virus based on its association with a variety of cancers and its ability to immortalize B lymphocytes in vitro [1].

PRIMARY INFECTION AND THE INFECTIOUS MONONUCLEOSIS SYNDROME

Epidemiology

The prevalence of EBV infection approaches 95% by early adulthood [4]. However, in developing countries and in the lower socioeconomic population in the United States, EBV seropositivity rates reach 60 to 80% during childhood. The rate in the higher socioeconomic population does not reach this level until late adolescence (Fig. 6–2) [5]. In preadolescent children, primary infection with EBV is asymptomatic or occasionally results in a mild, nonspecific, febrile illness. After adolescence, approximately 50% of primary EBV infections result in the syndrome of infectious mononucleosis. Thus, with the majority of primary EBV infections in the United States occurring later in life, the incidence of infectious mononucleosis in the United States is 45.2 cases per 100,000 population per year [6]. Conse-

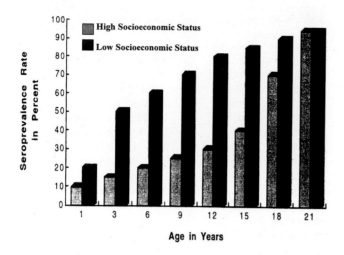

Figure 6–2. EBV seroprevalence rate as a function of age and socioeconomic status.

quently, infectious mononucleosis has its largest public health impact on young college student and military recruit populations but may occur at any age.

Pathogenesis

EBV is transmitted person-to-person by infectious virions that are produced at mucosal surfaces and shed into body fluids [7]. Oral mucosal contact with infectious saliva is the most common route of transmission. The presence of EBV in breast milk [8] and in genital secretions [9,10] suggests additional modes of transmission. Congenital EBV infection has been documented [11–13]. EBV may also be transmitted via organ transplantation or blood transfusion if these tissues contain EBV-infected lymphocytes [14].

Primary EBV infection usually occurs at the oropharyngeal epithelium (Fig. 6–3). The mechanism by which EBV

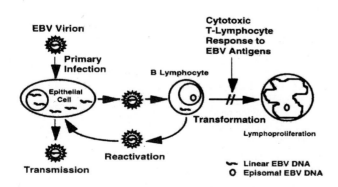

Figure 6–3. A simplified model of EBV infection and pathogenesis.

enters epithelial cells is not known but may involve a cell surface receptor. In epithelial cells, EBV infection typically results in productive viral replication in a cell differentiation-dependent manner. The EBV genome is replicated and packaged into protein nucleocapsids with lipid envelopes generated by the nuclear membrane. After processing through the Golgi apparatus, secretory vesicles fuse with the cell membrane and release mature infectious virions to the environment to transmit the infection (Fig. 6–3).

At least two EBV genes may be important to the pathogenesis of productive infection. The EBV gene *BCRF1* encodes a viral homologue of human interleukin 10. Expression of *BCRF1* may down-regulate the TH1 immune response of the host, thereby prolonging the duration of productive replication [15]. The EBV gene *BHRF1* encodes a viral homologue of human *Bcl-2,* an inhibitor of apoptosis or programmed cell death [16]. Expression of *BHRF1* and inhibition of apoptosis may preserve the cellular machinery necessary to support productive viral replication as the squamous epithelial cell differentiates.

Eventually, the host immune response succeeds in terminating EBV replication in the oropharynx. Although it is uncertain if EBV establishes latent infection in oropharyngeal epithelial cells [17], circulating B lymphocytes do become latently infected with EBV (Fig. 6–3).

EBV enters the B lymphocyte by specific binding to the cell surface complement receptor CR2 or CD21 [18]. The EBV genome circularizes, briefly replicates, and is maintained in the cell nucleus as multiple episomes (Fig. 6–3).

Expression of the EBV *EBNA-1* gene product is required to replicate and partition the EBV genomes as the B lymphocyte divides [19]. The *EBNA-1* protein also contains elements that inhibit antigen processing and major histocompatibility complex (MHC) class I–restricted antigen presentation. Thus, cytotoxic T-lymphocyte responses are not generated against this critical EBV protein [20]. Expression of the viral *LMP-2* gene also aids in the maintenance of EBV latency [21]. With restricted gene expression and evasion of the cellular immune system, latent infection of B lymphocytes may explain how EBV maintains a persistent infection [22].

Cytotoxic T lymphocytes and natural killer cells constitute the primary form of host defense against EBV (Fig. 6–3) [23]. MHC class I–restricted cytotoxic T lymphocytes are largely directed toward antigens involved in the regulation of cell growth of viral proteins (*EBNA-2, EBNA-3, EBNA-4, EBNA-5, EBNA-6, LMP-1,* and *LMP-2*). Thus, transformation and immortalization of B lymphocytes by these EBV proteins are severely curtailed in the presence of an effective immune response (Fig. 6–3). In the infectious mononucleosis syndrome, the atypical lymphocytes seen on peripheral blood smear are activated cytotoxic T lymphocytes responding to EBV-infected B lymphocytes.

In the absence of an effective cellular immune response, EBV-induced B-cell lymphoproliferations may occur (Fig. 6–3). In some cases, EBV infection of T lymphocytes may result in T-cell lymphoproliferations [24]. This may trigger the autoimmune reactivity seen in the neurological manifestations of infectious mononucleosis or the EBV-associated hemophagocytic syndrome [25].

The humoral response to EBV infection generates antibodies against a variety of EBV antigens. However, the role of these antibodies in the pathogenesis of, and recovery from, disease is not clear. EBV-specific antibodies are not protective against EBV superinfection, and multiple EBV types and strains may be found in the oropharynx and peripheral blood lymphocytes of some individuals. Immunoglobulin A (IgA) against EBV may actually facilitate virion entry into epithelial cells [26]. During the infectious mononucleosis syndrome, autoreactive antibodies against erythrocytes and platelets may contribute to the pathogenesis of complications such as autoimmune hemolytic anemia and thrombocytopenia [27,28].

Finally, long after the resolution of infectious mononucleosis, EBV reactivation from latency in B lymphocytes results in viral reinfection of the oropharyngeal epithelium (Fig. 6–3). Subsequent productive replication and shedding of infectious virions into saliva occurs completely asymptomatically [29]. Whereas latency is a strategy by which EBV persists for the life of the host, periodic reactivation allows the virus to be transmitted to new human hosts.

Clinical Manifestations

After an incubation period of 3 to 7 weeks, the EBV-associated infectious mononucleosis syndrome presents with a triad of fever, pharyngitis, and lymphadenopathy [30]. In some cases, one or more of these signs may be absent. The most frequent manifestations of infectious mononucleosis are listed in Table 6–2.

Table 6–3. Potential Complications of Infectious Mononucleosis

Neurological	Hematological
Encephalitis and seizures	Neutropenia
Meningoencephalitis	Thrombocytopenia
Transverse myelitis	Aplastic anemia
Cranial neuritis	Hemolytic anemia
Optic neuritis	Hemophagocytic
Peripheral neuropathy	syndrome
Mononeuritis multiplex	Splenic rupture
Guillain-Barré acute	Lymphoproliferative
syndrome	disease
Reye's syndrome	Hepatic
Respiratory	Hepatitis
Airway obstruction	Hepatic necrosis
Pneumonitis	Reye's syndrome
Cardiac	Renal
Myocarditis	Glomerulonephritis
Pericarditis	Interstitial nephritis
Hematological	

Serious complications may occur with infectious mononucleosis. Substantial edema of the oropharyngeal lymphoid tissue may lead to encroachment of the airway, with stridor and breathing difficulties. Splenic rupture occurs in 0.2% of affected adults. This complication most frequently occurs during the second week of the illness and typically results from trauma, including mild incidents. Other potential complications of the infectious mononucleosis syndrome are listed in Table 6–3.

Although most childhood EBV infections are asymptomatic or mild, infants and children who develop the infectious mononucleosis syndrome may present with signs and symptoms similar to those in adults. However, they are more likely to exhibit splenomegaly, hepatomegaly, and respiratory tract infections [31]. Other clinical presenta-

Table 6–2. Signs and Symptoms of Infectious Mononucleosis

Present in ≥ 50% of patients	Present in 10–0% of patients	Present in ≤ of patients
Fever	Anorexia	Palatal enanthem
Pharyngitis and sore throat	Nausea	Cutaneous exanthems
Lymphadenopathy	Abdominal discomfort	Jaundice
Malaise and fatigue	Hepatomegaly	Vomiting
Headache	Hepatic tenderness	Cough
Splenomegaly	Myalgias	Arthralgias
	Chills	

festations are seen with infectious mononucleosis (Table 6–5).

Dermatopathology

There are no pathognomonic histopathological findings that characterize the mucocutaneous lesions associated with primary EBV infection. Nonspecific exanthems demonstrate nonspecific pathologies. Specific cutaneous manifestations may be identified by their characteristic pathologies, but none is specific for EBV infection as the etiology. Although the subject has not been well studied, most EBV-associated cutaneous manifestations likely arise through immune-mediated events. However, direct EBV infection of cutaneous epithelial or vascular endothelial cells may account for some manifestations [42,53,55,56].

Laboratory Findings

Hepatocellular transaminase levels are frequently mild-to-moderately elevated in patients with infectious mononucleosis, but significant hyperbilirubinemia and clinically detectable jaundice occur in only 5% of cases [30]. The white blood cell count commonly demonstrates a lymphocytosis of greater than 50% with at least 10% atypical lymphocytes (Fig. 6–5). However, the absence of atypical lymphocytes does not exclude the diagnosis of infectious mononucleosis. Importantly, atypical lymphocytosis is not pathognomonic for EBV infection and may also be seen during infections with CMV, human herpesvirus 6 (HHV-6), toxoplasmosis, acute viral hepatitis, rubella, and mumps, and with drug hypersensitivity reactions. Mild thrombocytopenia may occur in up to one half of patients with infectious mononucleosis [57], but platelet counts below

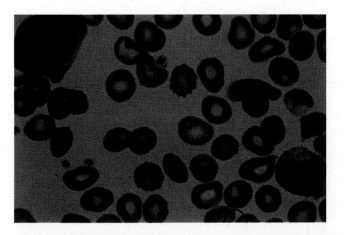

Figure 6–5. Atypical lymphocytes ($1000\times$)—Wright-stained peripheral blood smear showing infectious mononucleosis.

$20,000/mm^3$ are rare and are associated with potentially life-threatening hemorrhages [58].

Diagnosis

The diagnosis of primary EBV infection must be differentiated (Table 6–6) from a variety of other conditions of infectious and noninfectious etiologies [59], and is best made by serological testing. Heterophile antibodies capable of agglutinating sheep, horse, or bovine erythrocytes are present at titers of greater than 1:40 in approximately 90% of adolescent and adult patients with the infectious mononucleosis syndrome [60]. They may also be positive in patients with mild or asymptomatic primary EBV infection. False-positive tests are rare. Heterophile antibodies

Table 6–6. Differential Diagnoses of Infectious Mononucleosis

Group A streptococcal infection: Infection is similar with pharyngitis, fever, and submandibular adenopathy, but is not associated with hepatosplenomegaly.

Acute viral hepatitis (hepatitis A, B or C virus): Infection may be similar with fever, hepatomegaly and elevated hepatic enzymes, but negative heterophile antibody test and specific serologies.

Primary cytomegalovirus infection: Fever, lymphadenopathy, and malaise, but negative heterophile antibody test and specific serologies.

Primary human herpesvirus-6 infection: Fever, lymphadenopathy, and malaise, but negative heterophile antibody test and specific serologies.

Human immunodeficiency virus (HIV): May sometimes appear clinically similar, with fever, lymphadenopathy, and malaise, but negative heterophile antibody test and specific serologies.

Toxoplasmosis: Fever, lymphadenopathy, and malaise, but negative heterophile antibody test and specific serologies.

Lymphoma: May have a similar presentation, but negative heterophile antibody test and specific serologies.

Rubella: May rarely present with fever, malaise, adenopathy, maculopapular skin rash, and palatal petechiae, but negative heterophile antibody test and specific serologies.

Phenytoin hypersensitivity reaction: This reaction may present with fever, lymphadenopathy, hepatitis, and skin rash. The patient may develop leukocytosis with atypical lymphocytes. Unlike infectious mononucleosis, facial and periorbital edema are common and there is a history of phenytoin use (or other aromatic anticonvulsants), often begun in the previous 2–6 wk.

may persist after the onset of illness for 3 to 6 months and up to 18 months in some cases. However, in young children, heterophile antibodies are positive in only a small minority with primary EBV infection [61]. The greatest utility of the heterophile antibody test is as a rapid screen for primary EBV infection in young adults with a compatible clinical presentation. Several commercially produced rapid spot or slide tests for the presence of heterophile antibodies are currently available.

Specific EBV serologies are required to make a definitive diagnosis of EBV infection, especially when the heterophile antibody test is negative [30]. Titers of three different antibodies are needed determine the stage of EBV infection (Fig. 6–6). IgG and IgM against EBV viral capsid antigen (VCA) appear concurrently, at or before the onset of clinical symptoms in primary EBV infection. VCA IgG remains positive for life. VCA IgM reverts to negative within 2 or 3 months, usually after the clinical symptoms have resolved. Between 1 and 6 months after the onset

of symptoms, IgG against EBV nuclear antigens (EBNA) appear and then remain positive for life. Antibodies to EBV early antigens (EA) lack sensitivity and specificity for primary EBV infection and are rarely helpful in determining the stage of EBV infection. Thus, primary EBV infection is diagnosed by the presence of VCA IgG and VCA IgM antibodies in the absence of EBNA IgG antibodies (Table 6–7). The presence of antibodies to EBNA indicates that primary EBV infection occurred 1 or more months in the past and usually suggests that a patient's present clinical syndrome is unrelated to primary EBV infection. Thus, EBV serological tests are most useful to differentiate between acute primary infection and the chronic state of past, persistent infection.

Treatment

In the majority of cases, infectious mononucleosis is a self-limited disease, and patients need only supportive medical

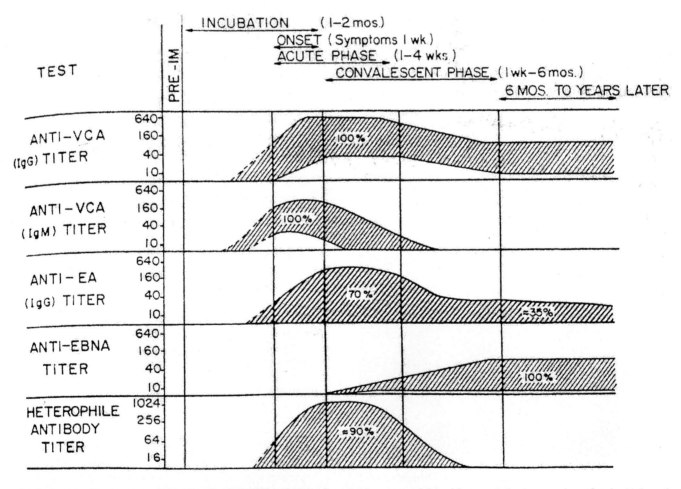

Figure 6–6. Characteristic EBV-specific antibody responses observed in young adults with acute infectious mononucleosis. (Adapted from Ref. 5 with permission.)

Table 6–7. Serological Diagnoses of EBV Infection

Antibody	Viral capsid antigen immunoglobulin G (VCA IgG)	VCA IgM	EBV nuclear antigens (EBNA) IgG
Acute primary infection	Positive	Positive	Negative
Past persistent infection	Positive	Negative	Positive

care (Table 6–8). Antiviral agents such as acyclovir inhibit EBV replication, but they do not influence the clinical course of infectious mononucleosis [62]. Acyclovir therapy does not eliminate the latent form of EBV infection and does not reduce the number of EBV-infected lymphocytes in the peripheral blood [63]. Combination therapy with oral acyclovir and oral corticosteroids provided no significant benefit over placebo in one large randomized, prospective clinical trial [64].

Corticosteroids do not negatively influence the clinical

Table 6–8. Treatment of Infectious Mononucleosis

Symptom	Treatment
General	Rest, proper nutrition, and adequate hydration
Fever	Antipyretics (aspirin should be avoided in children)
Headache	Analgesics (acetaminophen or nonsteroidal anti-inflammatory drugs)
Myalgias	Analgesics
Sore throat	Analgesics and salt water gargle
Cutaneous manifestations	Topical steroids for exanthems and oral antihistamines as needed for pruritus
Splenomegaly	Patients should be cautioned against physical activities that may traumatize the abdomen and cause splenic rupture.
Major complications:airway encroachment, hemolytic anemia, or severe thrombocytopenia	Prednisone 0.5 mg/kg per dose twice daily (maximum of 60 mg/24 hr tapered over a 1–2 wk period if clinical response is prompt)

outcome of infectious mononucleosis, but the associated risks of corticosteroid therapy cannot justify their routine use in uncomplicated cases. There are three clear indications for the use of corticosteroids in infectious mononucleosis: (1) lymphadenopathy and edema of the neck and throat causing respiratory compromise or airway obstruction, (2) hemolytic anemia, and (3) severe thrombocytopenia [30]. The role is less clear for corticosteroids in the neurological complications of EBV infection, but some experts advocate their use in more serious cases.

It is believed that the majority of the signs and symptoms of infectious mononucleosis result from the host immune response to the EBV infection, especially against the transformation-associated EBV antigens expressed in B lymphocytes. Thus, persistent cell-mediated immunity to EBV is protective against developing the symptoms of the infectious mononucleosis syndrome with EBV superinfection later in life. A vaccine to prevent primary EBV infection is not yet available.

LYMPHOPROLIFERATIVE DISEASE AND MALIGNANCY

Epidemiology

EBV-associated lymphoproliferative diseases occur in immunocompromised patients such as those with human immunodeficiency virus (HIV) infection, those receiving iatrogenic immunosuppression, or those with certain congenital immunodeficiency syndromes (Table 6–9). In the United States, the incidence of lymphoproliferative disease is between 2 and 10% for organ transplant recipients and between 10 and 30% for patients with the acquired immunodeficiency syndrome (AIDS) [65–67]. Hodgkin's lymphoma, African Burkitt's lymphoma, certain T-cell lymphomas, and nasopharyngeal carcinoma are EBV-associated malignancies that typically occur in otherwise non-immunocompromised patients (Table 6–1).

A prior history of infectious mononucleosis is a risk factor for developing Hodgkin's lymphoma [68]. African Burkitt's lymphoma is epidemiologically associated with malarial infection in sub-Saharan Africa. Nasopharyngeal

Table 6–9.   Immunocompromised Patients at Risk for EBV-associated Lymphoproliferative Disease

I.   Acquired immunodeficiency
   A.   Acquired immunodeficiency syndrome (AIDS) secondary to human immunodeficiency virus (HIV) infection
   B.   Iatrogenic immunosuppressive therapy
      1.   Organ transplant recipients
         a)   Anti–T-lymphocyte antibodies
         b)   Multiple high-dose steroid pulses
         c)   Cyclosporine
         d)   Azothiaprine
      2.   Autoimmune disease patients
         a)   Cyclosporine
         b)   Methotrexate
         c)   Azothiaprine
II.   Congenital immunodeficiency
   A.   Wiskott-Aldrich syndrome
   B.   Ataxia-telangiectasia syndrome
   C.   Common variable immunodeficiency syndrome
   D.   Severe combined immunodeficiency syndrome
   E.   X-linked lymphoproliferative syndrome (Duncan's syndrome)

carcinoma occurs commonly in certain ethnic groups and geographical regions, including southern China, Southeast Asia, Mediterranean Africa, and populations indigenous to Alaska. The epidemiology is still unclear for the recently recognized EBV-associated T-cell lymphomas, but most reports originate from east Asia [69]. Other EBV-associated malignancies are rare or contain EBV in only a small percentage of lesions (Table 6–1).

Pathogenesis

In patients with deficient cytotoxic T-lymphocyte activity against EBV, the number of EBV-infected lymphocytes in the peripheral blood rises dramatically, heralding the risk of lymphoproliferative disease [70]. Expression of the EBV proteins *EBNA-2, EBNA-3, EBNA-4, EBNA-5, EBNA-6,* and *LMP-1* is associated with the transformation and immortalization of B lymphocytes in vitro and in vivo [71]. As a group, these viral proteins transactivate the expression of cellular genes and interact with cellular proteins involved in the regulation of cell growth. The viral proto-oncogene *LMP-1* is especially important to the process of B-lymphocyte transformation, influencing cell surface receptor signaling pathways, interacting with cellular transcription factors, and inhibiting cell apoptosis. Several different patterns of expression of these latent,

transformation-associated EBV genes have been described for different EBV-associated malignancies. Although the biology of EBV latency and transformation is complex, it is believed that these EBV genes are important to the oncogenic process of all EBV-associated neoplasia [71,72]. Clearly, multiple other factors are involved as well, including host genetic susceptibility, host immune status, host age and route of infection, dietary and environmental influences, and EBV genetic variation. The exact role of EBV in the process of oncogenesis remains an important area of active investigation.

Clinical and Dermatological Manifestations

EBV-associated lymphoproliferative diseases and malignancies may involve any organ system of the body and may present with an enormous range of clinical findings. The most common cutaneous manifestation of EBV-associated lymphoproliferation or malignancy is subcutaneous lymphadenopathy secondary to invasion of, or metastases to, pre-existing lymph nodes. Less commonly, EBV-associated lymphoproliferation may involve the skin and subcutaneous tissues directly. The dermatological manifestations of EBV-associated lymphoproliferative disease and malignancy are listed in Table 6–10.

The primary tumor of nasopharyngeal carcinoma is often asymptomatic, and the disease frequently presents with metastases to lymph nodes in the head and neck (Fig. 6–7). Hodgkin's lymphoma may present primarily with palpable lymphadenopathy, including the cervical and sub-

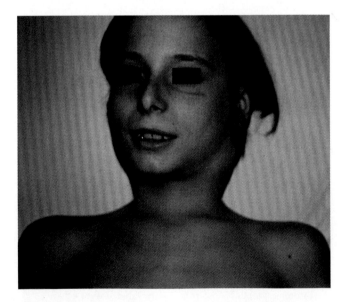

Figure 6–7.   Nasopharyngeal carcinoma with marked cervical lymphadenopathy.

Table 6–10. Dermatologic Manifestations of EBV-associated Lymphoproliferative Disease and Malignancy

I. Solid tumors
   A. Nasopharyngeal carcinoma
      1. Cervical lymphadenopathy from metastases
II. B-cell lymphoproliferative disorders
   A. Hodgkin's lymphoma
      1. Cervical and submandibular lymphadenopathy
   B. Burkitt's lymphoma
      1. Submandibular lymphadenopathy
      2. Parotid salivary gland enlargement
   C. Lymphoproliferative diseases of immunocompromised patients
      1. Diffuse subcutaneous lymphadenopathy
      2. Primary cutaneous lymphoma
         a) Nodules and ulceration
      3. Oral lymphoma in HIV-infected patients
         a) Swelling, ulceration, and necrosis
III. T-cell lymphoproliferative disorders
   A. Oral lymphoma in HIV-infected patients
      1. Swelling, ulceration, and necrosis
   B. Angiocentric cutaneous lymphoma
      1. Violaceous plaques
      2. Papules
      3. Nodules
      4. Bullae
      5. Chronic ulcers
      6. Subcutaneous tumors
   C. Subcutaneous lymphoma
      1. Panniculitis
   D. Histiocytoid cutaneous lymphoma
      1. Papules with necrosis
   E. Vesiculopapular lesions of the face
      1. Vesiculopapular eruptions
      2. Subcutaneous nodules

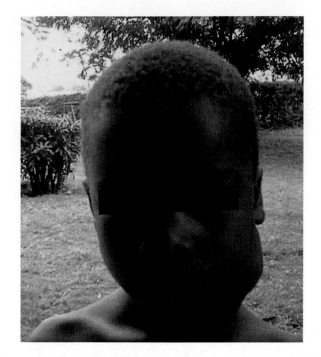

Figure 6–8. African Burkitt's lymphoma with marked cervical lymphadenopathy. (Courtesy of Barbara Lepard, M.D., Moshi, Tanzania.)

occur in the oral cavity with manifestations including swelling (Fig. 6–9) and ulcerations of the gingivae, hard palate, or tongue [74–77].

Recently, cutaneous T-cell lymphomas in otherwise immunocompetent patients have been found to contain EBV

mandibular lymph nodes. African Burkitt's lymphoma typically arises in lymphoid tissue associated with the oropharyngeal mucosa or gastrointestinal tract and may present in salivary glands or submandibular lymph nodes (Fig. 6–8). Lymphoproliferative diseases and malignant lymphomas occurring in immunocompromised patients may involve any of the groups of subcutaneous lymph nodes.

Primary cutaneous B-cell lymphomas containing EBV may occur in iatrogenically immunosuppressed patients after solid organ transplantation [73]. These cases presented clinically with multiple ulcerative cutaneous nodules in the absence of peripheral lymphadenopathy or internal organ involvement. In HIV-infected patients with AIDS, EBV-associated B-cell and T-cell lymphomas may

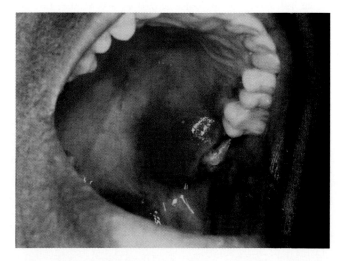

Figure 6–9. Lymphoma of the palate in an HIV-seropositive patient. (Courtesy of J. K. Maniar, M.D., Department of Dermatovenereology and AIDS Medicine, G. T. Hospital, Grant Medical College, Mumbai, India.)

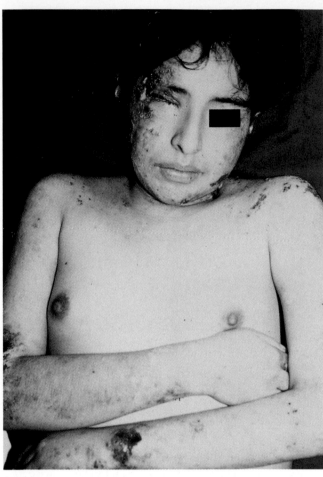

(a)

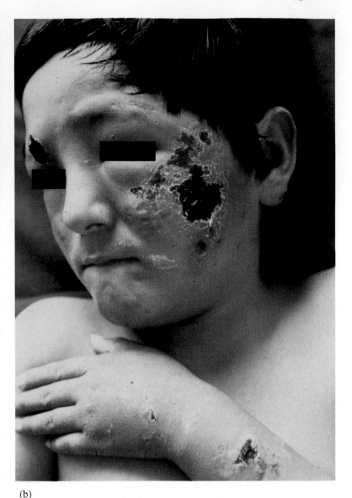

(b)

Figure 6–10. (a,b) Cutaneous facial and edematous T-cell lymphoma of childhood. The classic findings include a recurrent facial edema, along with the presence of papules and nodules that ulcerate and scar. It is associated with a fatal outcome, despite therapy. (Courtesy of Francisco Bravo Puccio, M.D., Instituto Dermatologico, Lima, Peru.)

in some cases [78–83]. In these reports, the dermatological manifestations included multiple violaceous plaques, papules, nodules, bullae, chronic ulcers (Fig. 6–10), and subcutaneous tumors on the trunk and extremities. Interestingly, a history of hypersensitivity to mosquito bites (intense erythematous swelling and skin ulceration, fever, and hepatitis) was noted for some patients with cutaneous EBV-associated lymphoproliferative disease. Notably, EBV is not associated with classical mycosis fungoides or with human T-cell lymphotropic virus (HTLV)–I–associated cutaneous adult T-cell lymphoma.

Laboratory Findings

There are no laboratory findings that are specific for, or even characteristic of, EBV-associated lymphoproliferative diseases or malignancies.

Dermatopathology

Histologically, nasopharyngeal carcinoma is a lymphoepithelial carcinoma characterized by either squamous, non-kerxatinizing, or undifferentiated epithelial cells, and a prominent desmoplastic lymphoid infiltration [84]. In nasopharyngeal carcinoma, EBV is present in the malignant epithelial cells but not the infiltrating lymphocytes. Hodgkin's lymphoma manifests a variety of histologic subtypes, but the mixed cellularity and nodular lymphocyte predominance subtypes are most likely to be EBV-associated [85]. In Hodgkin's lymphoma, EBV is detected only within the Reed-Sternberg cells [86]. Cutaneous B-cell lymphomas associated with EBV demonstrate a dense infiltrate of abnormal lymphocytes of varying morphology, including immunoblasts, plasmacytoid cells, and reactive lymphocytes. In some cases, the abnormal lymphocytes may maintain an angiocentric distribution [73].

A recent review from Japan has described four distinct EBV-associated cutaneous lymphoproliferative disorders involving T-cells and/or natural killer (NK) cells [87].

1. Angiocentric cutaneous lymphoma is characterized by angiocentric infiltration of atypical lymphoid cells and has similar histopathology to peripheral T-cell lymphomas arising within the nasal cavity (lethal midline granuloma).

2. Subcutaneous lymphoma is characterized by atypical lymphocyte infiltration into subcutaneous tissue, including fat lobules. Phagocytizing cells called "beanbag cells" are described. This disorder presents as a panniculitis and is associated with hemophagocytosis.

3. Histiocytoid lymphoma is described as a diffuse infiltration of the skin of phagocytizing histiocytoid cells and atypical lymphoid cells. This disorder is also associated with hemophagocytosis.

4. Vesiculopapular eruptions on the face, mimicking hydroa vacciniforme, have been described only in children. Histologically, this disorder is characterized by dermal angiocentric infiltration of atypical lymphoid cells with dermal necrosis. Although not initially malignant, this disorder may eventually evolve into malignancy [87].

Diagnosis

EBV serological tests have a very limited role in the diagnosis of EBV-associated lymphoproliferations and malignancies. Antibody titers may be difficult to interpret in immunocompromised patients with EBV reactivation [88–90]. VCA IgG titers may be quite high, but the titer level itself has no clinical utility. VCA IgM titers may intermittently return to positive, and the EBNA titer may revert to negative. This phenomenon confounds the differentiation between acute and past EBV infection. Except in cases of primary EBV infection and seroconversion, EBV antibody titers have no role in the diagnosis of EBV-associated lymphoproliferative diseases in immunocompromised patients.

The utility of EBV serological tests has been demonstrated in one situation. In the case of nasopharyngeal carcinoma, high titers of IgA to EBV VCA and EA often indicate the presence of the tumor before it becomes clinically apparent [91]. In the southern Chinese and Southeast Asian populations at risk for nasopharyngeal carcinoma, these serologies are often used as screening tests.

For all EBV-associated lymphoproliferations and malignancies, the definitive diagnosis is best made from biopsy tissue histopathology. The diagnosis of EBV infection within pathological tissues may be accomplished by a vari-

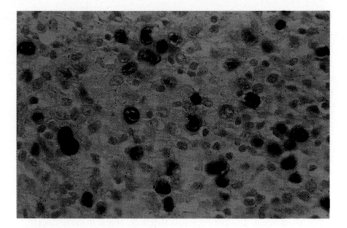

Figure 6–11. EBV-encoded RNA transcript–1 (EBER-1) in situ hybridization (600×) of a lymph node that contained EBV-positive B lymphocytes of posttransplant lymphoma.

ety of methods. In situ techniques can identify the specific cells infected and even the subcellular location of the viral genome or gene products. Several kits are commercially available for in situ nucleic acid hybridization to EBV DNA or to the EBV-encoded RNA transcripts EBER-1 and EBER-2, which are expressed in latent EBV infection (Fig. 6–11) [92]. Monoclonal antibodies (MAb) against EBV proteins are commercially available, including a MAb against ZEBRA, an EBV immediate early gene product of productively infected cells; a MAb against EA-D, an early gene product of productively infected cells; and a MAb against *LMP-1,* an EBV protein expressed in a variety of EBV-associated pathologies (Fig. 6–12) [17]. Electron microscopy (EM) may demonstrate intracellular virions with

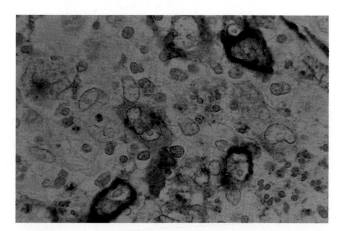

Figure 6–12. LMP-1 immunoperoxidase (1000×) of a lymph node that contained EBV-positive Reed-Sternberg cells characteristic of Hodgkin's disease.

characteristic herpesvirus morphology, but EBV cannot be specifically identified by EM [93].

Extraction and purification of DNA from tissue specimens permits the identification of EBV DNA by blot nucleic acid hybridization. This assay is useful to quantitate the number of EBV genomes present and to determine the clonality and state of infection of the EBV present in the tissue [94]. Amplification of EBV DNA by polymerase chain reaction is an extremely rapid and sensitive method of detecting the virus [95]. Direct viral culture of EBV is technically difficult, low in sensitivity, and available in only a few research laboratories. EBV culture has no role in routine clinical practice. With any method of detecting EBV in clinical tissue, caution must be used in interpreting the results. As with all persistent viruses, the presence of EBV in a pathological tissue does not necessarily imply causality of disease.

Treatment

Nearly all EBV-associated malignancies are latently infected, usually in a monoclonal manner with respect to the EBV genome. Therefore, antiviral drugs that inhibit EBV productive replication have no role in the therapy of EBV-associated lymphoproliferations and malignancies. Specific therapies vary with the type and stage of the disease and may include cytotoxic chemotherapy, radiation therapy, and surgical excision. The prognosis of many forms of EBV-associated malignancy is poor, especially for metastatic nasopharyngeal carcinoma and malignant non-Hodgkin's lymphomas of immunocompromised patients. Hodgkin's lymphoma in a nonimmunocompromised patient is an exception to this rule and often has a good prognosis with appropriate therapy.

Lymphoproliferative disorders in iatrogenically immunosuppressed patients are not malignant in many cases. They occur by the polyclonal proliferation of EBV-transformed B lymphocytes in the absence of an effective cytotoxic T-lymphocyte immune response [96]. In these cases, the EBV latency and transforming genes are expressed at high levels [97]. Successful therapy of these lymphoproliferative disorders requires at least partial restoration of cytotoxic T-lymphocyte immune function by a reduction in the immunosuppressive chemotherapy. In organ transplant recipients, the degree of reduction must be balanced against the increased risk of graft rejection. In some cases, a subset of the proliferating lymphocytes also exhibits productive EBV replication [98]. Although controlled data are lacking, high-dose parenteral acyclovir is often used as adjunctive therapy for these lymphoproliferative disorders [99]. Alpha interferon and intravenous immunoglobulin have also been used for their antiviral and immunomodulatory properties.

Perhaps the most promising new therapeutic approach to lymphoproliferative disorders in iatrogenically immunosuppressed patients involves the ex vivo expansion of host cytotoxic T lymphocytes against EBV-infected host target cells, followed by reinfusion of the activated cytotoxic T cells back into the patient. Preliminary data are encouraging from bone marrow transplant patients with EBV-associated lymphoproliferations for this still experimental therapy [100].

KIKUCHI'S HISTIOCYTIC NECROTIZING LYMPHADENITIS

Epidemiology

Kikuchi's histiocytic necrotizing lymphadenitis (Kikuchi's disease) is a rare disorder of unknown origin, although an association with primary EBV infection as well as other infectious etiologies has been suggested [101]. Kikuchi's disease most frequently affects females ages 20 to 30 years, but may affect any individual. First reported in Japan in 1972 [102,103], Kikuchi's disease has subsequently been recognized worldwide.

Pathogenesis

The etiology of Kikuchi's disease is not known, but the clinical and pathological features of the disease are suggestive of a hyperimmune reaction to an infectious agent. Several infectious agents including EBV [104] have been postulated, such as *Yersinia enterocolitica* [105], HIV [106,107], parvovirus B19 [108], HHV-6 [109], and *Toxoplasma gondii* [110]. The demonstration of transformation-associated EBV gene products within the abnormal lymphocytes suggests an etiological role for EBV in at least some cases [101]. Other studies have found no association between Kikuchi's disease and EBV or other specific infections [111–113]. The fact remains that a consistent etiological factor has yet to be discovered, and some authors have postulated that the hyperimmune pattern of Kikuchi's disease may be a reaction to a wide variety of etiological factors, possibly infectious, physical, chemical, or neoplastic [112,113].

Clinical Manifestations

The characteristic symptoms of Kikuchi's disease include regional lymph node enlargement with associated symptoms (Table 6–11). Lymphadenopathy of the cervical chain is most common, particularly the posterior cervical chain [114]. Other nodal regions may be involved, such as the supraclavicular, axillary, or inguinal nodes, and general-

Table 6.11. Clinical Manifestations of Kikuchi's Histiocytic Necrotizing Lymphadenitis

Time course of disease	Clinical manifestations	Laboratory analyses	Other notes
Incubation period unknown	Prodrome of upper respiratory symptoms may occasionally occur ↓	Positive serologies for primary EBV infection are supportive of a diagnosis.	The lymphadenopathy is typically painless, but may be tender in some cases
Over the course of weeks	Slow-growing, localized lymphadenopathy, sometimes with fever, chills, night sweats, fatigue, malaise, headache, sore throat, nausea, vomiting, weight loss, or arthralgias ↓	Definitive diagnosis is made only by lymph node biopsy and histological interpretation	
1–6 mo	Benign, self limited-course ↓ Resolution of all symptoms		In some cases, the disease may recur and then spontaneously resolve again

ized lymphadenopathy occasionally occurs [115]. Spleno-megaly develops in less than 10% of cases, and hepatomeg-aly is even more uncommon. Cutaneous lesions are present in up to 40% of patients and may include facial erythema, erythematous papules, plaques, nodules, cutaneous ulcers, and oral mucosal ulcers (Figs. 6–13 and 6–14) [116,117]. The signs and symptoms of Kikuchi's disease resolve spon-taneously within 1 to 6 months of onset, and often rapidly after excisional lymph node biopsy. The differential diag-nosis of Kikuchi's disease is listed in Table 6–12.

Dermatopathology

The histological findings of the skin lesions and the af-fected lymph nodes in Kikuchi's disease may mimic those of malignant lymphoma, causing occasional misdiagnosis. Characteristically, there is a dense dermal lymphohistio-cytic infiltrate with histiocytic aggregates, atypical lymphoid cells, karyorrhectic debris, and patchy necrosis. These features may extend into the outer root sheaths of hair follicles and deep into the reticular dermis. In affected lymph nodes, pathological foci appear as pale, wedge-shaped areas with atypical lymphoid cells, phagocytic his-tiocytes, and karyorrhectic debris. A characteristic histo-logical feature of Kikuchi's disease is the absence of neu-trophils despite the presence of necrosis [118].

Histopathologically, Kikuchi's disease may be difficult to differentiate from malignancy [101]. Immunohisto-chemical demonstration of a predominance of B lympho-cytes suggests lymphoma cutis, and chloroacetate esterase staining suggests leukemia cutis. Other diagnostic consid-erations include regressing atypical histiocytosis, malig-

Table 6–12. Differential Diagnoses of Kikuchi's Histiocytic Necrotizing Lymphadenitis

Atopic dermatitis: The skin manifestations may occasionally mimic this condition, but atopic dermatitis lacks the associated constitutional symptoms or lymphadenopathy.

Systemic lupus erythematosus: May also cause regional lymphadenopathy, but is normally associated with other autoimmune signs and symptoms (e.g., butterfly rash, photosensitivity). Can be differentiated by positive ANA titers and histology.

Scrofula (chronic tuberculous adenitis): Causes cervical lymphadenopathy, with nodes becoming harder and matted during the course of disease. Can be differentiated by histology.

Cat-scratch disease: May appear similar and require histological differentiation. History of recent cat exposure.

Malignant lymphoma: May have an identical presentation, but can be differentiated by histology.

Sarcoidosis: May also cause lymphadenopathy, but respiratory symptoms (e.g., cough, dyspnea, or chest discomfort) are typical.

Toxoplasmosis: Also causes lymphadenopathy and fatigue, but associated fever is uncommon. Can be differentiated by histology.

Kawasaki's disease: May also cause lymphadenopathy, but has other symptoms of conjunctival injection, oral mucosal findings, edema and erythema of the distal hands and feet, fine desquamation of the skin, etc.

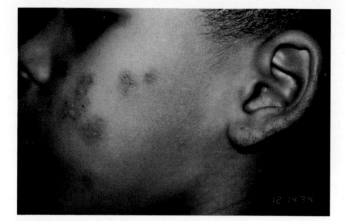

(a)

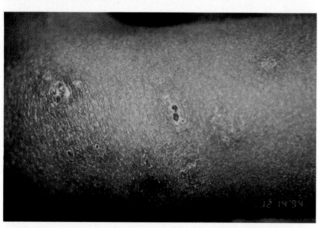

(b)

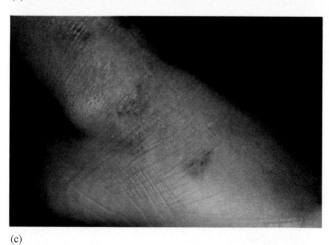

(c)

Figure 6–13. (a,b,c) Erythematous papules and plaques of Kikuchi's disease. (From Ref. 101. Used with permission.)

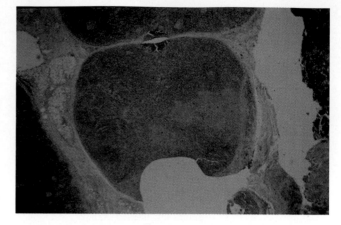

Figure 6–14. Lymph nodes of a patient with Kikuchi's disease. (From Ref. 101. Used with permission.)

nant histiocytosis, anaplastic large cell lymphoma, lymphoid papulosis, and lymphomatoid granulomatosis.

Diagnosis

Serological evidence of primary EBV infection (Table 6–7) is supportive of the diagnosis of Kikuchi's disease. As described in the section on EBV-associated lymphoproliferative disorders and malignancies, in situ histopathological techniques to detect EBV within the pathological tissue would be highly suggestive of the diagnosis of Kikuchi's disease. EBV has been demonstrated within the atypical immunoblasts by immunohistochemical staining for the EBV latent membrane protein (LMP-1) and by in situ nucleic acid hybridization to the EBV latency-associated transcript EBER-1 (Fig. 6–15). Definitive diagnosis

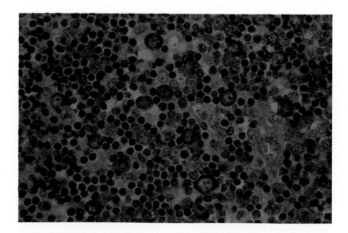

Figure 6–15. LMP-1 immunoperoxidase (600×) of a lymph node showing EBV-positive B immunoblasts in Kikuchi's disease. (From Ref. 101. Used with permission.)

Table 6–13. Treatment of Kikuchi's Histiocytic Necrotizing Lymphadenitis

Symptom	Treatment
General	Rest, good nutrition, and symptomatic treatment, as needed. Nonsteroidal anti-inflammatory agents have been helpful in many cases.
Fever	Antipyretics

of Kikuchi's disease can be made by histological examination of an excisional lymph node biopsy.

Treatment

Kikuchi's disease is a benign clinical entity that resolves without specific therapy (Table 6–13) [101]. It does not respond to chemotherapy or radiation therapy. The presence of latent EBV infection within B lymphocytes suggests that antiviral therapy is not indicated.

ORAL HAIRY LEUKOPLAKIA

Epidemiology

Oral hairy leukoplakia is an oral mucosal lesion common in EBV-seropositive patients who are infected with HIV [93]. The point prevalence may be as high as 25% in HIV-infected patients, and the lesion often appears early in the clinical course prior to the onset of AIDS [119,120]. Antiretroviral and/or antiherpesviral therapy reduces the prevalence of HIV-associated oral hairy leukoplakia [121]. In HIV-infected patients, oral hairy leukoplakia is more common in men [122,123] and in patients who smoke cigarettes [124,125]. Although the reasons are not clear, oral hairy leukoplakia is rarely reported in children who are infected with HIV [126–128]. Oral hairy leukoplakia is also relatively common in patients receiving immunosuppressive therapy such as organ transplant recipients, especially patients receiving the drug cyclosporine [129]. Oral hairy leukoplakia has also been described in several HIV-seronegative individuals who appeared to be otherwise immunocompetent [130–132].

Pathogenesis

Oral hairy leukoplakia is the only EBV-associated pathology characterized by high-level productive viral replication and is the only nonmalignant lesion of epithelial cell infection [93]. Inhibition of viral replication results in resolution of the lesion [133]. However, in all patients, the prevalence of EBV replication in the oropharyngeal epithelium far exceeds the incidence of oral hairy leukoplakia [134,135]. Thus, EBV replication itself is insufficient for the pathogenesis of oral hairy leukoplakia. The presence of oral hairy leukoplakia in otherwise healthy individuals suggests that severe immunodeficiency is not required for the pathogenesis of the lesion. Contrary to early reports, human papillomavirus is not routinely found in oral hairy leukoplakia and plays no apparent role in its pathogenesis.

Oral hairy leukoplakia is a unique form of EBV infection for the frequent presence of multiple coinfecting EBV types, strains, and recombinant variants within the lesion [136–139]. Intrastrain recombination results in juxtaposition, duplication, or deletion of specific gene sequences. Interstrain recombination between two or more strains coinfecting within the same cell may create new hybrid EBV genotypes. Genetic variation may contribute to EBV pathogenesis if critical viral protein functions are altered or if specific viral epitopes are mutated to permit evasion of cytotoxic T-lymphocyte immune surveillance. Oral hairy leukoplakia is also characterized by the expression of EBV gene products involved in the regulation of cell growth and apoptosis, including BHRF1, EBNA-2 and LMP-1 [138,140,141]. Thus, a convergence of factors may be necessary for the pathogenesis of oral hairy leukoplakia. These factors include EBV coinfection, replication, recombination, and expression of specific EBV gene products in tongue epithelium in the setting of an ineffective cytotoxic T-lymphocyte immune response to EBV.

Clinical Manifestations

The gross appearance of the oral hairy leukoplakia lesion may be variable (Table 6–14), and the lesion may easily be misdiagnosed (Table 6–15) [142]. Although oral hairy leukoplakia most often presents on the lateral borders of the tongue, it may spread to the ventral surface of the tongue where it can become flat and lack the characteristic "hairy" appearance (Figs. 6–16 to 6–18). Rarely, the lesion may occur on the dorsal surface of the tongue (Fig. 6–19) or the buccal mucosa (Fig. 6–20) [143]. Oral hairy leukoplakia often presents with bilateral involvement of the tongue, although the size of the corresponding plaques is not usually equal. The lesions are adherent and only the superficial layers can be scraped and removed from the mucosal surface. There is no associated erythema or edema of the surrounding tissue. Oral hairy leukoplakia does not appear to be a premalignant lesion, but some patients are disturbed by the cosmetic appearance of this condition.

Laboratory Findings

There are no laboratory findings that are specific or even characteristic of oral hairy leukoplakia. EBV serologies are

Table 6–14. Clinical Manifestations of Oral Hairy Leukoplakia

Time course of disease	Clinical manifestations	Laboratory analyses	Other notes
"Incubation" period unknown	Superficial white, raised plaque with corrugated or "hairy" appearance presents on the oral mucosa, most commonly on the lateral borders of the tongue ↓	EBV-specific serologies and cultures are not helpful Definitive diagnosis, if needed, by combination of histological examination and demonstration of EBV DNA or EBV gene products in epithelial cells	The lesions are typically asymptomatic, but some patients describe mild pain, discomfort, or alteration in taste
Weeks to months	Self-limited course, with resolution within weeks in immunocompetent persons and within months in immunocompromised persons ↓		
Weeks to months	Lesions may sometimes recur and remit repeatedly in immunocompromised persons		The natural history of oral hairy leukoplakia is variable in immunocompromised persons

Table 6–15. Differential Diagnoses of Oral hairy Leukoplakia

Oral candidiasis: Oral hairy leukoplakia is most often confused with candida (thrush) in HIV-infected patients. Candida typically occurs as a plaque-like lesion that is easily removed by scraping with a blunt instrument, revealing an erythematous base. Resolution if lesions after topical antifungal therapy also suggests candidiasis, whereas failure of the lesions to resolve suggests hairy leukoplakia. However, these clinical maneuvers are unreliable, and oral hairy leukoplakia lesions are commonly superinfected with candida.

Frictional keratosis: When located on the lateral borders of the tongue, this lesion may mimic oral hairy leukoplakia. There may be an obvious source of irritation, and the lesion typically resolves after removal of the provoking stimulus.

Tobacco-induced leukoplakias: Frequently seen in smokers and in individuals who chew smokeless tobacco. These lesions are often premalignant and should be carefully evaluated.

Lichen planus or lichenoid reactions: This condition of the oral mucosa may resemble oral hairy leukoplakia, but most commonly has a reticulated pattern and may be associated with the characteristic cutaneous lesions.

Syphilis: Oral manifestations of secondary syphilis usually present as atrophic patches on the tongue but elevated variations mimicking oral hairy leukoplakia have been described. Syphilis serology can be used to distinguish those entities.

usually indicative of past persistent infection and do not differ from those of individuals without oral hairy leukoplakia [144]. Oral hairy leukoplakia associated with primary EBV infection has not been described.

Dermatopathology

Histologically, oral hairy leukoplakia demonstrates a hyperplastic and irregular tongue epithelium resulting from parakeratosis and hyperkeratosis of the upper epithelial

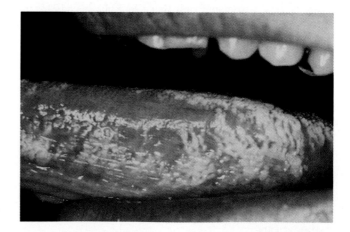

Figure 6–16. Oral hairy leukoplakia on the lateral border of the tongue demonstrating a discontinuous, patchy distribution of the lesion. (Courtesy of Catherine M. Flaitz, D.D.S., M.S., University of Texas–Houston Dental Branch, Houston, TX.)

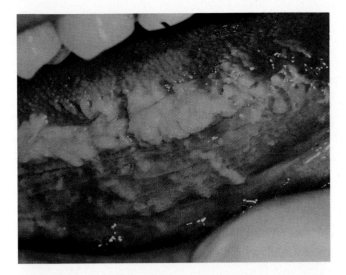

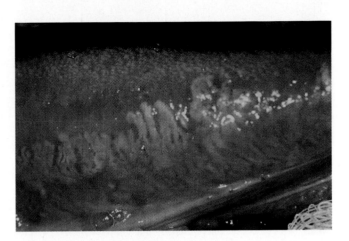

Figure 6–17. Oral hairy leukoplakia on the lateral border and ventral surface of the tongue demonstrating marked hyperkeratinization on the lateral border and a flatter, less keratinized appearance on the ventral surface. (Courtesy of Catherine M. Flaitz, D.D.S., M.S., University of Texas–Houston Dental Branch, Houston, TX.)

Figure 6–18. Oral hairy leukoplakia on the ventral surface of the tongue demonstrating a finer, more subtle appearance of the lesion. (Courtesy of Catherine M. Flaitz, D.D.S., M.S., University of Texas–Houston Dental Branch, Houston, TX.)

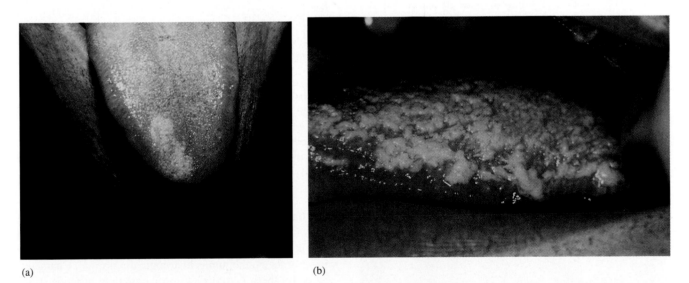

(a)   (b)

Figure 6–19. (a,b) Oral hairy leukoplakia involving the dorsal surface of the tongue with marked hyperkeratinization. (a, courtesy of Karen Wiss, M.D., Department of Dermatology, University of Massachusetts School of Medicine, Worcester, MA; b, courtesy of Catherine M. Flaitz, D.D.S., M.S., University of Texas–Houston Dental Branch, Houston, TX.)

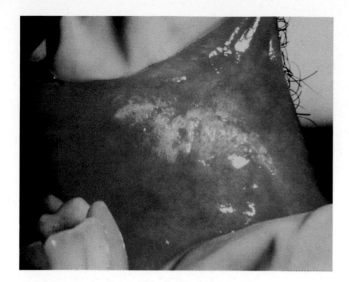

Figure 6–20. Oral hairy leukoplakia involving the buccal mucosa. (Courtesy of Catherine M. Flaitz, D.D.S., M.S., University of Texas–Houston Dental Branch, Houston, TX.)

layers (Fig. 6–21) [142,145]. The hyperkeratosis is largely responsible for the characteristic gross appearance of the lesion. Superficial infections of the hyperkeratinized epithelium with bacteria or fungal hyphae may also be seen (Fig. 6–22). The prickle cell layer in the midzone of the epithelium demonstrates acanthosis with foci or layers of cells resembling koilocytes (Fig. 6–23). These ballooning cells have a homogenous ''ground-glass'' appearance to

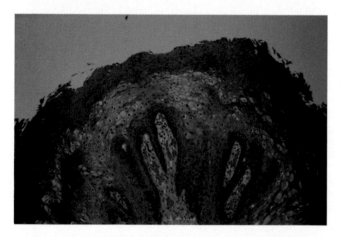

Figure 6–21. Oral hairy leukoplakia biopsy from tongue demonstrating epithelial hyperplasia with hyperkeratosis and parakeratosis of the superficial layer of the epithelium. Hematoxylin and eosin stain at 20× magnification. (Courtesy of Catherine M. Flaitz, D.D.S., M.S., University of Texas–Houston Dental Branch, Houston, TX.)

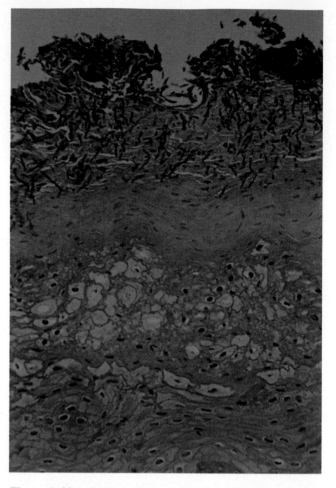

Figure 6–22. Oral hairy leukoplakia biopsy from tongue demonstrating fungal superinfection of the lesion. Magenta-staining fungal hyphae are abundant within the superficial, hyperkeratinized epithelium of the lesion. The epithelial midzone of the lesion demonstrates acanthosis. Periodic acid–Schiff stain at 40× magnification. (Courtesy of Catherine M. Flaitz, D.D.S., M.S., University of Texas–Houston Dental Branch, Houston, TX.)

the nuclei. Some authors have reported the presence of Cowdry type A intranuclear inclusions in these cells, but this is not a consistent or even common finding. The basal layer of the epithelium is histologically normal. Characteristically, there is a minimum or complete absence of inflammatory infiltrate associated with oral hairy leukoplakia. In HIV-infected patients, Langerhans cells are reported to be absent from oral hairy leukoplakia, but the pathogenic implications of this finding are not clear [146].

Diagnosis

Although the major histopathological features of oral hairy leukoplakia are highly suggestive of the diagnosis, none

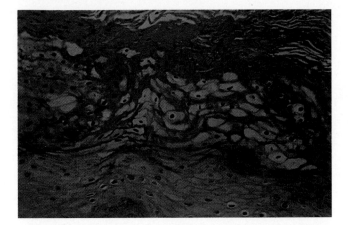

Figure 6–23. Oral hairy leukoplakia biopsy from tongue demonstrating marked acanthosis of the prickle-cell layer. The epithelial midzone contains palisades of ballooning cells with perinuclear cytoplasmic clearing and a homogeneous "ground-glass" appearance of the nuclei. Hematoxylin and eosin stain at 80× magnification. (Courtesy of Catherine M. Flaitz, D.D.S., M.S., University of Texas–Houston Dental Branch, Houston, TX.)

is unique to the lesion. Depending on the plane of tissue sectioning, hyperplasia, parakeratosis, and acanthosis appear in autopsy specimens of grossly normal tongues [147]. In both immunocompromised and immunocompetent patients, pseudo-hairy leukoplakia lesions may have the gross appearance and the histological features of oral hairy leukoplakia without the presence of EBV [148–150]. Therefore, the definitive diagnosis of oral hairy leukoplakia requires both an appropriate histopathological appearance and the demonstration of EBV DNA or EBV gene products within the epithelial cells of the lesion. EBV may be demonstrated using the detection techniques described in the section on EBV-associated lymphoproliferative disorders and malignancies. In oral hairy leukoplakia, EBV is detected within ballooned and nonballooned cells of the prickle cell layer, as well as the keratinized cells of the superficial epithelium (Fig. 6–24). EBV has not been convincingly demonstrated within the basal epithelial layer. In an HIV-infected patient with typical-appearing oral hairy leukoplakia, cytological examination of exfoliated cells from the lesion may support the diagnosis of oral hairy leukoplakia, and the demonstration of EBV in these cells is sufficient to make the diagnosis without a biopsy [142,151].

Treatment

Several therapeutic options exist for oral hairy leukoplakia, but treatment is usually not necessary. Some patients with

oral hairy leukoplakia describe mild pain, discomfort, paresthesias, or alteration in the sensation of taste, but many patients are unaware of the presence of their lesions. Although it has not been well studied, treatment of the lesion usually brings resolution of the symptoms as well. Treatment of oral hairy leukoplakia for cosmetic indications must be decided between the patient and the health care provider on an individual basis. The variable natural history of the lesion and its tendency toward spontaneous resolution should be considered in that decision (Table 6–16).

Systemic antiviral therapy with oral or parenteral agents active against EBV usually results in resolution of the lesion after 1 to 2 weeks of therapy. The response of oral hairy leukoplakia to acyclovir is well documented [133], but oral therapy with acyclovir requires high doses (800 mg five times/day) to achieve therapeutic levels. Valacyclovir (an acyclovir prodrug) and famciclovir are newer antiviral drugs with higher oral bioavailability than acyclovir and can be dosed less often. In many HIV-infected patients receiving parenteral ganciclovir, foscarnet or cidofovir for cytomegalovirus disease, oral hairy leukoplakia will resolve as well. All of these antiviral drugs inhibit EBV productive replication but do not eliminate the latent state of infection. Therefore in immunocompromised patients, oral hairy leukoplakia often recurs after the cessation of antiviral therapy [133].

Topical therapy for oral hairy leukoplakia with podophyllin resin 25% solution is effective in achieving partial or total resolution in most patients after only one or two treatment applications [152]. The treatments may tempo-

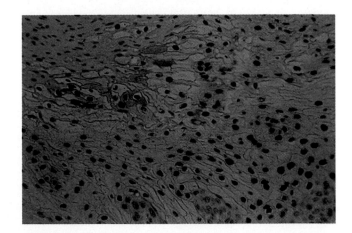

Figure 6–24. Oral hairy leukoplakia biopsy from tongue demonstrating the presence of EBV within the lesion using an immunohistochemical stain for the EBV early gene product EA-D. Hematoxylin counterstain at 80× magnification. (Courtesy of Catherine M. Flaitz, D.D.S., M.S., University of Texas–Houston Dental Branch, Houston, Texas.)

Table 6–16.   Treatment of Oral Hairy Leukoplakia

Symptoms	Treatment
Pain	**Topical therapy**
Paresthesias	Podophyllin resin 25% solution: applied
Altered taste	to lesion for 5 min.
Unsightly	Treatment may need to be repeated once,
appearance	and the lesions typically recur after
	treatment.
	Topical retinoids (reported by some
	authors)
	Cryotherapy with liquid nitrogen
	(reported by some authors)
	Systemic therapy
	Antiviral therapy with oral acyclovir,
	valacyclovir, or famciclovir. The lesion
	usually resolves in 1–2 wk.
	(Intravenous ganciclovir, foscarnet, or
	cidofovir given for CMV infection has
	led to resolution of oral hairy
	leukoplakia.)
	Surgical therapy
	Complete excision is rarely performed,
	but has been reported by some authors

rarily cause local pain, discomfort, and alteration of taste. In one study, 17% of patients treated had recurrence of oral hairy leukoplakia with a mean interval to recurrence of 17 weeks [153]. Cases have also been reported of lesions resolving following topical application of retinoids [154] or following liquid nitrogen cryotherapy [155]. Surgical excision of oral hairy leukoplakia eliminates the lesion and resolves the associated pain [156]. Interestingly, the lesion does not recur at the excision site but may reappear at adjacent sites on the lateral tongue. Therapeutic surgical excision is more invasive than other treatments but provides the opportunity to also make a histopathological diagnosis of oral hairy leukoplakia.

CONCLUSION

EBV is a ubiquitous human herpesvirus that is responsible for a significant amount of morbidity and mortality worldwide. The biology and pathogenesis of EBV infections are complex and incompletely understood. Antiviral drugs inhibit EBV productive replication, but many EBV-associated diseases result from EBV latency and the expression of EBV genes with the ability to transform cells. Important clinical manifestations of EBV infection include the infectious mononucleosis syndrome, lymphoproliferative disor-

ders, oral hairy leukoplakia, and a variety of malignancies. The cutaneous manifestations of EBV infection may arise through various immunological mechanisms or from direct EBV involvement of mucocutaneous and subcutaneous tissues. Cutaneous manifestations of EBV infection are common, especially in certain patient populations.

REFERENCES

1. D Liebowitz, E Kieff. Epstein-Barr virus. In: B Roizman, RJ Whitley, C Lopez, eds. The Human Herpesviruses. New York: Raven Press, 1993, pp 107–172.
2. MA Epstein, BG Achong, YM Barr. Virus particles in cultured lymphocytes Burkitt's lymphoma. Lancet 1: 702–703, 1964.
3. G Henle, W Henle, V Diehl. Relation of Burkitt tumor associated herpes-type virus to infectious mononucleosis. Proc Natl Acad Sci U S A 59:94–101, 1968.
4. MS Pereira, JM Blake, AD Macrae. EB virus antibody at different ages. BMJ 4:526–527, 1969.
5. G Henle, W Henle, CA Horowitz. Epstein-Barr virus specific diagnosis tests in infectious mononucleosis. Hum Pathol 5:551–565, 1974.
6. CW Heath Jr, AL Brodsky, AI Potolsky. Infectious mononucleosis in a general population. Am J Epidemiol 95: 46–52, 1972.
7. G Miller, JC Niederman, LL Andrews. Prolonged oropharyngeal excretion of Epstein-Barr virus after infectious mononucleosis. N Engl J Med 288:229–232, 1973.
8. AK Junker, EE Thomas, AGI Radcliffe, RB Forsyth, AG Davidson, L Rymo. Epstein-Barr virus shedding in breast milk. Am J Med Sci 302:220–223, 1991.
9. V Israele, P Shirley, JW Sixbey. Excretion of the Epstein-Barr virus from the genital tract of men. J Infect Dis 163: 1341–1343, 1991.
10. JW Sixbey, SM Lemon, JS Pagano. A second site for Epstein-Barr virus shedding: the uterine cervix. Lancet 2: 1122–1124, 1986.
11. M-C Meyohas, V Marechal, N Desire, J Bouillie, J Frottier, JC Nicolas. Study of mother-to-child Epstein-Barr virus transmission by means of nested PCRs. J Virol 70: 6816–6819, 1996.
12. JH Joncas, C Alfieri, M Leyritz-Wills, P Brochu, G Jasmin, I Boldogh, ES Huang. Simultaneous congenital infection with Epstein-Barr virus and cytomegalovirus. N Engl J Med 304:1399–1403, 1981.
13. GN Goldberg, VA Fulginiti, CG Ray, P Ferry, JF Jones, H Cross, L Minnich. In utero Epstein-Barr virus (infectious mononucleosis) infection. JAMA 246:1579–1581, 1981.
14. H Cen, MC Breinig, RW Atchison, M Ho, JLC McKnight. Epstein-Barr virus transmission via the donor organs in solid organ transplantation: polymerase chain reaction and restriction fragment length polymorphism analysis of IR2, IR3, and IR4. J Virol 65:976–980, 1991.
15. S Swaminathan, R Hesselton, J Sullivan, E Kieff. Epstein-

Barr virus recombinants with specifically mutated BCRF1 genes. J Virol 67:7406–7413, 1993.

16. S Henderson, D Huen, M Rowe, C Dawson, G Johnson, A Rickinson. Epstein-Barr virus–coded BHRF1 protein, a viral homologue of Bcl-2, protects human B cells from programmed cell death. Proc Natl Acad Sci U S A 90: 8479–8483, 1993.

17. R Pathmanathan, U Prasad, R Sadler, K Flynn, N Raab-Traub. Clonal proliferations of cells infected with Epstein-Barr virus in preinvasive lesions related to nasopharyngeal carcinoma. N Engl J Med 333:693–698, 1995.

18. NR Cooper, MD Moore, GR Nemerow. Immunobiology of CR2, the B lymphocyte receptor for the Epstein-Barr virus and C3d complement fragment. Annu Rev Immunol 6:85–113, 1988.

19. J Yates, N Warren, D Reisman, B Sugden. A cis acting element from the Epstein-Barr viral genome that permits stable replication of recombinant plasmids in latently infected cells. Proc Natl Acad Sci U S A 81:3806–3810, 1984.

20. J Levitskaya, M Coram, V Levitsky, S Imreh, PM Steigerwald-Mullen, G Klein, MG Kurilla, MG Masucci. Inhibition of antigen processing by the internal repeat region of the Epstein-Barr virus nuclear antigen-1. Nature 375: 685–688, 1995.

21. CL Miller, AL Burkhardt, JH Lee, B Stealey, R Longnecker, JB Bolen, E Kieff. Integral membrane protein 2 of Epstein-Barr virus regulates reactivation from latency through dominant negative effects on protein-tyrosine kinases. Immunity 2:155–166, 1995.

22. JW Gratama, MAP Oosterveer, FE Zwaan, J Lepoutre, G Klein, I Ernberg. Eradication of Epstein-Barr virus by allogeneic bone marrow transplantation: implications for sites of viral latency. Proc Natl Acad Sci U S A 85: 8693–8696, 1988.

23. MG Masucci, I Ernberg. Epstein-Barr virus: adaptation to a life within the immune system. Trends Microbiol 2: 125–130, 1994.

24. JF Jones, S Shurin, C Abramowsky, RR Tubbs, CG Sciotto, R Wahl, J Sands, D Gottman, BZ Katz, J Sklar. T-cell lymphomas containing Epstein-Barr viral DNA in patients with chronic Epstein-Barr virus infections. N Engl J Med 318:733–741, 1988.

25. H Kikuta. Epstein-Barr virus–associated hemophagocytic syndrome. Leuk Lymphoma 16:425–429, 1995.

26. J Sixbey, Q Yao. Immunoglobulin A–induced shift of Epstein-Barr virus tissue tropism. Science 255:1578–1580, 1992.

27. LS Wilkinson, LD Petz, G Garraty. Reappraisal of the role of anti-i in haemolytic anemia in infectious mononucleosis. Br J Haematol 25:715–722, 1973.

28. LM Kernoff. Demonstration of increased platelet bound IgG in infectious mononucleosis complicated by severe thrombocytopenia. Scand J Infect Dis 12:67–69, 1980.

29. JW Sixbey, JG Nedrud, N Raab-Traub, RA Hanes, JS Pagano. Epstein-Barr virus replication in oropharyngeal epithelial cells. N Engl J Med 310:1225–1230, 1984.

30. RT Schooley. Epstein-Barr virus (infectious mononucleosis). In: GL Mandell, JE Bennett, R Dolin, eds. Principles and Practice of Infectious Diseases. New York: Churchill Livingstone, Inc, 1995, pp 1364–1377.

31. CV Sumaya. Epstein-Barr virus infection: the expanded spectrum. Adv Pediatr Infect Dis 1:75–97, 1986.

32. JT McCarthy, RJ Hoagland. Cutaneous manifestations of infectious mononucleosis. JAMA 187:153, 1964.

33. U Baldari, C Cancellieri, B Celli, R Zanelli, AA Raccagni. Skin disorders and Epstein-Barr virus primary infection: results of a 31 month survey. J Eur Acad Dermatol Venereol 4:239–247, 1995.

34. AW Contratto. Infectious mononucleosis: a study of one hundred and ninety-six cases. Arch Intern Med 73: 449–459, 1944.

35. JA Africk, KM Halprin. Infectious mononucleosis presenting as urticaria. JAMA 209:1524–1525, 1969.

36. BM Andersen Lund, T Bergan. Temporary skin reactions to penicillins during the acute stage of infectious mononucleosis. Scand J Infect Dis 7:21–28, 1975.

37. H McKenzie, D Parratt, RG White. IgM and IgG antibody levels of ampicillin in patients with infectious mononucleosis. Clin Exp Immunol 26:214–221, 1976.

38. R Mulroy. Amoxicillin rash in infectious mononucleosis. BMJ 1:554, 1973.

39. F Drago, F Crovato, A Rebora. Gianotti-Crosti syndrome as a presenting sign of EBV-induced acute infectious mononucleosis. Clin Exp Dermatol 22:300–304, 1997.

40. L Lowe, AA Hebert, M Duvic. Gianotti-Crosti syndrome associated with Epstein-Barr virus infection. J Am Acad Dermatol 20:336–338, 1989.

41. A Taieb, P Plantin, P Du Pasquier, G Guillet, J Maleville. Gianotti-Crosti syndrome: a study of 26 cases. Br J Dermatol 115:49–59, 1986.

42. F Drago, M Romagnoli, A Loi, A Rebora. Epstein-Barr virus–related persistent erythema multiforme in chronic fatigue syndrome. Arch Dermatol 128:217–222, 1992.

43. DM Williamson. Erythema multiforme in infectious mononucleosis. Br J Dermatol 91:345–346, 1974.

44. HJ Bodansky. Erythema nodosum and infectious mononucleosis. BMJ 2:1263, 1979.

45. SC Cowdrey, JS Reynolds. Acute urticaria in infectious mononucleosis. Ann Allergy 27:182–187, 1969.

46. CJ Tyson, D Czarny. Cold induced urticaria in infectious mononucleosis. Med J Aust 1:33–35, 1981.

47. SE Straus, JI Cohen, G Tosato, J Meier. Epstein-Barr virus infections: biology, pathogenesis, and management. Ann Intern Med 118:45–58, 1993.

48. H Hammar. Erythema annulare centrifugum coincident with Epstein-Barr virus in an infant. Acad Pediatr Scand 63:788–792, 1974.

49. JM Boss, JD Boxley, R Summerly, RN Sutton. The detection of Epstein-Barr virus antibody in exanthematic dermatoses with special reference to pityriasis lichenoides. A preliminary survey. Clin Exp Dermatol 3:51–56, 1978.

50. JW Petrozzi. Infectious mononucleosis manifesting as palmar dermatitis. Arch Dermatol 104:207–209, 1971.

51. SA Spencer, NA Fenske, CG Espinoza, JR Hamill, LE Cohen, LR Espinoza. Granuloma annulare–like eruption due to chronic Epstein-Barr virus infection. Arch Dermatol 124:250–255, 1988.

52. F Drago, A Parodi, A Rebora. Gloves-and-socks syndrome in a patient with Epstein-Barr virus. Dermatology 194:374, 1997.

53. J Portnoy, GA Ahronheim, F Ghibu, B Clecner, JH Joncas. Recovery of Epstein-Barr virus from genital ulcers. N Engl J Med 311:966–968, 1984.

54. U Baldari, AA Raccagni, B Celli, MG Righini. Chronic bullous disease of childhood following Epstein-Barr virus seroconversion: a case report. Clin Exp Dermatol 21: 123–126, 1996.

55. F Drago, E Ranieri, A Pastorino, S Casazza, F Crovato, A Rebora. Epstein-Barr virus–related cutaneous amyloidosis. Successful treatment with acyclovir and interferon-alpha. Br J Dermatol 134:170–174, 1996.

56. J-P Fermand, J Gozlan, A Bendelac, MC Delauche-Cavallier, JC Brouet, F Morinet. Detection of Epstein-Barr virus in epidermal skin lesions of an immunocompromised patient. Ann Intern Med 112:511–515, 1990.

57. RL Carter. Platelet levels in infectious mononucleosis. Blood 25:817–821, 1964.

58. ML Pipp, ND Means, JW Sixbey, KL Morris, CL Gue, LM Baddour. Acute Epstein-Barr virus infection complicated by severe thrombocytopenia. Clin Infect Dis 25: 1237–1239, 1997.

59. RS Tomsick. The phenytoin syndrome. Cutis 32:535–541, 1983.

60. AS Evans, JC Niederman, LC Cenabre, B West, VA Richards. A prospective evaluation of heterophile and Epstein-Barr virus–specific IgM antibody tests in clinical and subclinical infectious mononucleosis: specificity and sensitivity of the tests and persistence of antibody. J Infect Dis 132:546–554, 1975.

61. CV Sumaya, Y Ench. Epstein-Barr virus mononucleosis in children. II. Heterophile antibodies and viral specific responses. Pediatrics 75:1011–1019, 1985.

62. C Van der Horst, J Joncas, G Ahronheim, N Gustafson, G Stein, M Gurwith, G Fleisher, J Sullivan, J Sixbey, S Roland, et al. Lack of effect of peroral acyclovir for the treatment of acute infectious mononucleosis. J Infect Dis 164:788–792, 1991.

63. QY Yao, P Ogan, M Rowe, M Wood, AB Rickinson. Epstein-Barr virus–infected B cells persist in the circulation of acyclovir-treated virus carriers. Int J Cancer 43:67–71, 1989.

64. E Tynell, E Aurelius, A Brandell, I Julander, M Wood, QY Yao, A Rickinson, B Akerlund, J Andersson. Acyclovir and prednisolone treatment of acute infectious mononucleosis: a multicenter, double-blind, placebo-controlled study. J Infect Dis 174:324–331, 1996.

65. AM Levine. Acquired immunodeficiency syndrome–related lymphoma. Blood 80:8–20, 1992.

66. E Brusamolino, G Pagnucco, C Bernasconi. Secondary lymphomas: a review on lymphoproliferative diseases arising in immunocompromised hosts: prevalence, clinical features and pathogenetic mechanisms. Haematologica 74: 605–622, 1989.

67. JI Cohen. Epstein-Barr virus lymphoproliferative disease associated with acquired immunodeficiency. Medicine 70: 137–160, 1991.

68. N Mueller, A Evans, NL Harris, GW Comstock, E Jellum, K Magnus, N Orentreich, BF Polk, J Vogelman. Hodgkin's disease and Epstein-Barr virus: altered antibody pattern before diagnosis. N Engl J Med 320:689–695, 1989.

69. IJ Su. Epstein-Barr and T cell lymphomas. Epstein-Barr Virus Report 3:1–6, 1996.

70. SA Ridler, MC Breinig, JC McKnight. Increased levels of circulating Epstein-Barr virus (EBV)–infected lymphocytes and decreased EBV nuclear antigen antibody responses are associated with the development of posttransplant lymphoproliferative disease in solid-organ transplant recipients. Blood 84:972–984, 1994.

71. PJ Farrell. Epstein-Barr virus immortalizing genes. Trends Microbiol 3:105–109, 1995.

72. SA Henderson, D Huen, M Rowe. Epstein-Barr virus transforming proteins. Semin Virol 5:391–399, 1994.

73. JM McGregor, CC-W Yu, QL Lu, FE Cotter, DA Levison, DM MacDonald. Posttransplant cutaneous lymphoma. J Am Acad Dermatol 29:549–554, 1993.

74. S Piluso, S Di Lollo, G Baroni, F Leoncini, D Gaglioti, A Saccardi, G Ficarra. Unusual clinical aspects of oral non-Hodgkin lymphomas in patients with HIV infection. Eur J Cancer B Oral Oncol 30B:61–64, 1994.

75. GD Palmer, PR Morgan, SJ Challacombe. T-cell lymphoma associated with periodontal disease and HIV infection: a case report. J Clin Periodontol 20:378–380, 1993.

76. HJ Delecluse, I Anagnostopoulos, F Dallenbach, M Hummel, T Marafioti, U Schneider, D Huhn, A Schmidt-Westhausen, PA Reichart, U Gross, H Stein. Plasmablastic lymphomas of the oral cavity: a new entity associated with the human immunodeficiency virus infection. Blood 89: 1413–1420, 1997.

77. JA Thomas, F Cotter, AM Hanby, LQ Long, PR Morgan, B Bramble, BM Bailey. Epstein-Barr virus–related oral T-cell lymphoma associated with human immunodeficiency virus immunosuppression. Blood 81:3350–3356, 1993.

78. I Anagnostopoulos, M Hummel, P Kaudewitz, P Korbjuhn, L Leoncini, H Stein. Low incidence of Epstein-Barr virus presence in primary cutaneous T-cell lymphoproliferations. Br J Dermatol 134:276–281, 1996.

79. CA Angel, DN Slater, JA Royds, SNP Nelson, SS Bleehen. Absence of Epstein-Barr viral encoded RNA in primary cutaneous T-cell lymphoma. J Pathol 178:173–175, 1996.

80. N Misago, K Ohshims, S Aiura, M Kikuchi, H Kohda. Primary cutaneous T-cell lymphoma with an angiocentric growth pattern: association with Epstein-Barr virus. Br J Dermatol 135:638–643, 1996.

81. CK Park, YH Ko. Detection of EBER nuclear RNA in T-cell lymphomas involving the skin: an in situ hybridization study. Br J Dermatol 134:488–493, 1996.

82. IJ Su, TF Tsai, AL Cheng, CC Chen. Cutaneous manifestations of Epstein-Barr virus–associated T-cell lymphoma. J Am Acad Dermatol 29:685–692, 1993.

83. TF Tsai, IJ Su, YC Lu, HP Yeh, HC Hsieh, HF Tien, JS Chen, WC Uen. Cutaneous angiocentric T-cell lymphoma associated with Epstein-Barr virus. J Am Acad Dermatol 26:31–38, 1992.

84. R Pathmanathan, U Prasad, G Chandrika, R Sadler, K Flynn, N Raab-Traub. Undifferentiated, nonkeratinizing, and squamous cell carcinoma of the nasopharynx: variants of Epstein-Barr virus–infected neoplasia. Am J Pathol 146:1355–1367, 1995.

85. AF Jarrett, AA Armstrong, E Alexander. Epidemiology of EBV and Hodgkin's lymphoma. Ann Oncol 7(suppl 4): 5–10, 1996.

86. LM Weiss, LA Movahed, RA Warnke, J Sklar. Detection of Epstein-Barr viral genomes in Reed-Sternberg cells of Hodgkin's disease. N Engl J Med 320:502–506, 1989.

87. K Iwatsuki, M Ohtsuka, H Harada, G Han, F Kaneko. Clinicopathologic manifestations of Epstein-Barr virus–associated cutaneous lymphoproliferative disorders. Arch Dermatol 133:1081–1086, 1997.

88. WA Andiman. EBV-associated syndromes: a critical reexamination. Pediatr Infect Dis 3:198–203, 1984.

89. W Henle, G Henle. Epstein-Barr virus–specific serology in immunologically compromised individuals. Cancer Res 41:4222–4225, 1981.

90. M Okano, GM Thiele, JR Davis, HL Grierson, DT Purtilo. Epstein-Barr virus and human diseases: recent advances in diagnosis. Clin Microbiol Rev 1:300–312, 1988.

91. JHC Ho, MH Ng, HC Kwan, JCW Chau. Epstein-Barr virus specific IgA and IgG serum antibodies in nasopharyngeal carcinoma. Br J Cancer 34:655–659, 1976.

92. EM MacMahon, RF Ambinder. EBER in situ hybridization: sensitive detection of latent Epstein-Barr virus in individual cells. Rev Med Virol 4:251–260, 1994.

93. JS Greenspan, D Greenspan, E Lennette, DI Abrams, MA Conant, V Petersen, UK Freese. Replication of Epstein-Barr virus within the epithelial cells of oral ''hairy'' leukoplakia, an AIDS-associated lesion. N Engl J Med 313: 1564–1571, 1985.

94. N Raab-Traub, K Flynn. The structure of the termini of the Epstein-Barr virus as a marker of clonal cellular proliferation. Cell 47:883–889, 1986.

95. L Pedneault, BZ Katz. Comparison of polymerase chain reaction and standard Southern blotting for the detection of Epstein-Barr virus DNA in various biopsy specimens. J Med Virol 39:33–43, 1993.

96. DW Hanto. Classification of Epstein-Barr virus–associated posttransplant lymphoproliferative diseases: implications for understanding their pathogenesis and developing rational treatment strategies. Annu Rev Med 46:381–394, 1995.

97. L Young, C Alfieri, K Hennessy, H Evans, C O'Hara, KC Anderson, J Ritz, RS Shapiro, A Rickinson, E Kieff, et al. Expression of Epstein-Barr virus transformation-associated genes in tissues of patients with EBV lymphoproliferative disease. N Engl J Med 321:1080–1085, 1989.

98. BZ Katz, N Raab-Traub, G Miller. Latent and replicating forms of Epstein-Barr virus DNA in lymphomas and lymphoproliferative diseases. J Infect Dis 160:589–598, 1989.

99. JL Sullivan, P Medveczky, SJ Forman, SM Baker, JE Monroe, C Mulder. Epstein-Barr virus–induced lymphoproliferation: implications for antiviral chemotherapy. N Engl J Med 311:1163–1167, 1984.

100. CM Rooney, CA Smith, CYC Ng, S Loftin, C Li, RA Krance, MK Brenner, HE Heslop. Use of gene-modified virus-specific T lymphocytes to control Epstein-Barr virus–related lymphoproliferation. Lancet 345:9–13, 1995.

101. A Yen, P Fearneyhough, SS Ramier, SD Hudnall. EBV-associated Kikuchi's histiocytic necrotizing lymphadenitis with cutaneous manifestations. J Am Acad Dermatol 36: 342–346, 1997.

102. M Kikuchi. Lymphadenitis showing focal reticulum cell hyperplasia with nuclear debris and phagocytes: a clinicopathological study. Nippon Ketsueki Gakkai Zassho 35: 379–380, 1972.

103. Y Fujimoto, Y Kojima, K Yamaguchi. Cervical subacute necrotizing lymphadenitis. Naika 30:920–927, 1972.

104. Y Sumiyoshi, M Kikuchi, T Minematu, K Ohshima, M Takeshita, Y Minamishima. Analysis of herpesvirus genomes in Kikuchi's disease. Virchows Arch 424:437–440, 1994.

105. AC Feller, K Lennert, H Stein, HD Bruhn, HH Wuthe. Immunohistology and etiology of histiocytic necrotizing lymphadenitis. Report of three instructive cases. Histopathology 7:825–839, 1983.

106. S Pasquinucci, M Conisi, F Cavinato, F Bolussi. Kikuchi's disease in a patient infected with AIDS (letter). AIDS 5: 235, 1991.

107. SA Pileri, E Sabattini, P Costigliola, S Poggi, E Ricchi, F Tumietto, F Chiodo. Kikuchi's lymphadenitis and HIV infection. AIDS 5:459–461, 1991.

108. O Meyer, P Ribard, N Belmatoug, MF Kahn, M Grossin, JC Fournet, C Darne, F Morinet. Trois cas de lymphadenite de Kikuchi au cours du lupus erythemateux systemique: role du parvovirus B19. Ann Med Interne (Paris) 142: 259–264, 1991.

109. Y Eizuru, T Minematsu, Y Minamishima. Human herpesvirus 6 in lymph nodes. Lancet 1:40, 1989.

110. M Kikuchi, M Yoshizumi, H Nakamura. Necrotizing lymphadenitis: possible acute toxoplasmic infection. Virchows Arch A Pathol Anat Histol 376:247–253, 1977.

111. Y Takano, M Saegusa, M Okudaira. Pathologic analyses of non-overt necrotizing type Kikuchi and Fujimoto's disease. Acta Pathol Jpn 43:635–645, 1993.

112. HC Hollingsworth, SC Peiper, LM Weiss, M Raffeld, ES Jaffe. An investigation of the viral pathogenesis of Kikuchi-Fujimoto disease. Lack of evidence for Epstein-Barr virus or human herpesvirus type 6 as the causative agents. Arch Pathol Lab Med 118:134–140, 1994.

113. J Huh, HS Chi, SS Kim, G Gong. A study of the viral etiology of histiocytic necrotizing lymphadenitis (Kikuchi-Fujimoto disease). J Korean Med Sci 13:27–30, 1998.

114. CE Garcia, HV Girdhar-Gopal, DM Dorfman. Kikuchi-Fujimoto disease of the neck: update. Ann Otol Rhinol Laryngol 102:11–15, 1993.

115. JK Chan, KC Wong, CS Ng. A fatal case of multicentric Kikuchi's histiocytic lymphadenitis. Cancer 63: 1856–1862, 1989.

116. T Kuo. Cutaneous manifestations of Kikuchi's histiocytic necrotizing lymphadenitis. Am J Surg Pathol 14:872–876, 1990.

117. A Seno, R Torigoe, K Shimoe, J Tada, J Arata, M Suwaki. Kikuchi's disease (histiocytic necrotizing lymphadenitis) with cutaneous involvement. J Am Acad Dermatol 30: 504–506, 1994.

118. GC Ejeckam, B Azadeh, I Matar, O Aboud. Kikuchi's lymphadenitis in Qatar. East Afr Med J 70:575–577, 1993.

119. AR Lifson, JF Hilton, JL Westenhouse, AJ Canchola, MC Samuel, MH Katz, SP Buchbinder, NA Hessol, DH Osmond, S Shiboski, et al. Time from HIV seroconversion to oral candidiasis or hairy leukoplakia among homosexual and bisexual men enrolled in three prospective cohorts. AIDS 8:73–79, 1994.

120. PA Reichart, A Langford, HR Gelderblom, HD Pohle, J Becker, H Wolf. Oral hairy leukoplakia: observations in 95 cases and review of the literature. J Oral Pathol Med 18:410–415, 1989.

121. S Jahn, HW Busch, P Altmeyer. Oral hairy leukoplakia in HIV-positive patients. J Am Acad Dermatol 38:284–285, 1998.

122. R Husak, C Garbe, CE Orfanos. Oral hairy leukoplakia in 71 HIV-seropositive patients: clinical symptoms, relation to immunologic status, and prognostic significance. J Am Acad Dermatol 35:928–934, 1996.

123. CH Shiboski, JF Hilton, JM Neuhaus, A Canchola, D Greenspan. Human immunodeficiency virus–related oral manifestations and gender. Arch Intern Med 156: 2249–2254, 1996.

124. AW Boulter, N Soltanpoor, AV Swan, W Birnbaum, NW Johnson, CG Teo. Risk factors associated with Epstein-Barr virus replication in oral epithelial cells of HIV-infected individuals. AIDS 10:935–940, 1996.

125. LJ Conley, TJ Bush, SP Buchbinder, KA Penley, FN Judson, SD Holmberg. The association between cigarette smoking and selected HIV-related medical conditions. AIDS 10:1121–1126, 1996.

126. JS Greenspan, MT Mastrucci, PJ Leggott, UK Freese, YG De Souza, GB Scott, D Greenspan. Hairy leukoplakia in a child. AIDS 2:143, 1988.

127. FS Ferguson, H Archard, GJ Nuovo, S Nachman. Hairy leukoplakia in a child with AIDS—a rare symptom: case report. Pediatr Dent 15:280–281, 1993.

128. D Nadal, B De Roche, M Buisson, RA Seger. Oral hairy leukoplakia in vertically and horizontally acquired HIV infection. Arch Dis Child 67:1296–1297, 1992.

129. GN King, CM Healy, MT Glover, JT Kwan, DM Williams, IM Leigh, MH Thornhill. Prevalence and risk factors associated with leukoplakia, hairy leukoplakia, erythematous candidiasis, and gingival hyperplasia in renal transplant recipients. Oral Surg Oral Med Oral Pathol 78:718–726, 1994.

130. E Eisenberg, D Krutchkoff, H Yamase. Incidental oral hairy leukoplakia in immunocompetent persons. Oral Surg Oral Med Oral Pathol 74:332–333, 1992.

131. DH Felix, K Watret, D Wray, JC Southam. Hairy leukoplakia in an HIV-negative, nonimmunosuppressed patient. Oral Surg Oral Med Oral Pathol 74:563–566, 1992.

132. F Lozada-Nur, J Robinson, JA Regezi. Oral hairy leukoplakia in nonimmunosuppressed patients: report of four cases. Oral Surg Oral Med Oral Pathol 78:599–602, 1994.

133. L Resnick, JS Herbst, DV Ablashi, S Atherton, B Frank, L Rosen, SN Horwitz. Regression of oral hairy leukoplakia after orally administered acyclovir therapy. JAMA 259: 384–388, 1988.

134. CV Sumaya, RN Boswell, Y Ench, DL Kisner, EM Hersh, JM Reuben, PW Mansell. Enhanced serological and virological findings of Epstein-Barr virus in patients with AIDS and AIDS-related complex. J Infect Dis 154: 864–870, 1986.

135. GR Alsip, Y Ench, CV Sumaya, RN Boswell. Increased Epstein-Barr virus DNA in oropharyngeal secretions from patients with AIDS, AIDS-related complex, or asymptomatic human immunodeficiency virus infections. J Infect Dis 157:1072–1076, 1988.

136. DM Walling, SN Edmiston, JW Sixbey, M Abdel-Hamid, L Resnick, N Raab-Traub. Coinfection with multiple strains of the Epstein-Barr virus in human immunodeficiency virus–associated hairy leukoplakia. Proc Natl Acad Sci U S A 89:6560–6564, 1992.

137. DM Walling, N Raab-Traub. Epstein-Barr virus intrastrain recombination in oral hairy leukoplakia. J Virol 68: 7909–7917, 1994.

138. DM Walling, AG Perkins, J Webster-Cyriaque, L Resnick, N Raab-Traub. The Epstein-Barr virus EBNA-2 gene in oral hairy leukoplakia: strain variation, genetic deletion, and transcriptional expression. J Virol 68:7918–7926, 1994.

139. DM Walling, NM Clark, DM Markovitz, TS Frank, DK Braun, E Eisenberg, DJ Krutchkoff, DH Felix, N Raab-Traub. Epstein-Barr virus coinfection and recombination in non-human immunodeficiency virus–associated oral hairy leukoplakia. J Infect Dis 171:1122–1130, 1995.

140. CW Dawson, AG Eliopoulos, J Dawson, L Young. BHRF1, a viral homologue of the Bcl-2 oncogene, disturbs epithelial cell differentiation. Oncogene 10:69–77, 1995.

141. K Gilligan, P Rajadurai, L Resnick, N Raab-Traub. Epstein-Barr virus small nuclear RNAs are not expressed in permissively infected cells in AIDS-associated leukoplakia. Proc Natl Acad Sci U S A 87:8790–8794, 1990.

142. JS Greenspan, D Greenspan. Oral hairy leukoplakia: diagnosis and management. Oral Surg Oral Med Oral Pathol 67:396–403, 1989.

143. S Kabani, D Greenspan, Y de Souza, JS Greenspan, E Cataldo. Oral hairy leukoplakia with extensive mucosal involvement. Oral Surg Oral Med Oral Pathol 67:411–415, 1989.

144. E Lucht, P Biberfeld, A Linde. Epstein-Barr virus (EBV) in saliva and EBV serology of HIV-1–infected persons with and without hairy leukoplakia. J Infect 31:189–194, 1995.

145. E Brehmer-Andersson, E Lucht, S Lindskog, M Ekman, P Biberfeld. Oral hairy leukoplakia: pathogenetic aspects and significance of the lesion. Acta Derm Venereol 74: 81–89, 1994.

146. TE Daniels, D Greenspan, JS Greenspan, E Lennette, M Schiodt, V Petersen, Y de Souza. Absence of Langerhans cells in oral hairy leukoplakia, an AIDS-associated lesion. J Invest Dermatol 89:178–182, 1987.

147. L Anderson, HP Philipsen, PA Reichart. Macro- and microanatomy of the lateral border of the tongue with special reference to oral hairy leukoplakia. J Oral Pathol Med 19: 77–80, 1990.

148. TL Green, JS Greenspan, D Greenspan, YG de Souza. Oral lesions mimicking hairy leukoplakia: a diagnostic dilemma. Oral Surg Oral Med Oral Pathol 67:422–426, 1989.

149. DA Fisher, TE Daniels, JS Greenspan. Oral hairy leukoplakia unassociated with human immunodeficiency virus: pseudo oral hairy leukoplakia. J Am Acad Dermatol 27: 257–258, 1992.

150. S Euvrard, J Kanitakis, C Pouteil-Noble, Y Chardonnet, JL Touraine, J Thivolet. Pseudo oral hairy leukoplakia in a renal allograft recipient. J Am Acad Dermatol 30: 300–303, 1994.

151. CA Migliorati, AC Jones, PA Baughman. Use of exfoliative cytology in the diagnosis of oral hairy leukoplakia. Oral Surg Oral Med Oral Pathol 76:704–710, 1993.

152. G Gowdey, RK Lee, WM Carpenter. Treatment of HIV-related hairy leukoplakia with podophyllum resin 25% solution. Oral Surg Oral Med Oral Pathol Oral Radiol Endod 79:64–67, 1995.

153. CM Nichols, CM Flaitz, MJ Hicks. Role of podophyllin resin therapy in oral hairy leukoplakia in HIV infection: clinicopathologic study (abstr). Proceedings of the XI International Conference on AIDS, Vancouver, Canada, 1996.

154. H Schoffer, FR Ochsendorf, EB Helm, R Milbradt. Treatment of oral ''hairy'' leukoplakia in AIDS patients vitamin A acid (topically) or acyclovir (systemically). Dermatologica 174:150–151, 1987.

155. BT Goh, RKW Lau. Treatment of AIDS-associated oral hairy leukoplakia with cryotherapy. Int J STD AIDS 5: 60–62, 1993.

156. JS Herbst, J Morgan, N Raab-Traub, L Resnick. Comparison of the efficacy of surgery and acyclovir therapy in oral hairy leukoplakia. J Am Acad Dermatol 21:753–756, 1989.

7

Cytomegalovirus

Istvan Boldogh, Janak A. Patel, and Tasnee Chonmaitree
University of Texas Medical Branch, Galveston, Texas, USA

Stephen K. Tyring
*University of Texas Medical Branch, Galveston, Texas, USA
and University of Texas Medical Branch Center for Clinical Studies, Houston, Texas, USA*

Cytomegalovirus (CMV), otherwise known as human herpesvirus 5, belongs to the subfamily of Betaherpesvirinae that is characterized by a narrow host range and a long replicative cycle. Human CMV is a ubiquitous virus which, for the most part, causes asymptomatic infection. This human pathogen silently infects an overwhelming majority of humans (60–100%). However, clinical disease in certain groups, such as neonates and immunocompromised individuals, can lead to significant morbidity and mortality. The range of clinical manifestations in these populations is broad and may impact nearly every medical subspecialty. As is characteristic of all herpesviruses, CMV persists in the host following primary infection and remains latent in infected individuals for life (Fig. 7–1).

HISTORY

In 1881, Ribbert first histologically observed "protozoan-like cells" in the organs of a stillborn with presumed congenital syphilis [1]. Goodpasture and Talbot later suggested in 1921 that the enlarged cells, or "cytomegalia," could be due to injury by a viral agent [2]. This disease became known as "cytomegalic inclusion disease" before a viral

Work performed and represented by the authors was supported by research grants from the National Institute of Environmental Health Sciences (Grant No. ESO6676) and UTMB Environmental Toxicology (Grant No. 4-14544-578780).

etiology was ever discovered, based on the characteristic large cells and intranuclear inclusions [3]. In 1956, Rowe et al. [4], Smith [5], and Weller et al. [6] each independently isolated human CMV strains in tissue culture. The virus was initially known as "salivary gland virus" or "salivary inclusion disease virus." Weller and his colleagues later proposed the term "cytomegalovirus" in 1960 [7].

STRUCTURE AND ORGANIZATION OF THE VIRAL GENOME

The genome of CMV is extremely large and is more complex than that of any other DNA virus. This genome can be divided into two segments, referred to as long (L) and short (S) components, which are flanked by terminal repetitive sequences (Fig. 7–2). The junction between the L and S component is composed of internal repeat (IR) sequences (designated IRL, 11 kb and IRS, 2 kb), which are flanked by terminal repetitive sequences (designated TR_L and TR_s); (see Fig. 7–2). The sequences between the repeat regions are unique (U) and are referred to as unique long (UL, 175 kb) and unique short (US, 38 kb) regions [8].

The various clinical isolates of CMV may differ in both size and number of terminal additions. The junction between the UL and L repeat is a major site of interstrain sequence variation. Oligonucleotide probes designed for this region can be used to differentiate one strain of CMV from another. The restriction endonuclease profiles of the

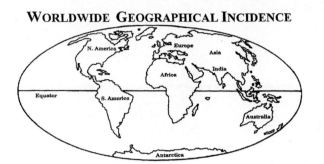

WORLDWIDE GEOGRAPHICAL INCIDENCE

TAXONOMY
Herpesviridae family
Betaherpesvirinae subfamily
(Human herpes virus 5)

TRANSMISSION

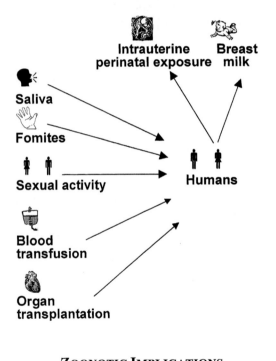

Intrauterine **Breast**
perinatal exposure **milk**

Saliva

Fomites

Sexual activity **Humans**

**Blood
transfusion**

**Organ
transplantation**

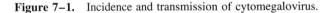

ZOONOTIC IMPLICATIONS
None

No known animal reservoirs for
human cytomegalovirus

Figure 7–1. Incidence and transmission of cytomegalovirus.

various strains of CMV have many similarities, but no two profiles are identical. Because of genomic variation, CMV may gain the ability to avoid neutralization; thus, some individuals may become reinfected with an epidemiologically (genotypically) unrelated isolate [9] that is resistant to one or more antiviral drugs [10]. Drug resistance appears particularly problematic for immunocompromised patients. However, the absence or gain of restriction enzyme sites that results in genomic polymorphism has not yet been linked to pathological differences among the CMV strains.

INCIDENCE

CMV infection is endemic in all parts of the world, and the prevalence of CMV-infected individuals is related to the socioeconomic status of the population. For instance, 60–70% of the population is seropositive for CMV in Central and Western Europe and the United States compared with 80–100% of the African population. The acquisition of CMV in developing countries also occurs at a younger age than in industrialized countries. This earlier and increased seroprevalence in lower socioeconomic environments has been attributed to crowded and communal living conditions, poor hygienic standards, and greater numbers of people (extended family) caring for an infant [11,12]. In the United States, age-related CMV prevalence studies have demonstrated that there is an increased risk of acquisition during early childhood, adolescence, and the reproductive years [13–15].

PATHOGENESIS

CMV is transmitted primarily by intimate person-to-person contact. Potential sources of infectious virus include oral secretions, urine, breast milk, semen, cervical and vaginal secretions, blood, and transplanted organs. Indirect transmission via contaminated fomites, such as toys, is also possible. CMV infection can occur as primary infection in those with no prior exposure to the virus or as a recurrent infection in those with previous exposure. In those with immunosuppression, reactivation of latent virus may also occur. Following primary or recurrent CMV infection in a pregnant woman, the virus may be transmitted to the fetus in utero in 40–50% of primary cases but in less than 1% of recurrent cases [16]. The rate of congenital CMV infection ranges from 0.2–2.5% of newborns [17,18], although most cases are asymptomatic. Pregnant women with primary infection frequently excrete CMV in cervical and vaginal secretions during the last trimester of pregnancy, which significantly increases the risk of perinatal transmission

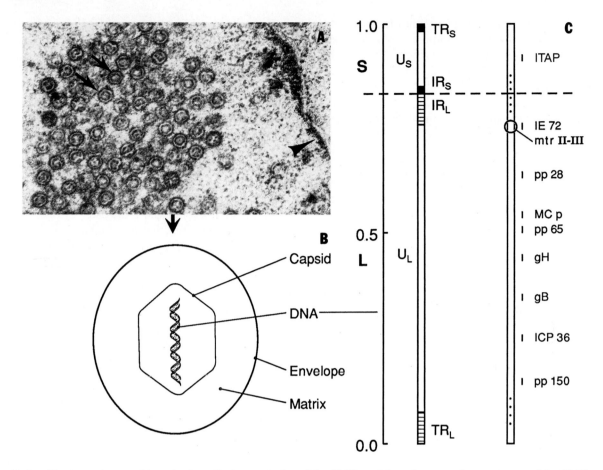

Figure 7–2. Electron micrographic and schematic demonstration of the CMV particle and structural arrangement of the CMV genome. (A) Section of a CMV-infected cell containing CMV particles (arrows) and nuclear membrane (arrowhead) ($\times 23,000$); (B) main components of CMV virion; (C) Physical organization of CMV DNA. U, unique region; TR, terminal repeats; IR, internal repeats; S, L, short and long region, respectively. Positions of open reading frames in the CMV genome encoding for proteins that are most important in human infections. ITAP, inhibitors of transporter-associated antigen processing; IE 72, regulatory phosphoprotein; pp28, pp65, pp150, structural virion components; MCp, major capsid protein; gH and gB, glycoprotein components of the envelope; ICP36, DNA binding protein. Mtr (morphological transforming region) II–III found in various human malignancies. Dotted region of the DNA found to be most variable among CMV isolates.

during delivery [8]. Infected mothers who breast-feed may also transmit the virus to their offspring.

CMV infection during early childhood often occurs as a result of horizontal spread among children, usually through exposure to infected saliva or urine. The incidence of CMV seropositivity in day-care centers is high, particularly among children ages 1 to 3 [19–21]. Beyond childhood, CMV is most frequently acquired through intimate physical contact and sexual transmission. The risk of CMV infection after transfusion of one unit of blood is approximately 3–4% [22,23]. Since CMV is transported in the bloodstream via leukocytes, leukocyte-depleted or cryopreserved blood carries less risk of transmission. CMV is not transmitted through fresh frozen plasma transfusions.

The incubation period for CMV is not exactly known but is estimated to be 4 to 8 weeks from study of cases acquired through perinatal transmission and blood transfusions [24,25]. Upon entering the human host, CMV disseminates throughout the body via the bloodstream and utilizes the blood leukocytes as transport media. CMV is rarely found free in plasma but can be isolated from the cellular fraction, particularly the polymorphonuclear cells. During the acute phase of CMV invasion, viral DNA and proteins can be demonstrated in both polymorphonuclear cells and monocytes. Although most infections with CMV remain latent and asymptomatic, the virus can also cause productive and symptomatic infection through cell lysis. During viremia, the virus may spread and infect various organs.

The target organs involved with lytic infection vary with the age of the host. CMV infection in the fetus or neonate typically involves the salivary glands (submandibular, sublingual) and neurons, among other organs [26]. Infection in otherwise healthy individuals most commonly affects the lymphoid tissues [27], whereas the lungs and other organs are frequently involved in immunocompromised persons [28].

CMV is a cytotoxic virus that alters the metabolic biochemical cascade of cells, resulting in cell enlargement (cytomegaly) and condensation of nuclear mass (nuclear inclusion). Consequently, CMV can produce cell injury and tissue destruction (lysis) during productive, symptomatic infection [29]. In organ disease, an inflammatory response ensues. Numbers of lymphocytes and plasma cells may vary in degree and distribution. This inflammatory response, along with alteration of cellular biochemical cascade events and/or cytotoxic effects of CMV replication, contributes to organ dysfunction [30].

Viremic spread of CMV often results in renal involvement and excretion of infectious CMV particles in urine (viruria). In immunocompetent individuals, CMV exposure of the kidneys is seldom associated with renal dysfunction. In immunocompromised patients (e.g., renal transplant recipients), hypertrophy and necrosis of endothelial cells may produce an accumulation of fibrillar material in the glomerular capillaries. Cytomegalic cells with nuclear inclusions are seen in the convoluted proximal tubules and occasionally in the glomeruli. CMV-specific macromolecules (DNA, RNA, IE, E, and L proteins) can be detected by in situ nucleic acid hybridization or by immunochemistry in the inflammatory mononuclear cells of the interstitial spaces of kidney biopsies. During glomerulopathy, there are deposits of immune complexes (IgG, IgM) on the basal membranes of glomeruli and mesangial areas, which may result in immune complex–associated diseases [30,31].

As stated previously, the lungs are frequently affected by CMV infection in immunosuppressed individuals, particularly after bone marrow transplantation. In the lungs, enlarged cells with late nuclear inclusion bodies and associated mononuclear cell inflammation are found primarily in the alveolar and bronchial epithelia [32]. These findings are rarely seen in the mucous membranes of the tracheobronchial region.

Histological studies of cutaneous ulcerations have often documented nuclear inclusions in capillary endothelial cells during CMV infection. When kidney, gastrointestinal tract, lung, and brain ulcerations are examined, endothelial cells are also cytomegalic and contain nuclear inclusions. Infectious CMV and CMV-specific macromolecules have been detected in the walls of blood vessels of patients afflicted with atherosclerosis [33].

Gastrointestinal involvement of CMV is commonly reported in human immunodeficiency virus (HIV)-infected individuals, infected neonates, and other immunosuppressed persons. An important complication is gastrointestinal hemorrhage, with occasional perforation and development of pneumatosis intestinalis. The colon, particularly the cecum, is the usual site of these lesions. However, the esophagus, stomach, pancreas, and proximal small bowel may also be affected. The induced lesions may vary from punctate superficial ulcerations to deep ulcerations. In untreated cases, perforation of the gut may occur. CMV-associated gastrointestinal lesions can appear in the absence of other manifestations of CMV disease.

Abnormal liver function test findings are common in CMV infection, with mild to moderately severe hepatitis occurring in 30–50% of organ transplant patients. By using in situ cytohybridization or immunofluorescent staining, the presence of CMV can be demonstrated in liver biopsies of these patients. Biopsy studies of immunocompetent individuals with CMV mononucleosis syndrome have also demonstrated histological abnormalities, such as increased hepatocellular mitotic activity, mild hepatocellular necrosis, granuloma formation, and bile duct epithelial damage. In addition, mononuclear portal/sinusoidal infiltrates can be seen in the absence of typical cytomegalic cells (Fig. 7–3). In the livers of infected newborns, cytomegalic cells are seen commonly in the bile duct epithelium, less frequently in capillary endothelium, and rarely in the parenchymal cells. In adults, however, hepatocytes may contain nuclear inclusions [34].

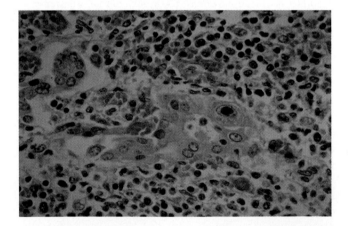

Figure 7–3. Cholangiole (bile duct) with CMV cytopathic effect in one cell and prominent portal infiltration with lymphocytes, plasma cells, macrophages, and eosinophils. (H & E stain.) (Photograph courtesy of Jerome H. Smith, M.D., Department of Pathology, University of Texas Medical Branch at Galveston, Galveston, TX.)

CMV infections disseminate and can be identified in neonates with congenital infection as well as in burned and immunocompromised adults. The physical findings include granulated tissues, localized ulcers, vesiculobullous lesions, hyperpigmentation, and induration. Despite the clinical variability, the histopathologic appearance of CMV skin lesions is similar—dilated dermal vessels with irregularly shaped periendothelial and endothelial cells containing large hyperchromatic, basophilic intranuclear inclusions [35–37].

Congenital CMV infection often adversely affects the central nervous system of the fetus and causes microcephaly, periventricular calcification, hydrocephaly, chorioretinitis, and optic atrophy [38,39]. Glial and neural cells may be productively and abortively infected. Pathologic manifestations may include microglial nodules, focal parenchymal necrosis, necrotizing ventriculitis, hemorrhages, astrocytic proliferation, perivascular inflammation, and ependymal granulation. Sensorineural hearing loss is a common feature of both clinical and subclinical congenital CMV infections. In the inner ear, enlarged cells with nuclear inclusions are often detected in epithelial cells of the cochlea, stria vascularis, limbus spiralis, Reissner's membrane, saccule, and utricle. Congenital CMV infections with diffuse inflammation, villitis, plasma cell infiltration, focal necrosis, and hemorrhage, with or without detectable cytomegalic cells in the placenta, have also been observed [39].

In vitro data suggest that CMV may be immunosuppressive. Primary CMV infection produces a decrease in the ratio of helper to suppressor lymphocytes. The decrease in this ratio is caused by an increase in the circulating suppressor cells. Immunocompetent adults with CMV mononucleosis also have impaired immunoproliferative responses of lymphocytes to mitogens [40]. CMV infection may lead to other transient immunological aberrations, such as the presence of immune complexes, cold agglutinins, rheumatoid factor, a positive Coombs' test result, or monoclonal gammopathies [41–43].

Similar to oncogenic viruses, CMV has been demonstrated to promote host DNA and RNA synthesis in infected cells. Both CMV particles (live or inactivated) and viral DNA (e.g., morphological transforming regions mtrI, mtrII, and mtrIII; see Fig. 7–2) can transform animal and human cells in vitro and are tumorigenic in animal models [44,45]. In addition, CMV or its macromolecules have been found in various human tumors, including prostatic carcinoma, adenocarcinoma of the colon, cervical carcinoma, and Kaposi's sarcoma [45]. The significance of these associations and the etiological role of CMV in malignancy are yet to be determined [46,47].

CELLULAR PATHOLOGY OF CMV INFECTIONS

A large number of cell types have receptors for CMV but only a few permit productive virus replication. After entry into the cells, the CMV genome may either remain in a quiescent (latent) state or progress to a productive state. In productive infection, there is a temporarily regulated sequential expression of the viral genome. The synthesized viral proteins can be classified into three broad categories: (1) immediate early (IE, alpha) proteins specified by viral mRNA whose synthesis does not require prior viral protein synthesis; (2) early (E, beta) proteins translated from mRNAs transcribed prior to the onset of viral DNA synthesis; and (3) late (L, gamma) proteins directed by mRNAs transcribed predominantly after synthesis of viral DNA. In vitro, CMV infection results in changes in cell shape and size (Fig. 7–4) and a relatively high production of progeny in fibroblast cells of human origin. CMV replication is a slow process, and more cell-associated virus than extracellular virus is produced. The ratio of infectious to defective particles is usually in the range of 1:500 to 1:5000. Cultured epithelial cell types (e.g., kidney), endothelial cells, or cells of lymphoid origin permit low CMV replication when treated with a chemical agent, such as phorbol-12-myristate-13-acetate, 5-azacytosine, iododeoxyuridine, or interleukin-2 (IL-2). In vivo, however, CMV replicates productively in a broad range of cells (mainly epithelial) in various organs, and the virus can be isolated from saliva, urine, tears, semen, vaginal secretions, milk, and other specimens [48].

The restricted expression of one or more of the gene classes results in an abortive infection. The molecular mechanisms that influence permissiveness are currently unclear. They appear to be related to cell activation cascade events that are involved in virus replication [49]. Restricted virus gene expression appears to be important to the development and maintenance of persistent or latent infection in vivo. For example, evidence suggests that cultured T and B lymphocytes are semipermissive for CMV, and gene expression is limited to the IE region(s). In contrast, monocytes of peripheral blood origin permit IE, E, and L gene expression and production of infectious virus at a very low level. The restriction of CMV replication in monocytes and lymphocytes may be eliminated by immunosuppression (e.g., HIV infection) which allows productive infection of these cells [50].

As noted above, CMV persists in the host for life following primary infection and remains latently associated with infected individuals for life [50]. The precise sites and mechanism of CMV latency remain unknown, although latent virus appears to have a broad tissue distribution as indicated by the transmission of CMV following organ

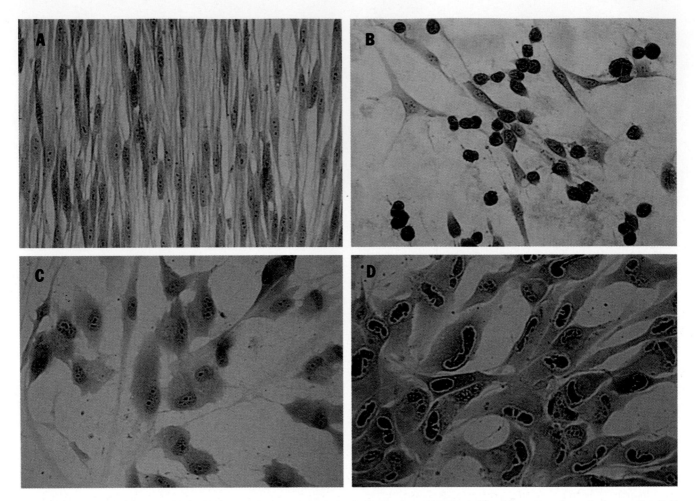

Figure 7–4. Morphological changes of CMV-infected permissive cells in vitro. (A) Noninfected human embryonic lung cells. Cell cultures in panels (B), (C), and (D) are infected with a multiplicity of infection (MOI) of 5 plaque forming units (PFU) per cell. (B) Cells are rounded and smaller in size at about 6 hr. (C) Cells demonstrate early nuclear inclusions between 24 hr and 36 hr. (D) Nuclei of enlarged (cytomegaly) cells show late type A nuclear inclusions from 72 hr on, after infection.

transplantation. Salivary glands, blood cells, spleen, uterus, and kidneys are often observed to harbor CMV. To date, very little is known about the molecular events directed by the virus and/or cell that control persistence and/or latency. CMV has mechanisms whereby the infected cells or the released CMV can protect itself from immune surveillance and can produce a productive infection in the presence of intact humoral and cellular immunity [51]. Spread of virus within tissues occurs mainly via the budding of CMV particles from one cell into adjacent cells. This avoidance of the extracellular milieu may be one of the important mechanisms of the virus for escaping neutralization by antibody. Virus shedding in many body fluids, such as saliva, urine, cervical secretions, and breast milk, may persist for months, which suggests that anti-CMV antibodies neutralize CMV in plasma but not in other body fluids.

Another mechanism by which CMV may avoid host defenses is by the induction of a receptor for the Fc portion of IgG antibody in infected cells (Fig. 7–5). The production of this glycoprotein appears during the early stage of CMV replication and it incorporates into the cell membrane but has not been found on virus particles. These molecules could provide a protective coat for the infected cells, preventing lysis by specific cytolytic antibody or lysis by cytotoxic T cells through binding of immunoglobulins by the Fc portion. The Fc receptors associated with CMV-infected cells may bind antibody-coated bacteria or immune complexes and may cause secondary inflammation in a CMV-infected organ [52].

Beta-2 microglobulin (β_2-microglobulin; light chain of class I HLA molecules) has a high binding affinity to CMV and provides another unique mechanism that may be im-

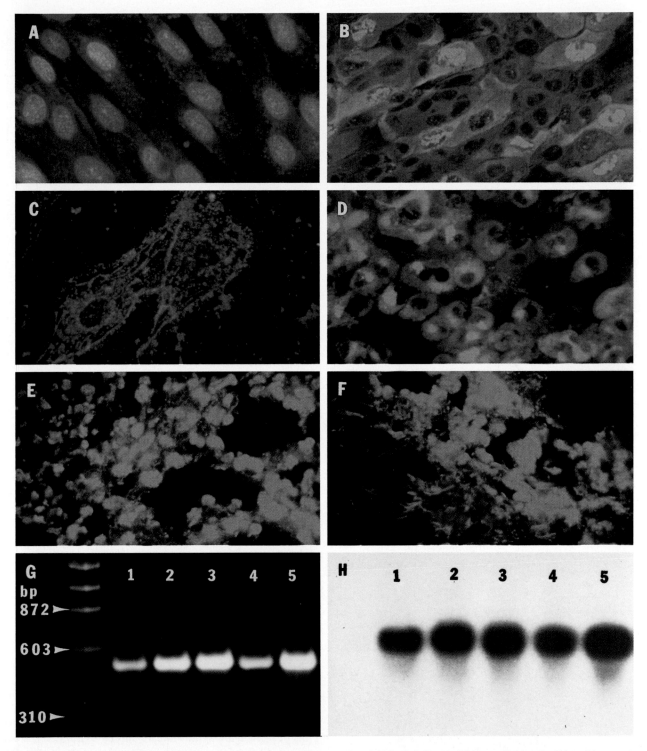

Figure 7–5. Detection of CMV-specific macromolecules at cellular and molecular levels. (A, B) Immediate early (A) and late antigens (B) demonstrated in CMV-infected cells by indirect immunofluorescent assay. (C, D) CMV-induced cellular Fc-binding receptors on the (C) membrane and in the (D) cytoplasm of the infected cells. (E, F) CMV-specific proteins in sections of CMV-induced skin lesions by immunohistochemistry. (G) Amplification of a 541 base pair segment of CMV immediate early 2 region of CMV DNA by polymerase chain reaction. (H) Autoradiogram demonstrates hybridization of ^{32}P-labeled oligonucleotide probe to polymerase chain reaction–amplified sequences shown in panel (G) (lanes 1 and 2, skin biopsies from HIV-infected patients; lanes 3 and 4, HIV-associated Kaposi's sarcoma; lane 5, Kaposi's sarcoma unrelated to HIV infection).

portant in avoiding neutralization by blocking the attachment of antibody to extracellular virions. On the other hand, β_2-microglobulin may mask CMV proteins, preventing efficient neutralization antibody production. Since β_2-microglobulin-free virus suspension demonstrates decreased infectivity in comparison to virus with β_2-microglobulin bound to its surface [53], β_2-microglobulin may also be a component in the process of binding of CMV to the cell membrane.

CLINICAL MANIFESTATIONS

Infection in Normal Children and Adults

The most commonly acquired CMV disease in immunocompetent individuals is CMV-induced mononucleosis. This illness causes fewer than 10% of all cases of mononucleosis [54] and is clinically indistinguishable from Epstein-Barr virus (EBV)–induced mononucleosis (Tables 7–1, 7–2, and 7–3). In addition to the characteristic fever and malaise with this illness, atypical lymphocytosis (Fig. 7–6) and mild elevation of liver enzymes usually occur [55,56]. A small percentage of patients develop a rubelliform or maculopapular cutaneous eruption. However, when ampicillin is administered during this illness, 80–100% of cases develop a maculopapular, morbilliform rash within a week or so (Fig. 7–7).

The disease course of CMV-induced mononucleosis is typically self-limited and benign, with only occasional complications. These may include interstitial pneumonia, hemolytic anemia, splenic infarction, thrombocytopenia, hepatitis, Guillain-Barré syndrome, meningoencephalitis, myocarditis, arthritis, pleuritis, and gastrointestinal and genitourinary syndromes. A mononucleosis syndrome caused by CMV has also been observed in immunocompe-

Table 7–1. Diseases and Complications Associated with Cytomegalovirus Infections

Congenital (Transplacental), Perinatal Infection
  Symptomatic
    Intrauterine growth retardation
    Prematurity
    Hepatosplenomegaly
    Jaundice
    Thrombocytopenia with petechiae
    Microcephaly with or without cerebral calcification
    Chorioretinitis
  Asymptomatic disease with neurological impairments
    Hearing loss
    Disorders of hearing, language, and learning
    Mental retardation with or without seizures
    Blindness
    Paraparesis
    Diplegia
Infection in Children and Adults
    Mononucleosis (fever, malaise, splenomegaly, hepatitis, peripheral and atypical lymphocytosis)
    Hemolytic anemia, thrombocytopenia
    Immunological abnormalities such as production of autoantibodies, cold agglutinins, rheumatoid factor, cryoglobulins
    Interstitial pneumonia
    Myocarditis
    Postperfusion syndrome
    Granulomatous hepatitis
    Guillain-Barré syndrome
    Meningoencephalitis (rare)
    Myocarditis
    Gastrointestinal syndromes (colitis, esophagitis)
    Genitourinary syndromes (cervicitis, urethral syndromes)
Proliferative Diseases Associated with CMV infection*
    Colon carcinoma
    Cervical carcinoma
    Prostate carcinoma
    Kaposi's sarcoma
    Atherosclerosis

* A causal relationship has not been definitively established.

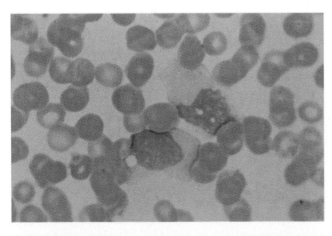

Figure 7–6. Atypical lymphocytes seen in peripheral blood smear in CMV mononucleosis.

tent individuals after blood transfusion. The symptoms of this postperfusion syndrome are similar to those described above and manifest several weeks to several months after the contaminated transfusion.

Congenital Infections

Congenital CMV infection occurs in an average of 1% of all newborn infants in the United States as a result of

Table 7–2. Clinical Manifestations of CMV-induced Mononucleosis

Time After exposure	Clinical manifestations	Laboratory analyses	Other notes
4–8 weeks	Syndrome of fever (+/− chills) and severe malaise. Some patients may have headache, myalgias, sore throat, rash, abdominal pain, splenomegaly, or, rarely, hepatomegaly ↓	Viral culture of body secretions CMV-specific serologies, with seroconversion or significant rise in antibody titers	This illness most often affects persons aged 20–40 years but can also be seen in children and adolescents
5–12 weeks (1–4 weeks later)	Resolution of symptoms. Some patients may have postviral asthenia for several more months	Heterophil antibody negative	CMV excretion in saliva, urine, and genital secretions may persist for months to years after acute infection

transplacental transmission of CMV. Most of the infected newborns are asymptomatic at birth. However, 5–17% may later demonstrate unilateral or bilateral deafness and/or other neurodevelopmental sequelae [57–59].

Symptomatic congenital CMV infection occurs in up to 10% of infected infants (see Table 7–1). The syndrome is characterized by intrauterine growth retardation, hepatosplenomegaly, pneumonitis, jaundice, thrombocytopenia with petechiae, and central nervous system involvement such as microcephaly, intracerebral calcifications (Fig. 7–8, A, B), chorioretinitis, other ocular defects, and sensorineural hearing loss. Other less common manifestations include long bone osteitis, cutaneous vasculitis, hemolytic anemia, ascites, and chronic hepatitis. Symptomatic congenital CMV infection is distinct from other congenitally

transmitted infections such as rubella, herpes simplex, enteroviral infection, congenital toxoplasmosis, and congenital syphilis.

Perinatal Infections

Perinatal CMV infection may be acquired from exposure of the newborn to virus in the maternal genital tract at delivery, from breast milk, or through multiple blood transfusions. The disease may manifest between 4 weeks and 16 weeks of age, but most infections are asymptomatic. In a small percentage of infants, there may be signs and

Table 7–3. Differential Diagnoses of Cytomegalovirus Mononucleosis

Epstein-Barr virus–induced mononucleosis: Generally, CMV-induced mononucleosis produces less severe and less frequent pharyngitis, lymphadenopathy, and splenomegaly. Exudative pharyngitis is rare with CMV disease. Heterophil antibody test and specific serologies can differentiate the two etiologies

Toxoplasmosis: This illness most frequently manifests with posterior cervical lymphadenopathy and fatigue without fever or pharyngitis

Viral Hepatitis: Patients typically have jaundice and tender hepatomegaly but may also have low-grade fever, fatigue, atypical lymphocytosis, and occasional lymphadenopathy

Lymphoma: Nontender fixed adenopathy is most characteristic

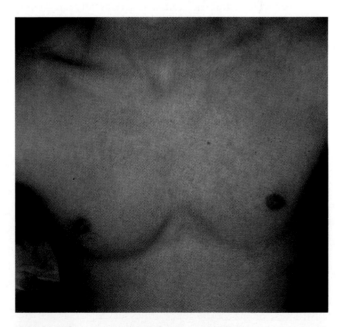

Figure 7–7. Ampicillin-induced morbilliform rash during the course of CMV mononucleosis.

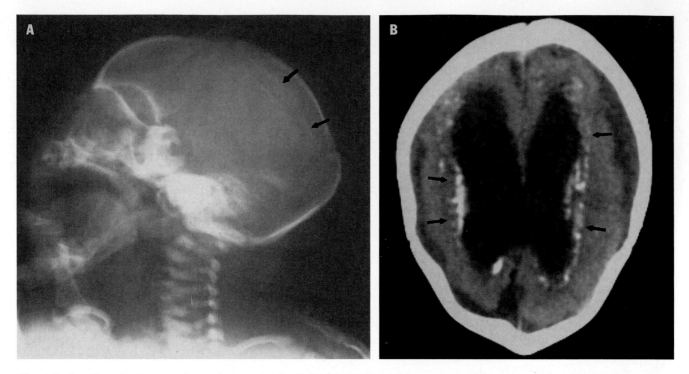

Figure 7–8. Neurodevelopmental sequelae associated with CMV infection. (A) Lateral view demonstrates microcephaly and curvilinear paraventricular calcification (arrows). (B) An axial computed tomographic scan of microcephaly, brain atrophy, enlargement of the ventricles, and a classic distribution of periventricular calcifications (arrows). (Radiograph courtesy of Susan D. John, M.D., and Leonard E. Swischuk, M.D., Department of Radiology, University of Texas Medical Branch at Galveston, Galveston, TX.)

symptoms of self-limited lymphadenopathy, hepatospleno-megaly, or pneumonitis. CMV pneumonitis is generally associated with an afebrile course. It is clinically and radio-graphically indistinguishable from other types of afebrile pneumonia caused by agents such as *Chlamydia trachom-atis, Pneumocystis carinii,* or respiratory viruses [58,59]. Occasionally, severe protracted pneumonitis occurs in pre-mature infants with bronchopulmonary dysplasia [59].

Infection in the Immunocompromised Host

The population of immunocompromised hosts has incre-sed, largely due to the increase in HIV infection and the use of immunosuppressive chemotherapy for malignancies or organ transplantation. Thus, the incidence of dissemi-nated CMV infection with significant morbidity and mor-tality has also increased [60].

The typical susceptible individual may have an underly-ing defect in the cellular (T-cell) and humoral (B-cell) im-mune responses. The CMV-infected host may remain asymptomatic, with prolonged viral shedding from mu-cosal sites, or may experience illnesses characterized by fever and mononucleosis syndrome, as seen in the normal

host. However, these patients are at risk for persistent vire-mia with systemic dissemination to distant organs, where continued viral replication results in tissue injury. The brain, lungs, eyes (Figs. 7–8 to 7–11), intestines, bone marrow, and blood vessels are the target tissues most fre-quently involved. The various disease manifestations are listed in Table 7–4.

Synergistic Interaction Between CMV and HIV

CMV is considered to be one of the most important viral infection among HIV-infected patients, as there are high morbidity and mortality rates in this population [61,62]. For example, in the HIV-infected patient, the following may occur: (1) CMV may produce a number of clinical syndromes, inducing retinitis, pneumonitis, encephalitis, and gastroenteritis; (2) CMV may potentiate cellular im-munodeficiency, either directly or in association with en-hanced HIV replication; and (3) after primary infection, CMV alone may depress T-lymphocyte helper/suppressor ratios and predispose the patient to opportunistic infections.

The synergistic and cofactorial roles of CMV in AIDS can be assessed by the following in vitro and in vivo obser-

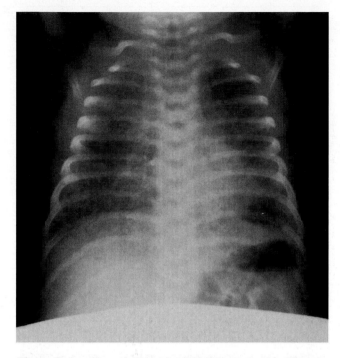

Figure 7–9. Chest radiograph of CMV pneumonitis. Note the bilateral reticulonodular infiltrates with mild overaeration of the lungs. (Radiograph courtesy of Susan D. John, M.D., and Leonard E. Swischuk, M.D., Department of Radiology, University of Texas Medical Branch at Galveston, Galveston, TX.)

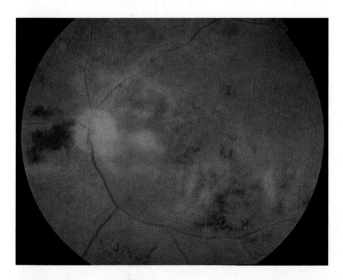

Figure 7–10. CMV-induced chorioretinitis in an HIV-infected patient. (Photograph courtesy of Helen Li, M.D., Department of Ophthalmology, University of Texas Medical Branch at Galveston, Galveston, TX.)

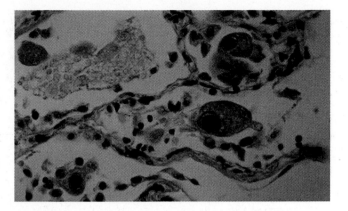

Figure 7–11. Photomicrograph of pneumocytes demonstrating CMV-induced cytopathic effect (cytomegaly and Cowdry type A nuclear inclusion) (Mallory's trichrome stain). (Photograph courtesy of Jerome H. Smith, M.D., Department of Pathology, University of Texas Medical Branch at Galveston, Galveston, TX.)

vations. Transactivation of the HIV genome by immediate early (IE) proteins of CMV occurs through enhancer-promoter sequences located within the HIV long terminal repeat (LTR). Transactivation by IE proteins is mediated either directly or by the induction of increases in the intracellular levels of transcription factors, such as NFκB and Sp1. CMV IE genes are usually expressed during latent infection. Thus, transactivation could occur in the absence of active virus replication at any time during the course of HIV disease. Recent molecular studies suggest that CMV and HIV act in synergy within the same cell. Indeed, infection of semipermissive cell types (e.g., lymphoblastoid, neural, endothelial) by HIV allows productive CMV replication. This demonstrates further evidence for a bidirectional interaction between CMV and HIV in vivo. Moreover, this synergism could provide a mechanism for the observed increase in the degree of viremia for both of these viruses in AIDS patients [63].

CMV infection can enhance expression of cell membrane molecules that are involved in HIV binding to the cell surface and introduction of HIV particles into cells [64]. Entry of immunoglobulin-coated HIV into CD4-negative cells (neural cells, and endothelial cells) has been shown to occur via receptors for the Fc portion of IgG molecules expressed on the cell membrane of CMV-infected cells. CMV infections induce the expression of Fc receptors on the plasmalemma of cells that normally do not display this molecule. As a result of these CMV-induced cellular changes, HIV can coinfect a broad range of cell types in vivo, possibly explaining the wide variety of clinical syndromes described in acquired immunodeficiency syndrome (AIDS) patients.

Table 7–4. Manifestations of CMV Infections in Immunocompromised Patients

Bone Marrow
  Leukopenia
  Anemia
  Thrombocytopenia
  Atypical lymphocytosis
Endocrine
  Adrenalitis
  Pancreatitis
Renal
  Glomerulonephritis
  Rejection of kidney graft
Skin
  Ulcers
  Papules
  Plaques
  Purpura
  Morbilliform rash
  Maculopapular rash
Gastrointestinal Tract
  Stomatitis
  Esophagitis
  Gastritis
  Duodenitis
  Ileitis/colitis
  Bowel ulcers
  Choleocystitis
  Cholangitis
  Papillary stenosis
Central Nervous System and Eye
  Encephalitis
  Transverse myelitis
  Guillain-Barré Syndrome
  Chorioretinitis
Lung
  Interstitial pneumonitis

Table 7–5. Cutaneous Manifestations of CMV Infections

Normal Host
  Congenital infections
    Blueberry-muffin lesions (dermal erythropoiesis)
    Petechiae and purpura
    Cutaneous vesicles
    Ichthyosis
  Mononucleosis-associated
    Ampicillin-induced rash
    Erythema nodosum
    Urticaria
    Cutaneous vasculitis
Immunocompromised Host
  Ulcer
  Purpura
  Petechiae
  Morbilliform and maculopapular rash
  Vesicles
  Verrucous or indurated plaques
  Nodules

CMV infection stimulates production of cellular factors that support HIV replication [63]. For example, CMV-infected cells (e.g., monocytes, macrophages) express enhanced quantities of tumor necrosis factor alpha, transforming growth factor beta, IL-1 beta, colony-stimulating factor-1, monocyte-derived neutrophil chemotactic factor, and neutrophil-activating factor. These cytokines, in turn, may be able to induce HIV expression and replication in chronically infected cells or release the HIV from latency.

Cutaneous Manifestations of CMV Infection

Cutaneous manifestations of CMV in the normal host are uncommon but well described (Table 7–5). Those seen in

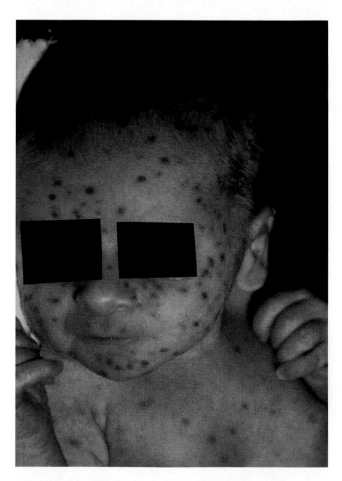

Figure 7–12. Blueberry-muffin lesions (from dermal erythropoiesis) in congenital CMV infection.

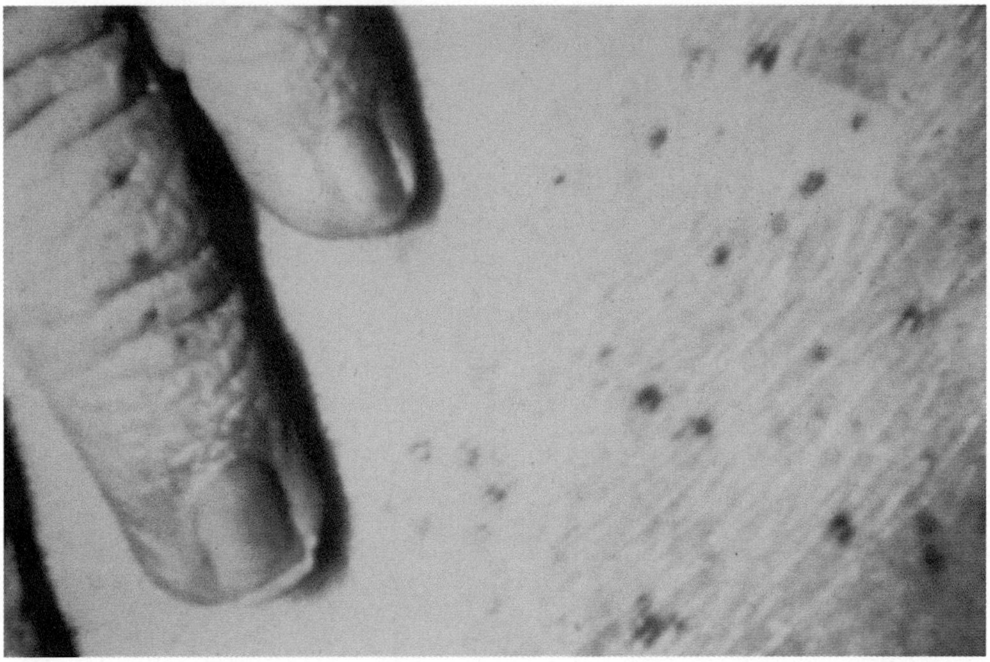

Figure 7–13. Petechial lesions in congenital CMV infection.

congenital CMV infection include blueberry muffin lesions (Fig. 7–12), which represent dermal erythropoiesis [65]; also seen are petechiae (Fig. 7–13) and purpura [66], cutaneous vesicles [67], and ichthyosis of the skin found in conjunction with keratitis and deafness [68]. Reports of

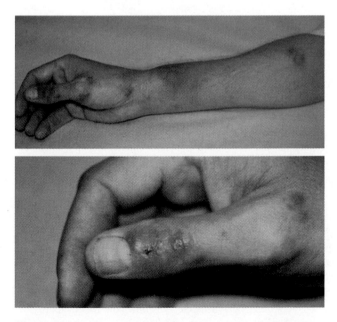

Figure 7–14. Cutaneous nodules associated with CMV in an HIV-infected patient.

rashes associated with CMV mononucleosis syndrome include the maculopapular rubelliform rash, the ampicillin-induced rash (Fig. 7–7), and erythema nodosum [69]. Cutaneous vasculitis has also been reported as a presenting symptom of acute CMV infection in a 4-month-old child [70].

CMV-associated skin lesions in the immunocompromised host (Figs. 7–14 and 7–15) are rare compared with the prevalence of CMV infection of other organs. Although several case reports have been published, the true incidence of cutaneous CMV is unknown. Various forms of cutaneous CMV have been described (Table 7–5). Ulcers are the predominant lesions and occur most frequently over the perianal area and buttocks (30% of reported cases) [66,71,72]. These lesions frequently contain other microorganisms, such as herpes simplex virus or *Staphylococcus aureus.* Other less commonly reported cutaneous lesions include purpura, petechiae, morbilliform and maculopapular rash, vesicles, and verrucous or indurated plaques and nodules. Although CMV does not appear to play a direct role in the pathogenesis of bacillary angiomatosis and Kaposi's sarcoma, CMV nucleic acids and antigens have been detected in these tissues [73].

CMV-associated ulcers and nodules seem to arise from infection of the endothelium of cutaneous blood vessels during the viremic phase of illness. These lesions may progress to vasculitis [64], with the appearance of purpuric nodules that may undergo infarction and sloughing of the

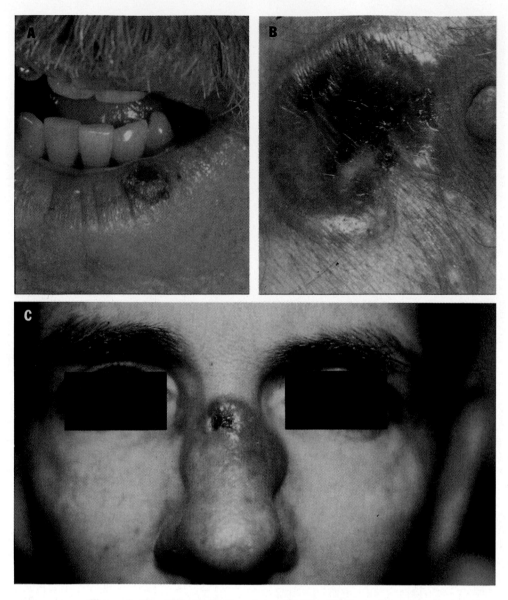

Figure 7–15. Cutaneous ulcerations. (A) Lip; (B) chest; (C) nose.

overlying epidermis. However, there is also evidence that the endothelial infection may not necessarily progress to skin lesions [66,71].

The immunocompromised host with cutaneous CMV usually has concurrent systemic CMV disease [70,71]. Therefore, prognosis with cutaneous CMV is poor, and the mortality rate is approximately 85% [70]. Nonetheless, the skin lesions of patients may show a beneficial response to CMV-specific antiviral chemotherapy [74].

Dermatopathology

Histological diagnosis of CMV has a high specificity but its sensitivity can be two to six times less than that of viral isolation [75]. The characteristic histological feature of CMV infection is the "owl's-eye" appearance owing to viral inclusion bodies found in infected endothelial cells (Fig. 7–16) [76]. These cells are typically enlarged one- to threefold and have large intranuclear inclusions with a surrounding clear halo. The cytoplasm also contains purplish, granular inclusions. The intranuclear inclusions seen in CMV infection appear identical to but slightly larger than those of herpes simplex virus and varicella zoster virus infection, which may at times cause confusion in diagnosis [77]. A sparse perivascular lymphocytic infiltrate in the upper dermis, along with spongiosis, is also seen with CMV infection. Involvement of the vascular endothelium

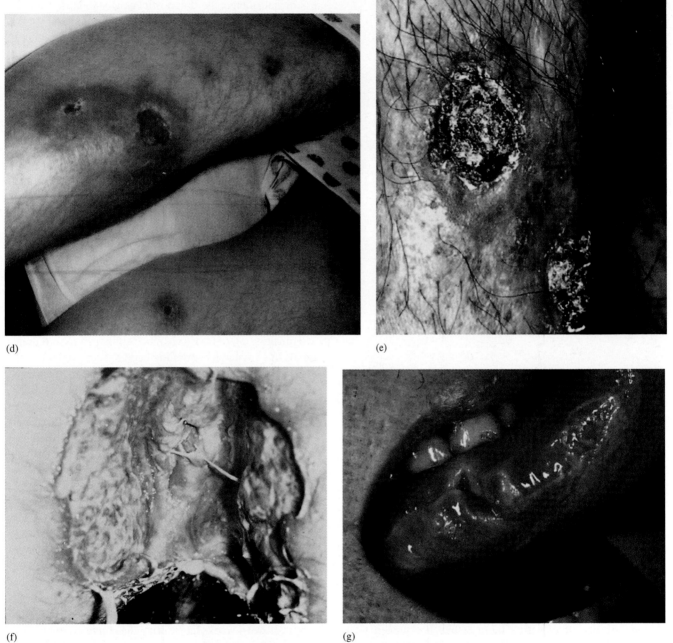

(d)

(e)

(f)

(g)

Figure 7–15. (Continued.) (d) Leg associated with CMV in HIV-positive patients. CMV ulcers may be (e) verrucous; (f) may become large in the perianal area; (g) or may appear on the tongue. [(d) Courtesy of James C. Shaw, M.D., Section of Dermatology, University of Chicago, Chicago, IL, (e), (g), courtesy of Siri Chiewchanvit, M.D., Chiang Mai, Thailand; (c) courtesy of Rocio Orozco-Scholtes, M.D., Department of Dermatology, National Institute of Nutrition, Tlalpan, Mexico.)]

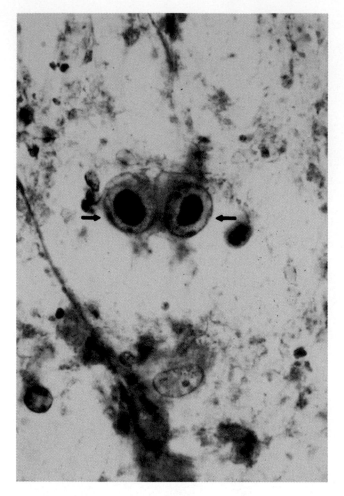

Figure 7–16. CMV-infected cells with prominent nuclear inclusions producing the typical "owl's-eye" appearance in vivo.

with vasculitis may be evident in some cases and is indicative of disseminated infection.

Diagnosis

The possibility of effective therapy has heightened the need for accurate and rapid laboratory methods for diagnosis of CMV infection. Current diagnostic tools include virus isolation in tissue culture (shell vial culture/immunochemistry/nucleic acid hybridization), histological-cytological detection of typical CMV cytopathology, immunological methods to detect seroconversion, and the detection of CMV antigens and/or nucleic acids within cells of infected organs and tissues [78–80]. The usual clinical specimens used for culture diagnosis of CMV are urine and saliva. The virus can also be isolated from stool, breast milk, semen, cervical secretions, and peripheral

blood cells. Although culture of CMV in human fibroblasts is still considered the diagnostic gold standard, isolation of infectious virus may take a few days to several weeks. Use of the shell vial culture, in conjunction with staining with monoclonal antibodies directed at immediate early CMV antigens, has made it possible to detect CMV in culture within 24 to 48 hours. For direct demonstration of the virus or inclusion-containing cells (Fig. 7–17), a urine sample is the most appropriate specimen. Patients with CMV infection excrete the virus consistently and in high quantity in the urine.

Immunofluorescence using monoclonal antibodies is a frequently used method to detect CMV-specific antigens in clinical specimens, such as peripheral blood cells, biopsies, autopsies, and amniotic cells. Radio- or biotin-labeled DNA or RNA probes are also used to detect CMV-related nucleic acid sequences (using in situ cytohybridization, Southern-, slot/dot-blot hybridization) directly in cells of clinical specimens. DNA amplification using polymerase chain reaction (PCR) achieves a high level of sensitivity in CMV nucleic acid detection in single cells (in situ PCR), body fluids, and tissue sections.

Transmission of CMV via blood transfusions and donor organs has created a continuing need for serological methods that are suitable for screening donors and recipients, in an effort to avoid adverse clinical outcomes of CMV infection in immunocompromised recipients. Numerous modalities for serological diagnosis are available and include (1) complement fixation; (2) enzyme-linked immunosorbent assay (ELISA); (3) immunofluorescence assay; (4) hemagglutination inhibition; (5) neutralization tests; and (6) latex agglutination assay. The presence of CMV-specific IgG antibody indicates past or present infection but has no diagnostic significance for acute infection unless a recent seroconversion can be documented. A fourfold or greater rise in CMV-specific IgG antibody titers is indicative of current active infection, but this does not differentiate between a primary or recurrent process. To document a rise in IgG antibodies, a blood sample should be drawn as soon as possible during the acute phase and a second sample drawn 4 weeks later during the convalescent period. CMV-specific IgM antibody levels can also be useful in the diagnosis of illness. If the test is performed properly, the presence of this antibody indicates recent or current CMV infection. In immunocompetent adults, IgM antibody usually persists for 6 weeks but may remain detectable for 3 to 6 months after primary infection [81]. The antibody may persist for 1 year or more in immunosuppressed individuals. False-positive reactions occur in the presence of rheumatoid factor, so this factor should be removed from the serum specimen prior to IgM testing.

Unfortunately, the variety of diagnostic methods avail-

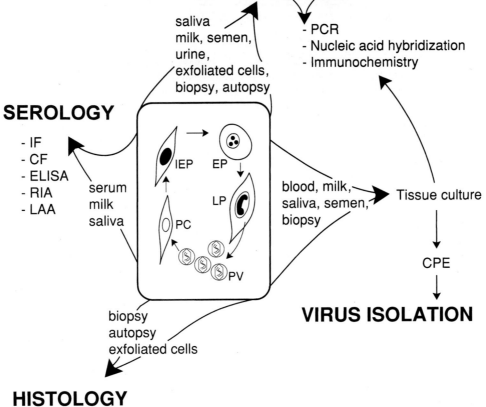

DIRECT DETECTION OF CMV MACROMOLECULES

saliva
milk, semen,
urine,
exfoliated cells,
biopsy, autopsy

- PCR
- Nucleic acid hybridization
- Immunochemistry

SEROLOGY

- IF
- CF
- ELISA
- RIA
- LAA

serum
milk
saliva

IEP   EP

LP

PC

PV

blood, milk,
saliva, semen,
biopsy

Tissue culture

CPE

VIRUS ISOLATION

biopsy
autopsy
exfoliated cells

HISTOLOGY

Figure 7–17. Diagnostic approach to detect primary or reactivated CMV infection. The central area demonstrates the phasing of CMV replication in the infected host (PC, permissive cell; IEP, immediate early; EP, early and LP, late proteins; PV, progeny virus). Main arrows: examples for clinical specimens most frequently used to detect CMV infection. PCR, polymerase chain reaction; IF, immunofluorescence; CF, complement fixation assay; RIA, radioimmunoassay; ELISA, enzyme-linked immunosorbent assay; LAA, latex agglutination assay; CPE, cytopathic effect.

able may still frequently fail to definitely establish CMV as the etiology of clinical problems, for various reasons. For instance, diagnosis of acute infection may be distorted because patients may shed CMV in urine, saliva, blood, and genital secretions for months to years following primary infection or virus reactivation.

CONTROL OF CMV INFECTION

Approaches that could ultimately control CMV infection include prevention, immunoprophylaxis, and therapy with antiviral drugs (Tables 7–6 and 7–7). Preventive therapy is practical for immunocompromised individuals who are not yet infected but are at risk for infection from a defined exposure, such as blood transfusion or organ transplanta-

Table 7–6. Treatment of CMV-Induced Monoucleosis

Symptom	Treatment
Fever	Antipyretics (e.g., acetaminophen); increase fluid intake to prevent dehydration
Malaise	Bed rest
Sore throat	Warm saltwater gargle 3–4 times a day
Splenomegaly	Avoid strenuous activity or contact sports for 4–6 weeks to lessen the risk of splenic injury
Elevated liver enzymes	Avoid alcohol consumption for 4–6 weeks to lessen the work of the liver

Table 7–7. Drugs Effective in Treatment and Prophylaxis of CMV Infection

Drug	Mechanism of action	Therapeutic effect
Idoxuridine Vidarabine Trifluridine	Inhibition of viral DNA polymerase; termination of viral DNA synthesis	Poor
Ribavirin	Inhibition of inosine monophosphate dehydrogenase; depletion of guanosine 5′- triphosphate (GTP) pool; alteration of mRNA capping	Moderate
Interferons	Inhibition of viral protein synthesis through degradation of viral RNA; inactivation of the initiating factor eIF2alpha	Moderate
Foscarnet*	Inhibition of pyrophosphate receptor site of the viral DNA polymerase	Good
Cidofovir*	Inhibition of CMV DNA polymerase	Good
Ganciclovir*	Selective inhibition of CMV DNA polymerase; termination of CMV DNA elongation	Good
Valganciclovir*	Selective inhibition of CMV DNA polymerase; termination of CMV DNA elongation	Good
Fomivirsen*	Inhibition of viral protein synthesis and thus of replication through binding with specific viral mRNA	Good

* FDA approved for use in treatment of CMV infections.

tion. The best preventive measure is to use tissues and blood from CMV antibody—negative donors for this specific population. Other modalities consist of pre- and posttransplant prophylaxis with antiviral drugs such as interferon [82], acyclovir [83], and ganciclovir [84] as well as use of intravenous immunoglobulins, particularly high titer CMV immunoglobulins [85]. For the treatment of CMV infection in immunocompromised persons, antiviral agents (Table 7-7) have been used with limited success. All of the currently available drugs are virustatic and not virucidal, and chronic administration is required to suppress the effects of the disease.

Ganciclovir

Ganciclovir is the first antiviral agent licensed specifically for the treatment of life-threatening and sight-threatening CMV infections. It is a synthetic acyclic nucleotide analogue of guanine that can be administered intravenously, orally, or by intravitreal implant. Ganciclovir is virustatic, providing suppression of active CMV infection but not complete cure. The disease process of CMV continues to progress after discontinuation of the medication. Ganciclovir is indicated for the treatment of CMV retinitis in immunocompromised patients [86] and for CMV prophylaxis in transplant recipients [87,88]. It may also be effective in CMV colitis, esophagitis, hepatitis, meningoenceph-

alitis, and pneumonitis [89]. Neither ganciclovir nor any other antiviral agent is currently recommended for the treatment of symptomatic congenital CMV. This subject remains controversial. Several case reports describe the benefit of ganciclovir treatment in children with urgent life-threatening complications of this illness [90,91], and further efficacy trials are currently in progress [92].

Because of poor oral bioavailability (8–9%), ganciclovir is usually given intravenously, particularly for induction treatment. Oral ganciclovir is more convenient for long-term maintenance but is not as effective as intravenous ganciclovir. Recently, the oral prodrug of ganciclovir, valganciclovir, became the first orally administered CMV therapy approved for both induction and maintenance therapy of CMV. The intravitreous implant is useful for localized CMV retinitis. However, this modality provides no protection against CMV for the remaining eye or other organs, and it requires surgical insertion every 6 months. A recent study combining treatment with the intraocular implant and oral ganciclovir demonstrated further delay in the progression of retinitis and reduction in the incidence of new CMV disease [93]. Adverse effects of ganciclovir include reversible neutropenia, thrombocytopenia, azoospermia, renal insufficiency, and central nervous system symptoms [94]. Resistance to ganciclovir and subsequent progression of the disease may develop in some strains of CMV through mutations in the viral DNA polymerase [10,95].

Foscarnet

The cellular actions of foscarnet (trisodium phosphonoformate) result in inhibition of CMV DNA synthesis and the subsequent production of late proteins. This virustatic drug has a consistent impact on virus shedding, and its effectiveness appears to be related to the time of initiation of therapy and particularly to the extent of tissue involvement [96]. Foscarnet has been successfully used for the treatment of CMV retinitis in AIDS patients and with some success in transplant recipients with life-threatening CMV infection [97,98]. This antiviral agent has two attributes that make it an attractive alternative to ganciclovir: it is not toxic to the bone marrow, and it is effective against ganciclovir-resistant CMV strains [99]. However, foscarnet must also be given intravenously because of poor oral bioavailability, and its common side effect, renal dysfunction, is often dose-limiting. Other adverse effects include electrolyte imbalances, genital ulceration (Fig. 7–18), nausea and vomiting, central nervous system disturbances, and deposits of the drug in bone, teeth, and cartilage. An in vitro study [100] suggests synergistic action between lower doses of ganciclovir and foscarnet, which may help to reduce toxicities and the development of drug resistance [80].

Cidofovir

Cidofovir has been approved for the treatment of CMV retinitis in HIV-infected patients who are unable to tolerate ganciclovir or foscarnet therapy. The drug must be given intravenously, but it has a more convenient dosing regimen of once every 2 weeks after the initial induction regimen of once every week (for 2 weeks). One HIV-infected patient with CMV retinitis, encephalitis, and esophagitis re-

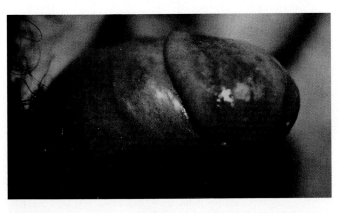

Figure 7–18. Penile erosion resulting from excretion of foscarnet in the urine.

sponded well to this therapy after becoming resistant to ganciclovir and foscarnet [101]. Large-scale clinical studies for the treatment of other CMV diseases have not yet been initiated. Adverse effects, such as nephrotoxicity, neutropenia, metabolic acidosis, and ocular hypotonia, require treatment discontinuation in approximately 25% of recipients.

Fomivirsen

Fomivirsen is the first antisense oligonucleotide approved by the FDA for antiviral use [102]. It is indicated as an intravitreal injection for CMV retinitis in HIV-infected patients who are unable to receive more conventional therapies because of intolerance or insufficient response. The drug is administered by monthly in-office injections, and the most common side effects include ocular inflammation and increased intraocular pressure [103].

Cytomegalovirus Immune Globulin

Cytomegalovirus immune globulin (CMVIG) may be used for the prevention of CMV disease in certain immunocompromised patients, particularly transplant recipients. Prophylactic treatment with CMVIG in at-risk renal transplant recipients significantly reduces the rate and severity of CMV disease as well as the risk of complications from fungal superinfection [85,104]. However, although CMVIG greatly impacts clinically evident disease, it has no effect on the rates of viral isolation or seroconversion [104]. More recently, application of pooled monoclonal antibodies to the major epitopes of CMV surface glycoproteins has been shown to prevent clinical disease.

Data from several studies indicate that regimens consisting of high-dose CMVIG combined with ganciclovir, acyclovir, foscarnet, or interferon are more effective than monotherapy of CMV-induced syndromes in transplant patients [105]. A combination of ganciclovir and CMV-specific or polyvalent immune globulin has been reported to improve survival significantly in CMV pneumonitis in recipients of allogeneic bone marrow transplants [106]. Combination therapy may also have a role in bone marrow transplant recipients with gastrointestinal CMV disease [89] as well as in renal transplant patients with fulminant CMV disease.

Vaccine

A live, attenuated vaccine, which is a high passage strain of CMV (Towne), has been given to healthy volunteers and transplant recipients [107]. This vaccine strain is reported not to produce latency, not to induce alterations of the CD4/CD8 ratio, and does not affect other T-lymphocyte subsets. Rather, it induces an excellent humoral immune response [107] with a neutralizing antibody production that persists for over 4 years. Vaccination has been shown to protect against the severity of symptomatic illness but not against infection in transplanted individuals with CMV-bearing organs [108,109]. In addition, when studying the efficacy of the vaccine in preventing child-to-mother transmission of CMV acquired in day-care centers, the results were disappointing. The rate of acute CMV infection for vaccinated mothers was no different than that for placebos, whereas naturally seropositive mothers were protected from infection [110]. Development of improved versions of the Towne strain vaccine are currently under way [111,112].

Subunit vaccines containing the viral envelope or structural component(s) of this envelope (gA/gB glycoprotein) or recombinant formulations (e.g., adenovirus-CMV, vaccinia-CMV) have also been developed to induce specific antibodies and CMV-specific cellular (cytotoxic T cells) sensitization [108,109]. Further studies are currently under way to determine the efficacy of these alternative vaccines.

CONCLUSION

CMV is the most common cause of intrauterine infection in humans. It is also of increasing importance in the immunocompromised host although a rare cause of symptomatic infection in the normal host. Up to 10% of infants with congenital CMV infection have severe symptoms at birth, and 5–17% of infants born with asymptomatic congenital infection suffer late sequelae, mostly deafness and other neurological problems. CMV infection in the immunocompromised host has a broad range of clinical manifestations, including a variety of skin diseases. Drug therapy for CMV has improved dramatically in the last few years but still remains far from optimal. Several drugs are effective in controlling CMV disease in most patients, but relapse is common and is expected after discontinuation of long-term therapy. In addition, adverse effects associated with these drugs are not benign. Prevention of CMV infection may be achieved by serological screening of blood and organ donors as well as the use of leukocyte-free blood in transfusions. Immunoglobulin prophylaxis may also be effective in ameliorating disease in renal allograft patients. Use of combinations of therapy, including antivirals, immunoglobulins, and cytokines, has been reported to decrease the morbidity and mortality associated with CMV disease; however, these therapeutic regimens require further study.

REFERENCES

1. H Ribbert. Ueber protozoanartige zellen in der neire eines syphilitischen neugeborenen und in der parotis von kindern. Zentralbl Allg Pathol 15:945–948, 1904.
2. EQ Goodpasture, FB Talbot. Concerning the nature of "protozoan-like" cells in certain lesions of infancy. Am J Dis Child 21:415–425, 1921.
3. KE Bowers. Cytomegalovirus infection. In: IM Freedberg, AZ Eisen, K Wolff, et al. Dermatology in General Medicine, 5th ed. New York: McGraw-Hill, 1999, pp 2450–2457.
4. WP Rowe, JW Hartley, S Waterman, HC Turner, RJ Huebner. Cytopathogenic agent resembling human salivary gland virus recovered from tissue cultures of human adenoids. Proc Soc Exp Biol Med 92:418–424, 1956.
5. MG Smith. Propagation in tissue cultures of a cytopathogenic virus from human salivary gland virus (SGV) disease. Proc Soc Exp Biol Med 92:424–430, 1956.
6. TH Weller, JC Macauley, JM Craig, P Wirth. Isolation of intranuclear inclusion producing agents from infants with illnesses resembling cytomegalic inclusion disease. Proc Soc Exp Biol Med 94:4–12, 1957.
7. HD Riley Jr. History of the cytomegalovirus. Southern Med J 90:184–190, 1997.
8. MS Chee, AT Bankier, S Beck, R Bohni, CM Brown, R Cerny, T Horsnell, CA Hutchison 3rd, T Kouzarides, JA Martignetti et al. Analysis of the protein-coding content of the sequence of human cytomegalovirus strain AD169. Curr Top Microbiol Immunol 154:125–169, 1990.
9. CA Alford, WJ Britt. Cytomegalovirus. In: B Roizman, RJ Whitley, C Lopez, eds. The Human Herpesviruses. New York: Raven Press, 1993, pp 227–255.
10. V Sullivan, KK Biron, C Talarico, SC Stanat, M Davis, LM Pozzi, DM Coen. A point mutation in the human cytomegalovirus DNA polymerase gene confers resistance to ganciclovir and phosphonylmethoxyalkyl derivatives. Antimicrob Agents Chemother 37:19–25, 1993.
11. DJ Lang, RM Garruto, DC Gajdusek. Early acquisition of cytomegalovirus and Epstein-Barr virus antibody in several isolated Melanesian populations. Am J Epidemiol 105: 480–487, 1977.
12. U Krech. Complement-fixing antibodies against cytomegalovirus in different parts of the world. Bull World Health Organ 49:103–106, 1973.
13. MD Yow, NH White, LH Taber, AL Frank, WC Gruber, RA May, HJ Norton. Acquisition of cytomegalovirus infection from birth to 10 years: a longitudinal serologic study. J Pediatr 110:37–42, 1987.
14. NH White, MD Yow, GJ Demmler, HJ Norton, J Hoyle, K Pinckard, C Mishaw, S Pokorny. Prevalence of cytomegalovirus antibody in subjects between the ages of 6 and 22 years. J Infect Dis 159:1013–1017, 1989.
15. CA Alford, S Stagno, RF Pass et al. Epidemiology of cytomegalovirus infections. In: AJ Nahmias, WR Dowdle, RD Schinazi, eds. The Human Herpesviruses: An Interdisciplinary Perspective. New York: Elsevier, 1987, pp 159–171.

16. S Stagno, RF Pass, ME Dworsky, RE Henderson, EG Moore, PD Walton, CA Alford. Congenital cytomegalovirus infection: the relative importance of primary and recurrent maternal infection. N Engl J Med 306:945–949, 1982.

17. S Saigal, O Lunyk, RP Larke, MA Chernasky. The outcome in children with congenital cytomegalovirus infection. A longitudinal follow-up study. Am J Dis Child 136:896–901, 1982.

18. RP Larke, E Wjeatley, S Saigal, MA Chernesky. Congenital cytomegalovirus infection in an urban Canadian community. J Infect Dis 142:647–653, 1980.

19. RF Pass, AM August, M Dworsky, DW Reynolds. Cytomegalovirus infection in a day-care center. N Engl J Med 307:477–479, 1982.

20. RF Pass, SC Hutto, DW Reynolds, RB Polhill. Increased frequency of cytomegalovirus infection in children in group day care. Pediatrics 74:121–126, 1984.

21. JR Murph, JF Bale Jr. The natural history of acquired cytomegalovirus infection among children in group day care. Am J Dis Child 142:843–846, 1988.

22. RA Bowden. Transfusion-transmitted cytomegalovirus infection. Hematol Oncol Clin North Am 9:155–166, 1995.

23. RC Kane, WE Rousseau, GR Noble, GE Tegtmeier, H Wulff, HB Herndon, TD Chin, WL Bayer. Cytomegalovirus infection in a volunteer blood donor population. Infect Immun 11:719–723, 1975.

24. DW Reynolds, E Huang, SD Thames. Cytomegalovirus excretion and perinatal infection. N Engl J Med 289:1–5, 1973.

25. DF Lang, JB Hanshaw. Cytomegalovirus infection and the post-perfusion syndrome: recognition of primary infections in four patients. N Engl J Med 280:1145–1149, 1969.

26. MG Smith, F Vellios. Inclusion disease or generalized salivary gland virus infection. Arch Pathol 50:862–884, 1950.

27. K Ii, K Hizawa, R Katsuse. Generalized cytomegalic inclusion disease presenting an infectious mononucleosis syndrome (so called cytomegalovirus mononucleosis) in a previously healthy adult: an autopsy study. Acta Pathol Jpn 22:723–737, 1972.

28. TW Wong, NE Warner. Cytomegalic inclusion disease in adults: report of 14 cases with review of literature. Arch Pathol 74:403–422, 1962.

29. T Albrecht, I Boldogh, MP Fons, T Valyi-Nagy. Activation of proto-oncogenes and cell activation signals in the initiation and progression of human cytomegalovirus infection. Front Virol 2:384–411, 1993.

30. JE Grundy. Virologic and pathogenic aspects of cytomegalovirus infection. Rev Infect Dis 12 (suppl 7):S711–S719, 1990.

31. R Colimon, S Michelson. Human cytomegalovirus: pathology, diagnosis, treatment. Adv Nephrol 19:333–356, 1990.

32. J vanZanten, L de Leij, J Prop, MC Harmsen, TH The. Human cytomegalovirus: a viral complication in transplantation. Clin Transplant 12:145–158, 1998.

33. E Adam, JL Melnick, ME DeBakey. Cytomegalovirus infection and atherosclerosis. Centr Eur J Publ Health 5:99–106, 1997.

34. J Mendez, M Espy, TF Smidt, J Wilson, R Weisner, CV Paya. Clinical significance of viral load in the diagnosis of cytomegalovirus disease after liver transplantation. Transplantation 65:1477–1481, 1998.

35. N Minars, JF Silverman, MR Escobar, AJ Martinez. Fatal cytomegalic disease. Arch Dermatol 113:1569–1571, 1977.

36. SB Boppana, KB Fowler, Y Vaid, G Hedlund, S Stagno, WJ Britt, RF Pass. Neuroradiographic findings in the newborn period and long term outcome in children with symptomatic congenital cytomegalovirus infection. Pediatrics 99:409–414, 1997.

37. I Bournerias, S Boisnic, O Patey, P Deny, S Gharakhanian, B Duflo, M Gentilini. Unusual cutaneous cytomegalovirus involvement in patients with acquired immunodeficiency syndrome. Arch Dermatol 125:1243–1246, 1989.

38. GJ Demler. Congenital cytomegalovirus infection and disease. Adv Pediatric Infect Dis 11:135–162, 1996.

39. CT Nelson, GJ Demler. Cytomegalovirus infection in the pregnant mother, fetus, and newborn infant. Clin Perinatol 24:151–160, 1997.

40. MS Pasternack, DN Medearis, RH Rubin. Cell-mediated immunity in experimental cytomegalovirus infections: a perspective. Rev Infect Dis 12(suppl 7):S720–S725, 1990.

41. GL Kantor, LS Goldberg, BL Johnson Jr, MM Derechin, EV Barnett. Immunological abnormalities induced by postperfusion cytomegalovirus infection. Ann Intern Med 73:553–558, 1970.

42. H Vodopick, SJ Chaskes, A Solomon, JA Stewart. Transient monoclonal gammopathy associated with cytomegalovirus infection. Blood 44:189–195, 1974.

43. S Stagno, JE Volanakis, DW Reynolds, R Stroud, CA Alford. Immune complexes in congenital and natal cytomegalovirus infections of man. J Clin Invest 60:838–845, 1977.

44. S Muralidhar, J Doniger, E Mendelson, JC Araujo, F Kashanchi, N Azumi, JN Brady, LJ Rosenthal. Human cytomegalovirus mtrII oncoprotein binds to p53 and downregulates p53-activated transcription. J Virol 70:8691–8700, 1996.

45. ES Huang, I Boldogh, EC Mar. Human cytomegalovirus: evidence for possible association with human cancer. In: LA Philips, ed. Viruses Associated with Human Cancer. New York: Marcel Dekker, 1983, pp 161–194.

46. DH Spector, SA Spector. The oncogenic potential of human cytomegalovirus. Prog Med Virol 29:45–89, 1984.

47. F Rapp. Cytomegalovirus and carcinogenesis. J Natl Cancer Inst 72:783–787, 1983.

48. T Albrecht, I Boldogh, M Fons, CH Lee, S AbuBakar, JM Russell, WW Au. Cell-activation responses to cytomegalovirus infection: relationship to the phasing of CMV replication and to the induction of cellular damage. Subcell Biochem 15:157–202, 1989.

49. T Albrecht, MP Fons, I Boldogh, S AbuBakar, CZ Deng, D Millinoff. Metabolic and cellular effects of human cytomegalovirus infection. Transplant Proc 23:48–55, 1991.

50. S Michelson. Interaction of human cytomegalovirus with monocytes/macrophages: love-hate relationship. Pathol Biol 45:146–158, 1997.

51. HT Reyburn, O Mandelboim, M Vales-Gomez, DM Davis, L Razmany, JL Strominger. The class I MHC homologue of human cytomegalovirus inhibits attack by natural killer cells. Nature 386:514–517, 1997.

52. PA Mackowisk, M Marling-Cason, JW Smith, JP Luby. Antibody-mediated bacterial adhesion to cytomegalovirus-induced Fc receptors. J Clin Invest 73:987–991, 1984.

53. JA McKeating, PD Griffiths, JE Grundy. Cytomegalovirus in urine specimens has host beta-2-microglobulin bound to the viral envelope. A mechanism of evading the host immune response? J Gen Virol 68:785–792, 1987.

54. AS Evans. Infectious mononucleosis and related syndromes. Am J Med Sci 276:325–339, 1978.

55. A Lajo, C Borque, F del Castillo, A Martin-Ancel. Mononucleosis caused by Epstein-Barr virus and cytomegalovirus in children: a comprehensive study of 124 cases. Pediatr Infect Dis J 13:56–60, 1994.

56. ML Kumar, GA Nankervis, AR Cooper, E Gold. Postnatally acquired cytomegalovirus infections in infants of CMV-excreting mothers. J Pediatrics 104:669–673, 1984.

57. Y Daniel, I Gull, MR Peyser, JB Lessing. Congenital cytomegalovirus infection. Eur J Obstet Gynecol Reprod Biol 63:7–16, 1995.

58. S Stagno. Cytomegalovirus. In: JS Remington, JO Klein, eds. Infectious Diseases of the Fetus and Newborn Infant, 4th ed. Philadelphia: WB Saunders, 1995, pp 312–353.

59. GJ Demmler. Cytomegalovirus. In: RD Feigin, JD Cherry, eds. Textbook of Pediatric Infectious Diseases, 4th ed. Philadelphia: WB Saunders, 1998, pp 1732–1751.

60. T Iwasaki, T Sata, T Kurata. Pathology of human cytomegalovirus infection in immunocompromised host. Jpn J Clin Med 56:115–120, 1998.

61. M Fiala, JD Mosca, P Barry, PA Luciw, HV Vinters. Multi-step pathogenesis of AIDS: role of cytomegalovirus. Res Immunol 142:87–95, 1991.

62. RT Schooley. Cytomegalovirus in the setting of infection with human immunodeficiency virus. Rev Infect Dis 12 (suppl 7):S811–S819, 1990.

63. ES Huang, TF Kowalik. The pathogenicity of human cytomegalovirus: an overview. Front Virol 2:3–45, 1993.

64. L Homsy, M Meyer, M Tateno, S Clarkson, JA Levy. The Fc and not CD4 receptor mediates antibody enhancement of HIV infection in human cells. Science 244:1357–1360, 1988.

65. JB Bowden, AA Hebert, RP Regina. Dermal hematopoiesis in neonates. Report of five cases. J Am Acad Dermatol. 20:1104–1110, 1989.

66. JL Lesher, GA Augusta. Cytomegalovirus infections and the skin. J Am Acad Dermatol 18:1333–1338, 1988.

67. J Blatt, O Kastner, DS Hodes. Cutaneous vesicles in congenital cytomegalovirus infection. J Pediatrics 92:509, 1978.

68. K Helm, AT Lane, J Orosz, L Metlay. Systemic cytomega-

lovirus in patients with the Keratitis, Ichthyosis, and Deafness (KID) Syndrome. Pediatr Dermatol 7:54–56, 1990.

69. JB Spear, HA Kessler, A Dworin, J Semel. Erythema nodosum associated with acute cytomegalovirus mononucleosis in an adult. Arch Intern Med 148:323–324, 1988.

70. A Sandler, JD Snedeker. Cytomegalovirus infection in an infant presenting with cutaneous vasculitis. Pediatr Infect Dis J 6:422–423, 1987.

71. LY Lee. Cytomegalovirus infection involving the skin in immunocompromised host. J Clin Pathol 92:96–100, 1989.

72. AS Colsky, SM Jegasothy, C Leonardi, RS Kirsner, FA Kerdel. Diagnosis and treatment of a case of cutaneous cytomegalovirus infection with a dramatic clinical presentation. J Am Acad Dermatol 38:349–351, 1998.

73. I Boldogh, E Beth, ES Huang, K Kyalwazi, G Giraldo. Kaposi's sarcoma. IV. Detection of CMV DNA, CMV RNA, and CMNA in tumor biopsies. Int J Cancer 28: 469–474, 1981.

74. MN Charthaigh, B Crowley, M Lynch, F Mulchay. Successful treatment of cutaneous cytomegalovirus. Int J STD AIDS 4:52–53, 1993.

75. S Naraqi. Cytomegaloviruses. In: RB Belshe, ed. Textbook of Human Virology, 2nd ed. St. Louis: Mosby, 1991, pp 889–924.

76. RJ Pariser. Histologically specific skin lesions in disseminated cytomegalovirus infection. J Am Acad Dermatol 9: 937–946, 1983.

77. FF Macasaet, KF Holley, TF Smith, TF Keys. Cytomegalovirus studies of autopsy tissue. II. Incidence of inclusion bodies and related pathologic data. Am J Clin Pathol 63: 859–865, 1975.

78. MP Landini. New approaches and perspectives in cytomegalovirus diagnosis. Prog Med Virol 40:157–177, 1993.

79. RL Hodinka. The clinical utility of viral quantitation using molecular methods. Clin Diagn Virol 10:25–47, 1998.

80. K Numazaki, S Chiba. Current aspects of diagnosis and treatment of cytomegalovirus infections in infants. Clin Diagn Virol 8:169–181, 1997.

81. GJ Demmler, HR Six, SM Hurst, MD Yow. Enzyme-linked immunosorbent assay for the detection of IgM-class antibodies to cytomegalovirus. J Infect Dis 153: 1152–1155, 1986.

82. MJ Wood. Antivirals in the context of HIV disease. J Antimicrob Chemother 37(suppl B):97–112, 1996.

83. F Baldanti, KK Biron, G Gerna. Interpreting human cytomegalovirus antiviral drug susceptibility testing: the role of the mixed virus populations. J Infect Dis 177:823–824, 1998.

84. JL Perez. Resistance to antivirals in human cytomegalovirus: mechanisms and clinical significance. Microbiologia 13:343–352, 1997.

85. DR Snydman. Prevention of cytomegalovirus-associated diseases with immunoglobulin. Transplant Proc 23: 131–135, 1991.

86. PF McAuliffe, MJ Hall, H Castro-Malspina, MH Heinemann. Use of the ganciclovir implant for treating cytomegalovirus retinitis secondary to immunosuppression after bone marrow transplantation. Am J Ophthalmol 123: 702–703, 1997.

87. M Halme, I Lautenschlager, L Halme, P Tukiainen, S Mattila. Ganciclovir prophylaxis after lung and heart-lung transplantation. Transpl Int 11(suppl 1):S499–S505, 1998.

88. SV Jassal, JM Rosco, JS Zaltzman, T Mazzulli, M Krajden, M Gadawski, DC Cattran, CJ Cardella, SE Albert, EH Cole. Clinical practice guidelines: prevention of cytomegalovirus disease after renal transplantation. J Am Soc Nephrol 9:1697–1708, 1998.

89. S Noble, D Faulds. Ganciclovir. An update of its use in the prevention of cytomegalovirus infection and disease in transplant recipients. Drugs 56:115–146, 1998.

90. JR Hocker, LN Cook, G Addams, GP Rabalais. Ganciclovir therapy of congenital cytomegalovirus pneumonia. Pediatr Infect Dis J 9:743–745, 1990.

91. JG Vallejo, JA Englund, JA Garcia-Prats, GJ Demmler. Ganciclovir treatment of steroid-associated cytomegalovirus disease in a congenitally infected neonate. Pediatr Infect Dis J 13:239–241, 1994.

92. HL Brown, MP Abernathy. Cytomegalovirus infection. Semin Perinatol 22:260–266, 1998.

93. DF Martin, BD Kuppermann, RA Wolitz, AG Palestine, H Li, CA Robinson. Oral ganciclovir for patients with cytomegalovirus retinitis treated with a ganciclovir implant. The Roche Ganciclovir Study Group. N Engl J Med 340:1063–1070, 1999.

94. E Farrugia, TR Schwab. Management and prevention of cytomegalovirus infection. Mayo Clin Proc 67:879–890, 1992.

95. A Erice, S Chou, KK Biron, SC Stanat, HH Balfour Jr, MC Jordan. Progressive disease due to ganciclovir-resistant cytomegalovirus in immunocompromised patients. N Engl J Med 320:289–293, 1989.

96. ML Levinson, PA Jacobson. Treatment and prophylaxis of cytomegalovirus diseases. Pharmacotherapy 12:300–318, 1992.

97. P Lehoang, B Giarard, M Robinet, P Marcel, L Zazoun, S Matheron, W Rozenbaum, C Katlama, I Morer, JO Lernestedt, et al. Foscarnet in the treatment of cytomegalovirus retinitis in acquired immunodeficiency syndrome. Ophthalmology 96:865–874, 1989.

98. O Ringden, B Lonnqvist, T Paulin, J Ahlmen, G Klintmalm, B Wahren, JO Lernestedt. Pharmacokinetics, safety and preliminary clinical experiences using foscarnet in the treatment of cytomegalovirus infections in bone marrow and renal transplant recipients. J Antimicrob Chemother 17:378–387, 1986.

99. JD Meyers. Prevention and treatment of cytomegalovirus infection. Ann Rev Med 42:179–187, 1991.

100. JF Manischewitz, GV Quinnan Jr, HC Lane, AE Wittek. Synergistic effect of ganciclovir and foscarnet on cytomegalovirus replication in vitro. Antimicrob Agents Chemother 34:373–375, 1990.

101. G Blick, T Garton, U Hopkins, L La Gravinese. Successful use of cidofovir in treating AIDS-related cytomegalovirus retinitis, encephalitis, and esophagitis. J Acquir Immune Defic Syndr 15:84–85, 1997.

102. Fomivirsen sodium approved to treat CMV retinitis. J Am Pharm Assoc 39:84–85, 1999.

103. CM Perry, JA Balfour. Fomivirsen. Drugs 57:375–380, 1999.

104. DR Snydman, BG Werner, B Heinze-Lacy, VP Berardi, NL Tilney, RL Kirkman, EL Milford, SI Cho, HL Bush Jr, AS Levey et al. Use of cytomegalovirus immune globulin to prevent cytomegalovirus disease in renal transplant recipients. N Engl J Med 317:1049–1054, 1987.

105. F Ginevri, G Losurdo, I Fontana, AM Rabagliati, L Bonatto, R Valente, P Venzano, A Nocera, GC Basile, U Valente, R Gusmano. Acyclovir plus CMV immunoglobulin prophylaxis and early therapy with ganciclovir are effective and safe in CMV high-risk renal transplant pediatric recipients. Transpl Int 11(suppl 1):S130–S134, 1998.

106. EC Reed. Treatment of cytomegalovirus pneumonia in transplant patients. Transplant Proc 23(suppl 1):8–12, 1991.

107. SA Plotkin, ML Smiley, HM Friedman, SE Starr, GR Fleisher, C Wlodaver, DC Dafoe, AD Friedman, RA Grossman, CF Barker. Towne-vaccine-induced prevention of cytomegalovirus disease after renal transplant. Lancet 1:528–530, 1984.

108. E Gonczol, K Berencsi, S Pincus, V Endresz, C Meric, E Paoletti, SA Plotkin. Preclinical evaluation of an AL:VAC (canarypox) human cytomegalovirus glycoprotein B vaccine candidate. Vaccine 13:1080–1085, 1995.

109. E Gonczol, SA Plotkin. Progress in vaccine development for prevention of human cytomegalovirus infection. Curr Top Microbiol Immunol 154:255–274, 1990.

110. SP Adler, SE Starr, SA Plotkin, SH Hempfling, J Buis, ML Manning, AM Best. Immunity induced by a primary cytomegalovirus infection protects against secondary infection among women of childbearing age. J Infect Dis 171:26–32, 1995.

111. SP Adler, SH Hempfling, SE Starr, S Plotkin, S Riddell. Evaluation of the safety and immunogenicity of the Towne strain of cytomegalovirus among women of childbearing age and children. Pediatr Infect Dis 17:200–206, 1998.

112. TA Cha, E Tom, GW Kemble, GM Duke, ES Mocarski, RR Spaete. Human cytomegalovirus clinical isolates carry at least 19 genes not found in laboratory strains. J Virol 70:78–83, 1996.

8

Human Herpesvirus 6

Samuel A. Shube
Boca Raton Community Hospital, Boca Raton, Florida, USA

Andrea M. Dominey
Rockwood Clinic, Spokane, Washington, USA

Tricia J. Brown
University of Oklahoma Health Sciences Center, Oklahoma City, Oklahoma, USA

Human herpesvirus 6 (HHV-6) was first isolated from peripheral blood mononuclear cells of patients with lymphoproliferative diseases in 1986 [1]. It is a 200-nm, enveloped, double-stranded DNA virus with a genome of more than 110,000 base pairs and molecular and morphological characteristics distinct from other members of the Herpesviridae family [2–4]. In vitro, HHV-6 can infect B and T lymphocytes, megakaryocytes, fibroblasts, and glial cells [4]. In vivo, the host range of HHV-6 broadens to include salivary glands, kidney endothelial cells, lymph nodes, and central nervous system tissue (neurons and oligodendrocytes) [5]. HHV-6 has been shown to be an etiological agent of exanthem subitum, a common childhood exanthem characterized by several days of high fever followed by the abrupt onset of a diffuse rash coinciding with defervescence [6]. See Figure 8–1 for more details.

HISTORY

Through the years, exanthem subitum has been known by several different names, such as roseola infantum, exanthem criticum, 3-day fever, fourth disease, pseudorubella, rose-rash, sixth disease, Filatov-Dukes disease, and Dukes' syndrome. This disease process may have been described

as early as 1870 [7]. However, early reports probably represent descriptions of a variety of exanthems, and credit for the first description of exanthem subitum is given to Zahorsky, who separated this disease from other exanthems in 1910 [8]. In 1941, Breese unsuccessfully attempted to culture a viral agent from three children with exanthem subitum [9]. In 1950, Kempe observed that the peak age of infection coincided with the ebb of passive maternal antibodies, and he predicted that a ubiquitous virus carried by healthy individuals was responsible for the infections [10]. He postulated that infection occurred through contact with nasal and pharyngeal secretions and suggested that a member of the Herpesviridae family would be an ideal candidate. In 1986, Salahuddin isolated a new virus from the peripheral blood leukocytes of six patients with lymphoproliferative disorders [1]. Host range, in vitro biological effects, and antigenic features distinguished this virus from the known human and nonhuman primate herpesviruses, and it was named human B-lymphotropic virus (HBLV). In the following year, experiments demonstrated that the cellular tropism of HBLV extended beyond B lymphocytes, and the taxonomic designation of human herpesvirus-6 (HHV-6) was proposed [11]. In 1988, Yamanishi isolated and cultured HHV-6 from the peripheral blood leukocytes of four patients with exanthem subitum, and he

TAXONOMY

Herpesviridae family
Betaherpesvirinae subfamily

GEOGRAPHIC WORLDWIDE INCIDENCE

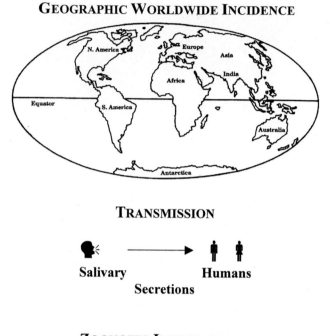

TRANSMISSION

Salivary
Secretions → Humans

ZOONOTIC IMPLICATIONS

None

Figure 8–1. Incidence and transmission of human herpesvirus 6.

confirmed by serological testing that HHV-6 was the cause of exanthem subitum [6]. Subsequent restriction enzyme analysis of DNA obtained from patients has demonstrated two separate strains of HHV-6 [12], now classified as variant A (HHV-6A) and variant B (HHV-6B). These two strains differ in biological, immunological, and molecular characteristics, although current serologic tests cannot easily distinguish between the two. Variant B is known to be the etiological agent of exanthem subitum, whereas variant A has not as yet been found to cause any specific disease process [5]. With DNA analysis of peripheral blood lymphocytes in healthy donors, variant B has been demonstrated to be three times more common than variant A [13]. Variant A appears to be more common in samples of uninvolved skin [5], in Kaposi's sarcoma [14], and in HIV-1–infected individuals (both symptomatic and asymptomatic) [15,16].

INCIDENCE

HHV-6 is one of the most ubiquitous viral agents infecting humans [17] and has been reported in patients worldwide [18–28]. Seroprevalence studies have shown that antibody to HHV-6 is present in 60–95% of the general population [29–37]. The majority of infections occur in the first 3 years of life [36,38]. It has been shown that between 0 to 4 weeks of age, IgG antibody to HHV-6 is present in 72–97% of infants tested because of transfer of maternal antibodies. By 6 months of age, seroprevalence decreases to 21–60% as a result of the waning of maternal antibodies. By 1 year of age, the seroprevalence again rises to 70–90%. Seroprevalence peaks at 80–100% in children ages 3 to 5 years old and then declines to 66–94% in the adult population [37,39]. Many clinical studies demonstrate a decline in HHV-6 antibodies with advancing age [32,39–41].

Exanthem subitum (roseola infantum) is one of most common exanthems encountered in young children [42]. It is rarely seen before 3 months of age or after 4 years of age, and 95% of cases occur between the ages of 6 months and 3 years. Fifty-five percent of cases occur within the first year of life and 90% occur within the first 2 years of life [43]. The sex ratio of affected individuals is equal in most large studies. In a prospective study of 70 newborn babies, approximately 16% developed classic clinical signs of exanthem subitum during the first year of life [9]. According to an age distribution curve, the author concluded that approximately 30% of all children eventually develop the disease. One particular study found that HHV-6 could be cultured from the peripheral blood of 14% of children 2 years of age or less who were brought to the emergency room with a febrile illness [42]. Of those patients 85% had at least a fourfold increase in IgG antibody titers against HHV-6, and an exanthem was noted at some time during the disease in 35% of children with positive cultures. The characteristic clinical feature of exanthem subitum, a rash that appears as the fever subsides, was noted in only 9% of these cases. The apparent discrepancy between a seroprevalence rate of 90–100% at 3 years of age and a clinical incidence rate of 30% is explained by the fact that the infection is associated with varied clinical manifestations, including subclinical infection. The infection has been described as having seasonal variation with the highest incidence in spring, summer, and fall [8,9,42,44,45]. In one study, 55% of cases occurred in February, March, and April [44]. Epidemics of exanthem subitum have been reported [46–49].

PATHOGENESIS

Kempe, in 1950, proposed that the route of transmission was probably nasopharyngeal viral shedding from healthy adults [10]. This hypothesis was supported by the fact that case-to-case transmission was extremely rare and that infection occurred in infants who were carefully protected against exposure to sick children or adults [10,36]. In 1988, HHV-6 was isolated from saliva of 9 out of 9 healthy individuals [20]. Subsequently, 63–95% of people tested were shown to have HHV-6 in their saliva [36,50,51]. Serial collections of saliva in healthy adults showed that viral shedding was intermittent and was not associated with specific antibody titer changes [36]. HHV-6 DNA and proteins have been demonstrated in submandibular, parotid, bronchial, and labial gland biopsies [52,53]. It is assumed that transfer of infected saliva from mother to infant is the most common source of HHV-6 transmission. Other tissues may serve as viral reservoirs as well. Okuno et al. [54] detected HHV-6 antigen in the tubular epithelium of rejected renal transplants. However, viral shedding in the urine is rare, both during the acute phase of exanthem subitum and after disease resolution [55,56]. There is also serological evidence that HHV-6 can be transmitted to transplant patients in their grafted tissues [57,58]. In utero transmission is a rare but can be a potential source of HHV-6 infection. One retrospective study of 799 cord-blood specimens demonstrated HHV-6–specific IgM antibodies in 0.28% of newborns [59]. A separate study of 305 newborns demonstrated HHV-6–specific DNA in uncultured cord blood mononuclear cells in 1.6% of cases [60]. Spontaneous abortions associated with HHV-6-positive placental or fetal tissue [61,62] and symptomatic congenital infection [63] have also been described. The possibility of perinatal transmission has been suggested after HHV-6 DNA was isolated from cervical tissue and secretions in women [64–66]. However, children born to mothers with positive cervical swabs did not acquire early HHV-6 infection in these studies. Viral secretion of HHV-6 in breast milk is doubtful, since HHV-6 DNA has not been found in breast milk [67], and 10 out of 11 babies withheld from breast milk seroconverted at the same age range as their breast-fed counterparts [68].

Like other members of the Herpesviridae family, HHV-6 is suspected to establish a latent infection in lymphocytes and may be reactivated at a later time, particularly in immunosuppressed patients [57,69]. In 1991 Kusuhara et al. [70] reviewed 23 otherwise healthy patients with previous exanthem subitum who developed a second episode of this disease. IgM and paired IgG serological examination revealed that 30% of the cases involved primary HHV-6 infection; therefore the initial episode of exanthem subitum must have been caused by another virus. Fifty-seven percent of the cases had no evidence of current HHV-6 infection, and these second episodes were probably due to another cause.

Seventeen percent of the cases were suggestive of reinfection or reactivation of HHV-6.

HHV-6 has been implicated in the pathogenesis of several other diseases (Table 8–1). Patients with systemic lupus erythematosus, Sjögrens syndrome, sarcoidosis, multiple sclerosis, and chronic fatigue syndrome have elevated seroprevalence and/or antibody titers to HHV-6 [71–76], but whether HHV-6 is the causal agent or the elevated titers represent an epiphenomenon remains to be elucidated. Patients with Hodgkin's, non-Hodgkin's, Burkitt's, and follicular large cell lymphoma, as well as those with angioimmunoblastic lymphadenopathy and acute myelogenous leukemia, have higher anti–HHV-6 antibody titers than normal [77–80]. A causal relationship between HHV-6 and any of these disorders remains unproved; however, it has been hypothesized that HHV-6 may induce polyclonal B-cell activation, alter the immune system, and lower the body's threshold for oncogenesis.

Transplant patients may undergo viral reactivation of HHV-6 as a result of immunosuppression [54,57,81–86].

Table 8–1. Disorders Possibly or Definitely Attributed to HHV-6

Childhood Illness
    Exanthem subitum
    Fever
    Lymphadenopathy
    Encephalitis
    Meningitis
    Hepatitis
    Intussusception
    Interstitial pneumonitis
    Immune thrombocytopenic purpura
Adult Illness
    Mononucleosis
    Lymphadenopathy
    Encephalitis
    Multiple sclerosis
    Chronic fatigue syndrome
    Autoimmune diseases
    Sinus histiocytosis with massive lymphadenopathy
      (Rosai-Dorfman syndrome)
Post-transplantation disorders
    Bone marrow suppression
    Skin eruptions
    Interstitial pneumonitis
    Encephalitis
Malignancy
    Leukemia
    Lymphoma
    Oral carcinoma

Significant increases in HHV-6 IgG titers associated with clinical findings have been reported in recipients of cardiac, bone marrow, liver, and renal transplants [54,57,82,83,85]. Overall, 40–50% of transplant recipients have HHV-6 infection. Almost half of these patients have symptomatic disease, most commonly manifesting as bone marrow suppression [87]. HHV-6 infection or reactivation in this population can lead to serious illness, including hepatitis [85], fever and rash [83], pneumonitis [84,88], encephalitis [89,90], bone marrow suppression [91,92], and graft dysfunction or rejection [95]. HHV-6 is also known to have a synergistic deleterious effect with cytomegalovirus in transplant recipients [94,95].

The role of HHV-6 in human immunodeficiency virus-1 (HIV-1)–infected patients is not completely clear. It has been suggested that HHV-6 may play a role in HIV-1–related disease, since both viruses are tropic for CD4+ cells [96,97]. Studies of HHV-6 seroprevalence in HIV-1–positive individuals have yielded conflicting results, showing increased seroprevalence [15,71], decreased seroprevalence [98,99] or seroprevalence similar to that of the general population [36,39,98,100,101]. In vitro studies have produced equally conflicting data. One group found that the replication of HIV-1 increased when cells were coinfected with HHV-6 [96,102], while another group found that HIV replication was inhibited by HHV-6 [20,103,104]. More specifically, HHV-6 has been found to transactivate HIV [105–107], upregulate the expression of CD4 cells [102], and induce particular cytokines that can switch HIV from a latent to replicative state [108,109]. It has been proposed that coinfection with HIV and HHV-6 may lead to further immunosuppression in the AIDS patient [15]. More research is needed to further dissect this intriguing relationship. With the advent of highly active retroviral therapy, the incidence of clinical HHV-6 disease in this population has significantly decreased. However, this virus may lead to widespread organ dissemination of the disease, pneumonitis, retinitis, and central nervous system involvement in patients with acquired immunodeficiency syndrome (AIDS) [110–112].

CLINICAL MANIFESTATIONS

Although HHV-6 has been implicated in a number of human illnesses, it has been proved to be the etiological agent of only one disease, exanthem subitum. The incubation period for this condition ranges from 5 to 15 days, with an average of 10 days [46–49]. The fever that heralds the abrupt onset of exanthem subitum is often as high as 38.4 to 40.6°C (102–105°F), may be constant or intermittent, and typically peaks in the early evening. Oropharyn-

Table 8–2. Clinical Features of Exanthem Subitum

	%
High fever	98
Maculopapular rash	30-98
Mild diarrhea	68
Nagayama's spots (erythematous papules on the soft palate)	65
Cough	50
Cervical lymphadenopathy	31
Edematous eyelids	30
Bulging anterior fontanelle	26
Seizures	8

geal lesions may precede the onset of the viral exanthem. Pharyngeal injection, round to linear erythematous macules, lymphoid hyperplasia, and tonsillar exudate have been described [8,10,42,44]. Mild injection of the tympanic membranes is frequently observed and conjunctival injection may be seen. Rare signs and symptoms include splenomegaly, abdominal pain, nausea, vomiting, and headache. Just before the onset of the exanthem, the patient may show a "sleepy" or "droopy" appearance resulting from localized palpebral edema [113]. This physical sign typically appears on the first to third day of fever and remits 24 hours after the onset of rash (see Table 8–2).

The appearance of the rash usually coincides with defervescence, although it has been noted to occur before the patient's temperature has returned to normal or up to 2 days after subsidence of the fever. The rash usually lasts 24–48 hours but has been reported to be as fleeting as 2 to 4 hours or as persistent as 9 days. The lesions are described as discrete, circular or elliptical, erythematous, 2–5 mm, "rose-red" macules or maculopapules that are occasionally surrounded by a white halo (Figs. 8–2 to 8–7). The eruption may look very similar to that seen in rubella or rubeola [114]. The classic form of exanthem subitum occurs in approximately 30% of HHV-6–infected individuals. HHV-6 infection may also appear as fever alone, exanthem alone, or asymptomatic infection [115,116]. An atypical eruption with oral and perineal lesions in a 13-month-old immunocompetent patient has also been described [117] (Table 8–3).

Exanthem subitum is generally a benign disease and complications are infrequent. Neurological complications may include convulsions, which accompany the abrupt rise of fever [7,10,42,118–121]. There have been occasional descriptions of increased cerebrospinal fluid pressure as well as bulging of the anterior fontanelle [120,122,123]. Encephalitis has also been reported with prolonged convulsions followed by coma and hemiparesis [124–129]. Sev-

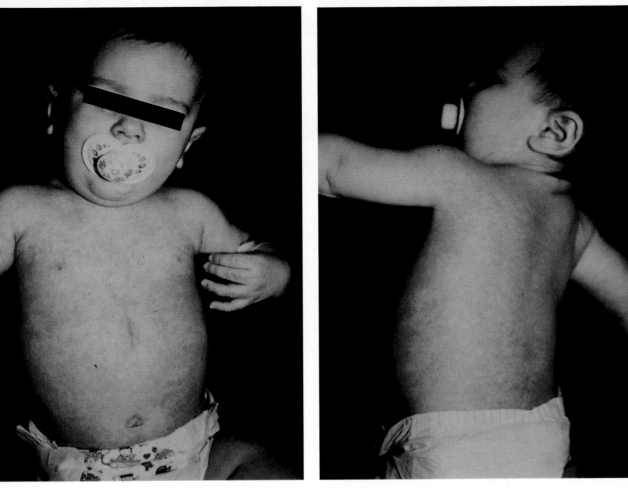

(a)   (b)

Figure 8–2. (a,b) Diffuse truncal eruption consisting of blanching erythematous macules appearing shortly after defervescence in an asymptomatic infant. (Photograph courtesy of Karen Wiss, M.D., Department of Dermatology, University of Massachusetts School of Medicine, Worcester, MA.)

Table 8–3. Clinical Manifestations of Exanthem Subitum

Time after exposure	Clinical manifestations	Laboratory analyses	Other notes
10 days	Abrupt onset of high fever lasting 3–5 days	Serology: IgM or fourfold increase in IgG; PCR detection of HHV-6 DNA in cell-free serum or plasma; viral culture; electron microscopy	Child is typically asymptomatic during the febrile stage
13–15 days	Appearance of a rose-pink maculopapular or macular eruption on neck and trunk lasting 1–2 days. May sometimes spread to face and proximal extremities		Slight irritability and malaise may be associated with higher elevations of temperature
14–17 days	Blanching and then fading of rash		Rash is not pruritic and does not desquamate

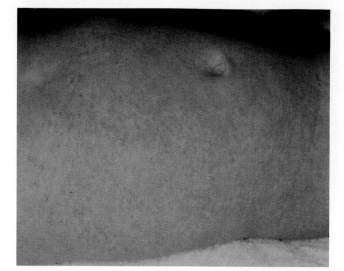

Figure 8–3. Rose-red macules on the abdomen of a young child. (Photograph courtesy of Susan Boiko, M.D., San Marcos, CA.)

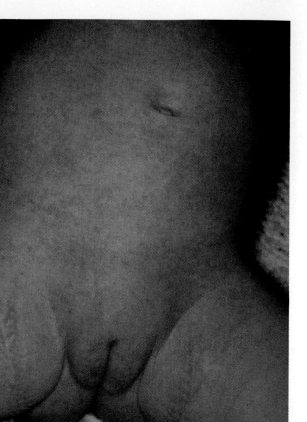

Figure 8–4. Discrete 1–3 mm erythematous oval macules and maculopapules on the lower abdomen. Some of the lesions are surrounded by a white halo. (Courtesy of Susan Boiko, M.D., San Marcos, CA.)

eral infants have died as a result of HHV-6 pneumonitis [130–132]. Thrombocytopenic purpura has been reported in association with primary HHV-6 infection on several occasions [133–136]. In addition, the virus has been shown to cause hepatitis, sometimes with fatal outcomes [23,137–140]. A mononucleosis-like syndrome not attributable to cytomegalovirus or Epstein-Barr virus has been linked to increased titers or seroconversion to HHV-6 in both children and adults [141–146].

DERMATOPATHOLOGY

Ultrastructural features of HHV-6 in lymphocytes from an infant with exanthem subitum have been described. The most characteristic ultrastructural feature is the coating of intracytoplasmic and extracellular nucleocapsids by a thick tegument, similar to human cytomegalovirus. However, the two viruses can be differentiated by the lack of beaded viral cores and lack of formation of dense bodies in cells infected by HHV-6 [147]. Histological features of a skin biopsy taken from one exanthem subitum patient with an atypical eruption included interface dermatitis with scattered necrotic keratinocytes, epidermal hyperplasia, and a lichenoid infiltrate composed of lymphocytes and histiocytes [117].

LABORATORY FINDINGS

Common laboratory examinations are generally not helpful in making the diagnosis of exanthem subitum. The only

Figure 8–5. Discrete 1–3 mm erythematous oval macules and maculopapules on the lower abdomen. Some of the lesions are surrounded by a white halo. (Courtesy of Karen Wiss, M.D., Department of Dermatology, University of Massachusetts School of Medicine, Worcester, MA.)

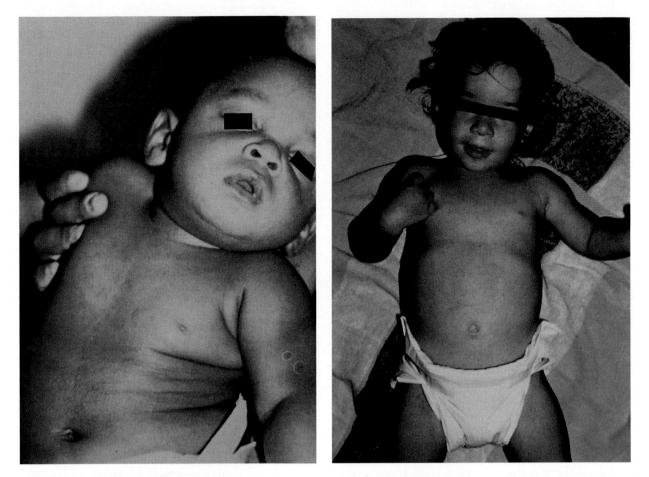

Figure 8–6, 8–7.   Widespread exanthem consisting of discrete erythematous papules. Note relative sparing of the face and extremities.

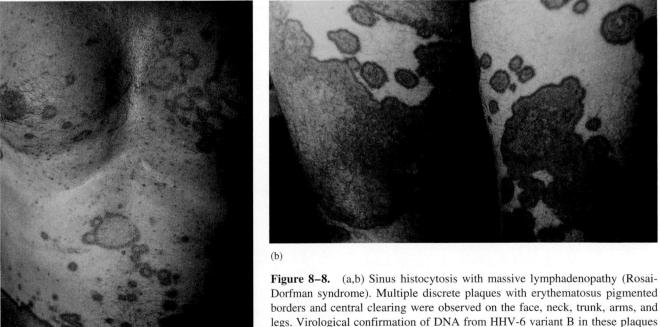

(a)

(b)

Figure 8–8.   (a,b) Sinus histocytosis with massive lymphadenopathy (Rosai-Dorfman syndrome). Multiple discrete plaques with erythematosus pigmented borders and central clearing were observed on the face, neck, trunk, arms, and legs. Virological confirmation of DNA from HHV-6 variant B in these plaques was obtained by using PCR. (Photographs courtesy of Amit Pandya, M.D., Department of Dermatology, University of Texas Southwestern School of Medicine, Dallas, TX.)

consistent abnormality seen is in the white blood cell count (WBC) [10,38,49]. In the majority of cases the total WBC count is low, although higher counts have been recorded early in the febrile period. The counts usually reach their nadir (as low as 3000 cells/mm^3) between days 3 and 6 of the illness and gradually normalize over a period of days. Concomitantly, the percentage of lymphocytes increases from 50–60% to 80–90%. In a study that compared emergency room visits of children with acute febrile illnesses, the HHV-6–positive group had a significantly lower WBC count than that of the HHV-6–negative group (8.9 × 10^3/mm^3 vs 13.2 × 10^3/mm^3), but no difference was seen between the two groups in the percentage of lymphocytes

[38]. Another study of 25 patients with exanthem subitum found that the majority of cases showed no leukopenia nor leukocytosis [121]. These results suggest that even WBC counts may be variable.

DIAGNOSIS

Exanthem subitum is a benign, self-limited disease with rare long-term sequelae. In the majority of cases, the diagnosis of exanthem subitum is based on the clinical findings of an otherwise asymptomatic young infant or child with abrupt onset of high fever followed by the appearance of

---

Table 8–4. Differential Diagnosis of Human Herpesvirus 6

Measles: Begins as fever accompanied by upper respiratory symptoms, such as cough, coryza, and palpebral conjunctivitis. Koplik's spots are also characteristic. The skin eruption in measles develops as the fever rises, not as it remits, and the lesions are dark red macules and papules. In addition, discrete papules become more numerous and merge to form large, irregular blotchy patches or plaques

Enteroviruses (e.g, Coxsackie, ECHO): These viruses infect infants and young children, particularly during the summer. Associated exanthems may be rubelliform, morbilliform, scarlatiniform, vesicular, urticarial, petechial, or pustular. Boston exanthem, caused by Echo 16, has a similar presentation to that of exanthem subitum in that the exanthem may appear with or shortly after defervescence. However, associated signs and symptoms such as upper respiratory tract symptoms, conjunctivitis, vomiting, diarrhea, and aseptic meningitis frequently occur with this disease

Adenovirus: The viral infections typically affect children ages 6 months to 5 years and most commonly occur during the winter and spring months. In addition to fever and upper respiratory symptoms, maculopapular, morbilliform, rubelliform, or petechial eruptions have been described

Epstein-Barr virus This virus can cause exanthems in up to one third of infected children. Maculopapular, petechial, papulovesicular, scarlatiniform, urticarial, and erythema multiforme-like exanthems have all been described. Fever, upper respiratory tract symptoms, hepatosplenomegaly, and adenopathy are often present at the time of the skin eruption.

Rubella: Begins with general malaise and a skin eruption that may vary from morbilliform on the chest to scarlatiniform over the abdomen and nodular on the extensor surfaces. Occipital adenopathy is prominent. Arthritis, encephalitis, and fetal damage may occur

Fifth disease (erythema infectiosum): Generally affects children older than 5 years of age. The infection begins with general malaise and low-grade fever, which is followed by malar erythema, or a "slapped-cheek" appearance. Subsequently, a reticular erythema develops over the extensor surfaces of the extremities. Arthralgias may be prominent in adults. Aplastic crisis may occur in individuals with hemoglobinopathies

Scarlet fever: Patients typically have fever, headache, malaise, marked pharyngitis, and adenopathy. While the patient is febrile, a "sandpaper-like" maculopapular eruption will appear, often accentuated in the skin folds. Circumoral pallor is common. Linear petechial lesions in the antecubital fossae and axillary folds, known as Pastia's lines, as well as subsequent acral desquamation, are helpful in making the diagnosis

Rocky Mountain Spotted Fever (and other rickettsial infections): Begins with an abrupt onset of fever, headache, and malaise with subsequent development of distal blanching macules that progress to involve the proximal extremities and trunk. The eruption ranges from blanching erythema to petechial and purpuric lesions. A history of tick bite is helpful but often not available.

Kawasaki's disease: Five of six criteria must be met for the diagnosis of this disease: fever persisting for 5 days or more, polymorphous eruption, conjunctival injection, oral mucosal changes, acral changes, and cervical lymphadenopathy. The major complication is coronary artery vasculitis

a rash and defervescence. It has been shown that these clinical findings correlate with a positive virological result in 86% of cases. It must be remembered, however, that only approximately 30% of children with HHV-6 infection have classic exanthem subitum. In cases that are equivocal or atypical, serological studies may prove useful. Differential diagnoses are listed in Table 8–4.

Serological assays for HHV-6 antibody are available. They can be useful in primary infection with detection of IgM titers or a fourfold increase in IgG titers among acute and convalescent serum samples. Although the presence of IgM in infants and children is a reliable marker for primary infection, its detection in adults can also appear during reactivation of HHV-6 [148]. The detection of IgG titer increases in paired serum samples can only provide retrospective information. Other laboratory investigations include viral culture, electron microscopic studies, detection of viral DNA using Southern blot techniques, in situ hybridization, and polymerase chain reaction (PCR) [18]. Viral culture, PCR, and electron microscopy are highly accurate and can be used reliably during the febrile phase of the disease when detectable viremia can reach 100%. Viral culture is not routinely feasible because it is technically demanding and may take over 1 week for results. Detection of HHV-6 DNA in cell-free plasma or serum by PCR is a definitive marker of active HHV-6 replication [149,150]. It must be remembered, however, that detectable virus decreases to 20% by day 4 of the illness and to 7% by days 5 to 7. Since the infection is permanent and intermittent shedding of viral particles may occur, there are doubts about the usefulness of these tests beyond the identification of primary infection. One study found that rapid microbiological diagnosis of acute HHV-6 infection is best performed with a combination of IgM serological methods and PCR detection of DNA in serum [151]. Quantitation of HHV-6 may prove to be useful in the future, with an increased viral burden suggesting acute illness. This method may then afford the opportunity to confirm the association of HHV-6 with various other disease syndromes.

TREATMENT AND PROPHYLAXIS

Although HHV-6 infection is usually a benign disease that requires no treatment, the potential for serious infections in both immunocompetent and immunocompromised hosts raises the need for antiviral therapy. HHV-6 lacks thymidine kinase, as does cytomegalovirus, and the antiviral susceptibilities of these two human herpesviruses are similar [152]. In vitro studies show that HHV-6 is susceptible to inhibition by pyrophosphate analogues, phosphonoacetic

acid, foscarnet, and ganciclovir [153–155]. The virus is relatively resistant to acyclovir [156]. HHV-6A appears to be relatively resistant to ganciclovir, while HHV-6B is susceptible [130,157]. No in vivo clinical trials have yet been undertaken to explore the therapeutic options for HHV-6. Only a few case reports have described the successful treatment of serious HHV-6 infection with foscarnet and/or ganciclovir, and the appropriate dosage is not known [90,158]. Several authors recommend the use of antiviral therapy for the treatment of serious HHV-6 infections, such as meningoencephalitis [90,159], or for the treatment of actively infected transplant recipients with bone marrow suppression, encephalitis, or pneumonitis [87]. No effective prophylaxis is available at this time. Further studies are needed before appropriate treatment of significant disease or prophylaxis for high risk individuals can be recommended.

CONCLUSION

HHV6 was first isolated in 1986 and was identified as the etiological agent for exanthem subitum in 1988. Since that time the virus has been shown to be ubiquitous, infecting 90–95% of the worldwide population. Although associations with many different syndromes have been noted, the only disease for which HHV-6 has been proved as the etiological agent is exanthem subitum. This disease, previously thought to infect about 30% of children, has now been shown to have several forms, including the classic presentation of fever followed by rash, fever alone, rash alone, or a subclinical syndrome defined only by isolation of the virus or detection of antibodies to the virus. By 3 years of age, 95% of children have contracted the virus. The virus appears to remain in the salivary glands of infected patients for life and has been reported to become reactivated if the patient becomes immunosuppressed. Additional reports of the occurrence of hepatitis, pneumonitis, and transplant graft rejection, among others, are commonly associated with these patients.

HHV-6 has also been associated with several other disorders, including lymphoproliferative disorders, HIV infection, and more recently with sinus histiocytosis with massive lymphadenopathy (Fig. 8-8) [160]. Whether a definite association is found, and to what extent the role of HHV-6 plays in the pathogenesis of these other syndromes, remains to be elucidated after careful study.

REFERENCES

1. SZ Salahuddin, DV Ablashi, PD Markham, SF Josephs, S Sturzenegger, M Kaplan, G Halligan, P Biberfeld, F

Wong-Staal, B Kramarsky, et al. Isolation of a new virus, HBLV, in patient with lymphoproliferative disorders. Science 234:596–601, 1986.

2. SF Josephs, SZ Salahuddin, DV Ablashi, F Schacter, F Wong-Staal, RC Gallo. Genomic analysis of the human B-lymphotropic virus (HBLV). Science 234:601–603, 1986.

3. P Biberfield, B Kramarsky, SZ Salahuddin, RC Gallo. Ultrastructural characterization of a new human B-lymphotropic DNA virus (HBLV) isolated from patients with lymphoproliferative disease. J Natl Cancer Inst 79: 933–941, 1987.

4. DV Ablashi, SZ Salahuddin, SF Josephs, F Imam, P Losso, RC Gallo. HBLV (or HHV-6) in human cell lines. Nature (Lond) 329:207, 1987.

5. DK Braun, G Dominguez, PE Pellet. Human herpesvirus 6. Clin Microbiol Rev 10:521–567, 1997.

6. K Yamanishi, J Okuno, K Shiraki, M Takahashi, T Kondo, Y Asano, T Kurata. Identification of human herpesvirus-6 as a causal agent for exanthem subitum. Lancet 1: 1065–1067, 1988.

7. JF Meigs, W Peppen. A Practical Treatise of the Diseases of Children, 4th ed. Philadelphia: Lindsay and Blakiston, 1870, pp 701–703, 803–806.

8. J Zahorsky. Roseola infantilism. Pediatrics 22:60–64, 1910.

9. BB Breese Jr. Roseola infantum (exanthem subitum). NY State J Med 41:1854–1859, 1941.

10. CH Kempe, EB Shaw, JR Jackson, HK Silver. Studies on the etiology of exanthem subitum. J Pediatr 37:561–568, 1950.

11. P Lusso, SZ Salahuddin, DV Ablashi, RC Gallo, F di Marzo Veronese, PD Markham. Diverse tropism of human B-lymphotropic virus (human herpesvirus 6) [letter]. Lancet 2:743–744, 1987.

12. EC Schirmer, LS Wyatt, K Yamanishi, WJ Rodriguez, N Frenkel. Differentiation between two distinct classes of viruses now classified as human herpesvirus 6. Proc Natl Acad Sci USA 88:5922–5926, 1991.

13. D Di Luca, R Dolcetti, P Mirandola, V De Re, P Secchiero, A Carbone, M Boiocchi, E Cassai. Human herpesvirus 6: a survey of presence and variant distribution in normal peripheral lymphocytes and lymphoproliferative disorders. J Infect Dis 170:211–215, 1994.

14. P Bovenzi, P Mirandola, P Secchiero, R Strumia, E Cassai, D Di Luca. Human herpesvirus-6 (variant A) in Kaposi's sarcoma. Lancet 341:1288–1289, 1993.

15. DV Ablashi, S Marsh, M Kaplan, JE Whitman Jr, GR Pearson. HHV-6 infection in HIV-infected asymptomatic and AIDS patients. Intervirology 41:1–9, 1998.

16. KK Knox, DR Carrigan. Active HHV-6 infection in the lymph nodes of HIV infected patients: in vitro evidence that HHV-6 can break HIV latency. J Acquir Immune Defic Syndr 11:370–378, 1996.

17. AL Komaroff. Human herpesvirus 6 and human disease [editorial]. Am J Clin Pathol 93:836–837, 1990.

18. PE Pellett, JB Black, M Yamamoto. Human herpesvirus 6: the virus and the search for its role as a human pathogen. Adv Virus Res 41:1–53, 1992.

19. Y Asano, T Yoshikawa, S Suga, T Yazaki, T Hata, T Nagai, Y Kajita, T Ozaki, S Yoshida. Viremia and neutralizing antibody response in infants with exanthem subitum. J Pediatr 14:535–539, 1989.

20. GR Pietroboni, GB Harnett, MR Bucens, RW Honess. Isolation of human herpesvirus 6 from saliva [letter]. Lancet 1:1059, 1988.

21. D Wakefield, A Lloyd, J Dwyer, SZ Salahuddin, DV Ablashi. Human herpesvirus 6 and myalgic encephalomyelitis. Lancet 1:1059, 1988.

22. WL Irving, AL Cunningham. Serological diagnosis of infection with human herpesvirus type 6. BMJ 300:156–159, 1990.

23. LM Huang, CY Lee, KH Lin, WM Chuu, PI Lee, RL Chen, JM Chen, DT Lin. Human herpesvirus-6 associated with fatal haemophagocytic syndrome [letter]. Lancet 336: 60–61, 1990.

24. G Rodier, E Fox, NT Constantine, EA Abbatte. HHV-6 in Djibouti—an epidemiological survey in young adults. Trans R Soc Trop Med Hyg 84:148–150, 1990.

25. H Agut, D Guetard, H Collandre, C Dauguet, L Montagnier, JM Miclea, H Baurmann, A Gessain. Concomitant infection by human herpes virus 6, HTLV-1, and HIV-2 [letter]. Lancet 1:712, 1988.

26. RS Tedder, M Briggs, CH Cameron, R Honess, D Robertson, H Whittle. A novel lymphotropic herpesvirus. Lancet 2:390–392, 1987.

27. GR Krueger, DV Ablashi. Human B-lymphotropic virus in Germany [letter]. Lancet 2:694, 1987.

28. RG Downing, N Sewankambo, D Serwadda, R Honess, D Crawford, R Jarrett, BE Griffin. Isolation of human lymphotropic herpes virus from Uganda [letter]. Lancet 2:390, 1987.

29. M Andre, B Matz. Antibody responses to human herpesvirus 6 and other herpes viruses [letter]. Lancet 2: 1425–1426, 1988.

30. M Briggs, J Fox, RS Tedder. Age prevalence of antibody to human herpesvirus 6 [letter]. Lancet 1:1058–1059, 1988.

31. T Okuno, K Takahashi, K Balachandra, K Shiraki, K Yamanishi, M Takahashi, K Baba. Seroepidemiology of human herpesvirus 6 infection in normal children and adults. J Clin Microbiol 27:651–653, 1989.

32. K Yanagi, S Harada, F Ban, A Oya, N Okabe, K Tobinai. High prevalence of antibody to human herpesvirus-6 and decrease in titer with increase in age in Japan [letter]. J Infect Dis 161:153–154, 1990.

33. C Saxinger, H Polesky, N Eby, Grufferman S, R Murphy, G Tegtmeir, V Parekh, S Memon, C Hung. Antibody reactivity with HBLV (HHV-6) in U.S. populations. J Virol Methods 21:199–208, 1988.

34. K Balachandra, Pi Ayuthaya, W Auwanit, C Jayavasu, T Okuno, K Yamanishi, M Takahashi. Prevalence of anti-

body to human herpes virus 6 in women and children. Microbiol Immunol 33:515–518, 1989.

35. T Yoshikawa, S Suga, Y Asano, T Yazaki, T Ozaki. Neutralizing antibodies to human herpesvirus-6 in healthy individuals. Pediatr Inf Dis J 9:589–590, 1990.

36. JA Levy, F Ferro, D Greenspan, ET Lennette. Frequent isolation of HHV-6 from saliva and high seroprevalence of the virus in the population. Lancet 335:1047–1050, 1990.

37. CT Leach, CV Sumaya, NA Brown. Human herpesvirus-6: clinical implications of a recently discovered, ubiquitous agent. J Pediatr 121:173–181, 1992.

38. P Pruksananonda, CB Hall, RA Insel, K McIntyre, PE Pellett, CE Long, KC Schnabel, PH Pincus, FR Stamey, TR Dambaugh, et al. Primary human herpesvirus 6 infection in young children. N Engl J Med 326:1445–1450, 1992.

39. G Enders, M Biber, G Meyer, E Helftenbein. Prevalence of antibodies to human herpesvirus 6 in different age groups, in children with exanthem subitum, other exanthematous childhood diseases, Kawasaki syndrome, and acute infections with other herpesviruses and HIV. Infection 18:12–15, 1990.

40. NA Brown, CR Sumaya, Y Liu, Y Ench, A Kovacs, M Coronesi, MH Kaplan. Fall in human herpesvirus 6 seropositivity with age. Lancet 2:396, 1988.

41. JA Levy, F Ferro, D Greenspan, ET Lennette. Frequent isolation of HHV-6 from saliva and high seroprevalence of the virus in the population. Lancet 335:1047–1050, 1990.

42. W Berenberg, S Wright, CA Janeway. Roseola infantum (exanthem subitum). N Engl J Med 251:253–259, 1949.

43. M Juretic. Exanthem subitum: a review of 243 cases. Helv Paediatr Acta 18:80–95, 1963.

44. HH Clemens. Exanthem subitum (roseola infantum): report of eighty cases. J Pediatr 26:66–67, 1945.

45. J Zahorsky. Roseola infantum—The rose rash of infants. Arch Pediatr 42:610–613, 1925.

46. HB Cushing. An epidemic of roseola infantum. Can Med Assoc J 17:905–906, 1927.

47. T Okuno, T Mukai, K Baba, Y Ohsumi, M Takahashi, K Yamanishi. Outbreak of exanthem subitum in an orphanage. J Pediatr 119:5:759–761, 1991.

48. U James, MB Freier. Roseola infantum: an outbreak in a maternity hospital. Arch Dis Child 24:54–58, 1949.

49. LH Berenberg, L Greenspan. Exanthem subitum (roseola infantum). Am J Dis Child 58:983–993, 1939.

50. MR Gopal, BJ Thomson, J Fox, RS Tedder, RW Hones. Detection by PCR of HHV-6 and EBV DNA in blood and oropharynx of healthy adults and HIV-seropositives. Lancet 335:1598–1599, 1990.

51. GB Harnett, TJ Farr, GR Pietroboni, MR Bucens. Frequent shedding of human herpesvirus 6 in saliva. J Med Virol 30:128–130, 1990.

52. JD Fox, M Briggs, PA Ward, RS Tedder. Human herpesvirus 6 in salivary glands. Lancet 336:590–593, 1990.

53. GR Krueger, K Wasserman, LS De Clerck WJ, Stevens, N Bourgeois, DV Ablashi, SF Josephs, N Balachandran. Latent herpesvirus-6 in salivary and bronchial glands [letter]. Lancet 336:1255–1256, 1990.

54. T Okuno, K Higashi, K Shiraki, K Yamanishi, M Takahashi, Y Kokado, M Ishibashi, S Takahara, T Sonoda, K Tanaka, et al. Human herpesvirus 6 infection in renal transplantation. Transplantation 49:519–522, 1990.

55. A Gautheret-Dejean, JT Aubin, L Poirel, Huraux JM, JC Nicolas, W Rozenbaum, H Agut. Detection of human Betaherpesvirinae in saliva and urine from immunocompromised and immunocompetent subjects. J Clin Microbiol 35:1600–1603, 1997.

56. S Suga, T Yoshikawa, Y Kajita, T Ozaki, Y Asano. Prospective study of persistence and excretion of human herpesvirus-6 in patients with exanthem subitum and their parents. Pediatrics 102:900–904, 1998.

57. DJ Morris, E Littler, JR Arrand, D Jordan, NP Mallick, RW Johnson. Human herpesvirus 6 infection in renal-transplant recipients [letter]. N Engl J Med 320:1560–1561, 1989.

58. KN Ward, JJ Gray, S Efstathiou. Brief report: primary human herpesvirus 6 infection in a patient following liver transplantation from a seropositive donor. J Med Virol 28:69–72, 1989.

59. WM Dunne Jr, G Demmler. Serologic evidence for congenital transmission of HHV-6. Lancet 340:121–122, 1992.

60. O Adams, C Krempe, G Kogler, P Wernet, A Scheid. Congenital infections with human herpesvirus 6. J Infect Dis 178:544–546, 1998.

61. Y Ando, K Kakimoto, Y Ekuni, M Ichijo. HHV-6 infection during pregnancy and spontaneous abortion [letter]. Lancet 340:1289, 1992.

62. JT Aubin, L Poirel, H Agut, JM Huraux, C Bignozzi, Y Brossard, N Mulliez, J Roume, F Lecuru, R Taurelle. Intrauterine transmission of human herpesvirus 6. Lancet 340:482–483, 1992.

63. S Wiersbitzky, E Beyersdorf, C Burtzlaff, H Wiersbitzky, S Crusius, I Weinke. Pre- and perinatal infections due to human herpesvirus-6 and Epstein-Barr-virus with lethal outcome or severe residual encephalopathy Padiatr Grenzgeb 31:199–201, 1993.

64. CT Leach, ER Newton, S McParlin, HB Jenson. Human herpesvirus 6 infection of the female genital tract. J Infect Dis 169:1281–1283, 1994.

65. D Di Luca, P Mirandola, T Ravaioli, B Bigoni, E Cassai. Distribution of HHV-6 variants in human tissues. Infect Agents Dis 5:203–214, 1996.

66. T Okuno, H Oishi, K Hayashi, M Nonogaki, K Tanaka, K Yamanishi. Human herpesviruses 6 and 7 in cervixes of pregnant women. J Clin Microbiol 33:1968–1970, 1995.

67. WM Dunne Jr, M Jevon. Examination of human breast milk for evidence of human herpesvirus 6 by polymerase chain reaction [letter]. J Infect Dis 168:250, 1993.

68. K Takahashi, S Sonoda, K Kawakami, K Miyata, T Oki, T Nagata, T Okuno, K Kamanishi. Human herpesvirus 6 and exanthem subitum. Lancet 1:1463, 1988.

69. H Kikuta, N Itami, S Matsumoto, T Chikaraishi, M Togashi. Frequent detection of human herpesvirus 6 DNA in peripheral blood mononuclear cells from kidney transplant patients [letter]. J Infect Dis 163:925, 1991.

70. K Kusuhara, K Ueda, K Okada, C Miyazaki, K Tokugawa, M Hirose, K Takahashi, K Yamanishi. Do second attacks of exanthema subitum result from human herpesvirus 6 reactivation or reinfection? Pediatr Infect Dis J 10: 468–469, 1991.

71. DV Ablashi, SF Josephs, C Buchbinder, K Hellman, S Nakamura, T Llana, P Lusso, M Kaplan, J Dahlberg, S Memon, et al. Human B lymphotropic virus (human herpes virus 6). J Virol Methods 21:29–48, 1988.

72. P Biberfeld, AL Petren, A Eklund, C Lindemalm, T Barkhem, M Ekman, D Ablashi, Z Salahuddin. Human herpes virus 6 (HHV-6, HBLV) in sarcoidosis and lymphoproliferative disorders. J Virol Methods 21:49–59, 1988.

73. GR Krueger, B Koch, A Ramon, DV Ablashi, SZ Salahuddin, SF Josephs, HZ Streicher, RC Gallo, U Habermann. Antibody prevalence to HBLV (human herpes virus 6, HHV-6) and suggestive pathogenicity in the general population and in patients with immune deficiency syndromes. J Virol Methods 21:125–131, 1988.

74. M Patnaik, AL Komaroff, E Conley, EA Ojo-Amaize, JB Peter. Prevalence of IgM antibodies to human herpesvirus 6 early antigen (p41/38) in patients with chronic fatigue syndrome. J Infect Dis 172:1364–1367, 1995.

75. P Sola, E Merelli, R Marasca, M Poggi, M Luppi, M Montorsi, G Torelli. Human herpesvirus 6 and multiple sclerosis: survey of anti-HHV-6 antibodies by immunofluorescence analysis and of viral sequences by polymerase chain reaction. J Neurol Neurosurg Psychiatry 56:917–919, 1993.

76. F Wilborn, CA Schmidt, V Brinkmann, K Jendroska, H Oettle, W Siegert. A potential role for human herpesvirus type 6 in nervous system disease. J Neuroimmunol 49: 213–214, 1994.

77. DA Clark, FE Alexander, PA McKinney, BE Roberts, C O'Brien, RF Jarrett, RA Cartwright, DE Onions. The seroepidemiology of human herpes virus 6 (HHV-6) from a case-control study of leukemia and lymphoma. Int J Cancer 45:829–833, 1990.

78. G Torelli, R Marasea, M Luppi, L Selleri, S Ferrari, F Narni, MT Mariano, M Federico, L Ceccherini-Nelli, M Bendinelli, et al. Human herpes virus 6 in human lymphomas: identification of specific sequences in Hodgkin's lymphomas by polymerase chain reaction. Blood 77: 2251–2258, 1991.

79. RF Jarret, S Gledhill, F Qureshi, SH Crae, R Madhok, I Brown, I Evans, A Krajewski, CJ O'Brien, RA Cartwright, et al. Identification of human herpes virus 6-specific DNA sequences in two patients with non-Hodgkin's lymphoma. Leukemia 2:496–502, 1988.

80. SF Josephs, A Buchbinder, HZ Streicher, DV Ablashi, SZ Salahuddin, HG Guo, F Wong-Staal, J Cossman, M Raffeld, J Sundeen, et al. Detection of human B lymphotropic virus (human herpes virus 6) sequences in B-cell lymphoma tissues of three patients. Leukemia 2:132–135, 1988.

81. S Chou, KM Scott. Rises in antibody to human herpesvirus 6 detected by enzyme immunoassay in transplant recipients with primary cytomegalovirus infection. J Clin Microbiol 28:851–854, 1989.

82. WL Irving, AL Cunningham, A Keogh, JR Chapman. Antibody in both human herpesvirus 6 and cytomegalovirus [letter]. Lancet 2:630–631, 1988.

83. Y Asano, T Yoshikawa, S Suga, T Nakashima, T Yazaki, M Fukuda, S Kojima, T Matsuyama. Reactivation of herpesvirus type 6 in children receiving bone marrow transplants for leukemia. N Engl J Med 324:634–635, 1991.

84. DR Carrigan, WR Drobyski, SK Russler, MA Tapper, KK Knox, RC Ash. Interstitial pneumonitis associated with human herpesvirus-6 infection after marrow transplantation. Lancet 338:147–149, 1991.

85. KN Ward, JJ Gray, S Efstathiou. Brief report: primary human herpes virus 6 infection in a patient following liver transplantation from a seropositive donor. J Med Virol 28: 69–72, 1989.

86. H Wizos, J Gibbons, PL Abt, RR Gifford, HC Yang. Human herpes virus 6 in monocytes of transplant patients. Lancet 335:486–487, 1990.

87. N Singh, DR Carrigan. Human herpesvirus-6 in transplantation: an emerging pathogen. Ann Intern Med 124: 1065–1071, 1996.

88. RW Cone, RC Hackman, ML Huang, RA Bowden, JD Meyers, M Metcalf, J Zeh, R Ashley, L Corey. Human herpesvirus 6 in lung tissue from patients with pneumonitis after bone marrow transplantation. N Engl J Med 329: 156–161, 1993.

89. G De Almeida Rodrigues, S Nagendra, CK Lee, De M Magalhaes-Silverman. Human herpes virus 6 fatal encephalitis in a bone marrow recipient. Scand J Infect Dis 31: 313–315, 1999.

90. C Rieux, A Gautheret-Dejean, D Challine-Lehmann, C Kirch, H Agut, JP Vernant. Human herpesvirus-6 meningoencephalitis in a recipient of an unrelated allogeneic bone marrow transplantation. Transplantation 65: 1408–1411, 1998.

91. WR Drobyski, M Dunne, EM Burd, KK Knox, RC Ash, MM Horowitz, N Flomenberg, DR Carrigan. Human herpesvirus-6 (HHV-6) infection in allogeneic bone marrow transplant recipients: evidence of a marrow-suppressive role for HHV-6 in vivo. J Infect Dis 167:735–739, 1993.

92. DR Carrigan, KK Knox. Human herpesvirus-6 (HHV-6) isolation from bone marrow: HHV-6-associated bone marrow suppression in bone marrow transplant patients. Blood 84:3307–3310, 1994.

93. I Lautenschlager, K Höckerstedt, K Linnavuori, E Taskinen. Human herpesvirus-6 infection after liver transplantation. Clin Infect Dis 26:702–707, 1998.

94. JA DesJardin, L Gibbons, E Cho, SE Supran, ME Falagas, BG Werner, DR Snydman. Human herpesvirus 6 reactivation is associated with cytomegalovirus infection and syndromes in kidney transplant recipients at risk for primary cytomegalovirus infection. J Infect Dis 178:1783–1786, 1998.

95. VM Ratnamohan, J Chapman, H Howse, K Bovington, P Robertson, K Byth, R Allen, AL Cunningham. Cytomegalovirus and human herpesvirus 6 both cause viral disease after renal transplantation. Transplantation 66:877–882, 1998.

96. P Lusso, B Ensoli, PD Markham, DV Ablashi, SZ Salahuddin, E Tschachler, F Wong-Staal, RC Gallo. Productive dual infection of human CD4+ T-lymphocyte by HIV-1 and HHV-6. Nature 337:370–373, 1989.

97. K Takahashi, S Sonoda, K Higashi, T Kondo, H Takahashi, M Takahashi, K Yamanishi. Predominant CD4 T-lymphocyte tropism of human herpesvirus 6-related virus. J Virol 63:3161–3163, 1989.

98. TJ Spira, LH Bozeman, KC Sanderlin, DT Warfield, PM Feorino, RC Holman, JE Kaplan, DB Fishbein, C Lopez. Lack of correlation between human herpesvirus-6 infection and the course of human immunodeficiency virus infection. J Infect Dis 161:567–570, 1990.

99. H Chen, AM Pesce, M Carbonari, F Ensoli, M Cherchi, G Campitelli, D Sbarigia, G Luzi, F Aiuti, M Fiorilli. Absence of antibodies to human herpesvirus-6 in patients with slowly progressive human immunodeficiency virus type 1 infection. Eur J Epidemiol 8:217–221, 1992.

100. NA Brown, A Kovacs, CR Lui, C Hur, JA Zaia, JW Mosley. Prevalence of antibody to human herpesvirus 6 among blood donors infected with HIV [letter]. Lancet 2:1146, 1988.

101. J Fox, M Briggs, RS Tedder. Antibody to human herpes virus 6 in HIV-1 positive and negative homosexual men. Lancet 2:396–397, 1988.

102. P Lusso, A DeMaria, M Mainati, F Lori, SE DeRocco, M Baseler, RC Gallo. Induction of CD-4 and susceptibility to HIV-1 infection in human CD-8 + T-Lymphocytes by human herpes virus 6. Nature 349:533–555, 1991.

103. DR Carrigan, KK Knox, MA Tapper. Suppression of human immunodeficiency virus type 1 replication by human herpes virus-6. J Infect Dis 162:844–851, 1990.

104. JA Levy, L Landay, ET Lannette. Human herpes virus-6 inhibits human immunodeficiency virus type-1 replication in cell culture. J Clin Microbiol 28:2362–2364, 1990.

105. RT Horvat, C Wood, N Balachandran. Transactivation of human immunodeficiency virus promoter by HHV-6. J Virol 63:970–973, 1989.

106. B Ensoli, P Lusso, F Schachter, SF Josephs, J Rappaport, F Negro, RC Gallo, F Wong-Staal. Human herpes virus-6 increases HIV-1 expression in co-infected T-cell via nuclear factors binding to the HIV-1 enhancer. EMBO J 8:3019–3027, 1989.

107. J Thompson, S Chaudhury, F Kashanchi, J Doniger, Z Berneman, N Frenkel, LJ Rosenthal. A transforming fragment within the direct repeat of human herpesvirus-6 that transactivates HIV-1. Oncogene 9:1167–1175, 1994.

108. L Flamand, J Gosselin, M D'Addarrio, J Hiscott, DV Ablashi, RC Gallo, J Menezes. Human herpesvirus-6 induces interleukin 1 β and tumor necrosis factor—but not interleukin-6 in peripheral blood mononuclear cell cultures. J Virol 65:5105–5110, 1991.

109. T Matsuyama, N Kobayashi, N Yamamoto. Cytokines and HIV infections: is AIDS a tumor necrosis factor disease? AIDS 5:1405–1417, 1991.

110. DA Clark, M Ait Khaled, AC Wheeler, IM Kidd, JE McLaughlin, MA Johnson, PD Griffiths, VC Emery. Quantification of human herpesvirus 6 in immunocompetent persons and post-mortem tissues from AIDS patients by PCR. J Gen Virol 77:2271–2275, 1996.

111. P Lusso, RC Gallo. HHV-6 and CMV pneumonitis in immunocompromised patients. Lancet 343:1647–1648, 1994.

112. KK Knox, DR Carrigan. Disseminated active HHV-6 infections in patients with AIDS. Lancet 343:577–578, 1994.

113. BC Berlinger. A physical sign useful in diagnosis of roseola infantum before the rash. Pediatrics 25:1034, 1960.

114. A Letchner. Roseola infantum: a review of fifty cases. Lancet 2:1163–1165, 1995.

115. S Suga, Yoshikawa T, Asano Y, T Yazaki, S Hirata. Human herpes virus 6 infection (exanthem subitum) without rash. Pediatrics 83:1003–1006, 1989.

116. Y Asano, S Suga, T Yoshikawa, A Urisu, T Yazaki. Human herpes virus 6 infection (exanthem subitum) without fever. J Pediatr 115:264–265, 1989.

117. PJ Prezioso, J Congiarella, M Lee, GJ Nuovo, W Borkowsky, SJ Orlow, MA Greco. Fatal disseminated infection with human herpesvirus-6. J Pediatr 120:921–923, 1992.

118. RM Greenthal. Roseola infantum (exanthem subitum). Med J 40:25–27, 1941.

119. HK Faber, LB Dickey. The symptomatology of exanthem subitum. Arch Pediatr 44:491–496, 1927.

120. KL Moller. Exanthema subitum and febrile convulsions. Acta Pediatr 45:534–540, 1956.

121. K Linnavuori, H Peltola, T Hovi. Serology versus clinical signs or symptoms and main laboratory findings in the diagnosis of exanthem subitum (roseola infantum). Pediatrics 89:103–106, 1992.

122. FA Oski. Roseola infantum. Another case of bulging fontanelle. Am J Dis Child 101:376–378, 1961.

123. Y Asano, T Nakashima, T Yoshikawa, S Suga, T Yazaki. Severity of human herpes 6 viremia and clinical findings in infants with exanthem subitum. J Pediatr 118:891–895, 1991.

124. DB Posson. Exanthem subitum (roseola infantum) complicated by prolonged convulsions and hemiplegia. J Pediatr 35:235–236, 1949.

125. PB Holliday. Preeruptive neurological complications of common contagious diseases—rubella, rubeola, roseola and varicella. J Pediatr 36:185–198, 1950.

126. MJ Wallfield. Exanthem subitum with an encephalitic onset. J Pediatr 5:800–801, 1934.

127. PL Burnstine, RS Paine. Residual encephalopathy following roseola infantum. Am J Dis Child 98:144–152, 1959.

128. Friedman JH, Golomb J, Aronjon L. Hemiplegia associated with roseola infantum (exanthem subitum). NY State J Med 50:1749–1750, 1950.

129. J Rosenblum. Roseola infantum (exanthem subitum) complicated by hemiplegia. Am J Dis Child 69:234–236, 1945.

130. KK Knox, D Pietryga, DJ Harrington, R Franciosi, DR Carrigan. Progressive immunodeficiency and fatal pneumonitis associated with human herpesvirus 6 infection in an infant. Clin Infect Dis 20:406–413, 1995.

131. JA Hammerling, RS Lambrecht, KS Kehl, DR Carrigan. Prevalence of human herpesvirus 6 in lung tissue from children with pneumonitis. J Clin Pathol 49:802–804, 1996.

132. MP Hoang, KF Ross, DB Dawson, RH Scheuermann, BB Rogers. Human herpesvirus-6 and sudden death in infancy: report of a case and review of the literature. J Forensic Sci 44:432–437, 1999.

133. K Nishimura, M Igarashi. Thrombocytopenic purpura associated with exanthem subitum. Pediatrics 60:260, 1977.

134. M Saijo, H Saijo, M Yamamoto, M Takimoto, H Fujiyasu, K Murono, K Fujita. Thrombocytopenic purpura associated with primary human herpesvirus 6 infection [letter]. Pediatr Infect Dis J 14:405, 1995.

135. K Kitamura, H Ohta, T Ihara, H Kamiya, H Ochiai, K Yamanishi, K Tanaka. Idiopathic thrombocytopenic purpura after human herpesvirus 6 infection. Lancet 344:830, 1994.

136. T Yoshikawa, Y Asano, I Kobayashi, T Nakashima, T Yazaki. Exacerbation of idiopathic thrombocytopenic purpura by primary human herpesvirus 6 infection. Pediatr Infect Dis J 12:409–410, 1993.

137. Y Asano, T Yoshikawa, S Suga, T Yazaki, K Kondo, K Yamanishi. Fatal fulminant hepatitis in an infant with human herpes virus 6 infection (exanthem subitum) without fever. Lancet 335:862–863, 1990.

138. S Dubedat, N Kappagoda. Hepatitis due to human herpes virus 6. Lancet 2:1463–1464, 1989.

139. R Sobue, H Miyazaki, M Okamoto, M Hirano, T Yoshikawa, S Suga, Y Asano. Fulminant hepatitis in primary human herpes virus 6 Infection. N Engl J Med 324:1290, 1991.

140. H Tajiri, O Nose, K Baba, S Okada. Human herpesvirus-6 infection with liver injury in neonatal hepatitis. Lancet 335:863, 1990.

141. TA Steeper, CA Horwitz, DV Ablashi, SZ Salahuddin, C Saxinger, R Saltzman, B Schwartz. The spectrum of clinical and laboratory findings resulting from human herpes virus 6 (HHV-6) in patients with mononucleosis-like illnesses not resulting from Epstein-Barr virus or cytomegalovirus. Am J Clin Pathol 93:776–783, 1990.

142. JC Niederman, MH Kaplan, CR Liu, NA Brown. Clinical and serological features of human herpes virus 6 infection in three adults. Lancet 2:817–819, 1988.

143. A Hanukoglu, E Somekh. Infectious mononucleosis-like illness in an infant with acute herpesvirus 6 infection. Pediatr Infect Dis J 13:750–751, 1994.

144. CK Kanegane, S Katayama, H Kyoutani, H Kanegane, N Shintani, T Miyawaki, N Taniguchi. Mononucleosis-like illness in an infant associated with human herpesvirus 6 infection. Acta Paediatr Jpn 37:227–229, 1995.

145. JH Van Zeijl, CR Korver, JM Galama. Human herpesvirus 6 mononucleosis and seizures. Pediatr Infect Dis J 14:637, 1995.

146. K Akashi, Y Eizuru, Y Sumiyoshi, T Minematsu, S Hara, M Harada, M Kikuchi, Y Niho, Y Minamishima. Severe infectious mononucleosis-like syndrome and primary human herpesvirus 6 infection in an adult. N Engl J Med 329:168–171, 1993.

147. M Yoshida, F Uno, ZL Bai, M Yamada, S Nii, T Sata, T Kurata, K Yamanishi, M Takahashi. Electron microscopic study of a herpes-type virus isolated from an infant with exanthem subitum. Microbiol Immunol 33:147–154, 1989.

148. JD Fox, P Ward, M Briggs, W Irving, TG Stammers, RS Tedder. Production of IgM antibody to HHV6 in reactivation and primary infection. Epidemiol Infect 104:289–296, 1990.

149. LM Huang, PF Kuo, CY Lee, JY Chen, MY Liu, CS Yang. Detection of human herpesvirus-6 DNA by polymerase chain reaction in serum or plasma. J Med Virol 38:7–10, 1992.

150. P Secchiero, DR Carrigan, Y Asano, L Benedetti, RW Crowley, AL Komaroff, RC Gallo, P Lusso. Detection of human herpesvirus 6 in plasma of children with primary infection and immunosuppressed patients by polymerase chain reaction. J Infect Dis 171:273–280, 1995.

151. RM Bland, PL Mackie, T Shorts, S Pate, JY Paton. The rapid diagnosis and clinical features of human herpesvirus 6. J Infect 36:161–165, 1998.

152. UA Gompels, J Nicholas, G Lawrence, M Jones, BJ Thomson, ME Martin, S Efstathiou, M Craxton, HA Macaulay. The DNA sequence of human herpesvirus-6: structure, coding content, and genome evolution. Virology 209:29–51, 1995.

153. WH Burns, CR Sandford. Susceptibility of human herpes virus 6 to antivirals in vitro. J Infect Dis 162:634–637, 1990.

154. MS Hirsch, JC Kaplan. Antiviral agents. In: BN Fields, DM Knipe, RM Chanock, et al., eds. Virology, 2nd ed. New York: Raven, 1990, pp 441–468.

155. HZ Streicher, CL Hung, DV Ablashi, K Hellman, C Saxinger, J Fullen, SZ Salahuddin. In vitro inhibition of human herpesvirus-6 by phosphonoformate. J Virol Methods 21:301–304, 1988.

156. H Agut, H Collandre, JT Aubin, D Guetard, V Favier, D

Ingrand, L Montagnier, JM Huraux. In vitro sensitivity of human herpesvirus-6 to antiviral drugs. Res Virol 140: 219–228, 1989.

157. A Akesson-Johansson, J Harmenberg, B Wahren, A Linde. Inhibition of human herpesvirus 6 replication by 9-(4-hydroxy-2-(hydroxymethyl)butyl)guanine (2HM-HBG) and other antiviral compounds. Antimicrob Agents Chemother 34:2417–2419, 1990.

158. PD Cole, J Stiles, F Boulad, TN Small, RJ O'Reilly, D George, P Szabolcs, TE Kiehn, NA Kernan. Successful treatment of human herpesvirus 6 encephalitis in a bone marrow transplant recipient. Clin Infect Dis 27:653–654, 1998.

159. EG Hermione Lyall. Human herpesvirus 6: primary infection and the central nervous system. Pediatr Infect Dis J 15:693–696, 1996.

160. MM Scheel, PL Rady, SK Tyring, AG Pandya. Sinus histocytosis with massive lymphadenopathy. Presentation as a giant granuloma annulare and detection of human herpesvirus 6. J Am Acad Dermatol 37:643–646, 1997.

9

Human Herpesvirus 7

Tricia J. Brown
University of Oklahoma Health Sciences Center, Oklahoma City, Oklahoma, USA

Angela Yen-Moore
University of Texas Southwestern Medical Center, Dallas, Texas, USA

Human herpesvirus 7 (HHV-7) is a recently discovered lymphotropic herpesvirus that is ubiquitous across the globe (Fig. 9–1). No clinical disease has yet been definitely linked to HHV-7, although several different conditions, such as exanthem subitum and pityriasis rosea, have been attributed to the virus by some investigators.

HISTORY

In 1990, Frenkel et al [1] first isolated what is now known as HHV-7 from cultured and activated CD4+ T peripheral blood lymphocytes of a healthy young adult. DNA analysis revealed this virus to resemble HHV-6 and cytomegalovirus. HHV-7 belongs to the beta herpesvirus subfamily [2,3].

INCIDENCE

The epidemiology of HHV-7 appears similar to that of HHV-6. The majority of adults have serological evidence of previous HHV-7 infection [4,5,6], with a seroprevalence rate of more than 85% in the United States [7]. Primary infection occurs slightly later than that for HHV-6, although most infections develop in the first 5 years of life [8]. While the highest period for primary HHV-6 infection is 6 to 12 months of age, that for HHV-7 infection is 1 to 2 years of age [9]. An American study of 164 children by Lanphear et al [10] revealed that low income and black race were risk factors for the early acquisition of HHV-7. An increased rate of infection in November, when compared with those of September and October, indicates seasonal variability.

PATHOGENESIS

Little is known about the pathogenesis of HHV-7 infection. The portal of entry, site of primary infection, and mechanism of latency are yet to be determined [7]. The human salivary glands are the only host cells known to persistently produce infectious HHV-7 virions. Several investigators have shown that HHV-7 can be readily isolated from the saliva of adults and children over the age of 12 months [11–14]. Although not definitively proved, transmission of HHV-7 likely occurs through saliva. The epidemiological patterns of transmission suggest intimate family contact and exchange of the salivary excretions [9]. The possibility of perinatal transmission of HHV-7 is also a consideration since HHV-7 DNA has been detected in cervical swabs of pregnant women [15].

While little is known of the pathogenesis of HHV-7, CD4 has been identified as the cellular receptor for this

GEOGRAPHICAL INCIDENCE

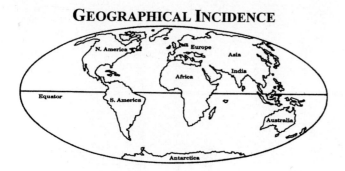

TAXONOMY

Herpesviridae family
Betaherpesvirinae subfamily

TRANSMISSION

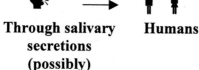

Through salivary   **Humans**
secretions
(possibly)

ZOONOTIC IMPLICATIONS

None

 } **Only known reservoir**
Humans

Figure 9–1. Incidence and transmission of human herpesvirus 7.

virus [16]. It has been suggested that HHV-7 may have an immunosuppressive effect, since CD4+ T lymphocytes play a crucial role in the development of immunity and HHV-7 down-modulates the expression of the CD4 receptor [17]. The interactions between human immunodeficiency virus (HIV) and HHV-7 are under investigation, as both viruses compete for the same cell receptor. It has been suggested that competition for the cell receptor by HHV-7 may down-regulate the infectivity of HIV on CD4+ T lymphocytes [16]. A T-lymphotropic vector has been developed from HHV-7 for potential use in gene therapy for diseases affecting CD4+ T lymphocytes, such as acquired immunodeficiency virus (AIDS), autoimmune diseases, and T-cell lymphomas [18].

HHV-7 typically remains latent in the infected human host [19]. This virus has been shown to establish latency in peripheral blood mononuclear cells and may be propagated in vitro in activated cord blood lymphocytes. The range of tissue hosts of HHV-7 has been considered more limited than that for HHV-6, although Kempf et al [20] demonstrated the persistence of HHV-7 antigen in human lungs, skin, and mammary glands. The infected cells were distinctly different from lymphocytes, and HHV-7 was not detected in brain, spleen, or large intestine tissues. These authors also suggest from their results that HHV-7 causes a persistent rather than a true latent infection. Compared with HHV-6, HHV-7 is more cell-associated, less cytopathic, and has a slower growth rate in culture [21]. The two viruses are serologically distinct, and prior infection with HHV-6 provides no protection against HHV-7 infection [2].

Little information is known regarding the effects of HHV-7 infection in immunocompromised individuals [22,23]. It has been shown that HHV-7 has been reactivated from latency in transplant recipients (kidney and bone marrow) [24,25]. One Japanese study of HHV-7 in bone marrow transplantation found no associated clinical symptoms that could be attributed to the virus [26]. Although the role of HHV-7 in transplantation is yet to be determined, this virus has been suspected as a cofactor for the development of other infections (cytomegalovirus) or the delay of engraftment [24].

Limited antigenic cross-reactivity has been reported between HHV-6 and HHV-7 [8,11], due to the significant homology between the two viruses. A study by Huang et al [9] revealed that almost 36% of positive anti–HHV-7 serological tests came from cross-reactions with HHV-6. These authors noted that primary HHV-6 infection can induce reactive HHV-7 antibodies although the titer is lower than that of primary HHV-7 infection. This reaction also has been observed by other authors [8,27]. However, a separate study has suggested that HHV-7 infection can induce HHV-6 antibodies but not the reverse [28]. In this investigation, several patients with documented HHV-7 seroconversion developed a simultaneous elevation of HHV-6 antibody titers, which resembled a booster effect. This HHV-6 antibody response has been seen in other studies of primary HHV-7 infections [27,29]. An in vitro study has demonstrated that HHV-7 has the potential to reactivate latent HHV-6 in activated peripheral blood mononuclear cells [30]. Although not proved, these authors hypothesize that in vivo primary infection with HHV-7 is linked to the reactivation of HHV-6, which subsequently causes the clinical manifestations of exanthem subitum.

CLINICAL MANIFESTATIONS

As previously stated, HHV-7 has not been definitively linked to any clinical disease (Table 9–1). Early on, HHV-7 was isolated from a patient with chronic fatigue syndrome [2], but no association was found in seroepidemiologic studies. HHV-7 has been isolated from one child with a chronic Epstein-Barr virus–like clinical infection [31]. Although no other viruses could be isolated in this patient, the definitive role of HHV-7 cannot be established from this one case report. Two children with minor upper respiratory tract infection were documented to have HHV-7 seroconversion, suggesting HHV-7 as the etiology [28]. Several authors have also linked HHV-7 infection with childhood febrile illnesses, sometimes complicated by seizures [29,32–34]. One study demonstrated that children with primary HHV-7 infection were more likely to have seizures (75%) when compared with children with primary HHV-6 infection (17%) [32].

The possible association of pityriasis rosea and HHV-7 was first proposed by Drago et al [35,36] in 1997 when they isolated HHV-7 DNA in skin biopsy specimens, peripheral blood mononuclear cells, and plasma specimens of 12 patients with this disease. However, these findings have not been confirmed by other studies of HHV-7 DNA and antigen detection in skin lesion specimens [37,38] or HHV-7 serological tests [39,40] in patients with pityriasis rosea.

Exanthem subitum is the most convincing clinical disease thought to be caused by HHV-7. While this illness is known to be caused by HHV-6, several studies have implicated HHV-7 as an etiological factor in a percentage of cases [27,28,41–44]. One specific study evaluated paired serological tests to both HHV-6 and HHV-7 from 49 patients with clinically diagnosed exanthem subitum [28]. Based on evidence of seroconversion, HHV-6 caused 73.5% of cases, while HHV-7 led to 10.2% of cases. While investigating the association of HHV-7 and exanthem subitum, Tanaka et al [27] have noted that the rash associated with HHV-7 infection is lighter in appearance and occurs slightly later during the course of disease than that of HHV-6 infection. They also observed that incomplete clinical features of exanthem subitum may occur with both viruses, producing only high fever and no rash. Neurological complications of HHV-7-induced exanthem subitum have been reported, such as acute hemiplegia and febrile convulsions [41]. Cerebrospinal fluid analysis from two of these cases were suggestive of encephalitis. Chapter 8 (Human Herpesvirus 6) provides an overview of the clinical features of exanthem subitum.

DIAGNOSIS

HHV-7 infection can be detected by several methods. Serological diagnosis is made with immunofluorescence assays, enzyme immunoassays, or immunoblot assays, with each using HHV-7 infected cells as the antigen source [2,8]. To decrease the rate of cross-reactivity with HHV-6 and to increase the specificity, absorption steps are essential with these tests. One longitudinal serological study noted that anti–HHV-7 titers, which were falsely elevated because of HHV-6 cross-reactivity, remained at a level less than 20 [9]. They concluded that a titer of at least 20 is appropriate for the serological diagnosis of HHV-7 infection.

HHV-7 DNA can be detected in specimens with polymerase chain reaction, most commonly from throat swabs or peripheral blood samples. Detection of antigens to HHV-7 can be detected by flow cytometry and immunohistochemical tests. The virus can also be isolated and cultured

Table 9–1. Clinical Manifestations of Exanthem Subitum

Time after exposure	Clinical manifestations	Laboratory analyses	Other notes
10 days	Abrupt onset of high fever, lasting 3–5 days	Serology: IgM or 4-fold increase in IgG; PCR detection of HHV-6 DNA in cell-free serum or plasma	Child is typically asymptomatic during the febrile stage
13–15 days	Appearance of a rose-pink maculopapular or macular eruption on neck and trunk, lasting 1–2 days. May sometimes spread to face and proximal extremities.	Viral culture Electron microscopy	Slight irritability and malaise may be associated with higher elevations of temperature
14–17 days	Blanching and then fading of the rash		Rash is not pruritic and does not desquamate

Table 9–2.   Differential Diagnoses of Exanthem Subitum

Measles: Begins as fever accompanied by upper respiratory symptoms, such as cough, coryza, and palpebral conjunctivitis. Koplik's spots are also characteristic. The skin eruption in measles develops as the fever rises, not as it remits, and the lesions are dark red macules and papules. In addition, discrete papules become more numerous and merge to form large, irregular blotchy patches or plaques with measles.

Enteroviruses (e.g, Coxsackie, ECHO): These viruses infect infants and young children, particularly during the summer. Associated exanthems may be rubelliform, morbilliform, scarlatiniform, vesicular, urticarial, petechial, or pustular. Boston exanthem, caused by ECHO 16, has a similar presentation to that of exanthem subitum in that the exanthem may appear with or shortly after defervescene. However, associated signs and symptoms such as upper respiratory tract symptoms, conjunctivitis, vomiting, diarrhea, and aseptic meningitis frequently occur with this disease

Adenovirus: These viral infections typically affect children ages 6 months to 5 years and most commonly occur during the winter and spring months. In addition to fever and upper respiratory symptoms, maculopapular, morbilliform, rubelliform, or petechial eruptions have been described

Epstein-Barr virus This virus can cause exanthems in up to one third of infected children. Maculopapular, petechial, papulovesicular, scarlatiniform, urticarial, and erythema multiforme-like exanthems have all been described. Fever, upper respiratory tract symptoms, hepatosplenomegaly, and adenopathy are often present at the time of the skin eruption.

Rubella: Begins with general malaise and a skin eruption that may vary from morbilliform on the chest to scarlatiniform over the abdomen and nodular on the extensor surfaces. Occipital adenopathy is prominent. Arthritis, encephalitis, and fetal damage may occur

Fifth disease (erythema infectiosum): Generally affects children older than 5 years of age. The infection begins with general malaise and low-grade fever, which is followed by malar erythema, or a "slapped-cheek" appearance. Subsequently, a reticular erythema develops over the extensor surfaces of the extremities. Arthralgias may be prominent in adults. Aplastic crisis may occur in individuals with hemoglobinopathies

Scarlet fever: Patients typically present with fever, headache, malaise, marked pharyngitis, and adenopathy. While the patient is febrile, a "sandpaper-like" maculopapular eruption will appear, often accentuated in the skin folds. Circumoral pallor is common. Linear petechial lesions in the antecubital fossae and axillary folds, known as Pastia's lines, as well as subsequent acral desquamation, are helpful in making the diagnosis

Rocky Mountain Spotted Fever (and other rickettsial infections): Begins with an abrupt onset of fever, headache, and malaise with subsequent development of distal blanching macules that progress to involve the proximal extremities and trunk. The eruption ranges from blanching erythema to petechial and purpuric lesions. A history of tick bite is helpful but often not available.

Kawasaki's disease: Five of six criteria must be met for the diagnosis of this disease: fever persisting for 5 days or more, polymorphous eruption, conjunctival injection, oral mucosal changes, acral changes, and cervical lymphadenopathy. The major complication is coronary artery vasculitis

---

from saliva or peripheral blood of infected patients. After preparation, the samples are inoculated onto mitogen-stimulated human cord blood lymphocytes. Cytopathic effects are typically seen in the culture within 2 to 4 weeks of cultivation, and the virus can be confirmed with an immunofluorescence assay. A variety of diseases may mimic exanthem subitum as shown in Table 9-2.

TREATMENT

No treatment is currently available or recommended specifically for HHV-7 infection (Table 9–3). The susceptibility

of the virus to antiviral agents is unknown. One in vivo small-scale study suggested that HHV-7 activity is suppressed with full therapeutic doses of both acyclovir and ganciclovir [24]. However, prophylactic or suppressive doses of these drugs had no noticeable impact on HHV-7 in this study. A handful of in vitro studies have demonstrated the inhibition of HHV-7 by various agents, such as ganciclovir, foscarnet, cidofovir, lobucavir, and others [45–47]. However, much more research will be necessary to characterize the optimal treatment for HHV-7 and when or if such treatment would be indicated.

Table 9–3. Treatment of Exanthem Subitum

Symptom	Treatment
Fever	Acetaminophen or nonsteroidal anti-inflammatory drugs
Cough	Antitussives
Exanthem	Reassurance. No treatment is needed
Neurologic complications	Anticonvulsants for seizures. Control of intracranial pressure and frequent neurological monitoring are indicated for meningitis

CONCLUSION

HHV-7 is a recently discovered virus with many unsolved puzzles. Medicine continues to search for a clinical disease to which it may be attributed. Our understanding of the pathogenesis, transmission, and development of latency of this virus remains limited. With further knowledge acquired through painstaking research, we may one day discover that HHV-7 has a much more important role in clinical medicine.

REFERENCES

1. N Frenkel, EC Schirmer, LS Wyatt, et al. Isolation of a new herpesvirus from human CD4 + T cells. Proc Natl Acad Sci USA 87:748–752, 1990.
2. ZN Berneman, DV Ablashi, G Li, et al. Human herpesvirus 7 is a T-lymphotropic virus and is related to, but significantly different from, human herpesvirus 6 and human cytomegalovirus. Proc Natl Acad Sci USA 89:10552–10556, 1992.
3. J Nicholas. Determination and analysis of the complete nucleotide sequence of human herpesvirus 7. J Virol 70:5975–5989, 1996.
4. P Secchiero, ZN Berneman, RC Gallo, P Lusso. Biological and molecular characteristics of human herpesvirus 7: in vitro growth optimization and development of a syncytia inhibition test. Virology 202:506–512, 1994.
5. GR Krueger, B Koch, N Leyssens, et al. Comparison of seroprevalences of human herpesvirus-6 and -7 in healthy blood donors from nine countries. Vox Sang 75:193–197, 1998.
6. F Wilborn, CA Schmidt, F Lorenz, et al. Human herpesvirus type 7 in blood donors: detection by the polymerase chain reaction. J Med Virol 47:65–69, 1995.
7. F Drago, A Rebora. The new herpesviruses: emerging pathogens of dermatological interest. Arch Dermatol 135:71–75, 1999.
8. LS Wyatt, WJ Rodriguez, N Balachandran, N Frenkel. Human herpesvirus 7: antigenic properties and prevalence in children and adults. J Virol 65:6260–6265, 1991.
9. LM Huang, CY Lee, MY Liu, PI Lee. Primary infections of human herpesvirus-7 and herpesvirus-6: a comparative, longitudinal study up to 6 years of age. Acta Paediatr 86:604–608, 1997.
10. BP Lanphear, CB Hall, J Black, P Auinger. Risk factors for the early acquisition of human herpesvirus 6 and human herpesvirus 7 infections in children. Pediatr Infect Dis J 17;792–795, 1998.
11. LS Wyatt, N Frenkel. Human herpesvirus 7 is a constitutive inhabitant of adult human saliva. J Virol 66:3206–3209, 1992.
12. JB Black, N Inoue, K Kite-Powell, S Zaki, PE Pellett. Frequent isolation of human herpesvirus 7 from saliva. Virus Res 29:91–98, 1993.
13. Y Hidaka, Y Liu, M Yamamoto, et al. Frequent isolation of human herpesvirus 7 from saliva samples. J Med Virol 40:343–346, 1993.
14. E Sada, M Yasukawa, C Ito, et al. Detection of human herpesvirus 6 and human herpesvirus 7 in the submandibular gland, parotid gland, and lip salivary gland by PCR. J Clin Microbiol 34:2320–2321, 1996.
15. T Okuno, H Oishi, K Hayashi, M Nonogaki, K Tanaka, K Yamanishi. Human herpesviruses 6 and 7 in cervixes of pregnant women. J Clin Microbiol 33:1968–1970, 1995.
16. P Lusso, P Secchiero, RW Crowley, A Garzino-Demo, ZN Berneman, RC Gallo. CD4 is a critical component of the receptor for human herpesvirus 7: interference with human immunodeficiency virus. Proc Natl Acad Sci USA 91:3872–3876, 1994.
17. M Furukawa, M Yasukawa, Y Yakushijin, S Fujita. Distinct effects of human herpesvirus 6 and human herpesvirus 7 on surface molecule expression and function of CD4 + T cells. J Immun 152:5768–5775, 1994.
18. H Romi, O Singer, D Rapaport, N Frenkel. Tamplicon-7, a novel T-lymphotropic vector derived from human herpesvirus 7. J Virol 73:7001–7007, 1999.
19. N Frenkel, LS Wyatt. HHV-6 and HHV-7 as exogenous agents in human lymphocytes. Dev Biol Stand 76:259–265, 1992.
20. W Kempf, V Adams, P Mirandola, et al. Persistence of human herpesvirus 7 in normal tissues detected by expression of a structural antigen. J Infect Dis 178:841–845, 1998.
21. DV Ablashi, ZN Berneman, B Kramarsky, J Whitman, Y Asano, GR Pearson. Human herpesvirus-7 (HHV-7): current status. Clin Diag Virol 4:1–13, 1995.
22. HK Osman, JS Peiris, CE Taylor, P Warwicker, RF Jarrett, CR Madeley. ''Cytomegalovirus disease'' in renal allograft recipients. Is human herpesvirus 7 a co-factor for disease progression. J Med Virol 48:295–301, 1996.
23. FZ Wang, H Dahl, A Linde, M Brytting, A Ehrnst, P Ljungman. Lymphotropic herpesviruses in allogeneic bone marrow transplantation. Blood 88:3615–3620, 1996.

24. PK Chan, JS Peiris, KY Yuen, et al. Human herpesvirus-6 and human herpesvirus-7 infections in bone marrow transplant recipients. J Med Virol 53:295–305, 1997.

25. HK Osman, JS Peiris, CE Taylor, JP Karlberg, CR Madeley. Correlation between the detection of viral DNA by the polymerase chain reaction in peripheral blood leukocytes and serological responses to human herpesvirus 6, human herpesvirus 7, and cytomegalovirus in renal allograft recipients. J Med Virol 53:288–294, 1997.

26. K Tanaka-Taya, S Okada. Human herpesvirus-6 and -7 infection and bone marrow transplantation (BMT) [abstract]. Nippon Rinsho 56:208–212, 1998.

27. K Tanaka, T Kondo, S Torigoe, S Okada, T Mukai, K Yamanishi. Human herpesvirus 7: another causal agent for roseola (exanthem subitum). J Pediatr 125:1–5, 1994.

28. Y Hidaka, K Okada, K Kusuhara, C Miyazaki, K Tokugawa, K Ueda. Exanthem subitum and human herpesvirus 7 infection. Pediatr Infect Dis J 13:1010–1011, 1994.

29. Y Asano, S Suga, T Yoshikawa, T Yazaki, T Uchikawa. Clinical features and viral excretion in an infant with primary human herpesvirus 7 infection. Pediatrics 95:187–190, 1995.

30. GC Katsafanas, EC Schirmer, LS Wyatt, N Frenkel. In vitro activation of human herpesviruses 6 and 7 from latency. Proc Natl Acad Sci USA 93:9788–9792, 1996.

31. K Kawa-Ha, K Tanaka, M Inoue, et al. Isolation of human herpesvirus 7 from a child with symptoms mimicking chronic Epstein-Barr virus infection. Brit J Haematol 84:545–548, 1993.

32. MT Caserta, CB Hall, K Schnabel, CE Long, N D'Heron. Primary human herpesvirus 7 infection: a comparison of human herpesvirus 7 and human herpesvirus 6 infections in children. J Pediatr 133:386–389, 1998.

33. M Caserta, CB Hall, K Schnabel, N D'Heron. Human herpesvirus-7 (HHV-7) infection in US children [Abstract 996]. Pediatr Res 39:168A, 1996.

34. M Porolani, C Cermelli, P Mirandola, D Di Luca. Isolation of human herpesvirus 7 from an infant with febrile syndrome. J Med Virol 45:282–283, 1995.

35. F Drago, E Ranieri, F Malaguti, ML Battifoglio, E Losi, A Rebora. Human herpesvirus 7 in patients with pityriasis rosea. Dermatology 195:374–378, 1997.

36. F Drago, E Ranieri, F Malaguti, E Losi, A Rebora. Human herpesvirus 7 in pityriasis rosea. Lancet 349:1367–1368, 1997.

37. W Kempf, V Adams, M Kleinhans, et al. Pityriasis rosea is not associated with human herpesvirus 7. Arch Dermatol 135:1070–1072, 1999.

38. W Kempf, V Adams, M Kleinhans, et al. Human herpesvirus 7 and pityriasis rosea [Abstract]. J Invest Dermatol 110:666,1998.

39. M Yasukawa, E Sada, H Machino, S Fujita. Reactivation of human herpesvirus 6 in pityriasis rosea [letter]. Br J Dermatol 140:169, 1999.

40. T Watanabe, M Sugaya, K Nakamura, K Tamaki. Human herpesvirus 7 and pityriasis rosea. J Invest Dermatol 113:288–289, 1999.

41. S Torigoe, W Koide, M Yamada, E Miyashiro, K Tanaka-Taya, K Yamanishi. Human herpesvirus 7 infection associated with central nervous system manifestations. J Pediatr 129:301–305, 1996.

42. S Torigoe, T Kumamoto, W Koide, K Taya, K Yamanishi. Clinical manifestations associated with human herpesvirus 7 infection. Arch Dis Child 72:518–519, 1995.

43. K Ueda, K Kusuhara, K Okada, et al. Primary human herpesvirus 7 infection and exanthema subitum [letter]. Pediatr Infect Dis J 13:167–168, 1994.

44. S Suga, T Yoshikawa, T Nagai, Y Asano. Clinical features and virological findings in children with primary human herpesvirus 7 infection. Pediatrics 99:E4, 1997.

45. Y Zhang, D Schols, E De Clercq. Selective activity of various antiviral compounds against HHV-7 infection. Antiviral Res 43:23–35, 1999.

46. K Takahashi. Recent advances in antiviral drugs—antiviral agents to HCMV, HHV-6, and HHV-7 [abstract]. Nippon Rinsho 56:140–144, 1998.

47. M Yoshida, M Yamada, T Tsukazaki et al. Comparison of antiviral compounds against human herpesvirus 6 and 7. Antiviral Res 40:73–84, 1998.

10

Human Herpesvirus 8

Tricia J. Brown
University of Oklahoma Health Sciences Center, Oklahoma City, Oklahoma, USA

Angela Yen-Moore
University of Texas Southwestern Medical Center, Dallas, Texas, USA

Stephen K. Tyring
*University of Texas Medical Branch, Galveston, Texas, USA
and University of Texas Medical Branch Center for Clinical Studies, Houston, Texas, USA*

Human herpesvirus 8 (HHV-8), previously called Kaposi's sarcoma-associated herpes virus (KSHV), was first detected in 1994 in Kaposi's sarcoma from patients with acquired immunodeficiency syndrome (AIDS). By using a modified form of polymerase chain reaction, all four types of Kaposi's sarcoma (KS) have been associated with HHV-8: (1) the classic form that typically occurs in elderly Mediterranean men, (2) the endemic form that affects persons of all ages in tropical Africa, (3) the immunosuppressive form that occurs in organ transplant recipients, and (4) the AIDS-associated form [1–4] (Fig. 10–1).

HISTORY

In 1872, Moriz Kaposi first described a rare cutaneous neoplasm that predominantly affected elderly men of Jewish and/or Mediterranean descent [5]. Intense medical interest did not develop until the AIDS epidemic when clusters of young homosexual men began to develop KS [6]. For many years, the cause of KS was suspected to be an infectious agent [7], but it was not until 1994 that Chang et al [8] identified herpes-like DNA sequences isolated from KS lesions of a patient with AIDS. This newly discovered virus was found to be closely related to the gammaher-

pesviruses, Epstein-Barr virus, and *Herpesvirus saimiri*, all of which infect lymphocytes and cause cell immortalization and transformation [9]. HHV-8 also has been associated with other cancers, such as Castleman's disease (an angiofollicular hyperplasia) [10–12] and body-cavity-based lymphomas (BCBL) [13–15] in patients with AIDS.

INCIDENCE

Classic KS occurs mainly in individuals of Mediterranean or Ashkenazi Jewish descent and is uncommon in countries with a small proportion of these ethnic groups. The average age of onset for classic KS is 65 years of age. Approximately 0.6% of organ transplant recipients (e.g., kidney, heart, and liver) develop KS, typically within 5 years of transplantation [16,17]. These tumors most frequently involve transplant recipients of Mediterranean, Jewish, Arabic, or African ancestry [18]. Human immunodeficiency virus (HIV)-positive homosexual men develop KS at a rate that is 20,000-fold higher than that of the general population [19]. African endemic KS is the cause of up to 10% of all histopathologically proven malignancies in southern equatorial Africa with a predominance in males of all ages.

HHV-8 has been found in the vast majority of all types

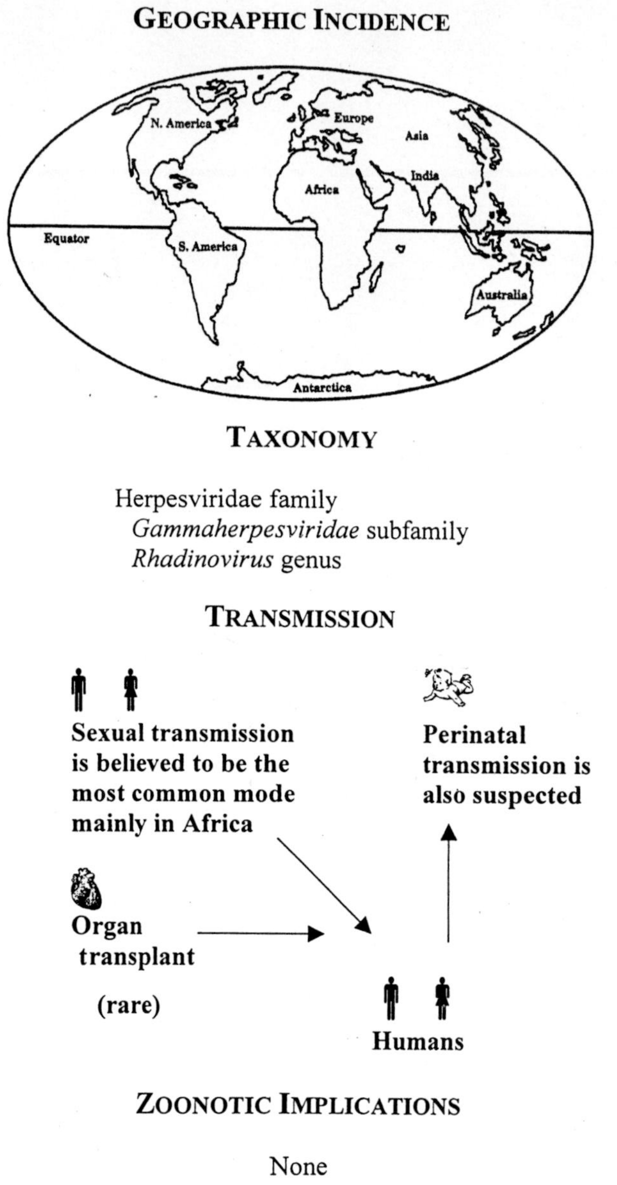

GEOGRAPHIC INCIDENCE

TAXONOMY

Herpesviridae family
Gammaherpesviridae subfamily
Rhadinovirus genus

TRANSMISSION

Sexual transmission is believed to be the most common mode mainly in Africa

Perinatal transmission is also suspected

Organ transplant

(rare)

Humans

ZOONOTIC IMPLICATIONS

None

Figure 10–1. Incidence and transmission of human herpesvirus 8.

of KS lesions across the globe and seroprevalence varies by geographic location. HHV-8 seropositivity is uncommon prior to puberty in the United States, as prevalence rates of antibodies to lytic and latent HHV-8 antigens vary from 0 to 5% in this population [20,21]. The prevalence of antibodies to lytic and latent HHV-8 antigens in otherwise healthy adults without KS in the United States has been reported as 25 to 27% [20,21]. Overall, the seroprevalence rates ranges from less than 5% in North America, Britain, and northern Europe to approximately 10% for southern

Europe [22–24]. In African countries, the HHV-8 seroprevalence rates range from 30 to 100% [22,25–28]. Approximately 30% of HIV-1 infected homosexual men in North America and Europe have evidence of HHV-8 infection [22,29–31]. The seroprevalence rates for HHV-8 closely correspond with the incidence rates for KS, as non–AIDS-related KS occurs more commonly in southern Europe and most frequently in Africa [19,32–34].

PATHOGENESIS

Several studies have evaluated the spread of HHV-8 infection, although our knowledge of this aspect is far from complete. The studies suggest that HHV-8 spreads mainly through sexual transmission among homosexual men in the United States [3,35], whereas mother-to-child transmission occurs most commonly in African countries [26,36,37]. In a study of perinatal transmission, approximately one third of HHV-8 infected mothers transmit the virus to their offspring [36]. Anal receptive intercourse appears to be a major mode of sexual transmission since the incidence of HHV-8 is higher in homosexual men than in HIV-infected women [20]. One study found HHV-8 seropositivity to be strongly associated with the number of homosexual male partners and the presence of HIV infection [35]. Infectious HHV-8 was recovered from the donated blood of one individual, indicating that HHV-8 could possibly be transmitted by blood transfusion [38]. However, no evidence or reports have yet supported this hypothesis. In Uganda, HHV-8 occurrence among prepubertal children suggests a horizontal pattern of transmission, perhaps similar to that of Epstein-Barr virus [27].

The isolation of HHV-8 in various body fluids has not proved to be the mode of transmission and remains controversial. In addition to KS skin lesions, the virus has been isolated in normal skin [39,40], peripheral blood mononuclear cells [39,41–46], seminal fluid [39,41,47–50] and saliva [39,51–53] from HHV-8 infected persons. Presence of HHV-8 in the blood is strongly predictive of later development of KS, with 75% of these patients developing KS within 5 years [42].

Nucleotide sequence analysis at five distinct loci across the 14 Kb genome of more than 60 HHV-8 samples from KS and lymphoma from North America, Africa, Middle East, Asia, and the Pacific have revealed that they cluster into four major subtypes (A, B, C, D). These can be further differentiated into 13 distinctive variants or clades, with B subtypes, found in Africa, being the original. Interestingly, it is hypothesized that the evolution of four distinct strains, each concentrated in different locales, correlates with models describing human migration out of Africa in three distinct waves [54]. The strong association between locales and subtype also indicate that HHV-8 is much more cryptic and much more difficult to transmit than other herpes viruses. [55,56]. This and other epidemiological data thus far strongly suggest that HHV-8 is less ubiquitous than other human herpesviruses [57].

KS is considered to be a vascular endothelial malignancy, although the origin of this tumor is not completely known [58]. Whether this tumor is a true malignancy or an intense cellular proliferation caused by angiogenic factors is not fully elucidated. The function of HHV-8 in the development of KS is not yet understood. Hypotheses include whether the virus is a coagent, has a causal role, or is an innocent bystander in the development of KS [35,59,60].

The role of HIV-1 infection in promotion of HHV-8 replication has been assumed to be due to immunosuppression of the host. Yet, HIV-2 infection is significantly less often associated than HIV-1 with KS despite a high prevalence of HHV-8 [28,61]. In addition, the risk of KS is much higher in those with HIV-1 infection when compared with organ transplant recipients receiving pharmacologic immunosuppression [19]. The promotion of aberrant cytokine production by the HIV-1 tat protein may play a causal role in the development of KS [62,63]. HIV-1 tat stimulates the activation and growth of endothelial cells as well as the expression and production of adhesion molecules and such angiogenic factors as basic fibroblast growth factor (b-FGF).

The 14 Kb genome of HHV-8 is bound at each end by multiple 85% G + C (guanine + cytosine) terminal repeat units. This HHV-8 genome has been sequenced in its entirety except for a 3 Kb sequence near the right end of the genome. Twenty five of the 95 genes of HHV-8 are unique to the Herpesviridae [58]. Those not common to genes found in the herpesviruses are referred to by open reading frame (ORF) number. Molecular studies have revealed a high number of viral oncogenes within the HHV-8 genome, most of which are not expressed in the latent state of HHV-8 infection [60].

Several of the genes believed to be most important in oncogenicity of the HHV-8, including ORF 71, ORF 72 and ORF 73, will be selectively discussed because they are consistently expressed in the latent state of HHV-8 infection [60]. The potential relevance of viral IL-6 will also be discussed. Although this gene is expressed in the lytic cycle, investigators believe it may be significant in a paracrine fashion [64–67].

ORF 71 encodes the viral homologue to cellular FLIP (Fas-ligand-interleukin-2-converting enzyme inhibitor protein) which can inhibit Fas-mediated apoptosis. Normally, when the CD95 or Fas-ligand is activated by natural killer and other effector cells, signal transduction is me-

diated through the Fas-associated death domain protein (FADD). This protein subsequently activates death effector domains (DED) of the protease also known as caspase-8. This activates cysteine proteases, which are responsible for activating the apoptosis cascade. Excessive expression of ORF 71 could be an obvious contributing factor to cell transformation.

ORF 72 is a viral encoded homologue of cellular cyclins that shares the greatest degree of homology with cyclin D2 [59]. Normally, cyclin D2 associates with CDK6 (cyclin dependent kinase 6) and has weaker associations with other CDKs. The cyclin D2-CDK6 complex has the responsibility of phosphorylating RB (retinoblastoma protein) and releasing E2F which activates the S phase genes. The complex formed between ORF 72 and CDK6 is immune to the CDK inhibitors, p16, p21 and p27, which normally inhibit the cyclin D2-CDK6 complex [68]. This could also lead to unregulated progression of the cell cycle and cell transformation.

ORF 73 is the latency-associated nuclear antigen (LANA) which may contribute to HHV-8 induced cell transformation by two distinct mechanisms. Through fluorescence in situ hybridization and immunofluorescence studies, LANA, as well as HHV-8 DNA, has been localized to the metaphase chromosome. It has been hypothesized that LANA tethers the HHV-8 DNA to the metaphase chromosome and maintains the latent state [69]. LANA also has the potential to inhibit the ability of P53 to induce cell death and to repress the transcriptional activity of the P53 gene [70].

Unlike the other genes described above, v-IL 6 is primarily expressed during lytic infection and has not been found to be expressed in the latent state [65]. This, however, does not exclude its capability to contribute in a paracrine fashion since KS lesions contain primarily latently infected cells, interspersed with a few lytically infected cells [60]. Despite expression of UL-6 during lytic infection, KS lesions do not seem to express IL 6 receptor-alpha [59,65]. This is one of the two subunits which form the IL 6 receptor, with the other one being gp 130. Osborne, et al have suggested that v-IL 6, unlike human IL 6, does not require the IL 6 receptor-alpha subunit but is capable of activating the JAK 1 and STAT 1/3 pathways with gp 130 alone [65]. Activation of the JAK1 and STAT 1/3 pathways would lead to increased cell division.

Variance in the expression of v-IL 6 may also be one of the key factors explaining the production of different pathological states from a single etiological agent. One important question, unanswered in HHV-8 research is, ''How is it possible that three distinct disease entities could arise from a single virus?'' These diseases include KS, primary effusion lymphoma (PEL) and multicentric Castleman's disease (MCD). Infection of different cell types and expression of a different genetic program is one theory. Many investigators have reported on differential expression of v-IL 6 as a significant factor [66,67]. For example, it has been determined that v-IL 6 is expressed in both PEL and MCD cells, but not in KS [64]. The explanation for this differential expression has not yet been determined. However, it has been shown that in both KS and PEL, HHV-8 infection is primarily of the latent type.

CLINICAL MANIFESTATIONS

AIDS-related KS typically presents as small macules or patches and/or plaques (Figs. 10–2 to 10–5) (Table 10–1). KS spreads to the oral or perioral areas in more than 50% of AIDS-related mucocutaneous KS and may sometimes be the presenting manifestation of HIV infection [68] (Fig. 10–6). Involvement of the oral mucosa causes significant discomfort, and problems with speech and eating may occur. Genital mucosa is also a common location for KS (Fig. 10–7). Approximately 80% of patients with AIDS-related KS have gastrointestinal involvement, particularly in the stomach and duodenum. Gastrointestinal involvement may lead to such clinical symptoms as nausea, vomiting, gastrointestinal bleeding or ulceration, perforation, and ileus. Pulmonary involvement may result in persistent cough, bronchospasm, or dyspnea with respiratory insufficiency and is associated with a poor prognosis. Overall, AIDS-related KS has a variable course, often with progres-

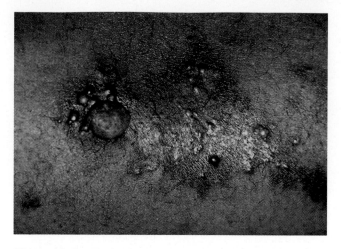

Figure 10–3. Both plaque and nodule stages of Kaposi's sarcoma are seen in this patient with acquired immunodeficiency syndrome.

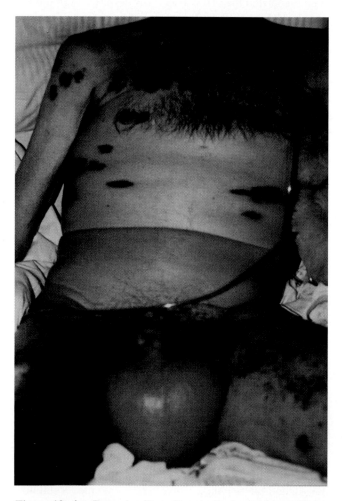

Figure 10–4. Extensive Kaposi's sarcoma in a patient with acquired immunodeficiency syndrome (Photograph courtesy of Axel Hoke, M.D., Novato, CA).

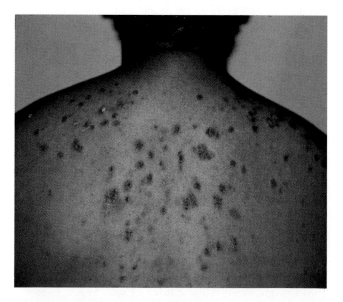

Figure 10–2. Plaques of Kaposi's sarcoma in a patient with acquired immunodeficiency syndrome.

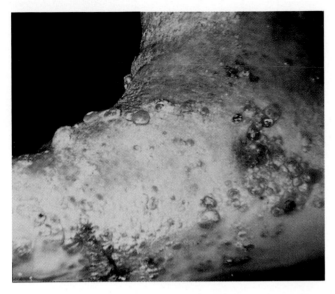

Figure 10–5. Kaposi's sarcoma may be very extensive and become verrucous as in this patient with acquired immunodeficiency syndrome. (Photograph courtesy of Axel Hoke, M.D., Novato, CA.)

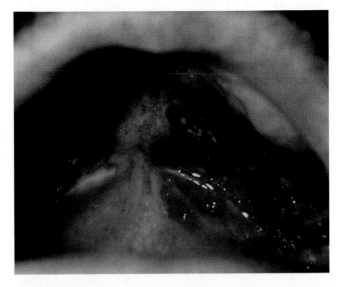

Figure 10–6. More than 50% of AIDS patients with acquired immunodeficiency syndrome with Kaposi's sarcoma will have oral lesions. (Photograph courtesy of Axel Hoke, M.D., Novato, CA.)

Table 10–1. Clinical Manifestations of Kaposi's Sarcoma

Time after exposure	Clinical manifestations	Laboratory analyses	Other notes
Incubation varies and is unknown	Development of small red to pink violaceous or brown macules (often elliptical), particularly in cleavage lines on the trunk. AIDS-related KS most commonly affects the face and trunk. Size varies from several millimeters to several centimeters. Classic KS more often presents as blue-red nodules on the lower legs These lesions may progress to form large plaques All types of KS lesions typically evolve through stages as patches, plaques, and nodules ↓	Histopathologic examination of lesional skin biopsy	AIDS lesions may become plaque-like and exophytic, sometimes with skin ulceration Classic lesions may become more brown, hyperkeratotic, eczematous, or ulcerated. Associated edema is often present is all types Multiple KS lesions of varying stages may be present
Several years	AIDS-related KS may slowly progress, often disseminating to lymph nodes, intestinal mucosa, and lungs. Patients with classic KS survive for at least 10–15 y Immunosuppressive KS may be either rapidly progressive or chronic and slow. In the African endemic form, children usually survive 2–3 yr, while young adults survive several years longer		AIDS-related KS often spreads to the oral mucosa, particularly the palate KS lesions may bleed easily. Pain may develop with large, edematous lesions

AIDS, acquired immunodeficiency syndrome.

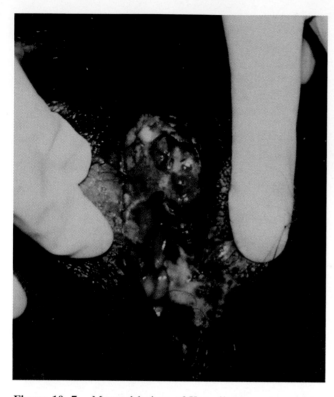

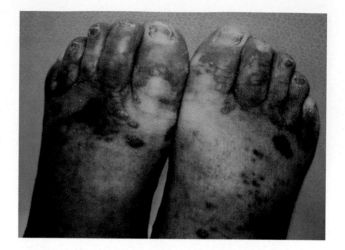

Figure 10–8. Classic Kaposi's sarcoma lesions most often affect the lower legs and feet as seen in this elderly man.

Figure 10–7. Mucosal lesions of Kaposi's sarcoma may also be observed in the vaginal canal in a patient with acquired immunodeficiency syndrome. (Photograph courtesy of Concepcion Arrastia, M.D., Department of Obstetrics and Gynecology, University of Texas Medical Branch at Galveston, Galveston, TX.)

sive deterioration after significant declines in CD4+ cell counts.

Classic KS typically has a slow progression and a benign and protracted course of disease. The early lesions have a spongy feel, but with time, they become firm. This variant classically involves the lower legs of elderly Mediterranean males, but it rarely develops on the oral mucous membranes and gastrointestinal tract [69] (Figs. 10–8 and 10–9).

KS associated with immunosuppression has a clinical course similar to classic or AIDS-related KS. This iatrogenic form of KS may have an aggressive course with rampant progression and dissemination unless the immunosuppressive agents are discontinued [70]. The lesions may improve or completely resolve with a reduction or withdrawal of immunosuppressive agents [71], and they may recur with resumption of immunosuppressive therapy [72].

The African endemic variant of KS has four subtypes: nodular, lymphadenopathic, florid, and infiltrative. The nodular form is most similar to classic KS and typically has a benign course lasting 5 to 8 years. A limited number

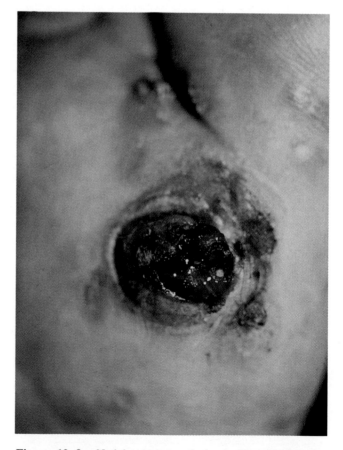

Figure 10–9. Nodular lesions of classic Kaposi's sarcoma made walking very difficult this elderly man, especially because of ulceration of some plantar lesions.

of cutaneous, well-circumscribed nodules are present with this form. The lymphadenopathic variant more commonly affects children and young adults and involves lymph nodes more often than skin. The florid type is more aggressive than the nodular form and may spread deeply to involve the dermis, subcutaneous tissue, muscle, and bone. The infiltrative form is even more aggressive. These two latter forms typically have extensive cutaneous lesions on one or more extremities.

KS is a highly vascular tumor, with some resemblance to angiosarcomas. Despite several case reports that indicate the presence of HHV-8 in angiosarcoma [73], most studies with large patient numbers have shown a low prevalence of 0 to 18% of HHV-8 in vascular tumors [74]. Lasota and Mittienem found a prevalence of 18% for HHV-8 in 33 cases of angiosarcoma [75]. Similar results have been found in other vascular tumors, including angiokeratomas, papillary haemangiomas, pyogenic granulomas, cavernous hemangiomas, arteriovenous hemangiomas, circumscribed lymphangioma, and hemangiopericytoma. In contrast to these vascular tumors, preliminary evidence supports a role for HHV-8 in angiolymphoid hyperplasia with eosinophilia (AHLE), which is an uncommon disorder characterized by soft angiomatous tumors on the face, ear, and scalp [76]. Subsequent studies confirming or disputing this evidence are needed.

With the discovery of HHV-8 in KS, researchers were quick to determine whether HHV-8 had a role in other more common epithelial lesions. KS is occasionally detected by polymerase chain reaction (PCR) in squamous cell caercinoma (SCC), actinic keratosis (AK), seborrheic keratosis (SK), basal cell carcinoma (BCC), leukoplakia, and Bowen's disease, leading some to believe that HHV-8 is much more ubiquitous than previously believed [77,78]. Furthermore, the virus becomes active and hence detectable in the immunocompromised, contributing to the development of the lesions described above. Most experts, however, feel that HHV-8 has little to do with the pathophysiology of these lesions [79]. In fact, extensive studies have been done on these and other epithelial lesions, including verruca vulgaris (VV), atypical squamous proliferation (ASP), Paget's disease, malignant melanoma, neurofibroma, sarcomas, histiocytofibroma, nevi, and chronic dermatitides. The presence of HHV-8 in these lesions was comparable to normal skin and consistently showed a lack of correlation between HHV-8 and all of the aforementioned lesions [79–84].

The reported presence of HHV-8 in 4 of 6 patients with pemphigus vulgaris and 6 of 6 patients with pemphigus foliaceus in 1997 was the first study to associate HHV-8 and pemphigus [85,86]. Since then, further studies regarding the prevalence of HHV-8 in paraneoplastic pemphigus, pemphigus vulgaris, and pemphigus foliaceus have been

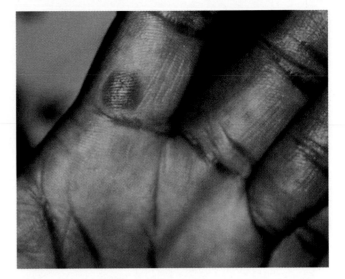

Figure 10–10. This angioma on the palm of a woman with POEMS (polyneuropathy, organomegaly, endocrinopathy, M protein, skin changes) syndrome and multicentric Castleman's disease contained human herpesvirus 8. (Photograph Courtesy of Tiffany Angel, M.D., Department of Dermatology, Baylor College of Medicine, Houston, TX.)

done using in situ hybridization, PCR, and serology. Most investigators have been unable to detect the presence of HHV-8 in pemphigus and doubt the existence of a causal relationship [87–90]. Other than KS, the malignancy most often associated with KS is Castleman's disease. POEMS syndrome (polyneuropathy, organomegaly, endocrinopathy, M protein, skin changes) is commonly coexistent with multicentric Castleman's disease. HHV-8 has been reported in POEMS syndrome coexisting with multicentric Castleman's disease (Fig. 10–10) [91].

DERMATOPATHOLOGY

The histology of the different variants of KS generally is identical. Histopathological examination reveals jagged vascular channels lined by atypical vascular endothelial cells (Fig. 10–11). These vessels are surrounded by a proliferation of spindle-shaped cells. KS lesions often progress through a series of three stages, each with characteristic histological changes. During the patch stage, the presence of a predominantly lymphocytic perivascular infiltrate (+/– plasma cells) may be minimal. Changes are limited typically to the reticular dermis early but progress to involve the entire dermis. A subtle proliferation of irregular, jagged endothelial-lined spaces around normal blood vessels may be seen microscopically.

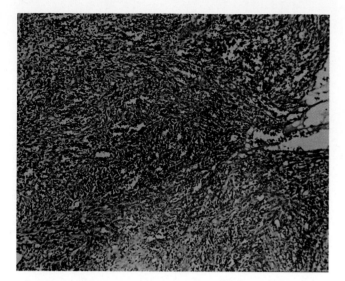

Figure 10–11. Histopathologic examination of Kaposi's sarcoma reveals jagged vascular channels lined by atypical vascular endothelial cells. These vessels are surrounded by a proliferation of spindle-shaped cells.

Table 10–2. Differential Diagnoses of Kaposi's Sarcoma (KS)

Insect bite: Lesions of KS are more violaceous than insect bites

Dermatofibroma: Lesions of KS are more violaceous than dermatofibromas

Ecchymosis: Lesions of KS may feel firm on palpation, whereas ecchymotic lesions tend to be flat and involve larger areas

Hemangioma: Lesions of KS are more violaceous than hemangiomas

Bacillary angiomatosis: Lesions of KS are generally less raised and less discrete than bacillary angiomatosis

Pyogenic granuloma: Lesions of KS are generally more violaceous than pyogenic granulomas

Melanocytic nevus: Lesions of KS are generally more erythematous: violaceous than melanocytic nevi

Verruga peruana: Lesions of KS are generally less raised and less discrete than those of verruga peruana, which is usually found only among people living in high elevations in Peru

During the plaque stage, there is a proliferation of spindle cells among dermal collagen bundles and vessels. Hemosiderin deposits and hyaline globules become prominent. The predominant lymphocytic perivascular infiltrate is still evident and remains throughout the course of disease. The neoplastic process begins to involve the superficial subcutaneous tissue.

The nodular stage of KS consists of a well-circumscribed intradermal nodule of cuboidal vascular endothelial cells arranged in fascicles and sheets, with slit-like vascular spaces between them. Single erythrocytes can be seen trapped within the vascular slits. Cytological atypia, ranging from mild to moderate, is present in the spindle cells. Mitotic figures may be scant or numerous.

DIAGNOSIS

Diagnosis of KS is confirmed by examination of a skin biopsy from the suspected lesion. Serology for HHV-8 is not indicated and is typically limited to the research environment. Table 10–2 lists possible differential diagnoses.

TREATMENT AND PREVENTION

A complete cure for KS is not available currently, and treatment is aimed at palliation and control of disease (Table 10–3). For iatrogenic KS, reduction or cessation of

immunosuppressive therapy generally leads to regression or resolution of disease, although the KS lesions often recur with reinstitution of immunosuppressive agents. With all forms of KS, inconspicuous, small, slow-growing cutaneous lesions may be monitored without treatment. Treatment is indicated if the lesions become cosmetically disturbing to the patient or if complications such as bleeding, lymphedema, or interference with functional activity develop. Classic KS lesions usually respond well to radiotherapy, and AIDS-associated KS lesions are extremely sensitive to this modality. Clinical studies have reported complete response with radiotherapy of KS lesions in 32 to 85% of patients [92,93]. Higher doses of radiation typically lead to higher response rates, and early lesions tend to respond more than mature lesions [94]. Surgery is generally not considered to be an effective therapy (Fig. 10–12). Intralesional vinblastine in localized lesions has a 60 to 90% response rate, which lasts for several months [95]. This modality is most effective for early small lesions. Side effects may include pain, alterations in skin pigmentation, and transient alopecia when vinblastine is injected in hair-bearing areas. Other intralesional agents also may be used (see Table 10–3). Intralesional interferon-α and tumor necrosis factor-α have high rates of complete response, although results are slow and side effects may include pain, local inflammation, and systemic symptoms [95,96]. Recently, the first topical at-home therapy for limited KS disease was approved for use in the United States [97,98].

Table 10–3.   Treatment of Kaposi's Sarcoma

Symptom	Treatment
Inconspicuous lesions	May be monitored without treatment
Limited disease	Cryotherapy for flat or superficial lesions, with two freeze thaw cycles Laser therapy (pulsed-dye laser) for small superficial lesions only Surgical excision for selected small solitary lesions only Radiotherapy is particularly good for facial lesions, lymphedema, or painful or bulky local lesions. Also indicated for confluent lesions involving a large surface area, large extremity lesions, or large oropharyngeal lesions Intralesional chemotherapy, with interferon-α, tumor necrosis factor -α, vinblastine, bleomycin, or the sclerosing agent, sodium tetradecyl sulfate (for oral lesions) Vinblastine is administered as 0.1 mg injected per square centimeter, which may be repeated in 3 weeks for recalcitrant lesions. Persistent lesions may be given incremental injections at doses of up to 0.2 mg per square centimeter Topical alitretinoin 0.1% gel, applied twice daily, and gradually increased to 3 to 4 applications daily, as tolerated Electrodessication Hyperthermia
Extensive disease	Systemic interferon-α, given at 30 million IU/m^2 3 times a wk until no further evidence of tumor, unless contraindications prevent continuation of therapy
Note: Single best treatment for HIV(+) KS is HAART	Systemic interferon-α with zidovudine but zidovudine is no longer used for monotherapy of HIV except where it is the only treatment available Systemic chemotherapy is most commonly performed with paclitaxel or with liposomal doxorubicin or daunorubicin Alternative chemotherapeutic agents include vinblastine, adriamycin, bleomycin, doxorubicin, daunorubicin, etoposide, retinoic acid, and teniposide. These agents may be used in combination or alone.

HIV, human immunodeficiency virus.

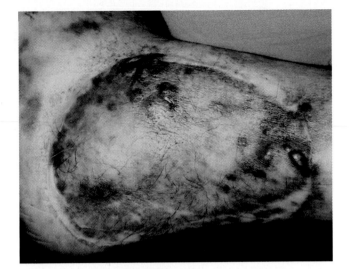

Figure 10–12.   Nodules of Kaposi's sarcoma (KS) are seen appearing in this graft that was used in the repair of the surgical site of a previous KS lesion. (Photograph courtesy of Luke Lewis, M.D., and Robert Purvis, M.D., Department of Dermatology, Texas Technological University Health Science Center, Lubbock, TX.)

Alitretinoin 0.1% gel is a 9-*cis*-retinoic acid that has a 35% response rate, typically seen within 12 to 16 weeks of therapy. Side effects include rash, pain, and paresthesia. This agent should not be applied to mucosal lesions.

Prior to the AIDS epidemic, systemic chemotherapeutic agents were traditionally administered for extensive classic and endemic KS disease [99]. With combination therapy, response rates are improved, although survival is not prolonged [95,100]. The liposomal encapsulated forms of doxorubicin and daunorubicin have shown more promising results in the treatment of classic and AIDS-related KS. These agents are more effective and significantly less toxic than their older counterparts [100–102].

With the advent of highly active antiretroviral therapy (HAART), the incidence of AIDS-associated Kaposi's sarcoma has been decreasing steadily [103]. This may be due to the supportive effect of HAART on KS via decreased HIV-related cytokines (rapid effect) on the immune system, the suppression of the HIV Tat protein, which stimulates KS spindle cell production [104,105], or other mechanisms. With the recent knowledge that KS is associated with HHV-8 infection, newer therapies have focused on the antiviral agents. In vitro susceptibility testing has shown HHV-8 to be insensitive to acyclovir, but sensitive to ganciclovir and foscarnet [106]. In vivo case reports and clinical trials have shown differing results in some cases. Improvement, remission, or prevention of KS lesions has been reported with foscarnet [107–110], ganciclovir [109,110], and cidofovir treatment [111], often administered for cytomegalovirus retinitis. However, reports of no improvement of KS or HHV-8 with cidofovir [112], foscarnet [45], and ganciclovir therapy [45,107] have been described.

Systemic interferon-α therapy has been studied more thoroughly than other antiviral agents for the treatment of KS. This modality is most successful for the treatment of extensive mucocutaneous disease or asymptomatic visceral involvement in patients who have an intact immune system. In clinical trials, overall response rates, including partial response, range from 30 to 46% [113–116]. In general, higher doses of interferon are more effective than lower doses in inducing tumor regression [114,115,117]. Patients who respond to interferon-α treatment have prolonged survival compared with nonresponders [114,115]. Many months of therapy are required before tumor response becomes evident, and patients must often discontinue therapy prior to improvement because of severe adverse effects. These side effects may include fever, chills, fatigue, malaise, nausea, vomiting, mental status changes, myalgias, anorexia, weight loss, diarrhea, hypotension, hepatotoxicity, and neutropenia [113–116]. Neutropenia and extreme fatigue are the most common dose-limiting factors. In patients with AIDS-associated KS, a combination of systemic interferon-α and zidovudine has been shown to be effective

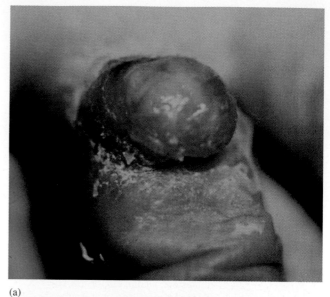

(a)

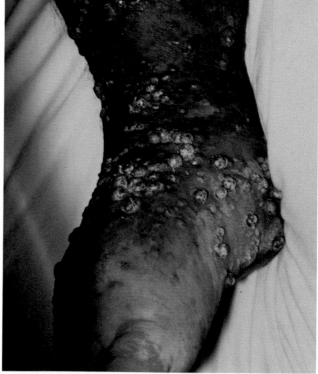

(b)

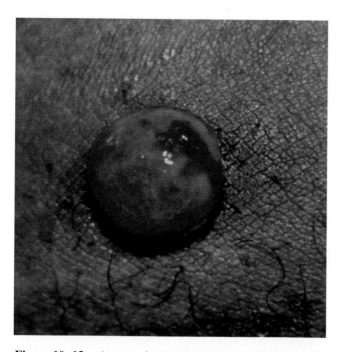

Figure 10–13. A pyogenic granuloma may have a clinical appearance very similar to that of nodular Kaposi's sarcoma.

Figure 10–14. (a) A solitary lesion of bacillary angiomatosis may mimic a progenic granuloma or nodular Kaposi's sarcoma (KS). (b) Rarely, bacillary angiomatosis lesions may be multiple and verrucous, thus mimicking KS (as seen in Fig. 10–5). (Photograph a courtesy of Timothy Berger, M.D., Department of Dermatology, University of California San Francisco School of Medicine, San Francisco, CA); photograph b courtesy of Axel Hoke, M.D., Novato, CA.)

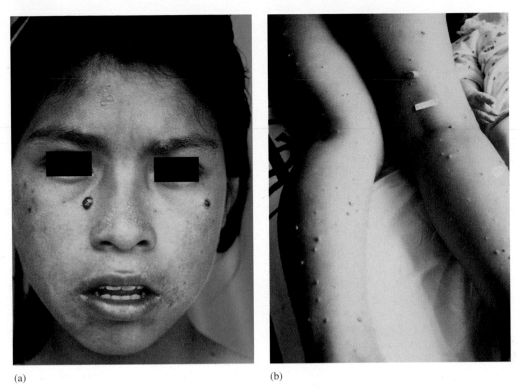

(a)   (b)

Figure 10–15. (a,b) Although rarely observed in persons living in locations other than the high elevations of Peru, verruga peruana may mimic nodular lesions of Kaposi's sarcoma, but it often may appear identical to bacillary angiomatosis. (Photographs courtesy of Francisco Bravo, M.D., Universidad Peruana Cayetano Heredia, Lima, Peru.)

[118–122]. Zidovudine is no longer used for monotherapy of HIV except when it is the only treatment available.

With the need for more effective treatment of KS, many novel therapies are currently under evaluation. Oral retinoic acid therapy, with either *trans*-retinoic acid [123] or 9-cis-retinoic acid [124], has demonstrated some promising results in clinical trials. Intralesional human chorionic gonadotropin (HCG) has been shown to induce regression of KS lesions in a dose-dependent manner [125,126]. Thalidomide [127] and intravenous immunoglobulin [128] also have produced regression of KS lesions in anecdotal reports.

Because the transmission of HHV-8 is not known entirely, methods of prevention have not been determined. If HHV-8 acquisition is associated with high-risk sexual behaviors, it is assumed, but not proved, that the practice of safe sex may decrease the risk of infection. Further studies are needed to expand our knowledge of this and other areas concerning KS and HHV-8.

CONCLUSION

HHV-8 is a recently discovered human herpesvirus with significant clinical implications because of its association with KS. The AIDS epidemic and its resulting dramatic increase in KS tumors have brought HHV-8 to the forefront of medicine. Although the various clinical stages are usually recognized easily, KS may be mimicked by a variety of other conditions, such as pyogenic granuloma (Fig. 10–13), bacillary angiomatosis (Fig. 10–14), or even verruga peruana (Fig. 10–15). Unfortunately, the understanding of HHV-8 is limited, and further studies are necessary to expand the knowledge base of the transmission, pathogenesis, and optimal treatment for this virus.

REFERENCES

1. B Safai, KG Johnson, PL Myskowski, B Koziner, SY Yang, S Cunningham-Rundles, JH Godbold, B Dupont. The natural history of Kaposi's sarcoma in the acquired immunodeficiency syndrome. Ann Intern Med 103: 744–750, 1985.
2. V Beral, H Jaffe, R Weiss. Cancer surveys: cancer, HIV, and AIDS. Eur J Cancer 27:1057–1058, 1991.
3. V Beral, TA Peterman, RL Berkelman, HW Jaffe. Kaposi's sarcoma among persons with AIDS: a sexually transmitted infection? Lancet 335:123–128, 1990.
4. Centers for Disease Control and Prevention. First 500,000

AIDS cases—United States, 1995. MMWR 44:849–853, 1995.

5. HW Haverkos. Factors associated with the pathogenesis of AIDS. J Infect Dis 156:251–257, 1987.

6. Centers for Disease Control and Prevention. Epidemiologic aspects of the current outbreak of Kaposi's sarcoma and opportunistic infection. N Engl J Med 306:248–252, 1982.

7. B Sigeal, S Levinton-Kriss, A Schiffer, J Sayar, I Engelberg, A Vonsover, Y Ramon, E Rubinstein. Kaposi's sarcoma in immunosuppression. Possibly the result of a dual viral infection. Cancer 65:492–498, 1990.

8. Y Chang, E Cesarman, M Pessin, F Lee, J Culpepper, DM Knowles, PS Moore. Identification of herpesvirus-like DNA sequences in AIDS-associated Kaposi's sarcoma. Science 266:1865–1869, 1994.

9. P Moore, SJ Gao, G Dominguez, E Cesarman, O Lungu, DM Knowles, R Garber, PE Pellett, DJ McGeoch, Y Chang. Primary characterization of a herpesvirus agent associated with Kaposi's sarcoma. J Virol 70:549–558, 1996.

10. N Dupin, I Gorin, J Deleuze, H Agut, JM Huraux, JP Escande. Herpes-like DNA sequences, AIDS-related tumors, and Castleman's disease. N Engl J Med 333:798–799, 1995.

11. J Soulier, L Grollet, E Oksenhendler, P Cacoub, D Cazals-Hatem, P Babinet, MF d'Agay, JP Clauvel, M Raphael, L Degos, et al. Kaposi's sarcoma-associated herpesvirus-like DNA sequences in multicentric Castleman's disease. Blood 86:1276–1280, 1995.

12. A Gessain, A Sudaka, J Briere, N Fouchard, MA Nicola, B Rio, M Arborio, X Troussard, J Audouin, J Diebold, et al. Kaposi sarcoma-associated herpesvirus-like virus (human herpesvirus type 8) DNA sequences in multicentric Castleman's disease: is there any relevant association in non-human immunodeficiency virus-infected patients? Blood 87:414–416, 1996.

13. E-Cesarman, Y Chang, PS Moore, JW Said, DM Knowles. Kaposi's sarcoma-associated herpesvirus-like DNA sequences in AIDS-related body-cavity-based lymphomas. N Engl J Med 332:1186–1191, 1995.

14. G Gaidano, C Pastore, A Gloghini, M Cusini, J Nomdedeu, G Volpe, D Capello, E Vaccher, R Bordes, U Tirelli, G Saglio, A Carbone. Distribution of human herpesvirus-8 sequences throughout the spectrum of AIDS-related neoplasia. AIDS 10:941–949, 1996.

15. MQ Ansari, DB Dawson, R Nador, C Rutherford, NR Schneider, MJ Latimer, L Picker, DM Knowles, RW McKenna. Primary body cavity-based AIDS related lymphomas. Am J Clin Pathol 105:221–229, 1996.

16. C Hiesse, F Kriaa, P Rieu, JR Larue, G Benoit, J Bellamy, P Blanchet, B Charpentier. Incidence and type of malignancies occurring after renal transplantation in conventionally and cyclosporine-treated recipients: analysis of a 20-year period in 1600 patients. Transplant Proc 27:972–974, 1995.

17. F Colina, F Lopez-Rios, C Lumbreras, J Martinez-Laso, IG Garcia, E Moreno-Gonzalez. Kaposi's sarcoma developing in a liver graft. Transplantation 61:1779–1781, 1996.

18. RJ Biggar, CS Rabkin. The epidemiology of AIDS-related neoplasms. Hematol Oncol Clin North Am 10:997–1010, 1996.

19. V Beral. Epidemiology of Kaposi's sarcoma. Cancer Surv 10:5–22, 1991.

20. ET Lennette, DJ Blackbourn, JA Levy. Antibodies to human herpesvirus type 8 in the general population and in Kaposi's sarcoma patients. Lancet 348:858–861, 1996.

21. A Blauvelt, S Sei, PM Cook, TF Schultz, KT Jeang. Human herpesvirus 8 infection occurs following adolescence in the United States. J Infect Dis 176:771–774, 1997.

22. SJ Gao, L Kingsley, M Li, W Zheng, C Parravicini, J Ziegler, R Newton, CR Rinaldo, A Saah, J Phair, R Detels, Y Chang, PS Moore. KSHV antibodies among Americans, Italians, and Ugandans with and without Kaposi's sarcoma. Nature Med 2:925–928, 1996.

23. GR Simpson, TF Schulz, D Whitby, PM Cook, C Boshoff, L Rainbow, MR Howard, SJ Gao, RA Bohenzky, P Simmonds, C Lee, A de Ruiter, A Hatzakis, RS Tedder, IV Weller, RA Weiss, PS Moore. Prevalence of Kaposi's sarcoma-associated herpesvirus infection measured by antibodies to recombinant capsid protein and latent immunofluorescence antigen. Lancet 348:1133–1138, 1996.

24. C Boshoff. Kaposi's sarcoma associated herpesvirus. Cancer Surv 33:157–190, 1999.

25. Y Chang, J Ziegler, H Wabinga, E Katangole-Mbidde, C Boshoff, T Schulz, D Whitby, D Maddalena, HW Jaffe, RA Weiss, PS Moore. Kaposi's sarcoma-associated herpesvirus and Kaposi's sarcoma in Africa. Arch Intern Med 156:202–204, 1996.

26. J He, G Bhat, C Kankasa, C Chintu, C Mitchell, W Duan, C Wood. Seroprevalence of human herpesvirus 8 among Zambian women of childbearing age without Kaposi's sarcoma (KS) and mother-child pairs of KS. J Infect Dis 178:1787–1790, 1998.

27. S Mayama, LE Cuevas, J Sheldon, OH Omar, DH Smith, P Okong, B Silvel, CA Hart, TF Schulz. Prevalence and transmission of Kaposi's sarcoma-associated herpesvirus (human herpesvirus 8) in Ugandan children and adolescents. Int J Cancer 77:817–820, 1998.

28. K Ariyoshi, M Schim van der Loeff, P Cook, D Whitby, T Corrah, S Jaffar, F Cham, S Sabally, D O'Donovan, RA Weiss, TF Schulz, H Whittle. Kaposi's sarcoma in the Gambia, West Africa is less frequent in human immunodeficiency virus type 2 than in human immunodeficiency virus type 1 infection despite a high prevalence of human herpesvirus 8. J Hum Virol 1:193–199, 1998.

29. DH Kedes, E Operskalski, M Busch, R Kohn, J Flood, D Ganem. The seroepidemiology of human herpesvirus 8 (Kaposi's sarcoma associated herpesvirus): distribution of infection in KS risk groups and evidence for sexual transmission. Nat Med 2:918–924, 1996.

30. N Renwick, T Halaby, GJ Weverling, NH Dukers, GR Simpson, RA Coutinho, JM Lange, TF Schulz, J Goudsmit. Seroconversion for human herpesvirus 8 during HIV infection is highly predictive of Kaposi's sarcoma. AIDS 12:2481–2488, 1998.

31. G Rezza, M Andreoni, M Dorrucci, P Pezzotti, P Monini, R Zerboni, B Salassa, V Colangeli, L Sarmati, E Nicastri, M Barbanera, R Pristera, F Aiuti, L Ortona, B Ensoli. Human herpesvirus 8 seropositivity and risk of Kaposi's sarcoma and other acquired immunodeficiency syndrome-related diseases. J Natl Cancer Inst 91:1468–1474, 1999.

32. RJ Biggar, J Horm, JF Fraumeni Jr, MH Greene, JJ Goedert. Incidence of Kaposi's sarcoma and mycosis fungoides in the United States including Puerto Rico, 1973–1981. J Natl Cancer Inst 73:89–94, 1984.

33. AE Grulich, V Beral, AJ Swerdlow. Kaposi's sarcoma in England and Wales before the AIDS epidemic. Br J Cancer 66:1135–1137, 1992.

34. H Hjalgrim, M Melbye, E Pukkala, F Langmark, M Frisch, M Dictor, A Ekbom. Epidemiology of Kaposi's sarcoma in the Nordic countries before the AIDS epidemic. Br J Cancer 74:1499–1502, 1996.

35. JN Martin, DE Ganem, DH Osmond, KA Page-Shafer, D Macrae, DH Kedes. Sexual transmission and the natural history of human herpesvirus 8 infection. N Engl J Med 338:948–954, 1998.

36. D Bourboulia, D Whitby, C Boshoff, R Newton, V Beral, H Carrara, A Lane, F Sitas. Serologic evidence for mother-to-child transmission of Kaposi sarcoma-associated herpesvirus infection. JAMA 280:31–32, 1998.

37. FC Kasolo, E Mpabalwani, UA Gompels. Infection with AIDS-related herpesviruses in human immunodeficiency virus-negative infants and endemic childhood Kaposi's sarcoma in Africa. J Gen Virol 78:847–855, 1997.

38. DJ Blackbourn, J Ambroziak, E Lennette, M Adams, B Ramachandran, JA Levy. Infectious human herpesvirus 8 in a healthy North American blood donor. Lancet 349:609–611, 1997.

39. JR LaDuca, JL Love, LZ Abbott, S Dube, AE Freidman-Kien, B Poiesz. Detection of human herpesvirus 8 DNA sequences in tissues and bodily fluids. J Infect Dis 178:1610–1615, 1998.

40. M Dictor, E Rambech, D Way, M Witte, N Bendsoe. Human herpesvirus 8 (Kaposi's sarcoma-associated herpesvirus) DNA in Kaposi's sarcoma lesions, AIDS Kaposi's sarcoma cell lines, endothelial Kaposi's sarcoma simulators, and the skin of immunosuppressed patients. Am J Pathol 148:2009–2016, 1996.

41. YQ Huang, JJ Li, BJ Poiesz, MH Kaplan, AE Friedman-Kien. Detection of the herpesvirus-like DNA sequences in matched specimens of semen and blood from patients with AIDS-related Kaposi's sarcoma by polymerase chain reaction and in situ hybridization. Am J Pathol 150:147–153, 1997.

42. D Whitby, MR Howard, M Tenant-Flowers, NS Brink, A Copas, C Boshoff, T Hatzioannou, FE Suggett, DM Aldam, AS Denton, et al. Detection of Kaposi's sarcoma associated herpesvirus in peripheral blood of HIV-infected individuals and progression to Kaposi's sarcoma. Lancet 346:799–802, 1995.

43. MS Smith, C Bloomer, R Horvat, E Goldstein, JM Casparian, B Chandran. Detection of human herpesvirus 8 DNA in Kaposi's sarcoma lesions and peripheral blood of human immunodeficiency virus-positive patients and correlation with serologic measurements. J Infect Dis 176:84–93, 1997.

44. SF Purvis, E Katongole-Mbidde, JL Johnson, DG Leonard, N Byabazaire, C Luckey, HE Schick, R Wallis, CA Elmets, CZ Giam. High incidence of Kaposi's sarcoma-associated herpesvirus and Epstein-Barr virus in tumor lesions and peripheral blood mononuclear cells from patients with Kaposi's sarcoma in Uganda. J Infect Dis 175:947–950, 1997.

45. RW Humphrey, TR O'Brien, FM Newcomb, H Nishihara, KM Wyvill, GA Ramos, MW Saville, JJ Goedert, SE Straus, R Yarchoan. Kaposi's sarcoma-associated herpesvirus-like DNA sequences in peripheral blood mononuclear cells: association with KS and persistence in patients receiving anti-herpesvirus drugs. Blood 88:297–301, 1996.

46. DA Rizzeri, J Liu, D Miralles, ST Traweek. Kaposi's-sarcoma associated herpesvirus is detected in peripheral blood mononuclear cells of HIV-infected homosexuals more often than in heterosexuals. Cancer J Sci Am 3:140–141, 1997.

47. P Monini, L de Lellis, M Fabris, F Rigolin, E Cassai. Kaposi's sarcoma-associated herpesvirus DNA sequences in prostate tissue and human semen. N Engl J Med 334:1168–1172, 1996.

48. DJ Blackbourn, JA Levy. Human herpesvirus 8 in semen and prostate. AIDS 11:249–250, 1997.

49. MR Howard, D Whitby, G Bahadur, F Suggett, C Boshoff, M Tenant-Flowers, TF Schulz, S Kirk, S Matthews, IV Weller, RS Tedder, RA Weiss. Detection of human herpesvirus 8 DNA in semen from HIV-infected individuals but not healthy semen donors. AIDS 11:F15–19, 1997.

50. P Gupta, MK Singh, C Rinaldo, M Ding, H Farzadegan, A Saah, D Hoover, P Moore, L Kingsley. Detection of Kaposi's sarcoma herpesvirus DNA in semen of homosexual men with Kaposi's sarcoma. AIDS 10:1596–1598, 1996.

51. I Boldogh, P Szaniszlo, WA Bresnahan, CM Flaitz, MC Nichols, T Albrecht. Kaposi's sarcoma herpesvirus-like DNA sequences in the saliva of individuals infected with human immunodeficiency virus. Clin Infect Dis 23:406–407, 1996.

52. DM Koelle, ML Huang, B Chandran, J Vieira, M Piepkorn, L Corey. Frequent detection of Kaposi's sarcoma-associated herpesvirus (human herpesvirus 8) DNA in saliva of human immunodeficiency virus-infected men: clinical and immunologic correlates. J Infect Dis 176:94–102, 1997.

53. J Viera, M Huang, DM Koelle, L Corey. Transmissible

Kaposi's sarcoma-associated herpesvirus (human herpesvirus 8) in saliva of men with a history of Kaposi's sarcoma. J Virol 71:7083–7087, 1997.

54. G Hayward. KSHV strains: the origins and global spread of the virus. Semin Cancer Biol 9:187–199, 1999.

55. S Engelbrecht, F Treurnicht, J Schneider, F Jordaan, J Steytler, PA Wranz, EJ van Rensburg. Detection of human herpes virus 8 DNA and sequence polymorphism in classical, epidemic, and iatrogenic Kaposi's sarcoma in South Africa. J Med Virol 52:168–172, 1997.

56. P Cook-Mozaffari, R Newton, V Beral, DP Burkitt. The geographical distribution of Kaposi's sarcoma and of lymphomas in Africa before the AIDS epidemic. Br J Cancer 78(11):1521–1528, 1998.

57. L Cahtlynne, D Ablashi. Seroepidemiology of Kaposi's sarcoma-associated herpesvirus (KSHV). Semin Cancer Biol 9:175–185, 1999.

58. C Boshoff, F Schultz, MM Kennedy, AK Graham, C Fisher, A Thomas, JO McGee, RA Weiss, JJ O'Leary. Kaposi's sarcoma-associated herpesvirus infects endothelial and spindle cells. Nat Med 1:1274–1278, 1995.

59. F. Neipel, B Fleckenstein. The role of HHV-8 in Kaposi's sarcoma. Semin Cancer Biol 9:151–164, 1999.

60. A Yen-Moore, SD Hudnall, PL Rady, RF Wagner Jr, TO Moore, O Memar, TK Hughes, SK Tyring. Differential expression of the HHV-8 vGCR cellular homolog gene in AIDS-associated and classic Kaposi's sarcoma: potential role of HIV-1 Tat. Virology 267:247–251, 2000.

61. R Sarid, S Olsen, P Moore. Kaposi's sarcoma-associated herpesvirus: Epidemiology, virology, and molecular biology. Adv Virus Res 52:139–232, 1999.

62. RC Gallo. The enigmas of Kaposi's sarcoma. Science 282:1837–1839, 1998.

63. MS Reitz, LS Nerurkar, RC Gallo. Perspective on Kaposi's sarcoma: facts, concepts, and conjectures. J Natl Cancer Inst 91:1453–1458, 1990.

64. C Parravinci, M Corbellino, M Paulli, U Magrini, M Lazzarino, PS Moore, Y Chang. Expression of a virus-derived cytokine, KSHV vIL-6, in HIV-seronegative Castleman's disease. Am J Pathol 151(6):1517–1522, 1997.

65. J Osborne, P Moore, Y Chang. KSHV-encoded viral IL-6 activates multiple human IL-6 signaling pathways. Human Immunol 60:921–927, 1999.

66. J Cannon, J Nicholas, J Orenstein, R Mann, P Murray, P Browning, JA DiGiuseppe, E Cesarman, GS Hayward, RF Ambinder. Herterogeneity of viral IL-6 expression in HHV-8-associated diseases. J Infect Dis 180:824–828, 1999.

67. K Staskus, R Sun, G Miller, P Racz, A Jaslowski, C Metroka, H Brett-Smith, AT Haase. Cellular tropism and viral interleukin-6 expression distinguish human herpesvirus 8 involvement in Kaposi's sarcoma, primary effusion lymphoma, and multicentric Castleman's disease. J Virol 73:4181–4187, 1999.

68. E Cannell, M Sibylle. Viral encoded cyclins. Semin Cancer Biol 9:221–229, 1999.

69. M Cotter II, E Robertson. The latency-associated nuclear antigen tethers the Kaposi's sarcoma-associated herpesvirus genome to host chromosomes in body cavity-based lymphoma cells. Virology 264:255–264, 1999.

70. J Fribor Jr, WP Kong, M Hottiger, G Nabel. P53 inhibition by the LANA protein of KSHV protects against cell death. Nature 402:889–894, 1999.

71. AC Wijnveen, H Persson, S Bjorck, I Blohme. Disseminated Kaposi's sarcoma—full regression after withdrawal of immunosuppressive therapy: report of a case. Transplant Proc 19:3735–3736, 1987.

72. I Penn. Incidence and treatment of neoplasia after transplantation. J Heart Lung Tranplant 12:S328–S336, 1993.

73. H Koizumi, A Ohkwara, O Itakura, H Kikuta. Herpesvirus-like DNA sequences in classic Kaposi's sarcoma and angiosarcoma in Japan. Br J Dermatol 135:1009–1010, 1996.

74. JA Martinez-Escribano, M del Pino Gil Mateo, J Miquel, E Ledesma, A Aliaga. Human herpesvirus 8 is not detectable by polymerase chain reaction in angiosarcoma. Br J Dermatol 138:546–547, 1998.

75. J Lasota, M Miettinen. Absence of Kaposi's sarcoma-associated virus (human herpesvirus-8) sequences in angiosarcoma. Virchows Arch 434:51–56, 1999.

76. R Gyulai, L Kemeny, M Kiss, S Nagy, E Adam, F Nagy, A Dobozy. Human herpesvirus 8 DNA sequences in angiosarcoma of the face. Br J Dermatol 137:467, 1997.

77. S Nashimoto, R Inagi, K Yamnishi, K Hosokawa, M Kakibuchi, K Yoshikawa. Prevalence of human herpesvirus-8 in skin lesions. Br J Dermatol 137:179–184, 1997.

78. PL Rady, A Yen, JL Rollefson I Orengo, S Bruce, TK Hughes, SK Tyring. Herpesvirus-like DNA sequences in non-Kaposi's sarcoma skin lesions of transplant patients. Lancet 345:1339–1340, 1995.

79. C Lebbe, R Tatoud, P Morel, F Calvo, S Euvrard, J Kanitakis, M Faure, A Claudy. Human herpesvirus 8 sequences are not detected in epithelial tumors from patients receiving transplants. Arch Dermatol 133:111, 1997.

80. N Dupin, I Gorin, JP Escande, V Calvez, M Grandadam, JM Huraux, H Agut. Lack of evidence of any association between human herpesvirus 8 and various skin tumors from both immunocompetent and immunosuppressed patients. Arch Dermatol 133:537–538, 1997.

81. V Adams, W Kempf, Schmid, B Muller, J Briner, G Burg. Absence of herpesvirus-like DNA sequences in skin cancer of non-immunosuppressed patients. Lancet 346:1715–1716, 1995.

82. A Uthman, C Brna, W Weninger, E Tschachler. No HHV-8 in non-Kaposi's sarcoma mucocutaneous lesions from immunodeficient HIV-positive patients. Lancet 347:1700–1701, 1996.

83. MP Mateo, FJ Miuel, E Ledesma, MI Ferber, C Tusset, A Aliaga. The absence of HHV-8 DNA sequences in skin tumors other than Kaposi's sarcoma from AIDS patients and transplant recipients. Br J Dermatol 139:918–919, 1998.

84. M Deichmann, M Thome, M Bock, A Jackel, V Wald-

mann, H Naher. The human herpesvirus-type 8 is not involved in malignant melanoma. Br J Cancer 80:67–69, 1999.

85. OM Memar, PL Rady, RM Goldblum, A Yen, SK Tyring. Human herpesvirus 8 DNA sequences in blistering skin from patients with pemphigus. Arch Dermatol 133: 1247–1251, 1997.

86. OM Memar, PL Rady, RM Goldblum, SK Tyring. Human herpesvirus-8 DNA sequences in a patient with pemphigus vulgaris, but without HIV infection or Kaposi's sarcoma. J Invest Dermatol 108:118–119, 1997.

87. G Bezold, CA Sander, MJ Flaig, RU Peter, G Messer. Lack of detection of human herpesvirus (HHV)-8 DNA in lesional skin of German pemphigus vulgaris and pemphigus foliaceus patients. J Invest Dermatol 114:739–741, 2000.

88. N Dupin, AG Marcelin, V Calvez, C Andr. Absence of a link between human herpesvirus 8 and pemphigus. Br J Dermatol 141:159–160, 1999.

89. G Cathomas, A Stalder, N Regamey, P Erb, PH Itin. No evidence of HHV-8 infection in patients with pemphigus vulgaris/foliaceus. Arch Dermatol 134:1162, 1998.

90. SS Cohen, MD Weinstein, BG Hendier, GH Anhalt, A Blauvelt. No evidence of human herpesvirus 8 infection inpatients with paraneoplastic pemphigus, pemphigus vulgaris, or pemphigus foliaceus. J Invest Dermatol 111: 781–783, 1998.

91. T Papo, M Soubrier, AG Marcelin, V Calvez, B Wechsler, JM Huraux, JC Piette, P Cacoub. Human herpesvirus 8 infection, Castleman's disease, and POEMS syndrome. Brit J Haematol 104:932–933, 1999.

92. P Piedbois, H Frikha, L Martin, E Levy, E Haddad, JP Le Bourgeois. Radiotherapy in the management of epidemic Kaposi's sarcoma. Int J Radiat Oncol Biol Phys 30: 1207–1211, 1994.

93. FH Saran, IA Adamietz, C Thilmann, S Mose, HD Bottcher. HIV-associated cutaneous Kaposi's sarcoma—palliative local treatment by radiotherapy. Acta Oncol 36:55–58, 1997.

94. DR Tomlinson, RJ Coker, M Fisher. Management and treatment of Kaposi's sarcoma in AIDS. Int J STD AIDS 7:466–470, 1996.

95. AK Morris, AW Valley. Overview of the management of AIDS-related Kaposi's sarcoma. Ann Pharmacother 30: 1150–1163, 1996.

96. E Sulis, C Floris, ML Sulis, S Zurrida, S Piro, A Pintus, L Contu. Interferon administered intralesionally in skin and oral cavity lesions in heterosexual drug addicted patients with AIDS-related Kaposi's sarcoma. Eur J Cancer Clin Oncol 25:759–761, 1989.

97. Clearance given for Panretin gel [news]. Oncologist 4:187, 1999.

98. M Duvic, AE Friedman-Kien, DJ Looney, SA Miles, PL Myskowski, DT Scadden, J Von Roenn, JE Galpin, J Groopman, G Loewen, V Stevens, JA Truglia, RC Yocum. Topical treatment of cutaneous lesions of acquired immu-

nodeficiency syndrome-related Kaposi sarcoma using alitretinoin gel. Arch Dermatol 136:1461–1469, 2000.

99. SE Krown, PL Myskowski, J Paredes. Medical management of AIDS patients. Kaposi's sarcoma. Med Clin North Am 76:235–252, 1992.

100. FC Lee, RT Mitsuyasu. Chemotherapy of AIDS-related Kaposi's sarcoma. Hematol Oncol Clin North Am 10: 1051–1068, 1996.

101. PS Gill, J Wernz, DT Scadden, P Cohen, GM Mukwaya, JH von Roenn, M Jacobs, S Kempin, I Silverberg, G Gonzales, MU Rarick, AM Myers, F Shepherd, C Sawka, MC Pike, ME Ross. Randomized phase III trial of liposomal daunorubicin verses doxorubicin, bleomycin, and vincristine in AIDS-related Kaposi's sarcoma. J Clin Oncol 14: 2353–2364, 1996.

102. AJ Coukell, CM Spencer. Polyethylene glycolliposomal doxorubicin. A review of its pharmacodynamic and pharmacokinetic properties, and therapeutic efficacy in the management of AIDS-related Kaposi's sarcoma. Drugs 53(3):520–538, 1997.

103. JL Jones, DL Hanson, JW Ward. Effect of antiretroviral therapy on recent trends in cancers among HIV-infected persons [abstr]. J Acquir Immune Defic Syndr Hum Retrovirol 17(Abstract S3):A38, 1998.

104. B Ensoli, G Barillari, SZ Salahuddin, RC Gallo, F Wong-Staal. Tat protein of HIV-1 stimulates growth of cells derived from Kaposi's sarcoma lesions of AIDS patients. Nature 345:84–86, 1990.

105. B Ensoli, R Gendelman, P Markham, V Fiorelli, S Colombini, M Raffeld, A Cafaro, HK Chang, JN Brady, RC Gallo. Synergy between basic fibroblast growth factor and HIV-1 Tat protein in induction of Kaposi's sarcoma. Nature 371:674–680, 1994.

106. DH Kedes, D Ganem. Sensitivity of Kaposi's sarcoma-associated herpesvirus replication to antiviral drugs. J Clin Invest 99:2082–2086, 1997.

107. R Robles, D Lugo, L Gee, MA Jacobson. Effect of antiviral drugs used to treat cytomegalovirus end-organ disease on subsequent course of previously diagnosed Kaposi's sarcoma in patients with AIDS. J Acquir Immune Defic Syndr 20:34–38, 1999.

108. L Morfeldt, J Torssander. Long time remission of Kaposi's sarcoma following foscarnet treatment in HIV-infected patients. Scand J Infect Dis 26:749–752, 1994.

109. MJ Glesby, DR Hoover, S Weng, NM Graham, JP Phair, R Detels, M Ho, AJ Saah. Use of antiherpes drugs and the risk of Kaposi's sarcoma: data from the Multicenter AIDS Cohort Study. J Infect Dis 173:1477–1480, 1996.

110. A Mocroft, M Youle, B Gazzard, J Morcinek, R Halai, AN Phillips. Anti-herpesvirus treatment and risk of Kaposi's sarcoma in HIV infection. AIDS 10:1101–1105, 1996.

111. Z Hammoud, DM Parenti, GL Simon. Abatement of cutaneous Kaposi's sarcoma associated with cidofovir treatment [letter]. Clin Infect Dis 26:1233–1234, 1998.

112. T Simonart, JC Noel, G De Dobbeleer, D Parent, JP Van Vooren, E De Clercq, R Snoeck. Treatment of classical

Kaposi's sarcoma with intralesional injections of cidofovir: report of a case. J Med Virol 55:215–218, 1998.

113. JE Groopman, MS Gottlieb, J Goodman, RT Mitsuyasu, MA Conant, H Prince, JL Fahey, M Derezin, WM Weinstein, C Casavante, et al. Recombinant alpha-2 interferon therapy for Kaposi's sarcoma associated with the acquired immunodeficiency syndrome. Ann Intern Med 100: 671–676, 1984.

114. RX Real, HF Oettgen, SE Krown. Kaposi's sarcoma and the acquired immunodeficiency syndrome: treatment with high and low doses of recombinant leukocyte A interferon. J Clin Oncol 4:544–551, 1986.

115. DI Abrams, PA Volberding. Alpha interferon therapy of AIDS-associated Kaposi's sarcoma. Semin Oncol 4(Suppl 2):43–47, 1987.

116. R De Wit, JK Schattenkerk, CA Boucher, PJ Bakker, KH Veenhof, SA Danner. Clinical and virologic effects of high-dose recombinant interferon-alpha in disseminated AIDS-related Kaposi's sarcoma. Lancet 2:1214–1217, 1988.

117. JE Groopman, DT Scadden. Interferon therapy for Kaposi's sarcoma associated with the acquired immunodeficiency syndrome (AIDS). Ann Intern Med 110:335–337, 1989.

118. JA Kovacs, L Deyton, R Davey, J Falloon, K Zunich, D Lee, JA Metcalf, JW Bigley, LA Sawyer, KC Zoon, et al. Combined zidovudine and interferon-alpha therapy in patients with Kaposi sarcoma and the acquired immunodeficiency syndrome (AIDS). Ann Intern Med 111:280–287, 1989.

119. SE Krown, JW Gold, D Niedzwiecki, D Bundow, N Flomenberg, B Gansbacher, BJ Brew. Interferon-alpha with zidovudine: safety, tolerance, and clinical and virologic effects in patients with Kaposi sarcoma associated with the acquired immunodeficiency syndrome (AIDS). Ann Intern Med 112:812–821, 1990.

120. MA Fischl, RB Uttamchandani, L Resnick, R Agarwal, MA Fletcher, J Patrone-Reese, L Dearmas, J Chidekel, M McCann, M Myers. A Phase I study of recombinant human interferon-alpha 2a or human lymphoblastoid interferon-alpha n1 and concomitant zidovudine in patients with AIDS-related Kaposi's sarcoma. J Acquir Immune Defic Syndr 4:1–10, 1991.

121. D Podzamczer, F Bolao, B Clotet, P Garcia, A Casanova, X Pagerols, F Gudiol. Low-dose interferon-alpha combined with zidovudine in patients with AIDS-associated Kaposi's sarcoma. J Intern Med 233:247–253, 1993.

122. S Mauss, H Jablonowski. Efficacy, safety, and tolerance of low dose, long-term interferon-alpha 2b and zidovudine in early-stage AIDS-associated Kaposi's sarcoma. J Acquir Immune Defic Syndr Hum Retrovirol 10:157–162, 1995.

123. P Saiag, M Pavlovic, T Clerici, V Feauveau, JC Nicolas, D Emile, C Chastang. Treatment of early AIDS-related Kaposi's sarcoma with oral all-*trans*-retinoic acid: results of a sequential nonrandomized phase II trial. Kaposi's Sarcoma ANRS Study Group. Agence Nationale de Recherches sur le SIDA. AIDS 12:2169–2176, 1998.

124. NA Rizvi, JL Marshall, E Ness, J Yoe, GM Gill, JA Truglia, GR Loewen, D Jaunakais, EH Ulm, MJ Hawkins. Phase I study of 9-*cis*-retinoic acid (ALRT1057 capsules) in adults with advanced cancer. Clin Cancer Res 4: 1437–1442, 1998.

125. PS Gill, Y Lunardi-Iskandar, S Louie, A Tulpule, T Zheng, BM Espina, JM Besnier, P Hermans, AM Levine, JL Bryant, RC Gallo. The effects of preparations of human chorionic gonadotropin on AIDS-related Kapsosi's sarcoma. N Engl J Med 335:1261–1269, 1996.

126. PJ Harris. Intralesional human chorionic gonadotropin for Kaposi's sarcoma. N Engl J Med 336:1187–1189, 1997.

127. RA Soler, M Howard, NS Brink, D Gibb, RS Tedder, D Nadal. Regression of AIDS-related Kaposi's sarcoma during therapy with thalidomide. Clin Infect Dis 23: 501–505, 1996.

128. Y Carmeli, D Mevorach, N Kaminski, E Raz. Regression of Kaposi's sarcoma after intravenous immunoglobulin treatment for polymyositis. Cancer 73:2859–2861, 1994.

11

Herpes B Virus

Paul Rockley
Cosmetic, Laser, and Classic Dermatology, North Miami Beach, Florida, USA
Stephen K. Tyring
University of Texas Medical Branch, Galveston, Texas, USA
and University of Texas Medical Branch Center for Clinical Studies, Houston, Texas, USA

The herpes virus B is the only nonhuman primate herpesvirus that causes definitive disease, usually fatal, in humans. Several terms have been ascribed to this virus, including monkey B virus, *Herpes simiae*, *Herpesvirus simiae*, and herpes B. The Herpesvirus Study Group for the International Committee on Taxonomy of Viruses has designated the name *Cercopithecine herpesvirus 1*, which is classified in the family Herpesviridae, subfamily Alphaherpesvirinae, and genus Simplexvirus [1]. However, the virus is most commonly known as B virus, the name given by original researchers. This pathogen is 1 of 35 simian herpesviruses that generally cause asymptomatic or mild, localized disease in nonhuman primates. It is indigenous in Asiatic Old World monkeys of the *Macaca* genus, and no other monkeys are known to naturally harbor the virus (Fig. 11–1). In the natural hosts, B virus infection closely resembles human herpes simplex virus type (HSV) 1 infection and frequently manifests clinically as recurrent gingivostomatitis. B virus in humans often manifests as a rapidly ascending, fulminant encephalomyelitis with a 70% fatality rate [2].

HISTORY

In 1932, a laboratory physician (W.B.) was bitten on the hand by a clinically normal rhesus monkey. Local inflammation rapidly evolved into lymphangitis, lymphadenitis, encephalomyelitis, respiratory paralysis, and death. Two virology laboratories independently analyzed autopsy specimens. Gay and Holden isolated a filterable agent from W.B.'s spinal cord and brain in 1933 [3]. Intradermal injection of the agent into rabbits produced a lethal disease similar to that observed in W.B. Cross-neutralization tests revealed that the agent was antigenically related to HSV and it was designated "W virus," after the first initial of the patient. Further work by Sabin and Wright in 1934 demonstrated that this agent was biologically distinct from HSV and they named it "B virus," after the patient's second initial [4].

The first primary isolation of B virus from a clinically normal rhesus monkey was reported by Reissig and Melnick in 1955 [5]. Suspensions of neurological tissue from this monkey produced disease after inoculation of monkeys, rabbits, hamsters, guinea pigs, rats, and mice. The virus grows in chick embryo cell lines, forming pock lesions on the chorioallantoic membrane, and in continuous cultures of monkey and rabbit kidney cells or human Hela cells. Experimentally infected animals can exhibit Cowdry type A intranuclear inclusions and multinucleated giant cells. Since intradermal inoculation of B virus into rabbits reliably causes fatal myelitis, the rabbit has become the animal model of choice for this virus.

EPIDEMIOLOGY

Seropositive macaques serve as a reservoir for transmission of B virus infection. Seroprevalence studies reveal that the

GEOGRAPHICAL INCIDENCE

The *Macaca* genus primates are enzootic
in Asia, but the incidence is likely
worldwide, since these macaques are
commonly used for laboratory research
and as house pets across the world.

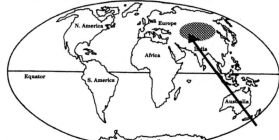

Macaca genus primates are enzootic in Asia

TAXONOMY

Herpesviridae family

Alphaherpesvirinae subfamily

Simplex virus

Cercopithecine herpesvirus 1
(B virus)

**Direct contact with an
infected macaque
or its body fluids or
tissue with exposure to a
break in the skin or a
mucocutaneous area. This
most commonly results from
monkey bites or scratches.**

**Fomites
(Cages)**

Humans

**One case of person-
to-person transmission
through direct contact
has been reported.**

**Two cases of possible
respiratory transmission
have been reported.**

ZOONOTIC IMPLICATIONS

Monkeys

**} Indigenous to Old World primates of
the *Macaca* genus, particularly rhesus
and cynomolgus monkeys.**

Figure 11–1.   Incidence and transmission of herpes B.

virus is common in adult monkeys housed in crowded
cages or residing in densely populated, wild habitats [6,7].
Seropositive rates in these populations range from 73 to
100% [2,6,8]. Prepubertal or isolated animals have a reduced prevalence of infection [9], while most monkeys
beyond 2 to 3 years of age are seropositive [10]. The majority of these animals acquire infection from sexual activity
or bites [11]. As with HSV, B virus establishes latency in
the infected macaques, and intermittent shedding of the
virus occurs with both symptomatic and asymptomatic
reactivation. Viral shedding may occur from the conjunctiva, buccal mucosa, and urogenital region [10]. The risk

of human infection after contact with seropositive monkeys
is low, since the overall frequency of B virus excretion in
these monkeys is less than 5% [12].

Since the initial report of B virus, almost 40 cases have
been described in the literature, most of which involve the
occupational exposure of research laboratory workers
[2,13–27]. Approximately two thirds of the cases have occurred in the United States, with the remaining reports from
Canada and Great Britain. No cases have been reported in
Asia, where Herpes B is enzootic in the macaques and
direct contact between the monkeys and humans is common. This paucity of reported cases in the enzootic region

likely may be due to the lack of adequate medical care or diagnostic methods for identifying B virus [14]. Even among laboratory workers, B virus infection is extremely uncommon, given the thousands of monkey bites, scratches, and other documented exposures that occur each year in these facilities.

Some investigators have suggested that HSV infection stimulates cross-reactive immunity to B virus. However, prior exposure to HSV does not appear to alter the clinical outcome of human B virus disease [13]. Undetected, asymptomatic B virus infection has been suggested to account for the apparent rarity of human cases despite frequent contact with infected laboratory monkeys. However, a large-scale, controlled seroprevalence survey comparing monkey handlers with those with no previous monkey exposure showed no significant seropositivity for B virus in either group [28].

PATHOGENESIS

Although several modes of transmission of human B virus infection have been reported, infection usually results from direct inoculation of contaminated macaque fluids or tissue, usually from a bite or scratch from the monkey or from contact with its cage [2,13–16]. Two cases have occurred from cuts from tissue culture bottles containing monkey kidney cells, and two additional cases were linked to contaminated needlestick injuries. One case was reported to be caused by contamination of a preexisting wound with monkey saliva. Acquired infection without known injury has been described in 6 cases: (1) a single case of fatal infection occurred via mucocutaneous (conjunctival) exposure [23]; (2) two cases have presented with respiratory symptoms and without ascending paralysis, suggesting possible respiratory transmission; (3) two cases occurred in laboratory workers without specific viral exposure; and (4) the wife, of a patient who died, developed herpetic vesicles on her finger after caring for her husband's lesions and applying the same medicated cream to her own dermatitis [14]. This final case is the only instance of human-to-human transmission that has been identified.

The incubation period of B virus is usually 3 to 5 days, but early clinical manifestations have occurred as late as 54 days after viral exposure. The B virus enters through the skin, producing erythema, edema, vesicles, and then necrosis of the involved area. At the site of inoculation of infectious material, B virus attaches to host epithelial surface receptors and penetrates through the plasma membrane. The naked capsid is transported to nuclear pores and viral DNA is released into the nucleus, causing viral replication. B virus can be recovered from the epidermal replication site during the first 2 weeks following infection [29].

Viral replication stimulates local inflammation, mononuclear infiltration, and the development of herpetic vesicles. These vesicles, however, are not always present with human infection [23]. Progression of disease is associated with lymphangitis, lymphadenopathy, and hemorrhagic, focal necrosis of the involved area. A viremia has been demonstrated in animal models but not in humans [13]. Viral spread occurs through neuronal and lymphatic routes. Neuronal spread is probably the primary route, as uptake of B virus by sensory and autonomic nerve endings, followed by axonal transport to the nucleus of nerve cell bodies, leads to acute neurologic findings in humans and latent infections in monkeys [30].

Although the majority of human B virus infections have demonstrated prominent neurological findings as the virus rapidly progresses from the peripheral nervous system (PNS) to the central nervous system (CNS), it is not known why B virus has a high affinity for human neuronal tissue. Whitley contrasted the generalized CNS disease characteristic of human B virus infection with the localized temporal lobe disease associated with HSV infection [31]. Human B virus infection frequently causes pontine and medullary lesions, but virtually any region of the CNS can be affected. Patients often develop combinations of transverse myelitis, encephalitis, encephalomyelitis, and myeloencephalitis [32,33]. Prominent pathologic features of CNS lesions include edema, neural degeneration, gliosis, and astrocytosis [14].

Autopsy data have revealed that B virus commonly infects the liver and lungs. The virus may also occasionally involve the heart, spleen, kidneys, and adrenals. The chief pathological feature of parenchymal involvement is focal, hemorrhagic necrosis.

CLINICAL MANIFESTATIONS

Four clinical syndromes of human infection reflect the different modes of B virus transmission. The progression of these infections can be influenced by several factors, such as the host's immunological status (particularly the level of antibodies to HSV), the patient's age, the site of viral entry, and the quantity of virus inoculated. By far, the most common syndrome of disease results from direct percutaneous inoculation of contaminated fluids or tissue. Typically days to weeks after viral inoculation, regional lymphadenitis and lymphadenopathy develop (Table 11–1). Local signs frequently develop at the site of inoculation, including vesicles, erythema, and edema (Figs. 11–2 to 11–4). Regional and secondary lymph nodes draining the

Table 11–1.   Clinical Manifestations of B Virus

Time after exposure	Clinical manifestations	Laboratory analysis	Other notes
3–5 days or more	Regional lymphadenopathy and lymphadenitis, +/− herpetic vesicular lesions at the site of inoculation, with erythema and edema ↓	Viral culture of vesicular fluid, tissue, or specimens (urine, CSF, stool) Identification of the virus in specimens, with polymerase chain reaction or in situ hybridization	Incubation may last for 2–5 weeks in some patients Some patients may develop fever, myalgia, cramping, and cranial nerve abnormalities during the lymphatic spread of disease
10–12 days	Sensorimotor abnormalities: dysesthesia, hyperesthesia, paresthesia ↓		
13–19 days	Progressive ascending paralysis, beginning as weakness and hyporeflexia ↓	Virus-specific serologies, although false positives may occur	
	Flaccid paralysis and areflexia ↓		
Rapid progression	Decreased consciousness, altered mentation, seizures, and respiratory depression ↓		
May occur within 2 weeks of symptom onset, or much later	Respiratory arrest and death		Late disease is often avoidable with antiviral treatment

CSF, cerebrospinal fluid.

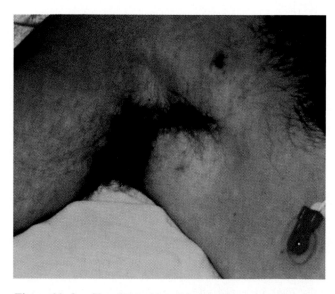

Figure 11–2.   Site of chest bite of rhesus macaque monkey from which B virus was recovered. (Photographs courtesy of Julia Hilliard, Ph.D., SW Foundation for Biomedical Research, San Antonio, TX.)

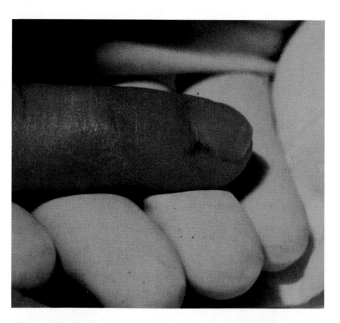

Figure 11–3.   Finger bite site from rhesus macaque monkey originally suspected of being site to which B virus was transmitted. No virus was recovered. (Photographs courtesy of Julia Hilliard, Ph.D., SW Foundation for Biomedical Research, San Antonio, TX.)

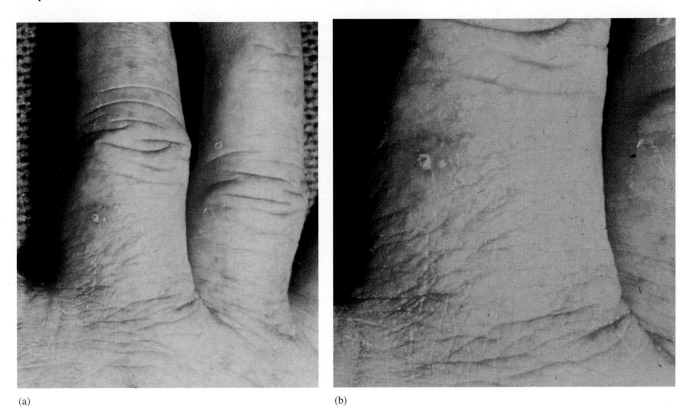

(a)   (b)

Figure 11–4. Inoculation site of scratch of finger on cage housing infected rhesus macaque. (a) Multiple sites appear in scratch areas. (b) Close-up of (a). (Photographs courtesy of Julia Hilliard, PhD, SW Foundation for Biomedical Research, San Antonio, TX.)

site of viral entry may become hemorrhagic and focally necrotic. Lymphatic spread of disease is often accompanied by fever, myalgias, fatigue, and other constitutional symptoms. Viral propagation in the PNS leads to sensory abnormalities, such as dysesthesias, hyperesthesias, and paresthesias. Neuronal spread of B virus from the PNS to the CNS leads to spinal cord involvement and acute ascending paralysis. This manifests itself as weakness and hyporeflexia, progressing to areflexia and flaccid paralysis. Widespread infection of the spinal cord causes transverse myelitis, which often results in bladder paralysis and subsequent urinary retention. CNS viral disease progresses to the brainstem giving rise to cranial nerve signs, such as nystagmus, diplopia, and dysphagia. Meningeal irritation is associated with headache, nausea, vomiting, and photophobia. In most patients, this is followed by meningoencephalomyelitis with involvement of the respiratory center. Eventually, inflammation and necrosis of the brain results in altered consciousness, depressed mentation, seizures, coma, respiratory failure, and death.

A second, much less common route of infection, is through possible aerosol inhalation of infectious airborne droplets (two cases reported). Upper respiratory tract flu-

like symptoms include low-grade fever, rhinorrhea, coryza, cough, pharyngitis, and laryngitis. Spread of B virus infection to the lower respiratory tract can produce persistent fever and respiratory distress owing to interstitial pneumonitis. The clinical course of two patients with B virus infection suggested respiratory exposure to infectious secretions. One of these patients developed neurologic symptoms and died [9,17].

A third uncommon manifestation of B virus infection is a recurrent vesicular eruption (Figs. 11–5 and 11–6). Only two patients have been reported with this form of B virus infection. One patient acquired herpetiform lesions by human-to-human transmission [15]. The second patient developed a zosteriform eruption from which B virus was isolated [18]. These recurrent forms of infection reveal that B virus shares with other herpesviruses the potential for latent infection and subsequent reactivation.

Asymptomatic infection is the fourth possible clinical manifestation of B virus (one case reported). This finding was reported in an animal handler who was stuck with a needle that was used to inject a B virus–infected monkey [19,33]. Physical examination and laboratory tests were unremarkable, except that B virus was isolated from cul-

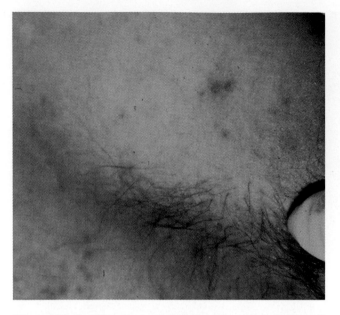

Figure 11–5. Secondary vesicular/papular eruption from B virus infection. (Photographs courtesy of Julia Hilliard, PhD, SW Foundation for Biomedical Research, San Antonio, TX.)

tures of skin biopsies taken from the puncture site of the patient. The patient was placed on empiric treatment with intravenous acyclovir followed by oral therapy, which may have prevented any of the expected manifestations of disease. This form of infection appears unusual but may be under-reported.

Once signs or symptoms of clinical disease develop, morbidity and mortality are extremely high. As previously stated, the overall mortality for clinical B virus infection in humans is 70%. The few survivors of the disease who experienced CNS involvement have often been left with neurological impairments, ranging from moderate to severe [2]. Fortunately, both the mortality and morbidity rates have been decreasing in recent years because of early institution of antiviral therapy [14].

DERMATOPATHOLOGY

Because of the small number of human cases and the biological hazards associated with B virus, very little information is available about the dermatopathologic findings of the associated skin lesions. It has been reported that a Tzanck smear of the herpetiform vesicles may show intranuclear inclusions and giant cells, although this is not a consistent feature. Skin biopsy specimens should be examined in the laboratory for evidence of B virus, but this virus

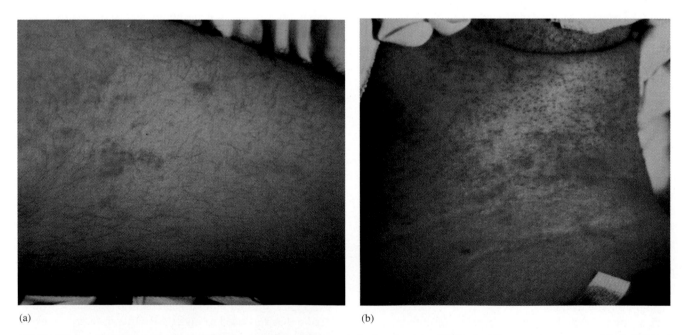

(a)   (b)

Figure 11–6. Secondary papular eruptions in patients with B virus infection. (a) Arm. (b) Neck. (Photographs courtesy of Julia Hilliard, Ph.D., SW Foundation for Biomedical Research, San Antonio, TX.)

is a biosafety level 4 pathogen that requires specific safety precautions. Any biopsy specimens should be shipped on ice to one of three laboratories (listed below) that are capable of isolating the virus from tissue.

DIAGNOSIS

Infection with B virus should be considered in animal handlers exposed to contaminated monkey secretions and tissues or any patient with a recent history of monkey bite, scratch, or needlestick injury. B virus infection should be strongly suspected if these individuals develop inflammation and vesicles at the inoculation site. Further support for B virus infection is provided by lymphatic spread, causing lymphangitis and lymphadenopathy as well as neuronal dissemination leading to PNS and CNS abnormalities. See Table 11–2 for differential diagnosis.

Confirmation of B virus infection can be difficult, since only three laboratories in the world (two in San Antonio, Texas, United States, and one in London, England) have been certified to handle this biohazard [34]. Laboratory diagnosis is best accomplished by culturing vesicular fluid or tissue homogenates from skin and mucous membranes on rabbit or monkey cell lines. B virus also has been detected in specimens of urine, stool, and cerebrospinal fluid from infected persons. Isolated B virus can be identified by a variety of virological techniques. Radiolabeled B virus DNA and proteins can be detected by restriction endonuclease analysis and electrophoretic patterns, respectively [35,36]. Although these approaches have standardized vi-

rological diagnosis of B virus infection in humans and nonhuman primates, their application is limited to settings in which sufficient quantities of B virus can be obtained for initial propagation on appropriate culture systems and subsequent interaction with permissive cells. Molecular methods, such as in situ hybridization and polymerase chain reaction, can directly detect amplified B virus DNA and are not subject to these limitations [37,38].

Serological diagnosis of B virus infection is greatly hindered by cross-reactivity between antibodies to B virus and those to HSV. The high prevalence of HSV antibodies among humans has further complicated efforts to use serology to confirm suspected cases of human B virus infection. In addition, low levels of antibodies to B virus are detectable in approximately half of the general adult human population irrespective of previous contact with monkeys. Investigators believe that these antibodies represent a heterotypical response attributable to HSV-directed immunoglobulins [39,40]. These findings reduce the sensitivity and specificity of serological tests, such as serum neutralization tests, complement fixation tests, cross-adsorption tests, plaque-reduction assays, and immunofluorescence tests. New serological approaches include competitive enzyme and monoclonal antibody assays, which have increased sensitivity, as well as immunoblot and dot-immunobinding assays, which have increased specificity [41–45]. Preabsorption of human sera with HSV antigens can greatly decrease, but not completely eliminate, the occurrence of false-positive serological results [28,46]. Despite all of these technological advances, there is currently no standard serological test that can reliably distinguish infection between B virus and HSV. However, properly performed serological studies in the patient with definite exposure or possible symptoms of disease may be helpful in the diagnosis of infection, provided there is cautious interpretation of results [34].

CONTROL AND PREVENTION

Formalin-inactivated B virus vaccines have been tested in a variety of experimental animals and more than 300 persons [9,32,47–49]. These studies showed that vaccination could stimulate production of low levels of neutralizing B virus antibodies in most species, including humans. The antibody levels produced in man were short in duration, which required 6 month interval boosters. While the vaccine had a protective effect in some animals, this finding could not be demonstrated in humans, and the vaccine was never licensed for general use [50].

Similarly, passive immunization with large doses of hyperimmune serum or gamma globulin administered si-

---

Table 11–2. Differential Diagnosis of B Virus

Herpes simplex virus: The early finding of herpetiform lesions of B virus infection may appear similar to this common infection. Encephalitis with herpes simplex virus may also present with neurological findings. Herpes simplex infection often has a history of recurrent lesions, particularly in the orolabial and genital areas, while B virus infection usually has a history of monkey exposure associated with the area of inoculation. Tzanck smear of B virus vesicles may also show giant cells with viral inclusions.

Herpes zoster infection: B virus may present with herpetiform lesions that spread in a region of the body and are not localized to the site of inoculation. The associated dyesthesias may also mimic the clinical picture of herpes zoster. The history of exposure to a macaque and the development of neurological manifestations strongly points to B virus infection.

multaneously with B viral challenge had transient protective effects in rabbits [51]. However, protection appeared to be due to destruction of epithelial cells as opposed to the direct neutralization of the B virus inoculum. Postexposure immunoprophylaxis has not proved useful for the treatment of patients infected with the B virus [50,51].

Since no B virus vaccine of proved efficacy is available, prevention is through meticulous laboratory handling techniques and proper animal colony management. The severity of human disease necessitates strict adherence to the B Virus Working Group recommendations and Center for Disease Control (CDC) guidelines for prevention of B virus infection in rhesus and macaque monkey handlers [34,52,53]. These guidelines include using macaque monkeys for research purposes only when clearly indicated and maintaining B virus–free monkeys under conditions that would preserve their disease-free state. Monkeys not known to be free of B virus infection should be regarded as infected. Direct handling of monkeys should be minimized and accomplished by using physical restraints, such as squeeze-back cages, tunnels, or chutes. Chemical restraints, such as ketamine hydrochloride injections, and behavioral conditioning are useful adjunctive measures.

All handlers should wear protective gear, such as long-sleeved clothing, face shields, and arm-length-reinforced leather gloves for unrestrained monkeys and latex or vinyl gloves for restrained animals. Cages and equipment must be free of sharp edges and kept in designated animal housing areas. Monkeys should be screened for evidence of B virus infection when laboratory studies may cause immunosuppression in the animals. Monkeys with lesions suggestive of active B virus infection need to be isolated until the lesions have healed. Animal handling requires education about the nature and risk of B virus infection as well as wound management protocols. Additional infection control measures include obtaining pre-employment and annual serum samples from handlers for analysis in the event of a suspected B virus infection as well as securing access to medical consultants for assistance in diagnosis and therapy of B virus infection [34,52,53].

TREATMENT

All wounds incurred by animal handlers that might be contaminated or that result in bleeding should be immediately and thoroughly scrubbed for 15 minutes, cleansed with soap and water, and treated with 10% iodine in alcohol or another concentrated detergent. Exposed mucosal surfaces of the eyes, mouth, and nose should be irrigated for at least 15 minutes with sterile saline solution or copious amounts of water. After initial culture specimens and serology sam-

ples have been obtained from the patient and monkey, the degree of risk for B virus infection should be determined. Detailed guidelines for the evaluation and management of this disease have been devised by the B Virus Working Group (Table 11–3) [34]. Superficial wounds caused by monkeys known to be B antibody negative probably require no further therapy, whereas wounds associated with monkeys of unknown B virus status are often treated with oral acyclovir for at least 2 weeks [54]. These cases can be monitored weekly by an occupational health service or animal care supervisor, but they require long-term follow-up (at least 2 months) since the use of prophylactic acyclovir can delay the onset of clinical disease [55]. It should be noted that the original bite may heal even in fatal cases (Fig. 11–7). B virus can be recovered long after healing has occurred (Julia Hilliard, personal communication).

Deep, penetrating or extensive wounds that cannot be adequately cleansed are also initially treated with oral acyclovir. These cases should be referred to a medical consultant who monitors the clinical status of the handler at weekly intervals for at least 2 months after exposure. If the handler develops signs or symptoms suggestive of B virus infection, then oral acyclovir is changed to intravenous acyclovir [34,52,53,55]. The reason that treatment is started with oral acyclovir is that early initiation of antiviral therapy takes precedence over the route of administration, and it is more practical to keep supplies of oral medication at monkey handling sites [54].

In vitro and in vivo studies with rabbits have demonstrated the effectiveness of both acyclovir and ganciclovir against B virus [54,56,57]. The few small-scale clinical reviews that monitored the human response to these antiviral agents have favored the use of acyclovir over ganciclovir [13,15,16,19,20,31,33]. Early administration of acyclovir slowed the progression of disease and allowed patients to return to normal function. Ganciclovir was less effective, but this medication was reserved for patients who either did not respond to acyclovir or had advanced disease prior to the initiation of therapy. In vitro studies with B virus have shown ganciclovir to have a slightly greater efficacy than acyclovir [54], but the associated toxicity with this drug is much greater. In view of these findings, including the low toxicity of acyclovir and the high mortality associated with B virus infection, it is logical to initiate prophylactic oral acyclovir immediately after exposure to B virus and therapeutic intravenous acyclovir for any clinical evidence of B virus infection. In the small number of patients who have received antiviral therapy, there has been a strong correlation between the patient's neurological condition at the start of therapy and the outcome of treatment [14]. For the most part, patients with no more than periph-

Table 11–3. Treatment of B virus infection in humans

Symptom	Treatment
Low risk of infection from exposure	No treatment needed. Monitor 2 to 3 times per week for 2 weeks, with follow up for at least 2 months, to ensure no development of signs or symptoms of disease.
Moderate to high risk of infection from exposure	Consider oral acyclovir 800 mg 5 times daily for at least 2 weeks. (Intravenous acyclovir may be considered for some high-risk exposures). Monitor 2–3 times per week for 2 weeks, with follow up for at least 2 months, to ensure no development of signs or symptoms of disease.
Asymptomatic culture-positive patient	Oral acyclovir 800 mg 5 times daily for 2 weeks. Therapy is then discontinued if the patient remains asymptomatic and remaining follow-up cultures and serologies are negative. Patient should be followed for at least 2 months, to ensure no development of signs or symptoms of disease.
Peripheral neuropathy symptoms or evidence of herpetiform lesions on the trunk or extremity	Intravenous acyclovir 10 mg/kg every 8 hours. Continue until symptoms resolve or significantly improve and serial cultures are negative for at least 10–14 days. Treatment may then be changed to oral acyclovir regimen.
Central neurological symptoms or evidence of herpetiform lesions on the head or neck	Intravenous acyclovir 15 mg/kg every 8 hours. Alternatively, ganciclovir 5mg/kg every 12 hours can be considered. Continue until symptoms resolve or significantly improve and serial cultures are persistently negative for at least 10–14 days. Treatment may then be changed to oral acyclovir regimen.

Source: Ref. 34.

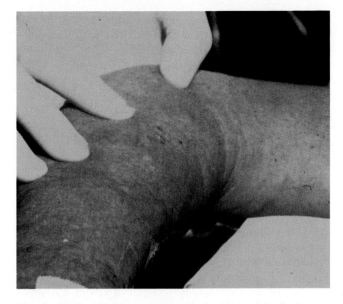

Figure 11–7. Healing arm bite in a subsequently fatal case. (Photographs courtesy of Julia Hilliard, Ph.D., SW Foundation for Biomedical Research, San Antonio, TX.)

eral neurological symptoms and/or skin lesions who begin treatment often have a good prognosis. Those patients who begin treatment after the demonstration of CNS involvement often have a fatal demise, despite high-dose intravenous therapy [13,15,20,21,23]. These findings underscore the need for expeditious management of potential disease and rapid initiation of antiviral therapy, if indicated.

Long-term oral suppressive acyclovir therapy has been recommended for those with documented B virus infection, although the necessary duration of treatment for these patients is not known [21]. Several surviving patients have been continued on this treatment for 4 to 7 years without adverse effects or recurrent disease [13,21]. If discontinuation of treatment is necessary, this process should be carefully monitored, such as in a hospital setting with isolation precautions. Cultures of genital, oropharyngeal, and conjunctival specimens should be obtained each week for at least 2 weeks after discontinuation of antiviral therapy. Authorities also advise obtaining B virus serologies at the time that treatment is stopped, as well as 3 and 6 weeks later [34]. A fourfold or greater rise in these specific antibody titers would signal the need for close monitoring for the development of disease symptoms or viral shedding.

CONCLUSION

Because clinical B virus infection in human hosts is extremely uncommon, the opportunities to study the pathogenesis and natural history of this disease in humans are quite limited. The risk of severe morbidity and mortality with this virus, which primarily affects exposed laboratory workers, has prompted several attempts to propagate B-virus negative macaque colonies for research laboratories. In any event, it is imperative to consider the diagnosis of B virus infection in any patient with known macaque exposure who presents with suspicious dermatological or neurological complaints, since early diagnosis and treatment can alter the often fatal course of this disease.

REFERENCES

1. B Roizman, LE Carmichael, F Deinhardt, G de-The, AJ Nahmias, W Plowright, F Rapp, P Sheldrick, M Takahashi, K Wolf. Herpesviridae. Definition, provisional nomenclature, and taxonomy. The Herpesvirus Study Group, the International Committee on Taxonomy of Viruses. Intervirology 16:201–217, 1981.
2. AE Palmer. B virus, Herpesvirus simiae: historical perspective. J Med Primatol 16:99–130, 1987.
3. FP Gay, M Holden. The herpes encephalitis problem. Int J Infect Dis 53:287–303, 1933.
4. AB Sabin, WM Wright. Acute ascending myelitis following a monkey bite, with the isolation of a virus capable of reproducing the disease. J Exp Med 59:115–136, 1934.
5. M Ressig, JL Melnick. The cellular changes produced in tissue cultures by herpes B virus correlated with the concurrent multiplication of the virus. J Exp Med 101:341–352, 1955.
6. KV Shah, JA Morrison. Comparison of three rhesus groups for antibody patterns to some viruses: absence of active simian virus 40 transmission in the free-ranging rhesus of Cayo Santiago. Am J Epidemiol 89:308–315, 1969.
7. HT Zwartouw, JA MacArthur, EA Boulter, JH Seamer, JH Marston, AS Chamove. Transmission of B virus infection between monkeys especially in relation to breeding colonies. Lab Anim 18:125–130, 1984.
8. RP Orcutt, GJ Pucak, HL Foster, JT Kilcourse, T Ferrell. Multiple testing for the detection of B virus antibody in specially handled rhesus monkeys after capture from virgin trapping grounds. Lab Anim Sci 26:70–74, 1976.
9. RN Hull. The simian herpesviruses. In: AS Kaplan, ed. The Herpesviruses. New York: Academic Press, 1973, pp 389–426.
10. BJ Weigler, DW Hird, JK Hilliard, NW Lerche, JA Roberts, LM Scott. Epidemiology of Cercopithecine Herpesvirus 1 (B Virus) infection and shedding in a large breeding cohort of rhesus macaques. J Infect Dis 167:257–263, 1993.
11. SR Ostrowski, MJ Leslie, T Parrott, S Abelt, PE Piercy. B-virus from pet macaque monkeys: an emerging threat in the United States? Emerg Infect Dis 4:117–121, 1998.
12. SA Keeble. B virus infection in monkeys. Ann NY Acad Sci 85:960–969, 1960.
13. GP Holmes, JK Hilliard, KC Klontz, AH Rupert, CM Schindler, E Parrish, DG Griffin, GS Ward, ND Bernstein, TW Bean, et al. B virus (Herpesvirus simiae) infection in humans: epidemiologic investigation of a cluster. Ann Intern Med 112:833–839, 1990.
14. BJ Weigler. Biology of B virus in macaque and human hosts: a review. Clin Infect Dis 14:555–567, 1992.
15. Centers for Disease Control. B virus infection in humans—Pensacola, Florida. MMWR Morb Mortal Wkly Rep 36:289–296, 1987.
16. Centers for Disease Control. B virus infection in humans—Michigan. MMWR Morb Mortal Wkly Rep 38: 453–454, 1989.
17. FP Nagler, M Klotz. A fatal B virus infection in a person subject to recurrent herpes labialis. Can Med Assoc J 79: 743–745, 1958.
18. J Fierer, P Bazeley, AI Braude. Herpes B virus encephalomyelitis presenting as ophthalmic zoster. Ann Intern Med 79:225–228, 1973.
19. AW Artenstein, CB Hicks, BS Goodwin, JK Hilliard. Human infection with B virus following a needlestick injury. Rev Infect Dis 13:288–291, 1991.
20. M Nanda, VT Curtin, JK Hilliard, ND Bernstein, RD Dix. Ocular histopathologic findings in a case of human herpes B virus infection. Arch Ophthalmol 108:713–716, 1990.
21. DS Davenport, DR Johnson, GP Holmes, DA Jewett, SC Ross, JK Hilliard. Diagnosis and management of human B virus (Herpesvirus simiae) infections in Michigan. Clin Infect Dis 19:33–41, 1994.
22. K Hummeler, WL Davidson, W Henle, AC LaBoccetta, HG Ruch. Encephalomyelitis due to infection with Herpesvirus simiae (Herpes B virus): report of two fatal laboratory acquired cases. N Engl J Med 261:64–68, 1959.
23. Centers for Disease Control and Prevention. Fatal Cercopithecine herpesvirus 1 (B virus) infection following a mucocutaneous exposure and interim recommendations for worker protection. MMWR Morb Mortal Wkly Rep 47: 1073–1076, 1998.
24. GE Breen, SG Lamb, AT Otaki. Monkey bite encephalomyelitis: report of a case with recovery. Br Med J 2:22–23, 1958.
25. BL Bryan, CD Espana, RW Emmons, N Vijayan, PD Hoeprich. Recovery from encephalomyelitis caused by Herpesvirus simiae: report of a case. Arch Intern Med 135: 868–870, 1975.
26. Centers for Disease Control. Herpes B encephalitis—California. MMWR Morb Mortal Wkly Rep 22:333–334, 1973.
27. FM Love, E Jungherr. Occupational infection with virus B of monkeys. JAMA 179:160–162, 1962.
28. A Freifeld, JK Hilliard, J Southers, M Murray, B Savarese, JM Schmitt, SE Straus. A controlled seroprevalence survey of primate handlers for evidence of asymptomatic herpes B virus infection. J Infect Dis 171:1031–1034, 1995.
29. HT Zwartouw, EA Boulter. Excretion of B virus in monkeys and evidence of genital infection. Lab Anim 18:65–70, 1984.
30. G Gosztonyi, D Falke, H Ludwig. Axonal-transsynaptic

spread as the basic pathogenetic mechanism in B virus infection of the nervous system. J Med Primatol 21:42–43, 1992.

31. RJ Whitley. Cercopithecine herpes virus 1 (B virus). In: BN Fields, DM Knipe, eds. Fields Virology. 2nd ed. New York: Raven Press, 1990, pp 2063–2075.

32. RN Hull. B virus vaccines. Lab Anim Sci 21:1068–1071, 1971.

33. PM Benson, SL Malane, R Banks, CB Hicks, J Hilliard. B virus (Herpesvirus simiae) and human infection. Arch Dermatol 125:1247–1248, 1989.

34. GP Holmes, LE Chapman, JA Stewart, SE Straus, JK Hilliard, DS Davenport. Guidelines for the prevention and treatment of B-virus infections in exposed persons. The B Virus Working Group. Clin Infect Dis 20:421–439, 1995.

35. JK Hilliard, RM Munoz, SL Lipper, R Eberle. Rapid identification of Herpesvirus simiae (B virus) DNA from clinical isolates in nonhuman primate colonies. J Virol Methods 13:55–62, 1986.

36. JK Hilliard, R Eberle, S Lipper, RM Munoz, SA Weiss. Herpesvirus simiae (B virus): replication of the virus and identification of viral polypeptides in infected cells. Arch Virol 93:185–198, 1987.

37. V Schuster, B Matz, H Wiegand, A Polack, B Corsten, D Neumann-Haefelin. Nucleic acid hybridization for detection of herpes viruses in clinical specimens. J Med Virol 19:277–286, 1986.

38. JK Hilliard, SS Kalter. Development of molecular probes for simian herpesvirus detection. Dev Biol Stand 59:79–86, 1985.

39. GL Van Hoosier, JL Melnick. Neutralizing antibodies in human sera to Herpesvirus simiae (B virus). Tex Rep Biol Med 19:376–380, 1961.

40. VJ Cabasso, WA Chappell, JE Avampato, JL Bittle. Correlation of B virus and herpes simplex virus antibodies in human sera. J Lab Clin Med 70:170–176, 1967.

41. D Katz, JK Hilliard, R Eberle, SL Lipper. ELISA for detection of group-common and virus-specific antibodies in human and simian sera induced by herpes simplex and related simian viruses. J Virol Methods 14:99–109, 1986.

42. LM Cropper, DN Lees, R Patt, IR Sharp, D Brown. Monoclonal antibodies for the identification of Herpesvirus simiae (B virus). Arch Virol 123:267–277, 1992.

43. JK Hilliard, R Eberle, D Katz, et al. Comparison of methods for identification of early signals of herpes B virus infections in humans and nonhuman primates. [Abstract no 284].

In: Abstracts of the 15th International Herpesvirus Workshop. Washington, D.C., 1990.

44. Munoz RM, Lipper SL, Hilliard JK. Identification of Herpesvirus simiae type specific polypeptides in a human outbreak of this virus [abstract no 198]. In: Abstracts of the 13th International Herpesvirus Workshop. Irvine, CA, 1988.

45. RL Heberling, SS Kalter. A dot-immunobinding assay on nitrocellulose with psoralen inactivated Herpesvirus simiae (B virus). Lab Anim Sci 37:304–308, 1987.

46. GW Gary, EL Palmer. Comparative complement fixation and serum neutralization antibody titers to herpes simplex virus type 1 and Herpesvirus simiae in Macaca mulatta and humans. J Clin Microbiol 5:465–470, 1977.

47. RN Hull. The significance of simian viruses to the monkey colony and laboratory investigator. Ann NY Acad Sci 162:472–482, 1969.

48. RN Hull, JC Nash. Immunization against B virus infection. I. Preparation of an experimental vaccine. Am J Hyg 71:15–28, 1960.

49. RN Hull, FB Peck Jr. Vaccination against herpesvirus infections. PAHO Sci Pub 147:266–275, 1967.

50. The B Virus Working Group. Guidelines for prevention of Herpesvirus simiae (B virus) infection in monkey handlers. J Med Primatol 17:77–83, 1988.

51. EA Boulter, HT Zwartouw, B Thorton. Postexposure immunoprophylaxis against B virus (Herpesvirus simiae) infection. Br Med J 283:1495–1497, 1981.

52. Center for Disease Control. Guidelines for prevention of Herpesvirus simiae (B virus) infection in monkey handlers. MMWR Morb Mortal Wkly Rep 36:680–689, 1987.

53. JE Kaplan. Guidelines for prevention of Herpesvirus simiae (B-virus) infection in monkey handlers. Lab Anim Sci 37:709–712, 1987.

54. HT Zwartouw, CR Humphreys, P Collins. Oral chemotherapy of fatal B virus (herpesvirus simiae) infection. Antiviral Res 11:275–284, 1989.

55. MH Wansbrough-Jones, B Cooper, N Sarantis. Prophylaxis against B virus infection. BMJ 297:909, 1988.

56. EA Boulter, B Thornton, EJ Bauer, A Bye. Successful treatment of experimental B virus (Herpesvirus simiae) infection with acyclovir. Br Med J 280:681–683, 1980.

57. KO Smith, KS Galloway, SL Hodges, KK Ogilvie, BK Radatus, SS Kalter, RL Heberling. Sensitivity of equine herpesviruses 1 and 3 in vitro to a new nucleoside analogue 9-{[2-hydroxy-1-(hydroxymethyl) ethoxy] methyl]} guanine. Am J Vet Res 44:1032–1035, 1983.

12

Human Papillomaviruses

Claire P. Mansur

Tufts University, Boston, and New England Medical Center, Boston, Massachusetts, USA

The papillomaviruses (PVs) are a large group of small DNA tumor viruses with a worldwide distribution (Fig. 12–1) that infect a number of species ranging from humans to fish. The bovine (BPV) and cottontail rabbit (CRPV) PVs have been historically important models for the genetic analysis of PV gene functions. The PVs, members of the Papovavirus class of viruses, are distantly related to other members of this class, including simian virus 40 and polyomavirus. The group of human papillomaviruses (HPVs) is very large, with over 80 different genotypes that are defined currently by differences in their nucleotide sequence (Table 12–1) [1]. Many of these genotypes correlate with a predilection to cause disease in distinct anatomical regions and clinical lesions with specific morphologies. However, the geographical and physical appearance of a papilloma does not always correlate with the HPV genotype. In the vast majority of cases, viral infection causes benign epithelial proliferations called warts or verrucae. Although these infections are benign, they are not insignificant. HPV infections are extremely common, can cause a significant morbidity, and at present represent one of the most common sexually transmitted diseases, causing warts of the penis, vulva, rectum, and cervix [2]. The medical cost of treatment of these benign lesions is enormous. Perhaps what has excited the most research interest in this virus is that a subset of the HPVs has been etiologically linked with the development of a number of epithelial malignancies. These cancer-associated HPV subtypes have been associated with over 99% of all cervical cancers and over 50% of vulvar, vaginal, anal, and penile cancers. The

importance of this relationship is clear, because cervical cancer is one of the most common causes of cancer death [3]. Also of note is the growing association of HPVs with other epithelial cancers, including those of the skin, larynx, and esophagus.

HISTORY

Warts were recognized by the ancient Greeks and Romans, and for centuries were thought to be a form of syphilis or gonorrhea. The viral etiology was first demonstrated in 1907 through experimental human inoculation of a cell-free extract of wart tissue from infected individuals [4]. The pathogenic virus was later confirmed in the 1940s by the visualization of viral particles in skin warts with electron microscopy. In the 1960s, it was assumed that there was only one type of HPV, and the morphological variation among lesions was due to the specific epithelium at a particular body site [5]. However, molecular biology techniques newly available in the 1970s demonstrated several types of HPV [6,7], and it became evident that each of the various clinical diseases is a result of infection with specific HPV types.

VIROLOGY

These spherical viruses are approximately 55 nm in diameter and, unlike many other viruses, lack an outer lipoprotein

247

TAXONOMY

Papovaviridae family
Papillomavirus genus

GEOGRAPHICAL INCIDENCE

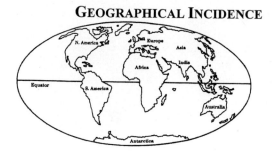

TRANSMISSION

Common warts, plantar warts, etc.: direct contact with infected individual or fomites.

Condyloma acuminata: direct genital contact, such as through sexual intercourse. Children may also acquire virus through intrapartum contact with mother's infected genitalia.

Respiratory papillomatosis: Intrapartum transmission from mother to child, likely with aspiration of the virus.

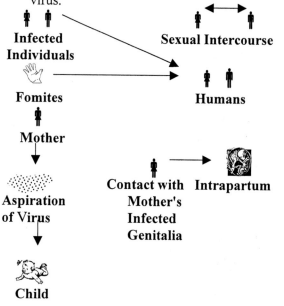

ZOONOTIC IMPLICATIONS

None for human papillomavirus infection.

Figure 12–1. Incidence and transmission of human papillomaviruses (HPVs).

envelope. Owing to the lack of this coat, PVs are quite stable in the environment and resistant to freezing or desiccation. These viruses show strict cellular tropism, infecting only the epithelial cells of their hosts. Molecular biological techniques have made it possible to clone complete viral genomes from the lesions of humans and animals and determine their nucleotide sequences.

The viral genome is small, about 8000 base pairs, and contains 10 open reading frames, or gene coding sequences (Fig. 12–2). The basic structure of the genome is the same for the different genotypes of PVs and consists of an upstream regulatory region (URR) that contains the origin of replication and many of the control elements for transcription and replication, an "early gene" (E) region, which encodes proteins that regulate viral function, and a "late gene" (L) region, which encodes the structural capsid proteins (Table 12–2). The viral capsid proteins encoded by the two L genes encode antigenic domains that are responsible for group-specific antisera to PVs. The viruses lack the full complement of genes required for DNA replication and so must recruit a number of cellular proteins for vegetative replication to occur. The regulation of viral gene expression is complex and incompletely understood, but evidence indicates regulation by both cellular and viral transcription factors. Cellular regulation of viral gene transcription is cell type–specific, and this may explain the marked epithelial tropism of the PVs [8–10].

PVs also show a strict species specificity, which means that they do not infect and undergo vegetative replication in cells of species other than their normal host. Thus, mature HPV virions cannot be produced in an animal model. Animal models of PV infection have been developed using specific animal PVs, in particular those using BPV and CRPV [11,12]. These animal models have taught us about the life cycle of these viruses. Although there are many similarities in the pathogenesis of the different PV genotypes, there are also distinct and important differences in the cellular functioning of their gene products, making extrapolation from animal models to HPV difficult. Because of these difficulties, it has been primarily through the application of molecular techniques that we have gained a better understanding of the functions of the HPVs.

With the cloning of a number of different PVs, the heterogeneity of these viruses, particularly the HPVs, became increasingly apparent. It was initially proposed that a new HPV genotype would be designated if this virus varied in nucleotide sequence by more than 50% from previously identified viruses using stringent DNA hybridization techniques. As more and more sequence data have become available for the viruses and the technology for identifying and sequencing these viruses has improved, a recent decision was made to require differences of 10% in nucleotide

Table 12–1. Disease Association of Human Papillomavirus (HPV) Genotypes

Characteristic HPV lesion	Associated HPV type
Palmoplantar warts	1
Common warts	2 (*4, 26, 27, 65, 78)
Flat warts	3, 10 (27, 28, 49)
Butcher's warts	7
Condylomata acuminata	6,11 (70, 83)
Bowenoid papulomatosis	16
Cervical intraepithelial neoplasia and cancers, anogenital cancers	16 & 18 most common; also 31, 33, 35, 39, 45, 51, 52, 58, 66, 69 (30, 34, 40, 42–44, 53–57, 59, 61, 62, 64, 67, 68, 71–74, 82)
Oral papillomas	6, 11
Oral focal epithelial hyperplasia	13, 32
Recurrent laryngeal papillomatosis	6,11
Cutaneous squamous cell carcinoma	41, 48 (29)
Laryngeal carcinoma	16,18
Verrucous carcinoma	16, 6, 11
Epidermodysplasia verruciformis (EV)	3, 5, 8, 9, 10, 12, 14, 15, 17, 19, 20, 21, 22,23, 24, 25, 36, 46, 47, 50 (37, 38)
Most EV-associated cancers	5, 8
Common warts in immunocompromised patients	EV types and 75, 76, 77
Epidermal cyst	60
Myrmecia wart	63

* = less frequent associations
Note: HPV types 79 and 81 have been designated but not reported; HPV type 80 has been found in histologically normal skin.

sequence in the late gene L1 open reading frame for the definition of a new type. Fully characterized HPV genotypes now number more than 80, and these are partially listed in Table 12–1. The continuing identification of new types suggests the actual number of existing genotypes will be greater than 100 [1].

Based on nucleotide sequence and clinical behavior, most HPVs can be placed into one of three categories. The first category contains those viruses that are most com-

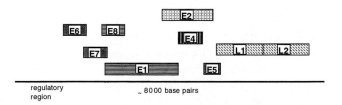

Figure 12–2. Schematic representation of the arrangement of the papillomavirus genome. The genome normally exists as a circular, double-stranded episome. E3 and E8 are not found in humans.

monly isolated from genital-mucosal lesions. Currently greater than 40 viruses belong to this category, but by far the most common isolates are HPV types 6, 11, 16, and 18. This group causes warts or condylomas on the genital skin and papillomas in oral and laryngeal epithelium, and is associated with the development of anogenital malignancies. The second category is composed of those viruses isolated from lesions on the nongenital keratinized skin in the general population, with HPV types 1, 2, and 3 being very common. This group is responsible for the common warts of hands and palmoplantar warts, the most common manifestations of HPV infection. The third category comprises those viruses isolated from the lesions of patients with the rare disease epidermodysplasia verruciformis (EV). These patients have a unique susceptibility to HPV infection and are infected with HPV subtypes rarely isolated in immunocompetent patients (discussed further later). Lastly, there are some remaining genotypes whose nucleotide sequences are heterogeneous and do not fit clearly with any of the previously discussed three categories, and these include HPV-63 and HPV-41.

Table 12–2.	HPV Proteins and Their Putative Functions
Viral protein	Proposed functions
E1	Forms a heterodimer with E2 and binds to the viral upstream regulatory region (URR) to function in viral DNA replication
E2	Participation with E1 in viral DNA replication
	Transcriptional regulation via binding sites in the URR, specifically transcriptional repression of E6 and E7
E3	Only in bovine papillomavirus
E4	Binds to and collapses the cellular cytokeratin network, allowing release of mature virions
E5	Enhances epidermal growth factor (EGF) and platelet-derived growth factor (PDGF) signaling via inhibition of turnover of the growth factor receptors
	Uncertain role in malignant transformation in HPV-related cancers
E6	High–cancer-risk E6 binds and mediates the rapid degradation of p53, inhibiting its cell cycle arrest and apoptotic responses to cellular DNA damage
	With high-risk E7, immortalizes primary keratinocytes and induces malignant transformation of cell lines
E7	High–cancer-risk E7 binds to the Rb family of growth regulatory proteins, inhibiting their negative regulation of the cell cycle
	Binds to and enhances the activity of AP-1 transcription factors
	Participates with E6 in cellular transformation
L1	Major capsid protein, alone or in combination with L2, can assemble into virus-like particles that have the antigenic epitopes that can stimulate the host's humoral response
L2	Minor capsid protein

Another important way to characterize these viruses is based on potential oncogenicity. Although there is a large array of genital-associated HPVs, each differs in its oncogenic potential. HPV-16 and HPV-18 are most commonly isolated from cervical cancers, whereas HPV-6 and HPV-11 are very common causes of benign genital warts only rarely associated with cervical cancers. This type of association within this group led to the concept of HPV types that could be characterized as being "high-risk" or "low-risk" for cancer development. Patients with EV very commonly develop squamous cell cancer (SCC) in warts located on sun-exposed skin. As seen with the anogenital HPV types, there are identifiable high-risk and low-risk types within the EV-associated group. Although approximately 17 HPV types have been associated with EV, the vast majority of the skin cancers in these patients are associated with HPV-5 and HPV-8. The mechanisms by which the high-risk HPVs participate in malignant transformation of cells is discussed further later.

EPIDEMIOLOGY

HPV infection, either mucosal or cutaneous, is very common, although the lack of reliable serological assays for detection of infection has prevented precise definition of lifetime cumulative incidence. Transmission of HPV is thought to occur through contact with individuals who have clinical or subclinical infection or contact with infectious virus present in the environment. The likelihood of developing a clinical infection is dependent on several factors including the quantity of virus, the nature of the contact, and the immunological state of the exposed individual. Warts are particularly common in patients with impairments in cell-mediated immunity (CMI) and occur in the majority of patients on immunosuppressive therapy following renal transplantation [13].

Cutaneous warts are uncommon in infancy, but the incidence in children and young adults may approach 10% [14]. Anogenital warts are uncommon in children, but are frequently seen in young adults. Anogenital warts are usually sexually transmitted, and they now represent one of the most common sexually transmitted diseases, with the incidence rising at a dramatic rate [2]. Anogenital warts do occur infrequently in infants and children and may be sexually transmitted, although infection may also occur from viral contact at birth from an infected mother or through spread from cutaneous warts. Although the presence of genital warts in children always raises concerns of sexual abuse, evidence indicates that a large proportion of these warts contain HPV types not usually associated with genital lesions. This suggests that transmission may occur via autoinoculation in children with cutaneous warts or contact with infected caretakers [15]. Similarly, laryngeal papillomas contain the same HPV types as genital warts, and approximately half of the cases occur in infants and children. In these cases, it is believed that infection frequently occurs through aspiration of the virus during birth.

In adults, genital HPV infections are usually transmitted sexually. The peak incidence of genital HPV infection occurs at 16 to 25 years of age, and the incidence increases with increasing numbers of sexual partners. After this age, the incidence of infection declines sharply. Depending on the assay used to detect HPV, the peak incidence of genital infection has been estimated to exceed 20% in sexually active women in this age group. The low-risk mucosal types, HPV-6 and HPV-11, are more likely to be isolated from genital warts of the external genital epithelium and less frequently isolated from cervical or vaginal lesions. These types are rarely isolated from genital cancers. The high-risk types, HPV-16 and HPV-18, are most frequently isolated from cervical and vaginal lesions. Asymptomatic genital infections and infections causing mild cervical dysplasia are very common, but the estimated prevalence rates vary substantially according to the assays used and the population studied. The incidence of both asymptomatic genital infection and mild dysplasia decreases dramatically after the ages of 20 to 25 years, suggesting that spontaneous clearing of infection is a common event. The incidence of HPV-associated cancer is much lower than the incidence of low-grade dysplasia, and the peak incidence of cancer occurs approximately 20 years later. This supports the concept that many infections clear spontaneously, and infection with high-risk HPV is not itself sufficient for the development of cancer. A worldwide study of the prevalence of HPV types found that over 90% of invasive cervical cancers contain HPV. Of these, 50% of the cancers contained HPV-16, 14% contained HPV-18, and less than 10% contained HPV-31 and HPV-45 [16]. The most important host factors that may increase the likelihood of progression from low-grade cervical lesions to carcinoma are probably immunological. Suspected environmental cofactors for the development of cervical cancer include smoking, nutritional status, and concurrent infection with other sexually transmitted agents, such as chlamydia, but studies do not unequivocally support a link. The incidence of high-risk HPV infection in men is more difficult to estimate, but because it is a sexually transmitted disease, it is likely to be similar to the incidence in women. High-risk HPV infections have been linked to a large proportion of anal and penile cancers [1,17].

PATHOGENESIS

Infection with HPV is thought to be acquired initially through inoculation of virus into the epidermis through epithelial defects. These may be microdefects, because infection often occurs in the absence of any history of injury to the skin, but skin maceration is probably an important predisposing factor. The HPVs infect only surface epithelial cells of the skin and mucous membranes. After infection, new warts may develop within a region or more dis-

tantly. Spread of infection can occur through direct infection of the skin or autoinoculation from infected skin cells, but not by blood-borne spread. It is common to see autoinoculation of virus on opposing body sites, such as on adjacent digits or in the anogenital region. In general, HPVs induce benign, self-limited proliferation in the skin. Although clinical morphology varies among HPV types, they share a similar histology showing localized epithelial hyperplasia above an intact basement membrane.

Specific HPV types are much more likely to infect specific body sites and, in particular, to show a preference for cutaneous versus mucosal sites. This is not invariably the case, however, because nongenital types have infrequently been isolated from genital lesions [15]. The clinical appearance of warts varies based on anatomical location, but infection is thought to proceed similarly in all sites. Little is known about the mechanisms of viral attachment and entry into the cell, but it has been demonstrated that PVs can attach to a number of nonepithelial cell types. Thus, it is not via attachment to an epithelial-specific receptor that PV cellular tropism is determined. It has been shown that attachment is mediated via the L1 protein, and it is believed that the receptor is likely to be a widely expressed and highly conserved cell surface protein [18]. Following infection of the basal cell compartment of the epidermis, the viral DNA exists as one or two copies of circular, episomal, double-stranded DNA. Through unknown mechanisms, the virus stimulates proliferation of basal cells, and the viral DNA is replicated and carried along with the epithelial cells as they stratify and differentiate. The lesion becomes acanthotic, presumably because of the stimulation of unscheduled cellular division. While infecting the basal cells, the virus does not undergo productive synthesis of virions, but rather viral early gene transcription and DNA replication are maintained at very low levels until higher strata of the epithelium are reached.

Following experimental inoculation of PVs in the skin, there is a long latency before clinical lesions develop, on the average of 6 to 9 months. This long period before the detection of clinical lesions implies that the viral genome may persist within the basal layer without stimulating cell proliferation or production of mature virus particles. In support of this, it has been shown that HPV DNA can be detected in normal mucosa of patients with laryngeal papillomatosis while the disease is in remission [19]. In epidemiological studies of genital HPV infection, HPV DNA is often detected in patients with no cytological or clinical abnormalities [20]. It is not clear whether this is a state of viral persistence with a low level of viral DNA replication or true viral latency (defined as nonreplicating, transcriptionally inactive virus). This restriction of viral gene expression in the basal layers makes it difficult for the immune system to detect the virus. Thus, it has been hypothesized that this may be a mechanism by which PVs evade the immune surveillance of the host [21].

Only in the terminally differentiating epithelial cells, presumably in response to differentiation-specific signals, do viral gene transcription and DNA synthesis accelerate and virions assemble. The viral capsid proteins assemble in the nucleus of the infected cell as differentiation moves toward the stratum corneum. Evidence indicates that the viral gene, E4 (which is probably more appropriately termed a *late gene*), attaches to and collapses the cytoplasmic keratin framework, presumably to allow release of infectious virions into the environment [22]. It is likely that in these outer levels of the epidermis, the virus is more protected from the immunological defenses of the host. The level of production of viral particles varies with the different types of warts, with levels being highest in patients with EV; in normal hosts, they are more plentiful in plantar warts and much lower in genital lesions (Fig. 12–3). In HPV-associated dysplasia and cancer, although the viral DNA is retained and genes are expressed, mature virion production is markedly decreased.

It is particularly important to note that it is within this progresively differentiating cellular environment that the virus must recruit the many cellular factors necessary for its own replication. The virus presumably does this by deregulating cell growth in the basal layer of the epithelium so it can utilize the cellular replicative machinery for its

own replication. Thus, even in benign infections, the viruses have some ability to stimulate cellular growth [23,24], and it is likely that acquisition of transforming function in the high-risk viruses may have come in part from a loss of regulation of this growth-promoting activity. Production of mature viral particles is seen only in the outer layers of the epidermis where the cells are terminally differentiated and no longer competent for cell division. Another important point is that the viruses require a differentiated environment for growth and it has not been possible to develop a simple means to culture HPVs in vitro. Very limited production of HPV virions has been achieved in vitro using infected human cells in an organotypic culture system [25,26]. However, introduction of cloned viral DNA into cultured cells has not led to synthesis of infectious viral particles.

Whereas there appear to be mechanisms by which PVs evade the host's immune response, there is also indirect evidence that the immune system plays an important role in controlling HPV infection [27,28]. Cutaneous warts frequently undergo spontaneous regression. Infrequently, treatment of a small number of warts may lead to resolution of many or all of the warts in a patient. The prevalence of genital HPV infections peaks in young adulthood and declines thereafter, implying spontaneous clearing of infection presumably by immune mechanisms. All of these phenomena suggest a role for the immune system in controlling HPV infection, but the precise mechanisms remain poorly understood. No consistent defect in the immune system in patients with warts has been demonstrated, but a number of lines of evidence point to the importance of CMI in the course of HPV infection. Patients with defects in CMI have a high incidence of warts, which occur in larger numbers and are more resistant to treatment. Furthermore, these warts frequently resolve spontaneously with correction of the immune defect. There is a higher incidence in HPV-associated cancers in renal transplant patients [29]. In immunocompetent patients, flat warts have been reported to undergo spontaneous resolution, and histologically, this is accompanied by a monocellular infiltrate of the skin.

The role that the humoral immune system plays in HPV infection is also unclear, but patients with humoral defects have not been found to be predisposed to HPV infection. In general, in benign infections the antibody response to early viral proteins is weak and declines over time. The incidence of type-specific reactions to HPV E6 and E7 proteins is somewhat higher in patients with cervical cancer, being detected in approximately half of these patients [29–31]. It is thought that this may be due to the increase in expression of E6 and E7 in progressively more dysplastic lesions (see Viral Oncogenesis). Improved detection of antibodies to viral capsid antigens has come with the synthe-

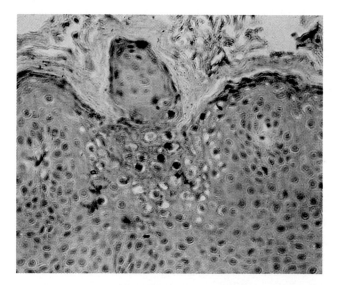

Figure 12–3. Immunoperoxidase staining of a lesion from a patient with epidermodysplasia verruciformis. The black dots represent clusters of mature HPV virions. (Photograph courtesy of Elliot Androphy, M.D., Department of Dermatology, Tufts/New England Medical Center, Boston, MA.)

sis of virus-like particles (VLPs). When the viral L1 or L1 and L2 proteins are expressed in eukaryotic cell lines, the proteins self-assemble into VLPs that are morphologically indistinguishable from native viral capsids [32]. Using VLPs, anticapsid antibodies are detected in over half of patients with low-grade or asymptomatic genital HPV-16 infections and in the majority of patients with HPV-16–associated cervical intraepithelial neoplasia (CIN) and invasive cancer, a somewhat surprising result given the rarity of mature virion production in these lesions. There is no evidence that these antibodies influence the course of the disease. Because these antigens are only produced in the outer layers of the epidermis, it has been hypothesized that these antibodies may be important in limiting reinfection rather than in inducing regression of active infection.

Viral Oncogenesis

Historically, PV infection was first linked to the development of cancer in studies that demonstrated the oncogenic potential of the BPV and CRPV. The first evidence for a iink between HPV infection and cancer in humans came from patients with EV in whom SCCs frequently develop in sun-exposed warty lesions. It is clear that among the over 80 different HPV genotypes, only a small subset of these are high-risk for malignant transformation. For example, whereas over 17 different HPV types have been associated with the lesions of EV, only HPV-5 and HPV-8 are associated with the majority of HPV-linked SCCs. Similarly, over 25 HPV types have been isolated from mucosal HPV lesions in normal hosts, but only HPV types 16, 18, 31, and 45 are detected at high frequency in cervical cancers. The association of this group of high-risk viruses with cervical cancers is well established, but recent evidence indicates that these viruses may be associated with even more cancers than previously suspected. The cancer-associated EV types have been isolated from skin cancers in immunocompromised patients, particularly renal transplant patients [29,33,34]. The high-risk genital types have been associated with other epithelial tumors, including those of the penis, vulva, anus, and oropharynx [35–40]. Now that sensitive methods for detecting a broad range of HPV subtypes have been developed, it has been reported that HPV DNA is detected in up to 30% of nonmelanoma skin cancers even in immunocompetent hosts [33]. These recent and surprising results suggest that the oncogenic potential of HPVs may be more far-reaching than first imagined. The mechanisms of HPV carcinogenesis are best understood with the high-risk genital HPV types. It is likely that the transforming effects of the EV-associated and skin cancer–associated HPV types may be somewhat different from the genital HPV types, but these potential differences are undefined at the present time.

As noted previously, although the vast majority of cervical cancers are associated with HPV infection, most viral infections, even with the high-risk viruses, do not lead to the development of cancer. In addition, there is a long latency between the initial infection and progression toward malignancy (on the order of decades), suggesting that the high-risk viruses predispose to malignancy but other events, such as mutations or oncogene activation, are required for full malignant transformation. HPV-containing cervical carcinoma cell lines and cancer specimens exhibit changes in the behavior of the viruses in these cells from what is seen in benign lesions. In benign infections, HPV DNA exists as a circular episome, whereas in cervical carcinoma cells, the viral DNA usually becomes integrated into the host DNA [41]. Importantly, with integration there is frequently a loss of the viral regulatory gene, E2, and sometimes E1, with subsequent dysregulation of E6 and E7 gene expression and increased levels of their protein products [42,43]. Integration may also disrupt cellular genes. Although integration does not consistently occur at the same sites in the cellular genome, integration near to cellular oncogenes has been reported [44]. As noted previously, production of mature virus particles is dependent upon a differentiated state of the cell, and in the poorly differentiated cells of CIN or frank malignancy, mature viral particles are infrequently detected.

Early evidence for a link between HPV infection and the development of cervical cancer came from identification of HPV-6 and HPV-11 DNA in benign genital warts and HPV-16 and HPV-18 DNA from cervical cancers and the precursor lesions of cervical dysplasia and carcinoma in situ. The detection of HPV DNA in human cancers did not prove that the viruses played an etiological role in the development of cancer, and evidence for this came from several lines of investigation. Several established HPV-positive cervical carcinoma cell lines such as HeLa and SiHa were found to continue to synthesize HPV proteins despite maintenance in culture for decades [45,46]. In specific, these cervical carcinoma cell lines were found to selectively retain and express the early viral genes E6 and E7 [47–49]. In addition, it was demonstrated that repression of HPV protein expression in cervical carcinoma cell lines led to decreased cell growth and loss of the transformed phenotype [50,51].

With the ability to clone the HPV genomes, a great deal of work has been done to examine the effect of HPV gene expression using in vitro cellular transformation assays. By introduction of HPV genomes or specific viral genes into cells grown in culture, various parameters of malignant transformation that are thought to mirror the in vivo transformation process have been measured [52]. It is now understood that malignant transformation is a multistep process with cellular dysplasia developing first, followed by carcinoma in situ, and finally development of invasive carcinoma. Using classic transformation assays, immortalization of cells corresponds to the early changes seen in carcinoma in situ, whereas measures of anchorage independent growth and tumorigenicity in mice corresponds to a more fully transformed phenotype. With numerous such assays, it was demonstrated that the high-risk HPV genotypes could induce immortalization of primary cells [53,54] and malignant progression of immortalized cell lines [42,51,52]. The morphological appearance of the immortalized cells closely mimics that which is seen in CIN. These cells are not tumorigenic but, when maintained for sustained periods in culture, will evolve a fully transformed phenotype. These effects can be achieved with expression of only the E6 and E7 genes, thus identifying these gene products as the major transforming proteins of the HPVs [53,56,57,58]. The E6 and E7 proteins from the low-risk HPVs show little or no activity in these transformation assays [59,60]. Studies with BPVs showed BPV E5 to be one of the major transforming proteins for BPV, but studies with HPV E5 indicate that it is only weakly transforming [61–63]. The fact that the high-risk HPVs, or the high-risk E6 and E7 gene products alone, induce immortalization of cells but not a fully transformed phenotype suggests that this HPV-mediated extension of lifespan allows time for additional genetic or epigenetic alterations that must accumulate for a fully malignant phenotype to be manifest. Better understanding of the functions of the individual HPV proteins has shown this to be the case.

As has been demonstrated for other viral oncogenes, the high-risk HPV E6 and E7 oncoproteins exert their transforming effects, at least in part, through interaction with cellular tumor suppressor genes. E6 binds to and mediates the rapid degradation of p53 via the cellular ubiquitin proteolysis pathway (Fig. 12–4). The high-risk E6 proteins bind to p53 in complex with a cellular factor called E6-AP, for E6-associated protein [64]. The low-risk E6 proteins do not induce degradation of p53 [65–67]. It has been reported that p53 is normally targeted and degraded through the ubiquitin pathway independent of E6 [68,69]. Thus, it appears that E6 stimulates accelerated turnover of p53 or perhaps stimulates degradation of p53 in the face of signals that would normally induce p53 stabilization. p53 mediates cellular growth arrest and apoptosis of cells particularly in response to DNA damage [70–74]. A critical mechanism by which p53 exerts its effects is through transcriptional activation [75–77]. Under conditions of cell stress and/or DNA damage, cellular levels of p53 rise primarily through a decrease in its degradation and p53-dependent transcrip-

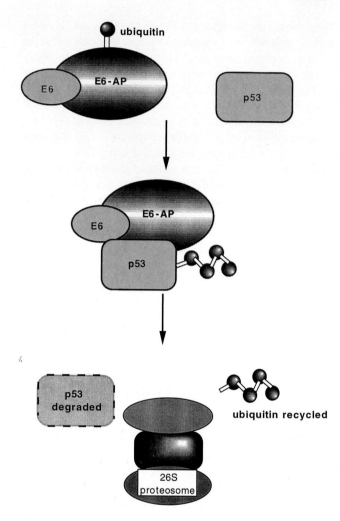

Figure 12–4. The high-risk E6 proteins bind to a cellular protein, E6-AP, and this complex binds to p53, which catalyzes the attachment of a chain of ubiquitin molecules to p53, resulting in its degradation via the cellular 26S proteosome.

tional activation increases [78–81]. An important transcriptional target of p53 is p21/WAF1 which is an inhibitor of cyclin-dependent kinases (CDKs) [78,81,82]. Through inhibition of CDKs, expression of genes necessary for progression through the cell cycle is inhibited, and there is a G1-mediated growth arrest that allows the cell time to repair damaged DNA. In other cases, presumably in response to more extensive damage to DNA, p53 signals cellular apoptosis, which is a programmed cell death [83]. Without the p53-mediated DNA damage response, the cell would be allowed to continue to divide, thereby perpetuating DNA mutations. Support for this theory has come from the demonstration of genomic instability and gene amplification in cells that lack p53 function [84,85]. Another mechanism by which p53 participates in the response to DNA damage is through binding to proteins such as RPA, TFIIH, and CSB, which have functions in both DNA replication and repair. Although the pathways are not completely worked out, it is thought that p53 may inhibit the DNA replication functions of these proteins but localize them to sites of DNA damage and perhaps participate directly in facilitating the DNA repair process [86–88]. The functional activities of p53 that are disrupted by interaction with the high-risk E6 proteins are depicted in Figure 12–5.

Like the high-risk E6 proteins, the high-risk E7 proteins interact with a cellular tumor suppressor. E7 binds to the retinoblastoma protein (Rb) and related proteins, p107 and p130, that, in cooperation with p53, also mediate cellular growth arrest [89–91]. Rb is a cellular growth regulator whose phosphorylation status is regulated through the cell cycle. It is activated in its hypophosphorylated state in G0 and G1 phases of the cell cycle. In this active, hypophosphorylated state, pRb binds to the cellular transcription factor E2F, inhibiting the transcription of genes necessary for cell cycle progression [92]. In the S and G2 phases, CDKs act to phosphorylate Rb, causing release of E2F and cell cycle progression. Thus, the p53 and Rb pathways converge: p53 increases levels of p21 that inhibits CDKs; with inhibition of CDKs, pRb is maintained in an active hypophosphorylated state. The high-risk E7 proteins bind preferentially to the hypophosphorylated form of Rb and

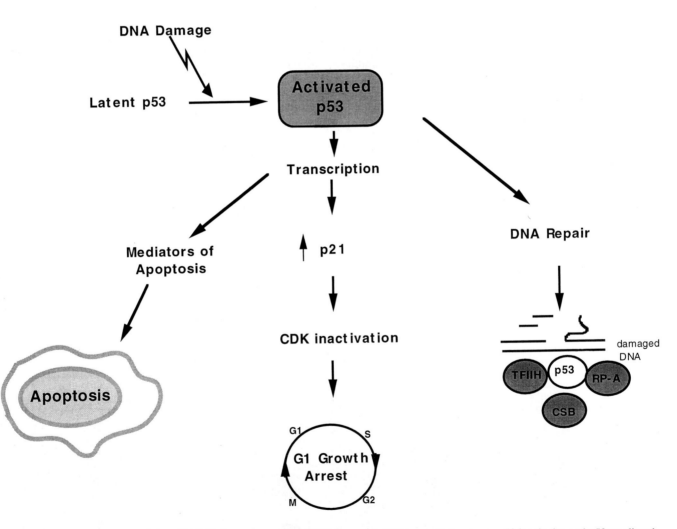

Figure 12–5. Mechanisms of the p53 DNA damage response. With damage to DNA or cellular stress, p53 levels rise and p53-mediated transcriptional activation increases. Through regulation of transcription, p53 mediates a G1 growth arrest. Through transcriptional-dependent and -independent mechanisms, under other conditions, p53 can signal cellular apoptosis. In addition, p53 can bind to proteins that function in DNA repair and through nonspecific DNA binding, localize them to sites of DNA damage.

induce the release of E2F [93], thereby providing another pathway to cell cycle progression and unscheduled DNA synthesis (Fig. 12–6). Again as seen with E6, the low-risk E7 proteins bind to Rb with much lower affinity than those of the high-risk HPVs [94,95]. Similarly, the related proteins, p107 and p130, complex with regulators of the cell cycle including other members of the E2F family, cyclin A and cyclin E [96,97], and participate in the regulation of both G1 and G2 cell cycle blocks. The interaction of high-risk E7 with these other Rb family members, as well as other mediators of cell cycle regulation, is thought to overcome inhibition of cell cycle arrest perhaps at both the G1 and the G2 phases of the cell cycle [91,98,99].

Inhibition of these tumor suppressors by E6 and E7 proteins is not sufficient for malignant transformation, but does lead to genetic instability, unregulated cellular growth, and the acquisition of additional mutations that presumably allow malignant progression [100]. Evidence indicates that there are other mechanisms by which E6 and E7 exert their transforming effects, such as through binding and/or mediating the degradation of other cellular proteins [101,102] and altering the function of other transcription factors [103], but these functions are at present less well defined. The HPV E2 protein also has an important role in regulating the transforming activity of the HPVs. As mentioned previously, the E2 proteins are regulators of viral gene transcription. Expression of E2 in cells that contain HPV-18 DNA has been shown to down-regulate the expression of E6 and E7 [104]. Disruption of the E2 gene leads to increased expression of the E6 and E7 proteins [42,43] and increases the immortalization capacity of HPV-16 [105]. Thus, the integration of the viral DNA into the host genome and frequent loss of expression of E2 in cervical neoplasias is likely to be an important mechanism by which expression of the viral transforming genes is deregulated. Evidence indicates that viral DNA integration and disruption of the E2 gene are neither necessary nor sufficient for malignant transformation because a number of cervical cancers with episomal viral DNA have been identified, and conversely, cells with integrated viral DNA and active viral gene expression do not always display a malignant phenotype [106,107]. Nonetheless, it is likely that loss of E2's regulatory function serves to enhance the transforming capability of these viruses.

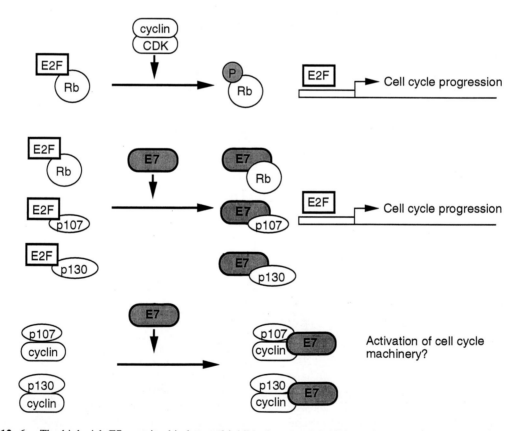

Figure 12–6. The high-risk E7 proteins bind to and inhibit the growth inhibitory functions of the Rb family of proteins.

Although BPV E5 is an important transforming protein, the role of HPV E5 in malignant conversion in vivo is uncertain. High levels of HPV E5 have been detected in lesions of CIN [108], but in cervical carcinoma the E5 gene is often deleted [42]. This has led to the hypothesis that the E5 gene may play a role early in viral infection, but is dispensable for the later stages of malignant transformation. The BPV E5 protein binds to and enhances the effect of the growth factors, platelet-derived growth factor (PDGF) and epidermal growth factor (EGF) [109,110]. The HPV-16 E5 protein has not been found to bind these growth factors or their receptors directly, but rather to enhance the activity of these receptors in part by decreasing their degradation rate through inhibition of the acidification of endocytic vesicles [111,112]. Presumably, without degradation, the growth factor receptors recycle to the cell surface and increase the responsiveness to growth stimulatory signals.

There is evidence that the cell has other defense mechanisms that protect against malignant transformation in addition to p53 and Rb. The majority of high-risk HPV infections never result in malignant transformation and, if so, occur only after a long latent period. This implies the existence of important cellular, immune, and/or viral modulators of HPV-transforming activities. During somatic cell hybridization studies, cells that have been immortalized by E6 and E7 and are hybridized with primary cells have their malignant phenotype suppressed, and they frequently undergo senescence. This modulating effect is likely to be due to down-regulation of E6 and E7 gene expression, but there is some evidence that this effect can be seen even with continued expression of the viral oncogenes [113,114]. When fully transformed cervical cells are grafted onto nude mice, they show no change in the expression of E6 and E7 genes. When immortalized, but not fully transformed, cells are grafted onto mice, expression of E6 and E7 genes is down-regulated [115]. These results suggest that the cell has mechanisms by which it can interfere with the function of the viral oncogenes and/or act to down-regulate their expression, mechanisms that the fully transformed cells have escaped. In order for malignant progression to occur, these cellular growth suppressive functions must be inactivated, and thus, other genetic or epigenetic events would be expected to have occurred. It is clear that the viral oncogenes do induce genetic instability, most profoundly through the interaction between high-risk E6 proteins and p53, but the exact mutations that occur to allow malignant progression have not been identified. In order to identify other likely mechanisms by which inhibition of cell growth is overcome, investigators have searched for genetic alterations that may be found in HPV-transformed cells and potential cofactors that may contribute to malignant progression. When cervical cancer cells have been subjected to cytogenetic analysis, a variety of chromosomal abnormalities at a number of different sites were found [116,117], although no one mutation has been consistently identified.

Despite this, a few candidate genes that may affect HPV function have been identified. It has been postulated that a tumor suppressor that may function in suppression of HPV-mediated transformation resides on the short arm of chromosome 11. Introduction of chromosome 11 into HPV-containing HeLa or SiHa cells suppresses the tumorigenic phenotype of these cells [118,119]. A locus on the short arm of chromosome 11 functions through down-regulation of viral gene transcription acting at the promoter of the viral URR [120,121]. Deletion of this region of chromosome 11 leads to overexpression of an inhibitory subunit of protein phosphatase 2A (PP2A) [122]. Through alteration of protein phosphorylation status, PP2A regulates the activity of a number of important cellular growth regulators and transcription factors (such as Rb, p53, and AP-1), and thus inhibition of PP2A may be a likely mechanism by which viral gene transcription is enhanced. Another candidate gene that has been proposed to be involved in malignant progression encodes the CDK inhibitor, $p16^{INK4}$. The function of $p16^{INK4}$ is not well understood, but it has been shown to up-regulate with inactivation of Rb and participate in the suppression of immortalization of cells. Spontaneous immortalization of Li Fraumeni fibroblasts (which have one mutant p53 allele) is associated with loss or mutation of the second p53 allele and loss of expression of $p16^{INK4}$ [123]. A subsequent study reported that loss of $p16^{INK4}$ may be necessary for immortalization of epithelial cells by HPV-16 E6 alone [124]. Further studies will be needed to clarify the relationship of $p16^{INK4}$ to HPV-induced transformation of cells.

Others have searched for paracrine effectors of HPV function. It has been reported that tumor necrosis factor (TNF)–α, interleukin-1, and transforming growth factor (TGF)–β can all induce down-regulation of viral early gene expression [125,126]. In other reports, it has been shown that HPV-transformed cells have evolved resistance to the growth suppressive effects of TGF-β [127], suggesting that with malignant progression, additional mutational events allow escape from this paracrine regulation. A cellular cofactor that may act in a positive way to stimulate HPV-transforming capability is glucocorticoids. The high-risk HPVs have glucocorticoid-responsive elements within the regulatory region of their genome, and addition of glucocorticoids to transformation assays is reported to enhance the immortalizing effects of HPV-16 [128]. Further,

Table 12–3.   Clinical Manifestations of HPV

Common warts (verruca vulgaris)	Present with single or grouped scaly, rough papules or nodules, especially on the hands. These commonly occur in children and young adults
Paronychial (periungual) warts	May occur at any age, with single or multiple confluent, keratotic lesions on the proximal periphery of the nails. These lesions are often painful, and may spread beneath the nail plate, causing separation of the nail plate and nail bed
Filiform warts	Consist of a tiny thin base with several keratotic thread-like projections. These occur most commonly on the face, neck, and genitalia. Warts may also take on the appearance of cutaneous horns
Flat warts (verruca plana)	Appear as grouped, minimally raised, flat-topped, skin-colored papules that are usually 2–4 mm in diameter. No papillomatosis or hyperkeratosis occurs with these lesions, so minimal scale is present. They occur most commonly on the face and hands of children, although they are also found in the beard area of men and the legs of women, where they are often spread by shaving. Multiple lesions may occur along a line of cutaneous trauma
Palmar and plantar warts	In the thick skin of the palms and soles, warts may have a number of clinical appearances. Simple palmar and plantar warts appear as minute punctate depressions. When they coalesce into large, thin, endophytic confluent plaques, they are referred to as mosaic warts. When they present as thick confluent plaques, they are known as myrmecia warts. The thickened, hyperkeratotic form is often painful with pressure. The borders are sharply demarcated, often with a surrounding border of thick callus
Butcher's warts	Present as verrucous papules, often multiple, on the hands and fingers of meat cutters
Anogenital warts (condyloma acuminata)	The appearance can vary from small verrucous papules, to discrete, sessile, smooth-topped papules or

	nodules, to large exophytic masses. These lesions are moist and fleshy and may become friable. Confluence into keratotic plaques is also seen. Their size usually varies from a few millimeters to a few centimeters, but they may reach several centimeters if they coalesce. Their color ranges from skin-colored to reddish-brown
Bowenoid papulosis	Usually presents as groups of 2–3 mm smooth-to-slightly verrucous papules on the external male or female genitalia. The lesions may be slightly reddish in color or hyperpigmented, and are often multiple in number
Respiratory papillomatosis	Consists of multiple benign verruca of the larynx, with possible extensions into the oropharynx or bronchopulmonary epithelium. Patients present with hoarseness or stridor, and in extreme cases, may have blockage of the airways
Oral papillomas	Appear as small, pink to white papules on the oral mucosa and hard palate. When found on the palate, they may become verrucous. Variants include oral florid papillomatosis and focal epithelial hyperplasia (Heck's disease). Oral condylomas may occur from orogenital sexual exposure
Verrucous carcinoma	Appear as large, exophytic tumors that range in size from a few to several centimeters. May develop on the genitals, oral mucosa, or soles of the feet [134]
Epidermodysplasia verruciformis	Present as widespread warts of the face, scalp, trunk, and extremities. These may appear either as flat warts or as red-brown macules resembling tinea versicolor or pityriasis rosea. These lesions usually appear in the first decade of life and may become very extensive and confluent. When present on the trunk, they may be fainter in color and more difficult to detect. Warty "seborrheic keratosis–like" lesions are often seen on the face, neck, and anogenital area. Mucosal lesions are unusual.

it was shown that HPV-16–mediated transformation is inhibited by exposure of cells to a glucocorticoid antagonist [129]. Clearly, the interaction between the host and high-risk HPVs is complex and incompletely understood. Evidence indicates that there are a number of lines of defense against the progression to malignancy and that these defenses are often successful in preventing the progression from infection to the development of cancer. A better understanding of these mechanisms and how they may fail is needed for the development of specific antiviral therapies for prevention and treatment of these common diseases.

CLINICAL MANIFESTATIONS

Warts may occur on any cutaneous or mucosal surface and are generally classified by their morphology and clinical location. As discussed previously, specific HPV subtypes have a predilection to cause warts in specific anatomical locations (Tables 12–1 and 12–3). As previously mentioned, common warts are most commonly associated with HPV-2, whereas flat warts are usually caused by HPV-3 or HPV-10 (Figs. 12–7 to 12–13). Palmar and plantar warts are most frequently due to infection with HPV-1 (Fig. 12–14), whereas butcher's warts are associated with HPV-7. The predilection for butcher's warts is believed to be due to associated trauma to the hands and not to transmission of an animal virus. Warts usually appear as hyperkeratotic papillomas that may occur on all cutaneous surfaces, and the appearance of warts may vary in different body sites. Close inspection of the papules, particularly after paring off the keratotic surface, often reveals "black dots," which

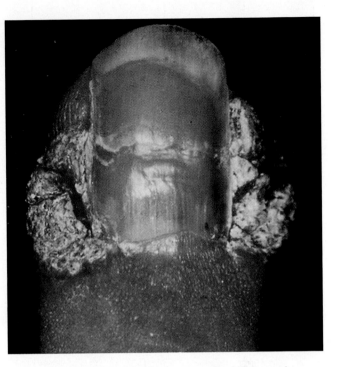

Figure 12–8. Paronychial warts with nail dystrophy.

represent thrombosed capillaries within the wart (Fig. 12–15).

Anogenital warts, or condyloma acuminata, may occur on the perineum, genitalia, crural folds, and anus and also may extend to involve the vagina, cervix, urethra, and rec-

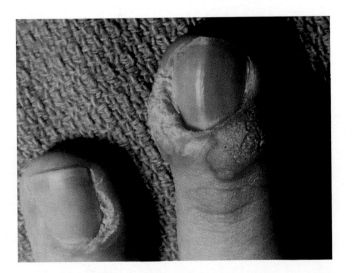

Figure 12–7. Periungual verruca vulgaris.

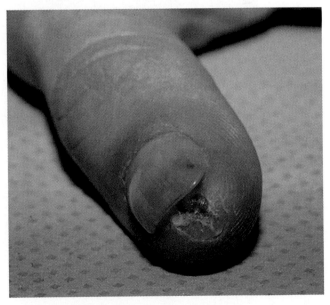

Figure 12–9. Subungual wart.

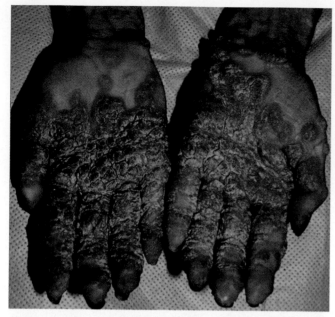

(a)

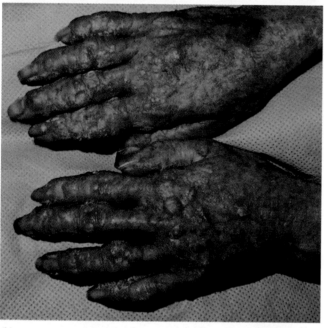

(b)

Figure 12–10. (a,b) Extensive verruca vulgaris covering both hands. (Photographs courtesy of Mario Marini, M.D., Department of Dermatology, University of Buenos Aires, Buenos Aires, Argentina.)

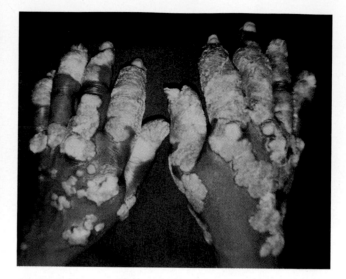

Figure 12–11. Extensive verruca vulgaris in another patient. (Photograph courtesy of Roberto Arenas, M.D., Mexico City, Mexico.)

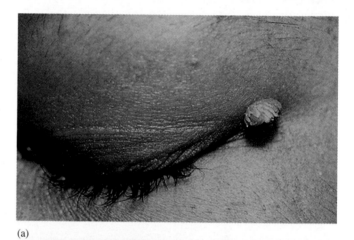

(a)

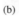

(b)

Figure 12–12. (a,b) Filiform warts.

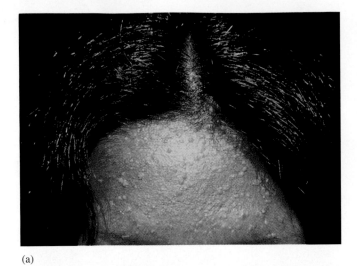

(a)

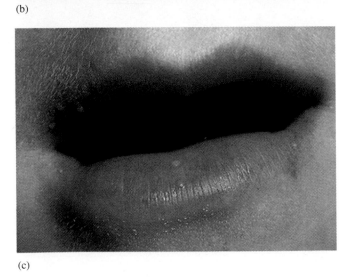

(b)

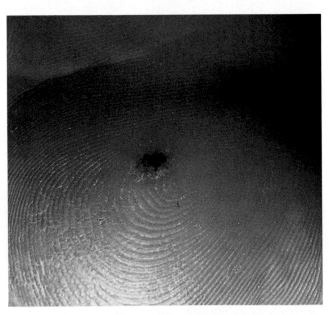

(c)

Figure 12–13. (a–c) Flat warts. (Photograph 13A courtesy of Axel Hoke, M.D., Novato, CA.)

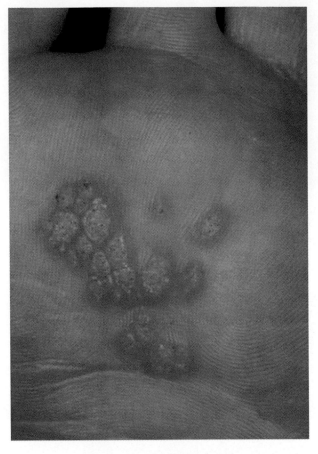

Figure 12–14. Plantar warts.

Figure 12–15. Simple punctate plantar wart showing capillary thromboses.

tum (Figs. 12–16 to 12–20). HPV-6 and HPV-11 are frequently isolated from anogenital warts, although over 25 different HPV types can cause mucosal lesions. On the cervix, condylomas may appear exophytic, endophytic, papillomatous, or flat or may be visible only by colposcopy. Condyloma are usually asymptomatic but occasionally cause itching or mild burning. During pregnancy, condyloma may enlarge and have been reported to obstruct vaginal delivery [130]. The detection of small condylomas can be enhanced by the application of a 5% acetic acid soak applied to the skin for a few minutes, after which small or previously undetectable lesions may appear as

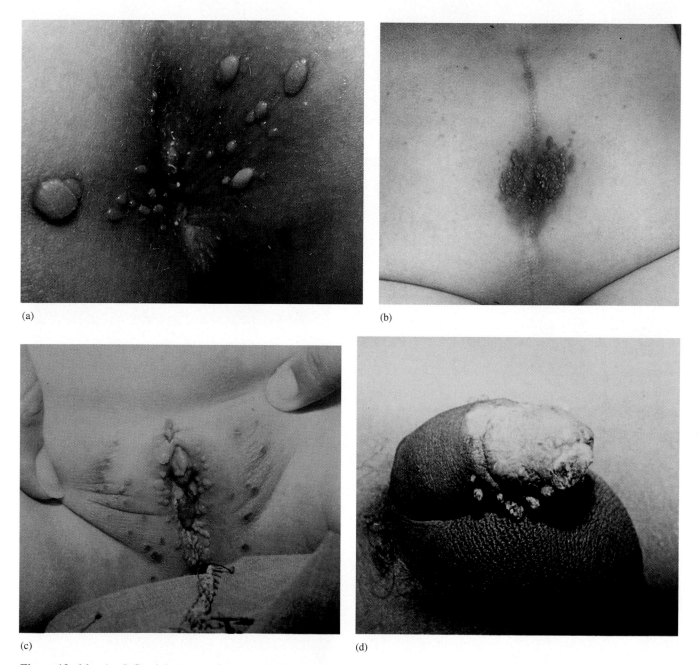

(a)

(b)

(c)

(d)

Figure 12–16. (a–d) Condyloma acuminata may be due to sexual abuse or may occur via nonsexual transmission. Perianal condylomata can have a variety of morphologies including (a) sessile smooth topped papules or (b) confluent "cauliflowerlike" exophytic masses. It may occur as (c) genital condyloma (in a small girl) or as a (d) penile condyloma (in a 15-yr-old boy with the acquired immunodeficiency syndrome [AIDS]).

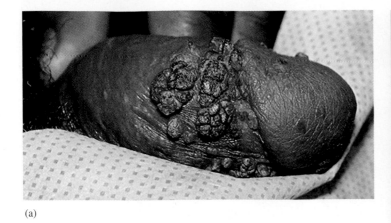

(a)

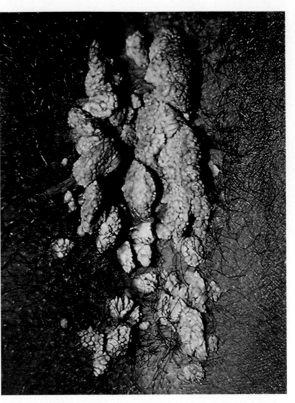

(b)

Figure 12–17. Verrucous condylomata on the (a) shaft of the penis and the (b) vulva.

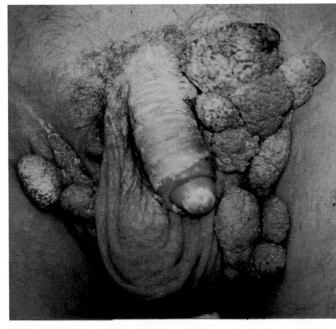

(a)

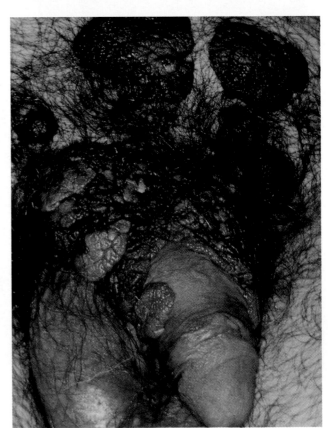

(b)

Figure 12–18. (a,b) Extensive condyloma of the male genitalia.

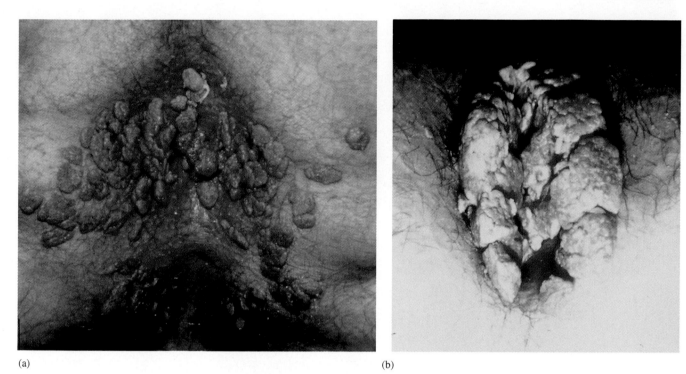

(a)   (b)

Figure 12–19.   (a,b) Extensive perianal condyloma.

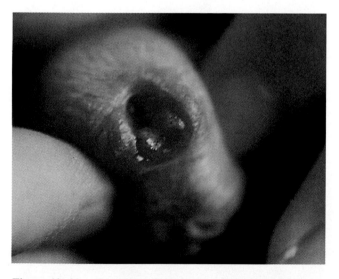

Figure 12–20.   Condyloma accuminata of the urethral meatus. (Photograph courtesy of Elliot Androphy, M.D., Department of Dermatology, Tufts/New England Medical Center, Boston, MA.)

whitish plaques. This method, however, is associated with high rates of both false positivity and false negativity.

Warts may present in locations other than the typical cutaneous and anogenital surfaces. For example, warts may produce major problems when they grow in the conjunctiva (Fig. 12–21). Another unusual location is around ostomy sites (Fig. 12–22).

Bowenoid papulosis is an unusual manifestation of HPV infection that involves the external male and female genitalia (Fig. 12–23). Histologically, these lesions reveal cellular dysplasia resembling squamous cell carcinoma in situ. Bowenoid papulosis is usually caused by the high-risk HPV-16, which would suggest that this is a precursor lesion to vulvar or penile cancer, but clinically these lesions usually behave in a benign manner. Nonetheless, these lesions need to be followed closely, because they are a potential source of HPV-16 and thus present an increased risk of cervical carcinoma to the patient or his or her sexual partners. In addition, cautious management is warranted because the actual incidence of malignant progression of these lesions, although low, is unknown (Fig. 12–24).

Bowen's disease refers to squamous cell carcinoma in situ (Figs. 12–25 and 12–26). When it presents on the penis, it is sometimes referred to as erythroplasia of

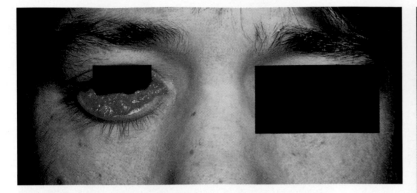

(a)

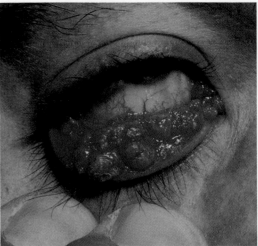

(b)

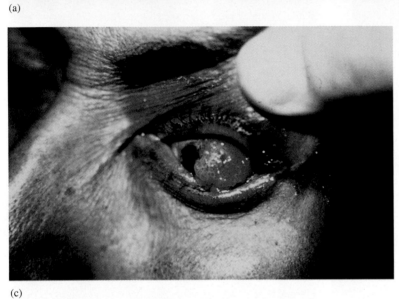

(c)

Figure 12–21. (a,b) Conjunctival warts. (c) More extensive warts of the eye in another patient. (Photograph 21a,b courtesy of Robert Brodell, M.D., Warren, Ohio; photograph 21C courtesy of Maria Gabriela Rodriguez, M.D., Mexico City, Mexico.)

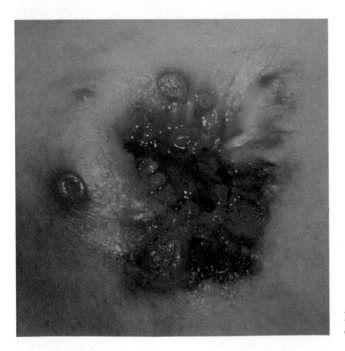

Figure 12–22. Warts and molluscum contagiosum surrounding an ostomy site.

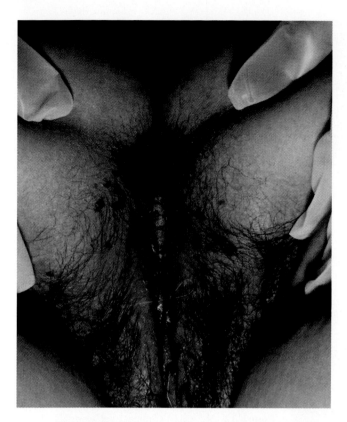

Figure 12–23.   Perianal Bowenoid papulosis.

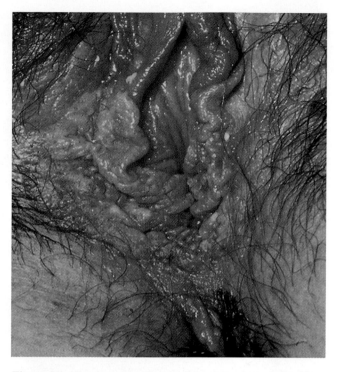

Figure 12–25.   Bowen's disease of the vulva that was found to contain HPV-16. (Photograph courtesy of Elliot Androphy, M.D., Department of Dermatology, Tufts/New England Medical Center, Boston, Massachusetts.)

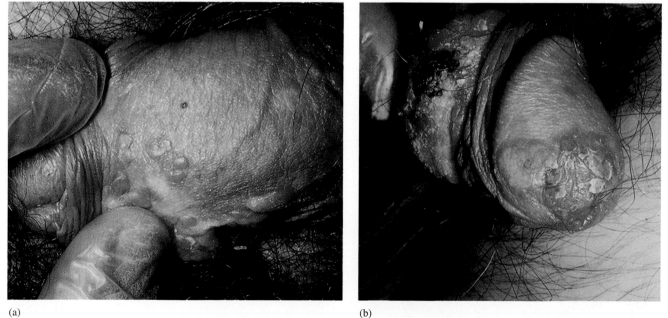

(a)   (b)

Figure 12–24.   (a) Skin-colored lesions of bowenoid papulosis on the shaft of the penis. (b) The other side of the penis revealed multicentric squamous cell carcinoma. Although this disease usually behaves in a benign manner, in very rare cases Bowenoid papulosis may progress to Bowen's disease or frank malignancy. (Photograph courtesy of Elliot Androphy, M.D., Department of Dermatology, Tufts/New England Medical Center, Boston, MA.)

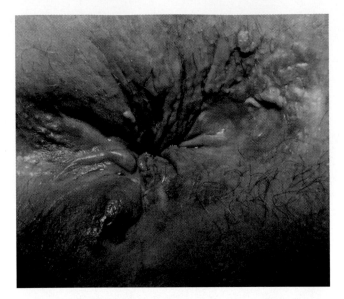

Figure 12–26. Perianal Bowen's disease.

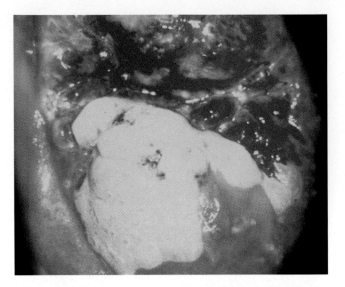

Figure 12–28. Cervical dysplasia. (Photograph courtesy of Kenneth Hatch, M.D., Department of Obstetrics and Gynecology, University of Arizona School of Medicine, Tucson, AZ.)

Queyrat (Fig. 12–27). Bowen's disease is usually associated with oncogenic HPV (e.g., HPV-16), especially when it presents in the anogenital area.

More than 50% of all anogenital malignancies are associated with oncogenic HPV. Cervical cancer is the second leading cause of cancer death in women in the world, with

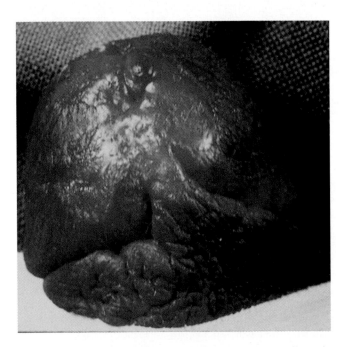

Figure 12–27. Erythroplasia of Queyrat (squamous cell carcinoma in situ of the penis).

approximately 500,000 cases and 200,000 deaths each year. Recent studies suggest that at least 99% of cervical cancers are associated with oncogenic HPV. Whereas HPV-16 appears most prevalent and is best studied, over 20 anogenital HPV types have malignant potential. The primary reason that cervical cancer is not even more prevalent is the use of the Pap smear in industrialized countries. If the Pap smear detects marked cellular atypia and dysplasia is confirmed (Fig. 12–28), treatment would be initiated (especially for high-grade dysplasia) that may help prevent progression to malignancy. Because cervical dysplasia is of viral etiology and standard therapy is usually not antiviral, recurrences are common.

A variety of anogenital SCCs are related to the presence of oncogenic HPV (e.g., HPV-16) (Figs. 12–29 to 12–35), but HPV alone is not thought to be sufficient for cancer to result. Other cofactors, termed *helper factors,* such as cigarette smoking, other infections, diet, genetic predisposition, play a role, but the interactions are not well understood. Less commonly adenocarcinoma may result from HPV oncogenesis (e.g., HPV-18) (Fig. 12–36).

Oncogenic HPV is found occasionally in cutaneous (nonanogenital) malignancies, but these reports are most frequent in immunocompromised persons, especially organ transplant recipients and persons with the acquired immunodeficiency syndrome (AIDS) (Fig. 12–37). In otherwise healthy persons, the nonanogenital malignancy most often associated with HPV (especially HPV-16) is subungual squamous cell carcinoma (Fig. 12–38), but cancers of the

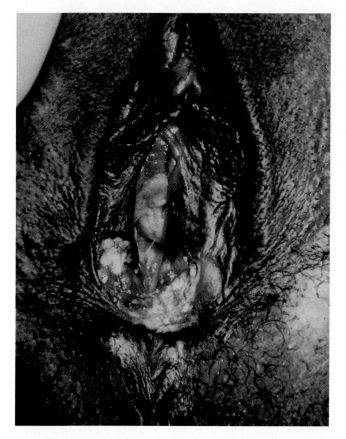

Figure 12–29. Vulvar squamous cell carcinoma associated with HPV-16. (Photograph courtesy of Concepcion Arrastia, M.D., Department of Obstetrics and Gynecology, University of Texas Medical Branch at Galveston, Galveston, TX.)

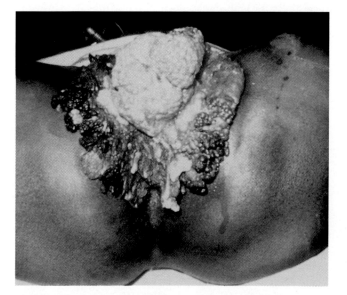

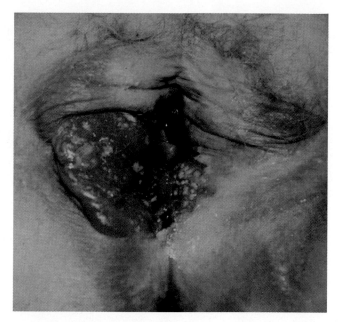

Figure 12–31. Vulvar squamous cell carcinoma associated with HPV-16. (Photograph courtesy of Concepcion Arrastia, M.D., Department of Obstetrics and Gynecology, University of Texas Medical Branch at Galveston, Galveston, TX.)

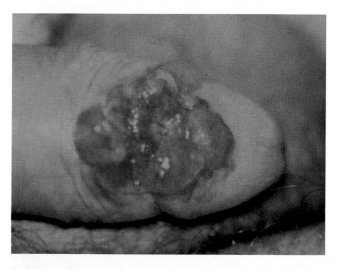

Figure 12–32. Squamous cell carcinoma of the penis associated with HPV-16. The patient was treated with a partial penectomy.

Figure 12–30. Vulvar squamous cell carcinoma associated with HPV-16. (Photograph courtesy of Kenneth Hatch, M.D., Department of Obstetrics and Gynecology, University of Arizona School of Medicine, Tucson, AZ.)

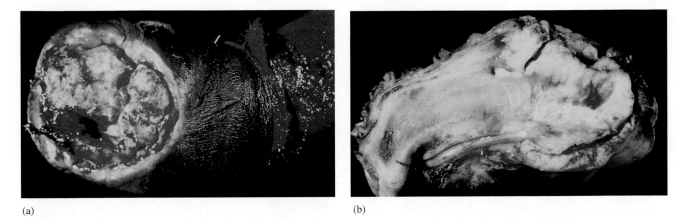

(a) (b)

Figure 12–33. (a) Squamous cell carcinoma of the penis associated with HPV-16. Metastases found in the inguinal lymph nodes also contained HPV-16 integrated into the host DNA. (b) Sagittal section of the penis.

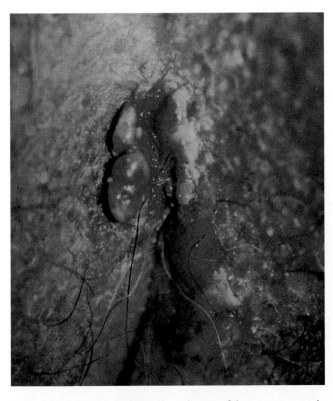

Figure 12–34. Squamous cell carcinoma of the scrotum associated with HPV-16.

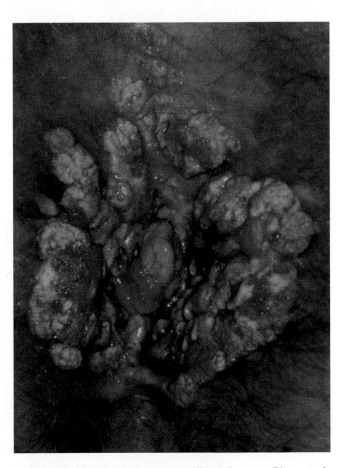

Figure 12–35. Anal squamous cell carcinoma. (Photograph courtesy of Margaret Muldrew, M.D., Denver, CO.)

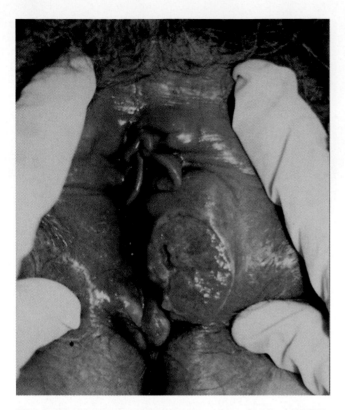

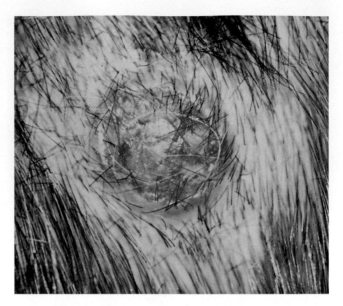

Figure 12–37. Squamous cell carcinoma of the scalp associated with HPV-16 in an AIDS patient.

Figure 12–36. Vulvar adenocarcinoma associated with HPV-18. (Photograph courtesy of Concepcion Arrastia, M.D., Department of Obstetrics and Gynecology, University of Texas Medical Branch at Galveston, Galveston, TX.)

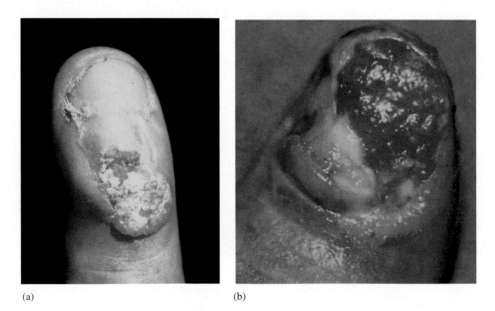

(a)   (b)

Figure 12–38. (a,b) Subungual squamous cell carcinoma associated with HPV-16. (Photograph 38A courtesy of Axel Hoke, M.D., Novato, CA; Photograph 38B courtesy of Roberto Cortez-Franco, M.D., Mexico City, Mexico.)

head and neck have recently been found to contain HPV (Fig. 12–39).

Respiratory, or laryngeal, papillomatosis is a rare disease in which patients develop multiple verruca of the larynx (Fig. 12–40), which may extend to the oropharynx or bronchopulmonary epithelium [131]. Although respiratory papillomatosis may occur at any age, it is most commonly seen in infants. These verrucae usually contain the HPV types associated with genital warts, and it is believed that virus is seeded to the larynx during birth from mothers with condyloma acuminata. Evidence to support this has come from studies that show an epidemiological correlation of condyloma in mothers of infants with the disease. These lesions often spontaneously remit during puberty, although recurrence is common and persistence of the viral DNA during remission has been demonstrated. Occasionally, respiratory papillomatosis may be due to oncogenic HPV types that may lead to cancer of the larynx (Fig. 12–41).

Oral papillomas are also associated with the HPV types isolated from condyloma acuminata (Fig. 12–42). Such lesions are frequently seen in immunocompromised persons (Fig. 12–43 to 12–45). Focal epithelial hyperplasia,

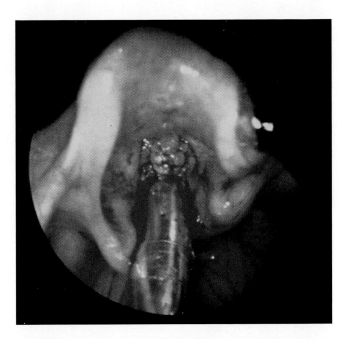

Figure 12–40. Laryngeal papillomatosis. (Photograph courtesy of Christopher Rassekh, M.D., Department of Otolaryngology, University of Texas Medical Branch at Galveston, Galveston, TX.)

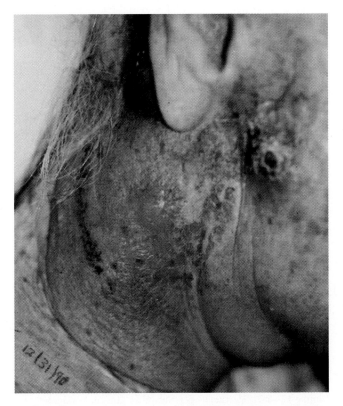

Figure 12–39. Verrucous carcinoma of the neck associated with HPV-16.

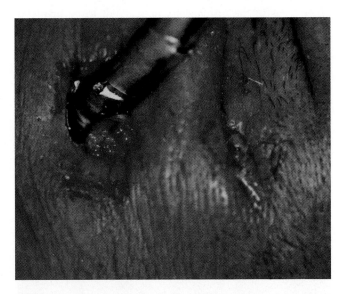

Figure 12–41. Squamous cell carcinoma of the larynx that eroded through the skin of the neck. (Photograph courtesy of Christopher Rassekh, M.D., Department of Otolaryngology, University of Texas Medical Branch at Galveston, Galveston, TX.)

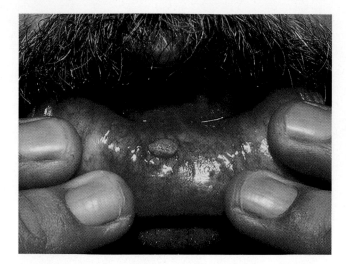

Figure 12–42. Condyloma acuminatum of the lower lip in a human immunodeficiency virus (HIV)–seronegative man.

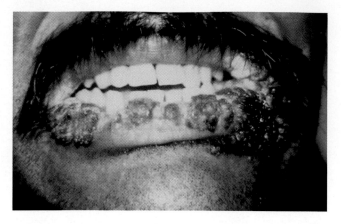

Figure 12–44. Verruca vulgarus of the lower lip in an AIDS patient.

also called Heck's disease, is an unusual HPV infection found mostly in children and is associated with HPV types 13, 32, and 57. It presents with multiple grouped or coalescent, pink to white, 1- to 5-mm, soft papules of the oropharynx that usually resolves spontaneously. It is seen most commonly on the lower lip but may occur on the buccal mucosa, tongue, or gums (Fig. 12–46). The palate and other areas of the oropharynx appear not to be involved

[132]. Heck's disease is most prevalent in certain ethnic groups that appear to be genetically susceptible to these HPV types. Another variant of oral papillomas is oral florid papillomatosis, in which patients develop multiple verrucous papillomas of the oral cavity which may progress to verrucous carcinoma (Fig. 12–47).

Verrucous carcinoma is a low-grade SCC and is commonly due to infection with HPV-6 and HPV-11, types not usually associated with malignancy [133]. Outside of the anogenital area, HPV-16 frequently has been associated

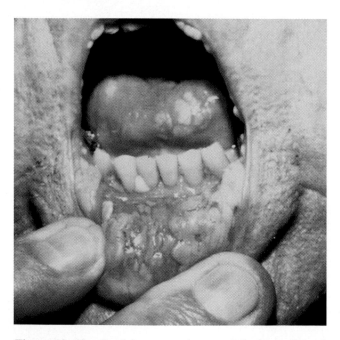

Figure 12–43. Condyloma acuminatum of the lower lip and tongue in an AIDS patient.

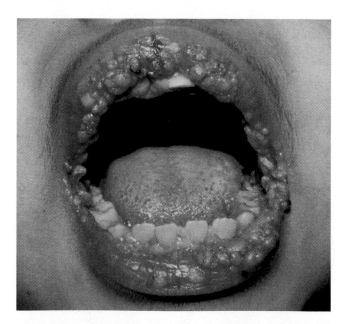

Figure 12–45. Verrucous papules of the lips and oral cavity in an 8-yr-old liver transplant recipient. These papules were found to contain HPV-16.

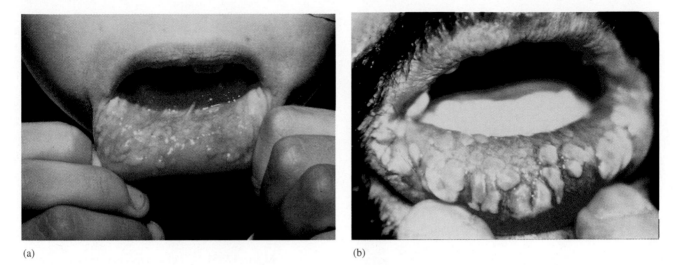

(a)   (b)

Figure 12–46. (a,b) Focal epithelia hyperplasia of the lips and buccal mucosa. (Photograph 46A from Cohen, et al. Pediatr Dermatol 10:245–51, 1993. Used with permission; Photograph a courtesy of Philip Cohen, M.D., Department of Dermatology, University of Texas Health Science Center, Houston, TX; Photograph b courtesy of Mario Marini, M.D., Department of Dermatology, University of Buenos Aires, Buenos Aires, Argentina.)

with verrucous carcinoma. It may represent an entity between a benign lesion and a frank malignancy in that it can be locally invasive and extremely destructive, but rarely metastasizes. When verrucous carcinoma occurs on the genitals, it has been termed a *giant condyloma acuminata of Buschke and Löwenstein* (Figs. 12–48 and 12–49). In the early stages, it resembles a large aggregate of condyloma acuminata; at later stages, a large verrucous tumor develops. It is most frequently located on the glans penis and

foreskin of uncircumcised males, but may also occur on the vulva and in the anal area. As mentioned previously, verrucous carcinoma may also develop in the lesions of oral florid papillomatosis. Clinically, the lesions evolve from whitish verrucous papules into large cauliflower–like lesions that may coalesce to involve a large area of the oral mucosa. Verrucous carcinoma can also occur on the soles of the feet where it is termed *epithelioma cuniculatum*

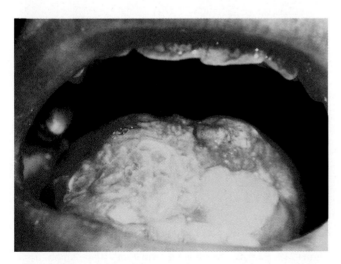

Figure 12–47. Verrucous carcinoma of the tongue. (Photograph courtesy of Mario Marini, M.D., Department of Dermatology, University of Buenos Aires, Buenos Aires, Argentina.)

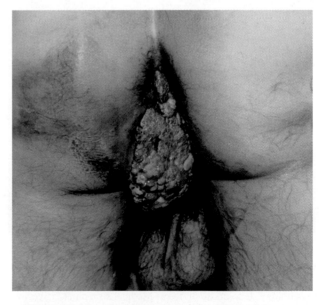

Figure 12–48. Buschke-Löwenstein tumor of the anus.

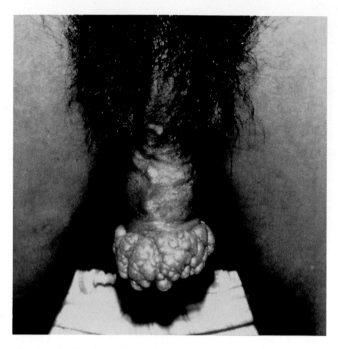

Figure 12–49. Buschke-Löwenstein tumor of the penis. (Photograph courtesy of Axel Hoke, M.D., Novato, CA.)

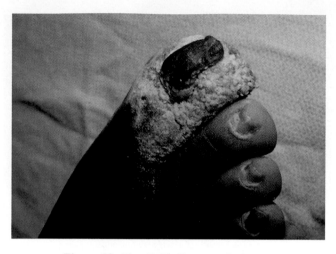

Figure 12–51. Epithelioma cuniculatum.

(Figs. 12–50 to 12–52). This lesion, which is thought to arise from a plantar wart, slowly evolves into a exophytic, verrucous, and fungating tumor that can invade deep into the underlying tissues. There is a tendency to form deep fistulae that are filled with horny material.

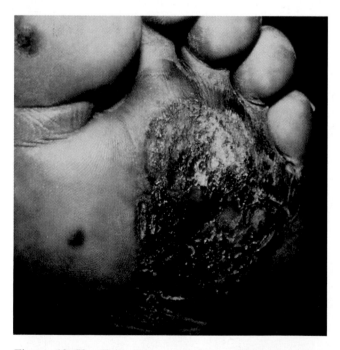

Figure 12–50. Epithelioma cuniculatum. (Photograph from Ho, et al. Arch Dermatol 136:547–552, 2000. Used with permission; Photograph courtesy of Dayna Diven, M.D., Department of Dermatology, University of Texas Medical Branch at Galveston, Galveston, TX.)

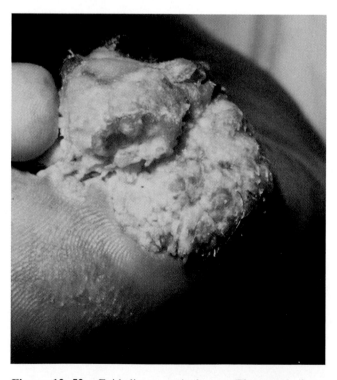

Figure 12–52. Epithelioma cuniculatum. (Photograph from Schell, et al. J Am Acad Dermatol 45:49–55, 2001. Used with permission; courtesy of Theodore Rosen, M.D., Department of Dermatology, Baylor College of Medicine, Houston, TX.)

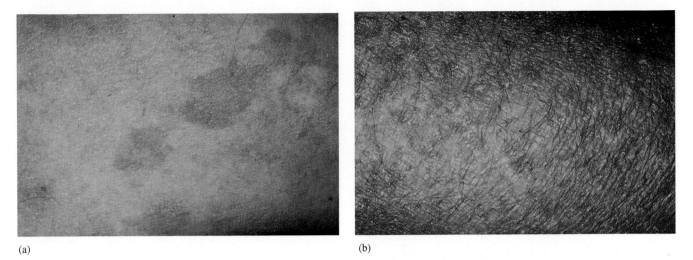

(a)   (b)

Figure 12–53. (a) Pityriasis versicolor–like lesions of the trunk and (b) extremities of a patient with epidermodysplasia verruciformis (EV).

EPIDERMODYSPLASIA VERRUCIFORMIS

EV is a rare lifelong disease with a worldwide distribution [134]. The patients are susceptible to infection with a specific group of HPV types, and they develop extensive infections with these types. These infections are never entirely cleared, and there is a high incidence of malignant conversion of these warty lesions (Fig. 12–53 to 12–55). These

patients are generally otherwise healthy, although an association with mental retardation has been seen. There are a number of HPV subtypes that are associated with EV (Table 12–1), and the incidence of these specific types is the same throughout the world. HPV-3 and HPV-10 cause flat warts in normal patients and also commonly cause flat warts in EV patients. Otherwise, the HPV types associated with EV are not usually found in the healthy population. Conversely, aside from HPV-3 and HPV-10, EV patients usually do not develop infection with the HPV types found

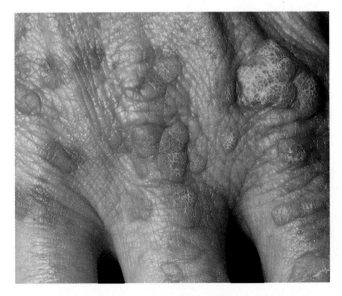

Figure 12–54. Flat warts in a patient with EV. In these patients, flat warts are often quite extensive and somewhat more verrucous than is commonly seen in a normal host. (Photograph courtesy of Elliot Androphy, M.D., Department of Dermatology, Tufts/ New England Medical Center, Boston, MA.)

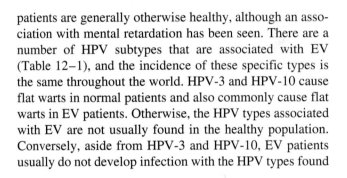
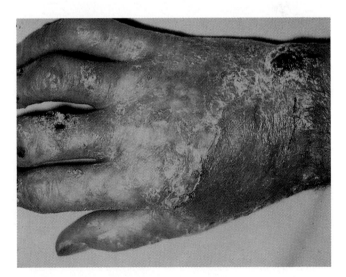

Figure 12–55. Multifocal squamous cell carcinoma in the sun-exposed skin of a patient with EV. HPV typing revealed HPV 8. (Photograph courtesy of Elliot Androphy, M.D., Department of Dermatology, Tufts/New England Medical Center, Boston, MA.)

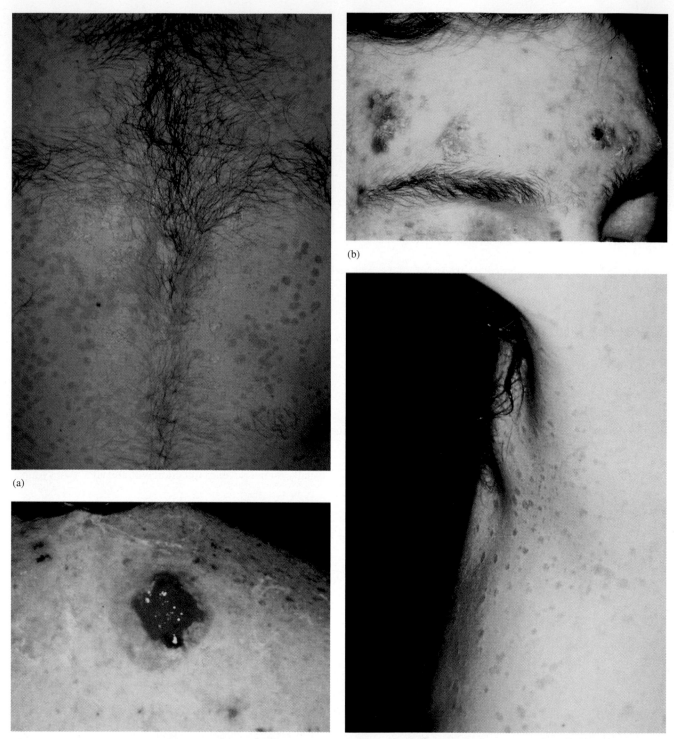

Figure 12–56. EV associated with HPV-8 (a) Erythematous macules containing the episomal form of HPV-8. (b) By age 24 yrs, the patient had developed multitudes of squamous cell carcinomas that contained both the episomal and the integrated forms of HPV-8. He had worked the previous six years in the oil fields of west Texas without sun protection. (c) He continued to develop aggressive squamous cell carcinomas, including this large ulcerated tumor on his back, seen at age 25 yr. (d) During the same clinic visit at which the ulcerated tumor on his back was observed, the patient was found to have marked left axillary lymphoadenopathy.

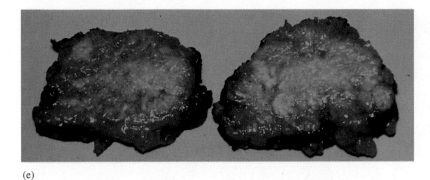

(e)

Figure 12–56. (Continued). (e) The metastatic squamous cell carcinoma from his left axilla is seen in the photograph. The patient died of metastatic squamous cell carcinoma at age 25 yr.

in normal hosts. Of this large group of EV-associated HPV genotypes, those most commonly isolated from these patients are HPV types 5, 8, 17, and 20. HPV-5 and HPV-8 are most commonly associated with the premalignant and malignant lesions found in these patients. Most patients are infected with more than one HPV type.

It is very likely that there are genetic factors involved in the pathogenesis of EV, because it is often familial and has been associated with parental consanguinity, but the nature of the genetic defect and precise mode of inheritance are not known. The pattern of inheritance usually suggests an autosomal recessive trait, but an X-linked recessive disease pattern has also been reported [135]. The predisposition to HPV infection is assumed to be caused by an immune defect, but again, the precise defect is not well defined. Most patients have a decreased number of T cells and T-helper cells, a lowered response to mitogens, and anergy to sensitization with dinitrochlorobenzene. The immune defect in EV patients leads to loss of the response of T cells and natural killer cells to EV-specific HPV antigens. The other tests of CMI responses and humoral immunity are normal [136,137]. Further supporting a role for an immune defect in the pathogenesis of EV, HPV-5 and HPV-8 have been associated with the development of benign lesions and skin cancers in immunocompromised patients, particularly renal transplant patients [33,138].

The clinical manifestations of EV fall into two broad categories; those caused by HPV-3 and those associated with the other EV-associated HPV types. HPV-3 causes verruca plana in the normal population and does the same in patients with EV. The main difference is that the flat warts in patients with EV may be more extensive, somewhat larger, more ill defined, and more confluent. Approximately one third to one half of these patients will develop premalignant and malignant change in the warty lesions on sun-exposed skin, beginning about the age of 30 years. These have the appearance of typical lesions of actinic keratosis, Bowen's disease, and SCC arising in the red-brown macules. The high association between the develop-

ment of these cancers and ultraviolet exposure suggests that this is an important cofactor in the development of these cancers (Fig. 12–56). The rate of degeneration of the premalignant lesions to carcinoma is much higher than in the general population. The number of viral particles is high in the benign lesions of EV; but with malignant degeneration, viral particles are rare or nondetectable. The viral DNA is present in high-copy number in the cells of primary and metastatic SCCs, but unlike most cases of cervical carcinoma, the DNA usually remains in an episomal, nonintegrated state [139].

The diagnosis of EV rests on the clinical picture of a lifelong history of extensive, intractable viral warts, usually with a history of familial involvement. On biopsy, the lesions of EV show the same histological changes as seen in the warts, actinic keratoses, and SCCs of normal hosts. The diagnosis can be confirmed by HPV typing by molecular amplification methods, because the EV-associated HPV types are rarely identified other than in patients with EV. The only distinction that must be made is from those patients who have an adult onset of an EV-like syndrome due to immunosuppression. Because there is no satisfactory treatment for this disease, the most important intervention is to ensure protection of the skin from the carcinogenic cofactors, ultraviolet and ionizing radiation (Fig. 12–57) and provide close follow-up to monitor the patient for the development of malignant changes.

HISTOPATHOLOGY

The histopathology of verrucae varies with the clinical location and HPV type involved. In general, most lesions show a certain degree of acanthosis, papillomatosis, and hyperkeratosis. A characteristic feature that distinguishes most warts is the presence of large vacuolated keratinocytes with pyknotic nuclei surrounded by a narrow clear halo and pale-staining cytoplasm. These are seen in the

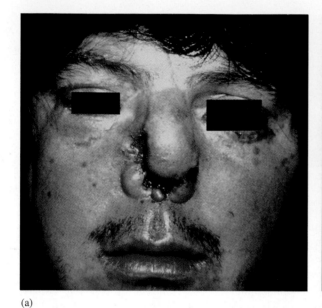

(a)

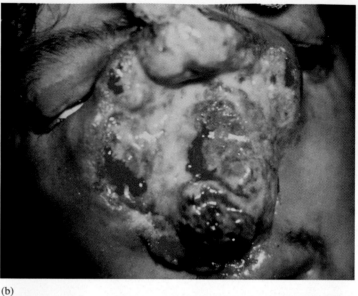

(b)

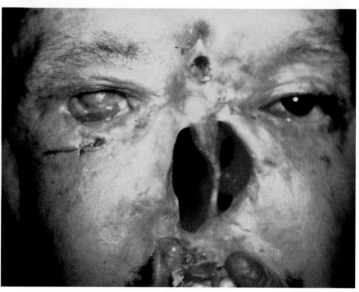

(c)

Figure 12–57. EV associated with HPV-5. (a) Squamous cell carcinomas from a patient in Mexico City were found to contain integrated HPV-5. (b) A few weeks after receiving radiation therapy, the patient's tumor became very aggressive. (c) Although the squamous cell carcinoma seen in "b" was removed, the patient continued to form new tumors. He subsequently died of metastatic squamous cell carcinoma. (Photographs courtesy of Roberto Cortez-Franco, M.D., Mexico City, Mexico.)

middle and outer layers of the epidermis and are called koilocytotic cells.

Common warts generally show marked acanthosis and hyperkeratosis. The elongated rete ridges are often bent inward toward the center of the wart. Koilocytes are usually prominent, and there are stacks of parakeratotic cells and foci of clumped basophilic keratohyalin granules. These granules are thought to be composed of or associated with the viral E4 protein. The dermal capillaries are dilated and may be thrombosed (Figs. 12–58 and 12–59). Filiform warts show much more elongated papillae with a thickened horny layer at the tip of the wart. Flat warts also show

hyperkeratosis and acanthosis but lack the papillomatosis and show only slight elongation of the rete ridges. Koilocytes are prominent in a thickened granular layer and the stratum corneum shows a "basket-weave" appearance. The superficial, mosaic-type, palmoplantar warts resemble other verrucae. In contrast, deep myrmecia warts show prominent cytoplasmic eosinophilic inclusion bodies surrounding the vacuolated nuclei of the koilocytes and prominent parakeratosis in the stratum corneum. On involution of verruca vulgaris, flat warts, or palmoplantar warts, the koilocytes and clumped keratohyalin granules become less prominent and there is a mononuclear cell infiltrate.

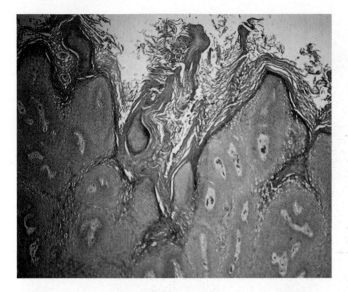

Figure 12–58. Verruca vulgaris showing prominent acanthosis, papillomatosis, and hyperkeratosis.

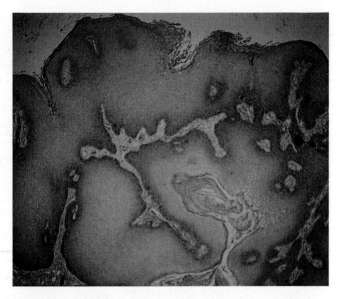

Figure 12–60. Condyloma accuminatum showing extensive acanthosis and large vacuolated keratinocytes and only minimal hyperkeratosis.

In condyloma acuminata, there is papillomatosis and marked acanthosis with elongation and branching of the rete ridges that may be extensive enough to resemble pseudocarcinomatous hyperplasia (Fig. 12–60). The stratum corneum is only slightly thickened. Large vacuolated keratinocytes with clumped keratohyalin granules are seen and are apt to be spread diffusely through the wart. The dermis is edematous with dilated capillaries, and there is usually a chronic inflammatory infiltrate. The histological appearance is similar in the lesions of oral papillomas.

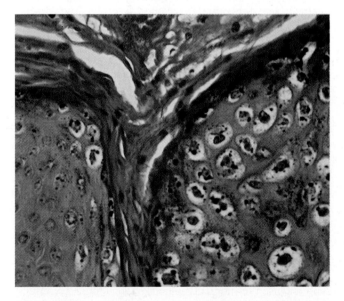

Figure 12–59. Verruca vulgaris with prominent koilocytosis.

The lesions of Bowenoid papulosis resemble Bowen's disease histologically. There is again marked acanthosis and elongation and thickening of the rete ridges, but throughout these lesions the epidermal cells lie in marked disorder and have a highly atypical appearance. Cells show large hyperchromatic nuclei, and multinucleated cells are commonly seen. The stratum corneum is parakeratotic with atypical, hyperchromatic nuclei. Dyskeratotic keratinocytes with dense eosinophilic cytoplasm are evident. Despite this resemblance to an SCC, the border between the epidermis and the dermis remains sharp and the basement membrane is intact. In the lesions of verrucous carcinoma, the superficial areas resemble a verruca, and throughout the lesion there is usually little cellular atypia. At the base of the lesion, the tumor has deep downward proliferations extending into the dermis and compressing the collagen bundles (Fig. 12–61).

The lesions associated with EV have a variable histological appearance. The benign verruca associated with HPV-3 are histologically identical to flat warts. With the lesions associated with HPV-5, there is a somewhat different appearance than is seen with common warts. The epidermal acanthosis is often markedly uneven and varies from very superficial to extremely deep extensions. The cells are swollen and irregular and, unlike typical koilocytes, have been noted to have foamy, pale-blue cytoplasm and lack the clear halo. Dyplastic-appearing keratinocytes with large, round, empty-appearing nuclei are seen. The changes typical of Bowen's disease are seen in more advanced lesions.

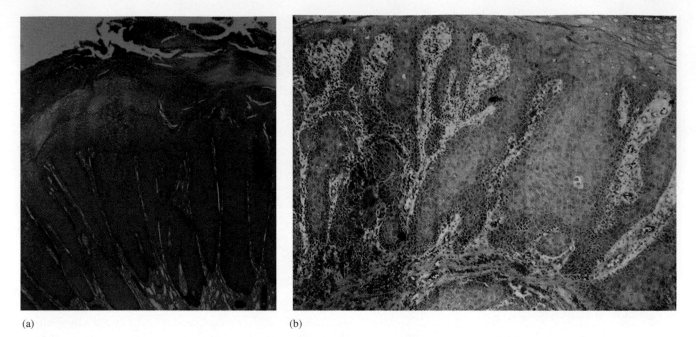

(a)   (b)

Figure 12–61. (a,b) Verrucous carcinoma. This lesion shows little cellular atypia but deep downward proliferations of the tumor extending into the dermis cuniculatum. (Photograph a from Ho, et al. Arch Dermatol 136:547–552, 2000. Used with permission; Photograph b courtesy of Dayna Diven, M.D., Department of Dermatology, University of Texas Medical Branch at Galveston, Galveston, TX.)

On electron microscopy, the various types of HPV-associated lesions all appear similar, but vary in the number of viral particles seen. The large dense intracytoplasmic and intranuclear inclusions are identifiable as keratohyalin granules and are associated with tonofilaments. Viral particles are detected only in the outer layers of the epidermis, first seen in the upper portion of the stratum malpighii. Whereas viral particles are often numerous in common, palmoplantar, and flat warts and the benign lesions of EV, they are very sparse or undetectable in condyloma acuminata and are only rarely detected in dysplastic or malignant lesions.

DIAGNOSIS

The diagnosis of HPV infection is generally straightforward and based on clinical appearance, but can be aided by histological examination (Table 12–4). Genital warts, particularly lesions of the uterine cervix, can be difficult to detect, and detection can be aided by the use of acetowhitening. A 5% acetic acid solution is applied to lesions with gauze or a cotton-tipped swab. In a few minutes after application, lesions may appear as whitish patches that were previously undetectable. The use of a magnifying lens or colposcopy further aids in the diagnosis of clinically inapparent lesions. These techniques are also useful for detecting genital warts in males. Acetowhitening, however, is associated with a high rate of both false-positive and false-negative findings. Immunohistochemical and molecular techniques can confirm the presence of HPV within a lesion but have been rarely used in the clinical setting. The presentation of multiple recalcitrant and recurrent warts with unusual morphology, particularly if familial, must suggest the diagnosis of EV.

The presence of HPV can be confirmed by detection of viral particles by electron microscopy, although this technique is not apt to be readily available, and more importantly, viral particles are usually very sparse in genital and dysplastic lesions. Immunohistochemical methods can be used to aid in the detection of HPV. The antibodies used are generally directed against viral capsid antigens and are cross-reactive with a broad spectrum of HPV types (Fig. 12–62). This method is again of limited usefulness, however, because mature virions expressing viral capsid antigens are not uniformly present and because these capsid antigens may be absent in HPV-related malignancies. Serum antibodies to viral early and capsid proteins are detected in only a minority of patients and thus there is no routinely used serological method for detecting HPV infection.

Table 12–4. Differential Diagnosis of HPV

Verruca vulgaris

Seborrheic keratosis: "Stuck-on"–appearing papules with verrucous friable surface

Nevi: Typically softer than warts with tan to brown to black pigment

Acrochordons: Typically are fleshy and soft, with no keratosis

Keratoacanthoma: Pink or red papule with central keratotic horn

Cutaneous horn: Conical, dense, hyperkeratotic nodule, often in elderly persons or sun-exposed skin

Squamous cell carcinoma: Indurated papule often with ulcerated or crusted center

Linear epidermal nevi: Linear, verrucous plaques, may have a warty appearance

Acanthosis nigricans: Hyperpigmented plaques may have a warty appearance

Acrokeratosis verruciformis and epidermolytic hyperkeratosis: Both show verrucous papules on the extremities, but can be distinguished by autosomal dominant inheritance in most cases

Molluscum contagiosum: May resemble common warts, but lesions are usually smooth-surfaced, flesh-colored, and often have a central punctum

Flat warts

Lichen planus: May sometimes have a slightly verrucous appearance, but distinguishing features include Wickham's striae, pruritus, and oral involvement

Paronychial warts

Squamous cell carcinoma: In older individuals, this carcinoma must be differentiated from benign warts

Plantar warts

Corns and calluses: Warts are distinguished by the presence of thrombosed capillaries and the disruption in the normal skin markings, features not found in calluses

Condyloma acuminata

Syphilitic condyloma lata: May appear similar, but can be distinguished by serology for syphilis and should be darkfield –positive for spirochetes

Molluscum contagiosum: May resemble genital warts, but lesions are usually smooth-surfaced, flesh-colored, and often have a central punctum

Pearly penile papules: Are 1–2-mm papules evenly distributed circumferentially around the corona of the glans penis

Bowenoid papulosis

Bowen's disease: Bowenoid papulosis can usually be distinguished by its onset at an earlier age, the reddishbrown color, somewhat verrucous surface, and the presence of multiple small lesions

Oral papillomatosis

Oral leukoplakia: Whitish patches usually macular, must be distinguished by biopsy

Epidermodysplasia verruciformis

Erythematous macules of the trunk and verrucous papules of the extremities; malignant transformation is often seen on sun-exposed skin

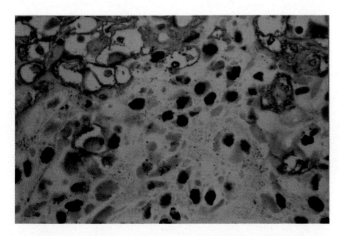

Figure 12–62. Positive immunohistochemical staining for HPV capsid antigens.

With the development of molecular biological techniques, there are now methods that are highly sensitive for the detection of HPV DNA and have allowed for the identification of the many different genotypes of PVs. These techniques identify HPV DNA directly and are much more sensitive than standard immunohistochemical methods. The techniques of Southern blot DNA hybridization and dot blot hybridization allow detection of HPV DNA in extracts of lesional tissue via hybridization with labeled complementary strands of known HPV DNA sequence [140]. Southern blot hybridization allows detection of specific HPV types with fairly high specificity and may also provide information on the integration state of the viral genome [141,142]. Another HPV DNA detection method is tissue in situ hybridization [143,144]. Cells or tissue sections mounted on slides are hybridized with labeled DNA or RNA probes to allow direct visualization of the location of the HPV genome within the tissue. When exon-specific probes are used, this test also allows localization of the expression of specific viral genes. The drawback of these tests is that all of these hybridization methods are relatively labor intensive, and with Southern and dot blotting, require more tissue than may be readily available.

The most sensitive and currently preferred method for detection of HPV in the research laboratory makes use of the polymerase chain reaction (PCR), a technique that allows primer-directed amplification of very small amounts of viral DNA [144–147]. With the most commonly employed PCR methods, the DNA primers are designed in such a way that they will hybridize with and amplify sequences in the L1 gene from a large number of HPV types (termed *degenerate primers*). The amplified product can then be more stringently hybridized with HPV type–specific probes to allow HPV typing. This method is both sensitive and specific. Using PCR methods, it is possible to detect as few as 10 to 100 copies of the viral genome with very small amounts of tissue, whereas the traditional blotting methods require 10^5 to 10^6 copies. The increased sensitivity of these methods has been of particular use in epidemiological studies to allow more accurate estimates of HPV incidence.

Whereas these methods are still mostly used in research laboratories, they are becoming commercially available and have been used in certain clinical settings. Clinical use of HPV typing has most commonly been used in conjunction with Pap smear for the detection of HPV infection. It has been shown that the histological criteria for HPV infection, such as koilocytosis and dyskeratosis, underestimate the incidence of infection and typing adds to the sensitivity of this screening. A method for detection of HPV DNA with sensitivity and specificity similar to that of PCR is the hybrid capture assay. An improved version of this assay, hybrid capture II, is generally acceptable for clinical use. Knowledge of the specific HPV type gives information on the risk for development of cervical cancer and can help in planning the frequency of follow-up for patients. At the present time, HPV typing is not routinely done, but has been implemented in cases with equivocal histological results. HPV typing has been used infrequently for the detection of high-risk HPV-5 in patients with EV. In the evaluation of children with condyloma acuminata, epidemiologists have used HPV typing to evaluate the likelihood of child abuse. These studies have shown that the incidence of child abuse in these cases may actually be lower than had previously been suspected [15].

TREATMENT

Unfortunately, there are no specific antiviral treatments for HPV infection (Table 12–5). Some warts prove very diffi-cult to eradicate, and recurrences are very common. Most current treatment regimens for warts involve physical destruction of the infected tissue. Decisions regarding treatment must take into account the type and location of warts, the age of the patient, and the immunological status of the patient. Because evidence indicates that in healthy children, two thirds of warts will spontaneously remit within 2 years [148], not every wart needs to be treated. If the warts are not physically or psychologically bothersome, a decision to postpone treatment may be made, particularly in younger children, because most of the treatment modalities involve some discomfort. The situation is somewhat different with genital warts because of their sexually transmitted nature and the risk of malignancy. In patients with anogenital warts, the sexual partners should be examined and treated, and women should have colposcopic examination of the uterine cervix and Pap smear. If there are anal warts, anoscopy should be considered. Patients need to be counseled as to the risks of transmission of the warts. An important consideration, particularly in the treatment of genital warts, is that the treatments currently available do not eliminate subclinical or latent infection [149]. HPV DNA has been detected in the clinically normal skin adjacent to treated genital warts, and the presence of HPV correlates with higher rates of wart recurrence [20]. Thus, patients need to be counseled as to the likelihood of recurrence. Long-term follow-up is recommended for patients with cervical or vaginal lesions. Although the lesions of Bowenoid papulosis will sometimes spontaneously remit, they represent a potential reservoir of HPV 16 and should be treated.

Topical Therapies

Topical acidic preparations are a commonly used first-line therapy for warts. Most commercial preparations use varying concentrations of salicylic acid in a number of different vehicles. The salicylic acid causes keratolysis of the infected tissue, and the success rate of this method is good with prolonged therapy. When hand warts, simple plantar warts, and mosaic warts are treated for 3 months, resolution has been seen in 45 to 84% [150]. The main drawback is that this method is time consuming and requires a high degree of patient motivation over a prolonged period of time. The application of caustic acids, such as 50% trichloroacetic acid, can be used for the destruction of warts in the office setting. These acids cause destruction of cellular proteins and induce inflammation and cell death. Another topical agent is cantharidin, which is a caustic extract from the green blister beetle that causes vesiculation and acantholysis of the skin. The major side effect of this treatment is that it can induce pronounced inflammation and discom-

Table 12–5. Treatment of Warts

Treatment	Method	Treatment	Method
Common warts		CO_2 laser	Expensive and typically reserved for recalcitrant warts
Salicylic acid	Available over the counter, and can be applied at home, once or twice daily, for several months. The wart is soaked in warm water to soften the tissue, followed by removal of the keratotic skin with an emory board or pumice stone. Salicylic acid is then applied to the wart. An adhesive bandage may be applied to enhance penetration. Patches or pads impregnated with salicylic acid are also available.	Bleomycin	Intralesional bleomycin can be used for the treatment of recalcitrant periungual and plantar warts. 0.5–1.0 U/ml concentration is injected directly into the wart tissue
		Surgical excision	Reserved for debulking large exophytic warts resistant to therapy
		Flat warts	
50% Tricholoacetic acid	Wart is pared down, then acid is applied in the office, either alone or under occlusion. The area should be rinsed off about 2 hr later. Therapy can be repeated at weekly intervals until resolution of the wart.	Retinoic acid 0.05%	Applied daily to warts until desquamation occurs, which is sometimes accompanied by mild local irritation
		Condylomata	
Cantharidin	This is applied to wart surface with or without occlusion, and left in place for 8–24 hr, after which a blister has usually formed. Therapy may be repeated after healing of the blister, at 1–3 wk intervals.	Podophyllin	Used primarily in the treatment of genital warts, because it is more effective on mucosal surfaces. (contains mutagens) (not standardized)
		Podophyllotoxin 0.5% solution or gel	Applied once or twice daily, stopping if marked irritation occurs (patient applied) (high recurrence rates)
Cryotherapy with liquid nitrogen	The keratotic material of the wart can be pared off, followed by freezing with liquid nitrogen, usually with two freeze-thaw cycles. The amount of time required for freezing varies with the thickness of the wart. Therapy often has to be repeated to clear the wart completely, usually at 2–3 wk intervals.	5-Fluorouracil (5%) solution	Primarily used for verruca plana and condyloma; (highly inflammatory) (teratogenic)
		Interferon-alpha	Given by injection; flu-like side effects
		Cidofovir	Not available in a topical preparation, but can be compounded as a cream or gel (e.g. 1–3%)
Electrodessication	Sometimes used for recalcitrant warts. The area must first be anesthetized, followed by electrodessication of the wart until a white crust appears. This crust is then curretted. Repeated treatments are usually required.	Imiquimod 5% cream	Applied (by patient) three times weekly overnight (low recurrence rates)

fort. Both trichloroacetic acid and cantharidin can cause marked epidermal destruction and potential scarring; thus, they are used only in the office setting.

Topical chemotherapeutic agents have also been employed in the treatment of warts. Podophyllin is a complex plant resin that is a potent antimitotic agent. This compound is contraindicated during pregnancy. Podophyllin is not a standardized preparation, and the concentration of its active ingredient, podophyllotoxin, can vary significantly. In addition, podophyllin contains two mutagens that have been epidemiologically implicated as being carcinogens. Purified solutions of podophyllotoxin are now available that have improved the safety profile and have been approved for treatment of genital warts. Podophyllotoxin 0.5% solution or gel is useful for the treatment of warts, but the local reaction can involve an erythema, burning, and superficial erosions. Because podophyllotoxin has no antiviral or immunodulatory activity, recurrences of anogenital warts are common. The antimetabolite 5-fluorouracil (5-FU) in a 5% solution has been used for the treatment of warts, primarily verruca plana and condyloma. Here again, this agent can induce inflammation, erosions, and postinflammatory hyperpigmentation and is teratogenic. 5-FU has also been used in combination with other destructive modalities to decrease the frequency of recurrences [151]. Intralesional therapy with the antimetabolite, bleomycin, is thought to act by inhibiting both cellular and viral DNA synthesis, but may also act by enhancing the host's immune response to the virus. Reported side effects include Raynaud's phenomena with periungual warts and extensive tissue necrosis, and thus this agent must be used cautiously.

A newer topical agent for the treatment of warts is imiquimod, an imidazoquinolin heterocyclic amine. This drug has been approved for topical treatment of anogenital condyloma. In a 5% cream formulation, imiquimod is applied by the patient overnight three times weekly. Although imiquimod has no specific antiviral effects, it is immunomodulatory and is thought to exert its effect against papillomavirus through induction of cytokines including interferon-alpha and TNF-α [152,153]. Clinical studies have shown clearance of genital warts in approximately 50% of patients (Fig. 12–63). There are no systemic adverse effects, and local irritation is the most common side effect [154]. Recurrences following complete clearance of condyloma acuminatum have been very low (e.g., 13% during a 3-month follow-up period in one study) [154]. Current studies have demonstrated the efficacy of imiquimod (often as adjunctive therapy) against nongenital warts.

Flat warts can be very resistant to therapy, but often respond well to the application of retinoic acid 0.05%. It probably works by acting as a keratolytic agent. Immuno-therapy has also been employed in the treatment of warts. Induction of an allergic reaction in the area of a wart may result in clearing. Dinitrochlorobenzene (DNCB) has traditionally been used for this, but concerns over its mutagenicity make its use controversial.

Destructive Procedures

Cryotherapy with liquid nitrogen is a commonly used treatment for warts on any part of the body. It works by destruction of the frozen tissue and induction of an immune response in the area. There is pain during treatment, and patients may note throbbing in the hours after the procedure. After several hours up to a few days, a clear or hemorrhagic blister develops that generally heals in 1 to 2 weeks. Occasionally, healing results in a clear area surrounded by a ring of new warts that produces a "halo" or "doughnut" effect (Fig. 12–64). Electrodessication has been used in the treatment of warts resistant to cryotherapy. This procedure is commonly associated with scarring after healing and thus should be avoided on plantar surfaces. The use of surgical excision of warts is usually reserved for debulking a large exophytic wart resistant to therapy and, because of high recurrence rates, must be used in conjunction with other treatment modalities. Mohs' micrographic surgery has been successfully used in the treatment of verrucous carcinoma. Treatment of verrucous carcinoma with ionizing radiation is strictly contraindicated because it is associated with recurrence of tumors with a greater invasive potential. The CO_2 laser has been used to treat warts, particularly those in which precise control of the extent of destruction of tissue is required and those refractory to other therapies. This is an expensive method of treatment, and reports of the success are highly variable. Infectious HPV particles have been identified in the vapor plume with laser therapy, and adequate protection with goggles and surgical mask is important [155].

Interferon

The interferons are a large family of proteins that are thought to have antiproliferative, antiviral, and immunomodulatory effects. Intralesional and parenteral interferon has been evaluated in the treatment of refractory genital warts. Intralesional therapy with interferon-α has led to clearing of warts in 36% of patients [156–158], but topical therapy with leukocyte interferon has not been shown to be effective [159]. Parenteral therapy with interferon-α or interferon-β led to clearing of genital warts in the majority of patients [160–162]. Intralesional therapy with interferon has also been investigated in the management of difficult cases of laryngeal and respiratory papillomatosis and EV.

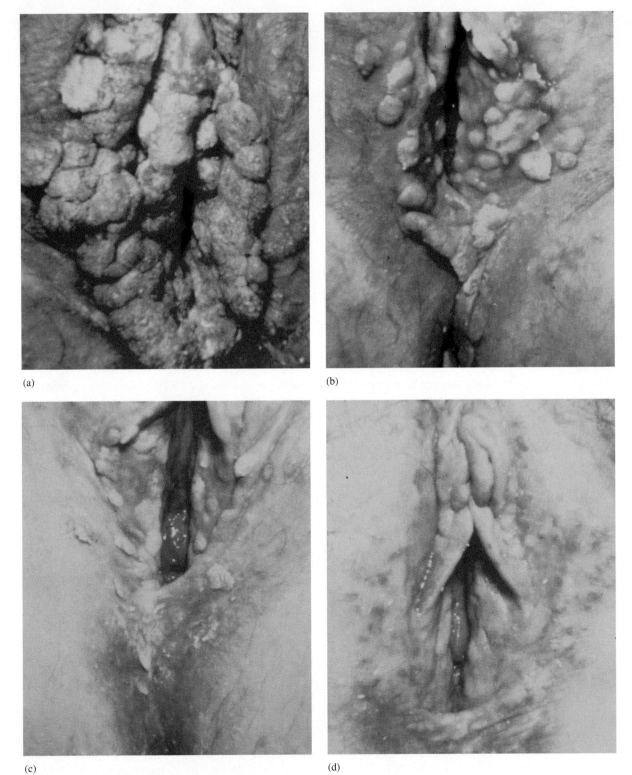

(a)

(b)

(c)

(d)

Figure 12–63. (a) Extensive condyloma acuminatum in a patient who had failed several nonantiviral therapies. (b) Four weeks after initiating therapy with 5% imiquimod cream overnight, three times/wk), a 50% decrease in the size and number of lesions was observed. (c) Six weeks after initiating therapy, a 90% reduction in the warts was noted. (d) Eight weeks after starting therapy, complete disappearance of all warts was seen. The patient remains clear six years after imiquimod therapy.

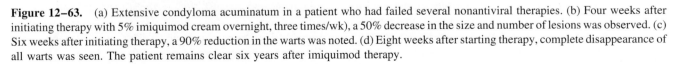

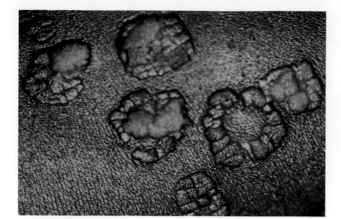

Figure 12–64. A ring of warts appeared around the site of previous warts treated with cryotherapy. (Photograph courtesy of Roberto Arenas, M.D., Mexico City, Mexico.)

Using a number of different treatment regimens, it has generally been shown to reduce warts in these patients, but recurrence is seen when therapy is stopped. In patients with severe respiratory papillomatosis, outcomes may be better if patients are treated with both surgery and interferon [163–165]. The most common side effects are pain at the injection site and flu-like symptoms, including fever, chills, headache, and nausea. In addition, laboratory abnormalities that may be seen include leukopenia, elevation of hepatic enzymes, anemia, and thrombocytopenia.

Cidofovir

Cidofovir is an antiviral drug approved only for the therapy of cytomegalovirus infections. It can, however, be compounded in a cream or gel and has been observed to have potential in the treatment of condyloma acuminatum. Results of controlled trials of topical cidofovir, however, have not been published.

THERAPY OF EPIDERMODYSPLASIA VERRUCIFORMIS

There is no effective treatment for this disorder; the locally destructive methods most commonly used for therapy of warts are not effective here, and systemic therapy may induce some improvement but is followed by recurrence. The use of systemic retinoids has been explored in EV and the long-term use of isotretinoin has been shown to decrease the number of benign lesions and slow the appearance of premalignant and malignant lesions. Interferons have been tried alone and in combination with retinoids,

but the improvement was transient [164]. The treatment of the premalignant and malignant lesions associated with EV is via the same methods as in the normal host. It is of primary importance to ensure protection of the skin from exposure to ultraviolet radiation and follow patients closely for the development of premalignant and malignant lesions. As with the treatment of verrucous carcinoma, any use of radiation therapy is contraindicated in these patients because ionizing radiation is a potent cocarcinogen for HPV-induced lesions. As with the normal host, treatment of HPV-associated cancers with x-radiation generally induces regression followed by recurrence, with a tumor showing a more malignant and aggressive phenotype.

Papillomavirus Vaccines

A very exciting area of PV research is in the development of potential therapeutic and prophylactic vaccines for HPV infection. Although there are several examples of vaccines that have had spectacular success in the prevention of other viral diseases, there are a number of features of HPV biology that make the development of a vaccine particularly difficult. The first problem is our poor understanding of the immune response to HPV infection. Despite the fact that spontaneous clearing of warts has commonly been seen, we do not understand the mechanism by which this specific immune response is generated and, therefore, cannot particularly target this pathway in the development of a vaccine. Another problem is that because there is no in vitro culture system nor an animal culture system for HPV, there is no ready source of live virus that might be exploited for a live attenuated viral vaccine, such as was used with poliovirus. A final problem is that, although most other viruses spend a portion of their life cycle in the systemic circulation where they are vulnerable to neutralizing antibodies, HPVs remain exclusively in the epithelium. Thus, antibodies must transverse the basement membrane and reach the outer layers of the skin or mucosa to be effective in preventing infection. Despite these and other confounding factors, significant progress is being made in the development of potential vaccine candidates.

Therapeutic Vaccines

There are currently no therapeutic vaccines against HPV approved for human use. A therapeutic vaccine is one that will result in clearing of an already established infection. Because of the significant mortality associated with cervical cancer, the earliest aims in this field would be toward development of a therapeutic vaccine for cervical carcinoma and its precursor lesions. The strategy behind the design of a therapeutic vaccine is to target cells for immune-mediated destruction that express a viral protein on their cell surface. These proteins may be viral cell surface proteins or viral proteins that are degraded intracellularly and presented on the cell surface as part of major histocompatibility complex (MHC) class I. The MHC I receptor/viral peptide complexes stimulate a cytotoxic response in CD8 + T cells. A candidate target for this type of vaccine would be the HPV early genes. Because the viral E6 and E7 genes are selectively retained and expressed in cervical dysplasia and cancer, they might be excellent candidates for the development of a therapeutic vaccine. Once a potential vaccine is designed, it is then necessary to address how such a vaccine would be delivered to the patient. One method for administering such a vaccine is through the use of recombinant viral vectors that would express the viral early genes. There are, however, a number of associated potential problems with such a vaccine, including the possibility that continuous expression of these viral oncogenes could promote tumorigenesis and that these genes might integrate into the host genome. Because of these concerns, the somewhat safer possibility of using purified E6 and E7 proteins with immunostimulating adjuvants is being explored.

Some data from trials of therapeutic vaccines in animals are available. Using a mouse model, it was shown that vaccination with killed HPV–containing tumor cells that were expressing HPV-16 E6 or E7 protected the mice when they were subsequently challenged with live tumor cells [166,167]. Immunization of mice with an immunogenic E7 peptide induced cytotoxic T lymphocytes that were able to lyse E7-expressing cells and inhibited tumor formation by an E7-expressing tumor cell line [168]. Using the cottontail rabbit, immunization with cells expressing CRPV E2 promoted the regression of established CRPV-induced papillomas [169]. At the present time, several therapeutic human trials have been planned. The details of what leads to an effective therapeutic immune response to HPV remains unclear, but likely immunogens that will be tested include bacterially produced E6 and E7 proteins, synthetic viral peptides, and recombinant viral vectors that express E6 and E7. Because of the potential risks of some of these vaccine strategies, the initial trials will probably be restricted to patients with invasive cervical carcinoma who have failed conventional therapy. Results of these first trials should be available within the next few years.

Prophylactic Vaccines

Unlike therapeutic vaccines, the goal of a prophylactic vaccine is to generate production of neutralizing antibodies to the viral capsid proteins that will block the virus before it can enter the cell. Because HPV does not enter the systemic circulation but rather remains in the epidermis, antibodies that are capable of reaching the skin must be generated. Antibody induction has been demonstrated in the mucus of the vaginal mucosa following systemic immunization, indicating that antibodies can traverse the basement membrane [170]. The preferred immunogens for this type of vaccine are the viral capsid proteins. Following synthesis of the capsid proteins, it is essential that they be folded as seen in the viral capsomere, because when they are synthesized in bacterial cells, they are denatured and, in this form, do not induce production of neutralizing antibodies. When the L1 and L2 proteins are generated in eukaryote cells, they self-assemble into the capsid structure, in particles called "virus-like particles" (VLPs), which are indistinguishable from mature virions except they lack the viral DNA. Using animal models, it has been shown that immunization with intact viruses does lead to production of neutralizing antibodies in cows, dogs, and other species. Cottontail rabbits immunized with CRPV VLPs had greatly reduced incidence of papilloma formation after challenge and developed no epithelial cancers [171]. Whereas dogs and rabbits are most commonly used as animal models to study PVs, a wide spectrum of animals are susceptible to the species-specific papillomavirus (Figs. 12–65 and 12–66).

Prophylactic vaccines are currently being developed for use in humans. Because the immune response generated to VLPs is type-specific, these vaccines will have to include a number of different HPV types and will likely include the

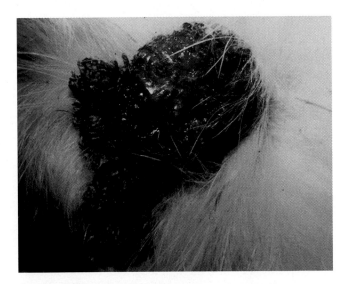

Figure 12–65. This squamous cell carcinoma on the back of a rabbit resulted from infection with the Shope papillomavirus. The rabbit has been used for many decades as an animal model for the study of papillomaviruses.

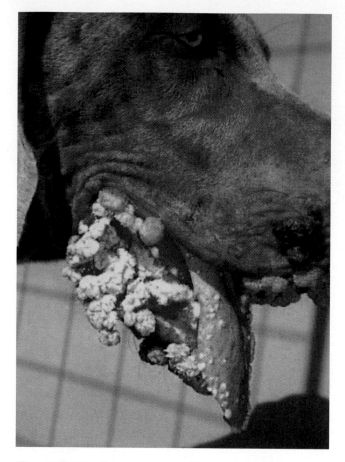

Figure 12–66. Extensive oral papillomatosis in a dog. The oral mucosa of the dog is commonly used for the study of papillomavirus vaccine.

HPV types most commonly associated with malignancy as well as those associated with benign genital disease (HPV-6 and HPV-11). The goal would be to administer this vaccine before the peak incidence of genital HPV infection at age 20 to 25 years, and thus a good target group would be women entering college. Because men are at much lower risk for the development of cancer, it is somewhat controversial whether they should be vaccinated. Because prevention of infection in men would also lower infection in women, it would be likely to lower the overall incidence of cervical cancers. Monitoring effectiveness would need to be through examining patients for HPV infection by a sensitive PCR-based DNA detection method (or hybrid capture assay) and also through long-term follow-up measuring the incidence of low-grade and high-grade CIN and other malignancies. Although it will obviously be a long time before the results of such trials are available, with the advent of new technology, such as the production of VLPs,

the prospects for an efficacious HPV vaccine are more hopeful than ever before.

CONCLUSION

The mucocutaneous manifestations of HPV range from benign warts to aggressive SCCs. These HPV-associated lesions often mimic (or are mimicked by) other non–HPV-associated lesions that have far different biological significance and/or therapies. In some cases, even the most well-trained and experienced clinicians cannot always distinguish among these possibilities. In case of doubt, a biopsy (and possibly other diagnostic procedures) should be considered. Owing to a lack of good in vitro culture systems or animal models for HPV, our understanding of the pathophysiology of HPV was very limited until the 1980s. During the past two decades, however, not only have sensitive molecular tools allowed detection of HPV DNA, they have also led to a markedly greater understanding of HPV viral oncogenesis. Much remains to be understood regarding the role of genetics, immunity, and cofactors in HPV infections (especially oncogenic HPV). Therapy for warts has evolved from surgical and cytodestructive techniques having no antiviral potential to immunomodulatory agents such as imiquimod (with indirect antiviral activity). Future interventions for HPV will include vaccines for warts as well as for anogential malignancies. Such vaccines will range from those purely for prophylactic use to those with therapeutic potential.

REFERENCES

1. H zur Hausen. Papillomavirus infections—a major cause of human cancers. Biochim Biophys Acta 1288:F55–F78, 1996.
2. KR Beutner, TM Becker, KM Stone. Epidemiology of human papillomavirus infections. Dermatol Clin 9: 211–218, 1991.
3. MH Schiffman. New epidemiology of human papillomavirus infection and cervical neoplasia. J Natl Cancer Inst 87: 1345–1347, 1995.
4. G Ciuffo. Innesto positivo con filtrato di verruca vulgare. G Ital Mal Venereol 48:12–17, 1907.
5. KE Rowson, BW Mahy. Human papova (wart) virus. Bacteriol Rev 31:110–131, 1967.
6. G Orth, M Favre, O Croissant. Characterization of a new type of human papillomavirus that causes skin warts. J Virol 24:108–120, 1977.
7. L Gissmann, H Pfister, H zur Hausen. Human papillomaviruses: characterization of four different isolates. J Virol 44:393–400, 1982.
8. TP Cripe, TH Haugen, JP Turk, F Tabatabai, PG Schmid

3rd, M Durst, L Gissmann, A Roman, LP Turek. Transcriptional regulation of the human papillomavirus-16 E6-E7 promoter by a keratinocyte-dependent enhancer, and by viral E2 trans-activator and repressor gene products: implications for cervical carcinogenesis. EMBO J 6: 3745–3753, 1987.

9. F Thierry, M Yaniv. The BPV-1 trans-acting protein can be either an activator or a repressor of the HPV 18 regulatory region. EMBO J 6:3391–3397, 1987.

10. MT Chin, TR Broker, LT Chow. Identification of a novel constitutive enhancer element and an associated binding protein: implications for human papillomavirus type 11 enhancer regulation. J Virol 63:2967–2976, 1989.

11. WD Lancaster, C Olson. Animal papillomaviruses. Microbiol Rev 46:191–207, 1982.

12. JW Kreider. The Shope papilloma to carcinoma complex of rabbits: a model system of neoplastic progression and spontaneous regression. Adv Cancer Res 35:85–110, 1981.

13. BB Barr, EC Benton, K McLaren, MH Bunney, IW Smith, K Blessing, JA Hunter. Human papilloma virus infection and skin cancer in renal allograft recipients. Lancet 1: 124–129, 1989.

14. R Laurent, JL Kienzler. Epidemiology of HPV infection. Clin Dermatol 3:64–74, 1985.

15. BA Cohen, P Honig, E Androphy. Anogenital warts in children. Clinical and virologic evaluation for sexual abuse. Arch Dermatol 126:1575–1580, 1990.

16. FX Bosch, M Manos, N Munoz, M Sherman, AM Jansen, J Peto, MH Schiffman, V Moreno, R Kurman, KV Shah. Prevalence of human papillomavirus in cervical cancer: a worldwide perspective. J Natl Cancer Inst 87:796–802, 1995.

17. MH Schiffman. Epidemiology of cervical human papillomaviruses. In: zur Hausen H, ed. Human Pathogenic Papillomaviruses. Heidelberg: Springer-Verlag, 1994, pp. 55–81.

18. R Roden, EM Weissinger, DW Henderson, F Booy, R Kirnbauer, JF Mushinski, DR Lowy, JT Schiller. Neutralization of bovine papillomavirus by antibodies to L1 and L2 capsid proteins. J Virol 68:7570–7574, 1994.

19. BM Steinberg, WC Topp, PS Schneider, AL Abramson. Laryngeal papillomavirus infection during clinical remission. N Engl J Med 308:1261–1264, 1983.

20. A Ferenczy, M Mitao, N Nagai. Latent papillomavirus and recurring genital warts. N Engl J Med 313:784–788, 1985.

21. JT Schiller, MM Okun. Papillomavirus vaccines: current status and future prospects. Adv Dermatol 11:355–381, 1996.

22. J Doorbar, S Ely, J Sterling, C McLean, L Crawford. Specific interaction between HPV-16 E1-E4 and cytokeratins results in collapse of the epithelial cell intermediate filament network. Nature 352:824–827, 1991.

23. A Storey, K Osborn, L Crawford. Co-transformation by human papillomavirus types 6 and 11. J Gen Virol 71: 165–171, 1990.

24. CL Halbert, GW Demers, DA Galloway. The E6 and E7 genes of human papillomavirus type 6 have weak immortalizing activity in human epithelial cells. J Virol 66: 2125–2134, 1992.

25. SC Dollard, JL Wilson, LM Demeter, W Bonnez, RC Reichman, TR Broker, LT Chow. Production of human papillomavirus and modulation of the infectious program in epithelial raft cultures. Genes Dev 6:1131–1142, 1992.

26. C Meyers, MG Frattini, JB Hudson, L Laimins. Biosynthesis of human papillomavirus from a continuous cell line upon epithelial differentiation. Science 257:971–973, 1992.

27. M von Knebel Doeberitz. Papillomaviruses in human disease: Part II. Molecular biology and immunology of papillomavirus infection and carcinogenesis. Eur J Med 1: 485–491, 1992.

28. H Kirchner. Immunobiology of human papillomavirus infection. Prog Med Virol 33:1–41, 1986.

29. I Penn. Cancers of the anogenital region in renal transplant recipients. Cancer 58:611–616, 1986.

30. M Muller, RP Viscidi, V Sun, E Guerrero, PM Hill, F Shah, FX Bosch, N Munoz, L Gissmann, KV Shah. Antibodies to HPV-16 E6 and E7 proteins as markers for HPV-16–associated invasive cervical cancer. Virology 187:508–514, 1992.

31. M Muller, RP Viscidi, V Ulken, JN Bavinck, PM Hill, SG Fisher, R Reid, N Munoz, A Schneider, KV Shah, et al. Antibodies to the E4, E6, and E7 proteins of human papillomavirus (HPV) type 16 in patients with HPV-associated diseases and in the normal population. J Invest Dermatol 104:138–141, 1995.

32. R Kirnbauer, J Taub, H Greenstone, R Roden, M Durst, L Gissmann, DR Lowy, JT Schiller. Efficient self-assembly of human papillomavirus type 16 L1 and L1 plus L2 into virus-like particles. J Virol 67:6929–6936, 1993.

33. V Shamanin, M Glover, C Rausch, C Proby, IM Leigh, H zur Hausen, EM de Villiers. Specific types of human papillomavirus found in benign proliferations and carcinomas of the skin in immunosuppressed patients. Cancer Res 54:4610–4613, 1994.

34. G Bens, U Wieland, A Hofmann, R Höpfl, H Pfister. Detection of new human papillomavirus sequences in skin lesions of a renal transplant recipient and characterization of one complete genome related to epidermodysplasia verruciformis–associated types. J Gen Virol 79:779–787, 1998.

35. S Hietanen, S Grénman, K Syrjänen, K Lappalainen, J Kauppinen, T Carey, S Syrjanen. Human papillomavirus in vulvar and vaginal carcinoma cell lines. Br J Cancer 72:134–139, 1995.

36. E Orihuela, SK Tyring, M Pow-Sang, S Dozier, R Cirelli, I Arany, P Rady, R Sanchez. Development of human papillomavirus type 16 associated squamous cell carcinoma of the scrotum in a patient with Darier's disease treated with systemic isotretinoin. J Urol 153:1940–1943, 1995.

37. DJ McCance, A Kalache, K Ashdown, L Andrade, F Men-

ezes. Human papillomavirus types 16 and 18 in carcinomas of the penis from Brazil. Int J Cancer 37:55–59, 1986.

38. KR Zachow, RS Ostrow, M Bender, S Watts, T Okagaki, F Pass, AJ Faras. Detection of human papillomavirus DNA in anogenital neoplasias. Nature 300:771–773, 1982.

39. L Gregoire, AL Cubilla, VE Reuter, GP Haas, WD Lancaster. Preferential association of human papillomavirus with high-grade histologic variants of penile-invasive squamous cell carcinoma. J Natl Cancer Inst 87:1705–1709, 1995.

40. PS Ramanujam, KS Venkatesh, TC Barnett, MJ Fietz. Study of human papillomavirus infection in patients with anal squamous carcinoma. Dis Colon Rectum 39:37–39, 1996.

41. AP Cullen, R Reid, M Campion, AT Lorincz. Analysis of the physical state of different human papillomavirus DNAs in intraepithelial and invasive cervical neoplasm. J Virol 65:606–612, 1991.

42. E Schwarz, UK Freese, L Gissmann, W Mayer, B Roggenbuck, A Stremlau, H zur Hausen. Structure and transcription of human papillomavirus sequences in cervical carcinoma cells. Nature 314:111–114, 1985.

43. S Jeon, PF Lambert. Integration of human papillomavirus type 16 DNA into the human genome leads to increased stability of E6 and E7 mRNAs: implications for cervical carcinogenesis. Proc Natl Acad Sci U S A 92:1654–1658, 1995.

44. M Durst, RT Dzarlieva-Petrusevska, P Boukamp, NE Fusenig, L Gissman. Molecular and cytogenic analysis of immortalized human primary keratinocytes obtained after transfection with human papillomavirus type 16 DNA. Oncogene 1:251–256, 1987.

45. MH Stoler, TR Broker. In situ hybridization detection of human papillomavirus DNAs and messenger RNAs in genital condylomas and a cervical carcinoma. Hum Pathol 17:1250–1258, 1986.

46. Y Tsunokawa, N Takebe, T Kasamatsu, M Terada, T Sugimura. Transforming activity of human papillomavirus type 16 DNA sequences in a cervical cancer. Proc Natl Acad Sci U S A 83:2200–2203, 1986.

47. L Banks, P Spence, E Androphy, N Hubbert, G Matlashewski, A Murray, L Crawford. Identification of human papillomavirus type 18 E6 polypeptide in cells derived from human cervical carcinomas. J Gen Virol 68:1351–1359, 1987.

48. EJ Androphy, NL Hubbert, JT Schiller, DR Lowy. Identification of the HPV-16 E6 protein from transformed mouse cells and human cervical carcinoma cell lines. EMBO J 6:989–992, 1987.

49. D Smotkin, FO Wettstein. Transcription of human papillomavirus type 16 early genes in a cervical cancer and a cancer-derived cell line and identification of the E7 protein. Proc Natl Acad Sci U S A 83:4680–4684, 1986.

50. M von Knebel Doeberitz, C Rittmuller, F Aengeneyndt, P Jansen-Durr, D Spitkovsky. Reversible repression of papillomavirus oncogene expression in cervical carcinoma cells: consequences for the phenotype and E6-p53 and E7-pRB interactions. J Virol 68:2811–2821, 1994.

51. T Tan, R Ting. In vitro and in vivo inhibition of human papillomavirus type 16 E6 and E7 genes. Cancer Res 55:4599–4605, 1995.

52. CP Mansur, EJ Androphy. Cellular transformation by papillomavirus oncoproteins. Biochim Biophys Acta 1155:323–345, 1993.

53. P Hawley-Nelson, KH Vousden, NL Hubbert, DR Lowy, JT Schiller. HPV16 E6 and E7 proteins cooperate to immortalize human foreskin keratinocytes. EMBO J 8:3905–3910, 1989.

54. K Munger, WC Phelps, V Bubb, PM Howley, R Schlegel. The E6 and E7 genes of the human papillomavirus type 16 together are necessary and sufficient for transformation of primary human keratinocytes. J Virol 63:4417–4421, 1989.

55. SL Watts, WC Phelps, RS Ostrow, KR Zachow, JA Faras. Cellular transformation by human papillomavirus DNA in vitro. Science 225:634–636, 1984.

56. S Yasumoto, AL Burkhardt, J Dongier, J DiPaolo. Human papillomavirus type 16 DNA–induced malignant transformation of NIH 3T3 cells. J Virol 57:572–577, 1986.

57. P Kaur, JK McDougall, R Cone. Immortalization of primary human epithelial cells by cloned cervical carcinoma DNA containing human papillomavirus type 16 E6/E7 open reading frames. J Gen Virol 70:1261–1266, 1989.

58. JB Hudson, MA Bedell, DJ McCance, LA Laiminis. Immortalization and altered differentiation of human keratinocytes in vitro by the E6 and E7 open reading frames of human papillomavirus type 18. J Virol 64:519–526, 1990.

59. A Storey, D Pim, A Murray, K Osborn, L Banks, L Crawford. Comparison of the in vitro transforming activities of human papillomavirus types. EMBO J 7:1815–1820, 1988.

60. R Schlegel, WC Phelps, YL Zhang, M Barbosa. Quantitative keratinocyte assay detects two biological activities of human papillomavirus DNA and identifies viral types associated with cervical carcinoma. EMBO J 7:3181–3187, 1988.

61. SL Chen, P Mounts. Transforming activity of E5a protein of human papillomavirus type 6 in NIH 3T3 and C127 cells. J Virol 64:3226–3233, 1990.

62. YP Tsao, TY Chu, TM Chen, YF Yang, SL Chen. Effects of E5a and E7 genes of human papillomavirus type 11 on immortalized human epidermal keratinocytes and NIH 3T3 cells. Arch Virol 138:177–185, 1994.

63. P Bergman, M Ustav, J Sedman, J Moreno-Lopez, B Venstrom, U Pettersson. The E5 gene of bovine papillomavirus type 1 is sufficient for complete oncogenic transformation of mouse fibroblasts. Oncogene 1:453–459, 1988.

64. JM Huibregtse, M Scheffner, PM Howley. Cloning and expression of the cDNA for E6-AP, a protein that mediates the interaction of the human papillomavirus E6 oncoprotein with p53. Mol Cell Biol 13:775–784, 1993.

65. BA Werness, AJ Levine, PM Howley. Association of human papillomavirus types 16 and 18 E6 proteins with p53. Science 248:76–79, 1990.

66. M Scheffner, BA Werness, JM Huibregtse, AJ Levine, PM Howley. The E6 oncoprotein encoded by human papillomavirus types 16 and 18 promotes the degradation of p53. Cell 63:1129–1136, 1990.

67. T Crook, JA Tidy, KH Vousden. Degradation of p53 can be targeted by HPV E6 sequence distinct from those required for p53 binding and trans-activation. Cell 67:547–556, 1991.

68. A Ciechanover, JA DiGiuseppe, B Bercovich, A Orian, JD Richter, AL Schwartz, GM Brodeur. Degradation of nuclear oncoproteins by the ubiquitin system. Proc Natl Acad Sci U S A 88:139–143, 1991.

69. DR Chowdary, JJ Dermody, KK Jha, HL Ozer. Accumulation of p53 in a mutant cell line defective in the ubiquitin pathway. Mol Cell Biol 14:1997–2003, 1994.

70. MB Kastan, O Onyekwere, D Sidransky, B Vogelstein, RW Craig. Participation of p53 protein in the cellular response to DNA damage. Cancer Res 51:6304–6311, 1991.

71. MB Kastan, Q Zhan, WS El-Deiry, F Carrier, T Jacks, WV Walsh, BS Plunkett, B Vogelstein, AJ Fornace Jr. A mammalian cell cycle checkpoint pathway utilizing p53 and GADD45 is defective in ataxia-telangiectasia. Cell 71:587–597, 1992.

72. SJ Kuerbitz, BS Plunkett, WV Walsh, MB Kastan. Wild-type p53 is a cell cycle checkpoint determinant following irradiation. Proc Natl Acad Sci U S A 89:7491–7495, 1992.

73. AR Clarke, CA Purdie, DJ Harrison, RG Morris, CC Bird, ML Hooper, AH Wyllie. Thymocyte apoptosis induced by p53-dependent and independent pathways. Nature 362:849–852, 1993.

74. SW Lowe, EM Schmitt, SW Smith, BA Osborne, T Jacks. p53 is required for radiation-induced apoptosis in mouse thymocytes. Nature 362:847–849, 1993.

75. GP Zambetti, J Bargonetti, K Walker, C Prives, AJ Levine. Wild-type p53 mediates positive regulation of gene expression through a specific DNA sequence element. Genes Dev 6:1143–1152, 1992.

76. SE Kern, KW Kinzler, A Bruskin, D Jarosz, P Friedman, C Prives, B Vogelstein. Identification of p53 as a sequence-specific DNA-binding protein. Science 252:1708–1711, 1991.

77. G Farmer, J Bargonetti, H Zhu, P Friedman, R Prywes, C Prives. Wild-type p53 activates transcription in vitro. Nature 358:83–86, 1992.

78. WS El-Deiry, T Tokino, VE Velculescu, DB Levy, R Parsons, JM Trent, D Lin, WE Mercer, KW Kinzler, B Vogelstein. WAF1, a potential mediator of p53 tumor suppression. Cell 75:817–825, 1993.

79. W Maltzman, L Czyzyk. UV irradiation stimulates levels of p53 cellular tumor antigen in nontransformed mouse cells. Mol Cell Biol 4:1689–1694, 1984.

80. P Hall, P McKee, H Menage, R Dover, D Lane. High levels of p53 protein in UV-irradiated normal human skin. Oncogene 8:203–207, 1993.

81. JW Harper, GR Adami, N Wei, K Keyomarsi, SJ Elledge. The p21 Cdk–interacting protein Cip1 is a potent inhibitor of G1 cyclin–dependent kinases. Cell 75:805–816, 1993.

82. Y Xiong, GJ Hannon, H Zhang, D Casso, R Kobayashi, D Beach. p21 is a universal inhibitor of cyclin kinases. Nature 366:701–704, 1993.

83. M Oren. Relationship of p53 to the control of apoptotic cell death. Semin Cancer Biol 5:221–227, 1994.

84. LR Livingstone, A White, J Sprouse, E Livanos, T Jacks, TD Tlsty. Altered cell cycle arrest and gene amplification potential accompany loss of wild-type p53. Cell 70:923–935, 1992.

85. Y Yin, MA Tainsky, FZ Bischoff, LC Strong, GM Wahl. Wild-type p53 restores cell cycle control and inhibits gene amplification in cells with mutant p53 alleles. Cell 70:937–948, 1992.

86. A Dutta, JM Ruppert, JC Aster, E Winchester. Inhibition of DNA replication factor RPA by p53. Nature 365:79–82, 1993.

87. R Drapkin, JT Reardon, A Ansari, JC Huang, L Zawel, K Ahn, A Sancar, D Reinberg. The dual role of TFIIH in DNA excision repair and in transcription by RNA polymerase II. Nature 368:769–772, 1994.

88. XW Wang, H Yeh, L Schaeffer, R Roy, V Moncollin, JM Egly, Z Wang, EC Freidberg, MK Evans, BG Taffe, et al. p53 modulation of TFIIH-associated nucleotide excision repair activity. Nature Genet 10:188–195, 1995.

89. K Munger, BA Werness, N Dyson, WC Phelps, E Harlow, PM Howley. Complex formation of human papillomavirus E7 proteins with the retinoblastoma tumor suppressor gene product. EMBO J 8:4099–4105, 1989.

90. N Dyson, PM Howley, K Munger, E Harlow. The human papillomavirus-16 E7 oncoprotein is able to bind to the retinoblastoma gene product. Science 243:934–937, 1989.

91. R Davies, R Hicks, T Crook, J Morris, K Vousden. Human papillomavirus type 16 E7 associates with a histone H1 kinase and with p107 through sequences necessary for transformation. J Virol 67:2521–2528, 1993.

92. S Shirodkar, M Ewen, JA DeCaprio, J Morgan, DM Livingston, T Chittenden. The transcription factor E2F interacts with the retinoblastoma product and a p107–cyclin A complex in a cell cycle-regulated manner. Cell 68:157–166, 1992.

93. Y Imai, Y Matsushima, S Takashi, M Terada. Purification and characterization of human papillomavirus type 16E7 protein with preferential binding capacity to the underphosphorylated form of retinoblastoma gene product. J Virol 65:4966–4972, 1991.

94. DV Heck, CL Yee, PM Howley, K Munger. Efficiency of binding the retinoblastoma protein correlates with the transforming capacity of the E7 oncoproteins of the human papillomaviruses. Proc Natl Acad Sci U S A 89:4442–4446, 1992.

95. BC Sang, MS Barbosa. Single amino acid substitutions in

low-risk human papillomavirus (HPV) type-6 E7 protein enhance features characteristic of the high-risk HPV E7 oncoproteins. Proc Natl Acad Sci U S A 89:8063–8067, 1992.

96. SH Devoto, M Mudryj, J Pines, T Hunter, JR Nevins. A cyclin A–protein kinase complex possesses sequence-specific DNA binding activity: p33cdk2 is a component of the E2F–cyclin A complex. Cell 68:167–176, 1992.

97. P Starostik, KN Chow, DC Dean. Transcriptional repression and growth suppression by the p107 pocket protein. Mol Cell Biol 16:3606–3614, 1996.

98. M Arroyo, S Bagchi, P Raychaudhuri. Association of the human papillomavirus type 16 E7 protein with the S-phase–specific E2F–cyclin A complex. Mol Cell Biol 13:6537–6546, 1993.

99. M Tommasino, JP Adamczewski, F Carlotti, CF Barth, R Manetti, M Contorni, F Cavalieri, T Hunt, L Crawford. HPV 16 E7 protein associates with the protein kinase p33–cdk2 and cyclin A. Oncogene 8:195–202, 1993.

100. A Almasan, SP Linke, TG Paulson, LC Huang, GM Wahl. Genetic instability as a consequence of inappropriate entry into and progression through S-phase. Cancer Metastasis Rev 14:59–73, 1995.

101. JJ Chen, CE Reid, V Band, EJ Androphy. Interaction of papillomavirus E6 oncoproteins with a putative calcium-binding protein. Science 269:529–531, 1995.

102. M Scheffner, K Munger, JM Huibregtse, PM Howley. Targeted degradation of the retinoblastoma protein by human papillomavirus E7-E6 fusion proteins. EMBO J 11: 2425–2431, 1992.

103. MJ Antinore, MJ Birrer, D Patel, L Nader, DJ McCance. The human papillomavirus type 16 E7 gene product interacts with and trans-activates the AP1 family of transcription factors. EMBO J 15:1950–1960, 1996.

104. C Desaintes, C Demeret, S Goyat, M Yaniv, F Thierry. Expression of the papillomavirus E2 protein in HeLa cells leads to apoptosis. EMBO J 16:504–514, 1997.

105. H Romanczuk, PM Howley. Disruption of either the E1 or the E2 regulating gene of human papillomavirus type 16 increases viral immortalization capacity. Proc Natl Acad Sci U S A 89:3159–3163, 1992.

106. T Matsukura, S Koi, M Sugase. Both episomal and integrated forms of human papillomavirus type 16 are involved in invasive cervical cancers. Virology 172:63–72, 1989.

107. F Bosch, E Schwarz, P Boukamp, NE Fusenig, D Bartsch, H zur Hausen. Suppression in vivo of human papillomavirus type 18 E6-E7 gene expression in nontumorigenic HeLa x fibroblast hybrid cells. J Virol 64:4743–4754, 1960.

108. MH Stoler, CR Rhodes, A Whitbeck, SM Wolinsky, LT Chow, TR Broker. Human papillomavirus type 16 and 18 gene expression in cervical neoplasias. Hum Pathol 23: 117–128, 1992.

109. BD Cohen, DJ Goldstein, L Rutledge, WC Vass, DR Lowy, R Schlegel, JT Schiller. Transformation-specific interaction of the bovine papillomavirus E5 oncoprotein with

the platelet-derived growth factor receptor transmembrane domain and epidermal growth factor receptor cytoplasmic domain. J Virol 67:5303–5311, 1993.

110. L Petti, LA Nilson, D DiMaio. Activation of the platelet-derived growth factor receptor by the bovine papillomavirus E5 transforming protein. EMBO J 10:845–855, 1991.

111. SW Straight, B Herman, DJ McCance. The E5 oncoprotein of human papillomavirus type 16 inhibits the acidification of endosomes in human keratinocytes. J Virol 69: 3185–3192, 1995.

112. M Conrad, VJ Bubb, R Schlegel. The human papillomavirus type 6 and 16 E5 proteins are membrane-associated proteins which associate with the 16-kilodalton pore-forming protein. J Virol 67:6170–6178, 1993.

113. EJ Stanbridge. Suppression of malignancy in human cells. Nature 260:17–20, 1976.

114. TM Chen, G Pecoraro, V Defendi. Genetic analysis of in vitro progression of human papillomavirus–transfected human cervical cells. Cancer Res 53:1167–1171, 1993.

115. M Durst, FX Bosch, D Glitz, A Schneider, H zur Hausen. Inverse relationship between human papillomavirus (HPV) type 16 early gene expression and cell differentiation in nude mouse epithelial cysts and tumors induced by HPV-positive human cell lines. J Virol 65:796–804, 1991.

116. PP Smith, EM Bryant, P Kaur, JK McDougall. Cytogenetic analysis of eight human papillomavirus immortalized human keratinocyte cell lines. Int J Cancer 44:1124–1131, 1989.

117. MR Mullokandov, NG Kholodilov, NB Atkin, RD Burk, AB Johnson, HP Klinger. Genomic alterations in cervical carcinoma: losses of chromosome heterozygosity and human papilloma virus tumor status. Cancer Res 56: 197–205, 1996.

118. M Koi, H Morita, H Yamada, H Satoh, JC Barrett, M Oshimura. Normal human chromosome 11 suppresses the tumorigenicity of human cervical tumor cell line SiHa. Mol Carcinog 2:12–21, 1989.

119. PJ Saxon, ES Srivatasan, J Stanbridge. Introduction of human chromosome 11 via microcell transfer controls tumorigenic expression of HeLa cells. EMBO J 5: 3461–3466, 1986.

120. F Rosl, M Durst, H zur Hausen. Selective suppression of human papillomavirus transcription in non-tumorigenic cells by 5-azacytidine. EMBO J 7:1321–1328, 1988.

121. PH Smits, HL Smits, MF Jebbink, J ter Schegget. The short arm of chromosome 11 likely is involved in the regulation of the human papillomavirus 16 early enhancer-promoter and in the suppression of the transforming activity of the viral DNA. Virology 176:158–165, 1990.

122. PH Smits, HL Smits, RP Minnaar, BA Hemmings, RE Mayer-Jaekel, R Schuurman, J van der Noordaa, J ter Schegget. The 55 kDa regulatory subunit of protein phosphatase 2A plays a role in the activation of the HPV 16 long control region in human cells with a deletion in the short arm of chromosome 11. EMBO J 11:460–4606, 1992.

123. EM Rogan, TM Bryan, B Hukku, BA Hemmings, RE Mayer-Jaekel, R Schuurman, J van der Noordaa, J ter Schegget. Alterations in p53 and p161NK4 expression and telomere length during spontaneous immortalization of Li-Fraumeni syndrome fibroblasts. Mol Cell Biol 15: 4745–4753, 1995.

124. CA Reznikoff, C Belair, E Savelieva, Y Zhai, K Pfeifer, T Yeager, KJ Thompson, S DeVries, C Bindley, MA Newton, et al. Long-term genome stability and minimal genotypic and phenotypic alterations in HPV16 E7-, but not E6-, immortalized human uroepithelial cells. Genes Dev 8:2227–2240, 1994.

125. S Kyo, M Inoue, N Hayasaka, T Inoue, M Yutsudo, O Tanizawa, A Hakura. Regulation of early gene expression of human papillomavirus type 16 by inflammatory cytokines. Virology 200:130–139, 1994.

126. L Braun, M Durst, R Mikumo, A Crowley, M Robinson. Regulation of growth and gene expression in human papillomavirus–transformed keratinocytes by transforming growth factor-beta: implications for the control of papillomavirus infection. Mol Carcinog 6:100–111, 1992.

127. JA Pietenpol, RW Stein, E Moran, P Yaciuk, R Schlegel, RM Lyons, MR Pittelkow, K Munger, PM Howley, HL Moses. TGF-beta 1 inhibition of c-myc transcription and growth in keratinocytes is abrogated by viral transforming proteins with pRB binding domains. Cell 61:777–785, 1990.

128. MM Pater, GA Hughes, DE Hyslop, H Nakshatri, A Pater. Glucocorticoid-dependent oncogenic transformation by type 16 but not type 11 human papilloma virus DNA. Nature 335:832–835, 1988.

129. MM Pater, A Pater. RU486 inhibits glucocorticoid hormone-dependent oncogenesis by human papillomavirus type 16 DNA. Virology 183:799–802, 1991.

130. NG Osborne, MD Adelson. Herpes simplex and human papillomavirus genital infections: controversies around obstetric management. Clin Obstet Gynecol 33:801–806, 1990.

131. P Mounts, H Kashima. Association of human papillomavirus subtype and clinical course in respiratory papillomatosis. Laryngoscope 194:28–33, 1984.

132. R Carlos, O Sedano. Multifocal papilloma virus epithelial hyperplasia. Oral Surg Oral Med Oral Pathol 77:631–635, 1994.

133. RA Schwartz. Verrucous carcinoma of the skin and mucosa. J Am Acad Dermatol 32:1–21, 1995.

134. G Orth, S Jablonska, M Jarzabek-Chorzelska, S Obalek, G Rzesa, M Favre, O Croissant. Characteristics of the lesions and risk of malignant conversion associated with the type of human papillomavirus associated with epidermodysplasia verruciformis. Cancer Res 39:1074–1082, 1979.

135. EJ Androphy, I Dvoretzky, DR Lowy. X-linked inheritance of epidermodysplasia verruciformis. Genetic and virologic studies of a kindred. Arch Dermatol 121:864–868, 1985.

136. S Majewski, J Malejczyk, S Jablonska, J Misiewicz, L Rudnicka, S Obalek, G Orth. Natural cell-mediated cytotoxicity against various target cells in patients with epidermodysplasia verruciformis. J Am Acad Dermatol 22: 423–427, 1990.

137. KD Cooper, EJ Androphy, D Lowy, SI Katz. Antigen presentation and T-cell activation in epidermodysplasia verruciformis. J Invest Dermatol 94:769–776, 1990.

138. LM Tieben, RJ Berkhout, HL Smits, JN Bouwes Bavinck, BJ Vermeer, JA Bruijn, FJ Van der Woude, J Ter Schegget. Detection of epidermodysplasia verruciformis–like human papillomavirus types in malignant and premalignant skin lesions of renal transplant recipients. Br J Dermatol 131: 226–230, 1994.

139. RS Ostrow, M Bender, M Nimura, T Seki, M Kawashima, F Pass, AJ Faras. Human papillomavirus DNA in cutaneous primary and metastasized squamous cell carcinomas from patients with epidermodysplasia verruciformis. Proc Natl Acad Sci U S A 79:1634–1638, 1982.

140. H Mark, Santoro K, Campbell W, Hann E, Lathrop J. Integration of human papillomavirus sequences in cervical tumor cell lines. Ann Clin Lab Sci 26:147–153, 1996.

141. C Gilles, J Piette, D Ploton, M Doco-Fenzy, JM Foidart. Viral integration sites in human papilloma virus-33–immortalized cervical keratinocyte cell lines. Cancer Genet Cytogenet 90:63–69, 1996.

142. JK McDougall, D Myerson, AM Beckmann. Detection of viral DNA and RNA by in situ hybridization. J Histochem Cytochem 34:33–38, 1986.

143. AJ Amortegui, MP Meyer. In-situ hybridization for the diagnosis and typing of human papillomavirus. Clin Biochem 23:301–306, 1990.

144. V Adams, C Moll, M Schmid, C Rodrigues, R Moos, J Briner. Detection and typing of human papillomavirus in biopsy and cytological specimens by polymerase chain reaction and restriction enzyme analysis: a method suitable for semiautomation. J Med Virol 48:161–170, 1996.

145. MA Bedell, JB Hudson, TR Golub, ME Turyk, M Hosken, GD Wilbanks, LA Laimins. Amplification of human papillomavirus genomes in vitro is dependent on epithelial differentiation. J Virol 65:2254–2260, 1991.

146. HU Bernard, SY Chan, MM Manos, CK Ong, LL Villa, H Delius, CL Peyton, HM Bauer, CM Wheeler. Identification and assessment of known and novel human papillomaviruses by polymerase chain reaction amplification, restriction fragment length polymorphisms, nucleotide sequence, and phylogenetic algorithms. J Infect Dis 170:1077–1085, 1994.

147. J Czegledy, M Evander, L Veres, L Gergely, G Wadell. Detection of transforming gene regions of human papillomavirus type 16 in cervical dysplasias by the polymerase chain reaction. Med Microbiol Immunol 180:37–43, 1991.

148. AM Messing, WL Epstein. Natural history of warts: a two year study. Arch Dermatol 87:306, 1963.

149. MR Ling. Therapy of genital human papillomavirus infections. Part I: Indications for and justification of therapy. Int J Dermatol 31:682–686, 1992.

150. MH Bunney, M Nolan, D Williams. An assessment of methods of treating viral warts by comparative treatment trials based on a standard design. Br J Dermatol 94: 667–672, 1976.

151. HB Krebs. Treatment of genital condylomata with topical 5-fluorouracil. Dermatol Clin 9:333–341, 1991.

152. M Stanley. Mechanism of action of imiquimod. Papillomavirus Rep 10:23–29, 1999.

153. SK Tyring, I Arany, MA Stanley, MA Tomai, RL Miller, MH Smith, DJ McDermott, HB Slade. A randomized, controlled, molecular study of condylomata acuminata clearance during treatment with imiquimod. J Infect Dis 178: 551–555, 1998.

154. L Edwards, A Ferenczy, L Eron, D Baker, ML Owens, TL Fox, AJ Hougham, KA Schmitt. Self-administered topical 5% imiquimod cream for external anogenital warts. HPV Study Group. Arch Dermatol 134:25–30, 1998.

155. WS Sawchuk, PJ Weber, DR Lowy, LM Dzubow. Infectious papillomavirus in the vapor of warts treated with carbon dioxide laser or electrocoagulation: detection and protection. J Am Acad Dermatol 21:41–49, 1989.

156. LJ Eron, F Jusdon, S Tucker, S Prawer, J Mills, K Murphy, M Hickey, M Rogers, S Flannigan, N Hien, et al. Interferon therapy for condyloma acuminata. N Engl J Med 315: 1059–1064, 1986.

157. JM Friedman-Kien, LJ Eron, M Conant, W Growdon, H Badiak, PW Bradstreet, D Fedorczyk, JR Trout, TF Plasse. Natural interferon alfa for treatment of condylomata acuminata. JAMA 259:533–538, 1988.

158. RC Reichman, D Oakes, W Bonnez, D Brown, HR Mattison, A Bailey-Farchione, MH Stoler, LM Demeter, SK Tyring, L Miller, et al. Treatment of condyloma acuminatum with three different interferon-α preparations administered parenterally: a double-blind, placebo-controlled trial. J Infect Dis 162:1270–1276, 1990.

159. S Keay, N Teng, M Eisenberg, B Story, PW Sellers, TC Merigan. Topical interferon for treating condyloma acuminata in women. J Infect Dis 158:934–939, 1988.

160. A Schonfeld, S Nitke, A Schattner. Intramuscular human interferon-β injections in treatment of condylomata acuminata. Lancet 1:1038–1042, 1984.

161. SA Gall, CE Hughes, K Trofatter. Interferon for the therapy of condyloma accuminatum. Obstet Gynecol 153: 157–163, 1985.

162. SA Gall. Human papillomavirus infection and therapy with interferon. Am J Obstet Gynecol 172:1354–1359, 1995.

163. S Haglund, P Lundquist, K Cantell, H Strander. Interferon therapy in juvenile laryngeal papillomatosis. Arch Otolaryngol 107:327–332, 1981.

164. EJ Androphy, I Dvoretzky, AE Maluish, HJ Wallace, DR Lowy. Response of warts in epidermodysplasia verruciformis to treatment with systemic and intralesional alpha interferon. J Am Acad Dermatol 11:197–202, 1984.

165. H Kashima, B Leventhal, K Clark, Cohen S, H Dedo, D Donovan, B Fearon, L Gardiner, H Goepfert, R Lusk, et al. Interferon alfa-N1 (Wellferon) in juvenile onset recurrent respiratory papillomatosis: results of a randomized study in twelve collaborative institutions. Laryngoscope 98: 334–340, 1988.

166. LP Chen, EK Thomas, SL Hu, I Hellstrom, KE Hellstrom. Human papillomavirus type 16 nucleoprotein E7 is a tumor rejection antigen. Proc Natl Acad Sci U S A 88:110–114, 1991.

167. L Chen, MT Mizuno, MC Singhal, SL Hu, DA Galloway, I Hellstrom, KE Hellstrom. Induction of cytotoxic T lymphocytes specific for a syngeneic tumor expressing the E6 oncoprotein of human papillomavirus type 16. J Immunol 148:2617–2621, 1992.

168. MC Feltkamp, GR Vreughenhil, MP Vierboom, E Ras, SH van der Burg, J ter Schegget, CJ Melief, WM Kast. Cytotoxic T lymphocytes raised against a subdominant epitope offered as a synthetic peptide eradicate human papillomavirus type 16–induced tumors. Eur J Immunol 25: 2638–2642, 1995.

169. R Selvakumar, LA Borenstein, YL Lin, R Ahmed, FO Wettstein. Immunization with nonstructural proteins E1 and E2 of cottontail rabbit papillomavirus stimulates regression of virus-induced papillomas. J Virol 69: 602–605, 1995.

170. JP Bouvet, L Belec, R Pires, J Pillot. Immunoglobulin G antibodies in human vaginal secretions after parenteral vaccination. Infect Immunol 62:3957–3961, 1994.

171. F Breitburd, R Kirnbauer, NL Hubbert. Immunization with virus like particles from cottontail rabbit papillomavirus (CRPV) can protect against experimental CRPV infection. J Virol 69:3959–3963, 1995.

13

Parvovirus B19

Karen Wiss
University of Massachusetts Medical School, Worcester, Massachusetts, USA

Tricia J. Brown
University of Oklahoma Health Sciences Center, Oklahoma City, Oklahoma, USA

Parvovirus B19 is the only member of the family Parvoviridae known to infect humans. The most characteristic cutaneous manifestation is erythema infectiosum (fifth disease). This illness is distinguished by a "slapped-cheek" appearance of the face and a pink, lacy eruption on the trunk and extremities. The B19 virus may also cause arthritis, aplastic crisis in individuals with hemoglobinopathies, chronic anemia in immunocompromised persons, and fetal hydrops after intrauterine infection. This virus has also been linked to the rare disorder, papular-purpuric gloves-and-socks syndrome (PPGSS).

HISTORY

Erythema infectiosum appears to be a recognized entity throughout the 1800s but was thought to represent a mild form of rubella or measles [1]. In 1889, Tschamer described an illness suggestive of erythema infectiosum that he called abortive rubella [2]. The illness was named fifth disease in 1905 during a time when childhood exanthems were designated first through sixth [3].

Interestingly, the virus was discovered a few years before it was associated with any specific illness. The virus was found during routine screening of serum samples from healthy blood donors for hepatitis B surface antigen [4]. Nine samples of blood from these donors were falsely positive for hepatitis by the technique of counter immunoelectrophoresis (CIE) but negative by hemagglutination and radioimmunoassay, which are more sensitive tests. Immunoelectron microscopy demonstrated viral particles resembling parvovirus, and these were designated B19 after one of the specimen labels [4]. The authors suspected that the virus was an infectious agent because 30% of serum from random adult samples had immunoglobulin G (IgG) antibody to the viral antigen. In 1983, B19 was confirmed to be a parvovirus [5].

The first report of a symptomatic parvovirus B19 infection was of two British soldiers with an acute febrile illness in 1980 [6]. B19 was also found in patients with sickle cell anemia and hypoplastic crisis in 1981 [7]. In 1983, there was an outbreak of fifth disease among London schoolchildren [8]. Serum samples from 31 schoolchildren and 6 adult exposures, all with the clinical signs of the disease, contained parvovirus-specific IgM antibody. No IgM was found in asymptomatic persons who were exposed. This was the first outbreak of erythema infectiosum to be examined for human parvovirus, and the findings of this study suggested B19 as the cause [9] (Fig. 13–1).

INCIDENCE

Although B19 can occur sporadically throughout the year, it tends to occur in epidemics in late winter and early spring [10]. The amount of infection within a community varies

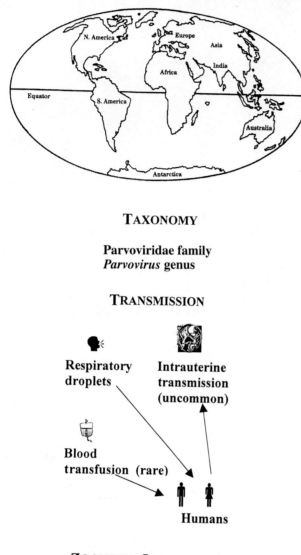

TAXONOMY

Parvoviridae family
Parvovirus **genus**

TRANSMISSION

Respiratory droplets

Intrauterine transmission (uncommon)

Blood transfusion (rare)

Humans

ZOONOTIC IMPLICATIONS

None

Figure 13–1.   Incidence and transmission of parvovirus B19.

from year to year. All ages can be affected and serological studies show increasing prevalence with age [10]. Studies have shown that 15 to 60% of children ages 5 to 19 years of age and 30 to 60% of adults are seropositive [4,11,12]. The seroprevalence increases to more than 90% in the elderly [12].

PATHOGENESIS

B19 virus is a member of the family Parvoviridae and the genus Parvovirus [13]. The other two genera in this family,

the Dependoviruses and the Densoviruses, infect other vertebrates and insects [14]. Other members of the genus Parvovirus include canine parvovirus and feline panleukopenia virus, as well as other animal parvoviruses [15]. The other animal parvoviruses are not thought to infect humans, and B19 is not believed to infect other animals [15].

B19 is the smallest known human pathogenic virus that contains single-stranded DNA encoding for at least two capsid or structural proteins and one nonstructural protein [14]. In contrast to some other parvoviruses and the other two genera, B19 is thought to be capable of autonomous replication (without coinfection of a helper virus) [14]. There is only one known serotype of parvovirus B19.

Transmission of B19 is primarily via the respiratory route by droplet aerosol [11] during the period of viremia [16]. Once the rash of erythema infectiosum appears, individuals are usually no longer infectious [11]. The rate of transmission among close household contacts is approximately 50% [17,18]. The virus may rarely be spread via blood transfusion [4] and blood products [19], although the risk of transmission with transfusion of one unit of blood is low [20]. Vertical transmission from mother to fetus may also occur [21]. Thirty percent of infected mothers transmit the virus to their offspring, as evidenced by IgM in cord blood or IgG present in the 9- to 12-month-old infant [22].

The pathogenesis of the characteristic rash of fifth disease is not known, but there is speculation that immune complexes play a role [10]. Both the rash and arthralgias are considered to be postinfectious phenomena that are due to immune-mediated defenses of the host. During infection, B19 virus primarily targets the erythroid cell line and is able to infect and lyse erythroid precursor cells [23]. Individuals with chronic hemolytic anemia or anemia associated with acute or chronic blood loss depend on compensatory increases in red cell production to maintain stable red cell indices. In these persons, B19 infection may lead to transient aplastic crisis [10]. In immunodeficient individuals, B19 infection may cause chronic red cell aplasia and associated chronic anemia [24]. Parvovirus B19 infection in the developing fetus may infect the erythroblasts, leading to hemolysis, anemia, and possibly hydrops and fetal death [25]. Because recurrent disease with B19 is rarely seen, it is assumed that infection confers long-term immunity [26].

CLINICAL MANIFESTATIONS

Parvovirus Infection in Children

Whereas most infections due to B19 are asymptomatic and unrecognized, erythema infectiosum (fifth disease) is the most common clinical syndrome associated with the virus (Figs. 13–2 to 13–6). This disease is most frequently seen in school-age children, although it may also occur in adults.

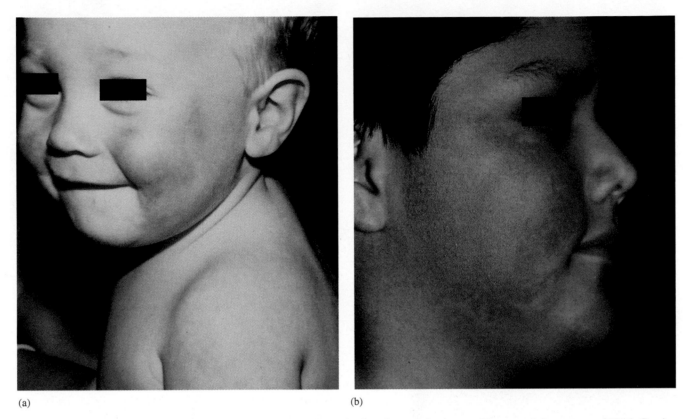

(a)   (b)

Figure 13–2. (a,b) The characteristic ''slapped-cheek'' malar rash of erythema infectiosum. (Photograph b courtesy of Edith Garcia-Gonzalez, M.D., Ph.D., and Lourdes Tamayo, M.D., Mexico City, Mexico.)

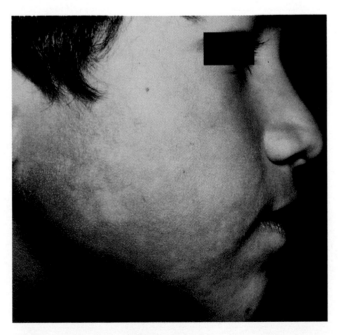

Figure 13–3. Facial erythema in a child with erythema infectiosum.

The clinical manifestations of erythema infectiosum are listed in Table 13–1.

Parvovirus B19 has also been associated with a variety of other clinical syndromes. There have been reports of children with parvovirus infection presenting with symptoms suggestive of juvenile rheumatoid arthritis [27]. Parvovirus B19 infection in children has also been associated with vascular purpura [28,29], including Henoch-Schönlein purpura [29]. Some patients develop only an enanthem, which consists of erythema of the tongue and pharynx or red macules on the buccal mucosa, hard palate, or soft palate [30]. Parvovirus B19 has also been responsible for obstructive respiratory disease such as bronchitis/bronchiolitis, laryngitis, and asthmatic attacks [31]. Differential diagnosis is shown in Table 13–2.

Parvovirus Infection in Adults

Adult B19 infection, in contrast to infection in children, is more likely to be asymptomatic, more commonly associated with arthropathy, and usually does not have the characteristic rash [32,33]. The usual course consists of fever, lymphadenopathy, mild arthritis of the hands, wrists, and knees, and no rash [34]. Pruritus can occur in some patients,

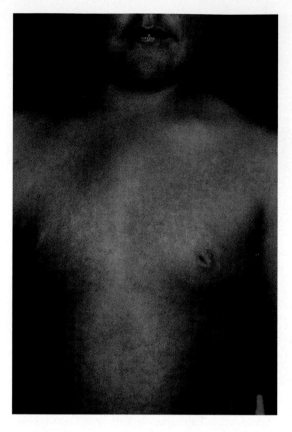

Figure 13–4. Facial eruption and extensive erythematous macules on chest and arms. (Photograph courtesy of Edith Garcia-Gonzalez, M.D., Ph.D., and Lourdes Tamayo, M.D., Mexico City, Mexico.)

Table 13–1. Clinical Manifestations of Erythema Infectiosum

Time after exposure	Clinical manifestations	Laboratory analyses	Other notes
7–11 days	Nonspecific symptoms of low-grade fever, mild coryza, and headache, lasting 2–3 days	Serology, particularly immunoglobulin M	This prodromal stage corresponds with the period of viremia. The constitutional symptoms tend to be more severe in adults
9–13 days	Characteristic rash on the malar eminences, with fiery–red, edematous, confluent plaques that have a "slapped-cheek" appearance (Figs. 13–2 and 13–3). With the rash, some patients may also develop pharyngitis, malaise, myalgias, diarrhea, nausea, cough, and conjunctivitis	Detection of B19 DNA by polymerase chain reaction, etc Viral isolation (difficult)	Relative circumoral pallor may occur during this stage of disease
10–17 days	Facial rash fades, while pink macules or papules appear on the trunk, neck, and extensor surfaces (Fig 13–4). The palms and soles are only rarely affected. The rash on the trunk and extremities often develops central clearing, giving it a lacy or reticulate appearance (Figs. 13–5 and 13–6)		About 7% of children develop arthralgias following the malar rash, whereas 80% of adults have joint involvement
15–26 days	Rash resolves after 5 days. Over the next several weeks, the rash may recur with certain stimuli, such as sunlight, exercise, temperature change, bathing, and emotional stress		The truncal exanthem can present in a variety of patterns, including morbilliform, confluent, circinate, and annular. Pruritus can occur in some patients, particularly adults

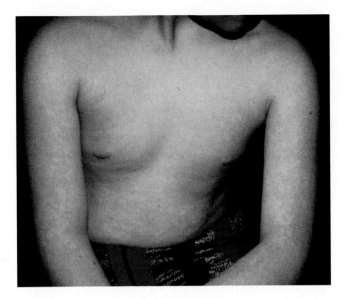

Figure 13–5. Lacy pink macules on the arms of a patient with parvovirus infection.

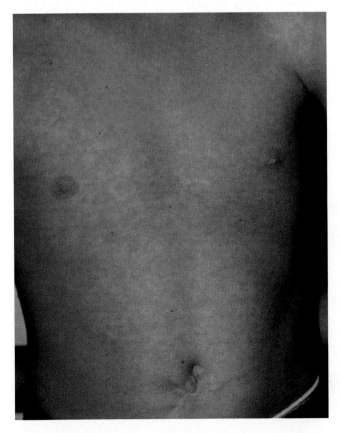

Figure 13–6. Reticulated pink macules and papules on the trunk of a child with erythema infectiosum. (Photograph courtesy of Claire Mansur, M.D., Department of Dermatology, Tufts University School of Medicine, Boston, MA.)

Table 13–2. Differential Diagnosis of Erythema Infectiosum

Rubella: The rash of rubella begins on the face and spreads inferiorly to the trunk and extremities. However, this exanthem progresses rapidly within 1 day, and fades over the next 2 days

Measles: The rash of measles begins on the forehead and spreads inferiorly, although at a slower pace. The rash reaches the feet by the third day, and lasts a total of 4–6 days. The lesions are more discrete papules. The facial exanthem is not limited to the malar eminences

Scarlet fever: Erythema infectiosum usually lacks pharyngitis, although this manifestation may be present. Culture for *Streptococcus pyogenes* can differentiate the two diseases. The rash of scarlet fever tends to be rough and accentuated in body folds

Drug reactions: May sometimes be difficult to differentiate and will require diagnostic testing for parvovirus B19

Erysipelas of the cheeks: This bacterial infection can also have erythematous, edematous, tender plaques involving the cheeks, but the area is typically hot to the touch and unilateral. This disease does not progress to a generalized cutaneous eruption

Collagen vascular disease (including juvenile rheumatoid arthritis and systemic lupus erythematosus): The arthralgias and malar rash of B19 infection can mimic various collagen vascular disorders. With acute B19 infection, the rheumatoid factor test can be positive, but joint destruction does not occur

---

particularly adults [35]. Infection is often asymptomatic (26% of adults in one study) [36]. Women are likely to have joint complaints and a rash, whereas men tend to have a flu-like illness [36]. Fatigue, malaise, and depression can persist for weeks after acute infection [34].

Acute arthropathy is the primary presentation of B19 infection in adults [35,36]. Women more so than men develop the arthropathy with synovitis, clinically manifested by joint swelling, stiffness, and pain [36]. The arthropathy is typically symmetrical and peripheral, involving multiple joints, and is of sudden onset and moderate severity [37]. The joint symptoms are usually brief, but can be persistent or recurrent for more than 2 months in 20% of adults [36,37]. The arthropathy usually involves the small joints of the hands, the feet, and the knees, but can affect almost any joint [36]. It can imitate Lyme arthritis [38], rheumatoid arthritis [39], or lupus arthritis [40].

B19 infection can cause severe pruritus with or without a rash. It has been suggested that parvovirus be considered in any patient with acute arthritis and pruritus [41]. Paresthesias of the fingers have also been described in association with parvovirus infection, with or without other features of the disease [42].

The rash, which is often not present in adults, usually consists of red macules that are occasionally lacy or blotchy, on the extremities [36]. The slapped-cheek appearance is rarely present. The rash is frequently pruritic and often severely affects the feet [36]. Other cutaneous presentations in adults include purpura [43], vesiculopustules [44], palmoplantar desquamation [45], polyarteritis nodosa [46], and a malar rash suggestive of lupus erythematosus [40].

Papular-Purpuric Gloves-and-Socks Syndrome

Papular-purpuric gloves-and-socks syndrome (PPGSS) is an unusual febrile dermatosis initially described by Harms et al in 1990 [47]. In 1991, the syndrome was first associated with acute parvovirus B19 infection [48]. Since that time, over 25 cases have been reported [47–62]. Although many possible viruses have been proposed as etiological agents [52,53,60–62], B19 is the only agent that has sufficiently been proved to cause the syndrome [59].

Although few details are known regarding PPGSS, this syndrome most commonly affects young adults and occurs most frequently during spring and summer. The characteristic clinical manifestations (Figs. 13–7 and 13–8) are described in Table 13–3. The disease course is generally self-limited, with no known sequelae. Differential diagnoses are described in Table 13–4.

Complications

The most widely reported complications of parvovirus B19 infection include transient aplastic crisis in patients with chronic hemolytic anemia, prolonged anemia in immunocompromised persons, and fetal hydrops with intrauterine infection. In addition, cases of aseptic meningitis and encephalitis have been reported with this virus [63–67]. Rare complications that have been attributed to parvovirus B19 infection include hemophagocytic syndrome [68], myocarditis [69], vasculitis [70], and recurrent agranulocytosis [71]. However, these case reports have not yet been substantiated by clinical studies.

Transient aplastic crisis due to B19 infection has been reported in sickle cell anemia [7,72], hereditary spherocy-

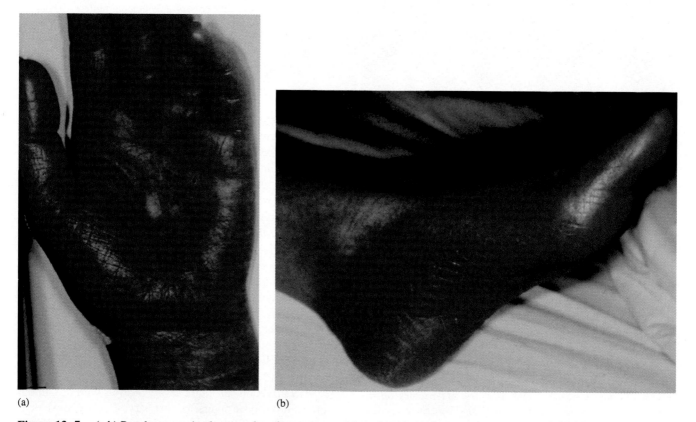

(a)   (b)

Figure 13–7. (a,b) Papular-purpuric gloves-and-socks syndrome. Marked erythema is seen covering the distal hands and feet. (Photographs courtesy of Linda de Raeve, M.D., Brussels, Belgium.)

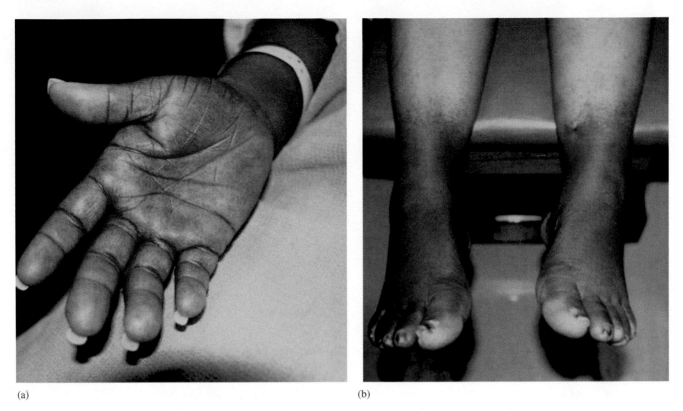

(a)   (b)

Figure 13–8. (a,b) Papular-purpuric gloves-and-socks syndrome. Marked erythema is seen covering the distal hands and feet. (Photographs courtesy of Soni Carlton, M.D., Department of Dermatology, University of Texas Medical Branch at Galveston, Galveston, TX.)

Table 13–3. Clinical Manifestations of Papular-Purpuric Gloves-and-Socks Syndrome

Time after exposure	Clinical manifestations	Laboratory analyses	Other notes
Overall time course of illness unknown	Mild transient prodromal symptoms in some patients, with low-grade fever, and less commonly fatigue, myalgias, anorexia, lymphadenopathy, and arthralgias	Serology, particularly immunoglobulin Detection of B19 DNA by polymerase chain reaction, etc	
	Rapidly progressive symmetrical swelling and erythema of distal hands and feet, which is painful and significantly pruritic	Viral isolation (difficult)	Less frequently involved areas include cheeks, elbows, knees, inner thighs, inguinal creases, buttocks, and glans penis
	Confluent papular-purpuric lesions involving the dorsal and ventral aspects of the distal extremities. The eruption has distinct margins ending at the wrists and ankles		
	Polymorphous enanthem of the hard and soft palate, buccal mucosa, and lips		Over 50% of patients also have diffuse erythema and edema of the lips, palatal vesicles, ulcerations, and/or petechiae, all of which are painful and pruritic
1–2 wk after onset of rash	Spontaneous resolution of entire syndrome		

Table 13–4. Differential Diagnosis of Papular-Purpuric Gloves and Socks Syndrome

Rocky Mountain spotted fever (and other rickettsial diseases): Rocky Mountain spotted fever is usually a more severe illness, with sudden onset of fever, significant headache, and myalgia. The characteristic exanthem begins on the wrists, forearms, and ankles, and later spreads to the palms and soles. The rash then progresses to involve the extremities, trunk, and face

Atypical measles: In atypical measles, the rash may appear first on the distal arms and legs rather than the face. However, the prodromal symptoms of measles are typically more prominent, and the exanthem of measles lasts only 4–6 days

Hand-foot-and-mouth disease: Low-grade fever, malaise and painful mucosal lesions occur with both diseases. However, the macules and papules that erupt on the distal extremities quickly progress to vesicles with hand-foot-and-mouth disease

Kawasaki disease: The erythema and edema usually begin on the palms and soles or the diaper area and spread to the trunk and extremities over the next 2 days. Also, this disease typically affects young children, and is uncommon after 8 years of age

tosis [73], pyruvate kinase deficiency [74], heterozygous beta-thalassemia [75], and autoimmune hemolytic anemia [76]. In some patients, the aplasia has been the initial manifestation of the underlying hematological disease [75,76]. Usually after 1 week of fever and constitutional complaints, patients develop pallor, fatigue, and worsening anemia [77]. Hypoplasia or aplasia of the erythroid series is seen with bone marrow examination [77]. Although most patients recover within 1 week, transfusion may be necessary [77]. The aplasia can be fatal if untreated [77]. Although usually asymptomatic, transient aplastic crisis can also occur in healthy individuals [15].

Chronic anemia due to persistent lysis of red cell precursors is another complication of parvovirus infection seen in immunocompromised persons [15]. This prolonged anemia has been described in congenital immunodeficiencies [24], in human immunodeficiency virus (HIV)–infected individuals [78], in acute leukemia [79], and in infancy without immunodeficiency [80].

The most common complication of intrauterine infection with parvovirus B19 is nonimmune fetal hydrops (hydrops fetalis) [21]. The virus infects erythroid precursors with resultant hemolysis in the fetus leading to anemia, tissue anoxia, and high-output heart failure [21]. The overall risk of fetal death is unknown, but studies have suggested that the risk is less than 10% after maternal infection

[21,22]. It has been postulated that infection between the 20th and the 28th weeks of gestation is of the greatest threat to the fetus [81]. In a woman with unknown serological status, the risk of fetal death is thought to be less than 2.5% after a household exposure and less than 1.5% after a work exposure [21]. There is no evidence that the rate of congenital anomalies is greater in B19-infected fetuses compared with background rates [21].

DERMATOPATHOLOGY

The histopathological changes in the skin of patients with fifth disease have not been well described and are not considered diagnostic [82]. Histological examination of various other tissues has shown homogeneous intranuclear inclusions in erythroid precursor cells [25,83]. These inclusions demonstrate parvovirus-like particles with electron microscopy [82].

Laboratory Findings

In most persons with erythema infectiosum, all laboratory results are normal [30,33]. Some healthy individuals do develop reticulocytopenia, anemia, lymphopenia, neutropenia, and thrombocytopenia, usually without clinical symptoms [16]. Immunocompromised patients with transient aplastic crisis have reticulocytopenia and anemia, the severity of which depends on the degree of the underlying anemia [11]. Rheumatoid factor can be positive in some patients with parvovirus-associated arthritis [37,39] and the erythrocyte sedimentation rate is occasionally elevated [27].

Diagnosis

The diagnosis of fifth disease is usually based on the clinical findings of a slapped-cheek eruption and a lacy rash on the extremities. In difficult cases, the detection of B19 IgM has been the mainstay for diagnosis. Antibody testing is usually performed with radioimmunoassay (RIA) or enzyme-linked immunosorbent (ELISA) techniques. IgM antibody can be detected within a few days after the onset of illness up to 6 months [84–86]. IgG antibody can usually be found by the 7th day of infection and lasts for years, and is most useful to confirm past infection [84,85]. It is often difficult to find antibody to parvovirus in immunodeficient individuals [78], and these cases will require other diagnostic methods. Table 13–2 highlights possible differential diagnoses.

Viral isolation is limited to a few research laboratories because there is no animal model and no easy tissue culture system for the virus. Testing can be arranged through state health departments when parvovirus is suspected in patients with aplastic crisis, immunodeficiency, pregnancy, or fetal hydrops [10].

B19 virus can be found in the serum during viremia with RIA, CIE, or ELISA. Dot-blot hybridization and polymerase chain reaction (PCR) are the most specific techniques to enable identification of B19 DNA in serum, urine, respiratory secretions, and other tissues [87,88]. B19 DNA can be found with PCR for 2 to 4 months after the onset of illness and can be a complement to specific antibody testing [86,89].

Treatment and Prophylaxis

Erythema infectiosum usually does not require any treatment, and no specific therapy is available. Supportive treatment, if needed, is the only therapy indicated for most cases. Currently, no vaccine is available to prevent parvovirus B19 infection, although potential candidates are currently in development and clinical trials [90,91]. The B19 virus is easily spread in circumstances of close contact such as day care facilities, schools, workplaces, and homes. Control measures directed toward individuals with erythema infectiosum are not effective, because persons are no longer infectious by the time they develop the clinical illness [11]. Patients with chronic anemia or aplastic crisis can be infectious for longer periods, and appropriate respiratory and contact isolation should be performed when these individuals are hospitalized [92]. Table 13–5 highlights symptomatic treatment of B-19.

CONCLUSION

Erythema infectiosum, with its distinct slapped-cheek eruption followed by a reticulate rash on the trunk and extremities, is the most characteristic presentation of human parvovirus infection. Whereas the disease has been known for a century, parvovirus B19 has only recently been identified as the etiological agent. B19 has now been associated with an increasing number of disorders including an acute polyarthropathy in adults, PPGSS, a wide spectrum of atypical cutaneous presentations, aplastic crisis, chronic anemia, and fetal hydrops. As techniques in identification and characterization of the virus improve, additional clinical syndromes associated with parvovirus B19 may be identified.

Table 13–5. Treatment of Parvovirus B19 Infection

Symptom	Treatment
Malaise and fatigue	Bed rest
Pruritus	Starch baths or antipruritics as needed
Arthralgia and arthritis	Nonsteroidal anti-inflammatory medications
Chronic anemia	Intravenous immunoglobulin: administration of either 400 mg/kg for 5 or 10 days, or 1 g/kg for 3 days has been reportedly successful
Transient aplastic crisis	May require blood transfusion and oxygen therapy, if severe [
Hydrops fetalis	Intrauterine blood transfusion has been successful in some cases, although treatment is controversial

REFERENCES

1. AM van Elsacker-Niele, MJ Anderson. First picture of erythema infectiosum? [letter]. Lancet 1:229, 1987.
2. A Tschamer. Ueber ortliche Rotheln. Jahrb Kinderheilkd 29:372–379, 1889.
3. L Shapiro. The numbered diseases: first through sixth [letter]. JAMA 194:210, 1965.
4. YE Cossart, B Cant, AM Field, D Widdows. Parvovirus-like particles in human sera. Lancet 1:72–73, 1975.
5. J Summers, SE Jones, MJ Anderson. Characterization of the genome of the agent of erythrocyte aplasia permits its classification as a human parvovirus. J Gen Virol 64: 2527–2532, 1983.
6. JM Shneerson, PP Mortimer, EM Vandervelde. Febrile illness due to a parvovirus. BMJ 280:1580, 1980.
7. JR Pattison, SE Jones, J Hodgson, LR Davis, JM White, CE Stroud, L Murtaza. Parvovirus infections and hypoplastic crisis in sickle-cell anaemia [letter]. Lancet 1:664–665, 1981.
8. MJ Anderson, SE Jones, SP Fisher-Hoch, E Lewis, SM Hall, CL Bartlett, BJ Cohen, PP Mortimer, MS Pereira. Human parvovirus, the cause of erythema infectiosum (fifth disease) [letter]. Lancet 1:1378, 1983.
9. MJ Anderson, E Lewis, IM Kidd, SM Hall, BJ Cohen. An outbreak of erythema infectiosum associated with human parvovirus infection. J Hyg 93:85–93, 1984.
10. Centers for Disease Control and Prevention. Risks associated with human parvovirus B19 infection. MMWR Morb Mortal Wkly Rep 38:81–97, 1989.
11. LJ Anderson. Role of parvovirus B19 in human disease. Pediatr Infect Dis J 6:711–718, 1987.
12. BJ Cohen, MM Buckley. The prevalence of antibody to

human parvovirus B19 in England and Wales. J Med Microbiol 25:151–153, 1988.

13. G Siegl, RC Bates, KI Berns, BJ Carter, DC Kelly, E Kurstak, P Tattersall. Characteristics and taxonomy of Parvoviridae. Intervirology 23:61–73, 1985.

14. MJ Anderson, JR Pattison. The human parvovirus: brief review. Arch Virol 82:137–148, 1984.

15. LJ Anderson. Human parvoviruses. J Infect Dis 161:603–608, 1990.

16. MJ Anderson, PG Higgins, LR Davis, JS Willman, SE Jones, IM Kidd, JR Pattison, DA Tyrrell. Experimental parvoviral infection in humans. J Infect Dis 152:257–265, 1985.

17. T Chorba, P Coccia, RC Holman, P Tattersall, LJ Anderson, J Sudman, NS Young, E Kurczynski, UM Saarinen, R Moir, et al. The role of parvovirus B19 in aplastic crisis and erythema infectiosum (fifth disease). J Infect Dis 154:383–393, 1986.

18. JG Tuckerman, T Brown, BJ Cohen. Erythema infectiosum in a village primary school: clinical and virological studies. J R Coll Gen Pract 36:267–270, 1986.

19. PP Mortimer, NLC Luban, JF Kelleher, BJ Cohen. Transmission of serum parvovirus-like virus by clotting-factor concentrates. Lancet 2:482–484, 1983.

20. BJ Cohen, AM Field, S Gudnadottir, S Beard, JA Barbara. Blood donor screening for parvovirus B19. J Virol Methods 30:233–238, 1990.

21. TJ Torok. Human parvovirus B19 infections in pregnancy. Pediatr Infect Dis J 9:772–776, 1990.

22. Public Health Laboratory Service Working Party on Fifth Disease. Prospective study of human parvovirus (B19) infection in pregnancy. BMJ 300:1166–1170, 1990.

23. N Young, M Harrison, J Moore, P Mortimer, RK Humphries. Direct demonstration of the human parvovirus in erythroid progenitor cells infected in vitro. J Clin Invest 74:2024–2032, 1984.

24. GJ Kurtzman, K Ozawa, B Cohen, G Hanson, R Oseas, NS Young. Chronic bone marrow failure due to persistent B19 parvovirus infection. N Engl J Med 317:287–294, 1987.

25. A Anand, ES Gray, T Brown, JP Clewley, BJ Cohen. Human parvovirus infection in pregnancy and hydrops fetalis. N Engl J Med 316:183–186, 1987.

26. LJ Anderson. Human parvovirus B19. In: DD Richman, RJ Whitley, FG Hayden, eds. Clinical Virology. New York: Churchill Livingstone, 1997, pp 613–631.

27. DM Reid, TM Reid, T Brown, JA Rennie, CJ Eastmond. Human parvovirus–associated arthritis: a clinical and laboratory description. Lancet 1:422–425, 1985.

28. JJ Lefrere, AM Courouce, JY Muller, M Clark, JP Soulier. Human parvovirus and purpura [letter]. Lancet 2:730, 1985.

29. JJ Lefrere, AM Courouce, JP Soulier, MP Cordier, MC Guesne Girault, C Polonovski, A Bensman. Henoch-Schönlein purpura and human parvovirus infection [letter]. Pediatrics 78:183–184, 1986.

30. FJ Condon. Erythema infectiosum—report of an area-wide outbreak. Am J Public Health 49:528–535, 1959.

31. S Wiersbitzky, TF Schwarz, R Bruns, EH Ballke, M Roggendorf, H Wiersbitzky, F Deinhardt. Acute obstructive respiratory diseases in infants and children associated with parvovirus B19 infection [letter]. Infection 19:252, 1991.

32. HM Feder, I Anderson. Fifth disease. A brief review of infections in childhood, in adulthood, and in pregnancy. Arch Intern Med 149:2176–2178, 1989.

33. FA Plummer, GW Hammond, K Forward, L Sekla, LM Thompson, SE Jones, IM Kidd, MJ Anderson. An erythema infectiosum–like illness caused by human parvovirus infection. N Engl J Med 313:74–79, 1985.

34. J Thurn. Human parvovirus B19: historical and clinical review. Rev Infect Dis 10:1005–1011, 1988.

35. EA Ager, TDY Chin, JD Poland. Epidemic erythema infectiosum. N Engl J Med 275:1326–1331, 1966.

36. AD Woolf, GV Campion, A Chishick, S Wise, BJ Cohen, PT Klouda, O Caul, PA Dieppe. Clinical manifestations of human parvovirus B19 in adults. Arch Intern Med 149:1153–1156, 1989.

37. DG White, AD Woolf, PP Mortimer, BJ Cohen, DR Blake, PA Bacon. Human parvovirus arthropathy. Lancet 1:419–421, 1985.

38. DR Mayo, DW Vance. Parvovirus B19 as the cause of a syndrome resembling Lyme arthritis in adults [letter]. N Engl J Med 324:419–420, 1991.

39. SJ Naides, EH Field. Transient rheumatoid factor positivity in acute human parvovirus B19 infection. Arch Intern Med 148:2587–2589, 1988.

40. RA Kalish, AN Knopf, GW Gary, JJ Canoso. Lupus-like presentation of human parvovirus B19 infection. J Rheumatol 19:169–171, 1992.

41. TA Jacks. Pruritus in parvovirus infection. J R Coll Gen Pract 37:210–211, 1987.

42. H Faden, GW Gary, M Korman. Numbness and tingling of fingers associated with parvovirus B19 infection [letter]. J Infect Dis 161:354–355, 1990.

43. PP Mortimer, BJ Cohen, MA Rossiter, SM Fairhead, AF Rahman. Human parvovirus and purpura [letter]. Lancet 2:730–731, 1985.

44. SJ Naides, W Piette, LA Veach, Z Argenyi. Human parvovirus B19–induced vesiculopustular skin eruption. Am J Med 84:968–971, 1988.

45. JL Dinerman, LC Corman. Human parvovirus B19 arthropathy associated with desquamation. Am J Med 89:826–828, 1990.

46. LC Corman, DJ Dolson. Polyarteritis nodosa and parvovirus B19 infection [letter]. Lancet 339:491, 1992.

47. M Harms, R Feldmann, JH Saurat. Papular-purpuric "gloves and socks" syndrome. J Am Acad Dermatol 23:850–854, 1990.

48. M Bagot, J Revuz. Papular-purpuric "gloves and socks" syndrome: primary infection with parvovirus B19? J Am Acad Dermatol 25:341, 1991.

49. CL Halasz, D Cormier, M Den. Petechial glove and sock syndrome caused by parvovirus B19. J Am Acad Dermatol 27:835–838, 1992.

50. E Vargas-Diez, GF Buezo, M Aragues, E Dauden, F De Ory. Papular-purpuric gloves-and-socks syndrome. Int J Dermatol 5:626–632, 1996.

51. JM Carrascosa. Sindrome de las papulas purpuricas en guante y calcetin: un peculiar patron de respuesta cutanea. Piel 10:115–117, 1995.

52. R Feldmann, M Harms, JH Saurat. Papular-purpuric "gloves and socks" syndrome: not only parvovirus B19. Dermatology 188:85–87, 1994.

53. A Pérez-Ferriols, A Martinez-Aparicio, A Aliaga-Boniche. Papular-purpuric "gloves and socks" syndrome caused by measles virus. J Am Acad Dermatol 30:291–292, 1994.

54. S Aractingi, D Bakhos, B Flageul, O Verola, M Brunet, L Dubertret, F Morinet. Immunohistochemical and virological study of skin in the papular-purpuric gloves and socks syndrome. Br J Dermatol 135:599–602, 1996.

55. A Trattner, M David. Purpuric "gloves and socks" syndrome: histologic, immunofluorescence, and polymerase chain reaction study. J Am Acad Dermatol 30:267–268, 1994.

56. L Borradori, P Cassinotti, D Perrenoud, E Frenk. Papular-purpuric "gloves and socks" syndrome. Int J Dermatol 33: 196–197, 1994.

57. L Puig, Diaz, R Alexandre, JM De Moragas. Petechial glove and sock syndrome caused by parvovirus B19. Cutis 54: 335–340, 1994.

58. PT Smith, ML Landry, H Carey, J Krasnoff, E Cooney. Papular-purpuric gloves and socks syndrome associated with acute parvovirus B19 infection: case report and review. Clin Infect Dis 27:164–168, 1998.

59. R Grilli, MJ Izquierdo, MC Fariña, H Kutzner, I Gadea, L Martin, L Requena. Papular-purpuric "gloves and socks" syndrome: polymerase chain reaction demonstration of parvovirus B19 DNA in cutaneous lesions and sera. J Am Acad Dermatol 41:793–796, 1999.

60. S Veraldi, G Rizzitelli, G Scarabelli, C Gelmetti. Papular-purpuric "gloves and socks" syndrome. Arch Dermatol 132:975–977, 1996.

61. JM Carrascosa, I Bielsa, M Ribera, C Ferrandiz. Papular-purpuric gloves and socks syndrome related to cytomegalovirus infection. Dermatology 191:269–270, 1995.

62. T Ruzicka, K Kalka. Papular-purpuric "gloves and socks" syndrome associated with human herpesvirus 6 infection. Arch Dermatol 134:242–244, 1998.

63. A Okumura, T Ichikawa. Aseptic meningitis caused by human parvovirus B19. Arch Dis Child 68:784–785, 1993.

64. P Cassinotti, D Schultze, P Schlageter, S Chevili, G Siegl. Persistent human parvovirus B19 infection following an acute infection with meningitis in an immunocompetent patient. Eur J Clin Microbiol Infect Dis 12:701–704, 1993.

65. JR Kerr. Parvovirus B19 infection. Eur J Clin Microbiol Infect Dis 15:10–29, 1996.

66. ED Heegaard, A Hornsleth. Parvovirus: the expanding spectrum of disease. Acta Paediatr 84:109–117, 1995.

67. PR Koduri, SJ Naides. Aseptic meningitis caused by parvovirus B19. Clin Infect Dis 21:1053, 1995.

68. SE Boruchoff, BA Woda, GA Pihan, WA Durbin, D Burstein, NR Blacklow. Parvovirus B19–associated hemophagocytic syndrome. Arch Intern Med 150:897–899, 1990.

69. T Peschgens, U Merz, K Steidel, et al. Parvovirus B19-assoziierte myokarditis bei einem 7-monate-alten kind. Pädiatr Grenzgeb 32:527–530, 1994.

70. TH Finkel, TJ Torok, PJ Ferguson, EL Durigon, SR Zaki, DY Leung, RJ Harbeck, EW Gelfand, FT Saulsbury, JR Hollister, et al. Chronic parvovirus B19 infection and systemic necrotising vasculitis: opportunistic infection or aetiological agent? Lancet 343:1255–1258, 1994.

71. J Pont, E Puchhammer-Stockl, A Chott, T Popow-Kraupp, H Kienzer, G Postner, N Honetz. Recurrent granulocytic aplasia as clinical presentation of a persistent parvovirus B19 infection. Br J Haematol 80:160–165, 1992.

72. GR Serjeant, JM Topley, K Mason, BE Serjeant, JR Pattison, SE Jones, R Mohamed. Outbreak of aplastic crises in sickle cell anaemia associated with parvovirus-like agent. Lancet 2:595–597, 1981.

73. T Tsukada, T Koike, R Koike, M Sanada, M Takahashi, A Shibata, T Nunoue. Epidemic of aplastic crisis in patients with hereditary spherocytosis in Japan [letter]. Lancet 1: 1401, 1985.

74. JR Duncan, CG Potter, MD Cappellini, JB Kurtz, MJ Anderson, DJ Weatherall. Aplastic crisis due to parvovirus infection in pyruvate kinase deficiency. Lancet 1:14–16, 1983.

75. JJ Lefrere, R Girot, AM Courouce, M Maier-Redelsperger, P Cornu. Familial human parvovirus infection associated with anemia in siblings with heterozygous B-thalassemia. J Infect Dis 153:977–979, 1986.

76. Y Bertrand, JJ Lefrere, G Leverger, AM Courouce, C Feo, M Clark, G Schaison, JP Soulier. Autoimmune haemolytic anaemia revealed by human parvovirus–linked erythroblastopenia. Lancet 2:382–383, 1985.

77. R Ware. Human parvovirus infection. J Pediatr 114: 343–348, 1989.

78. N Frickhofen, JL Abkowitz, M Safford, JM Berry, J Antunez-de-Mayolo, A Astrow, R Cohen, I Halperin, L King, D Mintzer, et al. Persistent B19 parvovirus infection in patients infected with human immunodeficiency virus type 1 (HIV-1): a treatable cause of anemia in AIDS. Ann Intern Med 113:926–933, 1990.

79. WC Koch, G Massey, CE Russell, SP Adler. Manifestations and treatment of human parvovirus B19 infection in immunocompromised patients. J Pediatr 116:355–359, 1990.

80. M Belloy, F Morinet, G Blondin, AM Courouce, Y Peyrol, E Vilmer. Erythroid hypoplasia due to chronic infection with parvovirus B19 [letter]. N Engl J Med 322:633–634, 1990.

81. TF Schwarz, A Nerlich, B Hottentrager, G Jager, I Wiest, S Kantimm, H Roggendorf, M Schultz, KP Gloning, T Schramm, et al. Parvovirus B19 infection of the fetus. Histology and in situ hybridization. Am J Clin Pathol 96: 121–126, 1991.

82. AB Ackerman. Superficial Perivascular Dermatitis in Histologic Diagnosis of Inflammatory Skin Diseases. Philadelphia: Lea & Febiger, 1978.

83. EO Caul, MJ Usher, PA Burton. Intrauterine infection with human parvovirus B19: a light and electron microscopy study. J Med Virol 24:55–66, 1988.

84. BJ Cohen, PP Mortimer, MS Pereira. Diagnostic assays with monoclonal antibodies for the human serum parvovirus–like virus (SPLV). J Hyg 91:113–130, 1983.

85. LJ Anderson, C Tsou, RA Parker, et al. Detection of antibodies and antigens of human parvovirus B19 by enzyme-linked immunosorbent assay. J Clin Microbiol 24:522–526, 1986.

86. DD Erdman, MJ Usher, C Tsou, EO Caul, GW Gary, S Kajigaya, NS Young, LJ Anderson. Human parvovirus B19 specific IgG, IgA, and IgM antibodies and DNA in serum specimens from persons with erythema infectiosum. J Med Virol 35:110–115, 1991.

87. MJ Anderson, SE Jones, AC Minson. Diagnosis of human parvovirus infection by dot-blot hybridization using cloned viral DNA. J Med Virol 15:163–172, 1985.

88. MM Salimans, S Holsappel, FM van de Rijke, NM Jiwa, AK Raap, HT Weiland. Rapid detection of human parvovirus B19 DNA by dot hybridization and the polymerase chain reaction. J Virol Methods 23:19–28, 1989.

89. G Patou, D Pillay, S Myint, J Pattison. Characterization of a nested polymerase chain reaction assay for detection of parvovirus B19. J Clin Microbiol 31:540–546, 1993.

90. GP Bansal, JA Gatfield, FE Dunn, AA Kramer, F Brady, CH Riggin, MS Collett, K Yoshimoto, S Kajigaya, NS Young. Candidate recombinant vaccine for human B19 parvovirus. J Infect Dis 167:1034–1044, 1993.

91. E Connor, G Folena-Wasserman, C Alfonso, et al. A phase I vaccine trial with recombinant parvovirus B19 virus–like particles in seronegative healthy adult volunteers [abstr]. Blood 86(suppl 1):135a, 1995.

92. LM Bell, SJ Naides, P Stoffman, RL Hodinka, SA Plotkin. Human parvovirus B19 infection among hospital staff members after contact with infected patients. N Engl J Med 321:485–491, 1989.

93. SJ Naides, LL Scharosch, F Foto, EJ Howard. Rheumatologic manifestations of human parvovirus B19 infection in adults. Initial two-year clinical experience. Arthritis Rheum 33:1297–1309, 1990.

94. JJ Nocton, LC Miller, LB Tucker, JG Schaller. Human parvovirus B19–associated arthritis in children. J Pediatr 122:186–190, 1993.

95. DA Corral, FS Darras, CW Jensen, TR Hakala, SJ Naides, JR Krause, TE Starzl, ML Jordan. Parvovirus B19 infection causing pure red cell aplasia in a recipient of pediatric donor kidneys. Transplantation 55:427–430, 1993.

96. JC Murray, MV Gresik, F Leger, KL McClain. B19 parvovirus–induced anemia in a normal child. Initial bone marrow erythroid hyperplasia and response to intravenous immunoglobulin. Am J Pediatr Hematol Oncol 15:420–430, 1993.

97. G Nigro, P D'Eufemia, M Zerbini, A Krzysztofiak, R Finocchiaro, O Giardini. Parvovirus B19 infection in a hypogammaglobulinemic infant with neurologic disorders and anemia: successful immunoglobulin therapy. Pediatr Infect Dis J 13:1019–1021, 1994.

98. V Sahakian, CP Weiner, SJ Naides, RA Williamson, LL Scharosch. Intrauterine transfusion treatment of nonimmune hydrops fetalis secondary to human parvovirus B19 infection. Am J Obstet Gynecol 164:1090–1091, 1991.

14

Cutaneous Manifestations of HIV Infection

Clay J. Cockerell
University of Texas Southwestern Medical Center, Dallas, Texas, USA

Philip R. Cohen
University of Texas–Houston Medical School, Houston, Texas, USA

The diagnosis and management of human immunodefiency virus (HIV) infection has evolved dramatically since the initial recognition of the acquired immunodeficiency syndrome (AIDS) (Fig. 14–1) [1]. The use of combination drug regimens that include protease inhibitors plus nucleoside and non-nucleoside reverse transcriptase inhibitors (highly active antiretroviral therapy [HAART]) can profoundly suppress viral replication with associated increases of CD4-positive lymphocyte counts and partial immune reconstitution [2–5]. With use of these new drug regimens, a significant drop in HIV-associated morbidity and mortality has been noted [6].

This trend has also been observed with many of the cutaneous manifestations of HIV infection, which are now less recalcitrant to therapy and have fewer unusual presentations. Nevertheless, strains of HIV have been isolated that are resistant to all current protease inhibitors, and reservoirs of HIV have been found in patients receiving HAART who have undetectable viral titers [7,8]. Thus, HAART profoundly suppresses viral replication but is not able to eliminate the virus completely.

Cutaneous disorders develop in over 90% of HIV-infected persons at some time during the course of the illness [9]. Table 14–1 lists these cutaneous manifestations and related disorders that may arise with HIV infection.

PATHOGENESIS OF HIV-RELATED SKIN DISEASES

We have a better understanding of the pathogenesis of skin diseases in patients with HIV infection. It is apparent that the effects of HIV on the immune system are much more complex than simple depletion of CD4 lymphocytes. Subsets of T-helper cells, referred to as Th1 and Th2, have been found to play significant roles in HIV infection and AIDS. Th1 cells predominate in the normal state in immunocompetent individuals. Th1 lymphocytes promote cellular immunity and produce interleukin (IL)-2, IL-12, and interferon gamma to eradicate infection. Th2 lymphocytes promote humoral immunity and produce IL-4, IL-5, IL-10, and allergic responses. Th1 cells suppress Th2 cells, and vice versa.

Patients infected with HIV initially manifest normal CD4 cell numbers, a low viral load, and a Th1-dominant immunological milieu. Later, with advanced infection, patients convert to low CD4 cell numbers, a high viral load, and a Th2-dominant immune state. Thus, many of the unusual cutaneous manifestations of HIV infection may be a result of conversion to a Th2 setting. For example, Th2 cytokines may promote the activity of associated angiogenic factors to stimulate Kaposi's sarcoma formation. In addition, HIV *tat* protein stimulates the growth of

Geographical Incidence

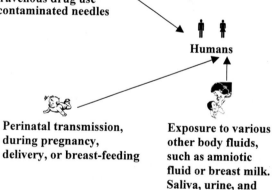

Worldwide Incidence

Taxonomy
Retroviridae family
Lentivirus group

TRANSMISSION

**Sexual intercourse,
through exposure
to infected semen,
cervical or vaginal
secretions, or blood**

**Exposure to infected
blood, such as through
transfusion, needle stick,
or intravenous drug use
with contaminated needles**

Humans

**Perinatal transmission,
during pregnancy,
delivery, or breast-feeding**

**Exposure to various
other body fluids,
such as amniotic
fluid or breast milk.
Saliva, urine, and
tears have not
yet been documented
to transmit HIV**

Figure 14–1. Incidence and transmission of HIV-1.

Kaposi's sarcoma cells *in vitro* as well as in mice. Other cytokines that may demonstrate angiogenic effects include IL-1, IL-6, and transforming growth factor (TGF)-beta. Similarly, bacillary angiomatosis may be a manifestation of an unusual response to *Bartonella* infection in a Th2 milieu.

Recently, deposition of fibrinogen, IgG, IgM, IgA, and C3, both at the dermoepidermal junction and around superficial blood vessels as shown by direct immunofluorescence, has been reported in cutaneous lesions of syphilis. This finding, as well as the presence of abundant plasma cells, suggests a Th2 immunological milieu and may explain the florid, unusual manifestations of syphilis in patients with HIV.

It is of interest that cutaneous manifestations were noted to develop when CD4 cell counts declined to certain levels with advancing HIV infection and have been noted to reappear at similar CD4 cell counts when the immune system of the host is being reconstituted with HAART.

VIRAL INFECTIONS

Acute Exanthem of HIV Disease

Definition
The acute reaction accompanied by HIV seroconversion refers to an acute viral prodrome accompanied by a cutaneous eruption seen in 10–50% of cases of acute infection with HIV 1.

Epidemiology
A study reported that the acute exanthem was observed in 81% of acute HIV-1 infections [10].

Pathogenesis
The pathogenesis of the development of the acute prodrome of HIV infection has not been fully elucidated, but widespread infection of cells with HIV most likely leads to release of cytokines and inflammatory mediators.

Clinical Manifestations
The clinical manifestations of the acute exanthem of HIV disease are listed in Table 14–2. Patients are highly infectious during the symptomatic period. The cutaneous eruption with this condition is similar to that seen with other viral illnesses or drug hypersensitivity reactions and may include urticaria, perlèche as well as palatal and esophageal ulcers, and candidiasis. Systemic manifestations include pneumonitis, esophagitis, meningitis, abdominal pain, and melena.

Histopathology
Histological evaluation of skin biopsy samples taken from the morbilliform eruption demonstrates an infiltrate consisting primarily of lymphocytes with occasional plasma cells around blood vessels of the superficial vascular plexus. There is also slight spongiosis, and occasional individually necrotic keratinocytes may be seen in the epidermis.

Table 14–1. Cutaneous Manifestations and Disorders Seen in HIV Infected Individuals

Viral
Acute exanthem of HIV disease
Herpes simplex virus
Varicella zoster virus
Cytomegalovirus
Oral hairy leukoplakia
Human papillomavirus
Molluscum contagiosum

Bacterial
Furuncles, abscesses, impetigo
Bacillary angiomatosis
Mycobacterial infections
Syphilis
Other venereal diseases, such as chancroid and
    granuloma inguinale

Ectoparasitic Infestations
Scabies
Demodicidosis
Acanthamebiasis

Parasitic Diseases
Pneumocystis carinii pneumonia
Leishmaniasis
Toxoplasmosis
Strongyloidiasis

Fungal
Candidiasis
Coccidioidomycosis
Cryptococcosis
Histoplasmosis
Paracoccidioidomycosis
Sporotrichosis
Penicilliosis

Noninfectious Skin Disorders
Seborrheic dermatitis
Psoriasis
Reiter's syndrome
Eosinophilic pustular folliculitis
Atopic dermatitis
Prurigo nodularis
Pityriasis rubra pilaris
Exfoliative erythroderma
Psoriasiform dermatitis of AIDS
Xerotic dermatitis
Erythema elevatum diutinum
Multiple dermatofibromas
Papular urticaria, chronic urticaria
Vasculitis and vascular-related diseases
Chronic actinic dermatitis of HIV
Porphyria cutanea tarda
Actinically aggravated rosacea
Granuloma annulare
Cutaneous drug eruptions
Hair and nail abnormalities
Vitiligo
Acquired ichthyosis

Neoplastic Disorders
Basal cell carcinoma
Kaposi's sarcoma
Lymphoreticular malignancies
Anal intraepithelial neoplasia
Cervical carcinoma
Cloacogenic carcinoma
Bowenoid papulosis
Epidermodysplasia verruciformis
Dysplastic nevi

Table 14–2. Clinical Manifestations of the Acute Exanthem of HIV Disease

Time after exposure	Clinical manifestations	Laboratory analyses	Other notes
3 to >6 weeks	Malaise, followed by fever as high as 102°F. Within one or more days, night sweats, pharyngitis, fatigue, lymphadenopathy, and a fine morbilliform rash may develop ↓	Demonstration of HIV p24 antigen HIV seroconversion typically occurs within 6 weeks of the acute illness. ELISA or Western blot can be used to detect antibodies	The rash generally involves the trunk, chest, back and upper arms Associated mucosal involvement (oropharyngeal, esophageal, or genital) has also been reported
4–8 weeks	Entire syndrome usually resolves, with complete recovery		

ELISA, enzyme-linked immunosorbent assay.

Laboratory Findings

Although the presence of HIV p24 antigen, HIV RNA, or antibodies directed to HIV can be found, no other specific laboratory finding demonstrates conclusive evidence of HIV infection.

Diagnosis

The diagnosis of the acute HIV exanthem is based on the presence of a characteristic clinical picture in an individual with risk factors for the development of HIV infection. Blood tests that reveal positive anti-HIV antibody (by the enzyme-linked immunosorbent assay [ELISA] and Western blot assay), circulating p24 antigen, or HIV RNA by polymerase chain reaction (PCR) are confirmatory.

Treatment

Antiretroviral agents have not been successful in the treatment of acute HIV exanthem.

Human Herpesvirus Infections

Definition

Herpesvirus infection refers to infection by any of the eight different viruses of the herpesvirus family.

Incidence

Herpesvirus infections are commonly encountered with patients infected with HIV and may be seen in up to 20–50% of patients at some point during the course of HIV infection [11]. Depending upon the degree of immunodeficiency, the likelihood of a patient's developing one of these eruptions can approach 95%, as in the case of cytomegalovirus (CMV) infection when CD4+ counts fall below 100 cells/mm³ [12]. The prevalence of infection with these viruses ranges from between 20 and 40% with herpes simplex virus (HSV) to virtually 100% with varicella zoster virus (VZV), CMV and Epstein-Barr virus (EBV) [13].

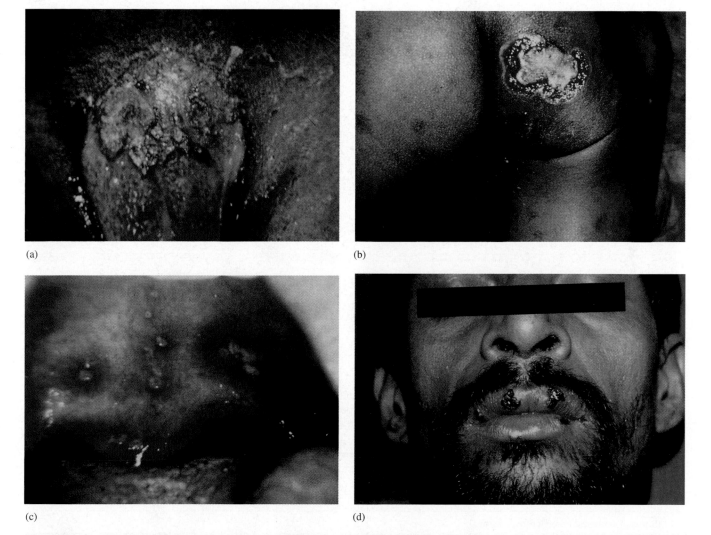

(a) (b) (c) (d)

Figure 14–2. Vesicles and ulcers of herpes simplex infections in HIV-seropositive patients: (a) chronic perianal ulcer, (b) chronic perianal ulcer, (c) vesicles of the hard and soft palate, and (d) labial eschars.

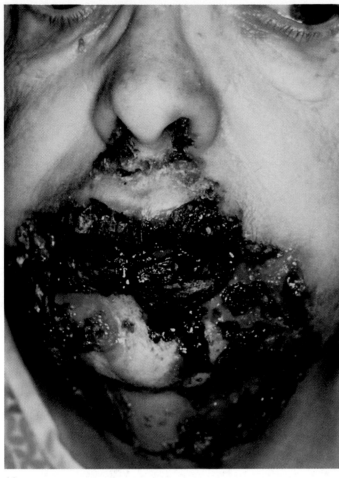

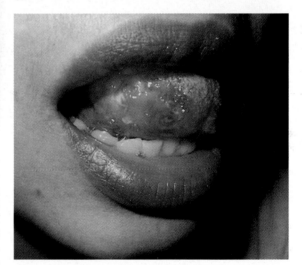

(e)

(f)

(g)

Figure 14–2. (*continued*). (e) Widespread labial and perioral eschars, (f) zosteriform herpes simplex, (g) aphthae major: Herpetic ulcers should be differentiated from other ulcerative diseases, such as aphthae major. (Photographed and reprinted with permission, Medical Aspects of Human Sexuality, 22:93, 1988; photograph b courtesy of J. K. Maniar, M.D., Department of Dermatovenereology and AIDS Medicine, G.T. Hospital, Grant Medical College, Mumbai, India; photograph g courtesy of Siri Chiewchanvit, M.D., Chiang Mai, Thailand.)

Pathogenesis

HSV-1 is the most common cause of oral herpetic infection, while HSV-2 is the most common etiological agent for anogenital herpes infections. It is well documented that genital ulcerations are risk factors for the acquisition of HIV infection [14]. Given that HSV-2 is the most common cause of genital ulcerations in the United States and Europe, HSV and HIV have important interactions that may have serious implications for patients with HIV infection. In vitro, HSV can potentiate HIV replication independent of HSV replication. This is caused by an early protein produced by HSV that results in enhanced HIV gene expres-

sion and replication. This is a result of intracellular transactivation of HIV [15].

Approximately 50% of HIV-1 seropositive patients develop herpes zoster (shingles). Patients treated with HAART whose CD4 lymphocyte counts rise from as low as 1 to 10 cells/mm^3 to between 200 and 500 cells/m^3 have a high risk of developing herpes zoster. The fact that herpes zoster develops preferentially when the CD4 lymphocyte number reaches a specific level suggests that a certain degree of immunity is required for this process. It may develop either when the CD4 cell number falls from a normal level or when it rises from a lower level.

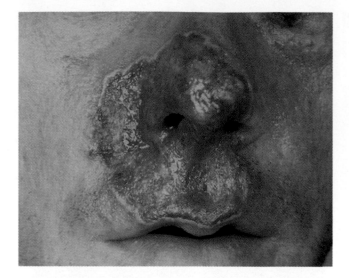

Figure 14–3. This chronic HSV infection had been under treatment with aciclovir at a dosage of 800 mg orally five times a day for 2 months at the time this photograph was taken. The condition responded to treatment with intravenous foscarnet.

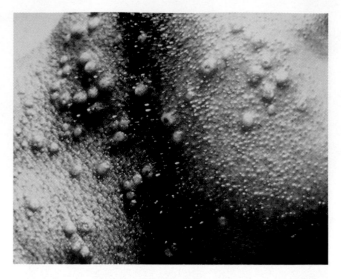

Figure 14–5. Kaposi's varicelliform eruption in an HIV-infected patient. (Reprinted with permission, Arch Int Med 151: 1295–1303, 1991.)

Clinical Manifestations

Herpes Simplex Infection. Oral, labial, and genital herpes simplex infections are commonly seen in immunocompetent patients and may be well localized in HIV-infected individuals who are relatively immunocompetent (see Chapter 4) (Figs. 14–2 to 14–7). Tender, painful ulcerative lesions of the penis, perianal area, and lip are characteristic, although other manifestations include perioral lesions and chronic ulcerative lesions on the glabrous skin such as that of the digits. Lesions that are untreated may continue to enlarge dramatically and become deeply situated and extremely painful. Other lesions may appear verrucous and hyperplastic. Epithelial sites other than mucocutaneous ones may be involved, including the cornea,

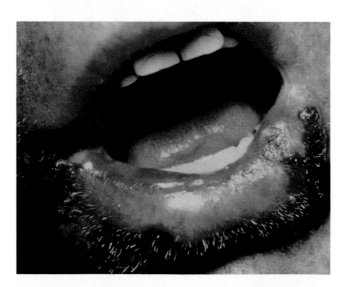

Figure 14–4. Nondescript eschars were the manifestation of HSV in this severely immunocompromised host, who died the day after this photograph.

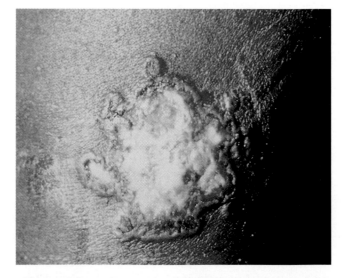

Figure 14–6. Occasionally, HSV infections may manifest as verrucous plaques such as seen here. Usually, numerous virally infected multinucleated epithelial giant cells are seen on microscopic examination of Tzanck preparations. In many cases, the causative virus is shown to be VZV.

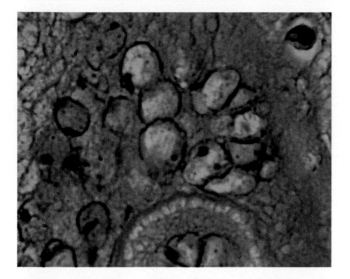

Figure 14–7. Microscopic appearance of multinucleated epithelial giant cells of HSV infection. Identical changes are seen in herpes zoster. (Hematoxylin and eosin, original magnification × 800.)

tracheobronchial tree, and esophagus as well as visceral sites such as the lung, pericardium, liver, and brain [16].

Varicella Zoster Virus (VZV). Varicella zoster, like other cutaneous infections in HIV-infected hosts, is thought by many to be predictive of progression from HIV infection to AIDS, having been associated with progression in 23% of HIV patients at 2 years, 46% at 4 years, and 73% at 6 years [17]. The virus exists in a dormant state in a dorsal root ganglion that becomes infected during prior varicella infection (see Chapter 5). With activation, the virus progresses down nerves of a solitary dermatome, leading to the characteristic zosteriform distribution of painful tense vesicles in the skin (Figs 14–8 and 14–9). If an HIV-infected patient is exposed to VZV for the first time, careful consideration should be given to the use of varicella zoster immunoglobulin or the administration of prophylactic acyclovir, valacyclovir, or famciclovir.

Complications, such as a second episode of varicella, repeat zoster infections, and multidermatomal forms, may occur. Varicella zoster may develop in HIV-infected children shortly after a course of primary varicella [18], and recurrent episodes of zoster have been documented in 5–23% of HIV-infected hosts, usually in those with advanced immunodeficiency syndrome. Blisters over large areas of the skin may develop concomitant with the characteristic zosteriform group of vesicles [19]. Crusted, punched-out ulcerations that leave painful atrophic scars may also be associated with postherpetic neuralgia [20]. Generally, these lesions develop a thick overlying eschar

and are remarkable for the lack of surrounding erythema. They occur most commonly on the buttocks and lower extremities but may be disseminated and are often resistant to therapy with acyclovir [21].

Cytomegalovirus. Up to 90% of patients with AIDS may develop acute active CMV infection at some point during their illness. CMV is the most common cause of serious opportunistic viral infection in AIDS [22]. As with other viral infections, HAART diminishes the frequency of this condition. Clinical manifestations may include ulcerations, keratotic verrucous lesions, palpable purpuric papules, and diffuse ulcerations (Fig. 14–10) (see Chapter 7). Vesicular, bullous, and generalized morbilliform eruptions as well as hyperpigmented indurated plaques and a generalized bullous toxic epidermal necrolysis-like eruption also may occur.

Prior to HAART, 50% of all AIDS patients had CMV viremia, with clinical manifestations of retinitis and gastroenteritis. Serious CMV retinitis may occur between 5 and 10% of patients and is found in 30% of AIDS patients at autopsy. Esophagitis and colitis as well as proctocolitis may develop in 5–10%.

Oral Hairy Leukoplakia (Epstein-Barr Virus). Epstein-Barr virus (EBV) selectively infects cells of the B-lymphocyte lineage and certain types of squamous epithelia (see Chapter 6). The majority of adults harbor a latent phase of EBV. Primary EBV infection is manifested as infectious mononucleosis. With advanced immunodeficiency in HIV-infected patients, EBV leads to oral hairy leukoplakia, Burkitt's lymphoma, or EBV-associated large-cell lymphoma.

Oral hairy leukoplakia (OHL) in the immunocompromised patient appears as one or more whitish plaques usually found on the lateral margins of the tongue (Fig. 14–11). OHL has also been correlated with progression from HIV infection to AIDS, as 48% of patients with OHL develop AIDS by 16 months and 83% by 31 months [23]. OHL is one of the mucocutaneous disorders that has been noted to regress with HAART.

Histopathology of HSV, VZV, and CMV

Herpes simplex and VZV infections may manifest as an intraepidermal acantholytic vesicular dermatitis associated with characteristic cytopathic effects in epithelial cells (see Chapters 4 and 5). In severely immunocompromised patients who develop infection with either HSV or VZV, there is extensive cytonecrosis of the epidermis associated with abundant viral infection of keratinocytes [24]. Often a complete syncytium of infected keratinocytes can be associated with involvement of follicles and adnexal struc-

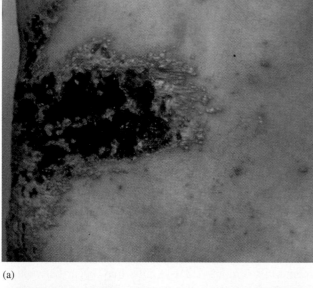

(a)

Figure 14–8. Herpes zoster may be an early manifestation of HIV infection or it may be seen in advanced AIDS, as depicted in (a). Herpes zoster in HIV-seropositive persons may be very aggressive and result in (b) loss of vision (V-1 distribution), or (c) Loss of teeth (V-2 distribution). Herpes zoster may produce (d) verrucous nodules, or (e) multidermatomal distribution, both usually seen only in immunocompromised persons, who have acyclovir-resistant herpes zoster. (Photograph a reprinted with permission, Clin Exp Dermatol 14:273, 1989; photographs b, c, and e courtesy of J. K. Maniar, M.D., Department of Dermatovenereology and AIDS Medicine, G.T. Hospital, Grant Medical College, Mumbai, India; photograph d courtesy of Jeffrey Callen, M.D., Division of Dermatology, Department of Internal Medicine, University of Louisville School of Medicine, Louisville, KY.)

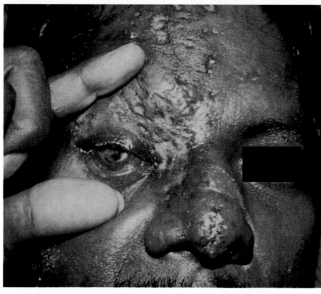

(b)

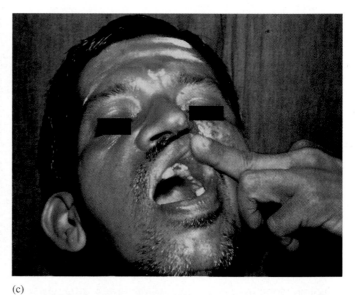

(c)

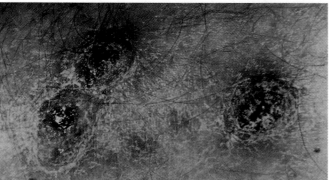

(d)

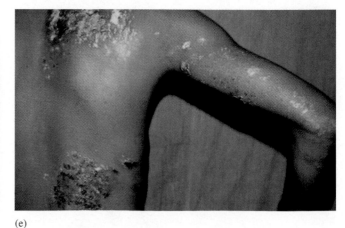

(e)

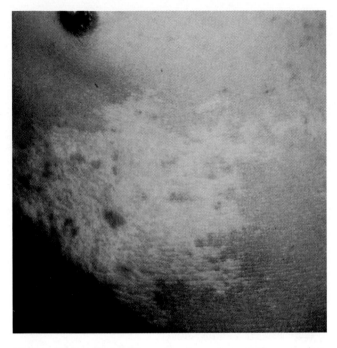

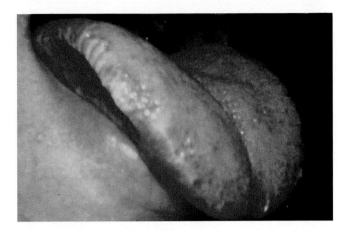

Figure 14–11. Whitish verrucous plaques of the sides of the tongue most commonly represent oral hairy leukoplakia, an EBV–induced lesion. (Reprinted with permission, Cutis 40: 406–409, 1987.)

Figure 14–9. Post-inflammatory hypopigmentation, scarring, and pain were complications of a severe episode of zoster in this immunocompromised host.

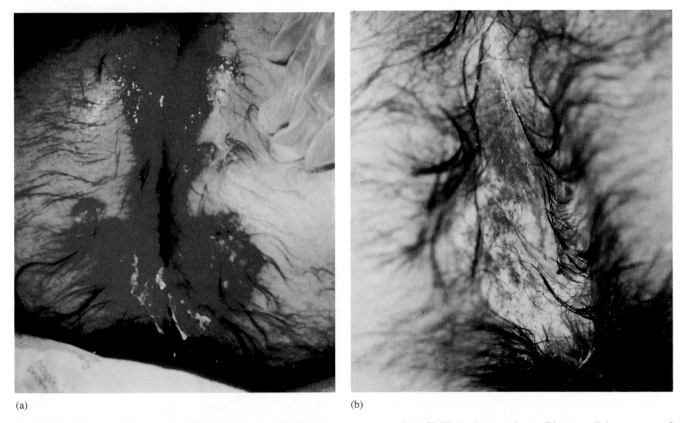

(a)   (b)

Figure 14–10. (a, b) Extensive perianal erosions and ulcerations were caused by CMV in these patients. (Photograph b courtesy of Mario Marini, M.D., Department of Dermatology, University of Buenos Aires, Argentina.)

tures. In some lesions, there may be extensive ulceration so that the herpetically infected cells cannot be visualized. In these cases, special immunoperoxidase stains and DNA probes may be useful in detecting viral antigens that may not be visible on routine microscopic examination. Skin lesions caused by both viruses appear identical histologically.

CMV characteristically infects fibroblasts and endothelial cells in the dermis associated with overlying ulceration (see Chapter 7). Mixed viral infections are not uncommon, and both HSV and CMV may occur within the same section.

OHL is manifest by marked epithelial hyperplasia with a verrucous corrugated appearance [25] (see Chapter 6). Electron microscopy as well as DNA in situ hybridization indicates viral particles in the epithelium, especially in the upper rather than lower portions.

Laboratory Findings

In general, no characteristic laboratory findings are associated with these infections, although patients with primary EBV infection show B-cell proliferation and exaggerated T-cell responses. CD4+ cell counts of less than 200 cells/mm^3 are typical. Zoster and OHL may occur in patients who are more immunocompetent.

Diagnosis

Diagnosis is made on the basis of culture, smears, biopsy, and clinical appearance of lesions (see Chapters 4 to 7).

Treatment

See Chapters 4 to 7 for the treatment of human herpesvirus infections. On occasion, patients with seemingly resistant herpes zoster or simplex may be suffering from atrophic gastritis that prevents absorption of acyclovir. A change to intravenous administration of acyclovir or to oral valacyclovir or famciclovir may be effective.

If an HIV-infected patient is exposed to VZV for the first time, either varicella zoster immunoglobulin and/or a prophylactic thymidine kinase inhibitor such as acyclovir, famciclovir, or valacyclovir should be administered. Administration of the varicella zoster virus vaccine should be considered for HIV-infected individuals who are still relatively immunocompetent and have not had previous infection with this virus.

Human Papillomavirus Infections

Definition

Human papillomavirus (HPV) infection refers to infections with viruses of the family of Papovaviridae (refer to Chapter 12).

Incidence

In HIV-infected individuals, coinfection with HPV is very prevalent. In one study, anogenital warts were demonstrated in 20% of HIV-infected homosexual men and 27% of homosexual men with AIDS. Using more sensitive studies, 48% of HIV-negative homosexual men and 54% of homosexual men with AIDS were shown to have evidence of HPV infection [26]. HPV types 6 and 11 are the most common viral isolates from anogenital condylomata, although oncogenic HPV types such as 16 and 18 are also often found in histologically benign lesions.

Pathogenesis

The human papilloma virus has a tropism for squamous epithelium and enters the cells of the basal cell layer probably through microscopic abrasions (see Chapter 12).

In addition to causing verrucae and papilloma, HPV infection may cause development of carcinoma, especially in patients with depressed cell-mediated immunity [27,28]. Furthermore, HIV *tat* protein transactivates HPV, leading to increased HPV expression.

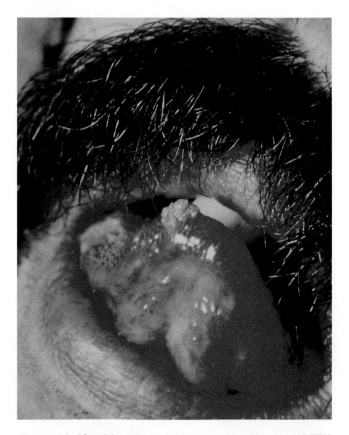

Figure 14–12. Lingual condyloma was an early sign of HIV infection in this patient. (Reprinted with permission, Arch Int Med 151:1295–1303, 1991.)

Clinical Manifestations of HPV Infection

Patients with HIV infection, especially those who are most immunocompromised, may have multiple verrucae vulgares, especially in periungual locations (Figs. 14–12 and 14–13). Multiple plantar warts, including mosaic warts, may cause pain on walking. Extensive flat and filiform warts on the bearded area of the face manifest by small verrucous papules are also seen in HIV-infected individuals and may be the first sign of HIV infection.

Epidermodysplasia verruciformis has been reported in patients with HIV infection and consists of a widespread papular eruption of reddish to skin-colored, flat, wartlike lesions involving mostly the sun-exposed areas of the skin (Fig. 14–14) [29].

Verrucous carcinoma manifest as a large verrucous plaque or tumor, most commonly in the perianal location, has also been reported in patients with HIV infection.

Histopathology
See Chapter 12.

Laboratory Findings

In general, routine laboratory findings are noncontributory in these cases, although patients with extensive disease often are found to have CD4+ cell numbers lower than 500 cells/mm^3 [30].

Diagnosis

The diagnosis of clinical HPV-induced lesions is based on clinical features in the context of histopathological find-

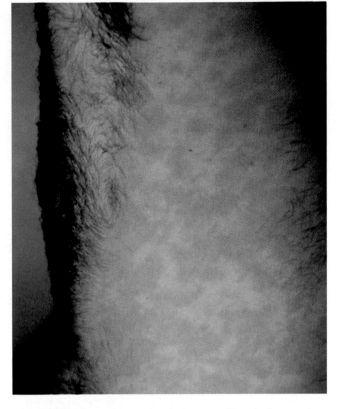

Figure 14–14. Epidermodysplasia verruciformis in a patient with HIV infection. This was severely pruritic and initially thought to represent a drug eruption.

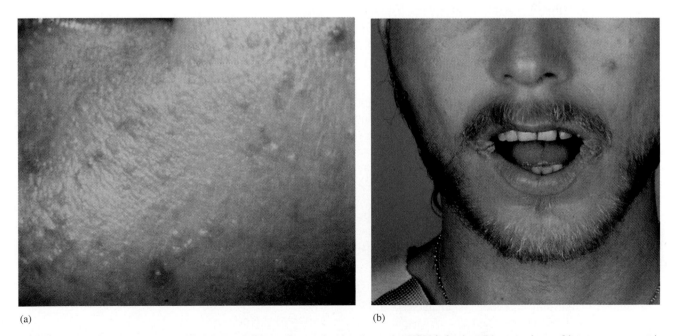

(a)   (b)

Figure 14–13. Multiple verrucae planae (a) and extensive perioral and angular HPV infection (b) were signs of immunocompromise in these patients. (Photograph (a) and reprinted with permission, Prim Care 16:421–444, 1989.)

ings. It is important to perform biopsies because any case could conceivably represent manifestations of a malignant HPV-induced condition (see Chapter 12).

Treatment

Treatment of HPV-induced lesions revolves around measures that result in diminution of clinical lesions, destruction of premalignant or malignant lesions, reduction of symptoms, and reduction of transmission to uninfected individuals (see Chapter 12). Successful therapy depends on the ability of the host's immune status to keep viral infection in check. Frequent recurrences are probably a consequence of reactivation of latent HPV infection, and therapy often must be extended to include normal-appearing tissue. Unfortunately, no treatment has been shown to eradicate HPV entirely.

Poxvirus Infections

Definition

Poxviruses are the largest of the animal viruses and, of these, two have been reported to infect HIV-seropositive patients, specifically molluscum contagiosum and vaccinia. These are complex DNA viruses that replicate in the cytoplasm and are especially adapted to epidermal cells (see Chapter 3) [31,32].

Incidence

Most patients who develop severe molluscum contagiosum have CD4+ cell counts of <200–250 cells/mm³. Vaccinia virus infection occurs sporadically in patients who have been occupationally exposed or are accidental hosts, such as a military recruit vaccinated for smallpox [31].

Pathogenesis

Molluscum contagiosum is spread by direct contact with epidermal epithelium. The virus replicates in the cytoplasm and produces molluscum or Henderson-Paterson bodies that fill the cytoplasm. The pathogenesis of molluscum contagiosum infection is thought to be related to an epidermal growth factor–like polypeptide induced by infection with the virus [33] (see Chapter 3).

Vaccinia causes a similar infection but rather than the nucleus being filled with molluscum bodies, prominent vacuolar or ballooning degeneration develops within cells. There is prominent inflammation and scarring.

Clinical Manifestations

Molluscum contagiosum infection is characterized by dome-shaped umbilicated translucent 2–4-mm papules that develop on any part of the body but preferentially affect the genital areas and the face in AIDS patients, especially

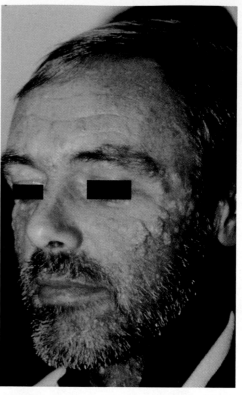

Figure 14–15. Extensive giant molluscum contagiosum of the face in patients with severe immunocompromise.

around the eyes (Figs. 14–15 and 14–16). Lesions are numerous and may become quite large in immunocompromised individuals. Individual lesions have a tendency to affect follicles and are therefore umbilicated with a central keratinous plug. In some cases, molluscum dermatitis occurs [32]. In HIV-infected patients, however, lesions may develop rapidly, i.e., over 2 to 4 weeks, and may persist for months to years. When HAART therapy is initiated and the CD4 lymphocyte count rises, lesions may undergo regression. Furthermore, the number of patients with multiple giant lesions is decreasing.

Vaccinia lesions are characterized by tense umbilicated vesicles and pustules that are similar to those described in other patients with widespread disseminated vaccinia infection (Fig. 14–17). Patients are usually clinically ill with fever and acute toxic symptoms associated with viremia.

Histopathology

See Chapter 3.

Laboratory Findings

Those patients with HIV infection generally have CD4+ counts below 250 cells/mm³.

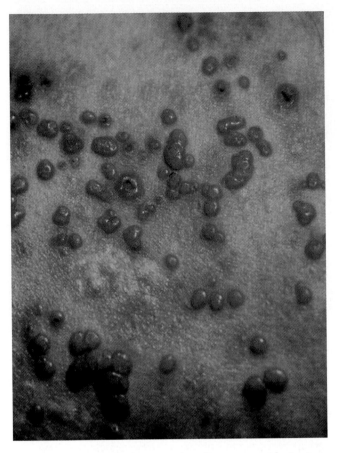

Figure 14–16. Extensive truncal molluscum papules. Lesions such as this must be differentiated from papules of disseminated cryptococcosis.

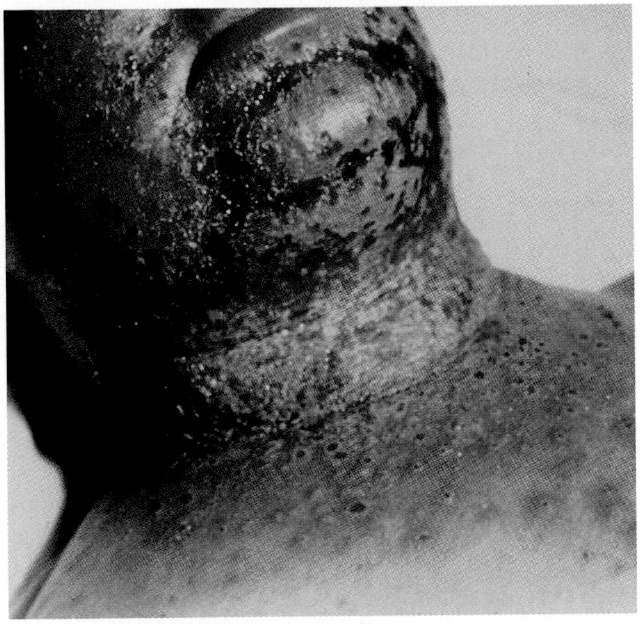

Figure 14–17. Eczema vaccinatum in an immunocompromised patient who received a smallpox vaccine for foreign travel.

Vaccinia infection may respond to treatment with semithiocarbazone, although this is generally not effective. Unfortunately, the condition is associated with a high mortality rate.

Diagnosis

Application of a small amount of liquid nitrogen or ethyl chloride will highlight the central umbilication of individual lesions, a finding that strongly suggests the diagnosis. In most cases, the diagnosis is readily established on the basis of clinical appearance and/or by histological evaluation of a skin biopsy specimen or a smear of contents of a papule. In AIDS patients, lesions may become very large and resemble cutaneous tumors [34]. Vaccinia is diagnosed on the basis of the clinical appearance of the eruption in the context of a history of exposure to the causative agent.

Treatment

Treatment of molluscum contagiosum generally employs destructive measures (see Chapter 3). Cryotherapy may induce dyspigmentation in dark-skinned individuals. Imiquimod and cidofovir have also been observed to be effective.

Other Viral Infections

Several other viral infections have been reported to develop with increased frequency in patients with HIV infection. Parvovirus B19, which is the cause of erythema infectiosum (fifth disease), may cause an exanthem in patients with HIV infection as well as fatal aplastic anemia [35]. The major target of the human parvovirus is the bone marrow erythroid progenitor cell. The exanthem and polyarthralgia that result in fifth disease are a result of antigen-antibody immune complexes and develop as bone marrow recovery is under way. In patients with immune deficits, however, persistent infection causing severe chronic anemia has been reported. Enteroviruses may also lead to florid morbilliform or vesicular eruptions.

Measles has been reported sporadically in patients with HIV infection with a variable course (see Chapter 16). Atypical-appearing exanthems associated with pneumonitis and encephalitis as well as more characteristic-appearing eruptions have been observed. Treatment consists of intravenous ribavirin and gamma globulin [36].

BACTERIAL INFECTIONS

Definition

Bacterial folliculitis, impetigo, bacillary epithelioid angiomatosis, botryomycosis, *Pseudomonas* infections, streptococcal axillary lymphadenitis, mycobacterial infections, syphilis, and other venereal diseases are some of the bacterial infections that may develop in patients with HIV infection. These disorders may be localized or widespread, involving many organs. There may be a number of different clinical morphological findings, many of which may be nondescript. For this reason, it is important that skin biopsies and cultures be performed in any immunocompromised patient in whom a skin lesion develops that could represent a manifestation of a serious bacterial infectious disease.

Epidemiology

Most banal bacterial infections, such as folliculitis and impetigo, are caused by *Staphylococcus* and *Streptococcus,* organisms commonly encountered in immunocompetent hosts. *Staphylococcus aureus* is the most common cutaneous and systemic bacterial pathogen in HIV-infected adults. The initial site of colonization with *S. aureus* is the nares. A nasal carriage rate of approximately 50% has been observed in HIV-infected hosts, twice that of HIV-seronegative homosexual and heterosexual men [37]. Multiple breaks in the skin from needle sticks, dermatoses, and immunodeficiency are risk factors for the development of *S. aureus* infection. Up to 83% of patients with AIDS may suffer from some form of *S. aureus* infecion at some point. Infection with *Pseudomonas* sp is also seen with some frequency in patients who are HIV infected, and up to 8% of all cases of bacteremia in patients with AIDS are caused by these organisms. Aggressive *Haemophilus influenzae* infection of the head and neck has also been observed [38].

Virtually any of the mycobacteria may induce skin lesions in up to 10% of patients with systemic mycobacterial infections. Extrapulmonary disease is commonly found in patients with AIDS. *Mycobacterium avium-intracellulare* occurs in the skin of patients with blood cultures positive for the same organism, and *M. haemophilum* causes skin lesions [39–40]. This is of importance as the latter organism is more difficult to culture than other mycobacteria.

Syphilis is common in patients with HIV infection and of all reported cases of syphilis, 25% develop in HIV-infected hosts [41]. Lymphogranuloma venereum, chancroid, granuloma inguinale, and *Neisseria gonorrhoeae* in-

fection may develop and be more severe as a consequence of immunocompromise.

Pathogenesis

In addition to low CD4 cell counts, dysfunctions in the B-cell arm of the immune response as well as with neutrophils and macrophages have been described in HIV patients with bacterial infections. HIV-infected patients may be neutropenic because of myelosuppression from medications and bone marrow infections such as those caused by *M. avium-intracellulare*. Furthermore, patients in later stages of HIV infection suffer from defective neutrophil chemotaxis as well as a decrease in the late stage oxidative burst with consequent diminished killing of *S. aureus*. Indwelling venous catheters that are commonly placed in patients with HIV infection serve as portals of entry and are a risk for systemic infection with bacteria as well as other pathogens. Elevated serum IgE levels are also associated with *S. aureus* infections and may play a role in the alteration of the immune system, leading to defective eradication of organisms.

A predisposition to the development of colonization and infection by bacterial microorganisms also relates to recrudescence or reactivation of latent infections. *M. tuberculosis* frequently produces infection in HIV-seropositive patients, probably as a result of reinfection or reactivation of pre-existing foci. An increasing number of infections with strains resistant to antituberculous medications have recently been reported, often with devastating consequences. Syphilis, too, has been shown to be associated with reactivation of presumed previously killed organisms in patients having prior disease treated with recommended antibiotic regimens.

Bacillary angiomatosis is a bacterial infection caused by organisms of the genus *Bartonella*, specifically *B. quintana, B. henselae,* and *B. elizabethae* [42]. The pathogenesis is not completely known, but it has been postulated that a vasoproliferative factor either is produced by the bacterium itself or is induced to be formed by the host as a consequence of bacterial infection.

Clinical Manifestations

In HIV-seropositive patients, mucocutaneous manifestations of bacterial infections may manifest multiple different morphological features. Pustules, ulcers, cellulitis, nodules, papules, and panniculitis may all be encountered. Clinical appearances may be nondescript and may mimic other disorders. Table 14–3 suggests treatments for bacterial infections associated with HIV infection.

Folliculitis, Abscesses, Furuncles, Impetigo and Related Infections.   Folliculitis generally manifests as widely distributed acneiform papules and pustules (Fig. 14–18). Al-

Table 14–3. Treatment of Bacterial Infections

Symptom	Treatment
Pyogenic bacterial infections	Oral dicloxacillin, cephalexin, or ciprofloxacin
	Chlorhexidine gluconate washes daily for 1 week, then every 1–2 weeks for 2–3 months. Application into the nostrils of topical antibiotics (e.g., polymyxin B sulfate, bacitracin, or mupirocin ointment) twice daily for 10–14 days may help to eradicate bacterial colonization
Bacillary angiomatosis	Erythromycin ethyl succinate, orally, 500 mg four times daily for 4 weeks to 6 months
	Doxycycline hydrochloride, 100 mg twice daily
	Rifampin, ciprofloxacin, trimethoprim-sulfamethoxazole, gentamicin, azithromycin, rozithromycin, and norfloxacin
	Trimethoprim-sulfamethoxazole daily can prevent relapse
Atypical mycobacterial infections	Clarithromycin, ansamycin, clofazimine, minocycline, and trimethoprim-sulfamethoxazole
	It is important to culture the organism to determine drug sensitivities for specific antibiotic treatment
Syphilis	Primary syphilis: penicillin G benzathine 2.4 million units injected intramuscularly once each week for up to three doses
	Secondary syphilis (in the absence of neurosyphilis): penicillin G benzathine 2.4 million units injected intramuscularly once each week for 3–4 weeks
	Tertiary syphilis and neurosyphilis: intravenous aqueous penicillin G, 3 million units every 4 hours for 10 days, followed by penicillin G benzathine 2.4 million units intramuscularly once each week for 3 more weeks
Chancroid	Erythromycin (oral), 500 mg four times daily for 7 days, or a single intramuscular injection of ceftriaxone 250 mg
Lymphogranuloma venereum	Doxycycline, 100 mg orally twice daily for 7 days
	Ofloxacin, 300 mg twice daily for 7 days
	Erythromycin, 500 mg 4 times daily for 7 days
Granuloma inguinale	Erythromycin or trimethoprim-sulfamethoxazole
Gonorrhea	Penicillin, spectinomycin, or ceftriaxone

though in most cases infections are confined to the skin, occasionally sepsis may develop. In some cases the bacterial density may lead to botryomycosis or ecthyma. These disorders appear as nondescript verrucous papules or as necrotizing ulcerations, respectively. Soft-tissue and deep-seated bacterial infections such as cellulitis, pyomyositis, deep soft-tissue abscesses, and necrotizing fasciitis may also develop in HIV-infected hosts. These are generally manifest as diffuse, red, warm tender areas in the skin. Extreme toxemia, associated with deeper infections, requires early recognition. Streptococcal axillary lymphadenitis presents as diffuse, usually bilateral painful swelling of lymph nodes in the axillae (Fig. 14–19) [43]. When the nodes are incised, copious pustular drainage is noted.

Impetigo is manifested as localized or widespread edematous crusted areas of the skin associated with yellowish surface crusts. It is seen more often in the axillary, inguinal, and other intertriginous locations in patients with HIV infection. Painful red macules may develop superficial vesicles that rupture and ooze serious and purulent fluid that contains potentially infective HIV. A characteristic honey-colored surface crust usually forms, and satellite lesions may develop. In some cases, intact bullae and pustules may be observed.

Botryomycosis is most commonly caused by *S. aureus* and represents a manifestation of extension of staphylococcal folliculitis with the formation of bacterial colonies in the dermis. Clinically, this is often manifested as a nonde-

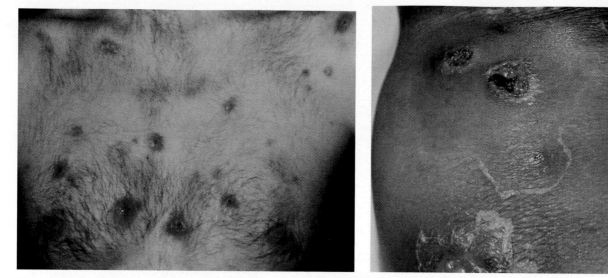

(a)   (b)

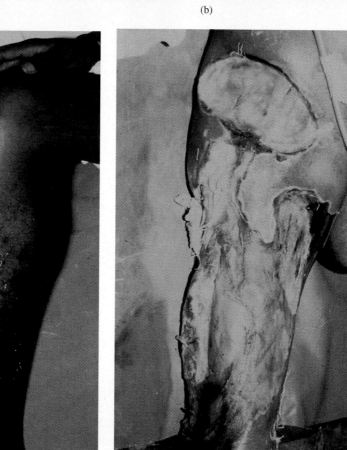

(c)   (d)

Figure 14–18.   Widespread furunculosis and bacterial folliculitis (a, b) may be an early sign of HIV infection. Cutaneous bacterial infections also include (c) ecthyma (a deep-seated infection that may be caused by either *S. aureus* or *P. aeruginosa*) may become very aggressive and progress to (d) pyomyositis. (Photographs c, d courtesy of J. K. Maniar, M.D., Department of Dermatovenereology and AIDS Medicine, G.T. Hospital, Grant Medical College, Mumbai, India.)

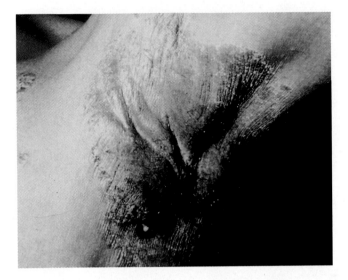

Figure 14–19. Streptococcal axillary lymphadenitis in an HIV-infected immunocompromised host.

script papule or plaque in the skin that may be surrounded by pustules on the trunk, neck, or extremities. Nonmenstrual toxic shock syndrome, most commonly associated with the use of nasal packing, infected wounds, or surgical sites, has also been reported in patients with advanced HIV disease. Patients have fever, shock, diffuse cutaneous erythema, and conjunctival injection with subsequent desquamation. Recurrent episodes of pyoderma-associated fever, hypotension, and erythroderma may also supervene. This is caused by a toxin-producing variant of *S. aureus*. A similar eruption has been reported caused by *Streptococcus pyogenes* known as the toxic strep syndrome.

Folliculitis, otitis externa, and ecthyma gangrenosum (both primary and secondary to septicemia) may be caused by *Pseudomonas aeruginosa* or *P. cepacia* and may be acquired from hot tub use [44]. When caused by *Pseudomonas* sp., the clinical manifestations of these disorders appear similar to those caused by other pyogenic bacteria, namely, firm, erythematous nodules as papulopustules with necrosis; therefore cultures are essential in making this distinction.

A condition with features similar to Job's syndrome is associated with recurrent staphylococcal abscesses, markedly increased serum IgE levels, and diminished polymorphonuclear leukocyte chemotaxis. Chronic diffuse dermatitis associated with elevated serum IgE levels and eosinophilia associated with recurrent *S. aureus* and *Candida albicans* infection have also been observed [45].

Haemophilus influenzae cellulitis manifest as diffuse erythema, and edema, often on the head and neck area, may develop in patients with HIV infection [38]. This infection may be aggressive, with a greater tendency to become disseminated or to involve deeper soft tissues and vital structures. Infections with *Streptomyces, Nocardia,* and *Actinomyces* may manifest as thickened verrucous plaques and chronic draining sinuses [46]. Deeply seated abscesses caused by *Rhodococcus equi* have been observed on multiple occasions [47]. *Corynebacterium diphtheriae* may cause bullous lesions that ulcerate and became covered with a greyish pseudomembrane [48]. Infections caused by "diphtheroids" may lead to pustular, folliculitis-like lesions, while salmonellosis may be associated with an eruption of faint pink macules on the skin. Multiple infectious agents may be found within a given skin lesion in patients with HIV infection and AIDS (Fig. 14–20). Mixed infections with pyogenic bacteria and acid-fast bacilli as well as viruses and fungi have been reported.

Bacillary Angiomatosis. Pinpoint reddish to purple papules are the earliest lesions of bacillary angiomatosis (Figs. 14–21 and 14–22). These may assume an appearance similar to that of pyogenic granulomas and are seen in two thirds of patients with cutaneous disease [49]. They range in number from one to several thousand and in size from 1 mm to several centimeters. Lesions may ulcerate and/or be covered by a crust. The second most common skin lesion is the subcutaneous nodule. These may be located deep in the subcutis and involve soft tissue and bone or occur as deeply seated skeletal muscle pyomyositis. When bone is involved, lesions are generally osteolytic in nature. Nondescript crusted ulcerations, plaques, and cellulitis may also be seen.

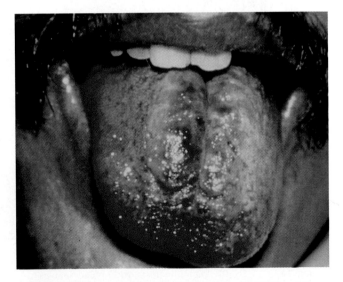

Figure 14–20. A case of a mixed infection with HSV and *Pseudomonas* in a patient with AIDS. (Reprinted with permission, Cutis 40:406–409, 1987.)

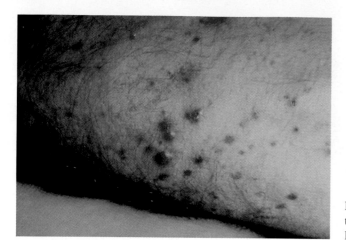

Figure 14–21. Bacillary angiomatosis, localized ''zosteriform'' type in an immunocompetent host. (Reprinted with permission, Arch Dermatol 126:787–790, 1990.)

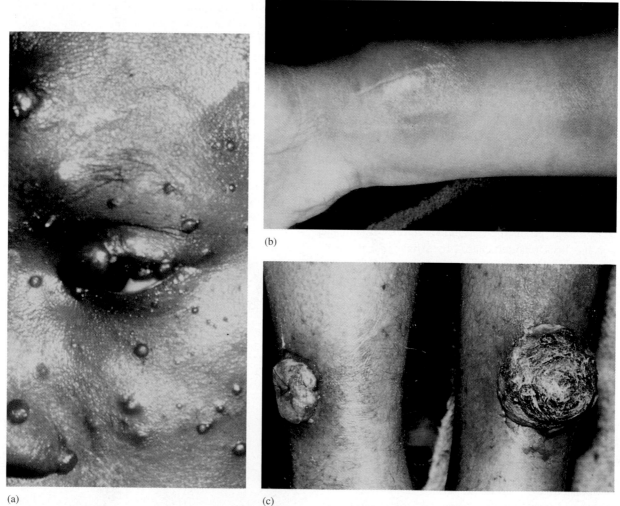

Figure 14–22. Bacillary angiomatosis, widespread nodules (a), deep dermal and osseous lesions (b), and crusted nodules (c) demonstrate that, in some cases, the characteristic vascular appearance of lesions may not be present. (Photograph b courtesy of Timothy Berger, M.D., Department of Dermatology, UC San Francisco, San Francisco, CA; photograph c courtesy of Walmar Roncalli P. DeOliveira, M.D., Sao Paulo, Brazil.)

Viscera may be involved either as disseminated vascular lesions or as bacillary peliosis hepatitis of the liver. Although virtually every organ system may be affected, the liver and spleen are the most common sites of involvement. Liver disease may develop in patients without skin lesions and is usually evidenced by elevated levels of circulating liver enzymes. Fever, weight loss, and night sweats are common. These symptoms usually resolve with institution of antibiotic therapy.

Mycobacterial Infections. Mycobacteria, especially *Mycobacterium avium-intracellulare* and *M. haemophilum,* may induce skin lesions in up to 10% of patients with systemic mycobacterial infections [39,40]. Other mycobacteria that may induce skin infections in HIV-infected patients include *M. marinum, M. chelonae, M. bovis* following bacille calmettie guerin (BCG) vaccination, and *M. thermoresistible. M. marinum* may cause classic swimming-pool granulomas that manifest as verrucous nodules in a sporotrichoid distribution. Most reported infections behave in a relatively indolent fashion, demonstrating good response to appropriate antibiotic therapy. *M. haemophilum* is a ubiquitous bacterium that may cause cutaneous infections in AIDS patients. *M. leprae* may be seen in AIDS patients in endemic areas.

Mycobacterial skin lesions may appear (Figs. 14–23 and 14–24) as small papules and pustules that resemble folliculitis, atopic dermatitis-like eruptions, localized cutaneous abscesses, suppurative lymphadenitis, nonspecific ulcerations, palmar and plantar hyperkeratoses, and sporotrichoid nodules. Lesions may take the form of painful erythematous papules and nodules on the distal extremities and ears [39]. Tuberculous lymphadenitis, in particular, is a characteristic finding of disseminated tuberculosis in intravenous drug users with AIDS and is manifested as suppurative draining lymph nodes in the neck, axillae, or groin. *M. leprae* may produce annular lesions (Fig. 14–25). The incidence of mycobacterial infections and related skin lesions has declined with the widespread use of prophylactic antibiotics and HAART.

Syphilis. Syphilis manifestations range from classic papulosquamous forms with involvement of the palms and soles and mucous membranes to unusual forms that may defy diagnosis (Figs. 14–26 and 14–27). Unusual manifestations of syphilis include rapid progression from the primary chancre to gummatous tertiary lues in a matter of months, lues maligna (syphilis with vasculitis), sclerodermiform lesions, rupial verrucous plaques, extensive oral ulcerations, keratoderma, deep cutaneous nodules, rubeoliform eruptions, and widespread gummas [50]. Central nervous system disease occurs more frequently and with greater severity in patients with HIV infection, and painful meningovascular syphilis may develop after treatment of secondary syphilis.

OTHER VENEREAL DISEASES

Granuloma inguinale caused by *Calymmatobacterium granulomatis* may develop in HIV-infected individuals as vegetating lesions on the penis or vulva associated with pseudobuboes in the inguinal crease. Lymphogranuloma venereum is manifested by generalized lymphadenopathy accompanied by vulvar or penile edema with ulcerations and erosions. Nonspecific genital ulcerations from which a number of bacteria may be isolated may be observed in which the precise etiology remains unclear. A common sexually transmitted disease in some parts of the world is chancroid, which has been increasing in incidence in the United States. The causative organism is a gram-negative coccobacillus, *Haemophilus ducreyi.* Cases have been reported in patients with HIV infection, especially those from Africa. Gonococcocemia with oligoarticular gonococcal arthritis of the hips and sternoclavicular joints also may develop [51].

Histopathology

Histopathological findings of folliculitis generally include collections of neutrophils within infundibula of hair follicles and a mixed perifollicular inflammatory cell infiltrate. Botryomycosis is characterized by a diffuse inflammatory cell infiltrate in the dermis associated with colonies of gram-positive bacteria forming grains in the skin. Ecthyma is manifested histologically as a deep ulcer that often extends to the subcutaneous fat, with extensive degeneration of dermal collagen. There is a mixed inflammatory cell infiltrate of neutrophils, eosinophils, and histiocytes.

Histopathological findings in bacillary angiomatosis are characterized by a lobular proliferation of capillaries associated with enlarged epithelioid-appearing endothelial cells. The background stroma is usually edematous in superficial lesions and more compact in deeper ones.

The histopathological appearance of cutaneous syphilis is usually similar to that of immunocompetent hosts, demonstrating the characteristic superficial and deep psoriasiform lichenoid pattern of inflammation associated with plasma cells and histiocytes.

Laboratory Findings

In pyogenic bacterial infections, laboratory findings may be similar to what would be expected in an immunocompetent host. In the setting of immunocompromise, however, patients may suffer from serious systemic bacterial infections and yet not mount significant elevations in white blood cell counts or demonstrate characteristic ''left shifts.'' Patients with syphilis may be truly seronegative for serological tests for syphilis despite the presence of demonstrable spirochetes in biopsy specimens. Seronega-

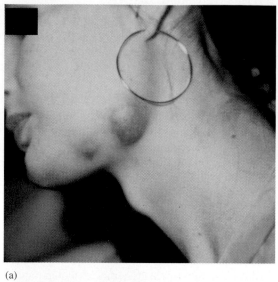

(a)

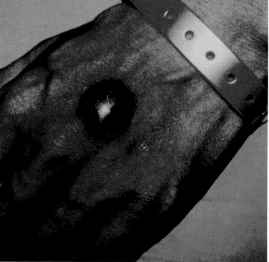

(b)

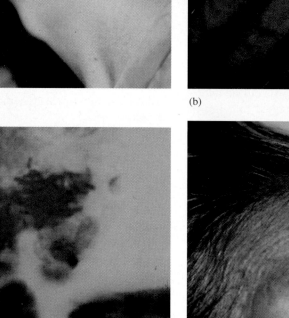

(c)

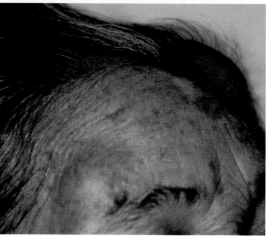

(d)

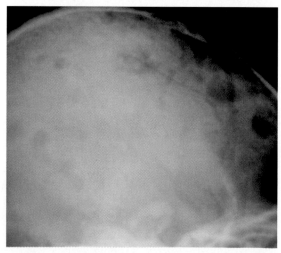

(e)

Figure 14–23. *Mycobacterium avium-intracellulare* abscesses in AIDS patients (a, b) with systemic mycobacterial infection. These mycobacteria can be found in the (c) bone marrow and can produce (d, e) lytic bone lesions. (Photograph c courtesy of Axel Hoke, M.D., Novato, CA; photographs d, e courtesy of J. K. Maniar, M.D., Department of Dermatovenereology and AIDS Medicine, G.T. Hospital, Grant Medical College, Mumbai, India.)

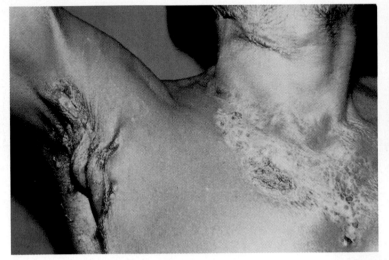

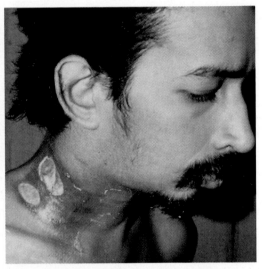

(a)

(b)

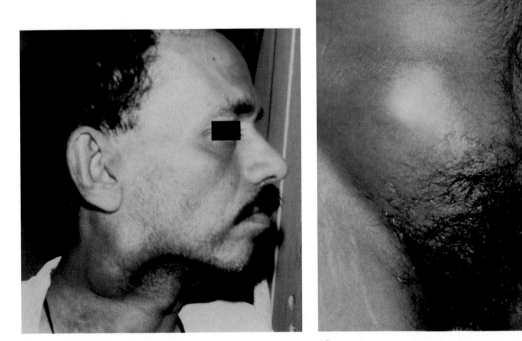

(c)

(d)

Figure 14–24. Scrofuloderma in HIV infection may be present in many forms (a, b). Mycobacterial infections may also manifest subcutaneously as (c) lymphadenopathy, or (d) cold abscesses. (Photographs b, c, d courtesy of J. K. Maniar, M.D., Department of Dermatovenereology and AIDS Medicine, G.T. Hospital, Grant Medical College, Mumbai, India.)

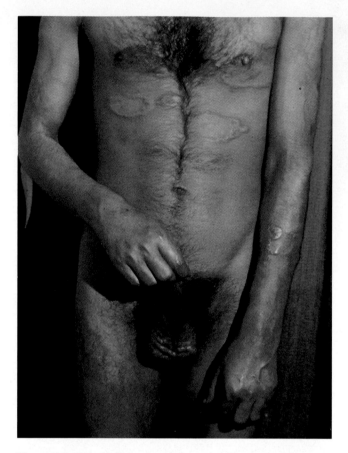

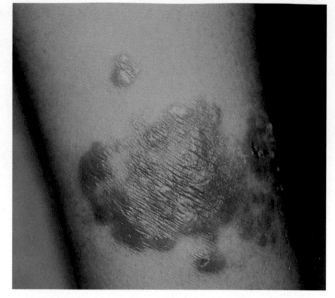

Figure 14–26. An unusual reddish plaque that proved to be syphilis when biopsied from an HIV-infected patient who was seronegative for syphilis.

Figure 14–25. *Mycobacterium leprae* is observed in HIV-seropositive patients in endemic areas and may produce annual lesions. (Photographs courtesy of J. K. Maniar, M.D., Department of Dermatovenereology and AIDS Medicine, G.T. Hospital, Grant Medical College, Mumbai, India.)

tivity may be caused either by a prozone phenomenon, the consequence of improperly diluted very high antibody titers, or as a consequence of true absence of antibody. Patients with bacillary angiomatosis usually have CD4+ cell counts less than 250 cells/mm³. Serological tests for anti-*Bartonella* antibody are usually positive by the time the clinical diagnosis has been made. *B. henselae* can be isolated from blood, and *B. quintana* can be isolated from cutaneous lesions [52,53].

In attempting to isolate *M. haemophilum,* cultures are often negative unless the culture is kept at low temperatures and supplemental iron is added in the form of hemolyzed red blood cells.

Diagnosis

Diagnosis of these infections is generally made on the basis of clinical findings and the results of smears, biopsies, and cultures. A battery of special stains and, in some cases,

immunoperoxidase stains for acid-fast bacilli may increase speed and sensitivity of diagnosis. Use of Gram's stain as well as periodic acid–Schiff and acid-fast stains ensures that more serious infections will not be missed. Cultures, complement fixation studies, and the polymerase chain reaction may be used in the rapid diagnosis of these infections. Although serological testing is generally reliable, HIV-infected patients with active syphilis may have negative VDRL (Venereal Disease Research Laboratories) and FTA-ABS (fluorescent treponemal antibody absorption test) results. In such cases, biopsy with special stains for spirochetes may be required. Granuloma inguinale is characteristically diagnosed by crush preparations of a friable skin lesion followed by histological examination. Chancroid is diagnosed by microscopic examination of gram-stained smears of lesions that demonstrate clusters of thin gram-negative rods, the characteristic "schools of fish."

Treatment

Treatment is based on accurate diagnosis and identification of causative microorganisms and their sensitivities to antibiotics. Table 14–3 outlines the recommended treatment for bacterial infections. Unfortunately, recurrence is the rule for pyogenic bacterial infections in immunocompromised hosts.

Cutaneous atypical mycobacterial infections demonstrate variable responses to antibiotics; therefore it is important to culture the organisms and determine sensitivities.

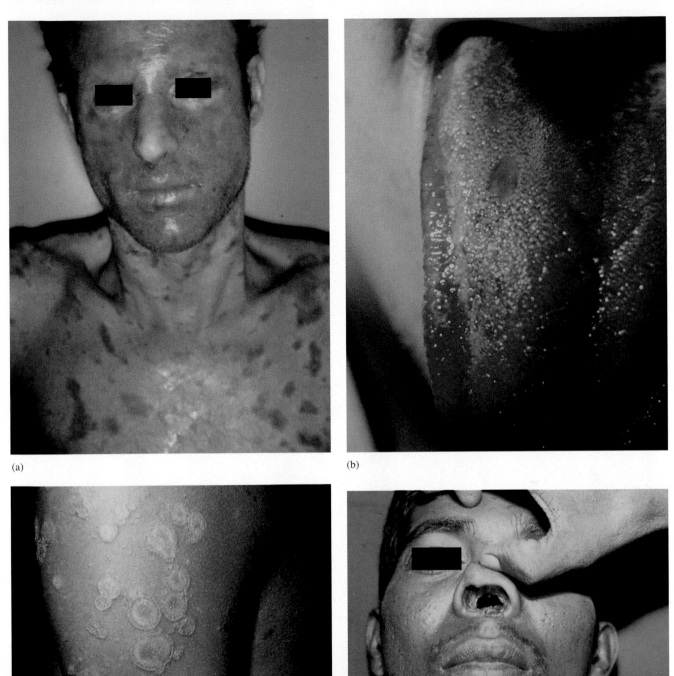

(a)

(b)

(c)

(d)

Figure 14–27. Secondary syphilis may show a wide spectrum of clinical manifestations. (a) This erythematous sclerodermiform eruption was also a manifestation of secondary syphilis in this HIV-infected individual. (b) Mucous patches of secondary syphilis. (c) Annular syphilides with mucosal involvement. (d) Gummas may be produced if syphilis is left untreated. (a, Reprinted with permission, Arch Dermatol 128:530–534, 1992. Photograph d courtesy of J. K. Maniar, M.D., Department of Dermatovenereology and AIDS Medicine, G.T. Hospital, Grant Medical College, Mumbai, India.)

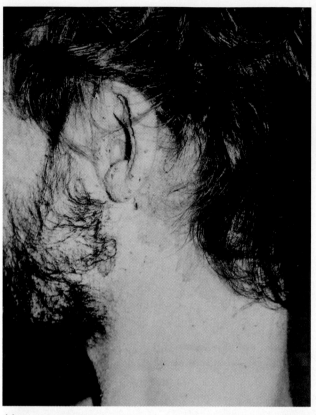

(a)

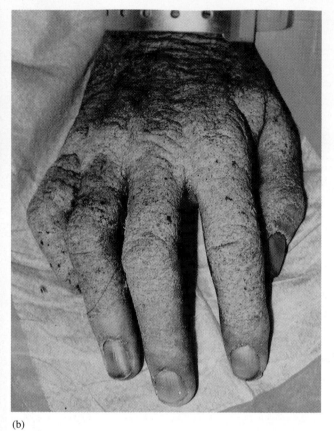

(b)

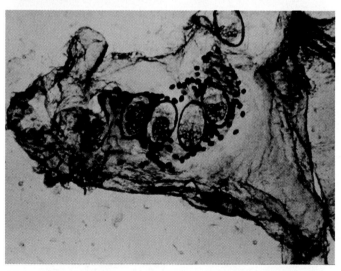

(c)

Figure 14–28.   Severely crusted scabies in a patient with AIDS (a, b). Head and neck involvement is common. (c) Scrapings of skin lesions usually demonstrate numerous live mites, eggs, and scybala.

Multiple-drug–resistant tuberculosis may not respond to any medication currently available, but regimens employing pyrazinamide, amikacin, olfloxacin, and ciprofloxacin have met with some success [54].

PARASITIC INFESTATIONS

Ectoparasites

Definition

Scabies, both classic and crusted types, demodicidosis, and acanthamebiasis may infect HIV-infected patients. Clinical morphologies may be unusual, and skin biopsies and cultures are often necessary to establish an accurate diagnosis.

Epidemiology

Scabies is one of the most frequent ectoparasitic infections in patients with HIV infection. The causative agent is the mite *Sarcoptes scabiei var. humanus.* Papular demodicidosis occurs sporadically in patients with HIV infection.

Pathogenesis

Severe infestation with scabies in patients with HIV infection develops as a consequence of the impaired immunity in these individuals. Patients with altered neurological status may fail to scratch away mites. HIV-infected patients with crusted scabies may have millions of mites. A proliferation of *Demodex folliculorum* within follicles causes papular demodicidoses.

Clinical Manifestations

Scabies in patients with HIV infection (Figs. 14–28, 14–29) may appear as hyperkeratotic plaques on the palms, soles, trunk, or extremities. In other patients, only scattered pruritic papules accompanied by slight scaling of the trunk and extremities may be seen. Any patient with a scaly persistent pruritic eruption should have skin lesions scraped and examined histologically in search of mites. Patients complain of intractable pruritus that is worse at night. Usually contacts are infested, especially in the context of the number of mites present on the skin of these individuals. Severe forms of scabies may be associated with secondary infection, bacteremia, and fatal septicemia, especially in severely compromised hosts, but this has decreased in incidence in patients receiving HAART [55].

Demodicidosis generally consists of a persistent pruritic follicular eruption that may be confused with other responses to arthropods, including scabies as well as folliculitis (Fig. 14–30). Lesions may involve the face, trunk, and extremities.

Acanthamebiasis consists of painful nodular lesions

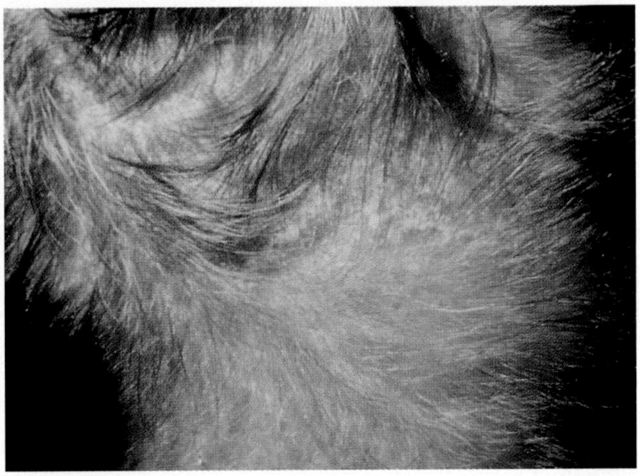

Figure 14–29. Crusted (Norwegian) scabies that mimicked seborrheic dermatitis.

with ulcerations, usually on the trunk or extremities; it can also be sexually transmitted (Fig. 14–31).

Histopathology

In crusted scabies there is usually a superficial and mid-to-deep perivascular and interstitial infiltrate of lymphocytes with numerous eosinophils. The epidermis is hyperplastic, with prominent crusting and many mites visible in the cornified layer.

Demodicidosis characteristically shows abundant *Demodex* mites within follicular infundibula associated with a mixed infiltrate of neutrophils and eosinophils within and around the infundibula of hair follicles.

Acanthamebiasis shows diffuse infiltrates of amebic cysts and trophozoites throughout the skin, especially around blood vessels and in the subcutaneous fat. Careful inspection is required, as these infiltrates may appear similar to histiocytes or other normal-appearing structures in the skin. Erythrophagocytosis may be noted.

Laboratory Findings

No specific laboratory findings are seen with any of these infestations, although elevated eosinophil counts are commonly noted.

Diagnosis

The diagnosis of scabies and demodicidosis depends primarily on the clinical appearance of skin lesions and demonstration of mites on microscopic examination of scrapings. Skin biopsies evaluated in the context of clinical history and appearance are important in the diagnosis of acanthamebiasis.

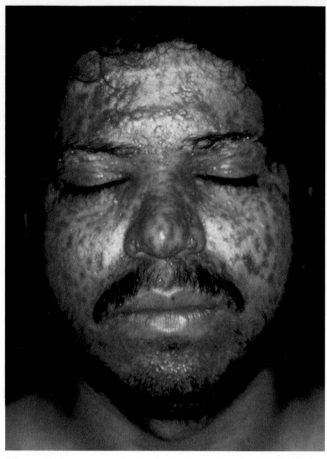

(a)

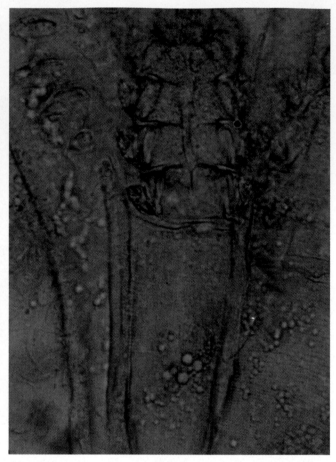

(b)

Figure 14–30. (a, b) Papular demodicidosis with scraping. (a) Note the similarity of the morphology of the lesions to acne rosacea and eosinophilic folliculitis. (b) *Demodex folliculorum* mites are visualized in large numbers. (Photographs courtesy of J. K. Maniar, M.D., Department of Dermatovenereology and AIDS Medicine, G.T. Hospital, Grant Medical College, Mumbai, India.)

Treatment

The treatment of ectoparasite infestations is listed in Table 14–4. After treatment of scabies in some patients, recurrences may occur as a consequence of failure to treat areas under the fingernails and the intertriginous zones, although resistance to scabicidal medications may develop. Some have recommended alternating treatment with lindane and permethrin. Multiple treatments may be required. Oral ivermectin is very effective in the therapy of crusted scabies. Postscabetic id reactions must be treated with antihistamines such as doxepin, 10 to 25 mg orally three to four times daily, with topical application of corticosteroid preparations to diminish inflammation. In cases of nodules, injection of triamcinolone acetonide may be required. Careful laundering of linen and clothing is necessary, and household and other contacts should be treated as well.

Internal Parasites

Definition

A number of parasites may produce cutaneous manifestations of systemic disease. These include *Pneumocystis carinii* infection, leishmaniasis, strongyloidiasis, and toxoplasmosis.

Epidemiology

P. carinii infection, disseminated strongyloidiasis caused by *Strongyloides stercoralis,* and disseminated toxoplasmosis, caused by *Toxoplasma gondii,* are rarely seen now that HAART and oral prophylaxis are given [56]. In contrast, multiple cases of leishmaniasis in HIV-infected hosts have been diagnosed in India, Southeast Asia, Spain, and South America (especially Brazil) [57]. The most common infecting organism is *Leishmania don-*

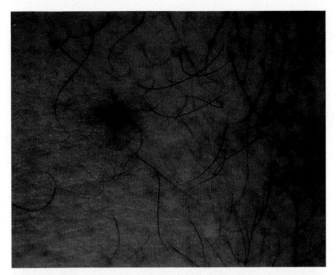

(a)

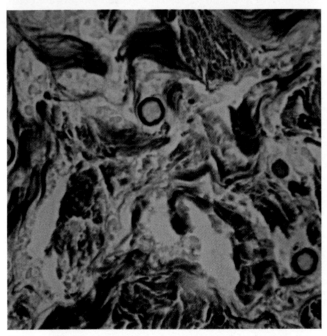

(b)

Figure 14–31. (a) Amebiasis in immunocompromised persons may appear as papules, pustules, or nodules and can be associated with liver abscesses. (b) Histological confirmation may be achieved by finding amoebic cysts in tissue. (Photographs a, b, courtesy of James Conners, M.D., Department of Dermatology, Yale University School of Medicine, New Haven, CT.)

Table 14–4. Treatment of Parasitic Infestations

Symptom	Treatment
Scabies	Lindane cream or lotion applied from head to toe and washed off after 8–12 hours of treatment. This regimen is repeated in 1 week
	Permethrin 5% cream applied in the same manner
	5% precipitated sulfur in petrolatum applied from the neck down nightly for 3 nights may also be effective
	Oral ivermectin, 200 μg/kg, is highly effective and is considered the treatment of choice for crusted scabies
Demodicidosis	Metronidazole gel, applied 2–3 times daily, with or without the addition of topical benzoyl benzoate
	Systemic metronidazole, 250 mg to 750 mg orally three times daily, may be required in cases not responsive to topical treatment
Amebiasis	Metronidazole, 750 mg orally twice daily for 10 days
	Response may be poor in severely immunocompromised persons
Pneumocystosis	Intravenous pentamidine, which is the usual treatment for *P. carinii* pneumonia
Strongyloidiasis	Thiabendazole, 25 mg/kg twice daily, lasting 4–5 days to several weeks, depending on the immune status of the host
Leishmaniasis	Stibogluconate sodium, 20 mg/kg each day for 3–4 weeks
	Ketoconazole or other imidazole antifungal medications may also be effective
Pruritus associated with these infestations	Topical application of corticosteroids or antipruritic agents containing menthol and phenol, pramoxine, and antihistamines may be required
	Doxepin, 10% in aquaphor ointment, is a valuable antipruritic agent that may be used in patients with refractory pruritus
	Exposure to ultraviolet B irradiation and psoralen plus ultraviolet A are also helpful

ovani, the protozoan responsible for the visceral form of the disease.

Pathogenesis

Cutaneous *P. carinii* infection is enhanced by the use of aerosolized pentamidine for the prophylaxis of *P. carinii* pneumonia. By creating a more unfavorable environment in the lung, organisms spread more widely to involve visceral organs as well as the skin.

Clinical Manifestations

P. carinii may have several different clinical manifestations. The most commonly reported form is that of friable reddish papules or nodules seen in the ear canal or the nares. Small translucent molluscum contagiosum-like papules (Fig. 14–32), bluish cellulitic plaque-like lesions, and deep-seated abscesses have also been observed. Given the diminishing frequency of systemic *P. carinii* infection secondary to administration of prophylactic antibiotics and HAART, skin lesions will be seen even less frequently.

Leishmaniasis does not have a uniform or specific appearance but often appears symmetrically on acral zones. Manifestations have included erythematous papules, hypopigmented macules, small subcutaneous nodules, scaly violaceous plaques, and ulcers (Fig. 14–33) [57].

Histopathology

P. carinii in the skin has an appearance similar to that in the lung, with a diffuse infiltrate of foamy-appearing cells that highlight the microorganisms, resulting in the "teacup-and-saucer" appearance when they are stained with Gomori's methenamine silver or Steiner's stain. Strongyloidiasis generally shows a diffuse infiltrate of lymphocytes and eosinophils scattered throughout the dermis.

Laboratory Findings

No specific laboratory findings are seen with any of these infestations, although elevated eosinophil counts are commonly noted.

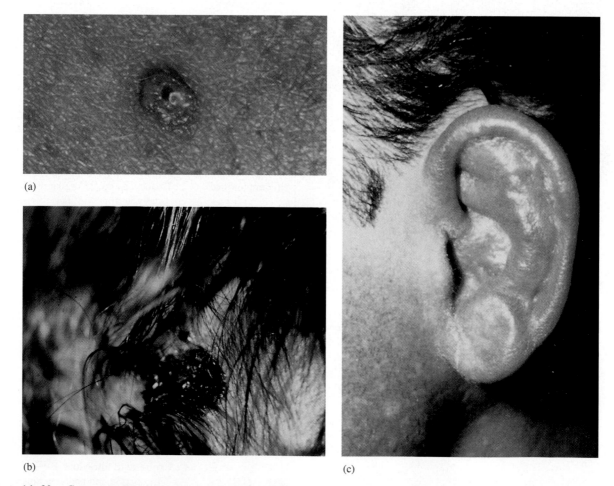

(a)

(b)   (c)

Figure 14–32. Cutaneous *Pneumocystis carinii* infection. The lesions may be nondescript and simulate molluscum contagiosum (a). (Reprinted with permission, Arch Dermatol, 127:1699–1701, 1991.) (b) Nodular, and (c) plaque-like presentations have also been described. (Photograph c courtesy of Timothy Berger, M.D., Department of Dermatology, UC San Francisco, San Francisco, CA.)

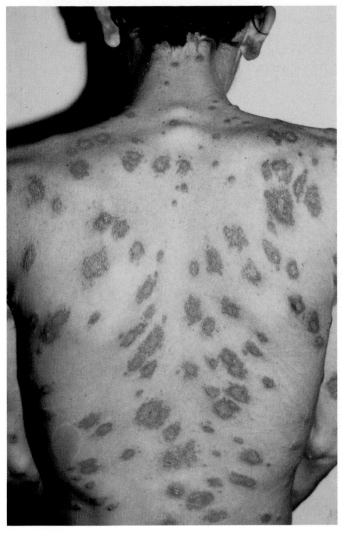

(a)

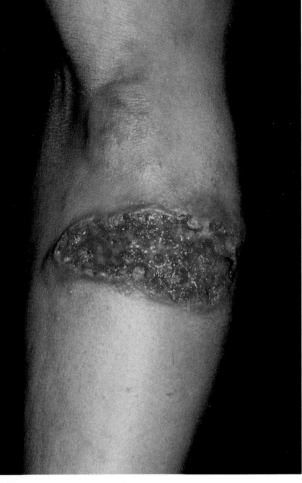

(b)

Figure 14–33.   Widespread plaques (a) and ulcers (b) of disseminated leishmaniasis. (Photographs courtesy of Walmar Roncalli P. DeOliveira, M.D., Sao Paulo, Brazil.)

Diagnosis

Skin biopsies evaluated in the context of clinical history and appearance are important in diagnosis of these conditions. Special serological and complement fixation tests may be helpful in confirming diagnoses. Treatment of parasitic infestations is shown in Table 14–4.

SYSTEMIC FUNGAL INFECTIONS

Definition

Blastomycosis, candidiasis, coccidioidomycosis, cryptococcosis, histoplasmosis, paracoccidioidomycosis, and sporotrichosis are some of the systemic fungal infections that occur in HIV-infected individuals (Table 14–5). These infections may occur in localized fashion involving a single tissue or as disseminated multiple-organ disease. Mucosal and cutaneous lesions may have many different clinical morphologies in HIV-seropositive patients, many of which may be unusual and challenge accurate clinical diagnosis.

Epidemiology

The most common opportunistic fungal infections to involve the skin in HIV-seropositive patients are histoplasmosis and cryptococcosis. Nearly 20% of HIV-seropositive individuals with disseminated histoplasmosis and up to

Table 14–5. Mucocutaneous Manifestations of Systemic Fungal Infections in Human Immunodeficiency Virus–Seropositive Patients

Manifestation	Occurrence	Morphological appearance
Blastomycosis		
Acute pulmonary infection–associated reactive erythema	Rare	Erythema nodosum
Primary cutaneous (inoculation) infection	Rare	Solitary indurated chancre-like ulcer that can subsequently be accompanied by lymphangitis, lymphadenitis, and subcutaneous nodules extending along the involved lymphatic vessel
Disseminated infection: cutaneous lesions in 70% of patients; oral lesions in 25% of patients	Most common	Centrifugally enlarging plaques with a scarred area of central healing and a raised verrucous pustule–containing border
	Less common	Ulcers with granulating bases that rapidly develop from pustules; subcutaneous abscess
	Rare	Widespread or acrally distributed pustules Oral ulcers and friable masses of heaped-up tissue
Coccidioidomycosis		
Acute pulmonary infection–associated reactive erythemas	50% of patients	Erythema multiforme, erythema nodosum, and "toxic" erythema (an erythematous, macropapular, morbilliform, or urticarial diffuse exanthem)
Primary cutaneous (inoculation) infection	Rare	Same as primary cutaneous blastomycosis
Disseminated infection: only occurs in about 1/10,000 cases; of these 15–20% have cutaneous lesions	Most common	A solitary verrucous plaque or granulomatous nodule on the face, multiple papules, modules, or pustules; subcutaneous abscesses (with or without overlying skin changes); sinuses, ulcers, and scars
Cryptococcosis		
Primary cutaneous infection	Rare	Variable
Disseminated infection	Usually seen in immunosuppressed individuals; mucocutaneous lesions occur in 10–20% of these patients	Erythematous papules that may develop into pustules or ulcerating nodules Other morphologies: abscesses, acneiform lesions, cellulitis, cutaneous ulcers, ecchymoses Oral ulcers (rare), purpura, pyoderma gangrenosum-like lesions, vasculitis, and verrucous lesions
Histoplasmosis		
Acute pulmonary infection–associated reactive erythemas		Erythema multiforme, erythema nodosum
Primary cutaneous (inoculation) infection	Rare	Same as primary cutaneous blastomycosis
Disseminated infection	Occurs in 1/1,000 to 1/500,000 cases; of these, 3% have cutaneous lesions and 21% have mucosal lesions	Acneiform or follicular lesions, exfoliative erythroderma, macules and patches, papules and nodules, petechiae, purpura, and ecchymoses, and plaques and ulcers (cutaneous and mucosal)

(continued)

Table 14–5. *(continued)*

Manifestation	Occurrence	Morphological appearance
Paracoccidioidomycosis		
Disseminated infection	Common	Mucosal lesions of the larynx, month, nose, and pharynx, that begin as papules and nodules and subsequently enlarge to become infiltrated, granulomatous, and ulcerated (and often extend onto the adjacent skin of the face)
	Rare	Cutaneous lesions may appear as widely scattered nodules, papules, pustules, or ulcers
Sporotrichosis		
Lymphocutaneous infection	Most common	A painless papule or pustule at the site of inoculation that develops into an ulcerated nodule; subsequently, asymptomatic subcutaneous nodules develop in an ascending direction along the corresponding lymphatic with or without accompanying lymphangitis and lymphadenopathy
Fixed cutaneous infection		Lesion or group of lesions, of variable morphology, localized to the site of inoculation, cellulitis (facial), erosions (pyodermatous), papules (infiltrated), plaques (large and warty or scaly and psoriasiform), and ulcers (thick and crusted or pyoderma gangrenosum-like)
Disseminated cutaneous infection	Rare	Polymorphous lesions similar in morphological appearance to fixed cutaneous sporotrichosis infection
Multifocal systemic infection	Rare	Widespread, scattered nodules or subcutaneous abscesses that subsequently ulcerate

10% of those with disseminated cryptococcosis develop mucocutaneous lesions. Systemic and cutaneous coccidioidomycosis are both being recognized more frequently in HIV-infected patients, although they are still seen only sporadically. HIV-infected hosts with blastomycosis, paracoccidioidomycosis, or sporotrichosis have also been observed, although rarely. Similarly, although mucocutaneous candidiasis occurs commonly in HIV-seropositive individuals, disseminated candidiasis is seldom reported.

Clinical Manifestations

Mucocutaneous lesions associated with systemic fungal infections may assume a number of different features (Table 14–6). The most common lesions are pustules and ulcers, although papules and nodules are also frequently observed. Less often, patches, plaques, and mucosal ulcerations are seen.

Blastomycosis.   Progressive disseminated blastomycosis is characterized by *B. dermatitidis*-related pustules, nodules, and cutaneous ulcers.

Candidiasis.   Oral thrush involving either the tongue and/or buccal mucosa, with or without esophageal infection, is the most common manifestation of candidiasis in HIV-seropositive patients (Fig. 14–34) and may be the initial sign of HIV infection. As an individual's immune status improves with HAART, oral candidiasis often resolves. Other manifestations that may develop include chronic paronychia and onychodystrophy, chronic refractory vaginal candidiasis, distal urethritis, and persistent monilial infection of the axilla, glans penis, groin, and/or inframammary area.

Disseminated candidiasis has been reported in a small number of HIV-infected patients. Administration of broad-spectrum antibiotics and total parenteral nutrition, extended placement of central intravenous catheters during prolonged hospitalizations, and, in children, previous oral candidiasis, are predisposing factors for systemic infection in these individuals [58].

Coccidioidomycosis.   Although an increasing number of HIV-infected patients with coccidioidomycosis are being described, only a few have been reported with associated skin lesions [59]. These lesions may include ulcers, abscesses, nodules, purpura, and papulopustules.

Cryptococcosis.   Cryptococcosis is a common infection to develop in HIV-infected individuals with low incidence of cutaneous involvement [60]. Mucocutaneous lesions of cryptococcosis are polymorphous and may appear as erythematous papules, nodules, pustules, and/or ulcers

Table 14–6. Cutaneous and Mucosal Lesions of Systemic Fungal Infections in Human Immunodeficiency Virus–Infected Patients

Morphology	Blasto-mycosis	Coccidioido-mycosis	Crypto-coccosis	Histo-plasmosis	Paracoccid-ioidomycosis	Sporo-trichosis
Macule				+		
Nodule		+	+			+
Abscess		+				
Herpes-like			+	+		
Fistulas				+		
Kaposi's sarcoma–like			+			
Molluscum contagiosum–like			+			
Purpura		+				
Papule		+	+	+		+
Patch		+		+		
Plaque				+		+
Pustule	+	+	+	+		+
Cutaneous ulcer	+		+	+	+	+
Mucosal ulcer			+	+		

of the skin and mucosa (Fig. 14–35). Cutaneous cryptococcosis, like other opportunistic infections that develop in these patients, may mimic the cutaneous morphology of other disorders, such as herpes simplex virus infection, cellulitis, or molluscum contagiosum infection as well as of soft-tissue hypertrophic lesions such as rhinophyma and Kaposi's sarcoma.

Histoplasmosis.   A review of 280 HIV-infected individuals with disseminated histoplasmosis identified 48 patients (17%) with histologically and/or culture-proven mucocutaneous lesions of *H. capsulatum* [61]. Clinically, the lesions may appear as cutaneous and mucosal ulcers, erythematous macules and patches, fistulas, papules and nodules, pustules, and verrucous plaques [62] (Table 14–6) (Fig. 14–36). *H. capsulatum* and Kaposi's sarcoma may coexist in a single skin lesion, and cases of concomitant psoriasis and histoplasmosis also have been described [62,63].

Paracoccidioidomycosis.   Descriptions of disseminated paracoccidioidosis in HIV-infected individuals are increasing in Brazil (Fig. 14–37). *P. brasiliensis* organisms

can be observed on hematoxylin and eosin stained sections prepared from a biopsy of the cutaneous ulcers.

Sporotrichosis.   Clinical forms of sporotrichosis include lymphocutaneous, fixed cutaneous, disseminated cutaneous, and systemic. The last may present as either localized pulmonary disease or as widespread involvement of numerous organs. In patients with HIV infection, skin lesions may be ulcers, papules, nodules, plaques, and/or pustules (Fig. 14–38). These may be widespread, and internal organ involvement may develop that often proves fatal.

Histopathology

The epidermis in mucocutaneous lesions of systemic fungal infections usually exhibits pseudocarcinomatous hyperplasia. There is almost always a supporative and granulomatous inflammatory infiltrate in the dermis in blastomycosis, coccidioidomycosis, paracoccidioidomycosis, and sporotrichosis. There may be transepidermal elimination of fungal spores. Histoplasmosis may exhibit a diffuse dermal infiltrate of histocytes, neutrophils, and leukocytoclasis. Cryptococcosis has a characteristic histopathological appearance in most cases. There is diffuse

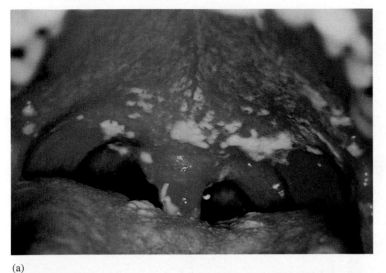

(a)

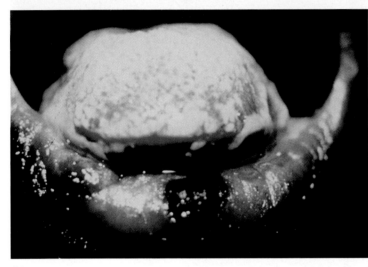

(b)

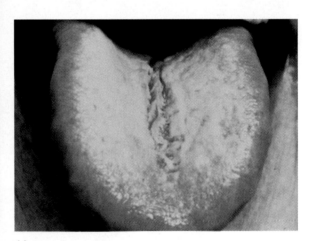

(c)

Figure 14–34. Hyperplastic and erosive candidiasis of the mouth (a–c) in HIV-infected patients. (Photograph b reprinted with permission, Cutis 40:406–409, 1987.)

pallor of the dermis that correlates with the mucoid capsular material of the organisms, which are usually present in abundance. The organisms can often be identified on hematoxylin and eosin stained sections, although special stains such as the periodic acid–Schiff and Gomoris methenamine silver can be used to facilitate their detection.

Diagnosis

When the possibility exists that a mucocutaneous lesion in an HIV-infected patient is secondary to dissemination of a systemic fungal infection, a tissue biopsy of that lesion should be prepared for histological evaluation and microbiological cultures. The growth of a fungal organism in culture is definitive evidence that the lesion is caused by an opportunistic fungus. Unfortunately, several of these organisms require several days to weeks to grow in culture so that more rapid methods to establish a definitive diagnosis are often required. In cases in which the number of microorganisms is small, the sensitivity of diagnosis can be increased by immunoperoxidase staining using antibodies directed to fungi or mycobacteria that cross-react with them. The polymerase chain reaction technique has expedited the diagnosis of some of these infections, but currently diagnostic molecular mycology is still a research methodology that is not routinely available. Finally, since fungal infection–associated lesions in HIV-seropositive individuals have been reported to harbor more than one pathogen, a diligent search for concurrent infectious organisms is warranted.

Treatment

Amphotericin B and imidazoles remain the drugs of choice for many systemic fungal infections, but many newer

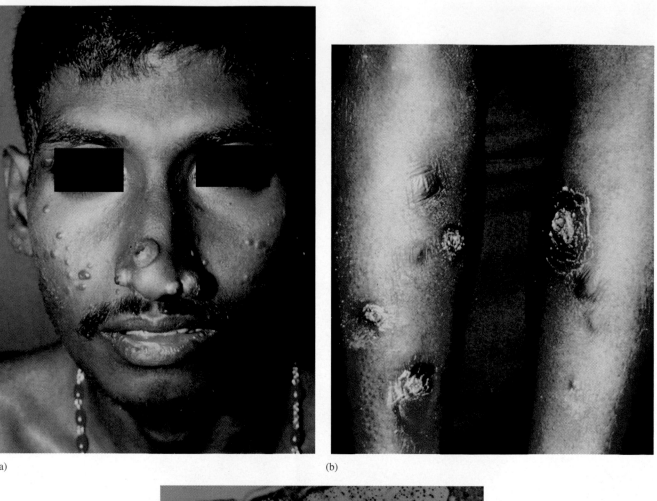

(a)   (b)

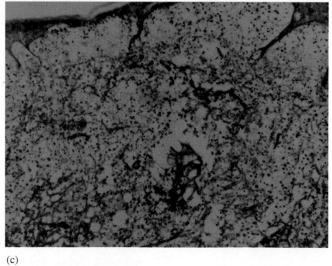

(c)

Figure 14–35. Widespread lesions of disseminated cryptococcosis may have different clinical appearances and may simulate (a) molluscum contagiosum or may be (b) nodular. (c) Histological diagnosis is necessary. (Photographs a and c courtesy of J. K. Maniar, M.D., Department of Dermatovenereology and AIDS Medicine, G.T. Hospital, Grant Medical College, Mumbai, India.)

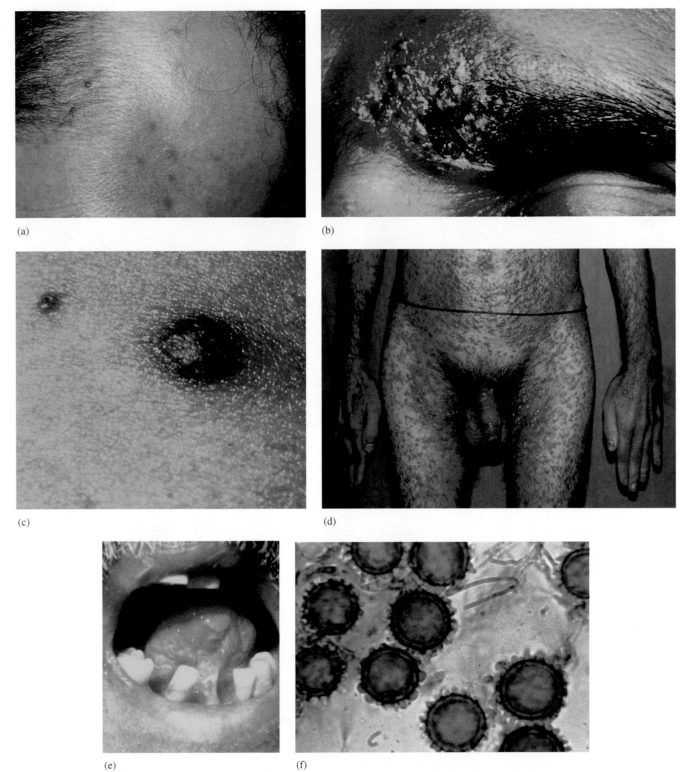

(a)

(b)

(c)

(d)

(e)

(f)

Figure 14–36. (a–d) Lesions of disseminated histoplasmosis may have multiple morphologies, including nondescript papules, plaques, ulcers, and psoriasiform lesions. (e) Oral ulcerations caused by disseminated *Histoplasma capsulatum* infection. (f) Histological diagnosis is necessary and may be confirmed by culturing the organism. (Photographs d and f courtesy of J. K. Maniar, M.D., Department of Dermatovenereology and AIDS Medicine, G.T. Hospital, Grant Medical College, Mumbai, India.)

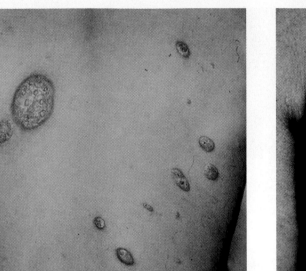

Figure 14–37. Paracoccidioidomycosis in Brazilian AIDS patient. This mycosis can appear with cutaneous plaques. (Photograph courtesy of Walmar Roncalli P. DeOliveira, M.D., Sao Paulo, Brazil.)

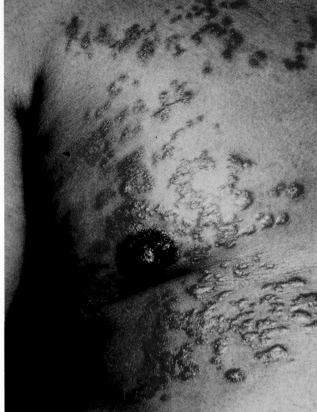

Figure 14–38. Sporotrichosis in AIDS patients may produce widespread papules, nodules, and plaques. (Photograph courtesy of Walmar Roncalli P. DeOliveira, M.D., Sao Paulo, Brazil.)

agents are under study [64] (Table 14–7). Fortunately, as more patients receive HAART, the incidence of these already rare complications may decrease.

OTHER FUNGAL INFECTIONS IN PATIENTS WITH HIV INFECTION

In addition to the fungal infections described previously, disseminated *Scedosporium inflatum, Pseudallescheria boydii,* and *Microsporum canis* occur, as have infections with other saprophytic fungi. Mycetomas, which may be either fungal or bacterial, may be found in AIDS patients as nodules with draining sinus tracts, most often on the feet (Fig. 14–39). Disseminated *Aspergillus* infection can manifest as facial palsy as a consequence of involvement of the mastoid sinus or as a retrobulbar lesion (Fig. 14–40). *Zygomycosis* infection of the head and neck may develop

and manifest as local pain, cutaneous necrosis, and necrotizing ulcerations. Deep soft-tissue muscular aspergillosis has also been noted. These infections are being encountered more frequently as a consequence of better prophylaxis against other opportunistic infections and because of abnormal neutrophil function that has been demonstrated in these patients.

Penicillium marneffei, a fungus that is endemic in Asia, causes a common infection in patients with AIDS in Thailand. Some of the cutaneous manifestations include umbilicated papules that could be confused with those of molluscum contagiosum, ecthyma-like lesions, folliculitis, subcutaneous nodules, and morbilliform eruptions (Fig. 14–41). The diagnosis is established by histological evaluation of skin biopsies and by the performance of cultures.

Infection by dermatophytes in HIV-infected individuals may occur on any cornified epithelial surface (Fig. 14–42). Dermatophyte infection of the feet, toenails, or fingernails also occurs commonly in HIV infection, with proximal white subungual onychomycosis of the toenails frequently observed. In contrast to the classic form of distal subungual

Table 14–7. Treatment of Systemic Fungal Infections

Disease	Treatment
Blastomycosis	Amphotericin B
Disseminated candidiasis	Amphotericin B
	Fluconazole or itraconazole may be effective for initial and maintenance therapy
Localized superficial candidiasis	Topical antifungal preparations
	Systemic therapy with imidazoles may be required in refractory cases
Coccidioidomycosis	Amphotericin B, intravenously
	Concomitant intrathecal amphotericin B may be required in some cases
Cryptococcosis	Amphotericin B
	Imidazoles
	Flucytosine (rarely)
Disseminated histoplasmosis	Amphotericin B
	Imidazoles have been shown to be effective in both prophylaxis and therapy
Paracoccidioidomycosis	Amphotericin B
	Imidazoles have been shown to be effective in both prophylaxis and therapy
Systemic sporotrichosis	Amphotericin B
	Ketoconazole, fluconazole, or itraconazole are also effective
Lymphocutaneous sporotrichosis	Potassium iodide. (Careful monitoring is necessary to avoid recurrences, as this drug is not fungicidal)

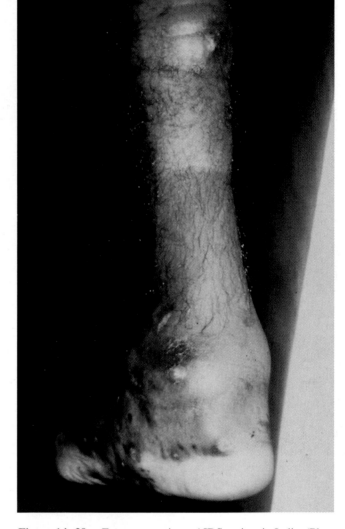

Figure 14–39. Eumycetoma in an AIDS patient in India. (Photograph courtesy of J. K. Maniar, M.D., Department of Dermatovenereology and AIDS Medicine, G.T. Hospital, Grant Medical College, Mumbai, India.)

onychomycosis in which the fungus infects the nail distally and spreads proximally, proximal white subungual onychomycosis is characterized by involvement of the proximal nail plate beginning under the posterior nail groove and extending distally. *Tinea corporis* may be manifested as extensive widespread involvement of the trunk and extremities. In any individual with extensive tinea corporis, the possibility of underlying HIV should be entertained.

Pityrosporum ovale and *P. orbiculare* are normal residents of the hair follicles of the scalp and may cause or exacerbate seborrheic dermatitis in patients with HIV infection. The density of *P. ovale* of the involved skin may correlate with the severity of seborrheic dermatitis. Pityrosporum folliculitis characterized by pruritic papules and pustules on the trunk and extremities also may develop in

HIV-infected hosts. Histological evaluation of potassium hydroxide preparations of scrapings from lesions shows yeasts and pseudohyphal forms of the organisms, and histopathological examination of skin biopsy specimens also demonstrates numerous organisms within hair follicles. In patients with HIV infection, extensive overgrowth of *P. ovale* of the glabrous skin leads to tinea versicolor, evidenced by scaling patches and plaques of the trunk. Treatment with oral imidazole antifungal medications such as fluconazole, itraconazole, or ketoconazole for 14 days is effective, although the condition tends to recur following its discontinuation.

Trichosporonosis caused by infection with *Tri-*

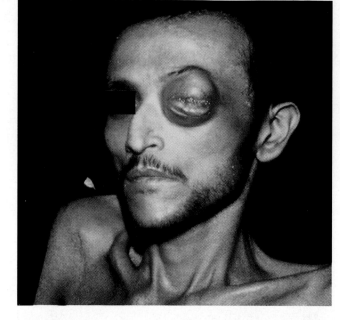

Figure 14–40. Retrobulbar aspergillosis. (Photograph courtesy of J. K. Maniar, M.D., Department of Dermatovenereology and AIDS Medicine, G.T. Hospital, Grant Medical College, Mumbai, India.)

chosporon beigelii generally causes white piedra, a superficial infection of the hair endemic to tropical and subtropical regions and parts of the southeastern United States. *Cladosporium cladosporioides* can cause pustular nodules. Cutaneous alternariosis presenting as an eschar on the leg and *Curvularia* phaeohyphomycosis causing a keratotic lesion on the scrotum have both been observed in HIV-infected individuals.

NONINFECTIOUS SKIN DISORDERS

In addition to infectious disorders, one or more of the following noninfectious cutaneous signs may point to HIV infection as a possible underlying cause of these conditions.

Seborrheic Dermatitis, Psoriasis, and Reiter's Syndrome

Definition

Seborrheic dermatitis and psoriasis are papulosquamous disorders associated with epidermal hyperplasia, increased epidermal turnover, and scaling. Reiter's syndrome is a condition consisting of urethritis, conjunctivitis, arthritis, and psoriasiform lesions of the glans penis and other parts

of the body. Seborrheic dermatitis has a characteristic distribution involving the scalp, nasolabial folds, and presternal areas and occasionally intertriginous sites. Psoriasis occurs in a number of different forms and is seen most commonly as scaly plaques of extensor surfaces. All three of these conditions are increased in incidence in patients with HIV infection.

Epidemiology

Seborrheic dermatitis is one of the most common skin conditions to affect patients with HIV infection, previously occurring at least once in nearly 85% of all HIV-infected individuals. HIV-associated psoriasis and arthritis as well as Reiter's syndrome occur more frequently in HIV patients than in the general population.

Pathogenesis

The pathogenesis of seborrheic dermatitis remains unknown, although it has been postulated to be caused by a reaction to *P. ovale.* Dysregulation of the immune system may cause the skin of HIV-infected hosts to become acanthotic and psoriasiform, possibly owing to cytokine release or an exaggerated inflammatory reaction. Why psoriasis develops in patients with HIV infection remains unknown, although several studies have postulated that the pathogenesis of psoriasis may be related to underlying vascular proliferation. Infections may also cause psoriasis to flare in patients with HIV disease, especially those caused by *Candida, Staphylococcus,* and *Streptococcus.* Reiter's syndrome in immunocompetent hosts is commonly triggered by infections with *Shigella flexneri, Campylobacter fetus,* and *Ureaplasma urealyticum.* These organisms are rarely found in HIV-infected patients with Reiter's syndrome, although some patients do have a culture-negative diarrheal illness or culture-negative urethritis at the time of the onset of the disorder. In that HLA-B27 is significantly associated with Reiter's disease, autoimmunity associated with this allele may be important.

Clinical Manifestations

Seborrheic dermatitis occurs as slightly indurated, diffuse or confluent, pinkish-red scaly plaques involving the face and scalp (Fig. 14–43). These may be large, thickened, and heavily crusted and may be present on other areas such as the upper anterior chest, back, groin, and extremities. In some patients, the condition may involve large areas of the skin, leading to erythroderma. Still other cases may be associated with alopecia. With the advent of HAART, however, the incidence of refractory cases seems to be diminishing.

Psoriasis may have a number of different manifestations. The classic cases consist of reddish plaques with superficial micaceous scale on the extensor surfaces and

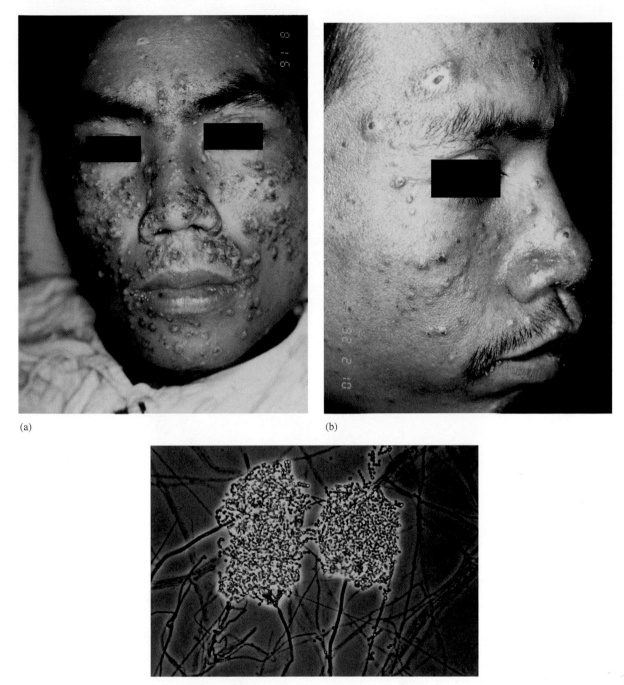

(a)

(b)

(c)

Figure 14–41. *Penicillium marneffei* in (a, b) Thai AIDS patients as (c) confirmed by culture. (Photographs courtesy of Siri Chiewchanvit, M.D., Chiang Mai, Thailand.)

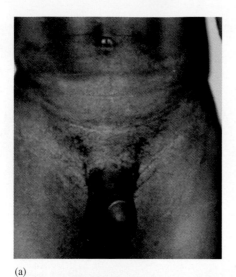

(a)

Figure 14–42. (a) Widespread dermatophytosis in a patient shown to be the first manifestation of HIV infection. (b, c) Severe manifestation of dermatophytosis in a patient with AIDS. Note the similarity to crusted scabies in Figure 14-28. (d) Proximal white subungual, and (e) total nail onychomycosis in patients with HIV infection. (Photograph d courtesy of J. K. Maniar, M.D., Department of Dermatovenereology and AIDS Medicine, G.T. Hospital, Grant Medical College, Mumbai, India.)

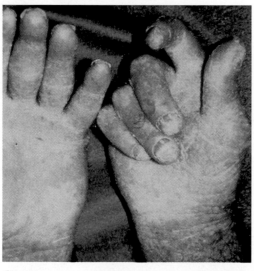

(b)

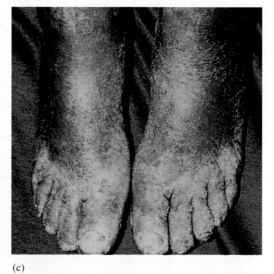

(c)

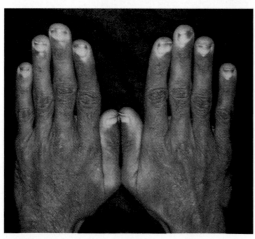

(d)

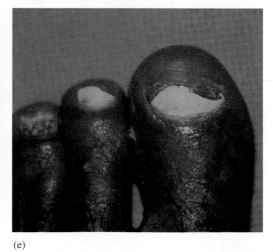

(e)

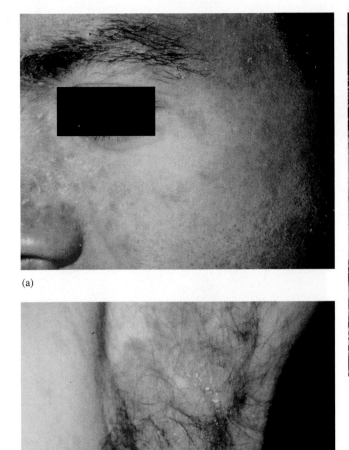

(a)

(c)

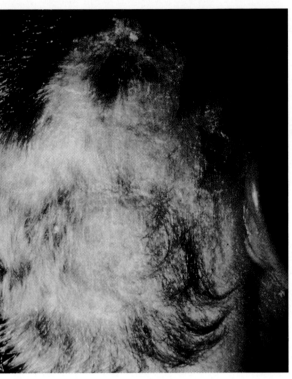

(b)

Figure 14–43. (a) Seborrheic dermatitis as an early manifestation of HIV infection. (b, c) Severe seborrheic dermatitis with alopecia and inverse distribution in an immunocompromised patient with AIDS.

nail changes of onycholysis, pitting, and subungual hyperkeratosis (Figs. 14–44 and 14–45). In other patients, severe psoriatic arthritis may be seen. Different forms of psoriasis may be found in the same patient, such as guttate psoriasis associated with classic psoriasis vulgaris. Severe exfoliative erythroderma may develop within several days, and acral pustular lesions of keratoderma blennorrhagicum coexisting with psoriasis or sebopsoriasis have been noted. Concomitant seborrheic dermatitis of the scalp is almost always seen. HIV-related psoriasis may develop in patients with mild pre-existing psoriasis that suddenly undergoes severe exacerbation once AIDS develops, or it may develop spontaneously at some point after HIV seroconversion in an individual who has never before had clinical disease.

Reiter's syndrome is characterized clinically by arthritis (especially sacroiliitis), urethritis, conjunctivitis, and pustular scaling lesions of the glabrous skin, glans penis, and scalp. Debilitating palmoplantar pustular disease is common, and there is generally striking nail dystrophy associated with periungual erythema, inflammation, and hyperkeratosis with prominent crusting (Fig. 14–46).

Histopathology

The histopathological findings of seborrheic dermatitis are similar to those seen in patients with non–HIV-associated disease, namely, psoriasiform hyperplasia of the epidermis with mounds of parakeratosis containing neutrophils near the ostia of hair follicular infundibula. An infiltrate of lymphocytes and scattered plasma cells are seen in the dermis. Seborrheic dermatitis in patients with HIV infection pro-

Figure 14–44. (a, b, c) Extensive eruptive psoriasis in HIV-infected hosts. (d) Inverse psoriasis.

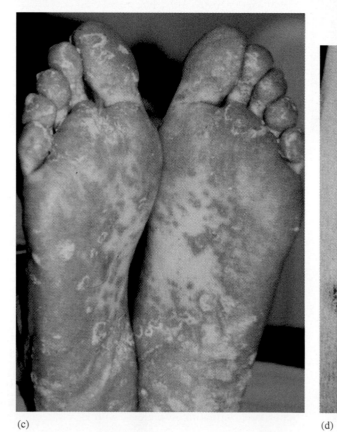

(a)

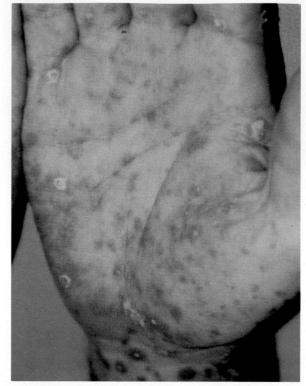

(b)

(c)

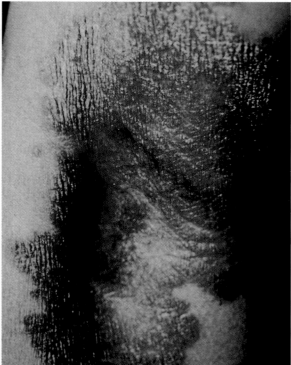

(d)

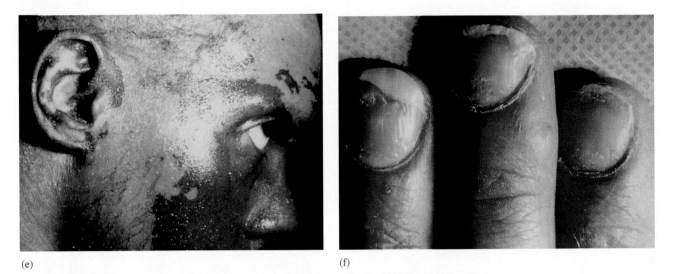

(e)   (f)

Figure 14–44. (continued). (e) Sebopsoriasis in an HIV-infected patient that progressed to widespread extensive involvement with erythroderma. (f) Nail changes of onycholysis and pitting with HIV-associated psoriasis.

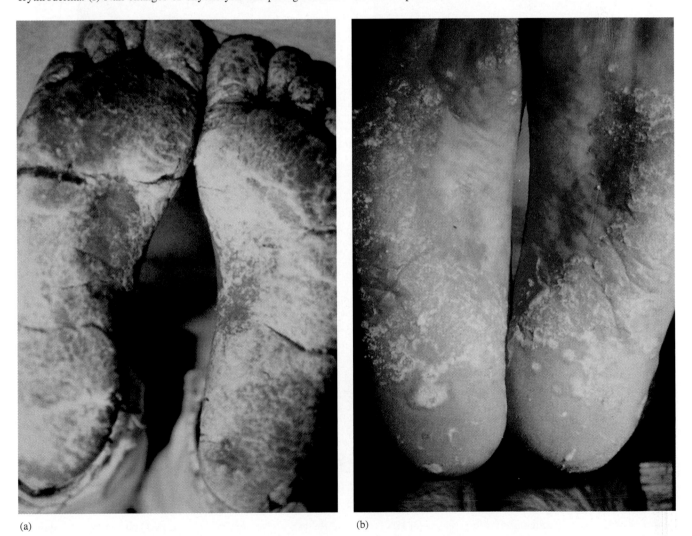

(a)   (b)

Figure 14–45. (a, b) Treatment may be effective with acitretin or low-dose methotrexate in this case of severe keratoderma.

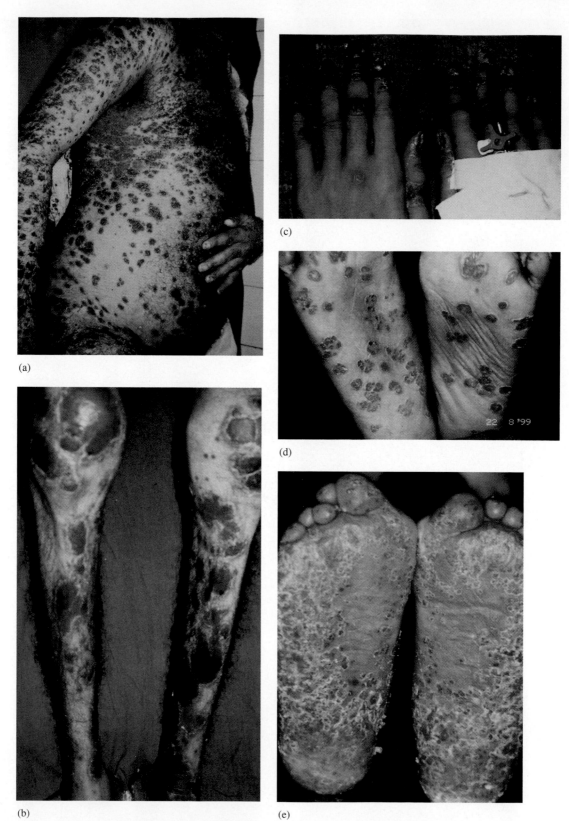

(a)

(b)

(c)

(d)

(e)

Figure 14–46.   (a–e) Pustular psoriasiform lesions of HIV-associated Reiter's syndrome. (Photographs a–d courtesy of J. K. Maniar, M.D., Department of Dermatovenereology and AIDS Medicine, G.T. Hospital, Grant Medical College, Mumbai, India.)

duces scattered individually necrotic keratinocytes, unlike its appearance in the general population. Some have likened this to cutaneous graft versus host disease.

Psoriasis, too, has histological features similar to those seen in non–HIV-infected patients. The pattern is generally that of marked acanthosis with regular elongation of epidermal retia associated with dilated tortuous blood vessels in the papillary dermis, thin suprapapillary plates, and mounds of parakeratosis containing neutrophils. In pustular cases, spongiform areas in the epidermis containing collections of neutrophils are noted. Reiter's disease has a histological picture similar to that of pustular psoriasis [65].

Laboratory Findings

No specific laboratory findings associated with these diseases have been reported other than the presence of HLA B27 in patients with Reiter's syndrome. CD4+ cell numbers may be at any level when seborrheic dermatitis develops; but when it becomes persistent and refractory to therapy, CD4+ cell numbers are generally lower than 250 cells/mm^3. Psoriasis, too, may develop at any point during the course of HIV infection but has been reported to be worse when CD4+ cell numbers are less than 500 cells/mm^3.

Diagnosis

The diagnosis of a psoriasiform dermatosis in HIV-infected hosts is generally based on evaluation of clinical and histological features of the disease in question. In most cases, diagnoses are not difficult to render. Scrapings for microscopic examination should be done to exclude the possibility of fungi and scabies if any question in the diagnosis persists.

Treatment

Table 14–8 lists the treatment for seborrheic dermatitis and psoriasis. Both topical antifungals and topical steroids are used for therapy of seborrheic dermatitis.

Both spontaneous remission of psoriasis and complete unresponsiveness to all forms of treatment have been observed in HIV-infected patients. In many cases, systemic drugs, systemic psoralen, and ultraviolet A therapy may be required. Methotrexate may be used with extreme caution. Concomitant administration of trimethoprim-containing compounds is contraindicated because the folate reductase–inhibiting effect is synergistic with that produced by methotrexate.

There has been concern that exposure to ultraviolet radiation may cause worsening of immunocompromise in patients with HIV disease, as in vitro exposure of HIV-infected cell lines to such radiation has been shown to lead to increased production of HIV from latently infected cells [66]. In spite of this, in clinical practice no evidence of

Table 14–8.　Treatment of Seborrheic Dermatitis and Psoriasis

Symptom	Treatment
Seborrheic dermatitis	Topical hydrocortisone, 2.5% ointment or cream, applied twice daily
	Topical antifungal creams, applied twice daily
	Ultraviolet B phototherapy is often effective as an adjunct
Psoriasis	Combination of hydrophilic petrolatum, applied several times daily, 3–5% salicylic acid ointment applied one to two times daily (for keratolytic effect), and triamcinolone acetonide ointment 0.025%–0.1% (or its equivalent) for localized short-term therapy, is partially effective
	2% crude coal tar and petrolatum followed by ultraviolet B phototherapy may also be beneficial
	Anthralin 0.1–1% cream or ointment applied either overnight or for short duration
	Acitretin, 25 mg to 50 mg orally each day, with or without the addition of dapsone, 100–200 mg orally each day
	Psoralen, taken orally, followed by ultraviolet A phototherapy
	Methotrexate (orally), starting at 5–7.5 mg/week and gradually increasing the dose by 2.5 mg/week as needed. Monitor carefully, as immunosuppression may occur
	Note: Concomitant administration of trimethoprim-containing compounds is contraindicated because the folate-inhibiting effect is synergistic with that induced by methotrexate

increased immunosuppression or worsening of HIV infection after exposure to ultraviolet radiation has been observed [67].

OTHER PAPULOSQUAMOUS DISORDERS

Pityriasis rubra pilaris is a papulosquamous dermatosis characterized by widespread scaly plaques that involve the scalp, trunk, extremities, palms, and soles, with characteristic follicular involvement and islands of skin that are spared by the disease (Fig. 14–47). Several HIV-infected patients

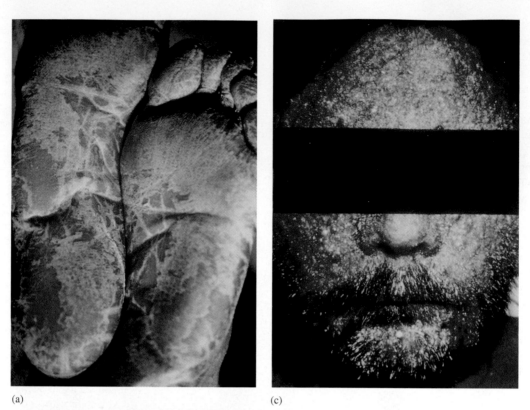

(a)

(c)

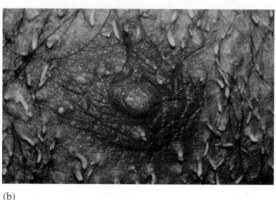

(b)

Figure 14–47. (a–c) Pityriasis rubra pilaris in patients with HIV infection. Note the prominent follicular involvement that led to the complication of explosive cystic acne. (Reprinted with permission, Br J Dermatol 126:617–620, 1992.)

with this disorder have been reported, some of whom developed explosive cystic acne vulgaris in association with the follicular abnormality [68]. Elongated cutaneous follicular spines have been observed, and at least once there was a report of histopathological evidence of mucin deposition [69]. Therapy with 13-*cis*-retinoic acid may be effective, and improvement following the administration of HAART may be noted.

Exfoliative erythroderma in patients with HIV infection is most commonly caused by psoriasis, although it may be caused by cutaneous T-cell lymphoma, atopic dermatitis, drug eruptions, and severe seborrheic dermatitis (Fig. 14–48). A hyperpigmented erythroderma associated with elevated immunoglobulin E levels has also been observed. Staphylococcal scalded skin syndrome as well as the toxic streptococcal syndrome are infectious causes of erythroderma and should be considered as these can be treated with antibiotics.

Histologically, patients with psoriasiform dermatitis have been shown to have findings similar to those of seborrheic dermatitis as well as of spongiotic dermatitis. Severe xerosis and acquired ichthyosis may develop as a consequence of abnormal nutrition as well as secondary to diminished autonomic nervous system function, with decreased

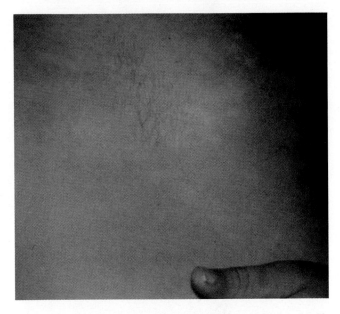

Figure 14–48. Erythroderma associated with AIDS. Many different factors may be etiological.

sweating and diminished sebaceous gland secretion. The problems may develop in 20–30% of HIV-infected patients (Fig. 14–49). Treatment consists of avoidance of soap and water and application of emollients, such as hydrophilic petrolatum or lotions containing 12% lactic acid. Pityriasis rosea may also occur in widespread fashion in patients with HIV disease.

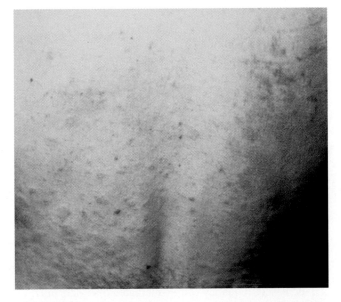

Figure 14–49. Severe asteatosis associated with HIV disease.

NONINFECTIOUS PAPULAR PRURITIC DISORDERS

Definition

Aside from infestations, a number of cutaneous disorders are pruritic and lead to extreme discomfort. Some conditions associated with itchy papular and pustular dermatoses in these individuals include eosinophilic (pustular) folliculitis, severe xerotic dermatitis, papular dermatitis of AIDS, papular urticaria, and atopic dermatitis. Eosinophilic (pustular) folliculitis is a condition of widespread follicular papules and pustules that is characterized by an influx of eosinophils in the infundibula of hair follicles (Fig. 14–50). Papular urticaria generally refers to responses to insect bite reactions or possibly to hypersensitivity "recall" reactions

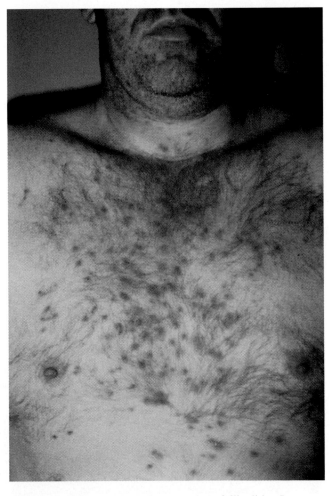

Figure 14–50. Eosinophilic (pustular) folliculitis. In some cases, the major presenting feature may be lichen simplex chronicus.

to insect bites suffered previously (Fig. 14–51). The papular dermatitis of AIDS is a condition of nondescript papules on the trunk and extremities in patients with HIV infection, the etiology of which has not been determined (Fig. 14–52).

Epidemiology

Pruritic conditions in patients with HIV infection are quite common, although the precise incidence and prevalence are unknown. Approximately 5–30% of HIV-infected patients develop eosinophilic folliculitis [70]. Other pruritic dermatoses, such as papular dermatitis of AIDS, papular urticaria, and atopic dermatitis, are seen in variable percentages, probably ranging between 1 and 2% or less. Atopic dermatitis may be seen more commonly in children with HIV infection. Xerotic dermatitis may be seen to some degree in up to 85% of patients.

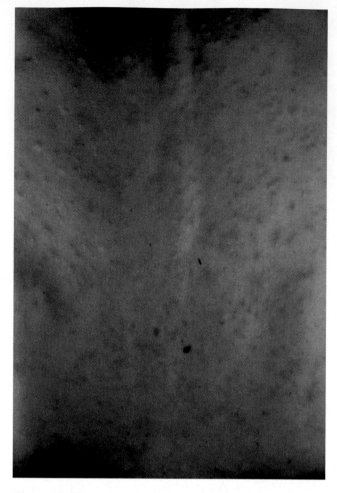

Figure 14–52. Acute papular urticarial reaction associated with acute seroconversion to HIV-1. Note the similarity to papular urticaria (Fig. 14–51).

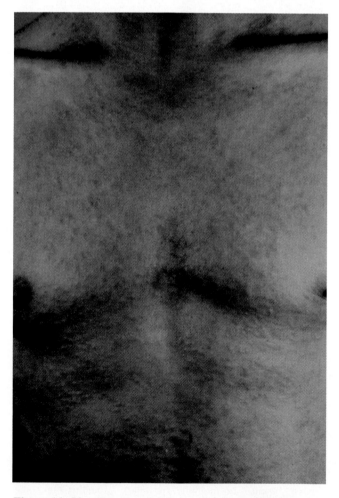

Figure 14–51. Papular urticaria associated with HIV infection.

Pathogenesis

The pathogenesis of pruritic dermatoses in patients with HIV infection is not entirely clear, although there are several theories that may be germane. All patients should be evaluated for the presence of ectoparasites and other pathogens such as scabies and fungi, as these may lead to itching. Systemic parasites also may lead to itching by inducing urticarial reactions or as a consequence of migration through the skin. Other causes of hypersensitivity, such as drug eruptions and underlying atopic dermatitis, may produce itching and should be excluded on clinical grounds. Patients with HIV infection commonly have circulating IgE antibodies to HIV, the levels of which increase as CD4+ cell numbers fall [71]. This may correlate with the increased frequency of IgE-mediated disorders in HIV-infected patients, such as worsened atopic dermatitis and other hypersensitivity disorders. Basophils have been shown to be hyper-releasable in patients with HIV disease, and it is presumed that mast cells are similarly hyper-releasable. Enhanced degranulation of basophils and mast cells results in increased release of mast cell mediators with attendant inflammatory reactions and pruritus. Patients with HIV disease may also have direct neural infection with neural irritation and enhanced sensations of itching. This may result in chronic excoriation, lichen simplex chronicus, and nodular prurigo. Sometimes, autonomic dysfunction is associated with diminished sweating and sebaceous gland secretion, worsening xerosis. In addition, patients infected with HIV are under severe stress for a number of reasons, and it is well known that stress may lead to urticaria and itching. Finally, patients with HIV infection may develop pruritus secondary to underlying circulating pruritogens associated with systemic disorders. Liver disease, renal disease, and systemic lymphoma all may be associated with pruritus. All these factors should be considered when dealing with an itchy HIV-infected patient.

The pathogenesis of eosinophilic (pustular) folliculitis is unknown but has been postulated to be a consequence of an exaggerated reaction to *Pityrosporum* yeasts normally present within follicular infundibula.

Clinical Manifestations

Eosinophilic (pustular) folliculitis (EF) is one of the most characteristic and common pruritic dermatoses to develop in patients with CD4 lymphocyte counts below 200 cells/mm^3. The frequency declined significantly with the advent of HAART, but EF may reappear in patients with low CD4 cell numbers.

Patients often have widespread excoriated follicular papules that commonly involve the trunk, extremities, and head and neck areas [70]. It is important to exclude the diagnosis of scabies, which may look quite similar to EF, by performing scrapings and biopsies if necessary. It is rare to find intact pustules because patients are usually so uncomfortable that by the time they see the dermatologist, lesions have been excoriated.

Papular dermatitis of AIDS is a nondescript papular eruption in patients with HIV infection. The original description was that of an eruption of urticarial papules present on the trunk and extremities associated with excoriation and rubbing. Many believe that this may represent a reaction to insect bites or eosinophilic (pustular) folliculitis.

Atopic dermatitis produces erythematous patches and plaques with fine papulovesicles associated with scaling, crusting, and lichen simplex chronicus. Patients often have associated hyperlinear palms, allergic rhinitis, and asthma.

HIV-infected individuals who develop atopic dermatitis may manifest severe forms of the disorder with erythroderma.

Xerotic dermatitis exhibits diffuse dryness of the skin with hyperpigmented scales and focal crusting. Many lesions may be fissured, and eczema craquelé may develop. This latter complication enhances localized infection, as the broken skin serves as a portal of entry for bacteria and fungi.

Prurigo nodularis appears as hyperpigmented dome-shaped papules and nodules usually associated with lichen simplex chronicus. Lesions are produced by chronic rubbing and scratching.

Papular urticaria and chronic urticaria are manifested by pinkish-red erythematous papules and plaques, initially with little surface change (Fig. 14–53). Edema and a peau d'orange appearance of the skin are noted. Angioedema may be seen. Although papular urticaria may be excoriated, primary urticaria generally is not.

Histopathology

EF has a characteristic histopathological appearance—within the infundibula of hair follicles there are clusters of eosinophils that may be numerous. There is often a perifollicular inflammatory infiltrate of lymphocytes, neutrophils, and some eosinophils, especially when the follicles have ruptured.

The papular dermatitis of AIDS is similar to that of insect bite reactions, with a superficial and deep perivascular and interstitial infiltrate of lymphocytes, some histiocytes, and eosinophils.

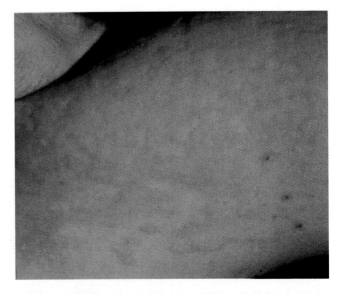

Figure 14–53. Acute urticaria in HIV-infected patients.

Atopic dermatitis has microscopic features of a superficial perivascular infiltrate of lymphocytes and eosinophils, with epidermal hyperplasia and foci of spongiosis. Late lesions have the morphological appearance of lichen simplex chronicus. Asteatotic or xerotic dermatitis shows very little inflammation in the dermis, with slight epidermal hyperplasia, tiny amounts of spongiosis, and small zones of parakeratosis.

Laboratory Findings

Most patients with EF have low CD4+ cell counts. Eosinophilia may be found in patients with atopic dermatitis or papular urticaria. Although IgE levels are often elevated, no laboratory test is specific for any of these disorders. Underlying liver or renal impairment may be present.

Differential Diagnosis

The differential diagnosis of EF includes a number of other pruritic dermatoses that may be found in both HIV-infected individuals and immunocompetent patients. Bacterial folliculitis may be associated with pruritis and has clinical features similar to those of EF. Insect bite reactions, scabies, and dermatitis herpetiformis must all be excluded. If skin scrapings show no evidence of scabies, in most cases the diagnosis can generally be assumed to be EF and treated accordingly, without a biopsy.

Papular urticaria is thought to be a manifestation of insect bite reactions so that it is important to exclude scabies and pediculosis by microscopic examination of skin scrapings. In some cases, careful histories reveal no evidence of insect bite reactions.

Atopic dermatitis must be differentiated from other psoriasiform dermatitides such as psoriasis, cutaneous T-cell lymphoma, and psoriasiform drug eruptions. In general, the presence of severe pruritus and a history of atopy aid in this diagnosis. Xerotic dermatitis should be excluded from other forms of dry, scaly dermatoses, such as the characteristic ''flaky-paint'' dermatitis seen with kwashiorkor. In individuals with advanced AIDS, evaluation of nutritional status is essential.

Diagnosis

The diagnosis of noninfectious papular pruritus is based on history, physical examination, and performance of biopsies and scrapings. Evaluation for causes of chronic urticaria is similar to that undertaken in immunocompetent hosts, although searches for underlying parasitic and protozoal infestations and drug hypersensitivity reactions should be undertaken in all cases, as these are seen more commonly in HIV-infected hosts.

Treatment

Therapy of EF has been the subject of a number of studies because of the high incidence of the disorder and the mor-

bidity it produces in HIV-infected individuals. Patients are generally treated with gradually increasing phototherapy units of ultraviolet B (UVB). Several studies have demonstrated that moderate exposure to UVB is safe in the treatment of HIV-related dermatoses if administered appropriately [67]. Therapy with itraconazole is also used, although its mechanism of action is unknown; it may act by diminishing the concentration of *Pityrosporum* yeasts within follicular infundibula. Other treatments are shown in Table 14–9. For papular urticaria, systemic antihistamines are generally used. In general, nonsedating antihistamines are not as effective as classic H-1 antagonists that induce somnolence, as these may aid in lessening the perceived sensation of itching. It is important to search for underlying causes of pruritus, such as ingestants that may be causing an allergic reaction. Chronic urticaria is often difficult to control in immunocompetent patients and may be especially problematic in HIV-infected hosts. It is usually difficult to establish an etiology. Atopic dermatitis usually responds to measures used for treatment in immunocompetent hosts.

VASCULITIS AND OTHER VASCULAR-RELATED ABNORMALITIES

Definition

Patients with HIV and AIDS develop a number of conditions that either involve primarily the blood vessels with inflammation or are associated with vascular proliferation. Kaposi's sarcoma is discussed in the section on neoplastic disorders. Some of the conditions associated with vascular abnormalities include vasculitis, idiopathic thrombocytopenic purpura, hyperalgesic pseudothrombophlebitis, diffuse facial and truncal telangiectasia, and erythema elevatum diutinum.

Epidemiology

All these conditions have been reported only sporadically in patients with HIV disease.

Pathogenesis

Vasculitis and erythema elevatum diutinum represent manifestations of immune complex-mediated disease. Antigen-antibody complexes collect within blood vessels, leading to deposition of fibrin in walls of blood vessels and attendant signs of inflammation. As the CD4+ cell count falls, the B-cell arm of the immune response may become hyperactive, leading to a relative overabundance of antibody secretion. The altered concentration of antigen to antibody in the circulation leads to precipitation and abnormal clearance of immune complexes [72]. This mechanism may be related to the development of idiopathic thrombocytopenic

Table 14-9. Treatment of Noninfectious Papular Pruritic Disorders

Symptom	Treatment
Eosinophilic pustular folliculitis	Ultraviolet B phototherapy or natural sunlight exposure Itraconazole 100–200 mg orally twice daily Metronidazole orally may also be effective Oral 13-*cis*-retinoic acid may also be effective Doxepin, 10–20 mg orally every 6 hours, or other antihistamines for pruritus Topical application of antipruritic agents, such as pramoxine and menthol and phenol-containing lotions, may also be beneficial in diminishing itching
Papular urticaria	Systemic antihistamines Topical corticosteroid preparations (e.g., triamcinolone acetonide 0.1% ointment or more potent steroids) are beneficial in lessening inflammation 10% doxepin compounded in aquaphor ointment is also effective
Xerotic dermatitis	Avoidance of excessive exposure to soap and water and other irritating factors Potent emollients, such as hydrophilic petrolatum and alpha-hydroxy acid–containing preparations 12% lactic acid lotions are effective in lessening the severe dryness
Atopic dermatitis	Avoidance of irritants Emollient application Topical corticosteroid preparations Tacrolimus ointment (0.03% or 0.1%)

purpura as well. Extravasated erythrocytes lead to the characteristic clinical picture of palpable purpura and petechiae.

Hyperalgesic pseudothrombophlebitis is thought to be related to deeply seated Kaposi's sarcoma, with associated secretion of cytokines and inflammatory mediators. Widespread telangiectasias may be associated with a circulating vascular proliferation factor that may be related to fibroblast growth factor or other vasoproliferative agents.

Clinical Manifestations

Leukocytoclastic vasculitis may progress clinically through several stages, beginning as urticarial papules or as small petechiae. In most cases, characteristic palpable purpuric papules develop most commonly on the extremities, although any body site may be involved. In patients with HIV infection, lesions may be more numerous and more florid than in immunocompetent hosts (Fig. 14–54). Pustules, ulcers, and bullae may also be seen. Erythema elevatum diutinum is a manifestation of chronic leukocytoclastic vasculitis that evolves into indurated reddish plaques, often over the joints (Figs. 14–55). The dorsal surfaces of the hands, especially over the knuckles and around the ankles and knees, are common sites of involvement. Plaques may assume a somewhat yellowish color as a consequence of the influx of numerous neutrophils and their degradation, which correlates with the clinical name of extracellular cholesterolosis that was previously applied to this condition. In time, plaques give way to firm, thick fibrotic nodules that may extend to involve volar skin surfaces. Generally, lesions are asymptomatic, but if they are located on weight-bearing sites, they may be painful [73]. Idiopathic thrombocytopenic purpura usually manifests as petechiae or palpable purpura and may simulate leukocytoclastic vasculitis.

Hyperalgesic pseudothrombophlebitis is associated with diffuse swelling of an extremity with extreme tenderness. Patients note marked sensitivity to even the lightest touch. No thrombophlebitic cords can be palpated. Diffuse telangiectasia has a clinical appearance somewhat similar to that of poikiloderma of Civatte (Figs. 14–56 and 14–57). The reddish telangiectatic areas on the cheeks, neck, chest, and trunk are not the result of sun exposure.

Histopathology

Leukocytoclastic vasculitis has a characteristic histopathological appearance that is usually diagnostic. Very early urticarial or petechial lesions are characterized by a perivascular and interstitial infiltrate that contains lymphocytes, neutrophils, and eosinophils, with abundant nuclear dust. Minimal involvement of actual blood vessels may be noted, so that no fibrin within the walls of vessels is appreciated. In time, inflammatory cells are noted within the walls of small and medium-sized blood vessels with abundant deposition of fibrin. In fully developed lesions, there may be significant thrombi within vascular lumina. Erythema elevatum diutinum is characterized by similar histological findings initially, but in due course, abundant fibrosis is noted around blood vessels and in the stroma.

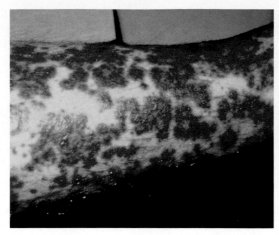

(a)

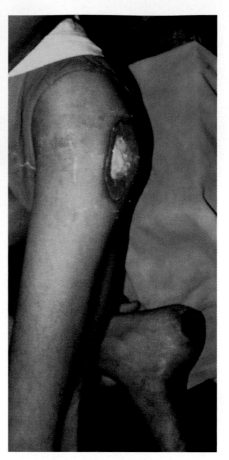

Figure 14–54. (a) Severe leukocytoclastic vasculitis of undetermined origin in an HIV-infected patient. (b) Severe vasculitis may result in deep ulcers. (a, Reprinted with permission, Arch Int Med 151:1295–1303, 1991; photograph b courtesy of J. K. Maniar, M.D., Department of Dermatovenereology and AIDS Medicine, G.T. Hospital, Grant Medical College, Mumbai, India.)

(b)

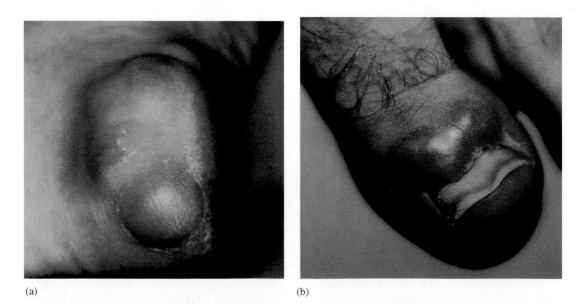

(a)   (b)

Figure 14–55. (a, b) Erythema elevatum diutinum in AIDS. (a, Reprinted with permission, J Am Acad Dermatol 28:919–922, 1993).

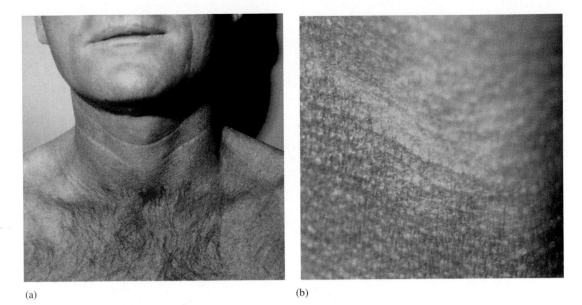

(a)　　　　　　　　　　　　　　　　　　(b)

Figure 14–56. (a, b) Widespread telangiectasia and poikiloderma in HIV infection.

An increase in the number of MAC-387 positive histiocytes as well as fibroblasts can be demonstrated with immunoperoxidase stains. Only minimal granulomatous inflammation is seen, although in some lesions, cholesterol clefts are observed in the interstitium. Collections of neutrophils and eosinophils are seen in late fibrotic lesions, even though vasculitis may have abated.

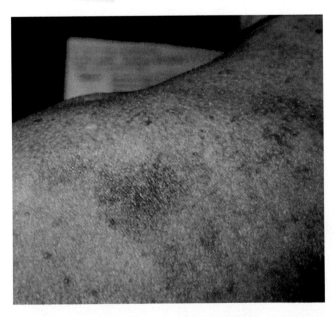

Figure 14–57. "Blotchy" matlike telangiectasia of the trunk.

Laboratory Findings

Elevated erythrocyte sedimentation rates may be found in patients with leukocytoclastic vasculitis and erythema elevatum diutinum. If an underlying cause of vasculitis is present, such as a connective tissue disease, characteristic laboratory findings of the underlying disease are found in most cases. CD4+ cell counts vary widely. Hypocomplementemia may be noted, and if vasculitis involves the kidneys, findings of renal dysfunction such as elevated serum creatinine levels may be present. Prolonged bleeding times will be noted in idiopathic thrombocytopenic purpura. Elevated antistreptolysin O titers or elevated immunoglobulin levels may be found in patients with erythema elevatum diutinum. No known abnormalities are found in patients with either hyperalgesic pseudothrombophlebitis or diffuse telangiectasia.

Diagnosis

Diagnosis of each of these conditions is based on characteristic clinical findings and exclusion of other diseases in combination with histopathological findings.

Treatment

The management of vascular-related disorders is outlined in Table 14–10. The treatment of vasculitis consists primarily of identifying the underlying cause and correcting associated abnormalities. Before cyclophosphamide, methotrexate, or other potentially immunosuppressive immunomodulators are administered, careful assessment of the immune status of the patient must be undertaken. All patients

Table 14–10. Treatment of Vasculitis and Vascular-related Abnormalities

Symptom	Treatment
Vasculitis	Nonsteroidal anti-inflammatory agents may be beneficial in some cases
	Colchicine, dapsone, or systemic corticosteroids such as prednisone may be required in severe cases
	Cyclophosphamide and methotrexate are occasionally needed in severe cases
	Splenectomy is effective for idiopathic thrombocytopenic purpura
Erythema elevatum diutinum	Dapsone therapy (oral)
	Surgical excision has been effective in some cases
Hyperalgesic pseudothrombophlebitis	Analgesics and nonsteroidal anti-inflammatory agents are the primary treatment
	Narcotic analgesics may be required, as the condition is extremely painful
	Bed rest, warm compresses, and leg elevation may be useful
Diffuse telangiectasis	Selective laser destruction using argon or tunable dye laser
	Electrocoagulation may also be beneficial
	Cosmetic camouflage using green-tinted makeup is helpful in masking the red appearance of the skin

who are to be treated with agents such as these must be monitored carefully. In HIV-infected patients the response of erythema elevatum diutinum to dapsone may be blunted or there may be no response at all.

PHOTOINDUCED AND PHOTOAGGRAVATED CONDITIONS

Definition

Several skin disorders that are worsened by light exposure may be associated with HIV infection. These include chronic actinic dermatitis, porphyria cutanea tarda (PCT), photoexacerbated drug eruptions, photoexacerbated rosacea, and granuloma annulare.

Epidemiology

No specific figures exist regarding the prevalence of these conditions in that most have been reported only sporadically. Porphyria cutanea tarda, however, is being reported with some frequency, although the overall prevalence of this condition remains low.

Pathogenesis

Chronic actinic dermatitis may be associated with HIV infection because of the exaggerated B-cell immunity that may be present in these individuals. Patients with HIV infection may develop allergies to drugs and other substances owing to alterations of the immune system and recall of underlying allergic phenomena. Patients with HIV infection produce greater concentrations of porphyrins, possibly as a consequence of abnormal liver function secondary to hepatitis, such as hepatitis C or other factors. This latter factor may be of prime importance, as over 50% of all patients with porphyria cutanea tarda (PCT) have been found to be coinfected with this virus.

Clinical Manifestations

Chronic actinic dermatitis of HIV infection characteristically is manifested by psoriasiform lichenified plaques in the sun-exposed areas of the body; these plaques are often hyperpigmented, scaly, and pruritic [74]. Lesions are generally located on the dorsal surfaces of the hands, forearms, face, upper anterior chest, and the posterior neck. Extensive lichenification is often seen, and patients may have an appearance similar to that described with actinic reticuloid. The appearance of PCT is virtually identical to that seen in immunocompetent hosts, with blisters on the dorsal surfaces of the hands and other sun-exposed areas (Fig. 14–58). These blisters are associated with crusting, milia formation, dyspigmentation, and scarring [75]. There is also often hyperpigmentation and hypertrichosis of the malar areas of the face. Patients may report the excretion of dark urine. Widespread granuloma annulare is manifested by small pinkish dermal papules distributed on sun-exposed areas. Photoexacerbated drug eruptions often appear lichenoid or erythematous and are distributed on photoexposed sites (Figs. 14–59 and 14–60). Actinically aggravated rosacea looks similar to acne rosacea in immunocompetent hosts, with an eruption of follicular papules and pustules on the face (Fig. 14–61). Extrafacial lesions may be seen. Dermal waxy papules may represent granulomatous rosacea, which may also be worsened by sunlight exposure.

Histopathology

Chronic actinic dermatitis is generally manifested by a superficial and often deep psoriasiform dermatitis with an infiltrate of lymphocytes and abundant eosinophils. In im-

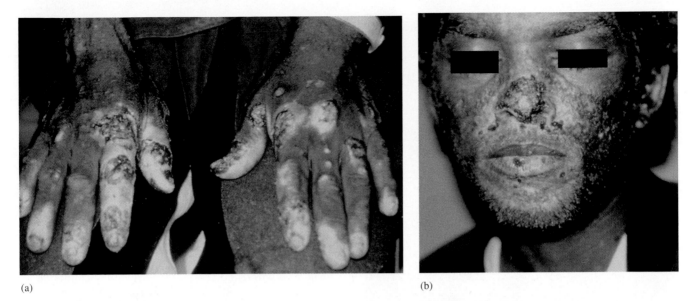

(a)   (b)

Figure 14–58.   Severe porphyria cutanea tarda in a patient with HIV infection. Most patients with this complication have been found to suffer from concomitant hepatitis C infection.

munocompetent individuals, PCT has histological findings that are characterized by a subepidermal blister with minimal inflammation in the dermis. Preservation of dermal papillae, so-called "festooning," is seen, and there are thick hyaline periodic acid-Schiff stained–positive rims surrounding blood vessels in the upper dermis. Elongated

aggregations of necrotic keratinocytes are often present in the epidermis, overlying the blister; these have been referred to as "caterpillar bodies" [76]. Granuloma annulare also has a histological pattern that resembles a diffuse infiltrate of palisaded histiocytes in the dermis, with mucin in the center of the palisade. Eruptive forms of granuloma annulare may be associated only with an interstitial infiltrate without significant palisading. Rosacea is manifested

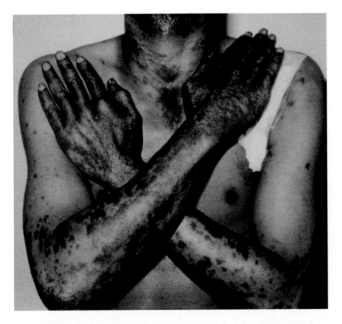

Figure 14–59.   Lichenoid photodermatitis of unknown origin in a patient with AIDS.

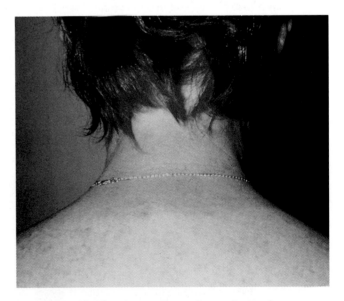

Figure 14–60.   Acute phototoxic reaction to dapsone.

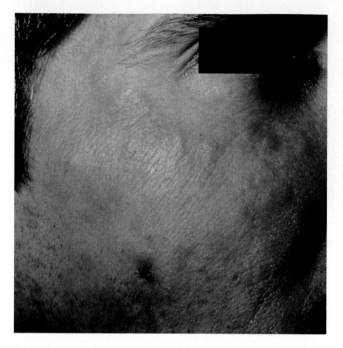

Figure 14–61. Acne rosacea may be photoexacerbated in HIV-infected hosts.

by a perifollicular infiltrate of lymphocytes, some neutrophils, and follicular pustules.

Laboratory Findings

The only significant laboratory findings associated with PCT are elevated circulating and urinary uroporphyrins ($\leq$ 9000 IU/ml) and coproporphyrins. CD4+ cell counts range from 3 to >500 cells/mm^3, which indicates that the disorder may develop at any stage of HIV infection. Elevated serum glutamic-oxaloacetic transaminase and serum glutamate pyruvate transaminase enzyme levels and, occasionally, hyperbilirubinemia occur. Many patients with HIV infection and PCT are anemic rather than polycythemic, and treatment with phlebotomy cannot be undertaken in such patients. CD4+ cell counts below 200 cells/mm^3 usually are associated with photoaggravated disorders.

Diagnosis

The diagnosis of chronic actinic dermatitis involves a history of recent exposure to potential photoallergens or phototoxins as well as a past history of exposure that may have been reactivated. PCT is diagnosed on the basis of clinical and histological findings as well as demonstration of elevated urinary uroporphyrin and coproporphyrin levels. Actinically exacerbated granulomatous disorders are diagnosed on the basis of exclusion of infectious diseases in the context of characteristic clinical findings.

Treatment

The management of photoaggravated conditions is outlined in Table 14–11. In some cases of chronic actinic dermatitis, complete light avoidance may be essential, as even light emitted from television monitors may be sufficient to worsen the condition. Paradoxically, the use of psoralen and ultraviolet A therapy may "harden" the skin and lead to remission.

PCT is classically treated by repeat phlebotomy. In patients with HIV infection who are often anemic, this treatment cannot be used. Low doses of hydroxychloroquine may be effective in mobilizing accumulated porphyrin in the liver [77]. Erythropoietin has been shown to be effective in treatment of PCT by enhancing heme biosynthesis [78]. This results in mobilization of porphyrins. Although expensive, this might be the most beneficial form of treatment, as it will tend to correct the hematological deficit as well as the metabolic one. The effect of HAART on the incidence of HIV-associated PCT is unknown at this time.

Table 14–11. Treatment of Photoinduced and Photoaggravated Conditions

Symptom	Treatment
Chronic actinic dermatitis	Avoidance of photoallergens and phototoxins
	Avoidance of ultraviolet light
	Application of topical corticosteroid preparations
	Hydroxychloroquine (Plaquenil) 200 mg orally one to two times daily, may also be beneficial
Porphyria cutanea tarda	Hydroxychloroquine starting at 25 mg/wk and gradually increased to 200 mg/wk
	Erythropoietin
Rosacea	Oral tetracycline and topical benzoyl peroxide combination
	Metronidazole gel applied twice daily is also effective
	Metronidazole, 250–750 mg orally three times daily
	Avoidance of ultraviolet light may be necessary in cases associated with photoexacerbation
Granuloma annulare	Nicotinamide may be effective
	Application of topical corticosteroid preparations may be effective
	Avoidance of ultraviolet light may be necessary in cases associated with photoexacerbation

Rosacea is often treated with the usual antirosacea regimen of tetracycline and topical benzoyl peroxide. Topical or systemic metronidazole may be beneficial, as *Demodex* mites are thought to play a role in the pathogenesis in some cases.

CUTANEOUS DRUG ERUPTIONS

Definition

Drug eruptions are cutaneous disorders caused by the oral or parenteral administration of therapeutic drugs. Most are hypersensitive in nature, although others are a consequence of direct toxicity or unusual idiosyncratic reactions.

Epidemiology

Cutaneous drug reactions are the most common manifestation of drug hypersensitivity. A study of 684 HIV-infected patients in Boston revealed that 79% had one or more dermatological diagnoses, 188 of which included cutaneous reactions to drugs [79]. The incidence of many of these reactions is higher in HIV-infected patients than in the general population, including hypersensitivity to multiple drugs. The best known example of a drug that causes hypersensitivity reactions in HIV-infected hosts is trimethoprim-sulfamethoxazole. In some studies, 50–60% of HIV-positive patients were shown to develop a cutaneous eruption due to this agent. Up to 45% of patients develop maculopapular eruptions, with variable numbers of other reactions being reported. African-American patients seem to have a lower risk of cutaneous trimethoprim-sulfamethoxazole reactions. Stevens-Johnson syndrome and toxic epidermal necrolysis occur sporadically [80]. Other antibiotics also are common offenders; as maculopapular eruptions often may be seen in patients taking antituberculous regimens, amoxicillin-clavulanic acid, a combination of clindamycin and primaquine, intravenous clindamycin, and fusidate. Thalidomide used for treatment of aphthous ulcers may cause a widespread maculopapular exanthem in HIV-positive patients [81]. Zidovudine also may cause an exanthematous eruption in 1% of patients, which may mandate its discontinuation. Other eruptions and toxic drug effects have been reported to occur sporadically [82].

Pathogenesis

Drug eruptions develop as a consequence of any of the classic hypersensitivity reactions described by Coombs and Gell. Immediate hypersensitivity mediated by immunoglobulin E may lead to anaphylactoid and urticarial reactions. Type 2 reactions involving IgG and IgM antibodies may induce hemolytic anemia and thrombocytopenia. Immune complex mediated–reactions may produce serum sickness–like eruptions or drug-induced lupus erythematosus. Morbilliform eruptions may be present, although they may also be the result of cell-mediated (type 4) immune reactions. The pathogenesis of some of these eruptions is unknown. Underlying infection with CMV or EBV may predispose the patient to adverse drug reactions analogous to those seen with EBV–induced infectious mononucleosis and ampicillin [83].

Clinical Manifestations

Trimethoprim-sulfamethoxazole is the best known and most common allergic drug eruption to develop in patients with HIV infection (Fig. 14–62). In most cases, a widespread eruption of fine pink to red macules and papules involving the trunk and extremities develops 8 to 12 days after initiating therapy and reaches maximal intensity 1 to 2 days later. In some cases, desquamation may supervene. The eruption may disappear within 3 to 5 days even though therapy is continued. In some cases, the eruption may persist for days to weeks following discontinuation of the medication. Cutaneous eruptions caused by trimethoprim-sulfamethoxazole do not always recur with drug rechallenge in HIV-infected patients. However, if the agent is to be reinstituted, it should be done under controlled circumstances to monitor for possible anaphylactoid reactions characterized by fever, urticarial papules and plaques associated with angioedema, shortness of breath, and bronchospasm, Stevens-Johnson syndrome, characterized by fever, widespread blistering of the skin and mucous membranes of the eye, mouth, and/or genitals, may also develop. Toxic epidermal necrolysis (TEN) is a more serious manifestation that involves widespread areas of the skin with confluent bullae that often leads to loss of skin in massive sheets. Many cases of TEN have been reported in HIV-infected individuals. Other antibiotics, such as cephalexin and rifabutin, may produce morbilliform eruptions (Fig. 14–63).

Zidovudine may induce several different cutaneous complications. Blue to brown-black nail discoloration has been reported in over 40% of patients [84] (Fig. 14–64). It is more common in Black patients and usually begins 4 to 8 weeks after initiating treatment or may occur as late as 1 year. Longitudinal streaks are most common, but diffuse pigmentation and transverse bands may occur. The thumbnails are affected most frequently. Zidovudine may also cause hyperpigmentation of the mucous membranes and the skin that may mimic a clinical picture seen with adrenal insufficiency [85]. In addition to pigmentary abnormalities, severe exanthematous eruptions, such as lichenoid reactions, that may appear almost identical to lichen planus may develop within 1 to 2 weeks following the initiation of zidovudine therapy. Other manifestations include acral and periarticular reticulate erythema that may simulate dermatomyositis.

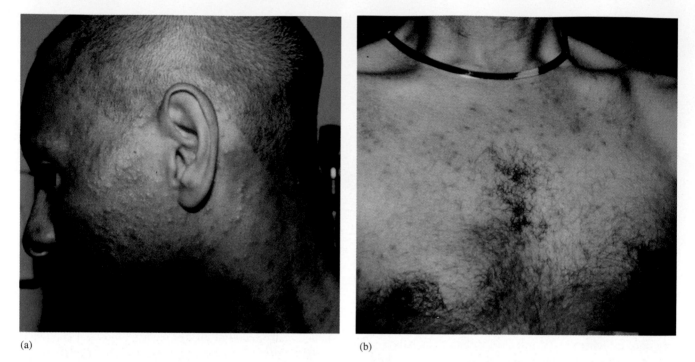

(a)   (b)

Figure 14–62. (a, b) Unusual papular drug eruption in response to trimethroprim-sulfamethoxazole, mimicking eosinophilic (pustular) folliculitis.

Indinavir use has been associated with a number of dermatological-abnormalities, including paronychia and pyogenic granuloma of the great toes [86], recurrent paronychia and ingrown toenails [87], hair loss of the lower extremities [88], and striae formation [89]. This drug, as well as the other protease inhibitors, has been associated with a form of lipodystrophy leading to abnormal fat accumulation in particular areas along with an overall wasting appearance in others [90,91]. The fat accumulation typically leads to the development of a cervicodorsal fat pad (''buffalo hump'') [92–96], and/or an increased abdominal girth (''protease pouch,'' ''crix belly'') [93,94,97], or breast development [97]. Some of these patients may also develop elevated triglyceride and cholesterol levels. The metabolic factors involved in this adverse effect are unknown at this time, although several potential mechanisms have been suggested [98].

Penile ulcerations caused by foscarnet develop about 11 to 16 days after initiation of therapy. Lesions range in number from two to five and are usually 1–5 cm in diameter and consist of erosive, bullous, tender ulcerations [99]. Sites of high deposits of urine concentration (urethral meatus and scrotum) are affected. Oral and esophageal ulcers may also develop. In addition to ulcerations, a generalized cutaneous eruption has been reported [100]. Widespread erythro-

derma has been reported in association with rifampin administration.

Parenteral pentamidine reactions range from morbilliform to urticarial eruptions. Sulfadoxine-pyrimethamine (Fansidar) may cause erythema multiforme and toxic epidermal necrolysis, while aerosolized pentamidine may cause a widespread erythematous maculopapular pruritic eruption. Other causes of toxic epidermal necrolysis include chlormezanone, fluoxetine, and thiacetazone. Unfortunately, patients sensitive to trimethoprim-sulfamethoxazole also often react to the most common substitute, dapsone. A sulfone syndrome has been observed when dapsone is used as a prophylaxis against *Pneumocystis carinii* infection. Finally, systemic treatment with methotrexate for psoriasis and with corticosteroids for vasculitis has precipitated both rapid proliferation and the sudden appearance of non-Hodgkin's lymphoma, opportunistic infections, and Kaposi's sarcoma.

Histopathology

The histopathology of morbilliform drug eruptions typically consists of a superficial perivascular inflammatory infiltrate of lymphocytes with scattered eosinophils associated with vacuolar alteration of the dermoepidermal junction and individually necrotic keratinocytes. Erythema

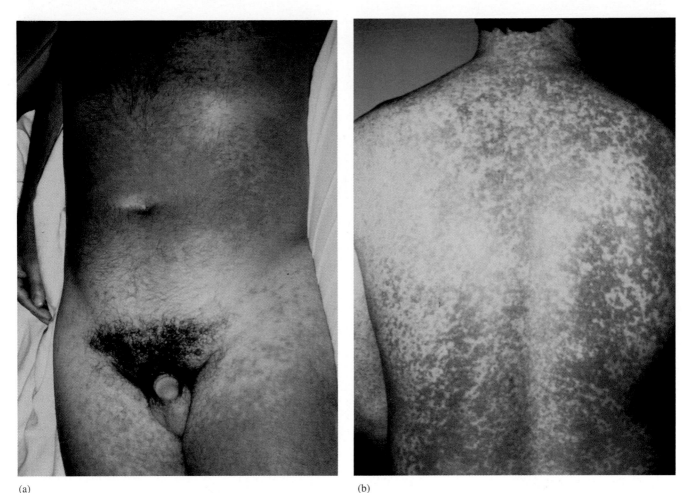

(a) (b)

Figure 14–63. (a, b) Morbilliform eruptions in response to cephalexin and rifabutin, respectively, in patients with HIV infection.

multiforme, Stevens-Johnson syndrome, and toxic epidermal necrolysis are all characterized by prominent vacuolar interface changes, with extensive keratinocytic necrosis of the epidermis. In toxic epidermal necrolysis, the number of inflammatory cells in the dermis may be minimal, although there is confluent epidermal necrosis with no parakeratosis, a consequence of the rapid progression of the eruption. Urticarial allergic eruptions are usually characterized by mixed infiltrates of inflammatory cells interstitially in the dermis with minimal epidermal change. Ulcerations caused by foscarnet generally show a mixed perivascular and interstitial infiltrate in the dermis with ulceration and epidermal necrosis, although inflammation may be minimal. Zidovudine-induced lichenoid eruptions may appear histologically identical to those of lichen planus, whereas zidovudine-induced nail pigmentation generally consists of an increase in the amount of melanin within melanocytes associated with scattered melanophages in the dermis.

Laboratory Findings

In most cases, laboratory findings are nonspecific, although patients with cutaneous drug eruptions have lowered $CD4+$ cell numbers (≤ 250 cells/mm^3). Eosinophilia may be noted as a general sign of hypersensitivity. As drugs may induce a number of other systemic problems, it is not uncommon to see accompanying changes such as neutropenia, thrombocytopenia, hypoglycemia, elevation of transaminase levels, and anemia.

Diagnosis

Diagnosis is generally made on the basis of the clinical appearance of the eruption correlated with the history of drug intake. As a general rule, antibiotics are the most common offenders, followed by anticonvulsants, nonsteroidal anti-inflammatory agents, and antiretrovirals [79]. Furthermore, patients may be sensitive to multiple drugs. Biopsies may be required and, in some cases, rechallenge

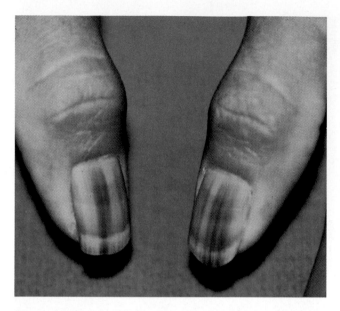

Figure 14–64. Longitudinal pigmented bands of multiple nails caused by zidovudine.

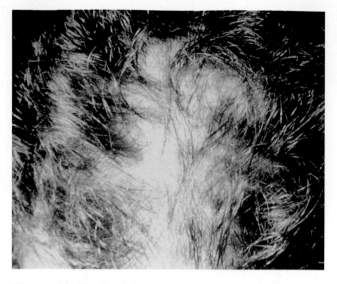

Figure 14–65. Noninflammatory alopecia associated with chronic HIV infection.

with the suspected offending allergen may be necessary to prove the diagnosis.

Treatment

The most serious cutaneous complication is epidermal necrolysis that may arise if the diagnosis is not made in timely fashion and the offending agent is not withdrawn. Other complications include systemic toxicity, such as hepatotoxicity or renal damage associated with the sulfone syndrome. Toxic epidermal necrolysis may lead to secondary infection with sepsis, volume depletion, and high output cardiac failure as a consequence of widespread denudation of the skin. Patients who develop this must be treated aggressively in intensive care settings. Whether systemic corticosteroids should be used remains controversial. Hypersensitivity to trimethoprim-sulfamethoxazole has been successfully treated with desensitization. Desensitization may also be attempted with other antibiotics when necessary.

Hair and Nail Abnormalities

A number of abnormalities of hair and nails may be encountered in patients with HIV infection. Chronic inflammatory and noninflammatory alopecia has been observed (Fig. 14–65). The hair may become lusterless and dull with straightening. Although these changes may be related to HIV infection and concomitant nutritional abnormalities, diffuse alopecia may also be associated with underlying

connective-tissue diseases or syphilis. Diffuse, fine, downy alopecia may occur in patients with end-stage AIDS. Finally, patients with HIV infection may develop serious infections with fever leading to true telogen effluvium.

In addition to loss of scalp hair, there may be elongation (trichomegaly) of the eyelashes, a sign of a prolonged anagen phase (Fig. 14–66) [101]. Other changes of the hair seen in HIV-infected patients include premature canities (Fig. 14–67) and alopecia areata [102].

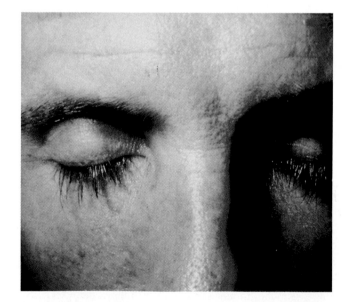

Figure 14–66. HIV-associated trichomegaly of the eyelashes.

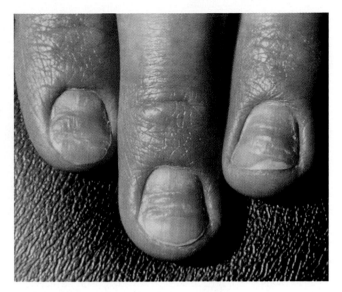

Figure 14–68. Beau's lines in a patient recently recovered from *Pneumocystis carinii* pneumonia.

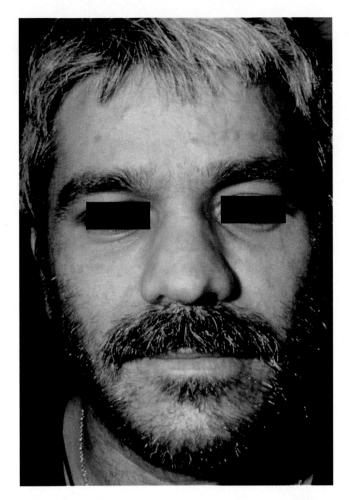

Figure 14–67. Premature canities in patients with AIDS.

Nail disorders may develop in patients with HIV infection. Nail plate thickening with subungual hyperkeratosis and dystrophy may be associated with fungal infections caused by dermatophytes as well as by *Candida, Hendersonula toruloidea,* and other nondermatophyte fungi. The yellow nail syndrome secondary to metabolic abnormalities, lymphedema, and hypoxia is characterized by transverse and longitudinal ridging. As in immunocompetent patients, Beau's lines may be seen 2 to 3 months after an episode of a serious infection (Fig. 14–68). Diminished thickness of the nail plate may also be seen. Increased nail plate opacity as well as both Muehrcke's and Terry's nails (Fig. 14–69) have been seen. Ridging and nail thickness changes are most likely a consequence of diminished matrix growth with decreased nail plate turnover. Involvement of the periungual tissues by infectious agents, psoriasis, and erythema with features similar to Gottron's papules may also be seen.

Miscellaneous Inflammatory and Metabolic Skin Disorders Associated with HIV Infection

Calciphylaxis is a disorder that represents a manifestation of hyperparathyroidism; it develops in association with renal failure [103]. Sensitivity to elevated circulating levels of parathyroid hormone leads to widespread calcification of the skin, soft tissues, blood vessels, and viscera. Diminished levels of protein C may be important in the pathogenesis of the disorder. Histopathologically, there is extensive calcification of small and medium-sized blood vessels throughout the dermis and subcutaneous fat, with secondary cutaneous necrosis and prominent thrombosis. Painful skin lesions may appear as livedo reticularis-like areas of the skin with hemorrhage, purplish discoloration, and erythema (Fig. 14–70). Necrosis and gangrene may appear within a few days. Treatment consists of correction of serum calcium and phosphorus abnormalities as well as emergency parathyroidectomy. Some patients may have no detectable abnormalities in either parathormone, calcium, or phosphorus. Calcinosis cutis has also been observed in an infant infected in utero with HIV (Fig. 14–71).

In addition to the diseases described, a host of poorly defined inflammatory skin disorders has been noted in patients with HIV disease. These are thought to occur as a consequence of cutaneous eruptions developing in the setting of an abnormal immune state that includes diminished neutrophil function, elevated serum levels of IgE, abnormal T-cell, B-cell, and macrophage function, and the presence of circulating antiepidermal antibodies. Widespread scaly

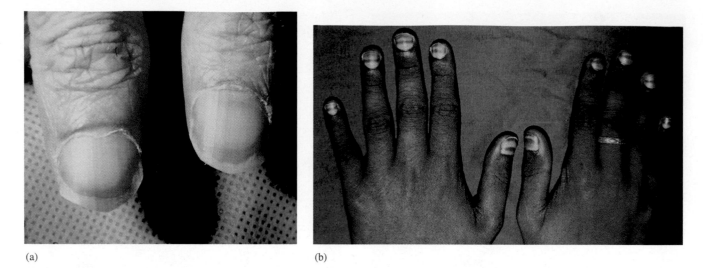

(a)   (b)

Figure 14–69. (a) Terry's nails in a patient with advanced AIDS. Such nail changes should be distinguished from (b) "half-and-half" nails, which are associated with uremia. (Photograph b courtesy of J. K. Maniar, M.D., Department of Dermatovenereology and AIDS Medicine, G. T. Hospital, Grant Medical College, Mumbai, India.)

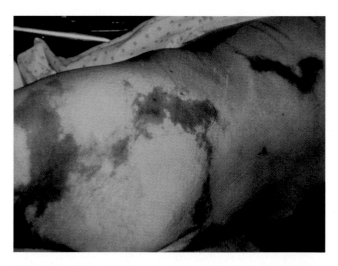

Figure 14–70. Calciphylaxis in an HIV-seropositive patient with chronic renal failure. (Reprinted by permission, J Am Acad Dermatol 26:559–562, 1992.)

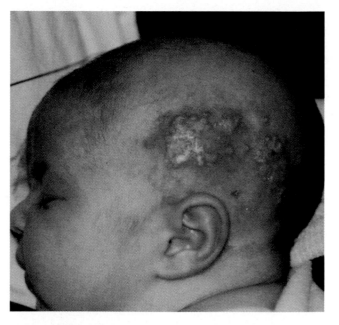

Figure 14–71. Calcinosis cutis in an infant infected with HIV in utero. (Photograph courtesy of San Chen, M.D., Department of Dermatology, University of Texas Medical Branch at Galveston, Galveston, TX.)

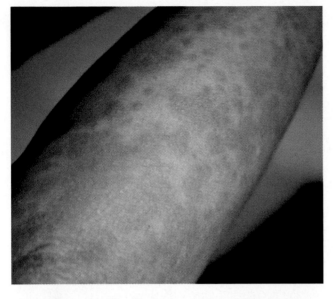

Figure 14–72. Evolving erythema multiforme.

dermatoses, erythema multiforme (Fig. 14–72), diffuse noninfectious granulomatous dermatitis, gyrate erythema-like eruptions (Fig. 14–73), and serum sickness–like eruptions (Fig. 14–74) correlate poorly if at all with classically described clinical disorders. In addition to the unusual clinical picture, histopathological findings correlate with clinical findings in only 30% of cases. Other unusual cutaneous conditions include lichenoid granulomatous dermatitis, exaggerated responses to insect bites, Sweet's syndrome (Fig. 14–75), disseminated granuloma annulare (Fig. 14–76), and nonspecific cellulitis [104].

Features of adult Kawasaki's disease include the age of onset, pneumonia, arthritis, aseptic meningitis, and the

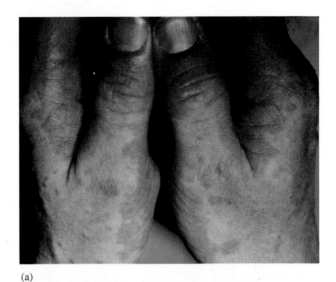

(a)

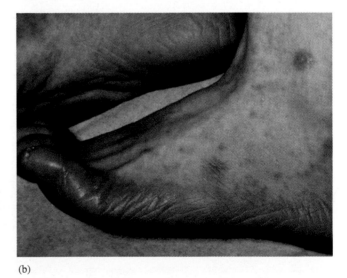

(b)

Figure 14–74. (a, b) Serum sickness–like eruption in HIV-infected patient that developed shortly after a wasp sting.

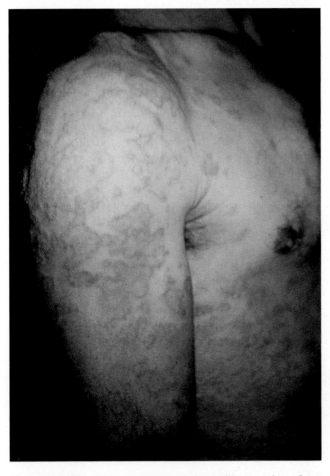

Figure 14–73. Unusual gyrate erythema-like eruption of unknown etiology in an HIV-infected patient.

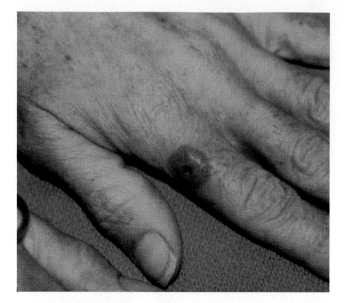

Figure 14–75. Sweet's syndrome associated with a squamous cell carcinoma of the lung in an HIV-infected host.

absence of cardiac involvement or thrombocytosis. Clinically, patients had fever of more than 5 days' duration that was unresponsive to antibiotics and that was associated with bilateral conjunctivitis, a generalized confluent macular eruption with edema of the hands that underwent desquamation, oral mucous membrane changes, and cervical adenopathy.

Acute allergic contact dermatitis and acute anaphylactic

reactions as a consequence of latex sensitivity have also been reported in HIV-infected patients [105].

Malnutrition becomes a common problem in individuals with HIV disease. Cutaneous manifestations of protein and vitamin deficiencies may be encountered. An eruption of multiple spiny follicular papules known as phrynoderma may be a manifestation of vitamin A deficiency. Vitamin C deficiency results in scurvy, which is manifested as bleeding gums and perifollicular petechiae. Pellagra (pyridoxine deficiency) is evidenced as a blistering photosensitive eruption with hyperpigmentation that is associated with diarrhea and dementia. Kwashiorkor presents with dry scaly areas of the skin, the so-called "flaky-paint" dermatitis. Diminished luster to the hair and a reddish-orange color may also be noted. Treatment with nutritional zinc replacement reduces periorificial erythema that is a manifestation of acrodermatitis enteropathica [106]. Advanced AIDS may also be associated with diffuse hyperpigmentation and necrotizing gingivitis (Fig. 14–77).

NEOPLASTIC DISORDERS

A number of different neoplastic disorders may develop in patients with HIV disease. These may be classified as epithelial, lymphoreticular, vascular, smooth muscle, and melanocytic.

Epithelial Cutaneous Neoplasms

Definition

Epithelial neoplasms are either benign or malignant proliferations, such as (1) neoplasms of the anorectal area, in-

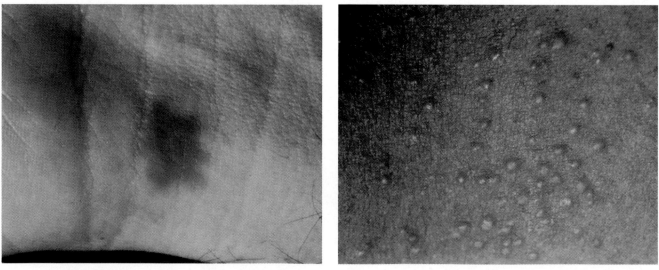

(a)   (b)

Figure 14–76. (a, b) Disseminated HIV-associated granuloma annulare. Plaques may mimic those of Kaposi's sarcoma.

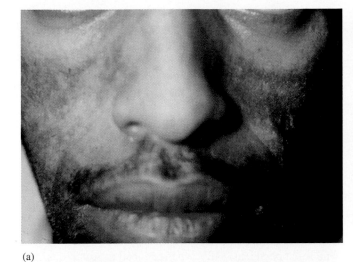

(a)

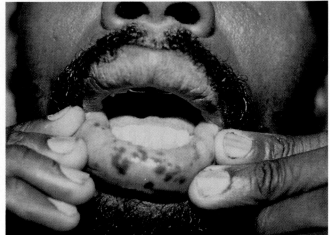

(b)

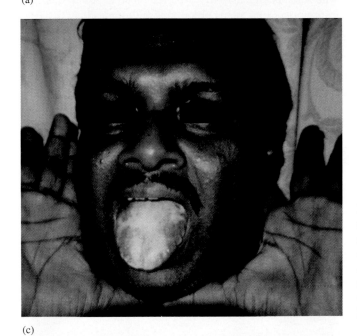

(c)

Figure 14–77. (a–c) Diffuse hyperpigmentation associated with advanced AIDS. (d, e) Necrotizing gingivitis with loss of teeth noted in E. (Photograph b courtesy of Jeffrey Callen, M.D., Division of Dermatology, Department of Internal Medicine, University of Louisville School of Medicine, Louisville, KY; photograph c courtesy of J. K. Maniar, M.D., Department of Dermatovenereology and AIDS Medicine, G.T. Hospital, Grant Medical College, Mumbai, India.)

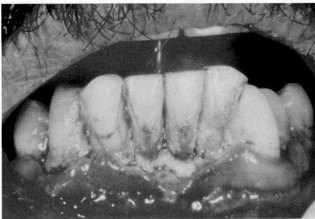

(d)

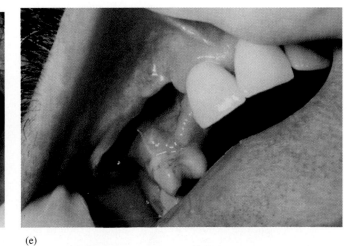

(e)

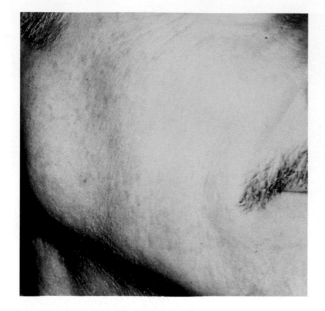

Figure 14–78. Parotid gland tumor in an HIV-seropositive patient. (Photograph courtesy of Axel Hoke, M.D., Novato, CA.)

cluding anal intraepithelial neoplasia, squamous cell carcinoma in situ, fully developed squamous cell carcinoma and cloacogenic carcinoma; (2) both cervical intraepithelial neoplasia and fully developed cervical carcinoma in HIV-infected women; (3) bowenoid papulosis; (4) basal cell carcinoma, both multiple, primary, and metastatic; (5) multiple cutaneous squamous cell carcinomas associated with epidermodysplasia verruciformis; and (6) multiple sebaceous gland tumors. Other noncutaneous epithelial neoplasms that have been observed in patients with HIV infection include small cell carcinoma of the lung, anaplastic carcinoma, testicular germ cell tumors, seminoma, transitional cell carcinoma of the bladder, and parotid gland tumors (Fig. 14–78).

Epidemiology

The incidence of epithelial neoplasms in patients infected with HIV is markedly increased, most commonly in oral, cervical, and anorectal locations [107]. Bowenoid papulosis, cloacogenic carcinoma, and transitional cell carcinoma are also increased in incidence. These neoplasms, as well as carcinoma of the cervix, are thought to be related to repeated trauma and human papillomavirus (HPV) infection.

HPV infection is highly prevalent as vulvar HPV infection, condyloma acuminata, and vulvar intraepithelial neoplasia. Invasive squamous cell carcinoma arising in HPV-induced anal intraepithelial neoplasia or cervical intraepithelial neoplasia has become a major clinical problem as

patients with HIV infection survive longer [108–110]. Epidermodysplasia verruciformis, a condition of widespread HPV infection with multiple carcinomas, has been reported in several patients with HIV infection.

Pathogenesis

HPV infection, deficient cell-mediated immunity, the HIV *tat* protein, and other, less understood factors interact to promote epithelial neoplasia in HIV-seropositive persons (see Chapter 12).

Clinical Manifestations

Invasive verrucous squamous cell carcinoma may occur either in the cervix or in the anorectal area (see Chapter 12). Bowenoid papulosis is generally manifested as brown-to-black flat-topped papules on the labia or penile skin. The same oncogenic HPV types can lead to squamous cell carcinoma of the penis or keratoacanthomas (Fig. 14–79). Epidermodysplasia verruciformis has a clinical appearance of widespread warty papules that are either pink or red. Metastases of basal cell carcinoma may occur, usually in draining lymph nodes and the lung.

Histopathology

The histopathological findings of these conditions range from subtle atypical intraepithelial proliferations within stratified squamous epithelial cells to full-thickness involvement of the epithelium by atypical neoplastic keratinocytes (see Chapter 12).

Laboratory Findings

HPV genomic DNA can be identified with neoplastic cells by the polymerase chain reaction in many cases (see Chapter 12).

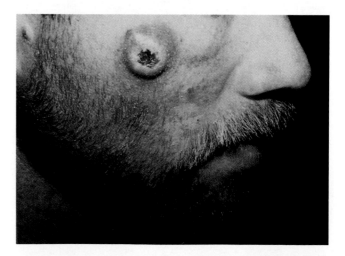

Figure 14–79. Keratoacanthoma associated with HPV infection.

Diagnosis

Diagnosis is established primarily on the basis of clinical appearance and skin biopsy (see Chapter 12).

Treatment

Treatment of squamous cell carcinoma usually requires excision or aggressive destructive measures (Table 14–12) (see Chapter 12).

Lymphoreticular Malignancies

Definition

A number of different lymphoreticular malignancies of both B- and T-cell lineage may involve lymph nodes and

Table 14-12.	Treatment of Neoplastic Disorders
Symptom	Treatment
Epithelial Cutaneous Neoplasms	
Squamous cell carcinoma	Surgical excision
	Carbon dioxide laser destruction
Bowenoid papulosis	Electrodesiccation and curettage
	Other destructive surgical methods
Basal cell carcinoma	Surgical excision, cryosurgery
Epidermodysplasia verruciformis	Surgical excision
	Destructive treatment methods
Lymphoreticular Malignancies	
Cutaneous T-cell lymphoma	Psoralen and ultraviolet A* therapy
	Total body electron beam
	Topical nitrogen mustard
Systemic lymphoma	Methotrexate, prednisone, bleomycin, doxorubicin, cyclophosphamide, vincristine
Kaposi's Sarcoma	Cryotherapy with liquid nitrogen
	Radiation therapy
	Electron beam therapy
	Intralesional injections of vinblastine sulfate, 0.2–0.4 mg/ml at biweekly intervals
	Intralesional interferon alpha-2b
	Alitretinoin gel
	Liposomally encapsulated doxorubicin and daunorubicin
	Photodynamic therapy
	Isotretinoin plus interferon

* Many of these agents may accelerate immunocompromise and accelerate death.

the reticuloendothelial system, although the skin may be involved primarily or secondarily. Non-Hodgkin's lymphoma, mostly high grade (small noncleaved cell and large cell immunoblastic) and intermediate grade (diffuse large cell) B-cell lymphomas, is seen most commonly in HIV patients, although cutaneous T-cell lymphomas, Hodgkin's disease, lymphomatoid granulomatous (angiocentric peripheral T-cell lymphoma), and adult T-cell leukemia-lymphoma caused by HTLV-1 (human T-cell lymphotropic virus) have been reported.

Incidence

Non-Hodgkin's and Hodgkin's lymphomas have increased in the greatest proportion in patients with HIV infection. Other lymphomas, such as cutaneous T-cell lymphoma, have been reported sporadically.

Pathogenesis

Approximately 25% of AIDS patients with non-Hodgkin's lymphoma have had histological findings of follicular hyperplasia observed on biopsy. These lymph nodes contain polyclonal proliferations of B lymphocytes, a finding similar to what is seen in African children with endemic Burkitt's lymphoma as well as in iatrogenically immunosuppressed patients. Polyclonal B-cell proliferation is thought to be caused directly by viral infection or as a consequence of loss of T-cell immunoregulation. Clonal immunoglobulin heavy-chain rearrangements, however, have been found in HIV-associated lymph node hyperplasia, suggesting a premalignant nature of such proliferations.

EBV infection is another factor of importance in the pathogenesis of HIV-related lymphoma, as this virus may be found in a high percentage of HIV-associated non-Hodgkin's lymphomas. Activation of the B-cell arm of the immune system develops in HIV-infected patients as a consequence of constant stimulation by foreign antigens. Concomitant infection by EBV may lead to immortalization of infected lymphocytes, resulting in uncontrolled lymphoproliferation and, eventually, malignancy.

Clinical Manifestations

Although lymphoma usually involves visceral sites, the skin may have pink to purplish papules or nodules with non-Hodgkin's lymphoma (Fig. 14–80). Deeply seated soft-tissue involvement may expand superficially, forming dome-shaped nodules that often ulcerate. Cutaneous Hodgkin's disease appears similar to non-Hodgkin's lymphoma either as diffuse nodular lesions or as a "panniculitis." HIV-related cutaneous T-cell lymphoma may have a clinical appearance similar to the widespread plaques of mycosis fungoides. HTLV-1 lymphoma may also resemble mycosis fungoides. Lymphomas can also result in osteolysis

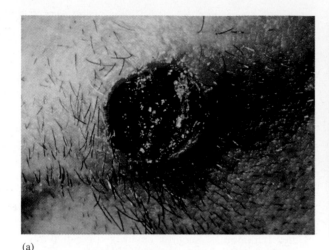

(a)

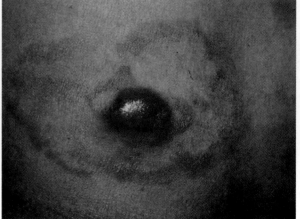

(b)

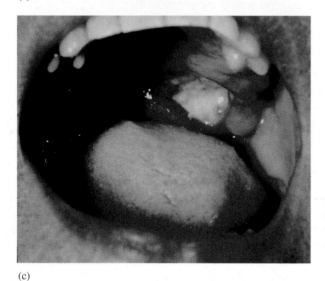

(c)

Figure 14–80. HIV-associated lymphoma presenting as (a) ulcers, or (b) nodules of the glabrous skin, and (c) mucosal ulcers. (Photograph b courtesy of Rajani Katta, M.D., Department of Dermatology, Baylor College of Medicine, Houston, TX.)

(Fig. 14–81). A unique malignancy described in HIV-seropositive persons is the CD30 + lymphoma (Fig. 14–82).

Histopathology

When the skin is involved by lymphoma, there is generally a diffuse infiltrate of atypical lymphoid cells that are monomorphous in appearance. Many of the cells are large, pleomorphic, and in mitosis. The infiltrate tends to be deeply situated, involving the lower portions of the dermis and subcutaneous fat, and there is often extensive necrosis as well as obliteration of pre-existing adnexal structures. Hodgkin's disease may have an appearance similar to that of an inflammatory infiltrate in the skin, although the diffuse nature of the infiltrate and the presence of large, atypical cells having a Reed-Sternberg–like morphology generally aid in making the diagnosis. Cutaneous T-cell

lymphoma is usually manifested histologically by psoriasiform hyperplasia of the epidermis with a band-like infiltrate of atypical lymphocytes; many have convoluted nuclei with a cerebriform appearance. These cells are also present in the epidermis, where they often form small collections. In cases of HTLV-1–associated lymphoma, neoplastic lymphocytes are often extremely large and multilobulated, with a "clover-leaf" appearance. There is also usually prominent exocytosis and, in that there is an associated leukemia, atypical lymphoid cells are often seen in blood vessels and lymphatics.

Laboratory Findings

Patients may have abundant circulating atypical lymphocytes that may number up to 600,000 cells/mm^3 in Sézary's syndrome and in adult T-cell lymphoma/leukemia. In con-

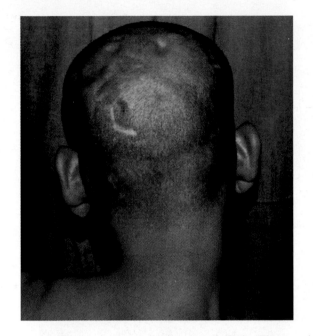

Figure 14–81. Lymphoma resulting in osteolysis. (Photograph courtesy of J. K. Maniar, M.D., Department of Dermatovenereology and AIDS Medicine, G. T. Hospital, Grant Medical College, Mumbai, India.)

trast, when hemophagocytosis or extensive bone marrow involvement supervenes, there may be profound anemia and pancytopenia.

Diagnosis

The routine diagnosis of these neoplasms is based on the characteristic clinical appearance taken in the context of histopathological features. In many cases, gene rearrangement studies, flow cytometric immunological analysis, and the use of DNA probes are necessary to further characterize and subtype the neoplasm. Immunophenotyping of mycosis fungoides–like cutaneous T-cell lymphoma in HIV patients may be characterized by an infiltrate of CD8 + lymphocytes in some cases. HTLV-1–associated leukemia-lymphoma is characterized by an infiltrate of CD4 + cells with absent CD2 + and CD7 + antigens [111].

Treatment

Treatment consists of the usual therapy for systemic lymphoma (methotrexate, prednisone, bleomycin, doxorubicin, cyclophosphamide, vincristine). Cutaneous T-cell lymphoma may respond to treatment with psoralen and ultraviolet A therapy, total body electron beam, and topical nitrogen mustard. As patients are already immunocompromised, administration of many of these agents may cause profound exacerbation of this condition with acceleration of death (Table 14–12).

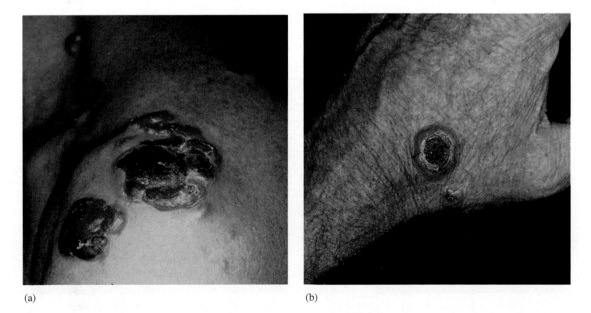

(a)   (b)

Figure 14–82. (a and b), CD30 + lymphoma producing cutaneous nodules. (Photographs courtesy of Jeffrey Callen, M.D., Division of Dermatology, Department of Internal Medicine, University of Louisville School of Medicine, Louisville, KY.)

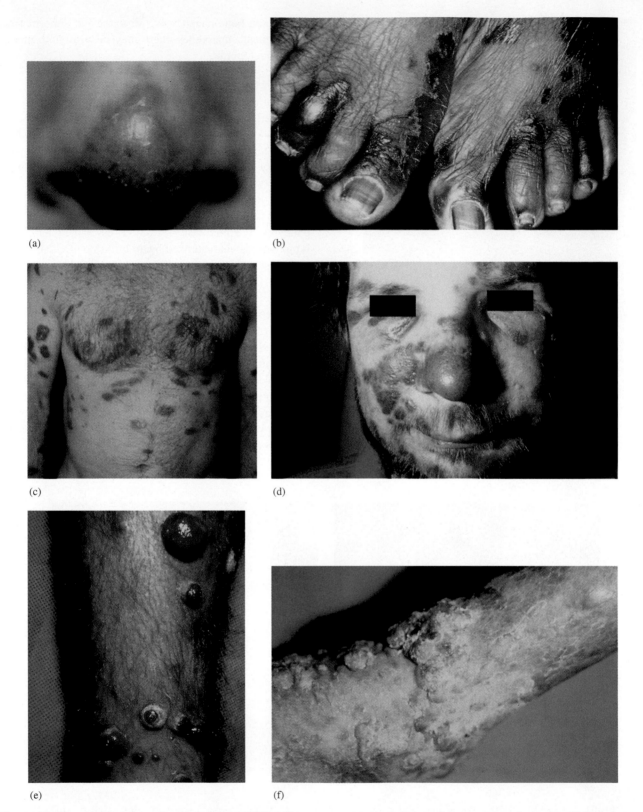

(a)

(b)

(c)

(d)

(e)

(f)

Figure 14–83. (a) Patch to early plaque stage of Kaposi's sarcoma. (b) Involvement of feet and legs in pattern similar to that of classic Kaposi's sarcoma. (c, d) Extensive disseminated plaques may be severely cosmetically disfiguring. (e, f) Nodular stage of Kaposi's sarcoma with f showing verrucous morphology.

KAPOSI'S SARCOMA

Definition

Kaposi's sarcoma (KS) is a vascular neoplastic disorder that normally occurs in an isolated subset of individuals. First described by Moritz Kaposi in 1872, it is the most frequent neoplastic disorder to develop in patients with AIDS.

Epidemiology

Shortly after the beginning of the AIDS epidemic, the frequency of occurrence of KS increased significantly. With the widespread use of HAART, the prevalence of KS dropped dramatically. The disorder has continued to be far less common among intravenous drug users and is rare in women, hemophiliacs and their sexual partners. In some regions of Africa, the incidence of KS in women approaches 40% of the total number of KS cases related to HIV infection [112]. In patients with KS but no HIV infection, the disease tends to have a more indolent course similar to that observed in elderly Italian and Jewish men [113].

Pathogenesis

Many features suggest that KS may be transmitted by a sexually transmissible agent [114], as human herpesvirus 8 (HHV8) DNA genomic sequences appear in almost 100% of KS lesions that have been studied [115] (see Chapter 10).

Clinical Manifestations

Clinically, KS skin lesions may be pink, red, brown, or purple macules, patches, plaques, nodules, or tumors (see Chapter 10) (Figs. 14–83 to 14–85).

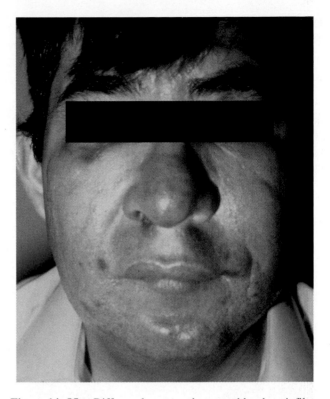

Figure 14–85. Diffuse edema may be caused by deep infiltrative involvement by Kaposi's sarcoma and lead to a vena cava-like syndrome.

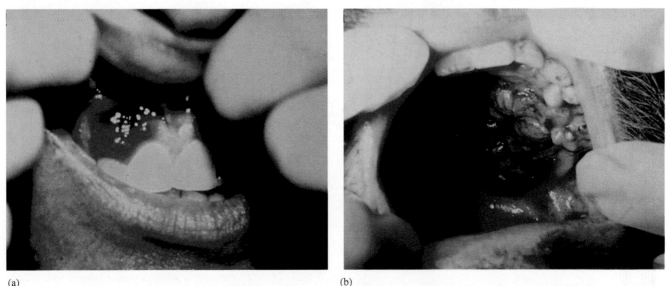

(a) (b)

Figure 14–84. (a, b) Oral mucosal involvement with Kaposi's sarcoma.

Histopathology

The histopathological findings of Kaposi's sarcoma vary with the stage of the lesion in question (see Chapter 10).

Laboratory Findings

No specific laboratory findings are seen in patients with AIDS-related KS, but degree of immunosuppression is a correlate. As a result of marked improvement of the immune status in most patients treated with HAART, KS has become much less common.

Diagnosis

Diagnosis is generally based on the characteristic clinical features of purplish skin lesions in the appropriate clinical setting in conjunction with histopathological findings. The neoplasm occurs only rarely in women and children.

Treatment

It is recommended that, unless medically necessary [116,117], no additional treatment be undertaken for KS until HAART has been administered for several months (see Chapter 10) (Fig. 14–86).

Other Cutaneous Neoplasms

Several other cutaneous malignancies have been reported in HIV-seropositive patients. Malignant melanoma may be quite aggressive, even those with Breslow thicknesses of 0.6–1.4 mm. One patient had an amelanotic malignant melanoma of the neck that clinically mimicked molluscum contagiosum (Fig. 14–87). In addition to melanoma, eruptive multiple dysplastic nevi have been observed in these individuals in some cases (Fig. 14–88).

Smooth muscle tumors including leiomyoma, leiomyosarcoma, and nodal myofibroblastoma have been described in children [118]. The synchronous development of multiple tumors in this age group is extremely rare; therefore the association with HIV infection is likely to be definitive.

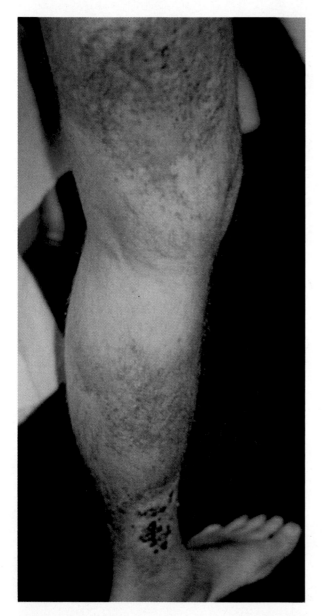

Figure 14–86. Kaposi's sarcoma following local irradiation. Often there is significant residual disease, as seen here.

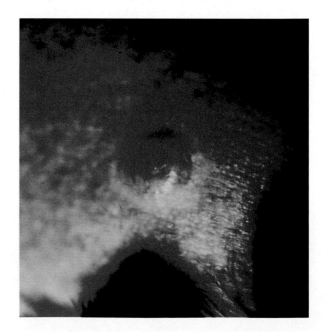

Figure 14–87. Amelanotic melanoma in a patient with AIDS. Note the similarity to either a basal cell carcinoma or a giant molluscum contagiosum lesion.

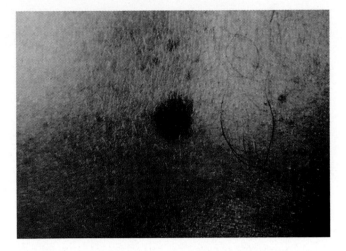

Figure 14–88. Dysplastic nevus in a patient with HIV infection.

ANTIRETROVIRAL THERAPY

Highly active antiretroviral therapy (HAART) is complex for both the physician and patient and usually consists of three or more antiretroviral drugs from two or three of the four different classes of drugs (Table 14–13). An HIV expert is required to carry out the complex task of combining drug classes, negotiating treatment regimens, and monitoring laboratory parameters.

Serious side effects, patient compliance, and risk of resistant strains emerging from suboptimal or inappropriate dosing complicate current antiretroviral therapy. The following antiretroviral drugs are currently available: (1) *Nucleoside Reverse Transcriptase Inhibitors (NRTIs):* zidovudine (Retrovir) [AZT]; lamivudine (Epivir) [3TC]; lamivudine/zidovudine (Combivir); stavudine (Zerit) [D4T]; didanosine (Videx) [ddI]; zalcitabine (Hivid) [ddC]; and abacavir (Ziagen); and abacavir + lamivudine + zidovudine (Trizivir). (2) *Non-Nucleoside Reverse Transcriptase Inhibitors (NNRTIs):* nevirapine (Viramune); delavirdine (Rescriptor); and efavirenz (Sustiva). (3) *Nucleotide Reverse Transcriptase Inhibitors:* tenofovir (Viread). (4) *Protease Inhibitors:* saquinavir (Fortovase); saquinavir (Invirase); ritonavir (Norvir); indinavir (Crixivan); nelfinavir (Viracept); amprenavir (Agenerase); and lopinavir + ritonavir (Kaletra).

Antiretroviral therapy is recommended for any symptomatic HIV-positive patient, for postexposure prophylaxis, and for pregnant women to prevent vertical transmission.

The decision to start treatment in asymptomatic patients is based on the patient's willingness to adhere to the complex drug regimen, both the immunological and virological parameters and a risk/benefit analysis. Patients with CD4 counts less than 350 CD4+ cells/mm^3 and an HIV RNA viral load greater than 30,000 copies/ml (bDNA assay) or 55,000 copies/ml (RT-PCR assay) are candidates for treatment [119].

Virological status is a better predictor of clinical outcome, although both viral load and CD4 counts are predictors of patient prognosis [119]. Maximal durable viral suppression, immunological restoration, and improved quality of life [119] are the ultimate goals of therapy. Combination therapy with a protease inhibitor plus two NRTIs usually achieves maximal durable viral suppression. Efavirenz, the NNRTI, may be used in place of a protease inhibitor (PI) [119]. Two PIs, ritonavir and saquinavir, in combination with two NRTIs [119], is another option.

Patients must be monitored for adverse events and treatment response following initiation of treatment. Optimal response is defined as (at least) a one log decrease in viral load at 8 weeks and no detectable virus (<50 copies/ml) at 4–6 months of therapy [119]. Viral load measurements should be monitored every 3–4 months once a patient is on therapy. An entirely new regimen with a minimum of two new agents not likely to demonstrate cross-resistance should be instituted following primary treatment failure.

Nucleoside Reverse Transcriptase Inhibitors (NRTIs)

Starting with AZT, NRTIs were the first class of antiretroviral drugs introduced in 1987. They are dideoxynucleoside analogues, which are phosphorylated intracellularly into the active triphosphate form. The triphosphate metabolite acts as an alternate substrate for the enzyme, competitively inhibiting reverse transcriptase. Once the metabolite is incorporated into the developing DNA strand, chain termination ensues (Fig. 14–89). A common adverse effect is lactic acidosis with hepatomegaly; hepatic steatosis is rare but is a potentially life-threatening toxicity seen with use of NRTIs (Table 14–13).

Zidovudine (Retrovir) [AZT]

The first NRTI introduced in 1987 was zidovudine, but it was synthesized in the 1960s as an antineoplastic drug. Monotherapy was the antiviral treatment of choice in HIV-infected patients when AZT was the only antiretroviral drug available, but zidovudine–specific resistant HIV strains have evolved. Delayed CD4 count decline and improved survival rates were observed among AZT recipients [120]. Reduced susceptibility isolates are recovered after only 6 months of monotherapy with zidovudine, and resistance increases with continued use [121]. When HAART is available, antiretroviral monotherapy is no longer a treatment option.

Table 14–13. Antiretroviral Therapy

Drug	Form	Dose	Dietary	Adverse events	Laboratory tests
Nucleoside Reverse Transcriptase Inhibitors (NRTIs)					
Zidovudine (Retrovir) AZT	100-mg caps 300-mg tabs 10 mg/ml IV solution 10 mg/ml oral solution	200 mg tid 300 mg bid	None	Bone marrow suppression: anemia or neutropenia GI: nausea, vomiting, hepatotoxicity, hepatic steatosis Others: fatigue, metabolic acidosis, myopathy, myositis, headache, insomnia, hyperpigmented and slow-growing nails, urticaria, pruritus, nonspecific maculopapular rash	CBC (monthly) Electrolytes, creatine kinase, and liver function tests (every 3 months)
Lamivudine (Epivir) 3TC	150-mg tabs 10 mg/ml solution	150 mg bid	None	Nausea, vomiting, anorexia, lactic acidosis, hepatic steatosis, peripheral neuropathy, headache, malaise, pancreatitis, hyperglycemia, fatigue, psychosis, and mania	Amylase, lipase
Stavudine (Zerit) D4T	15-mg caps 20-mg caps 30-mg caps 40-mg caps 1 mg/ml solution	40 mg bid	None	Peripheral neuropathy, lactic acidosis Hepatic steatosis, myopathy, and pancreatitis	Amylase, lipase, liver function tests
Didanosine (Videx) ddI	25-mg tabs 50-mg tabs 100-mg tabs 150-mg tabs 200-mg tabs 167-mg sachets 250-mg sachets 400-mg EC caps	200 mg tabs bid; 250 mg powder bid 400 mg tabs qd	30 min before meals	Nausea, vomiting, diarrhea, peripheral neuropathy, pancreatitis, hepatitis, lactic acidosis with hepatic steatosis, dry mouth, hypertriglyceridemia, hyperuricemia, optic neuritis, and rash	Amylase, lipase, liver function tests, lipids
Zalcitabine (Hivid) ddc	0.375-mg tabs 0.75-mg tabs	0.75 mg tid	Avoid aluminum magnesium antacids	Peripheral neuropathy, neutropenia, pancreatitis, aphthous ulcers, somatitis, esophageal ulcers, hepatomegaly, steatosis, lactic acidosis, reported urticaria, and one anaphylactoid reaction	CBC, amylase, lipase

(continued)

Table 14–13. *(continued)*

Drug	Form	Dose	Dietary	Adverse events	Laboratory tests
Nucleoside Reverse Transcriptase Inhibitors (NRTIs)					
Abacavir (Ziagen) ABC	300-mg tabs 20-mg/ml solution	300 mg bid	None; avoid alcohol	Hypersensitivity syndrome, fever, maculopapular rash, nausea, vomiting, fatigue, diarrhea, anorexia, malaise, myalgias, arthralgias, lactic acidosis with hepatic steatosis, hepatitis, respiratory symptoms such as sore throat, cough, and shortness of breath	Amylase, lipase, creatine kinase, liver function tests
Combivir	300-mg AZT, 150 mg 3TC	bid	None	As above	CBC, electrolytes, creatine kinase, liver function tests, amylase, lipase
Trizivir	300-mg AZT, 150 mg 3TC, 300 mg ABC	bid	None	As above	CBC, electrolytes, creatine kinase, liver function tests, amylase, lipase
Non-Nucleoside Reverse Transcriptase Inhibitors (NNRTIs)					
Nevirapine (Viramune)	200-mg tabs 50 mg/5 ml suspension	200 mg × 14 d then, 200 mg bid	No antacids within 1 hr	Rash, Stevens-Johnson syndrome, and hepatitis	Liver function tests
Delavirdine (Rescriptor)	100-mg tabs 200-mg tabs	400 mg tid in 3 oz water	No antacids within 1 hour; low-fat diet	Rash, Stevens-Johnson syndrome Hepatitis, headaches, increased liver function test values	Liver function tests
Efavirenz (Sustiva)	50-mg caps 100-mg caps 200-mg caps	600 mg at night	Low-fat diet	Dizziness, insomnia, nightmares, delusions, hallucinations, amnesia, confusion, impaired concentration, somnolence, agitation, euphoria, depersonalization, depression, maculopapular rash, increased liver function test values, false-positive cannabinoid test	Liver function tests
Nucleotide Reverse Transcriptase Inhibitor					
Tenofovir (Viread)	300-mg tablet	300 mg daily	With meal	Gastrointestinal (diarrhea, nausea, vomiting, flatulence), lactic acidosis, hepatomegaly with steatosis	Liver function tests

(continues)

Table 14–13. (*continued*)

Drug	Form	Dose	Dietary	Adverse events	Laboratory tests
Protease Inhibitors					
Saquinavir (Fortovase)	200-mg caps, soft gel	1200 mg tid, soft gel	With food (within 2 hours of a meal)	Nausea, vomiting, diarrhea, hepatitis, lipodystrophy, hyperlipidemia,	Liver function tests, lipids, glucose
(Invirase)	200-mg caps, hard gel	400 mg tid, hard gel		diabetes mellitus, hyperglycemia, headache, elevated liver function values, lipodystrophy	
Ritonavir (Norvir)	100-mg caps 600 mg/7.5 ml solution	600 mg bid or 7.5 ml bid	With food; refrigerate caps not in solution	Nausea, vomiting, diarrhea, hepatitis, pancreatitis, hyperlipidemia, hyperglycemia, peripheral neuropathy, circumoral paresthesias, asthenia, abnormal fat distribution, unpalatable taste, maculopapular rash, increased creatine kinase, uric acid, and liver function test values	Liver function tests, lipids, amylase, lipase, glucose
Indinavir (Crixivan)	200-mg caps 333-mg caps 400-mg caps	800 mg q8h; separate dosing with ddI by 1 h	With food (1 h before or 2 h after meals); drink plenty of water	Nausea, vomiting, diarrhea, hepatitis, nephrolithiasis, acute interstitial nephritis, acute renal failure, hyperglycemia, diabetes mellitus, hyperlipidemia, hemolysis, thrombocytopenia, rash, abnormal fat distribution, headache, asthenia, blurred vision, dizziness, and metallic taste	Liver function tests, lipids, glucose, urinalysis, creatinine
Nelfinavir (Viracept)	250-mg tabs 50 mg/g powder	750 mg tid; or 1250 mg bid	With food	Diarrhea, hepatitis, hyperlipidemia, hyperglycemia, and abnormal fat redistribution	Liver function tests, lipids, glucose

(*continued*)

Table 14–13. (*continued*)

Drug	Form	Dose	Dietary	Adverse events	Laboratory tests
Protease Inhibitors					
Amprenavir (Agenerase)	50-mg caps 150-mg caps 15 mg/ml solution	1200 mg bid; 1400 mg bid solution	Avoid high-fat meals	Nausea, vomiting, diarrhea, hepatitis, circumoral paresthesias, hyperlipidemias, diabetes mellitus, hemolytic anemia, rash, lipodystrophy	Liver function tests, amylase, lipase, glucose
Lopinavir + Ritonavir (Kaletra)	133.3 mg lopinavir + 33.3 mg ritonavir; 80 mg lopinavir + 20 mg ritonavir (solution)	400 mg lopinavir + 100 mg ritonavir bid	With food	Nausea, vomiting, diarrhea, asthenia, increased transaminases, hyperglycemia, lipodystrophy, hyperlipidemia	Liver function tests, lipids, amylase, glucose, lipase

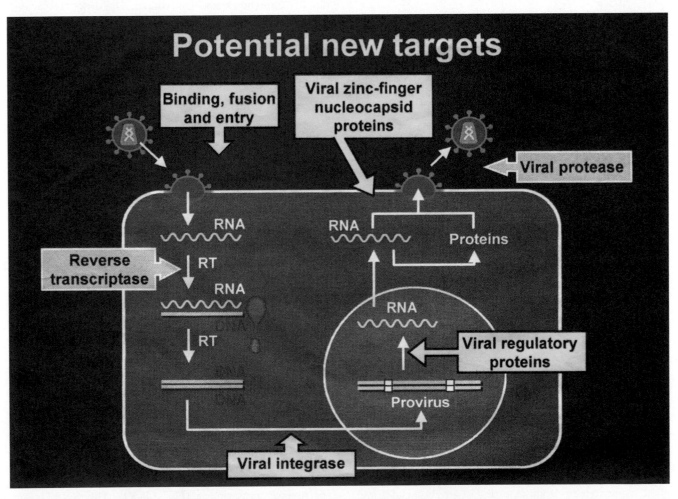

Figure 14–89. Sites of action of antiretroviral drugs. (Illustration courtesy of William O'Brien, M.D., Department of Internal Medicine, University of Texas Medical Branch at Galveston, Galveston, TX.)

The recommended dose of zidovudine is 300 mg bid with no dietary restrictions. Since zidovudine alters methadone levels, special care must be taken in the methadone-dependent patient.

Lamivudine (Epivir) [3T3]

Because lamivudine is active against both HIV and hepatitis B in HIV-infected patients with a concomitant hepatitis B infection receiving HAART therapy, it is the drug of choice. Significantly lower mortality rates and longer AIDS-free survival were observed in HIV-infected patients who received initial therapy with regimens including either lamivudine or stavudine than in those receiving initial therapies with regimens limited to zidovudine, didanosine, and zalcitabine [122]. The dose of lamivudine is 150 mg bid, but adjustment is recommended for renal impairment. No dietary restrictions or significant drug-drug interactions are noted.

Lamivudine/Zidovudine (Combivir)

A combination of lamivudine (150 mg) and zidovudine (300 mg) marketed as Combivir provides a convenient formulation that allows bid dosing with no dietary restrictions.

Stavudine (Zerit) [D4T]

Patients who have failed or are intolerant to other more common antiretroviral agents may be treated with stavudine [123], 40 mg bid. No dietary restrictions are recommended. A sensory neurological examination, routine liver function tests, and monitoring of amylase and lipase values are recommended every 3 months.

Didanosine (Videx) [ddI]

Patients unable to tolerate zidovudine or refractory to its effects may benefit from didanosine given as two 100-mg tablets bid. Didanosine must be taken 30 minutes prior to or 2 hours after a meal, since it is best absorbed in a nonacidic environment. Medications that require an acidic environment for absorption should not be given with it, as didanosine is formulated in an antacid buffer. Ketoconazole, itraconazole, dapsone, indinavir, delavirdine, pyrimethamine, quinolone antibiotics and related medications that require an acidic environment for absorption should be given at least 2 hours before or 6 hours after administration of didanosine.

Isolated elevated amylase levels may be observed [124], but the rare occurrence of pancreatitis is normally reversible upon termination of didanosine. Use of medications that affect the peripheral nerves, such as zalcitabine (ddC), isoniazid and chemotherapeutic drugs, may produce synergistic neurotoxicity. Routine testing of amylase and lipase levels, liver function tests, triglyceride checks, and a sensory neurological examination are recommended at least every 3 months.

Zalcitabine (Hivid) [ddC]

Zalcitabine is effective when used in combination therapy and is indicated in HIV infection demonstrating both immunological and virological failure. Probenicid increases the bioavailability of zalcitabine by 50%, but cimetidine, metoclopramide, and aluminum and magnesium hydroxide preparations decrease the bioavailability of zalcitabine. Amylase and lipase measurements, a complete blood count, and a sensory neurological exam must be performed every 3 months. The usual dose of zalcitabine is 0.75 mg tid.

Abacavir Sulfate (Ziagen)

Abacavir is a potent second-generation nucleoside analogue responsible for profound reductions in viral load and increases in CD4+ counts [125, 126]. Cross-resistance to abacavir is seen, with resistance among the nucleoside analogues zidovudine and lamivudine. The dose of abacavir is 300 mg tablets bid with no meal restrictions. Alcohol causes a synergistic increase in abacavir and is thus the only dietary restriction. An evolving maculopapular rash that is centripetal in distribution, urticarial in appearance, and becoming confluent characterizes the reversible hypersensitivity syndrome. Preceding the rash patients may experience fever, malaise, arthralgias, and myalgias. Patients should discontinue treatment if they experience a combination of these symptoms with a rash. They may continue the medication but must have close follow-up examination if a rash and fever are the only symptoms. The hypersensitivity syndrome usually resolves within 1 to 2 days of discontinuing the medication; a rechallenge with abacavir is contraindicated because hypotension or death could occur. Liver function tests and monitoring of creatine kinase, amylase, and lipase levels every 3 months are the recommended laboratory parameters for patients on abacavir.

Abacavir + Lamivudine + Zidovudine (Trizivir)

Trizivir combines 300 mg of zidovudine, 150 mg lamivudine, and 300 mg of abacavir (Table 14–13). One tablet is taken twice a day with no diet restrictions.

Non-Nucleoside Reverse Transcriptase Inhibitors (NNRTIs)

The NNRTIs are entirely unrelated to the nucleoside analogues but inhibit HIV replication at the same stage. These drugs are not incorporated into the developing viral DNA chain but noncompetitively bind directly to the active site of reverse transcriptase (Fig. 14–89). The NNRTIs are highly active against HIV-1 but not HIV-2. The NNRTIs do not require phosphorylation and are active in their native state [127]. Monotherapy is not an option since cross-resistance between other NNRTIs does occur [128,129]. Since their synergistic activity is more potent, these drugs are suited for combination therapy with nucleoside analogues and protease inhibitors. All of the NNRTIs are metabolized by the cytochrome P450 and may cause a rash and increases in transaminase levels (Table 14–13).

Nevirapine (Viramune)

Nevirapine, the first NNRTI introduced in 1996, binds to the HIV reverse transcriptase and blocks RNA and DNA-dependent DNA polymerase. Nevirapine is indicated in patients who have demonstrated immunological and virological failure and should be used in combination with nucleoside analogues. The usual dose is 200 mg bid. It is recommended that nevirapine be discontinued if the patient's clinical, immunological and virological status does not improve (because resistance develops quickly) [130]. The cytochrome P450 system, in particular the isozyme cytochrome P450 3A inducer (CYP3A), metabolizes nevirapine. Nevirapine's induction of CYP3A causes concentrations of other drugs such as protease inhibitors and rifampin to decrease, and dosage adjustment may be required because these drugs are similarly metabolized.

In about 50% of patients a transient and self-limiting pruritic erythematous, macular, papular eruption develops on the trunk, face, and extremities within 1 to 8 weeks [128,130,131]. In 6–7% of patients Stevens-Johnson syndrome can develop [132]. The clinician must terminate therapy with nevirapine if the rash that develops is noted to involve the mucous membranes, is moist, or becomes extensive and is accompanied by fever [133]. Nevirapine decreases methadone levels and should not be administered with cisapride. It is recommended that liver function tests be performed routinely every 3 months because liver toxicity is also a known side effect.

Delavirdine (Rescriptor)

The primary indication for delavirdine is in combination therapy [134]. The metabolism of delavirdine, like the other NNRTIs, depends on cytochrome P450 metabolism, specifically the 3A inhibitor isozyme. Since delavirdine inhibits the CYP3A enzyme, it inhibits the enzymatic metabolism of itself and other drugs; therefore, increased plasma levels of medications like cisapride, clarithromycin, terfenadine, astemizole, warfarin, protease inhibitors, benzodiazepines, and calcium channel blockers are observed and may cause life-threatening side effects if they are coadministered with delavirdine [135]. Since antacids and meals high in fat significantly reduce the absorption of delavirdine, a dose of four 100-mg tablets tid or four 100-mg tablets dissolved in at least 3 oz of water tid should be given 1 hour apart from these foods.

When delavirdine was administered with protease inhibitors, significant drug-drug interactions occurred. The concentrations of both saquinavir and indinavir are increased by delavirdine. The use of certain protease inhibitors like the soft gel saquinavir capsule (Fortovase) can cause potential synergistic liver toxicity. Liver function tests are recommended every 3 months.

Rash, Stevens-Johnson syndrome, and hepatitis are the most common side effects, as with other NNRTIs. Rashes develop within 1–3 weeks of starting treatment and resolve 3–14 days after onset in clinical studies [133,135].

Efavirenz (Sustiva)

Efavirenz, 600 mg qhs, must be administered in a combination cocktail with a protease inhibitor and/or NRTI [133]. Monotherapy is contraindicated because viral resistance can emerge.

As many as 50% of patients taking efavirenz reported mild side effects in clinical trials. Side effects were more common in patients with a history of psychiatric illness and substance abuse. Within the first few days of initiating therapy, the side effects appeared and then resolved within 7–14 days. In 27% of treated patients a macular papular eruption developed within the first 1–2 weeks of therapy. Liver function tests should be done every 3 months.

Taking certain drugs concomitantly is contraindicated because efavirenz is a mixed P450 3A inducer-inhibitor. The metabolism of some drugs is inhibited as a result of the enzyme competition, which increases their concentrations. Cisapride, midazolam, triazolam, clarithromycin, or ergot derivatives should not be administered with efavirenz, since life-threatening complications, such as cardiac arrhythmias, prolonged sedation, or respiratory depression can occur. Significant drug-drug interactions are possible with the protease inhibitors. When indinavir is coadministered with efavirenz, the levels of indinavir are decreased by 30%. Saquinavir levels are decreased by 60% with efavirenz.

Nucleotide Reverse Transcriptase Inhibitor

Tenofovir disoproxil fumarate (Viread) is the first nucleotide analogue that was approved (October 2001) for HIV-1 treatment. Nucleotides are similar to nucleoside analogues and block HIV replication in the same manner [136]. Tenofovir is to be used in combination with other antiretroviral drugs. It is available as a 300-mg tablet to be taken orally, with a meal.

Protease Inhibitors

Protease inhibitors (PIs), introduced in 1995, inhibit HIV protease, a virus-specific enzyme, which prevents the cleavage of viral polyproteins in the final stages of viral protein processing. This, in turn, prevents virus assembly, which results in a defective, noninfectious viral particle [137,138] (Fig. 14–89). PIs are effective in chronically infected cells and prevent replication in newly infected cells [139]. More effective in reducing the viral load than the nucleoside analogues, PIs are associated with increased body weight and improved quality of life [140–142]. However, they have been associated with a form of lipodystrophy resulting in abnormal fat accumulation in localized areas, commonly referred to as "protease pouch," "buffalo hump," and "crix belly" [143–146] (Table 14–13; Fig. 14–90). PIs have the disadvantages of high cost, common cross-resistance, poor central nervous system penetration, and significant drug-drug interactions [147]. All PIs are metabolized by the cytochrome P450 hepatic microsomal enzyme, CYP3A isozyme. Terfenadine, cisapride, triazolam, midazolam, or ergot derivatives cannot be given with PIs because plasma concentrations of either drug may require dosage adjustments to avoid potentially serious reactions.

Saquinavir (Fortovase) or Saquinavir (Invirase)

The first protease inhibitor approved for the treatment of HIV was saquinavir in the hard gel capsule in a dose of 600 mg tid. Saquinavir was reformulated shortly thereafter into the soft gel capsule, which resulted in a fivefold greater absorption and increased reduction in viral load [148].

Liver function tests, as well as glucose and lipid level determinations, are recommended every 3 months.

Since food increases drug levels six-fold, the standard dose of Fortovase is six 200-mg soft gel capsules three times a day (1200 mg) with a meal or within 2 hours after eating.

Ritonavir (Norvir)

The second PI to be approved for use in HIV patients was ritonavir [149]. A few cases of a maculopapular eruption and fever have been reported within a few days of treatment initiation. Several cases of hypermenorrhea also have been

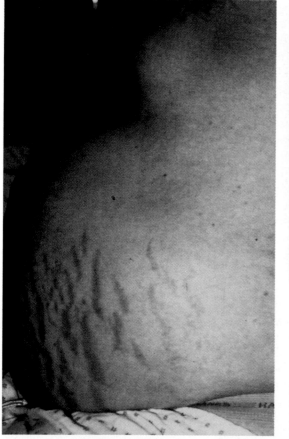

(a)

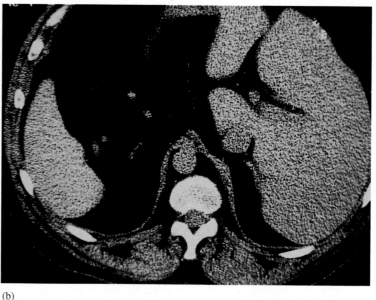

(b)

Figure 14–90. (a, b) Lipodystrophy in patients receiving HAART therapy for 5 years. (Photographs courtesy of Komal Chopra, M.D., Department of Dermatology, Columbia University School of Medicine, New York City, NY.)

reported [150]. A large meal must be taken with both the liquid and capsule preparations to decrease diarrhea and increase plasma levels 600-mg capsules bid or 7.5 ml bid. To enhance tolerance, gradual dose escalation is recommended over 10–14 days.

Liver function tests and glucose, lipid, amylase, and lipase level values are recommended every 3 months. When administering ritonavir to patients with chronic hepatitis B or C infection, care should be taken as with other drugs that may be potentially hepatotoxic.

Indinavir (Crixivan)

Indinavir was approved by the Food and Drug Administration (FDA) for use in HIV patients in 1997 (recommended dose is 800 mg tid) [151]. Nephrolithiasis may occur [142], since indinavir is poorly soluble in urine [152,153]. Patients are encouraged to drink at least 64 oz of water each day to maintain adequate hydration.

Food can decrease drug levels by 77%, so indinavir may be taken on an empty stomach or ingested with one of the 24 recommended dietary choices. Agents such as ddI, antacids, and sucralfate, which interfere with the gastric pH, should be avoided if taken concomitantly because indinavir requires an acidic pH for maximal absorption.

Nelfinavir (Viracept)

Prolonged viral suppression is observed when nelfinavir, approved for combination therapy in HIV patients in 1997, is used with two nucleoside analogues [133,154]. Nelfinavir should not be given with other protease inhibitors. The nelfinavir dose is three 250-mg tablets tid or 1250 mg bid, taken with food to increase levels two to threefold.

Amprenavir (Agenerase)

Amprenavir, which received FDA approval in 1999, must be administered as a cocktail with two nucleoside analogues [155]. A maculopapular rash occurs with rare progression to Stevens-Johnson syndrome. Amprenavir in 150-mg capsules, 1200 mg given twice a day, is administered with or without food. Liver function tests and amylase, lipase, and glucose level studies are recommended every 3 months. Each capsule of amprenavir contains 150 IU of vitamin E, but the long-term effect of 2400 IU (16 capsules) of vitamin E per day is not known.

Lopinavir + Ritonavir (Kaletra)

The coformulation of ritonavir and lopinavir (Kaletra) was FDA approved in 2000 for the treatment of HIV infection in adults and children 6 months and older in combination with other antiretroviral medications. This new treatment option, Kaletra, takes advantage of the ability of ritonavir to boost the levels of other PIs, creating a potent anti-HIV combination. The lopinavir-ritonavir (400/100 mg) combination given bid is the recommended regimen.

Antiretroviral Treatment Toxicities

Lactic Acidosis and Hepatic Steatosis

Obese females and persons with prolonged use of NRTIs are most at risk for lactic acidosis and hepatic steatosis, which are associated with high fatality rates [156,157]. The NRTIs may be at fault since they are thought to induce mitochondrial toxicity. Gastrointestinal complaints such as abdominal distention, nausea, vomiting, abdominal pain, diarrhea, anorexia, weight loss, and hepatomegaly are observed. An increased anion gap and elevated levels of aminotransferases, creatine phosphokinase, lactate dehydrogenase, lipase, and amylase may be seen [158]. Toxicities may spontaneously resolve following discontinuation of NRTIs, and an NRTI-sparing regimen is recommended. Progressive lactic acidosis, dyspnea, tachypnea, and ultimately respiratory failure may result from failure to suspend NRTI therapy in the presence of lactic acidosis and hepatic steatosis. Bicarbonate infusions and hemodialysis may be used for therapy [159].

Hyperglycemia

Hyperglycemia, diabetic ketoacidosis, exacerbation of preexisting diabetes, and new-onset diabetes mellitus are reported in patients receiving HAART. The protease inhibitors are usually involved, although poor glycemic control can occur with many of the antiretroviral agents [160]. Although the exact cause of the hyperglycemia is not known, it is suspected that beta cell dysfunction and peripheral insulin resistance could be the cause [160–162]. During the first year of therapy with protease inhibitors, it is recommended that fasting blood glucose levels be checked at least every 3–4 months.

Lipodystrophy

Changes in body fat distribution known as lipodystrophy are observed in patients on HAART therapy. Lipodystrophy can occur with any antiretroviral therapy and even in the absence of therapy, but it is often associated with the use of PIs and NRTIs [163–167]. The morphological changes of lipodystrophy may not be apparent for months after therapy initiation. Lipodystrophy appears clinically as central obesity secondary to visceral fat accumulation. Successful treatment standards have not been established [168–170], but therapy is aimed at halting the progression of the fat maldistribution.

Hyperlipidemia

During HAART therapy, there are increases in cholesterol and triglyceride levels. It is suspected that PIs interfere with normal cellular proteins involved in lipid metabolism, but the pathogensis of these lipid abnormalities is not known [171]. Long-term studies will provide evidence to determine whether PIs result in progression to premature cardiovascular disease [172]. Fasting laboratory lipid evaluations are recommended for patients receiving PIs every 3–4 months. The effectiveness of lipid-lowering agents, exercise, and diet modification to control hyperlipidemia is not clear. Potential enhanced hydroxymethyl-glutaryl coenzyme A reductase inhibitor–related toxicity also must be carefully monitored [119].

Increased Bleeding Episodes in Patients with Hemophilia

Increased episodes of spontaneous bleeding into joints, soft tissues, brain, and gastrointestinal system are noted in hemophiliacs using PIs [173]. Additional coagulation factor is required for some patients while on PI therapy.

Osteoporosis and Osteopenia

Patients on PI therapy have an increased risk of osteoporosis and osteopenia, but the pathogenesis of such adverse effects on bone metabolism is unknown.

Postexposure Prophylaxis

Postexposure prophylaxis is recommended for the management of health care workers who have been exposed to blood or body fluid that is tainted or is suspected as being from a patient with HIV.

Both basic and the expanded regimens are available for postexposure prophylaxis. For occupational HIV exposure for which there is a recognized transmission risk, the basic regimen is 4 weeks of zidovudine, 600 mg/day in divided doses, plus lamivudine, 150 mg bid [119]. For occupational HIV exposures that pose increased risk of transmission, such as a high viral load or a large volume of blood, the expanded regimen is recommended. A protease inhibitor, indinavir, 800 mg tid, or nelfinavir, 750 mg tid, is added to the basic regimen for the expanded regimen [119].

Investigational Drugs

Integrase inhibitors, fusion inhibitors, zinc finger inhibitors, and hydroxyurea are new drug classes under investigation.

Adefovir (Preveon) and the prodrug Bis-POC PMPA are nucleotide analogues that inhibit reverse transcriptase, and they both have broad-spectrum antiviral activity against HIV, several herpesviruses, and hepatitis B [174]. Adefovir is available through compassionate use programs. Nephrotoxicity has been noted in patients taking adefovir more than 20 weeks and resulted in the need for dialysis in two patients.

A once daily azapeptide protease inhibitor, BMS-232632, appears to be safe and well tolerated according to the results of a phase II study. It was as effective as five to ten times the amount of nelfinavir at reducing the HIV viral load [175] (Fig. 14–89). New classes of small molecules that specifically inhibit the incorporation of HIV DNA, called integrase inhibitors, have been isolated from the fungus, *Fusarium hetrosporum,* by randomly screening natural product extracts [176]. Strand transfer reactions in HIV-1 infected cells are inhibited by these compounds.

Fusion inhibitors are another entirely new class of compounds under development that inhibit viral fusion and specifically inhibit glycoprotein 41-mediated fusion and viral entry (Fig. 14–89) [177]. Clinical trials have shown that fusion inhibitors such as T-20, or petafuside, reduce viral loads faster than conventional therapy.

Halting glycoprotein 41 binding would stop HIV from infecting cells. Thus, a weak spot called the HIV "deep pocket" within the HIV glycoprotein 41 protein is a potential drug target.

Although indicated for the treatment of sickle cell anemia and certain types of malignancies, hydroxyurea is also currently being investigated for the treatment of HIV [178]. Reduced intracellular levels of deoxynucleoside triphosphates that are necessary for DNA synthesis [178] result from hydroxyurea inhibition of the cellular enzyme ribonucleotide reductase.

CONCLUSIONS

In summary, patients with HIV infection are prone to develop numerous cutaneous manifestations, especially if HAART is not available. The number of different expressions of disease in the skin is greater than that in any other organ and is the source of significant morbidity. By recognizing these signs and symptoms and performing appropriate diagnostic testing to establish correct diagnoses, these complications can be minimized significantly. It is possible, however, that the skin changes may be nonspecific, may be unique to one part of the world (such as fogo selvagem in Brazil) (Fig. 14–91), or may not be present. In the latter case, HIV seroconversion may still be associated with lymphadenopathy. In advanced AIDS, neurological defects may be caused by opportunistic infections that rarely have cutaneous manifestations (e.g., toxoplasmosis and the JC papovavirus causing progressive multifocal leukoencephalopathy). If, however, these clinical manifestations of HIV seroconversion are not present or noticed, many months or even years may pass before symptoms become obvious. In such cases, HIV infection will be diagnosed only if serological testing is carried out for reasons other than illness (e.g., blood donations, job or insurance physical examination).

Maximal viral suppression, sustained durability, decreased morbidity and mortality, increased CD4 count, decreased evolving resistance, and fewer side effects com-

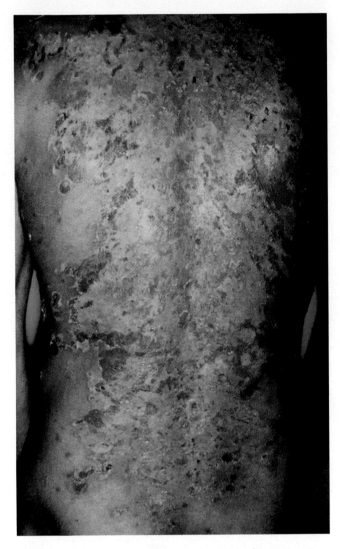

Figure 14–91. Fogo selvagem in a Brazilian AIDS patient. (Photograph courtesy of Walmar Roncalli P. DeOliveira, M.D., Sao Paulo, Brazil.)

control the epidemic include public awareness, education, condom use or abstinence, testing blood products, and not sharing needles. Despite these interventions, 16,000 people become infected with HIV every day. Therefore, it is clear that a safe and effective vaccine is needed to supplement these public health measures.

bined with increased compliance remain the goal of therapy among the different classes and complexity of antiretroviral regimens. The direction of therapy is best guided by serial viral load measurements, CD4 counts, and clinical assessments. Since HAART may cost $15,000 to $20,000 per year, it is not readily available to 99% of the estimated 40 million HIV-infected people in the world. Two NRTIs and a PI usually make up HAART, but other combination regimens exist. Since antiretroviral agents are not virucidal, viral eradication with HAART cannot be achieved. Viral loads return to pretreatment levels when HAART therapy is stopped. Drugs under investigation may prevent fusion between the HIV virus and healthy cells. Available tools to

REFERENCES

1. MS Gottlieb, R Schroff, HM Schanker, JD Weisman, PT Fan, RA Wolf, A Saxon. *Pneumocystis carinii* pneumonia and mucosal candidiasis in previously healthy homosexual men: evidence of a new acquired cellular immunodeficiency. N Engl J Med 305:1425–1431, 1981.
2. C Flexner. HIV—protease inhibitors. N Engl J Med 338: 1281–1291, 1998.
3. RM Gulick, JW Mellors, D Havlir, JJ Eron, C Gonzalez, D McMahon, D McMahon, DD Richman, FT Valentine, L Jonas, A Meibohm, EA Emini, JA Chodakewitz. Treatment with indinavir, zidovudine, and lamivudine in adults with human immunodeficiency virus infection and prior antiretroviral therapy. N Engl J Med 337:734–739, 1997.
4. B Autran, G Carcelain, TS Li, C Blanc, D Mathez, R Tubiana, C Katlama, P Debre, J Leibowitch. Positive effects of combined antiretroviral therapy on CD4 + T cell homeostasis and function in advanced HIV disease. Science 277:112–116, 1997.
5. S Staszewski, J Morales-Ramirez, KT Tashima, A Rachlis, D Skiest, J Stanford, R Stryker, P Johnson, DF Labriola, D Farina, DJ Manion, NM Ruiz. Efavirenz plus zidovudine and lamivudine, efavirenz plus indinavir, and indinavir plus zidovudine and lamivudine in the treatment of HIV-1 infection in adults. Study 006 Team. N Engl J Med 341: 1865–1873, 1999.
6. F Palella, K Delaney, AC Moorman, MO Loveless, J Fuhrer, GA Satten, DJ Aschman, SD Holmberg. Declining morbidity and mortality among patients with advanced human immunodeficiency virus infection. N Engl J Med 338:853–860, 1998.
7. JH Condra, WA Schleif, OM Blahy, LJ Gabryelski, DJ Graham, JC Quintero, A Rhodes, HL Robbins, E Roth, M Shivaprakash, et al. In vivo emergence of HIV-1 variants resistant to multiple protease inhibitors. Nature 374: 569–571, 1995.
8. D Finzi, M Hermankova, T Pierson, LM Carruth, C Buck, RE Chaisson, TC Quinn, K Chadwick, J Margolick, R Brookmeyer, J Gallant, M Markowitz, DD Ho, DD Richman, RF Siliciano. Identification of a reservoir for HIV-1 in patients on highly active antiretroviral therapy. Science 278:1295–1300, 1997.
9. BM Coldiron, PR Bergstresser. Prevalence and clinical spectrum of skin disease in patients infected with human immunodeficiency virus. Arch Dermatol 125:357–361, 1988.
10. B Tindall, S Barker, B Donovan, T Barnes, J Roberts, C Kronenberg, J Gold, R Penny, D Cooper. Characterization

of the acute clinical illness associated with human immunodeficiency virus infection. Arch Intern Med 148: 945–949, 1988.

11. S Safran, R Ashley, C Houlihan, PS Cusick, J Mills. Clinical and serologic features of herpes simplex virus infection in patients with AIDS. AIDS 5:1107–1110, 1991.

12. EC Klatt, D Shibata. Cytomegalovirus infection in the acquired immunodeficiency syndrome. Arch Pathol Lab Med 112:540–544, 1988.

13. H Masur. Clinical implications of herpes virus infections in patients with AIDS. Am J Med 92:1S–2S, 1992.

14. WE Stamm, HH Hansfield, AM Rompalo, RL Ashley, PL Roberts, L Corey. The association between genital ulcerative disease and acquisition of HIV infection in homosexual men. JAMA 260:1429–1433, 1988.

15. J Lawrence. Perspective. Molecular interactions among herpes viruses and human immunodeficiency viruses. J Infect Dis 162:338–347, 1990.

16. GL Marks, PE Nolan, KS Erlich, MN Ellis. Mucocutaneous dissemination of acylovir-resistant herpes simplex virus in a patient with AIDS. Rev Infect Dis 11:474–476, 1989.

17. AE Friedman-Kien, FL LaFleur, EC Gendler, NP Hennessey, R Montagna, S Halbert, P Rubinstein, K Krasinski, E Zang, B Poiesz. Herpes zoster: a possible early clinical sign for development of acquired immunodeficiency syndrome in high-risk individuals. J Am Acad Dermatol 14: 1023–1028, 1986.

18. S Pahwa, K Biron, W Lim, P Swenson, MH Kaplan, N Sadick, R Pahwa. Continuous varicella zoster infection associated with acyclovir resistance in a child with AIDS. JAMA 260:2879–2882, 1988.

19. IH Gilson, JH Barnett, MA Conant, OL Laskin, J Williams, PG Jones. Disseminated ecthymatous varicella-zoster virus infection in patients with acquired immunodeficiency syndrome. J Am Acad Dermatol 20:637–642, 1989.

20. PR Cohen, VP Beltranny, ME Grossman. Disseminated herpes zoster in patients with immunodeficiency virus infection. Am J Med 84:1076–1080, 1988.

21. MA Jacobson, TG Berger, S Fikrig, P Becherer, JW Moohr, SC Stanat, KK Biron. Acyclovir-resistant varicella zoster virus infection after chronic oral acyclovir therapy in patients with the acquired immunodeficiency syndrome (AIDS). Ann Intern Med 112:187–191, 1990.

22. KE Bowers. Cytomegalovirus infection. In: IM Freedberg, AZ Eisen, K Wolff, KF Austen, LA Goldsmiths, SI Katz, TB Fitzpatrick, eds. Fitzpatrick's Dermatology in General Medicine. McGraw-Hill NY, NY. Vol. II, 5th ed, 1999, pp 2540–2457.

23. D Greenspan, JS Greenspan, G Overby, H Hollander, DI Abrams, L MacPhail, C Borowsky, DW Feigal Jr. Risk factors for rapid progression from hairy leukoplakia to AIDS: a nested case-control study. J Acquir Immune Defic Syndr 4:652–658, 1991.

24. KJ Smith, HG Skelton, P Angritt. Histopathologic features of HIV-associated skin disease. Dermatol Clin 9:551–578, 1991.

25. CJ Cockerell. Cutaneous manifestations of HIV infection. In: AE Friedman-Kien, CJ Cockerell, eds. Color Atlas of AIDS. Philadelphia: WB Saunders, 1989, p 96.

26. JM Palefsky, J Gonzales, RM Greenblatt, DK Ahn, H Hollander. Anal intraepithelial neoplasia and anal papillomavirus infection among homosexual males with group IV HIV disease. JAMA 263:2911–2916, 1990.

27. MA Byrne, D Taylor-Robinson, PE Munday, JR Harris. The common occurrence of human papillomavirus in intraepithelial neoplasia in women infected by HIV. AIDS 3: 379–382, 1989.

28. JH Frazer, G Medley, RM Cratper. Association between anorectal dysplasia, human papillomavirus and immunodeficiency virus infection in homosexual men. Lancet 2: 657–660, 1986.

29. TG Berger, WS Sawchuk, C Leonardi, A Langenberg, J Tappero, PE Leboit. Epidermodysplasia verruciformis-associated papillomavirus infection complicating human immunodeficiency virus disease. Br J Dermatol 126:79–83, 1991.

30. A McMillan, PE Bishop. Clinical course of anogenital warts in man infected with HIV. Genitourin Med 65: 225–228, 1989.

31. RR Redfield, DC Wright, WD James, TS Jones, C Brown, DS Burke. Disseminated vaccinia in a military recruit with human immunodeficiency virus (HIV) disease. N Engl J Med 316:673–676, 1987.

32. TG Berger, I Greene. Bacterial, viral, fungal and parasitic infections in HIV disease and AIDS. Dermatol Clin 3: 465–492, 1991.

33. KJ Smith, HG Skelton, J Yeager, WD James, KF Wagner. Molluscum contagiosum. ultrastructure evidence for its presence in skin adjacent to clinical lesions in patients infected with human immunodeficiency virus type 1. Arch Dermatol 128:223–227, 1992.

34. CS Petersen, J Gerstoft. Molluscum contagiosum in patients with human immunodeficiency virus infection. Dermatology 184:19–21, 1992.

35. TJ Torok. Parvovirus and human disease. Adv Intern Med 37:431–455, 1992.

36. LA Ross, KS Kim, Z Comport. Successful treatment of disseminated measles in a patient with acquired immune deficiency syndrome: consideration of anti-viral and passive immunotherapy. Am J Med 88:313–314, 1990.

37. R Ganesh, D Castle, D Gibbon, I Phillips, C Bradbeer. Staphylococcal carriage in HIV infection. Lancet 2:558, 1989.

38. R Steinhart, AL Reingold, F Taylor, G Anderson, JD Wenger. Invasive *Haemophilus influenzae* infections in men with HIV infection. JAMA 268:3350–3352, 1992.

39. WL Strauss, SM Ostroff, DB Jernigan, TE Kiehn, EM Sordillo, D Armstrong, N Boone, N Schneider, JO Kilburn, VA Silcox, et al. Clinical and epidemiologic characteristics of *Mycobacterium haemophilum,* an emerging pathogen in immunocompromised patients. Ann Intern Med 120: 118–125, 1994.

40. PK Rohatgi, JV Palazzolo, NB Saini. Acute miliary tuberculosis of the skin in acquired immunodeficiency syndrome. J Am Acad Dermatol 26:285–287, 1992.

41. TC Quinn, RO Cannon, D Glasser, SL Groseclose, WS Brathwaite, AS Fauci, EW Hook 3rd. The association of syphilis with risk of human immunodeficiency virus infection in patients attending sexually transmitted disease clinics. Arch Int Med 150:1297–1302, 1990.

42. K Adal, CJ Cockerell, WP Petrie. Cat scratch disease, bacillary angiomatosis, and other infections due to *Rochalimaea*. N Engl J Med 330:1509–1515, 1994.

43. F Janssen, A Zelinsky-Gurung, E Caumes, JM Decazed. Group A streptococcal cellulitis-adenitis in a patient with the acquired immunodeficiency syndrome. J Am Acad Dermatol 24:363–365, 1991.

44. LK Dropulic, JM Leslie, LJ Eldred, J Zenilman, CL Sears. Clinical manifestations and risk factors of *Pseudomonas aeruginosa* infection in patients with AIDS. J Infect Dis 171:930–937, 1995.

45. LA Cone, DR Woodard, RG Byrd, K Schulz, SM Kopp, PM Schlievert. A recalcitrant, erythematous, desquamating disorder associated with toxin-producing staphylococci in patients with AIDS. J Infect Dis 165:638–643, 1992.

46. K Javaly, HW Horowitz, GP Wormser. Nocardiosis in patients with human immunodeficiency virus infection. Medicine 71:128–138, 1992.

47. M Drancourt, E Bonnet, H Gallais, Y Peloux, D Raoult. *Rhodococcus equi* infection in patients with AIDS. J Infect 24:123–131, 1992.

48. B Halioua, O Patey, D Casciani, JP Emond, A Dublanchet, JE Malkin, C Lafaix. Cutaneous diphtheria in a patient with HIV infection. Ann Dermatol Venereol 119:874–877, 1992.

49. CJ Cockerell, PE LeBoit. Bacillary angiomatosis. A novel pseudoneoplastic, infectious vascular disorder. J Am Acad Dermatol 22:501–519, 1990.

50. N Gregory, M Sanchez, MR Buchness. The spectrum of syphilis in patients with human immunodeficiency virus infection. J Am Acad Dermatol 22:1061–1067, 1990.

51. IS Strongin, SA Kale, MK Raymond, RL Luskin, GW Weisberg, JJ Jacobs. An unusual presentation of gonococcal arthritis in an HIV-positive patient. Ann Rheum Dis 50:572–573, 1991.

52. RL Regnery, BE Anderson, JE Clarridge 3d, MC Rodriguez-Barradas, DC Jones, JH Carr. Characterization of a novel *Rochalimaea* species, *R. henselae* sp. nov. isolated from blood of a febrile, human immunodeficiency virus-positive patient. J Clin Microbiol 30:265–274, 1992.

53. JE Koehler, FD Quinn, TG Berger, PE LeBoit, JW Tappero. Isolation of *Rochalimaea* species from cutaneous and osseous lesions of bacillary angiomatosis. N Engl J Med 327:1625–1631, 1992.

54. MD Geman. Treatment of multidrug resistant tuberculosis. N Engl J Med 329:784–791, 1993.

55. SM Skinner, RL DeVillez. Sepsis associated with Norwegian scabies in patients with acquired immunodeficiency syndrome. Arch Dermatol 50:213–216, 1992.

56. NP Hennessey, EL Parro, CJ Cockerell. Cutaneous *Pneumocystis carinii* infection in patients with acquired immunodeficiency syndrome. Arch Dermatol 127:1699–1701, 1991.

57. C Postigo, R Llamas, C Zarco, R Rubio, F Pulido, JR Costa, L Iglesias. Cutaneous lesions in patients with visceral leishmaniasis and HIV infection. J Infect 35:265–268, 1997.

58. E Leibovitz, M Rigaud, S Chandwani, A Kaul, MA Greco, H Pollack, R Lawrence, D Di John, B Hanna, K Krasinski, et al. Disseminated fungal infections in children infected with human immunodeficiency virus. Pediatr Infect Dis J 10:888–894, 1991.

59. DG Fish, NM Ampel, JN Galgiani, CL Dols, PC Kelly, CH Johnson, D Pappagianis, JE Edwards, RB Wasserman, RJ Clark, et al. Coccidioidomycosis during human immunodeficiency virus infection: a review of 77 patients. Medicine 69:384–391, 1990.

60. P Manrique, J Mayo, JA Alvarez, X Ganchegui, I Zabalza, M Flores. Polymorphous cutaneous cryptococcosis: Nodular, herpes-like, and molluscum-like lesions in a patient with the acquired immunodeficiency syndrome. J Am Acad Dermatol 26:122–124, 1992.

61. PR Cohen, ME Grossman, DN Silvers. Disseminated histoplasmosis and human immunodeficiency virus infection. Int J Dermatol 30:614–622, 1991.

62. MB Chaker, CJ Cockerell. Concomitant psoriasis, seborrheic dermatitis and disseminated cutaneous histoplasmosis in a patient infected with human immunodeficiency virus. J Am Acad Dermatol 29:311–313, 1993.

63. MC Cole, PR Cohen, KH Satra, ME Grossman. The concurrent presence of systemic disease pathogens and cutaneous Kaposi's sarcoma in the same lesion: *Histoplasma capsulatum* and Kaposi's sarcoma cocxisting in a single skin lesion in a patient with AIDS. J Am Acad Dermatol 26:285–287, 1992.

64. CL Terrell, CE Hughes. Antifungal agents used for deep-seated mycotic infections. Mayo Clin Proc 67:69–91, 1992.

65. J Romani, L Puig, E Baselga, JM De Moragas. Reiter's syndrome-like pattern in AIDS-associated psoriasiform dermatitis. Int J Dermatol 35:484–488, 1996.

66. RA Johnson. Cutaneous manifestations of human immunodeficiency virus disease. In: IM Freedberg, AZ Eisen, K Wolff, KF Austen, LA Goldsmith, SI Katz, TB Fitzpatrick, eds. Fitzpatrick's Dermatology in General Medicine, 5th ed. New York: McGraw-Hill, 1999, p 2312.

67. T Meola, NA Soter, R Ostrecher, M Sanchez, JA Moy. The safety of UVB phototherapy in patients with HIV infection. J Am Acad Dermatol 29:216–220, 1993.

68. AG Martin, CC Weaver, CJ Cockerell, TG Berger. Pityriasis rubra pilaris in the setting of HIV infection: clinical behaviour and association with explosive cystic acne. Br J Dermatol 126:617–620, 1992.

69. Le P Bozec, M Janier, P Reygagnee, L Pinquier, C Blanchet-Bardon, L Dubertret. Pityriasis rubra pilaris in a patient with AIDS. Acta Derm Venereol 118:862–864, 1991.

70. D Rosenthal, PE LeBoit, L Klumpp, TG Berger. Human immunodeficiency virus-associated eosinophilic folliculitis: a unique dermatitis associated with advanced human immunodeficiency virus infection. Arch Dermatol 127: 206–209, 1991.

71. NS Sadik, NS McNutt. Cutaneous hypersensitivity reactions in patients with AIDS. Int J Dermatol 32:621–627, 1993.

72. G Pantaleo, C Graziosi, AS Fauci. Immunopathogenesis of human immunodeficiency virus infection. N Engl J Med 328:327–335, 1993.

73. PE LeBoit, CJ Cockerell. Nodular lesions of erythema elevatum diutinum in patients with human immunodeficiency infection. J Am Acad Dermatol 28:919–922, 1993.

74. N Tojo, N Yoshimura, M Yoshizawa, M Ichioka, M Chida, I Miyazato, S Taniai, F Marumo, O Matubara, T Kato, et al. Vitiligo and chronic photosensitivity in human immunodeficiency virus infection. Jpn J Med 30:255–259, 1991.

75. MT Herranz, A el Amrani, P Aranegui, JF Jimenez-Alonso, JM Rodenas, RM Vivaldi. Porphyria cutanea tarda and acquired immunodeficiency syndrome: pathogenetic implications. Arch Dermatol 12:1585–1586, 1991.

76. BM Egbert, PE LeBoit, T McCalmont, CH Hu, C Austin. Caterpillar bodies: distinctive, basement membrane-containing structures in blisters of porphyria. Am J Dermatopathol June, 15:199–202, 1993.

77. CJ Cockerell. Successful treatment of HIV-related porphyria cutanea tarda with low-dose oral hydroxychloroquine. Poster Presentation, American Academy of Dermatology, Washington, DC. 1996.

78. KE Anderson, DE Goeger, RW Carson, SM Lee, RB Stead. Erythropoietin for the treatment of porphyria cutanea tarda in a patient on long-term hemodialysis. N Eng J Med 322:315–317, 1990.

79. SA Coopman, RA Johnson, R Platt, RS Stern. Cutaneous disease and drug reactions in HIV infection. N Engl J Med 328:1670–1674, 1993.

80. DW Metry, CJ Lahart, KL Farmer, AA Hebert. Stevens-Johnson syndrome caused by the antiretroviral drug nevirapine. J Am Acad Dermatol 44:354–357, 2001.

81. I Williams, IV Weller, A Malni, J Anderson, MF Waters. Thalidomide hypersensitivity in AIDS. Lancet 337: 436–437, 1991.

82. PJ Bayard, TG Berger, MA Jacobsen. Drug hypersensitivity reactions in human immunodeficiency virus disease. J Acquir Immune Defic Syndr 5:1237–1257, 1992.

83. PP Koopmans, AJ van der Ven, TB Vree, JW van der Meer. Pathogenesis of hypersensitivity reactions to drugs in patients with HIV infection: Allergic or toxic? AIDS 9: 217–222, 1995.

84. PC Don, F Fusco, P Fried, A Batterman, FP Duncanson, TH Lenox, NC Klein. Nail dyschromia associated with zidovudine. Ann Intern Med 112:145–146, 1990.

85. RG Greenberg, TG Berger. Nail and mucocutaneous hyperpigmentation with azidothymidine therapy. J Am Acad Dermatol 22:327–330, 1990.

86. F Bouscarat, C Bouchard. Paronychia and pyogenic granuloma of the great toes in patients treated with indinavir. N Engl J Med 338:1776–1777, 1998.

87. M Alam, RK Scher. Indinavir-related recurrent paronychia and ingrown toenails. Cutis 64:277–278, 1999.

88. F Bouscarat, MH Prevot, S Matheron. Alopecia associated with indinavir therapy. N Engl J Med 341:618, 1999.

89. A Darvay, K Acland, W Lynn, R Russell-Jones. Striae formation in two HIV-positive persons receiving protease inhibitors. J Am Acad Dermatol 41:467–469, 1999.

90. M Silva, PR Skolnik, SL Gorbach, Spiegelman D, IB Wilson, MG Fernandez-DiFranco, TA Knox. The effect of protease inhibitors on weight and body composition in HIV-infected patients. AIDS 12:1645–1651, 1998.

91. K Williamson, AC Reboli, SM Manders. Protease inhibitor-induced lipodystrophy. J Am Acad Dermatol 40: 635–636, 1999.

92. JC Lo, K Mulligan, VW Tai, H Algren, M Schambelan. "Buffalo hump" in men with HIV-1 infection. Lancet 351:867–870, 1998.

93. R Striker, D Conlin, M Marz, L Wiviott. Localized adipose tissue hypertrophy in patients receiving human immunodeficiency virus protease inhibitors. Clin Infect Dis 27: 218–220, 1998.

94. A Carr, DA Cooper. Images in clinical medicine. Lipodystrophy associated with an HIV-protease inhibitor. N Engl J Med 339:1296, 1998.

95. DM Aboulafia, D Bundow. Images in clinical medicine. Buffalo hump in a patient with the acquired immunodeficiency syndrome. N Engl J Med 339:1297, 1998.

96. VR Roth, S Kravcik, JB Angel. Development of cervical fat pads following therapy with human immunodeficiency virus type 1 protease inhibitors. Clin Infect Dis 27:65–67, 1998.

97. I Herry, L Bernard, P de Truchis, C Perronne. Hypertrophy of the breasts in a patient treated with indinavir. Clin Infect Dis 25:937–938, 1997.

98. MS Hirsch, A Klibanski. Editorial response: What price progress? Pseudo-Cushing's syndrome associated with antiretroviral therapy in patients with human immunodeficiency virus infection. Clin Infect Dis 27:73–75, 1998.

99. JW van der Pijl, PH Frissen, P Reiss, HJ Hulsebosch, JG Van Den Tweel, JM Lange, SA Danner. Foscarnet and penile ulceration. Lancet 335:286, 1990.

100. C Blanshard. Generalized cutaneous rash associated with foscarnet usage in AIDS. J Infect Dis 23:336–337, 1991.

101. MH Kaplan, NS Sadik, M Talmor. Acquired trichomegaly of the eyelashes—a cutaneous marker of acquired immunodeficiency syndrome. J Am Acad Dermatol 25: 801–804, 1991.

102. NS Sadick. Clinical and laboratory evaluation of AIDS trichopathy. Int J Dermatol 32:33–38, 1993.

103. CJ Cockerell, ET Dolan. Widespread cutaneous and sys-

temic calcification (calciphylaxis) in patients with the acquired immunodeficiency syndrome and renal disease. J Am Acad Dermatol 26:559–562, 1992.

104. CJ Cockerell. Noninfectious inflammatory skin diseases in HIV infected individuals. Dermatol Clin 9:531–541, 1991.

105. AA Fisher. Condom conundrums. Cutis 48:359–360, 1991.

106. M Reichel, TM Mauro, VA Ziboh, AC Huntley, MP Fletcher. Acrodermatitis enteropathica in a patient with the acquired immunodeficiency syndrome. Arch Dermatol 128:415–417, 1992.

107. Schulz TF, CH Boshoff, RA Weiss. HIV infection and neoplasia. Lancet 348:587–591, 1996.

108. D Caussy, JJ Goedert, J Palefsky, J Gonzales, CS Rabkin, RA DiGioia, WC Sanchez, RJ Grossman, G Colclough, SZ Wiktor, et al. Interaction of HIV and papillomaviruses: association with anal intraepithelial abnormality in homosexual men. Int J Cancer 46:214–219, 1990.

109. KJ Smith, HG Skelton, J Yeager, P Angritt, KF Wagner. Cutaneous neoplasms in a military population of HIV-1-positive patients. J Am Acad Dermatol 29:400–406, 1993.

110. ME Hagensee, N Kiviat, CW Critchlow, SE Hawes, J Kuypers, S Holte, DA Galloway. Seroprevalence of human papillomavirus types 6 and 16 capsid antibodies in homosexual men. J Infect Dis 176:625–631, 1997.

111. T Nagatani, M Miyazawa, T Matsuki. Adult T-cell leukemia/lymphoma (ATL)—clinical, histopathological, immunological and immunohistochemical characteristics. Exp Dermatol 1:248–252, 1992.

112. AE Friedman-Kien, BR Saltzman. Clinical manifestations of classical endemic African and epidemic AIDS-associated Kaposi's sarcoma. J Am Acad Dermatol 22:1237–1250, 1990.

113. AE Friedman-Kien, BR Saltzman, YZ Cao, MS Nestor, M Mirabile, JJ Li, TA Peterman. Kaposi's sarcoma in HIV-negative homosexual men. Lancet 335:168–169, 1990.

114. V Beral, TA Peterman, RL Berkelman, HW Jaffe. Kaposi's sarcoma among persons with AIDS: A sexually transmitted infection? Lancet 335:123–128, 1990.

115. Y Chang, E Cesarman, MS Pessin, F Lee, J Culpepper, DM Knowles, PS Moore. Identification of herpesvirus DNA sequences in AIDS-associated Kaposi's sarcoma. Science 266:1865–1869, 1994.

116. SF Krown, JWM Golft, D Niedzwicki. Interferon and zidovudine—safety tolerance and clinical and virological effects in patients with Kaposi's sarcoma associated with the acquired immunodeficiency syndrome (AIDS). Ann Intern Med 112:812–821, 1990.

117. S Walmsley, DW Northfelt, B Melosky, M Conant, AE Friedman-Kien, B Wagner. Treatment of AIDS-related cutaneous Kaposi's sarcoma with topical alitretinoin (9-cis-retinoic acid) gel. J Acquir Immune Defic Syndr 22:235–246, 1999.

118. SJ Orlow, H Kamino, RL Lawrence. Multiple subcutaneous leiomyosarcomas in an adolescent with AIDS. Am J Pediatr Hematol Oncol 14:265–268, 1992.

119. United States Department of Health and Human Services, Guidelines for the Use of Antiretroviral Agents in HIV-Infected Adults and Adolescents; February 5, 2001, available on the HIV/AIDS Treatment Information Service Website (*http://www.hivatis.org*).

120. PA Volberding, SW Lagakos, MA Koch, C Pettinelli, MW Myers, DK Booth, HH Bàlfour Jr, RC Reichman, JA Barlett, MS Hirsch, et al. Zidovudine in asymptomatic HIV infection: a controlled trial in persons with fewer than 500 CD4 positive cells per cubic millimeter. The AIDS Clinical Trial Group of the National Institute of Allergy and Infectious Diseases. N Engl J Med 332:941–949, 1990.

121. DD Richman. Resistance of clinical isolates of human immunodeficiency virus to antiretroviral agents. Antimicrob Agents Chemother 37:1207–1213, 1993.

122. RS Hogg, KV Heath, B Yip, KJ Craib, MV O'Shaughnessy, MT Schechter, JS Montaner. Improved survival among HIV infected individuals following initiation of antiretroviral therapy. JAMA 279:450–454, 1998.

123. BP Griffith, H Brett-Smith, G Kim, JW Mellors, TM Chacko, RB Garner, YC Cheng, P Alcabes, G Friedland. Effect of stavudine on HIV-1 virus load as measured by quantitative mononuclear cell culture, plasma RNA, and immune complex-dissociation antigenemia. J Infect Dis 173:1252–1255, 1996.

124. JO Kahn, SW Lagakos, DD Richman, A Cross, C Pettinelli, SH Liou, M Brown, PA Volberding, CS Crumpacker, G Beall, et al. A controlled trial comparing continued zidovudine with didanosine in HIV infection. The NIAID AIDS Clinical Trial Group. N Engl J Med 327:581–587, 1992.

125. SM Plauge, SS Good, WH Miller. Abacavir (1592), a second generation nucleoside HIV reverse transcriptase inhibitor. Int Antiviral News 6:7, 1998.

126. M Fishchl, F Greenberg, N Clumeck, et al. Abstracts of the 6th International Conference on Retroviruses and Opportunistic Infections; Chicago, Illinois, January 31–February 4, 1999. Abstract no. 19, p. 70.

127. SJ Smerdon, J Jager, J Wang, LA Kohlstaedt, AJ Chirino, JM Friedman, PA Rice, TA Steitz. Structure of the binding site for the non-nucleoside inhibitors of the reverse transcriptase of HIV-1. Proc Natl Acad Sci USA 26:3911–3915, 1994.

128. D Havlir, SH Cheesman, M McLaughlin, R Murphy, A Erice, SA Spector, TC Greenough, JL Sullivan, D Hall, M Myers et al. High-dose nevirapine: safety, pharmacokinetics, and antiviral effect in patients with HIV infection. J Infect Dis 171:537–545, 1995.

129. JH Nunberg, WA Schleif, EJ Boots, JA O'Brien, JC Quintero, JM Hoffman, EA Emini, ME Goldman. Viral resistance to HIV-1: Specific pyridinone reverse transcriptase inhibitors. J Virol 65:4887–4892, 1991.

130. D Richman, D Havlir, J Corbeil, D Looney, C Ignacio, SA Spector, J Sullivan, S Cheeseman, K Barringer, D Pauletti, et al. Nevirapine resistance mutations of HIV-1 selected during therapy. J Virol 68:1660–1666, 1994.

131. A Barner, M Myers. Nevirapine and rashes. Lancet 351: 1133, 1998.

132. RT D'Aquila, MD Hughes, VA Johnston, MA Fischl, JP Sommadossi, SH Liou, J Timpone, M Myers, N Basgoz, M Niu, MS Hirsch. Nevirapine, zidovudine and didanosine compared with zidovudine and didanosine in patients with HIV-1 infection. A randomized double blind, placebo-controlled trial. National Institute of Allergy and Infectious Diseases AIDS Clinical Trial Group Protocol 241 Investigators. Ann Intern Med 124:1019–1030, 1996.

133. DV Havlir, JMA Lange. New antiretrovirals and new combinations. AIDS 12(suppl A):S165–S174, 1998.

134. PC Bellman. Clinical experience with adding delavirdine to combination therapy in patients in whom multiple antiretroviral treatment including protease inhibitors has failed. AIDS 12:1333–1340, 1998.

135. R Murphy. Non-nucleoside reverse transcriptase inhibitors. AIDS Clin Care 9:75–79, 1997.

136. JSG Montaner, V Montessori, R Harrigan, M O'Shaughnessy, R Hogg. Antiretroviral therapy: "the state of the art." Biomed Pharmacother 53:63–72, 1999.

137. SG Deeks, M Smith, M Holodnity, JO Khan. HIV-1 protease inhibitors. A review for clinicians. JAMA 277: 145–153, 1997.

138. CK Mc Donald, DR Kurtzkes. HIV-1 protease inhibitors. Arch Intern Med 157:951–959, 1997.

139. C Debouck. The HIV-1 protease as a therapeutic target for AIDS. AIDS Res Human Retroviruses 8:153–164, 1992.

140. JC Schmit, B Weber. Recent advances in antiretroviral therapy and HIV infection monitoring. Intervirology 40: 304–321, 1997.

141. M Markowitz, M Saag, WG Powderly, AM Hurley, A Hsu, JM Valdes, D Henry, F Sattler, A La Marca, JM Leonard, et al. A preliminary study of ritonavir, an inhibitor of HIV-1 protease, to treat HIV-1 infection. N Engl J Med 333:1534–1539, 1995.

142. MN Chaudry, DH Shepp. Antiretroviral agents: current usage. Dermatol Clin 15:319–329, 1997.

143. M Silva, PR Skolnik, SL Gorbach, D Spiegelman, IB Wilson, MG Fernandez-DiFranco, TA Knox. The effect of protease inhibitors on weight and body composition in HIV infected patients. AIDS 12:1645–1651, 1998.

144. A Carr, DA Cooper. Images in clinical medicine. Lipodystrophy associated with an HIV protease inhibitor. N Engl J Med 339:1296, 1998.

145. DM Aboulafia, D Bundaw. Images in clinical medicine. "Buffalo hump" in a patient with HIV. N Engl J Med 339:1297, 1998.

146. K Williamson, AC Reboli, SM Manders. Protease inhibitor-induced lipodystrophy. JAAD 40:635–636, 1999.

147. JH Condra, WA Schleif, OM Blahy, et al. In vivo emergence of HIV-1 variants resistant to multiple protease inhibitors. Nature 374:569–571, 1995.

148. RT Mitsuyasu, PR Skolnik, SR Cohen, B Conway, MJ Gill, PC Jensen, JJ Pulvirenti, LN Slater, RT Schooley, MA Thompson, RA Torres, CM Tsoukas. Activity of the soft gelatin formulation of saquinavir in combination therapy in antiretroviral-naïve patients. NV 15355 Study Team AIDS 12:F103–F109, 1998.

149. DW Cameron, M Heath-Chiozzi, S Danner, C Cohen, S Kravcik, C Maurath, E Sun, D Henry, R Rode, A Potthoff, J Leonard. Randomized placebo-controlled trial of ritonavir in advanced HIV-1 disease. The Advanced HIV Disease Ritonavir Study Group. Lancet 351:543–549, 1998.

150. H Nielsen. Hypermennorrhea associated with ritonavir [letter]. Lancet 353:811–812, 1999.

151. LJ Martinez. Approval of new protease inhibitors. Res Init Treat Act 2:1–3, 1996.

152. K Boubaker, P Sudre, F Bally, G Vogel, JY Meuwly, MP Glauser, A Telenti. Changes in renal function associated with indinavir. AIDS 12:F249–F254, 1998.

153. H Hanabusa, H Tagami, H Hataya. Renal atrophy associated with long-term treatment with indinavir. N Engl J Med 340:392–393, 1999.

154. M Saag, M Knowles, Y Chang, et al. Durable effect of Viracept (nelfinavir mesylate, NFV) in triple combination therapy. Programs and abstracts of the 37th International Conference on Antimicrobial Agents and Chemotherapy, Toronto, Canada, September 28–October 1, 1997.

155. American Society for Microbiology's 39th Interscience Conference on Antimicrobial Agents and Chemotherapy (ICAAC), San Francisco, CA, September 26–29, 1999.

156. IS Fortgang, PC Belitsos, RE Chaisson, RD Moore. Hepatomegaly and steatosis in HIV-infected patients receiving nucleoside analog antiretroviral therapy. Am J Gastroenterol 90:1443–1436, 1995.

157. HJ Hofstede, S de Marie, NA Foudraine, SA Danner, K Brinkman. Clinical features and risk factors of lactic acidosis following long-term antiretroviral therapy: 4 fatal cases. Int J STD AIDS 11:611–616, 2000.

158. Lonergan JT, Behling C, Pfander H, TI Hassanein, WC Mathews. Hyperlactatemia and hepatic abnormalities in 10 human immunodeficiency virus-infected patients receiving nucleoside analogue combination regimens. Clin Infect Dis 31:162–166, 2000.

159. R Chodock, E Mylonakis, D Shemin, V Runarsdottir, P Yodice, R Renzi, K Tashima, C Towe, JD Rich. Survival of a human immunodeficiency patient with nucleoside-induced lactic acidosis: the role of hemodialysis treatment. Nephrol Dial Transplant 14:2484–2486, 1999.

160. K Mulligan, C Grunfeld, VW Tai, H Algren, M Pang, DN Chernoff, JC Lo, M Schambelan. Hyperlipidemia and insulin resistance are induced by protease inhibitors independent of changes in body composition in patients with HIV infection. J Acquir Immune Defic Syndr 23:35–43, 2000.

161. G Behrens, A Dejam, H Schmidt, HJ Balks, G Brabant, T Korner, M Stoll, RE Schmidt. Impaired glucose tolerance, beta cell function and lipid metabolism in HIV patients under treatment with protease inhibitors. AIDS 13: F63–F70, 1999.

162. CM Shikuma, C Waslien, J Mc Keague, N Baker, M Ara-

kaki, XW Cui, S Souza, A Imrie, R Arakaki. Fasting hyper-insulinemia and increased waist-to-hip ratios in non-wasting individuals with AIDS. AIDS 13:1359–1365, 1999.

163. KD Miller, E Jones, JA Yanovski, R Shankar, I Feuerstein, J Falloon. Visceral abdominal-fat accumulation associated with use of indinavir. Lancet 351:871–875, 1998.

164. JC Lo, K Mulligan, VW Tai, H Algren, M Schambelan. "Buffalo hump" in men with HIV-1 infection. Lancet 351:867–870, 1998.

165. A Carr, K Samaras, A Thorisdottir, GR Kaufmann, DJ Chisholm, DA Cooper. Diagnosis, prediction and natural course of HIV-1 protease-inhibitor associated lipodystrophy, hyperlipidemia and diabetes mellitus: a cohort study. Lancet 353:2093–2099, 1999.

166. T Saint-Marc, M Partisani, I Poizot-Martin, F Bruno, O Rouviere, JM Lang, JA Gastaut, JL Touraine. A syndrome of peripheral fat wasting (lipodystrophy) in patients receiving long-term nucleoside analogue therapy. AIDS 13:1659–1667, 1999.

167. A Carr, J Miller, M Law, DA Cooper. A syndrome of lipoatrophy, lactic acidaemia and liver dysfunction associated with HIV nucleoside analogue therapy: contribution to protease inhibitor-related lipodystrophy syndrome. AIDS 14:F25–F32, 2000.

168. Martinez E, Conget I, Lozano L, R Casamitjana, JM Gatell. Reversion of metabolic abnormalities after switching from HIV-1 positive protease inhibitor to nevirapine. AIDS 13:805–810, 1999.

169. P Barreiro, V Soriano, F Blanco, C Casimiro, JJ de la Cruz, J Gonzalez-Lahoz. Risk and benefits of replacing protease inhibitors by nevirapine in HIV-1 infected subjects under long-term successful triple combination therapy. AIDS 14:807–812, 2000.

170. R Roubenoff, L Weiss, A Mc Dermott, T Heflin, GJ Cloutier, M Wood, S Gorbach. A pilot study of exercise training to reduce trunk fat in adults with HIV-1 associated fat redistribution. AIDS 13:1373–1375, 1999.

171. A Carr, K Samaras, DJ Chisholm, DA Cooper. Pathogenesis of HIV-1 protease inhibitor associated peripheral lipod-ystrophy, hyperlipidemia, and insulin resistance. Lancet 351:1881–1883, 1998.

172. D Klein, L Hurley, S Sidney. Do protease inhibitors increase the risk of coronary heart disease among HIV-positive patients? Additional follow-up. Seventh Conference on Retroviruses and Opportunistic Infections (Abstract 33), San Francisco, CA, 2000.

173. JA Rascoosin, CM Kessler. Bleeding episodes in HIV-positive patients taking HIV protease inhibitors: A case series. Hemophilia 5:266–269, 1999.

174. SG Deeks, A Collier, J Lalezari, A Pavia, D Rodrigue, WL Drew, J Toole, HS Jaffe, AS Mulato, PD Lamy, W Li, JM Cherrington, N Hellmann, J Kahn. The safety and efficacy of adefovir dipivoxil, a novel anti-human immunodeficiency virus (HIV) therapy, in HIV infected adults: a randomized double blind, placebo-controlled trial. J Infect Dis 176:1517–1523, 1997.

175. K Squires. Once-a-day protease inhibitor appears safe and effective after 48 weeks. Eighth Conference on Retroviruses and Opportunistic Infections, San Francisco, CA, 2001.

176. D Hazuda, CU Blau, P Felock, J Hastings, B Pramanik, A Wolfe, F Bushman, C Farnet, M Goetz, M Williams, K Silverman, R Lingham, S Singh. Isolation and characterization of novel human immunodeficiency virus integrase inhibitors from fungal metabolites. Antivir Chem Chemother 10:63–70, 1999.

177. JM Kilby, S Hopkins, TM Venetta, B DiMassimo, GA Cloud, JY Lee, L Alldredge, E Hunter, D Lambert, D Bolognesi, T Matthews, MR Johnson, MA Nowak, GM Shaw, MS Saag. Potent suppression of HIV-1 replication in humans by T-20, a peptide inhibitor of gp-41 mediated virus entry. Nat Med 4:1302–1307, 1998.

178. OT Rutschmann, M Opravil, A Iten, R Malinverni, PL Vernazza, HC Bucher, E Bernasconi, P Sudre, D Leduc, S Yerly, LH Perrin, B Hirschel. A placebo-controlled trial of didanosine plus stavudine, with and without hydroxyurea, for HIV infection. The Swiss HIV Cohort study. AIDS 12:F71–F77, 1998.

15

Colorado Tick Fever

Michael R. Weir
Scott and White Clinic and Memorial Hospital, Temple, Texas, USA

Tracey E. Weir
Brackenridge Hospital, Austin, Texas, USA

Colorado tick fever (CTF) virus is a Coltivirus in the family Reoviridae. A spherical virion, it has a diameter of 80 μm. The genome has 12 segments in contrast to 10 segments in other orbiviruses. Humans are incidental hosts of the virus, and human disease is predominantly a self-limited febrile illness with rare encephalitic or hemorrhagic manifestations (Fig. 15–1).

HISTORY

In the 1850s, settlers of the Rocky Mountains first recognized the entity "Mountain fever," which described the clinical symptoms of a group of febrile diseases, mainly Rocky Mountain spotted fever, CTF, typhus, and others. In 1930, Becker was the first to clearly distinguish the clinical manifestations of CTF and he gave the disease its currently used name [1]. Florio et al, in 1944 [2], successfully transmitted the disease to adult volunteers and animals, and in 1950, isolated the virus from endemic *Dermacentor andersoni* ticks [3].

INCIDENCE

The epidemiology of CTF corresponds with the geographic distribution of its vector, the wood tick (*D. andersoni*), which is found only at elevations of 4000–10,000 feet in the western United States and southwestern Canada. Colorado and Idaho report most of the cases, occurring between March and September. The peak incidence occurs in May and June, when the ticks are most active. Hikers, campers, and forestry workers are most often affected. Second attacks are rare, and susceptibility is universal. Cases of CTF have only rarely been reported in non-endemic areas. One case of transfusion-related transmission has been reported [4], and CTF in persons exposed to ticks brought home on clothing of relatives has occurred [5].

PATHOGENESIS

A wide variety of mammals, principally rodents, are naturally infected with CTF, whereas only humans develop clinical disease. The golden-mantled ground squirrel, the Columbia ground squirrel, the porcupine, the yellow-pine chipmunk, and the least chipmunk are amplifying hosts for the virus [6–9], while larger mammals (e.g., deer and elk) have no known role in virus perpetuation. Uninfected ticks acquire the virus while feeding on a viremic mammal. The wood tick life span averages 2–3 years, and CTF infection remains for life in this species. Both male and female adult wood ticks may transmit the virus to humans and animals.

Soon after inoculation, the CTF virus invades the bone marrow and the host erythrocyte precursors. The CTF virus is unique among arboviruses in that it is harbored within

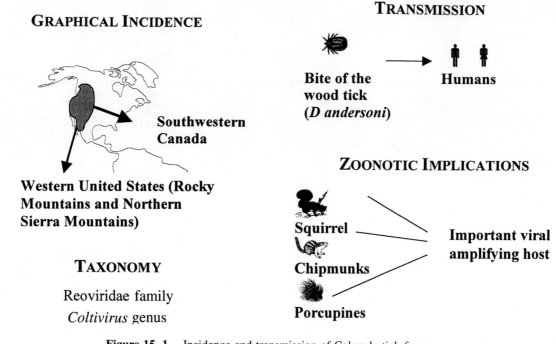

Figure 15–1. Incidence and transmission of Colorado tick fever.

erythrocytes during infection [10]. Persistence of the virus within peripheral erythrocytes prolongs the viremia long after acute infection has resolved [11]. Host immune mechanisms have little efficacy for the erythrocyte-sequestered virus. This evasion of immunity delays the development of complement fixation and neutralizing antibodies [10,11]. The involvement of bone marrow erythrocytic precursors is also associated with other marrow cell lines. Hemorrhagic and vasculitic manifestations may sometimes result from the bone marrow invasion.

CLINICAL MANIFESTATIONS

The clinical manifestations of CTF are described in Table 15–1. Neither respiratory nor gastrointestinal symptoms are prominent with this infection. Associated skin rash with CTF is not a prominent, common, or characteristic feature. In two large clinical series, the incidence of skin eruption ranged from 5 to 12% [12,13]. The associated exanthem is often transient and faint, and it may be limited to the trunk or become generalized [12–15]. Macular, maculo-

Table 15–1. Clinical Manifestations of Colorado Tick Fever

Time after exposure	Clinical manifestations	Laboratory analyses	Other notes
3–6 days	Acute onset of malaise, myalgia, high fever, chills, intense headache, painful skull, photophobia, retroorbital pain, and lumbar back pain. Nausea and vomiting may occur. This phase lasts for 5–10 days	Demonstration of viral antigens in erythrocytes by immunofluorescence Viral isolation from erythrocytes Serology (less useful)	A biphasic pattern occurs in half of patients, with initial febrile illness for 2–3 days, followed by an asymptomatic afebrile period for 1–2 days, then a second symptomatic febrile period lasting for 2 more days
8–16 days	Convalescent phase begins, with asthenia, weakness, and malaise resolving within a few weeks. Some patients may experience prolonged convalescence for months		

Table 15–2. Differential Diagnoses for Colorado Tick Fever

Rocky Mountain spotted fever: Fever, headache, and rash are typical manifestations of RMSF. It is seen predominately in children in the eastern United States, but a similar illness occurs in Brazil. A tick bite history is inconstant. Fever occurs 2–8 days later. The rash, a vasculitis due to endothelial cell involvement, blanches initially, then turns purpuric, perhaps hemorrhagic or even necrotic. It appears on the wrists and ankles frequently involving the palms and soles, then spreads centrally. Absence of the rash occurs in proven disease. The headache may be associated with meningeal signs, and altered mental status or coma may occur. Cardiac involvement results in failure and arrhythmias. Myositis and pneumonia are seen and edema may occur. Thrombocytopenia is common as is leukocytopenia, but leukocytosis occurs with secondary infectious complications. Treatment with chloramphenicol or tetracycline must be based on suspicion of diagnosis; untreated disease may be fatal

Lyme disease: A tick bite precedes the classic erythema migrans eruption early in the course of disease. Late manifestations are arthritis, aseptic meningitis, cranial nerve palsy, or heart block

Tularemia: Tularemia may be associated with a tick bite, but the site of inoculation becomes painful and ulcerated, with associated lymphadenopathy. The less common presentation with bacteremia or meningitis is similar to CTF but may be more severe

Enteroviral infections: Patients have fever, headache and nuchal rigidity. Cerebrospinal fluid studies show lymphocytic predominance with elevated protein. Enteroviral meningoencephalitis will be clinically indistinguishable from other central nervous system diseases. Serology, viral isolation, or where available, nucleic acid amplification testing will prove the etiology

Herpes simplex virus (HSV) encephalitis: HSV encephalitis should be excluded because of its severe outcome and response to antiviral therapy. Rapid testing for HSV is commonly employed. A hemorrhagic, necrotizing encephalitis of the temporal lobes is typical, but it may appear as meningitis or frank encephalitis with seizures and coma

Other Arboviral Infections:

ONN is suggested by sub-Sarahan travel, fever, arthritis, a morbilliform rash, and lymphadenopathy.

Sindbis is suggested by fever, rash, arthritis with travel in Europe, Asia, Africa, or Australia, and mosquito exposure

Mayaro is suggested by fever, chills, headache, myalgia, arthralgia, and a maculopapular rash as the fever fades and travel to Brazil or Trinidad, with mosquito exposure. Travel to Australia, mosquito exposure, fever, arthritis, and rash suggests Ross River virus or Barmah Forest disease

Oropouche is suggested by travel to Trinidad or northern South America, fever, myalgia, anorexia, headache, photophobia, leukopenia, with exposure to Culicoides midges or suggestive season and habitat

Sandfly fever is suggested by travel to Africa, southern Europe, central Asia or the Americas in the summer, exposure to small flies, or habitat with fever, myalgia, photophobia, retro-orbital pain, and conjunctival injection

Other Arboviral Encephalitis:

Eastern equine encephalitis is suggested by encephalopathy (altered mental status, coma, seizures), by salt marsh habitat in North and South America, deaths in horses and pheasants, and mosquito exposure in hot, damp months

Western equine encephalitis is suggested by encephalopathy with mosquito exposure in western United States and Canada and an equine epizootic

Venezuelan equine encephalitis is suggested by encephalopathy with travel in South and Central America, the Florida Everglades, Mexico or Texas, infection of conjunctivae or pharynx, flushed facies and muscular tenderness, an equine epizootic, and exposure to mosquitoes in wet, warm months

West Nile fever is suggested by travel to rural Africa, southern Europe, central or south Africa, or northeastern United States, mosquito exposure, symptoms of headache, myalgia, lymphadenopathy, leukopenia, and a nonpruritic maculopapular rash

California encephalitis is suggested by encephalopathy with rural midwest United States travel in July through September

Japanese encephalitis is suggested by severe encephalopathy in children in Asia in the monsoon season

St. Louis encephalitis is suggested by encephalopathy with central and western United States travel, mosquito exposure in late summer to early autumn

Tick-borne encephalitis is suspected by tick exposure in Russia or central Europe in late spring or summer after heavy rainfall or exposure to raw milk in a patient with altered mental status, fever, thrombocytopenia, and leukopenia

Powassan encephalitis occurs in Russia, Canada, and the United States. Young boys are more commonly affected, and tick exposure is frequent

papular, morbilliform, and petechial eruptions have been described [12].

Most cases of CTF resolve completely without sequelae, and complications may occur, but rarely. Hemorrhagic diathesis has been reported, particularly in children less than 10 years of age, and has led to death in 3 cases [12,13,16–19]. This manifestation is typically associated with thrombocytopenia and sometimes with disseminated intravascular coagulation. Central nervous system (CNS) involvement may occasionally develop, with signs and symptoms consistent with aseptic meningitis or encephalitis. This complication may be self-limited or progress to coma and death, and it may lead to residual neurologic dysfunction [12,16,20]. Other rare complications in adults include epididymoorchitis, pericarditis, hepatitis, and pneumonitis [4,16,21–23]. Differential diagnoses are shown in Table 15–2.

Table 15–3. Treatment of Colorado Tick Fever

Symptom	Treatment
Fever	Acetominophen. Antipyretics that interfere with coagulation (e.g., salicylates and non-steroidal anti-inflammatories) should be avoided because of the associated thrombocytopenia and the small risk of hemorrhage with this disease
Myalgia	Analgesics, as above
Nausea and vomiting	Maintain adequate hydration. Severe symptoms may require intravenous fluid and electrolyte replacement
Central nervous system involvement	Should be treated as for aseptic meningitis or encephalitis

LABORATORY FINDINGS

Leukopenia and thrombocytopenia are common, more so with hemorrhagic findings. CNS disease shows cerebrospinal fluid findings common for viral disease—slightly elevated protein and lymphocytic pleocytosis.

DIAGNOSIS

Appropriate clinical symptoms in the patient with recent tick exposure should lead the physician to suspect CTF. In a large case study, 90% of patients with CTF reported exposure to ticks prior to illness, while only 52% were aware of an actual tick bite [13]. Viral isolation from blood (specifically, erythrocytes) can confirm the diagnosis, and most patients remain viremic throughout the course of clinical symptoms [13]. Complement fixation and neutralizing antibodies appear late in the disease due to viral persistence and sequestration in red blood cells, which limits the use of serology. Paired antibody titers can document prior infection but are less useful than in other arboviral diseases. Immunoglobulin M is first detectable at the same time as neutralizing antibodies (14–21 days) and abruptly declines after 6 weeks [5,24]. Direct detection of viral antigens by immunofluorescence of erythrocyte smears is a rapid technique for diagnosis, and infected blood remains positive for up to 20 weeks after the onset of the illness. However, this method has low sensitivity during the first 7 days of disease, so a negative test should be repeated during the second week of clinical illness [25,26].

PREVENTION AND TREATMENT

Proper clothing, avoiding tick-infested areas, prompt tick removal, and limiting exposure provide the only truly effective strategies in preventing infection. No vaccine or specific antiviral treatment is currently available, and treatment for CTF is symptomatic. The expected outcome is good without sequelae, except in cases with CNS involvement [27]. Treatment of symptoms is listed in Table 15–3.

CONCLUSION

Colorado tick fever is the most benign illness transmitted by ticks in the United States. Because of significantly prolonged viremia with this infection, blood donation should be prohibited for 6 months to 1 year after clinical disease to prevent transfusion-acquired disease.

REFERENCES

1. FE Becker. Tick-borne infections in Colorado. I. The diagnosis and management of infections transmitted by the wood tick. Colo Med 27:36–43, 1930.
2. L Florio, M Stewart, ER Mugrage. The experimental transmission of Colorado tick fever. J Exp Med 80:165–188, 1944.
3. L Florio, MS Miller, ER Mugrage. Colorado tick fever. Isolation of the virus from Dermacentor andersoni in nature and a laboratory study of the transmission of the virus in the tick. J Immunol 64:257–263, 1950.
4. Centers for Disease Control. Transmission of Colorado tick

fever virus by blood transfusion—Montana. MMWR Morbid Mortal Wkly Rep 24:422–423, 1975.

5. TF Tsai. Arboviral infections in the United States. Infect Dis Clin North Am 5:73–102, 1991.

6. RG McLean, AB Carey, LJ Kirk, DB Francy. Ecology of porcupines (Erethizon dorsatum) and Colorado tick fever virus in Rocky Mountain National Park, 1975–1977. J Med Entomol 30:236–238, 1993.

7. W Burgdorfer. Colorado tick fever. II. The behavior of CTF virus in rodents. J Infect Dis 107:384–388, 1960.

8. W Burgdorfer, CM Eklund. Studies on the ecology of Colorado tick fever virus in Western Montana. Am J Hyg 69:127–137, 1959.

9. CM Eklund, GM Kohls, WL Jellison. Isolation of Colorado tick fever virus from rodents in Colorado. Science 128:413–414, 1958.

10. RW Emmons, LS Oshiro, HN Johnson, EH Lennette. Intra-erythrocytic location of Colorado tick fever virus. J Gen Virol 17:185–195, 1972.

11. LE Hughes, EA Casper, CM Clifford. Persistence of Colorado tick fever virus in red blood cells. Am J Trop Med Hyg 23:530–532, 1974.

12. SL Spruance, A Bailey. Colorado tick fever: a review of 115 laboratory confirmed cases. Arch Intern Med 131:288–293, 1973.

13. HC Goodpasture, JD Poland, DB Francy, GS Bowen, KA Horn. Colorado tick fever: clinical, epidemiologic, and laboratory aspects of 228 cases in Colorado in 1973–1974. Ann Intern Med 88:303–310, 1978.

14. RW Emmons. An overview of Colorado tick fever. Prog Clin Biol Res 178:47–52, 1985.

15. CM Eklund, GM Kohls, JM Brennan. Distribution of Colorado tick fever and virus-carrying ticks. JAMA 157:335–337, 1955.

16. CM Eklund, GM Kohls, WL Jellison, et al. The clinical and ecological aspects of Colorado tick fever. In: Proceedings of the 6th International Conference of Tropical Medicine and Malaria, Vol 5. Lisbon, 1959, pp 197.

17. DL Dawson, TM Vernon. Colorado tick fever—Colorado. MMWR Morbid Mortal Wkly Rep 21:374, 1972.

18. CM Eklund, RC Kennedy, M Casey. Colorado tick fever. Rocky Mt Med J 58:21–25, 1961.

19. HK Silver, G Meiklejohn, CH Kempe. Colorado tick fever. Am J Dis Child 101:30–36, 1961.

20. JL Ater, JC Overall, TJ Yeh, RT O'Brien, A Bailey. Circulating interferon and clinical symptoms in Colorado tick fever. J Infect Dis 151:966–968, 1985.

21. WJ Hierholzer, DW Barry. Colorado tick fever pericarditis. JAMA 217:825, 1971.

22. RV Loge. Acute hepatitis associated with Colorado tick fever. West J Med 142:91–92, 1985.

23. MP Earnest, JC Breckinridge, RJ Barr, DB Francy, CS Mollohan. Colorado tick fever. Clinical and epidemiologic features and evaluation of diagnostic methods. Rocky Mt Med J 68:60–62, 1971.

24. RW Emmons. Ecology of Colorado tick fever. Ann Rev Microbiol 42:49–64, 1988.

25. SY Gaidamovich, GA Klisenko, NK Shanovan. New aspects of laboratory techniques for studies of Colorado tick fever. Am J Trop Med Hyg 23:526–529, 1974.

26. RW Emmons, EH Lennette. Immunofluorescent staining in the laboratory diagnosis of Colorado tick fever. J Lab Clin Med 68:923–929, 1966.

27. CH Fraser, DW Schiff. Colorado tick fever encephalitis. Report of a case. Pediatrics 29:187–190, 1962.

16

Measles

Vera Y. Soong
University of Alabama at Birmingham School of Medicine, Birmingham, Alabama, USA

Tricia J. Brown
University of Oklahoma Health Sciences Center, Oklahoma City, Oklahoma, USA

Measles is an acute exanthematous and enanthematous disease caused by the rubeola virus. This highly communicable illness is characterized by fever, cough, coryza, and a maculopapular eruption. Although measles is generally self-limited, serious complications of the respiratory and central nervous systems may occur. Measles remains a worldwide problem, with significant morbidity and mortality in developing countries (Fig. 16–1).

HISTORY

The name measles is thought to be derived from the Latin *misellus* or *misella,* from the word miser, meaning miserable. *Morbilli,* the diminutive of *morbus,* was used to distinguish this minor illness from bubonic plaque, *morbus,* the major disease. The term morbilliform is still in common use to describe a measles-like exanthem [1]. Measles has been recognized for over 2000 years, although it was frequently thought to be a mild form of smallpox. Rhazes, an Arabic physician, is credited with the earliest written description of measles in the 10th century A.D. in which he distinguished measles from smallpox [2]. Rhazes quoted El Yehudi, a Hebrew physician, who described measles in Syria in the 7th century A.D [3]. Thomas Sydenham recorded a measles epidemic in London in 1670 [4,5]. Noah Webster wrote about the contagious nature of measles in 1799 after epidemics swept through the early American colonies. In 1846, Paul Panum, a Danish physician, published a landmark description of an outbreak in the Faroe Islands [6]. He described the incubation period, respiratory mode of transmission, and apparent lifetime immunity of previously infected persons. Koplik, in 1896, described the characteristic enanthem of measles that bears his name [7]. In 1905, Hektoen conclusively demonstrated the transmission of measles by infecting susceptible volunteers through the transfer of blood from acutely infected patients [8]. Goldberger and Anderson confirmed the viral etiology in 1911 after transmitting measles to rhesus monkeys by injection of filtered material from acutely ill human patients [9,10]. In 1954, Enders and Peebles were the first to report the propagation of wild measles virus in primary human renal tissue culture cells and to describe the characteristic cytopathic effects of this virus [11]. This work led directly to the development of the live attenuated measles vaccine currently in use today [12].

VIROLOGY

The measles virus is a single-stranded RNA virus of the family Paramyxovirus. Other members of this family include parainfluenza 1–5, mumps, and Newcastle disease viruses. Measles, canine distemper, and rinderpest viruses, members of the genus *Morbillivirus,* are closely related viruses termed medipest viruses [13]. The measles virus is

GEOGRAPHICAL INCIDENCE

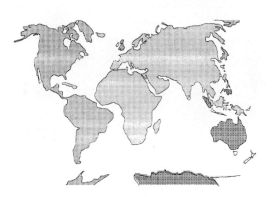

TAXONOMY

Paramyxoviridae family
Morbillivirus **genus**

TRANSMISSION

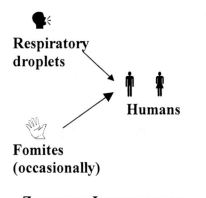

Respiratory droplets

Humans

Fomites (occasionally)

ZOONOTIC IMPLICATIONS

None

Figure 16–1. Incidence and transmission of measles.

distinctive owing to its ability to cause hemagglutination; the other members of its genus do not. The organism is very labile and easily inactivated [14]. Low relative humidity is the most important factor that determines viral survival [15]. Viral decay increases dramatically in the range of 50 to 70% humidity. This may account for the increased

incidence of measles in winter, when indoor relative humidity is low. The virus is also readily inactivated by lipid solvents and ionizing radiation [16].

Humans are the only natural hosts of the wild measles virus although other primates can be infected. There is no animal reservoir. Human or simian renal cell cultures are most widely used to isolate the virus from infected patients. Two types of cytopathic effects (CPE) are produced by measles virus in tissue culture: multinucleated giant cells and spindle cell transformation [17]. Multinucleated giant cells, analogous to Warthin-Finkelday cells seen in the reticuloendothelial system, appear in 6 to 10 days. Cell fusion is mediated via the F glycoprotein. These cells are associated with a high infectivity. Spindle cell transformation is produced by vaccine, rather than wild strains and is characterized by alteration of single cells into spindle or stellate shapes. Both forms of CPE may be present simultaneously in tissue culture. They provide reliable evidence of viral multiplication and are the basis for procedures for viral isolation, assays of infectivity, and determinations of neutralizing antibodies.

EPIDEMIOLOGY

Measles remains a global disease. For the year 1997, the World Health Organization (WHO) estimated 31 million cases and 1 million deaths worldwide due to measles [18]. It is hyperendemic in many developing countries, with over 500,000 deaths each year in sub-Saharan Africa. Prior to available vaccination, approximately 130 million cases and 7 to 8 million deaths occurred annually worldwide due to measles infection [19,20]. During the pre-vaccine era, more than 95% of the United States population contracted the disease before their 20th birthday, usually in early childhood. Epidemics in the late winter and early spring occurred every 2 to 3 years. Widespread measles vaccination began in the 1960s and has thus far reduced global measles morbidity and mortality by 74% and 85%, respectively [21]. Results of epidemiological data for 1998 suggest that measles is no longer an indigenous illness in the United States [22]. Of the record low number of 100 cases that occurred that year, 71 cases were internationally imported or importation-associated. A similar number of cases was reported in the United States in 1999, in 2000, and again in 2001. An international meeting of the WHO, the Pan American Health Organization, and Centers for Disease Control and Prevention (CDCP) has outlined strategies for the global eradication of measles by a target date between 2005 and 2010 [23,24].

Measles is one of the most communicable of infectious diseases. Transmission via respiratory droplets approaches

100% [25], although relatively close contact is required. Infection is typically acquired from inhalation of respiratory droplets as a consequence of face-to-face exposure to infected individuals who are coughing and sneezing during the prodromal stage [6,9,26]. The measles virus can survive for 2 hours in respiratory droplets [27], making occasional transmission by contact with fomites possible. Airborne transmission of measles in a physician's office [28–30] and an elementary school [31] have been documented. Patients shed measles virus from the nasopharynx and are considered infectious from the beginning of the prodrome until approximately 4 days after the appearance of the rash [32]. Immunocompromised persons may shed the measles virus for extended periods. These individuals should be kept in respiratory isolation during hospitalization [27].

Criteria for the clinical diagnosis of measles as defined by the CDCP [33] are: (1) a generalized maculopapular rash lasting 3 or more days, (2) a temperature of 38.3°C (101°F) or greater, and (3) the presence of cough, coryza (Fig. 16–2), or conjunctivitis (Fig. 16–3). Cases are further classified as suspect, probable, or confirmed. A confirmed case meets the clinical case definition and is serologically confirmed or epidemiologically linked to another confirmed or probable case. Only confirmed cases are reported to the CDCP. A programmatically preventable case occurs in a patient for whom vaccination was indicated but was not received. A programmatically unpreventable case occurs in a person: (1) less than 16 months of age, (2) born before 1957, (3) with adequate evidence of immunity, (4) with a

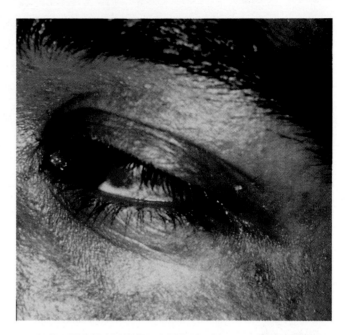

Figure 16–3. Conjunctivitis associated with measles. (Photograph courtesy of Mark Lebwohl, M.D., Department of Dermatology, Mt. Sinai School of Medicine, New York, NY.)

medical contraindication to receiving vaccine, or (5) with a religious or philosophical exemption under the law. Measles cases are also differentiated as indigenous, imported (out-of-state or international), or importation-spread.

PATHOGENESIS

The pathogenesis of measles has been described by Kempe and Fulginiti [34]. The portals of entry of infection are the nasopharynx and perhaps the conjunctiva. Spread to regional lymph nodes and primary viremia occurs by day 3. During days 3 to 5, the virus multiplies in the respiratory epithelium at the site of initial infection as well as throughout the reticuloendothelial system. A secondary viremia occurs during days 5 to 7, resulting in the establishment of generalized infection. During the second week of infection, the virus can be found in blood, skin, respiratory tract, and other organs. During days 11 to 14 after exposure, the prodromal period of measles occurs. It appears that prodromal measles corresponds to a period of intense viral multiplication and dissemination during which tissue damage occurs, resulting in the clinical illness. During days 15 to 17, viremia diminishes as viral multiplication slows. This rapid decline in tissue viral content coincides with the appearance of measles antibody during days 14 to 18. As serum antibody levels increase, the virus becomes unde-

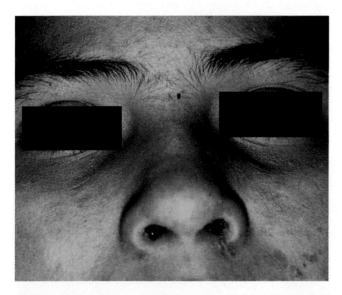

Figure 16–2. Coryza associated with measles. (Photograph courtesy Lourdes Tamayo, M.D., and Edith Garcia-Gonzalez, M.D., Ph.D., Department of Dermatology, Instituto Nacional de Perinatologie, Mexico City, Mexico.)

tectable in blood, urine, and nasopharyngeal secretions. Thus, the appearance of the measles exanthem coincides temporally with the appearance of serum antibody and the subsequent loss of communicability of the disease.

CLINICAL MANIFESTATIONS

Measles infection is only rarely associated with subclinical infection. The characteristic erythematosus macules and papules are present (Figs. 16–4 to 16–7), other clinical manifestations are listed in Table 16–1. Fever associated with measles infection may exceed 40°C (104°F), and the patient may appear extremely ill and toxic. Pharyngitis and cervical lymph node enlargement are common with measles; generalized lymphadenopathy also may be seen. Diarrhea, vomiting, laryngitis, croup, and abdominal pain may occur, particularly in children.

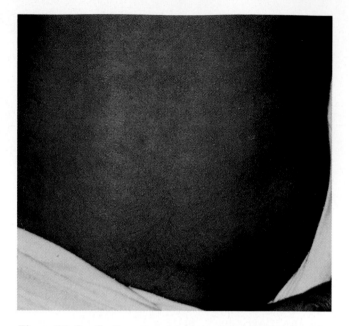

Figure 16–5. Erythematous macules and papules of acute measles.

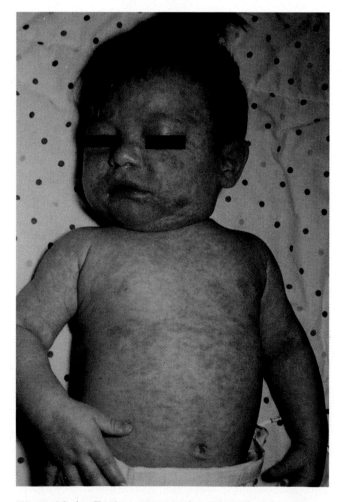

Figure 16–4. Erythematous macules and papules of acute measles.

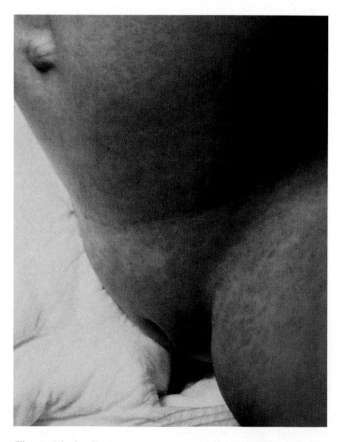

Figure 16–6. Erythematous macules and papules of acute measles.

Table 16–1. Clinical Manifestations of Measles

Time after exposure	Clinical manifestations	Laboratory analyses	Other notes
8–12 days	Prodromal symptoms, including fever, malaise, coryza, cough, conjunctivitis, photophobia, and periorbital edema	Serology, particularly IgM Detection of measles virus antigen in tissues Viral culture (difficult)	The cough has a brassy or barking quality, and may be severe Symptoms increase in severity over the next few days
10–14 days	Koplik's spots appear at the end of the prodromal period and remain discrete for 2–3 days		As the exanthem progresses, initially discrete lesions become confluent, especially on the face, neck and shoulders
11–16 days	Exanthem begins on the 3rd or 4th day of fever, beginning as prominent, blanchable, erythematous macules and papules on the neck, hairline, forehead and postauricular areas. The exanthem spreads to the trunk and extremities over the next 2–3 days, reaching the feet in 3 days		Fever peaks on the 2nd or 3rd day of the rash, followed by rapid defervescence (unless complications occur)
15–19 days	Exanthem reaches its peak after 3 days, which conicides with the peak of the prodromal symptoms		Fine desquamation may be seen with resolution of the rash. Conjunctivitis and coryza resolve at this time, but dry cough may persist for 10 days or more
16–20 days	Exanthem begins to clear, in order of appearance. As the rash fades, it becomes a copper color, then leaves a brown nonblanching discoloration		

IgM, immunoglobulin M.

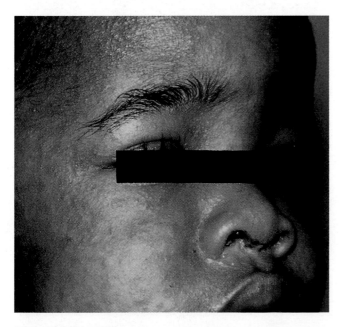

Figure 16–7. Erythematous macules and papules of acute measles.

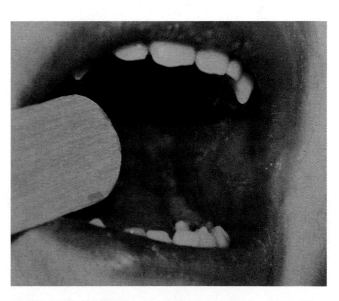

Figure 16–8. Koplik's spots seen on the buccal mucosa. (Photograph courtesy Lourdes Tamayo, M.D., and Edith Garcia-Gonzalez, M.D., Ph.D., Department of Dermatology, Instituto Nacional de Perinatologie, Mexico City, Mexico.)

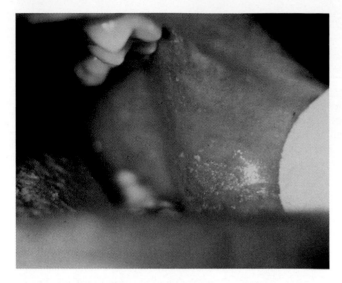

Figure 16–9. Koplik's spots seen on the buccal mucosa. (Photograph courtesy Lourdes Tamayo, M.D., and Edith Garcia-Gonzalez, M.D., Ph.D., Department of Dermatology, Instituto Nacional de Perinatologie, Mexico City, Mexico.)

Koplik's spots are pathognomonic for measles. They are initially seen as clusters of punctate blue-white papules on an erythematous base and are located on the buccal mucosa adjacent to the upper molars (Figs. 16–8 and 16–9). These lesions rapidly increase in number and can involve the entire buccal and lower labial mucosa. Initially about 1 mm in size, the lesions may coalesce as they become more numerous. The background oral mucosa has a characteristic red, granular appearance (Fig. 16–10).

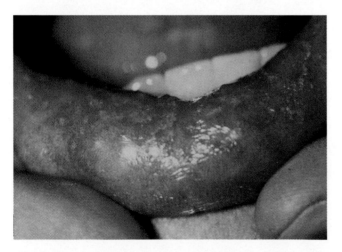

Figure 16–10. Red, granular, manifestations of measles on the oral mucosa. (Photograph courtesy Lourdes Tamayo, M.D., and Edith Garcia-Gonzalez, M.D., Ph.D., Department of Dermatology, Instituto Nacional de Perinatologie, Mexico City, Mexico.)

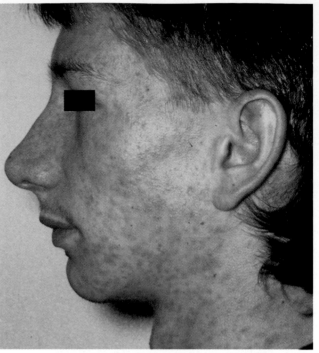

Figure 16–11. Exanthem of measles after resolution of fever and other symptoms.

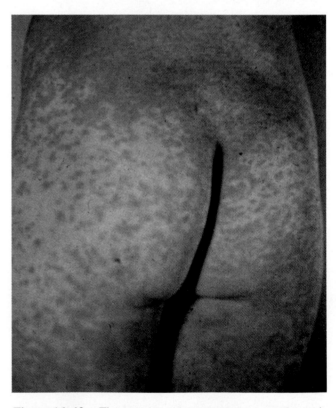

Figure 16–12. The exanthema becomes a copper color as it begins to fade (after two weeks).

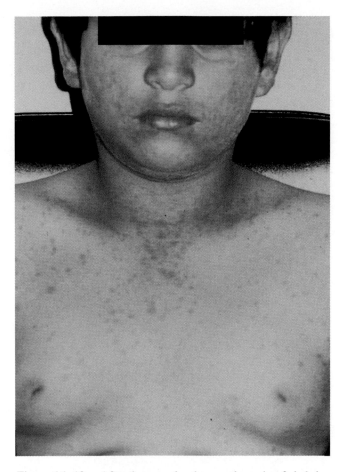

Figure 16–13. After three weeks, the exanthema has faded significantly, leaving a brown, nonblanching discoloration. (Photograph courtesy of Shirley Pren, M.D., Department of Pediatrics, University of Miami School of Medicine, Miami, FL.)

Koplik's spots are often described as having the appearance of a grain of salt on a red background.

Clinical recovery begins after the appearance of the rash in uncomplicated measles. In severe cases, the exanthem may have associated edema, particularly on the face. The brownish discoloration of the rash that develops as the exanthem fades is thought to be due to capillary hemorrhage (Figs. 16–11 to 16–13). In fair-skinned persons, the rash may become purpuric instead of fading, although this is not related to hemorrhagic manifestation of measles [35]. Table 16–2 lists possible differential diagnoses.

MODIFIED MEASLES

Modified measles is a milder form of measles that is seen in persons with passive immunity to the virus. It occurs

Table 16–2. Differential Diagnosis of Measles

Mycoplasma pneumoniae: The fever, cough, and other manifestations associated with this infection may mimic measles. An exanthem commonly occurs, typically as an erythematous maculopapular rash, most prominent on the trunk and back. This rash may either be rubelliform and discrete or morbilliform and confluent.

Infectious mononucleosis: This infection typically consists of fever, lymphadenopathy, hepatosplenomegaly, sore throat, and fatigue. A morbilliform or papular rash is present in 5–15% of cases, particularly in young children. This exanthem is typically present on the arms or trunk. The ampicillin-associated rash begins on the trunk and spreads to the face and extremities

Rubella: The rash and severity of this disease are less striking than that of measles, and the course of disease is of shorter duration. The rubella rash fades as it spreads and is associated with prominent posterior cervical lymphadenopathy

Erythema infectiosum: The infection typically has a prominent "slapped cheek" appearance to the rash on the face

Meningococcemia: The rash with this infection may be similar to that of measles, but it is usually petechial and purpuric. Also, cough and conjunctivitis are usually absent

Rickettsial infections: With these infections cough may be present, but the rash typically spares the face

Scarlet fever: The rash of this infection is typically diffuse and finely papular, with a "goose flesh" or sandpaper-like texture on an erythematous base. Scarlet fever is also usually accompanied by a sore throat and pharyngeal exudate

Exanthem subitum (roseola infantum): The rash of this disease appears as the high fever disappears. This exanthem begins on the trunk, neck, or behind the ears, and only occasionally spreads to the extremities

Enteroviral infections: The rash and severity of these diseases are less striking than that of measles.

Drug eruptions: There is an absence of cough and other characteristic prodromal symptoms with a drug eruption. A patient history of recent drug ingestion may explain rash

in infants less than 9 months of age with transplacentally acquired antibody to the virus, in susceptible patients given immune globulin after exposure to rubeola, after vaccine failure, or rarely in recurrent disease [36–40]. Patients with modified measles have an attenuated illness with a shortened prodromal period; fever, coryza, and cough are mild. Koplik's spots may not occur. The exanthem evolves as in typical measles, but the lesions do not become confluent.

The illness may not fulfill the CDCP clinical criteria for the diagnosis of measles, most often due to absent or low-grade fever. Undiagnosed modified measles occurring after secondary vaccine failure may lead to underreporting of measles cases and falsely elevated vaccine efficacy rates in highly vaccinated populations [38].

ATYPICAL MEASLES

The live attenuated measles vaccine available today affords most persons with effective immunity against natural measles infection. A killed vaccine, which was used in the United States during the years 1963 to 1967, was withdrawn after the emergence of the atypical measles syndrome patients exposed to wild measles virus [41–44]. Although atypical measles has rarely been reported in recipients of the live attenuated vaccine [45], this syndrome occurs almost exclusively in recipients of the killed vaccine. Atypical measles rarely occurs, and it is now an infrequent disease of young adults.

The pathogenesis of atypical measles remains unclear. The illness is characterized by the occurrence of excessively high measles antibody titers. Often immeasurable or low at the onset of the exanthem, antibody titers rise dramatically to levels as high as 1:128,000 within 2 weeks [46]. It has been found that the antigenicity of the F glycoprotein of the viral envelope is destroyed by the inactivation of the virus during preparation of the killed vaccine. Therefore, the killed measles vaccine does not induce an antibody response to the F protein, which mediates cell fusion and cell-to-cell spread of the virus. The spread of infection in recipients of the killed vaccine is unchecked due to lack of these neutralizing antibodies. In contrast, the antigenicity of the H glycoprotein is preserved and may simultaneously induce later hypersensitivity to natural measles infection. This results in the syndrome of atypical measles, with hypersensitivity responses in multiple organs, despite partial immunity [44].

After an incubation period of 7 to 14 days, atypical measles begins abruptly with high fever, headache, photophobia, myalgias, arthralgias, abdominal pain, tachypnea, pleuritic chest pain, nonproductive cough, and prostration. Coryza and conjunctivitis are absent. Koplik's spots are not seen. After 2 to 3 days, the exanthem appears. Unlike typical measles, the eruption begins peripherally on the hands, wrists, feet, and ankles and spreads centripetally (Figs. 16–14 to 16–16). The exanthem usually begins as erythematous macules and papules but may progress to vesicular or petechial lesions. The vesicular lesions appear singly or in crops, primarily on the trunk, and may resemble the exanthem of varicella. The petechial lesions may be

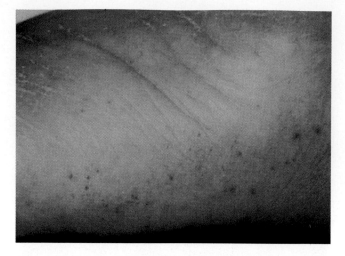

Figure 16–14. The eruption of atypical measles begins on the extremities and spreads centripetally. (Photograph courtesy of Mark Lebwohl, M.D., Department of Dermatology, Mt. Sinai School of Medicine, New York, NY.)

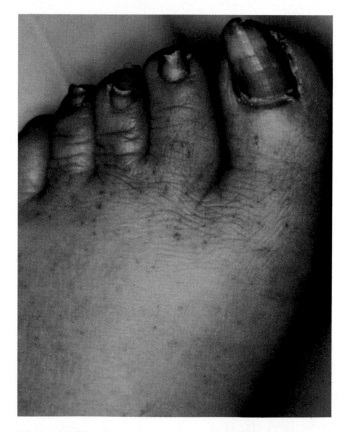

Figure 16–15. The eruption of atypical measles begins on the extremities and spreads centripetally. (Photograph courtesy of Mark Lebwohl, M.D., Department of Dermatology, Mt. Sinai School of Medicine, New York, NY.)

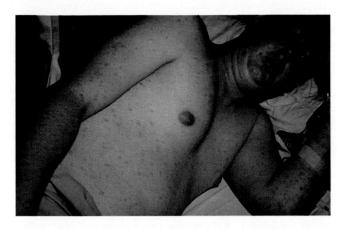

Figure 16–16. The eruption of atypical measles begins on the extremities and spreads centripetally. (Photograph courtesy of Monica McCrary, M.D., Department of Dermatology, Medical College of Georgia, Augusta, GA)

associated with purpura and occur predominantly on the trunk and extremities with relative sparing of the face. This cutaneous pattern may be confused with Rocky Mountain spotted fever, meningococcemia, Henoch-Schönlein purpura, or Gianotti-Crosti syndrome. The exanthem also may be predominantly an erythematous maculopapular eruption that has been confused with scarlet fever [44,47,48]. Erythematous papules coalescing into plaques in an inverse photodistribution has been reported [49]. Peripheral edema is commonly seen.

Involvement of the respiratory tract in atypical measles is prominent, with hilar adenopathy, pulmonary infiltrates, and pleural effusion frequently seen [44,48]. Pulmonary infiltrates may be diffuse, segmental, or nodular. Patients may present with hypoxemia, and acute respiratory failure has been documented. Pulmonary function tests reveal severe restrictive lung disease. Although pulmonary disease is self-limited, residual calcified nodular lesions may persist for years [50]. Transient hepatitis may complicate atypical measles [46]. Skin biopsy differs from that of classic measles in that a prominent mixed vasculitis is seen and the typical measles histologic complex is absent [44]. Although the morbidity of atypical measles is greater than that of classic measles, it is generally a self-limited illness with a good prognosis. Atypical measles is not thought to be contagious. However, viable measles virus has been cultured from the nasopharyngeal aspirate of one patient [49].

COMPLICATIONS

Respiratory Manifestations

The most common complication of measles is secondary bacterial infection, with otitis media being the most fre-

quent. Laryngitis and laryngotracheitis also occur frequently. Pneumonia is a common, often serious, complication of measles with reported rates of 3.5 to 50%. Pneumonia may be the result of direct viral invasion of the lungs or bacterial superinfection [51–54]. Primary measles pneumonitis is seen more frequently in children and is characterized by the presence of multinucleated giant cells with intranuclear and intracytoplasmic inclusion bodies [55,56]. Secondary bacterial pulmonary infection is more common in adults, occurring in 30 to 60% of military recruits with measles [53,54]. The most common organisms cultured include *Hemophilus influenza, Neisseria meningitides* and *Streptococcus pyogenes.* Radiographic findings are nonspecific, with a fine multilobular reticulonodular infiltrate as the most common finding (Fig. 16–17).

Pneumonia is the most common cause of death associated with measles, with the greatest mortality occurring in pediatric, malnourished, and immunocompromised patients. This complication accounted for 65% of measles-related deaths in infants less than 1 year of age and 60% of all deaths due to measles in the years 1964 to 1971 [57]. An immunocompromised child exposed to measles may

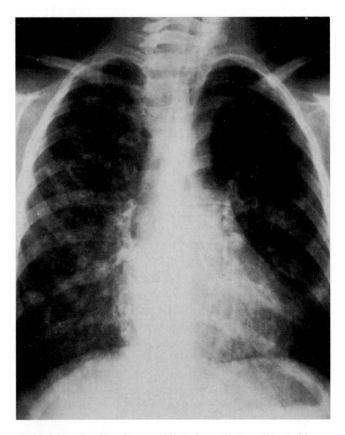

Figure 16–17. The fine, multilobular reticulonodular infiltrate of measles pneumonia.

develop fatal giant cell pneumonia with or without a rash [56,58]. Measles in human immunodeficiency virus (HIV)–infected children also has a higher case-fatality rate than in normal hosts [59–61]. In developing countries, malnourishment and intense exposure due to crowded living conditions contribute to high mortality rates [62]. Although measles pneumonia increases the morbidity of the disease in healthy adolescents and young adults, deaths are rare.

Natural measles infection causes prolonged depression of cell-mediated immunity and an extended period of impaired in vitro lymphoproliferative responses to mitogens [34,63,64]. Pulmonary tuberculosis may be precipitated or exacerbated by wild measles infection. In addition, measles infection or measles vaccination can cause transient depression of the tuberculin skin test.

ENCEPHALITIS

The incidence of post-infectious encephalitis is 0.5 to 1/1000 cases of measles infection [65]. The decline in measles encephalitis has paralleled the decline in the incidence of measles [66]. However, many patients with uncomplicated measles may have abnormal electroencephalographic changes, but viral invasion of the brain is not an obligate step in measles encephalomyelitis [67]. Measles encephalitis is an acute perivenular inflammatory and demyelinating disease that presents with an abrupt recrudescence of fever, seizures, headache, lethargy, irritability, and depressed level of consciousness, including coma [68,69]. Most cases occur within 7 days of the onset of the exanthem, often after the eruption has faded and fever has abated. The mortality rate of acute measles encephalitis is approximately 15%. Another 25% of patients have serious neurological sequelae, including mental retardation, seizures, deafness, behavioral disorders, hemiplegia, and paraplegia [66,70].

SUBACUTE SCLEROSING PANENCEPHALITIS

Subacute sclerosing panencephalitis (SSPE) is a chronic neurological disease caused by a persistent abortive infection with the measles virus. This late complication of measles was first described by Dawson in 1933, who proposed a viral etiology due to the presence of intranuclear inclusion bodies in brain tissue. [71] SSPE is rare, with an incidence of 5 to 10 cases per million cases of measles. SSPE occurs less frequently following measles vaccination [3]. Most cases occur in children between the ages 5 and 14 years. Nearly half of all patients have a history of acquiring measles before 2 years of age. The mean latent period between acute measles infection and the onset of SSPE is 7 years,

with a range of 6 months to 18 years [72]. The disease is 2 to 3 times more common in males than females. The incidence is higher in rural areas, especially farms, and in persons exposed to birds, pigs, and dogs with canine distemper, which suggests some form of associated zoonotic infection. A serious head injury also is a risk factor for SSPE [73]. The disease also has been reported in immunocompromised patients [58]. SSPE is not considered contagious [32].

SSPE is a progressive, degenerative neurological disease with an average survival of 6 to 9 months after onset. The onset is gradual, with intellectual decline and abnormal behavior that may initially be diagnosed as a psychological problem. After 1 to 2 months, seizures, mycolonic jerks, ataxia, dyskinesia, and visual impairment may suddenly develop without headache or fever [74]. The disease is relentlessly progressive in most cases, eventuating in coma, opisthotonus, emaciation, and death over the next few months. Patients who do not die remain in the fourth stage, characterized by severe loss of cerebral cortex function. Remission is rare but has been reported [75]. No effective treatment has been developed.

With laboratory evaluation, one finds that the electroencephalogram (EEG) is abnormal, showing periodic bursts of high voltage activity at 3 to 5 second intervals. An increased level of gamma globulin in the cerebrospinal fluid (CSF) is seen [74]. Antibody to measles virus is present both in the serum and CSF of patients with SSPE [74,76]. A significant titer of intrathecal measles antibody is the most valuable single test for establishing the diagnosis [77]. The measles virus has been cultured from the brain of patients with SSPE as well [78,79]. Isolation of infectious virus was accomplished only with cocultivation techniques, which suggests that the virus is present in a defective or latent form.

OTHER MANIFESTATIONS

Hepatitis occurs in measles, with 80% of cases reported in adults [80,81]. It is seen most commonly in severely ill patients. Jaundice may occur, but liver involvement is self-limited with no long-term sequelae. However, a clear correlation between the severity of hepatic involvement and the occurrence of secondary bacterial infections may occur.

Black measles, a rare form of rubeola, differs from typical measles in that confluent hemorrhagic exanthem, gastrointestinal and respiratory tract bleeding, and severe hyperpyrexia are seen. It is frequently complicated by pneumonia and encephalitis or encephalopathy and has a significant mortality. Little is known about the pathogenesis of black measles [1,40].

Measles complicating pregnancy has been associated with spontaneous abortions, premature delivery, and low-birth-weight infants. There is no convincing evidence that measles infection early in pregnancy causes congenital anomalies [34,82–84]. During the measles epidemic in Houston in 1988 to 1989, 13 patients with gestational measles were hospitalized. The most common maternal complication was pneumonia, and one patient died. Four of the thirteen patients had an adverse fetal outcome (premature labor, spontaneous abortion). The other mothers delivered healthy, full-term infants [85].

Transitory hypocalcemia of unknown etiology, with tetany as a rare complication, has been reported [86,87]. Transient development of a lupus anticoagulant after measles in an otherwise healthy child has been documented [88]. Noma-like post-measles ulcerations occur in African children after desquamation of the skin eruption. Ulcerations occur at the lips and in the perioral, perinasal, and periorbital areas with resultant scarring and mutilation [89]. Non-erosive stomatitis may result in severe oral stenosis that requires commissurotomy after natural measles and has been reported in the United States [90]. Other unusual manifestations of measles include myocarditis, pericarditis, thrombocytopenic purpura, Stevens-Johnson syndrome, pneumomediastinum, subcutaneous emphysema, appendicitis, ileocolitis, mesenteric lymphadenitis, acute glomerulonephritis, corneal ulceration leading to blindness, and gangrene of the extremities [40].

PATHOLOGY

The distinctive pathological feature of measles is multinucleated giant cells [58]. Two types have been described: reticuloendothelial giant cells (Warthin-Finkelday cells) and epithelial giant cells. The Warthin-Finkelday cells, first described in 1931, are found in tonsils (Fig. 16–18), lymph nodes, Peyer patches, appendix, thymus, spleen, and bone marrow. They are large, with up to 50 nuclei and scant cytoplasm. These cells are seen in prodromal measles and disappear within 2 to 4 days after the onset of the exanthem when serum antibodies appear. Epithelial giant cells are found predominantly in the respiratory mucosa but have been described in the oral mucosa, skin, salivary glands, liver, kidney, bladder, and gastrointestinal tract. They will be described in greater detail below. During the prodromal period these cells are sloughed from respiratory epithelium and can be found in pharyngeal smears.

The histological changes of measles in skin and oral mucosa are distinctive [91,92]. The most characteristic feature of the exanthem is syncytial-type multinucleated giant cells in the epidermis (Fig. 16–19). These cells have 3 to

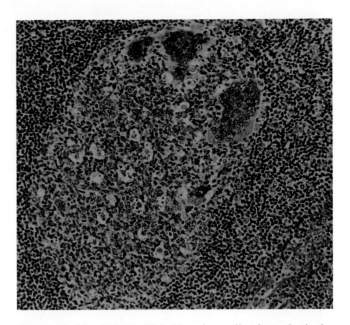

Figure 16–18. Warthin-Finkelday giant cells of measles in the tonsils.

26 nuclei, abundant cytoplasm, and contain pink intranuclear and intracytoplasmic inclusion bodies. Other epidermal changes include focal parakeratosis, dyskeratosis, and spongiosis associated with a few lymphocytes. Some epidermal cells show intracellular edema. Spongiosis progresses to intraepidermal vesiculation in a minority of cases. The epidermal changes are strikingly focal, associated primarily with hair follicles and eccrine sweat ducts. In the dermis, a sparse superficial perivascular lymphohistiocytic infiltrate is seen.

The histological changes seen in Koplik's spots are sim-

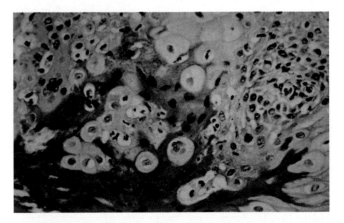

Figure 16–19. Syncytial-type multinucleated giant cells of measles in the epidermis.

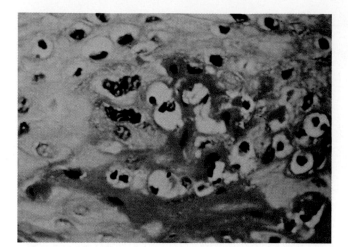

Figure 16–20. Multinucleated giant cells of measles in Koplik's spots.

ilar to those seen in skin. Giant cells are more numerous and contain more nuclei (Fig. 16–20). Intracellular edema is more prominent, whereas spongiosis and the dermal infiltrate are less pronounced. Electron microscopy reveals aggregates of microtubules characteristic of paramyxovirus within the cytoplasm and nuclei of giant cells (Fig. 16–21). These viral microtubular aggregates lend support to the hypothesis that direct viral invasion of the skin and oral mucosa causes the cutaneous manifestations of measles.

LABORATORY FINDINGS

Patients may have mild leukopenia, often with relative lymphocytosis. With measles encephalitis, the cerebral

spinal fluid typically shows an increase in protein and a slight increase in lymphocytes, while the glucose level remains normal.

DIAGNOSIS

The diagnosis of classic measles was easily made on clinical grounds during the pre-vaccine era when it was extremely common. However, many clinicians today are unfamiliar with the illness, as the incidence has declined with widespread vaccination. Also, measles occurring in immunocompromised hosts (Fig. 16–22) and modified or atypical measles can be difficult to diagnose on clinical criteria alone (Table 16–3). Laboratory confirmation of rubeola can be done by viral culture, demonstration of measles antigen in infected tissue, or serological testing. Viral isolation in tissue culture is technically difficult and used primarily in research settings. Examination of nasopharyngeal secretions or urinary sediment stained with fluorescent antibody, if available, also can establish the diagnosis [93].

Serological assays are the most widely used techniques to confirm the diagnosis of rubeola. The virus neutralization test based on neutralization of the viral cytopathic effect in cell culture is the serological standard but is not widely available [39]. The most sensitive test is the plaque reduction neutralization assay [94]. Until recently, the most commonly used assays were the hemagglutination inhibition (HI) and the complement fixation (CF) tests [95]. Classic and atypical measles infection can be confirmed by a fourfold rise in measles specific HI or CF antibody titers between acute and convalescent serum specimens collected

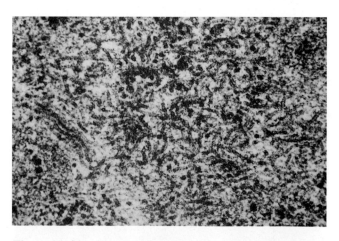

Figure 16–21. Electron microscopy showing aggregates of microtubules characteristic of paramyxovirus (e.g., measles) within the cytoplasm and nuclei of giant cells.

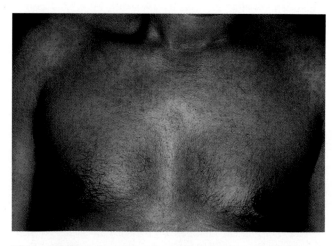

Figure 16–22. Acute measles in an human immunodeficiency virus seropositive male. (Photograph courtesy of Walmar Roncalli P. de Oliveira, M.D., Sao Paulo, Brazil.)

Table 16–3. Treatment of Measles

Symptom	Treatment
Fever	Antipyretics (acetaminophen or non-steroidal anti-inflammatory drugs)
	Maintain fluid balance, with ingestion of adequate liquids
	Bed rest and limited activity (Measles infection damages the ciliated respiratory epithelium, which can predispose for bacterial pneumonia in persons who resume activity too soon and are exposed to other persons.)
Cough	Antitussive medicines (narcotic cough suppressants should be avoided)
Conjuctivitis	Humidification of the room
	Daily rinsing of the eyes with sterile saline solution
Otitis media	Antibiotic therapy
Pneumonia	Antibiotics should be given, since bacterial and primary viral pneumonias are difficult to differentiate. Aerosolized ribavirin can be considered for the treatment of known primary viral pneumonia
Laryngotracheitis	Humidification of air
Encephalitis	Supportive care of symptoms, such as maintenance of fluids and electrolytes, and anticonvulsants for seizures
Malnutrition	Vitamin A supplementation

1 to 3 weeks apart. HI antibodies become detectable in the first several days after the exanthem appears, peak approximately 2 weeks later, and persist for years. The rise in complement fixation titers lag behind HI titers by 1 to 3 days but do not persist, becoming undetectable after 5 to 10 years. Thus, the HI assay can be used to determine the immune status of the patient, but the CF assay cannot be used for this purpose. An indirect fluorescent antibody (IFA) slide test is also available [96]. The HI and IFA assays correlate well and both can be used to determine the immune status of the patient. The enzyme linked immunosorbent assay (ELISA) is now in widespread use and is both highly sensitive and specific for the diagnosis of measles [97,98].

Measles-specific immunoglobulin M (IgM) antibodies appear shortly after the onset of the exanthem, peak within 10 days, and are undetectable by 30 days. Measurement of this antibody in one serum sample is useful in the diagnosis of acute measles during epidemics when rapid laboratory confirmation is crucial. IgM antibody determinations can be done with sucrose gradient ultracentrifugation, the HI test modified by staphylococcal protein A adsorption or 2-mercaptoethanol reduction, or by ELISA [36,95,97,99]. Sekla et al [99] found ELISA for the detection of specific IgM antibodies to be the most suitable method for rapid diagnosis during a measles outbreak. However, a convalescent serum sample should be tested if the acute serum is negative for IgM antibodies. It must be emphasized that a crucial factor in all methods of serological testing is the time of collection of the serum sample in relation to the time of appearance of antibodies. In practical terms, this requires knowledge of the time the serum was obtained with respect to the appearance of the exanthem.

PREVENTION

Since 1976, the live, further attenuated vaccine that has been used exclusively in the United States is the Moraten strain. It is available in a monovalent formulation or in combination with rubella (measles and rubella [MR]) or with mumps and rubella (measles-mumps-rubella [MMR]). Improper storage or handling may inactivate the vaccine virus and cause primary vaccine failure. The lyophilized vaccine must be reconstituted properly and used within 8 hours or discarded [32,100].

The measles vaccine produces a subclinical or mild, noncommunicable infection. A measles antibody response develops in at least 95% of susceptible children vaccinated at 15 months of age or older (i.e., the incidence of primary vaccine failure is 5% or less). Immunity appears lifelong in most individuals with occasional secondary vaccine failure [36–39].

Persons are considered immune to measles if they: (1) were born before 1957; (2) have documentation of physician-diagnosed measles; (3) have laboratory evidence of measles immunity; or (4) have documentation of adequate vaccination. All other persons, except for those with a medical contraindication or religious or philosophical exemption, should be vaccinated. The Advisory Committee on Immunization Practices (ACIP) currently recommends a two-dose vaccination regimen for measles, with the first dose given at 12 to 15 months of age [101]. The second dose should be given no earlier than 1 month later, but is typically given at 4 to 6 years of age. During a measles outbreak, the monovalent measles vaccine can be given to infants as young as 6 months of age. However, infants vaccinated before 12 months of age should be considered unvaccinated and should be vaccinated as outlined above.

The measles vaccine now in use has an excellent record of safety. Fever (temperature 39–40°C or greater) begins 5 to 12 days after vaccination and lasts several days in 5 to 15% of vaccinees. These patients are otherwise well. Transient rashes occur in 5% of vaccine recipients. It has been suggested that side effects are more common and severe in adults [102]. Serious neurological disease, including encephalitis, transverse myelitis, encephalopathy, aseptic meningitis, Reye's syndrome, cranial nerve palsy, cerebellar ataxia, and Guillain-Barré syndrome, occur in less than one per one million doses [103]. The incidence of encephalitis is lower than encephalitis of unknown etiology, which suggests that the vaccine is not the cause. Thrombocytopenic purpura [104] and toxic epidermal necrolysis [105] in vaccine recipients has been reported.

Medical contraindications to the measles vaccine include pregnancy, anaphylactic hypersensitivity to egg ingestion [106,107] or neomycin, and most cases of altered immunity. Immunocompromised patients (those with immunodeficiency diseases, those with malignancies, or those receiving immunosuppressive drugs or radiation) should not be given live measles vaccine because of the possibility of severe infection with the vaccine virus. Children with HIV infection are the exception. These children, including those with the acquired immunodeficiency syndrome (AIDS), should be vaccinated at 15 months of age [108]. This recommendation is based on the fact that measles is a severe, sometimes fatal, disease in these children and the incidence of complications from the vaccine is low [59,60].

The vaccine should be deferred in patients who have received immune globulin (IG) in the preceding 3 months and should be given at least 2 weeks before IG is administered. This is recommended because IG, and products such as whole blood or blood plasma, may contain sufficient measles antibody to neutralize the vaccine virus.

In susceptible persons exposed to measles, the administration of live measles vaccine within 72 hours may prevent the disease. For patients for whom contraindications exist for vaccination, prophylaxis with IG given within 6 days of exposure can prevent or modify the disease. Persons who may need passive immunization include susceptible household contacts (particularly infants less that 1 year of age), infants born to mothers with measles, and immunocompromised patients for whom the risk of complications is the greatest. The recommended dose of IG for the normal host is 0.25 mL/kg (max 15 mL) intramuscularly. Immunocompromised patients should receive 0.5 mL/kg (max 15 mL). IG is also indicated for susceptible asymptomatic household contacts with HIV infection, particularly infants less than 1 year of age, and pregnant women. It has been

proposed that all HIV-infected children exposed to measles, regardless of HIV symptomatology, vaccination status, or receipt of passive prophylaxis, be prophylactically immunized with IG [59,60].

TREATMENT

Treatment of measles is supportive, as there is no specific antiviral agent yet available (see Table 16–3). Antibiotic therapy should not be given unless the patient has bacterial superinfection. Prophylactic antibiotics during acute measles fail to prevent bacterial complications and may even predispose the person to infection with a resistant organism [109]. Although prophylactic IG can prevent or modify the illness, high-dose intravenous IG given during the acute stage of measles does not affect the clinical course of measles [110]. Ribavirin has been used to treat measles and has been shown to improve the clinical outcome in various studies [111,112]. However, other authors have reported that ribavirin given to patients with gestational measles showed no clear clinical benefit nor adverse outcome [85]. Although not consistently effective, aerosolized ribavirin may be indicated in immunocompromised patients because of the potential of severe illness and the absence of other available therapy [60]. In developing countries where malnutrition is common, vitamin A significantly reduces the mortality and morbidity of severe measles infections [113–116]. In countries with malnutrition, the WHO recommends vitamin A treatment for children with measles infection, with the dose based on the child's age. The American Academy of Pediatrics also has recommended vitamin A supplementation for certain circumstances in the United States, such as a child aged 6 months to 2 years who requires hospitalization [117]. Aerosolized-ribavirin may be considered for treatment of primary viral pneumonia [118].

CONCLUSION

Measles is an acute systemic viral illness that is self-limited in most cases; however, serious complications involving the respiratory and central nervous systems may occur. Measles remains a major public health concern around the world despite intensive efforts to eradicate the disease. The rapid diagnosis of measles and prompt containment of outbreaks is hampered by the fact that many health care providers today have never seen a patient with measles. Physicians must maintain a high index of suspicion when seeing a febrile patient with an exanthem and cough. Importation of measles from other countries where measles remains an endemic disease will continue. In addition, the typical features of this illness may be obscured in the setting of immunocompromised patients and in those with atypical or modified measles. Health care practitioners must remain vigilant in the coming years if the goal to eliminate measles is to be reached.

REFERENCES

1. LZ Cooper. Measles. In: IM Freedberg, AZ Eisen, K Wolff, et al, eds. Dermatology in General Medicine. 5th ed. New York: McGraw-Hill, 1999, pp 2398–2403.

2. GS Wilson. Measles as a universal disease. Am J Dis Child 103:219–223, 1962.

3. JF. Modlin, JT Jabbour, JJ Witte, NA Halsey. Epidemiologic studies of measles, measles vaccine, and subacute sclerosing panencephalitis. Pediatrics 59:505–512, 1977.

4. B Gastel. Measles: a potentially finite history. J Hist Med Allied Sci 28:34–44, 1973.

5. T Sydenham. The works of Thomas Sydenham, Vol 2. London:Sydenham Society, 1922, pp 250.

6. PL Panum. Observation made during the epidemic of measles on the Faroe Islands in the year 1846. Med Classics 3:829–886, 1939.

7. H Koplik. The diagnosis of the invasion of measles from a study of the exanthema as it appears on the buccal mucous membrane. Arch Pediatr 13:918–922, 1896.

8. L Hektoen. Experimental measles. J Infect Dis 2:238–255, 1905.

9. J Goldberger, JF Anderson. An experimental demonstration of the presence of the virus of measles in the mixed buccal and nasal secretions. JAMA 57:476–478, 1911.

10. JF Anderson, J Goldberger. The period of infectivity of the blood in measles. JAMA 62:113–114, 1911.

11. JF Enders, TC Peebles. Propagation in tissue cultures of cytopathogenic agents from patients with measles. Proc Soc Exp Biol Med 86:277–286, 1954.

12. JF Enders, SL Katz, MV Milovanovic, A Hollaway. Studies on an attentuated measles-virus vaccine; development and preparation of the vaccine: techniques for assay of effects of vaccination. N Eng J Med 263:153–159, 1960.

13. DT Imagawa. Relationships among measles, canine distemper and rinderpest viruses. Progr Med Virol 10:160–193, 1968.

14. FL Black. Growth and stability of measles virus. Virology 7:184–192, 1959.

15. JG DeJong. The survival of measles virus in air, in relation to the epidemiology of measles. Archiv Ges Virusforsch 16:97–102, 1965.

16. SJ Musser, GE Underwood. Studies on measles virus. J Immunol 85:292–297, 1960.

17. JF Enders. Measles virus, historical review, isolation, and behavior in various systems. Am J Dis Child 103:282–287, 1962.

18. World Health Organization. Measles: progress towards global control and regional elimination 1990–1998. Weekly Epidemiol Rec 50:389–393, 1998.

19. FL Black. Measles: viral infections of humans. In: AS Evans, ed. Epidemiology and Control. 3rd ed. New York: Plenum, 1989, pp 451.

20. FT Cutts, LE Markowitz. Successes and failures in measles control. J Infect Dis 70(Suppl 1):S32–S41, 1994.

21. FT Cutts, AM Henao-Restrepo, JM Olivé. Measles elimination: progress and challenges. Vaccine 17(Suppl 3): S47–S52, 1999.

22. Centers for Disease Control and Prevention. Epidemiology of Measles—United States, 1998. MMWR Morbid Mortal Wkly Rep 48:749–753, 1999.

23. Expanded Programme on Immunisation. Meeting on advances in measles elimination: conclusions and recommendations. Weekly Epidemiol Rec 71:305–312, 1996.

24. Centers for Disease Control and Prevention. Measles eradication: recommendations from a meeting cosponsored by the World Health Organization, the Pan American Health Organization, and CDC. MMWR Morbid Mortal Wkly Rep 46(No. RR-11):1–20, 1997.

25. BG Gellin, SL Katz. Putting a stop to a serial killer: measles. J Infect Dis 170(Suppl 1):S1–S2, 1994.

26. FL Babbott, JE Gordon. Modern measles. Am. J Med Sci 228:334–361, 1954.

27. WL Atkinson. Epidemiology and prevention of measles. Dermatol Clin 13:553–559, 1995.

28. PL Remington, WN Hall, IH Davis, A Herald, RA Gunn. Airborne transmission of measles in a physician's office. JAMA 253;1574–1577, 1985.

29. AB Bloch, WA Orenstein, WM Ewing. Measles outbreak in a pediatric practice: airborne transmission in an office setting. Pediatrics 75:676–683, 1985.

30. Centers for Disease Control and Prevention. Measles transmitted in a medical office building—New Mexico, 1986. MMWR Morbid Mortal Wkly Rep 36:25–27, 1987.

31. EC Riley, G Murphy, RL Riley. Airborne spread of measles in a suburban elementary school. Am J Epidemiol 107:421–432, 1978.

32. Committee on Infectious Disease, American Academy of Pediatrics. Measles (rubeola). In: Report of The Committee on Infectious Diseases. 21st ed. Elk Grove Village, 1988, pp 277–289.

33. Centers for Disease Control and Prevention. Classification of measles cases and categorization of measles elimination programs. MMWR Morbid Mortal Wkly Rep 31:707–711, 1983.

34. CH Kempe, VA Fulginiti. The pathogenesis of measles virus infection. Arch Ges Virusforsch 16:103–128, 1965.

35. JB Hudson, L Weinstein, TW Chang. Thrombocytopenic purpura in measles. J Pediatr 48:48–56, 1956.

36. JD Cherry, RD Feigin, PG Shackelford, DR Hinthorne, RR Schmidt. A clinical and serologic study of 103 children with measles vaccine failure. J Pediatr 82:802–808, 1973.

37. RG Mathias, WG Meekison, TA Arcand, MT Schechter. The role of secondary vaccine failures in measles outbreaks. Am J Public Health 79:475–478, 1989.

38. MB Edmonson, DG Addiss, JT McPherson, JL Berg, SR Circo, JP Davis. Mild measles and secondary vaccine failure during a sustained outbreak in a highly vaccinated population. JAMA 263:2467–2471, 1990.

39. LE Markowitz, SR Preblud, PE Fine, WA Orenstein. Duration of live measles vaccine-induced immunity. Pediatr Infect Dis J 9:101–110, 1990.

40. JD Cherry. Measles. In: RD Feigin, JD Cherry, eds. Textbook of Pediatric Infectious Diseases. 2nd ed. Philadelphia: WB Saunders, 1987, pp 1607–1628.

41. LW Rauh, R Schmidt. Measles immunization with killed virus vaccine; serum antibody titers and experience with exposure to measles epidemic. Am J Dis Child 109:232–237, 1965.

42. VA Fulginiti, JH Arthur. Altered reactivity to measles virus skin test reactivity and antibody response to measles virus antigens in recipients of killed measles virus vaccine. J Pediatr 75:609–616, 1969.

43. PR Nader, MS Horwitz, J Rousseau. Atypical exanthem following exposure to natural measles: eleven cases in children previously inoculated with killed vaccine. J Pediatr 72:22–28, 1968.

44. D Annunziato, MH Kaplan, WW Hall, H Ichinose, JH Lin, D Balsam, VS Paladino. Atypical measles syndrome: pathologic and serologic findings. Pediatrics 70:203–209, 1982.

45. JD Cherry, RD Feigin, LA Lobes Jr, PG Shackelford. Atypical measles in children previously immunized with attenuated measles virus vaccines. Pediatrics 50:712–717, 1972.

46. HM Frey, S Krugman. Case report atypical measles syndrome: unusual hepatic, pulmonary and immunologic aspects. Am J Med Sci 281:51–55, 1981.

47. MS Horwitz, C Grose, M Fisher. Atypical measles rash mimicking Rocky Mountain spotted fever. N Engl J Med 289:1203–1204, 1973.

48. WJ Hall, CB Hall. Atypical measles in adolescents: evaluation of clinical and pulmonary function. Ann Intern Med 90:882–886, 1979.

49. RJ Sharpe, LS Albert, MJ Imber, HA Haynes. Isolation of viable virus from a patient with atypical measles and rash in an inverse photodistribution. J Am Acad Dermatol 22:1107–1109, 1990.

50. J Mitnick, MH Becker, M Rothberg, NG Genieser. Nodular residua of atypical measles pneumonia. Am J Roentgenol 134:257–260, 1980.

51. L Weinstein, W Franklin. The pneumonia of measles. Am J Med Sci 217:314–324, 1949.

52. C O'Donovan, KN Barua. Measles pneumonia. Am J Trop Med Hyg 22:73–77, 1973.

53. RW Olson, GR Hodges. Measles pneumonia bacterial suprainfection as a complicating factor. JAMA 232:363–365, 1975.

54. DH Gremillion, GE Crawford. Measles pneumonia in young adults. An analysis of 106 cases. Am J Med 71:539–542, 1981.

55. RW Archibald, RO Weller, SR Meadow. Measles pneumonia and the nature of the inclusion-bearing giant cells: a light and electron-microscope study. J Pathol 103:27–34, 1971.

56. JF Enders, K McCarthy, A Mitus, WJ Cheatham. Isolation of measles virus at autopsy in cases of giant-cell pneumonia without rash. N Engl J Med 261:875–881, 1959.

57. RM Barkin. Measles mortality; analysis of the primary cause of death. Am J Dis Child 129:307–309, 1975.

58. V Breitfield, Y Hashida, FE Sherman, K Odagiri, EJ Yunis. Fatal measles infection in children with leukemia. Lab Invest 28:279–291, 1973.

59. Centers for Disease Control and Prevention. Measles in HIV-infected children, United States. MMWR Morbid Mortal Wkly Rep 37:183–186, 1988.

60. K Krasinski, W Borkowsky. Measles and measles immunity in children infected with human immunodeficiency virus. JAMA 261:2512–2516, 1989.

61. LE Markowitz, FW Chandler, EO Roldan, MJ Saldana, KC Roach, SS Hutchins, SR Preblud, CD Mitchell, GB Scott. Fatal measles pneumonia without rash in a child with AIDS. J Infect Dis 158:480–483, 1988.

62. P Aaby, J Bukh, M Lisse, AJ Smits. Measles mortality, state of nutrition, and family structure: a community study from Guinea-Bissau. J Infect Dis 147:693–701, 1983.

63. HC Whittle, J Dossetor, A Oduloju, AD Bryceson, BM Greenwood. Cell-mediated immunity during natural measles infection. J Clin Invest 62:678–684, 1978.

64. RL Hirsch, DE Griffin, RT Johnson, SJ Cooper, I Lindo de Soriano, S Roedenbeck, A Vaisberg. Cellular immune responses during complicated and uncomplicated measles virus infections of man. Clin Immunol Immunopathol 31:1–12, 1984.

65. AL Hoyne, EL Slotkowski. Frequency of encephalitis as a complication of measles; report of twenty cases. Am J Dis Child 73:554–558, 1947.

66. Centers for Disease Control and Prevention. Measles encephalitis—United States, 1962–1979. MMWR Morbid Mortal Wkly Rep 30:362–364, 1981.

67. HE Gendelman, JS Wolinsky, RT Johnson, NJ Pressman, GH Pezeshkpour, GF Boisset. Measles encephalomyelitis: Lack of evidence of viral invasion of the central nervous system and quantitative study of the nature of demyelination. Ann Neurol 15:353–360, 1984.

68. E Appelbaum, VB Dolgopol, J Dolgin. Measles encephalitis. Am J Dis Child 77:25–48, 1949.

69. AC LaBoccetta, AS Tornay. Measles encephalitis report of 61 cases. Am J Dis Child 107:247–255, 1964.

70. JA Aarli. Nervous complications of measles clinical manifestations and prognosis. Europ Neurol 12:79–93, 1974.

71. JR Dawson. Cellular inclusions in cerebral lesions of lethargic encephalitis. Am J Pathol 9:7–16, 1933.

72. MH Bellman, G Dick. Surveillance of subacute sclerosing panencephalitis. Br Med J 281:393–394, 1980.

73. NA Halsey, JF Modlin, JT Jabbour, L Dubey, DL Eddins, DD Ludwig. Risk factors in subacute sclerosing pa-

nencephalitis: a case-control study. Am J Epidemiol 111: 415–423, 1980.

74. JT Jabbour, JH Garcia, H Lemmi, J Ragland, DA Duenas, JL Sever. Subacute sclerosing panencephalitis. A multidisciplinary study of eight cases. JAMA 207:2248–2254, 1969.

75. JS Resnick, WK Engel, JL Sever. Subacute sclerosing panencephalitis. Spontaneous improvement in a patient with elevated measles antibody in blood and spinal fluid. N Engl J Med 279:126–129, 1968.

76. JH Connolly, IV Allen, LJ Hurwitz, JH Millar. Measles-virus antibody and antigen in subacute sclerosing panencephalitis. Lancet 1:542–544, 1967.

77. JL Sever, H Krebs, A Ley, LH Barbosa, D Rubenstein. Diagnosis of subacute panencephalitis. The value and availability of measles antibody determinations. JAMA 228:604–606, 1974.

78. FE Payne, JV Baublis, HH Itabashi. Isolation of measles virus from cell cultures of brain from a patient with subacute sclerosing panencephalitis. N Engl J Med 281: 585–589, 1969.

79. L Horta-Barbosa, DA Fuccillo, WT London, JT Jabbour, W Zeman, JL Sever. Isolation of measles virus from brain cell cultures of two patients with subacute sclerosing panencephalitis. Proc Soc Exp Biol Med 132:272–277, 1969.

80. H Shaley-Zimels, Z Weizman, C Lotan, D Gavish, Z Ackerman, A Morag. Extent of measles hepatitis in various ages. Hepatology 8:1138–1139, 1988.

81. D Gavish, Y Kleinman, A Morag, T Chajek-Shaul. Hepatitis and jaundice associated with measles in young adults; an analysis of 65 cases. Arch Intern Med 143:674–677, 1983.

82. E Gazala, M Karplus, JR Liberman, I Sarov. The effect of maternal measles on the fetus. Pediatr Infect Dis J 4: 203–204, 1985.

83. M Siegel, HT Fuerst. Low birth weight and maternal virus diseases. A prospective study of rubella, measles, mumps, chickenpox, and hepatitis. JAMA 197:680–684, 1966.

84. CS Jespersen, J Littauer, U Sagild. Measles as a cause of fetal defects. A retrospective study of ten measles epidemics in Greenland. Acta Paediatr Scand 66:367–372, 1977.

85. RL Atmar, JA Englund, H Hunter. Complications of measles in pregnancy. Clin Infect Dis 14:217–226, 1991.

86. R Sobel, S Einhorn, M Maislos, R Shainkin-Kestenbaum, S Shany, J Horowitz. Transitory hypocalcemia complicating measles. Arch Intern Med 145:2043–2044, 1985.

87. M Mouallem, E Friedman, R Pauzner, Z Farfel. Measles epidemic in young adults. Arch Intern Med 147: 1111–1113, 1987.

88. W Muntean, W Petek. Lupus anticoagulant after measles. Eur J Pediatr 134:135–138, 1980.

89. A Kozminska-Kubarska, D Talleyrand, M Bakatubia. Cutaneous complications during measles in Zairian children: noma-like postmeasles ulcerations. Int J Dermatol 21: 465–469, 1982.

90. N Guillozet. Oral stenosis in measles. Int J Dermatol 20: 262–263, 1981.

91. DW Suringa, LJ Bank, AB Ackerman. Role of measles virus in skin lesions and Koplik's spots. N Engl J Med 283:1139–1142, 1970.

92. AB Ackerman, DW Suringa. Multinucleate epidermal cells in measles. Arch Dermatol 103:180–184, 1971.

93. R Llanes-Rodas, C Liu. Rapid diagnosis of measles from urinary sediments stained with fluorescent antibody. N Eng J Med 275:516–523, 1966.

94. P Albrecht, K Herrmann, GR Burns. Role of virus strain in conventional and enhanced measles plaque neutralization test. J Virol Methods 3:251–260, 1981.

95. Centers for Disease Control and Prevention. Serologic diagnosis of measles. MMWR Morbid Mortal Wkly Rep 31: 396–402, 1982.

96. MB Kleiman, CA Bookhold, SE Zimmerman, C Griffin, ML French, C Barrett. Adaptation of a commercially available indirect fluorescent antibody slide test for measuring measles-specific immunoglobulins. Diagn Microbiol Infect Dis 4:285–290, 1986.

97. GP Rice, P Casali, MB Oldstone. A new solid-phase enzyme-linked immunosorbent assay for specific antibodies to measles virus. J Infect Dis 147:1055–1059, 1983.

98. KA Weigle, MD Murphy, PA Brunell. Enzyme-linked immunosorbent assay for evaluation of immunity to measles virus. J Clin Microbiol 19:376–379, 1984.

99. L Sekla, W Stackiw, G Eibisch, I Johnson. An evaluation of measles serodiagnosis during an outbreak in a vaccinated community. Clin Invest Med 11:304–309, 1988.

100. Centers for Disease Control and Prevention. Measles prevention: recommendations of the Immunization Practices Advisory Committee (ACIP). MMWR Morbid Mortal Wkly Rep 38:1–18, 1989.

101. Centers for Disease Control and Prevention. Measles, mumps, and rubella—vaccine use and strategies for elimination of measles, rubella, and congenital rubella syndrome and control of mumps: recommendations of the Advisory Committee on Immunization Practices (ACIP). MMWR Morbid Mortal Wkly Rep 47(RR-8):1–57, 1998.

102. PJ Krause, JD Cherry, J Deseda-Tous, JG Champion, M Strassburg, C Sullivan, MJ Spencer, YJ Bryson, RC Welliver, KM Boyer. Epidemic measles in young adults: clinical, epidemiologic, and serologic studies. Ann Intern Med 90:873–876, 1979.

103. PJ Landrigan, JJ Witte. Neurologic disorders following live measles-virus vaccination. JAMA 223:1459–1462, 1973.

104. AJ Bachand, J Rubenstein, AN Morrison. Thrombocytopenic purpura following live measles vaccine. Am J Dis Child 118:283–285, 1967.

105. RG Shoss, S Rayhanzadeh. Toxic epidermal necrolysis following measles vaccination. Arch Dermatol 110: 766–770, 1974.

106. MA Greenberg, DL Birx. Safe administration of mumps, measles, rubella vaccine in egg-allergic children. J Pediatr 113:504–506, 1988.

107. S Lavi, B Zimmerman, G Koren, R Gold. Administration

of measles, mumps, and rubella virus vaccine (live) to egg-allergic children. JAMA 263:269–271, 1990.

108. Centers for Disease Control and Prevention. Immunization of children infected with human immunodeficiency virus—supplementary ACIP statement. MMWR Morbid Mortal Wkly Rep 37:181–183, 1988.

109. L Weinstein. Failure of chemotherapy to prevent the bacterial complications of measles. N Engl J Med 253:679–683, 1955.

110. C Shieh, K Hsieh. Failure of intravenous immunoglobulin to affect the recovery of immune function after measles. Pediatr Infect Dis J 8:888–891, 1989.

111. G Banks, H Fernandez. Clinical use of ribavirin in measles: a summarized review. In: RA Smith, V Knight, JA Smith, eds. Clinical Applications of Ribavirin. Orlando:Academic Press, 1984, pp 203–209.

112. CV Uylangco, GJ Beroy, LT Santiago, VD Mercoleza, SL Mendoza. A double-blind, placebo-controlled evaluation of ribavirin in the treatment of acute measles. Clin Ther 3:389–396, 1981.

113. AJ Barclay, A Foster, A Sommer. Vitamin A supplements and mortality related to measles: a randomized clinical trial. BMJ 294:294–296, 1987.

114. GD Hussey, M Klein. A randomized, controlled trial of vitamin A in children with severe measles. N Engl J Med 323:160–164, 1990.

115. A Coutsoudis, M Broughton, HM Coovadia. Vitamin A supplementation reduces measles morbidity in young African children: a randomized, placebo-controlled, double-blind trial. Am J Clin Nutr 54:890–895, 1991.

116. A Coutsoudis, P Kiepiela, HM Coovadia. Vitamin A supplementation enhances specific IgG antibody levels and total lymphocyte numbers while improving morbidity in measles. Pediatr Infect Dis J 11:203–209, 1992.

117. American Academy of Pediatrics, Committee on Infectious Diseases, 1992–1993. Vitamin A treatment of measles. Pediatrics 91:1014–1015, 1993.

118. AL Forni, NW Schluger, RB Roberts. Severe measles pneumonitis in adults: evaluation of clinical characteristics and therapy with intravenous ribavirin. Clin Infect Dis 19:454–462, 1994.

17

Marburg and Ebola Hemorrhagic Fevers

Michael R. Weir
Scott and White Clinic and Memorial Hospital, Temple, Texas, USA

Tracey E. Weir
Brackenridge Hospital, Austin, Texas, USA

Marburg and Ebola viruses are the sole agents of the family Filoviridae, so named for the appearance of its filamentous, threadlike viral particles under electron microscopy [1]. Both viruses share a clinical pattern of human-to-human spread and hemorrhagic symptoms, as seen in Africa in Lassa fever and Crimean-Congo hemorrhagic fever (Fig. 17–1). A high case to infection ratio and high case fatality rate make these viruses particularly worrisome [1]. The filoviruses have the highest case fatality rates of all viral hemorrhagic fevers [2].

HISTORY

The first filovirus outbreaks occurred in 1967 in Germany and Yugoslavia [3,4]. Clinical symptoms of hemorrhagic fever developed in 35 laboratory workers who were exposed to blood and tissue samples from green monkeys imported from Uganda. The virus found to cause the epidemic was named after the city of first occurrence, Marburg. A handful of small outbreaks or isolated cases have been reported through the years, with a 28% fatality rate [5–9]. In 1976, two epidemics of hemorrhagic fever occurred simultaneously in Zaire and Sudan, involving more than 560 cases with a 71% mortality rate [10,11]. The causative virus isolated from both epidemics was found to be morphologically similar to but serologically different from the Marburg virus [11,12]. This separate virus was named

Ebola virus after a small river in northwestern Zaire. Since the original outbreaks, Africa has experienced several epidemics [13–16], while a handful of distant countries have seen cases of laboratory infection from imported monkeys [8]. Cynomolgus monkeys imported from the Philippines have been the predominant source of laboratory-associated infection [17–19].

EPIDEMIOLOGY

The search for the origin of filovirus outbreaks has been frustrating and futile for scientists. The original source of infection for all index cases is unknown. The source of infections in laboratory monkeys is unknown. In the 1967 Marburg outbreak, all monkey-related cases were linked to direct contact with blood, organs, or tissue of the infected animals. The Ebola laboratory outbreak in 1976 involved individuals in direct contact with monkey tissue but not animal handlers [20]. The source of all secondary infections has been identified as person-to-person transmission, usually through close contact, with exposure to infected blood or body fluids. Aerosol transmission among monkeys has been suggested by evidence during laboratory animal outbreaks [21–23]. However, aerosol transmission has never been documented in humans and appears rare by epidemiology studies [13,24]. This form of transmission may be considered as a faint possibility, but only perhaps

GEOGRAPHICAL INCIDENCE

All natural outbreaks have occurred in southern countries of Africa, while laboratory cases have occurred in the United States and Europe from importation from Africa or the Phillipines.

Isolated cases in United States and Europe

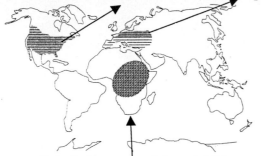

Sub-Sahara countries of Africa

TAXONOMY
Filoviridae family

TRANSMISSION

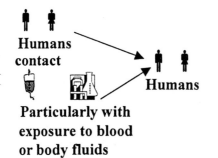

Humans contact

Humans

Particularly with exposure to blood or body fluids

ZOONOTIC IMPLICATIONS

Monkeys

} Source of isolated laboratory infections although not naturally infected.

Figure 17–1. Incidence and transmission of Marburg and Ebola hemorrhagic fevers

in extremely rare cases involving persons with advanced disease and pulmonary involvement [25]. High case fatality rates have occurred in outbreaks among primary infections, but less so in secondary infections. Serological surveillance of contacts has been unrewarding, evidence that most or all infections are symptomatic and primary infections are more severe than secondary infections.

PATHOGENESIS

The natural history and reservoir for the Ebola and Marburg viruses, as well as the details concerning the pathogenesis of these viruses, remain a mystery. No consistent vector or primate host has been identified [17]. Although monkeys have been identified as the source of infection in laboratory-associated disease, they have not been shown to be a natural reservoir of filoviruses. A common exposure to bats has been suggested, but studies provide no evidence of infection [1]. Spread of the virus in epidemics is through intimate human contact and mucous membrane or skin exposure to infected blood or bodily fluids [26]. Close contact in general is not exceptionally efficient in transmission, and secondary attack rates with this form of exposure do not typically exceed 10% [27]. The risk of transmission is highest during the late stages of illness, when vomiting, diarrhea, shock, and hemorrhage may occur [25]. The virus grows in many cell lines, particularly the reticuloendothelial system. Viremia occurs early, and cellular immunity appears with waning viremia. There is bleeding and shock, probably from vascular or endothelial injury due to the virus or to an immunological mechanism.

CLINICAL MANIFESTATIONS

The clinical manifestations of Ebola and Marburg hemorrhagic fever are listed in Table 17–1. On physical examination, the patient appears extremely ill, apathetic, dehydrated, and often disoriented. Injection of the conjunctivae and pharynx represent the predominant mucous membrane involvement (Fig. 17–2). The posterior pharynx may also contain exudative or ulcerative lesions. Non-pruritic erythematous patches may appear after 2 weeks on the trunk, with extension to the extremities and subsequent desquamation after 1 week. Petechiae, ecchymoses and bleeding may be noted, especially at pressure points. Relative bradycardia is commonly present. Some patients may have basilar rales, edema, or hepatic tenderness (Figs. 17–3 to 17–5). Jaundice is not a typical feature. Mild lymphadenopathy may be present in Marburg hemorrhagic fever, but it is not considered a feature of Ebola infection. Mucosal

Table 17–1. Clinical Manifestations of Marburg and Ebola Hemorrhagic Diseases

Time After exposure	Clinical manifestations	Laboratory analyses	Other notes
6–9 days	Abrupt onset of fever, severe headache, profound malaise, and myalgia	Antigen detection in blood or serum by IFA	Prostration and obtundation occur with progression of disease. A mask-like or ghost-like facies is described in the most severe cases, along with wasting
8–11 days	Clinical deterioration, with severe nausea and vomiting, pharyngitis, diarrhea (+/− blood), and abdominal pain. Bleeding occurs during the first week of disease, with ecchymoses, petechiae, and bleeding from gastrointestinal tract, mucous membranes, vagina, and venipuncture sites	Serology, with IgM or fourfold rise in IgG. Viral isolation from blood products. Positive direct Coombs tests	Cutaneous hemorrhage is unusual. The rash is a characteristic feature, and is useful for differential diagnosis. Abortion commonly occurs in pregnant women as a result of infection
13–15 days	A nonpruritic, maculopapular rash appears on the trunk and spreads to the extremities, and desquamates after 7 days		
16–20 days	Intractable shock with pulmonary insufficiency, often progressing to adult respiratory distress syndrome. This stage often progresses to death		
Over 5 more weeks	Slow recovery in survivors, with prostration and weigh loss. Sequelae may include uveitis, orchitis, deafness, arthralgia, pancreatitis, myelitis, psychosis, or myositis		

IgM, IgG, immunoglobulin M, G.

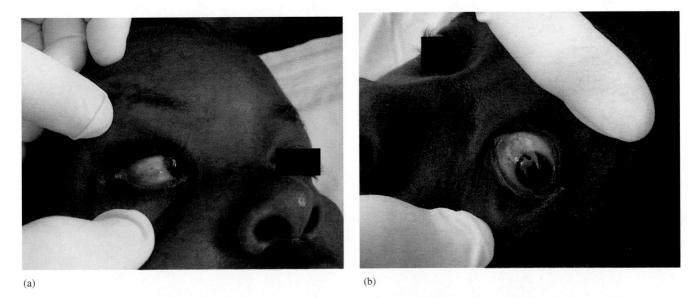

(a)

(b)

Figure 17–2. Conjunctivitis typically found in Ebola patients. (a) Early onset of Ebola conjunctivitis. (b) Latter manifestations of Ebola conjunctivitis. (Photographs courtesy of Dr. Ben Naafs.)

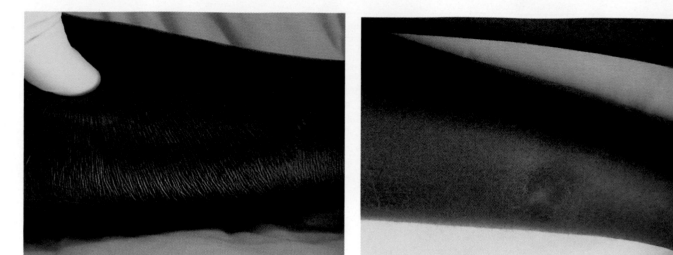

(a)   (b)

Figure 17–3.   View of Ebola-caused edema in leg. (a) Pressure being applied to leg. (b) View of edema pit after release of pressure. (Photographs courtesy of Dr. Ben Naafs.)

bleeding and persistent vomiting are specific but ominous symptoms [1]. Neurological involvement is also a poor prognostic indicator and is evidenced by nuchal rigidity, paresthesias, or changes in mentation.

LABORATORY FINDINGS

An early lymphopenia is suddenly replaced by significant neutrophilia with a left shift. Platelet numbers are modestly depressed, but function is profoundly abnormal, such that

platelet aggregation is impaired. The activated partial thromboplastin time (PTT) is lengthened, and the direct Coombs test is usually positive [6]. The plasma fibrinogen levels are variable, whereas fibrinogen degradation products are typically elevated after day 5 of clinical symptoms [6]. Hepatic transaminases are elevated, but other hepatic

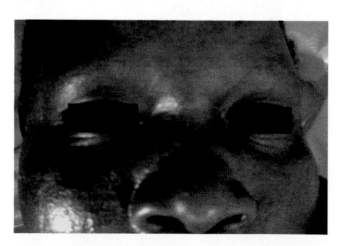

Figure 17–4.   View of Ebola patient showing facial edema. (Photograph courtesy of Dr. Ben Naafs.)

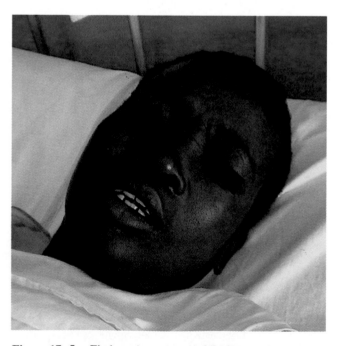

Figure 17–5.   Ebola patient with painful edema and tenderness of the face. (Photograph courtesy of Dr. Ben Naafs.)

function is preserved. Hepatic failure and disseminated intravascular coagulation (DIC) are not evident in most cases. Proteinuria is universal in these cases [28].

PATHOLOGY

Focal necrosis of multiple organs, including liver, gonads, kidney, and lymphoid tissues, are seen. The lesions are insufficient to explain the severe clinical manifestations, particularly the lethal cases. These seem to involve a pro-

found platelet dysfunction and an endothelial injury. In severe cases, widespread hemorrhage occurs, often into the visceral organs, the lumen of the stomach and intestines, the skin, and mucous membranes [2,28].

DIAGNOSIS

Indirect immunofluorescent assay for antigen detection in infected blood products is the test used initially, and it remains a basic and rapid diagnostic tool. Diagnosis by

---

Table 17–2. Differential Diagnoses for Marburg and Ebola Hemorrhagic Diseases

Yellow fever: The keys to diagnosis of yellow fever are exposure to mosquitoes and travel to tropics of Africa or the Americas toward the end of rainy season. Jaundice is profound with hemorrhagic manifestations

West Nile fever: Suggested by travel to rural Africa, southern Europe, central or south Africa, or northeastern United States, mosquito exposure, symptoms of headache, myalgia, lymphadenopathy, leukopenia, and a nonpruritic maculopapular rash

Rift Valley fever: This febrile influenza-like illness has infrequent occurrence of hemorrhagic disease, encephalitis, or retinitis. Jaundice is significant feature. Animal epizootics occur during periods of excessive rainfall. Patients have occupational animal exposure

Influenza: The coryza, cough, myalgia, and fever without rash, jaundice, frequent hemorrhage or encephalitis lead to the suspicion of influenza. Secondary bacterial complications—pneumonia and meningitis—compound the differential diagnosis and require specific antibiotic therapy

Malaria: Patients have periodic paroxysms of fever along with constitutional and gastrointestinal symptoms. Splenomegaly, pallor, and jaundice are common. *Plasmodium falciparum* in a nonimmune host may lead to cerebral malaria, blackwater fever, hepatic failure and respiratory failure

Typhoid fever: Insidious onset of fever, anorexia, abdominal pain, and constipation precede dramatic fever spikes. Rose spots may be evident. Liver function tests are abnormal. Low white cell and platelet counts are typical. Stool cultures document the etiology

Shigellosis: The acute onset of fever, toxic appearance, diarrhea (+/− blood), and abdominal pain are indicative of shigellosis. Shigellosis does not develop a skin eruption and has leukocytosis with leukocytes in the stool

Lassa fever and the South American hemorrhagic fevers: Suspect for travel to Nigeria, Argentina, Bolivia or Venezuela; rodent or nosocomial exposure; and in a patient with pharyngitis, retrosternal pain, and proteinuria. Fever, edema, conjunctivitis, and hemorrhage are also seen

Crimean-Congo hemorrhagic fever: Suggested by fever, prostration, hepatitis, hemorrhage, and tick or nosocomial exposure in Africa or eastern Europe, middle East, or Asia

Dengue: Suggested by worldwide travel in the tropics and mosquito exposure. Children predominantly affected with a capillary leak syndrome resulting in hemorrhage with shock

Kyanasur Forest disease: Suggested by tick or nosocomial exposure in India with resulting fever, myalgia, lymphadenopathy, hemorrhage, or encephalitis

Omsk hemorrhagic fever: Suggested by tick exposure in western Siberia in the spring, summer, or fall, or by muskrat hunting in the winter. The patient is usually male and may have hemorrhage and encephalopathy

Colorado tick fever: Suggested by exposure to ticks in western United States or Canada at altitudes above 4000 feet, in May to June, outdoor activities. Characterized by fever, rarely encephalitis or hemorrhage, with leukopenia and thrombocytopenia

Hantavirus hemorrhagic fever: Suggested by rodent exposure, travel to Asia or Korea, the Balkans, Scandanavia, Russia, and western Europe in the summer or fall. Characterized by a patient with fever, conjunctivitis, retro-orbital pain, hemorrhage, shock, proteinuria, and renal failure

Chikungunya fever: Suggested by severe arthralgia with hemorrhagic manifestations like dengue, yet milder. Most recognized disease is urban in the rainy season in sub-Sarahan Africa, India, southeast Asia, or the Philippines. A maculopapular rash, lymphadenopathy with conjunctival injection and periorbital edema are suggestive

serology involves the detection of immunoglobulin M (IgM) antibody, which appears as the viremia fades, or a fourfold rise in IgG titers from paired sera. This can be performed by immunofluorescence assay (IFA), Western blot, or radioimmunoprecipitation, although enzyme-linked immunosorbent assay (ELISA) is the superior and recommended assay for serology. Viral isolation is readily achieved from infected serum, plasma, or blood during the febrile stage. Other infected tissues have been used for viral isolation as well. Vero E-6 or SW-13 cells support growth, but blind suckling mice or guinea pig passage may be required for the more fastidious Sudan strain of virus. The viruses require special handling due to the biohazard level 4 classification [28]. Table 17–2 lists the differential diagnoses.

Table 17–3. Treatment of Marburg and Ebola Hemorrhagic Diseases

Symptom	Treatment
Fever	Antipyretics (avoid medications which interfere with platelet function, since the infection is already associated with thrombocytopenia and abnormal platelet aggregation)
Vomiting, diarrhea and dehydration	Oral rehydration is preferred to limit the potential for viral exposure to medical staff as well as to preserve the integrity of the skin (patients are at risk for hemorrhage from venepuncture sites). The electrolyte balance, particularly potassium, should be maintained. Antiemetics may be useful. With intractable vomiting and diarrhea, intravenous hydration is unavoidable, but special care should be exercised with these patients
Shock	Volume expanders (intravenous fluids or albumin) and blood transfusions are critical. Renal function should be monitored closely. Oliguric patients may benefit from mannitol, whereas anuric patients often need dialysis treatment
Hemorrhage	Fresh blood transfusions, platelets transfusions, fibrinogen, and/or clotting factor concentrates may be useful

TREATMENT AND PREVENTION

No specific treatment for filovirus infection is available. Ribavirin and interferon have no effect on these viruses. The administration of convalescent serum has been occasionally used, but it has no proved effect and its usefulness is doubtful. Prophylactic heparin has been recommended by some, but its use should be limited to the treatment of associated DIC. Symptomatic treatment remains the only management for filovirus infections (Table 17–3).

The development of inactivated filovirus vaccines has thus far yielded inadequate results [29,30]. Much more important and effective is the prevention of spread by strict barrier isolation and precautions for bodily fluids. The infected patient with symptoms of cough, vomiting, diarrhea, or hemorrhage should be placed in a negative pressure room, if available [25]. See Table 17-3 for more details.

CONCLUSION

Ebola and Marburg hemorrhagic fevers have a high disease rate and case fatality rate for primary infections. Secondary infections fare better. Transmitted by close human contact, these diseases are a present risk in Africa. Absence of an identified natural cycle limits precautions for primary human exposure. It is expected that the risk of importation of these diseases will increase as travel among Africa, Asia, and other continents continues to grow.

REFERENCES

1. JB McCormick. Diseases caused by hantaviruses. In: GT Strickland, ed. Hunter's Tropical Medicine. 7th ed. Philadelphia: WB Saunders, 1991, pp 244–248.
2. B Beer, R Kurth, A Bukreyev. Characteristics of Filoviridae: Marburg and Ebola viruses. Naturwissenschaften 86: 8–17, 1999.
3. R Siegert, HL Shu, W Slenzcka, D Peters, G Mueller. Zur Aetiologie einer unbekannten, von Affen ausgegangenen menschlichen Infektionskrankheit. Dtsch Med Wochensch 92:2341–2343, 1967.
4. W Stille, E Böhle, E Helm, W vanRey, W Siede. Ueber eine durch Cercopithecus aetiops uebertragene Infektionskrankheit. Dtsch Med Wochensch 93:572–582, 1968.
5. JL Conrad, M Issacson, EB Smith, H Wulff, M Crees, P Geldenhuys, J Johnston. Epidemiologic investigation of Marburg virus disease, Southern Africa, 1975. Am J Trop Med Hyg 27:1210–1215, 1978.
6. JS Gear, GA Cassel, AJ Gear, B Trappler, L Clausen, AM Meyers, MC Kew, TH Bothwell, R Sher, GB Miller, J Schneider, HJ Koornhof, ED Gomperts, M Isaacson, JH Gear. Outbreak of Marburg virus disease in Johannesburg. BMJ 4:489–493, 1975.

7. VV Nikiforov, IuI Turovskii, PP Kalinin, LA Akinfeeva, LR Katkova, VS Barmin, EI Riabchikova, NI Popkova, AM Shestopalov, VP Nazarov, et al. [A case of a laboratory infection with Marburg fever]. Zh Mikrobiol Epidemiol Immunobiol 3:104–106, 1994.

8. H Feldmann, W Slenczka, HD Klenk. Emerging and re-emerging of filoviruses. Arch Virol Suppl 11:77–100, 1996.

9. V Volchkov, V Volchkova, C Eckel, HD Klenk, M Bouloy, B LeGuenno, H Feldmann. Emergence of subtype Zaire Ebola virus in Gabon. Virology 232:139–144, 1997.

10. ET Bowen, G Lloyd, WJ Harris, GS Platt, A Baskerville, EE Vella. Viral haemorrhagic fever in southern Sudan and northern Zaire. Preliminary studies on the aetiological agent. Lancet 1:571–573, 1977.

11. KM Johnson, JV Lange, PA Webb, FA Murphy. Isolation and partial characterization of a new virus causing acute haemorrhagic fever in Zaire. Lancet 1:569–571, 1977.

12. S Pattyn, G van der Groen, G Courteille, W Jacob, P Piot. Isolation of Marburg-like virus from a case of haemorrhagic fever in Zaire. Lancet 1:573–574, 1977.

13. RC Baron, JB McCormick, OA Zubeir. Ebola virus disease in southern Sudan: hospital dissemination and intrafamilial spread. Bull World Health Organ 61:997–1003, 1983.

14. MC Georges-Courbot, CY Lu, J Lansoud-Soukate, E Leroy, S Baize. Isolation and partial molecular characterisation of a strain of Ebola virus during a recent epidemic of viral haemorrhagic fever in Gabon. Lancet 349:181, 1997.

15. Centers for Disease Control and Prevention. Outbreak of Ebola viral hemorrhagic fever Zaire, 1995. MMWR Morbid Mortal Wkly Rep 44:381–382, 1995.

16. Centers for Disease Control and Prevention. Update: outbreak of Ebola viral hemorrhagic fever Zaire, 1995. MMWR Morbid Mortal Wkly Rep 44:468–475, 1995.

17. H Hotta. Viral hemorrhagic fever—Ebola hemorrhagic fever, Marburg disease and Lassa fever. Rinsho Byori 46:651–655, 1998.

18. PB Jahrling, TW Geisbert, DW Dalgard, ED Johnson, TG Ksiazek, WC Hall, CJ Peters. Preliminary report: isolation of Ebola virus from monkeys imported to USA. Lancet 335:502–505, 1990.

19. ME Miranda, ME White, MM Dayrit, CG Hayes, TG Ksiazek, JP Burans. Seroepidemiological study of filovirus related to Ebola in the Philippines. Lancet 337:425–426, 1991.

20. B LeGuenno. Haemorrhagic fevers and ecological perturbations. Arch Virol Suppl 13:191–199, 1997.

21. CG Hayes, JP Burans, TG Ksiazek, RA Del Rosario, ME Miranda, CR Manaloto, AB Barrientos, CG Robles, MM Dayrit, CJ Peters. Outbreak of fatal illness among captive macaques in the Philippines caused by an Ebola-related filovirus. Am J Trop Med Hyg 46:664–671, 1992.

22. DW Dalgard, RJ Hardy, SL Pearson, GJ Pucak, RV Quander, PM Zack, CJ Peters, PB Jahrling. Combined simian hemorrhagic fever and Ebola virus infection in cynomolgus monkeys. Lab Anim Sci 42:152–157, 1992.

23. E Johnson, N Jaax, J White, P Jahrling. Lethal experimental infection of rhesus monkeys by aerosolized Ebola virus. Int J Exp Pathol 76:227–236, 1995.

24. Centers for Disease Control and Prevention. Management of patients with suspected viral hemorrhagic fever. MMWR Morbid Mortal Wkly Rep 37(Suppl 3):1–16, 1988.

25. Centers for Disease Control and Prevention. Update: management of patients with suspected viral hemorrhagic fever—United States. MMWR Morbid Mortal Wkly Rep 44:475–479, 1995.

26. PM Tukei. Threat of Marburg and Ebola viral haemorrhagic fevers in Africa. East Africa Med J 73:27–31, 1996.

27. CJ Peters, A Sanchez, PE Rollin, TG Ksiazek, FA Murphy. Filoviridae: Marburg and Ebola viruses. In: BN Fields, DM Knipe, PM Howley, et al, eds. Fields Virology. 3rd ed. Philadelphia: Lippincott-Raven Publishers, 1996, pp 1161–1176.

28. JB McCormick, S Fisher-Hock. Viral hemorrhagic fevers. In: KS Warren, AA Mahmoud, eds. Tropical and Geographical Medicine. 2nd ed. New York: McGraw-Hill, 1990, pp 700–728.

29. GM Ignatyev, AP Agafonov, MA Streltsova, EA Kashentseva. Inactivated Marburg virus elicits a nonprotective immune response in rhesus monkeys. J Biotechnol 44:111–118, 1996.

30. HW Lupton, RD Lambert, DL Bumgardner, JB Moe, GA Eddy. Inactivated vaccine for Ebola virus efficacious in guinea pig model. Lancet 2:1294–1295, 1980.

18

Bunyaviridae and Arenaviridae

Michael R. Weir
Scott and White Clinic and Memorial Hospital, Temple, Texas, USA

Tracey E. Weir
Brackenridge Hospital, Austin, Texas, USA

Numerous viruses are associated with the syndrome of viral hemorrhagic fever or encephalitis and occur worldwide (Fig. 18–1). The majority of these pathogens come from the following virus families: Arenaviridae, Bunyaviridae, Filoviridae, and Flaviviridae. Although the epidemiology and spectrum of disease varies among these infections, clinical features may sometimes be difficult to differentiate among them. The Bunyaviridae family consists of more than 200 different viruses, several of which are human pathogens. The Arenaviridae family has four well-described human pathogens among its 14 known virus members. All of these viruses have natural animal hosts, and most of these human infections are acquired through mosquito or tick transmission. Oropouche virus and sandfly fever viruses, members of the Bunyaviridae, are discussed in Chapter 21.

BUNYAVIRIDAE

California/La Crosse Encephalitis

Definition

The California encephalitis serogroup consists of mosquito-transmitted, enveloped RNA viruses that cause human encephalitis or milder disease. The prototype virus is La Crosse (LAC), which causes disease predominantly in children. Three viral subgroups, A, B, and C, are distinguished by RNA techniques. The La Crosse virus causes nearly all of the infections attributed to the California group viruses in the United States (Fig. 18–2).

Other viruses of the California serogroup that cause encephalitis in humans include the California virus, snowshoe hare virus, Inkoo and Tahyna viruses, trivittatus virus, and Jamestown Canyon virus. California virus is found in the southwestern United States. Jamestown Canyon virus is found in Alaska and the northeastern United States. It is transmitted by Culiseta mosquitoes and amplified in white-tail deer. Snowshoe hare virus, named after its mammalian host, is found in Canada, Alaska, and the Rocky Mountains. Trivittatus virus is present in the midwestern and southeastern United States. Tahyna occurs in southern Europe and Inkoo occurs in Finland. Reindeer and moose are natural hosts.

History

In 1960, La Crosse virus was first isolated from a 4-year-old patient who died from encephalitis in La Crosse, Wisconsin, hence the name. Epidemiological and serological studies demonstrated that the La Crosse virus was a significant cause of "rural encephalitis" that had inflicted a number of children in the upper Midwest, particularly Wisconsin and Minnesota. A virus previously isolated in 1943 in California (California virus) [1] proved to be a similar, but much less common, cause of encephalitis. Except for

GEOGRAPHICAL INCIDENCE

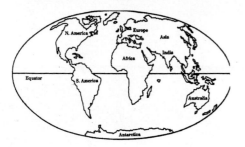

TAXONOMY

Bunyaviridae family

    Bunyavirus genus (California/LaCrosse)
    Hantavirus genus (Hantavirus)
    Nairovirus genus (Crimean-Congo)
    Phlebovirus genus (Rift Valley fever)
Arenaviridae family

    Arenavirus genus (Lassa and South American fevers)

Figure 18–1. Taxonomy and incidence of Bunyaviridae and Arenaviridae families.

epidemics due to St. Louis encephalitis virus, La Crosse virus is the most prevalent mosquito-borne arboviral infection and the most commonly identified cause of encephalitis in the United States [2].

Incidence

Most La Crosse infections result in subclinical infection or fever alone, while encephalitis with fever is much less frequent. Serological studies suggest that La Crosse virus may infect more than 300,000 humans each year in the United States, with more than 1000 subclinical or mildly symptomatic infections per reported clinical case [3]. Most cases of La Crosse occur in Wisconsin, Illinois, Ohio, and Minnesota. Sporadic infections have been found in 20 other states, predominantly in areas east of the Mississippi River. In endemic areas, the annual incidence of La Crosse encephalitis is 10 to 30 cases per 100,000 persons, which exceeds that for all types of bacterial meningitis [4]. An average of 73 cases of La Crosse encephalitis are reported to the Centers for Disease Control and Prevention (CDCP) in the United States each year [5]. The majority of cases occur between July and September when the specific mosquito vector is most active. Cases of encephalitis occur almost exclusively in children less than 15 years of age [6]. Boys develop infection twice as often as girls, likely because of increased outdoor exposure in this group [7].

GEOGRAPHICAL INCIDENCE

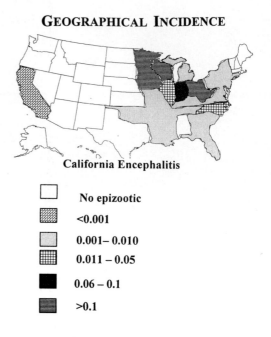

California Encephalitis

☐	No epizootic
▨	<0.001
▨	0.001– 0.010
▦	0.011 – 0.05
■	0.06 – 0.1
▤	>0.1

TRANSMISSION

Completion of a blood meal is not necessary for transmission, and probing alone is infectious.

Squirrels, other small mammals	Bite of an infected mosquito	Humans

ZOONOTIC IMPLICATIONS

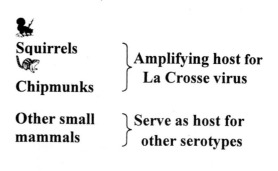

Squirrels

Chipmunks } **Amplifying host for La Crosse virus**

Other small mammals } **Serve as host for other serotypes**

Figure 18–2. Incidence and transmission of California/La Crosse encephalitis.

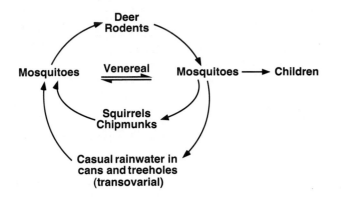

Figure 18–3. Transmission of La Crosse encephalitis among vectors and hosts.

Most cases occur in rural areas or forested suburbs and small mammals are potential amplifying hosts [8]. Seroprevalence rates rise with age, reaching about 20% by age 60 years. There are few deaths (0.3%), and low rates of sequelae.

Pathogenesis

Aedes triseriatus, the tree hole mosquito, is the mosquito vector of La Crosse virus and also a reservoir in nature. Once infected, these mosquitoes carry the virus for life. The female breeds in small collections of rain water, such as tree holes, cans, and discarded containers. She transmits the virus to offspring, constituting an over-wintering mechanism for the virus. There also is venereal transmission to uninfected females during mating. Small mammals, such as chipmunks and squirrels, serve as amplifying hosts [9]. Humans are dead-end hosts as they do not have a prolonged viremia with La Crosse infection. Related viruses have a

variety of natural hosts, mosquito vector species, and biotypes (Fig. 18–3).

After the virus is introduced into human skin and subcutaneous tissue by the feeding mosquito, viral replication occurs in nearby muscle tissue. This leads to dissemination into the blood. With viremia, further viral replication occurs in vascular endothelial cells, reticuloendothelial cells, and chondrocytes. This amplification results in further viremia with central nervous system (CNS) invasion. Access to the CNS is gained by infection of the vascular endothelial cells, followed by infection of neurons and glial cells [10,11].

Clinical Manifestations

La Crosse virus and related viruses share a common clinical pattern. Encephalitis is less common than inapparent or nonspecific mild infection. Symptomatic disease occurs in less than 1% of infections. Children have more severe disease, a higher frequency of encephalitis and more frequent sequelae (Table 18–1). Mild cases involve meningeal signs and disorientation. More severe cases have seizures and altered states of consciousness with paresis, aphasia, and abnormal reflexes. Only 25% of cases develop nuchal rigidity, and only 50% of cases have any signs of meningeal irritation. No associated cutaneous manifestations have been described. Seizure disorders constitute the principal sequelae. Less than 2% of patients have significant neurological sequelae, such as focal weakness or spasticity [8]. Common migraine headaches may occur after encephalitis, particularly in those children who developed localization-related epilepsy [12]. Poor school performance in some children is a possible consequence, but epidemiological studies have difficulty distinguishing this manifestation

Table 18–1. Clinical Manifestations of La Crosse Infection

Time after exposure	Clinical manifestations	Laboratory analyses	Other notes
3–7 days	Prodrome of fever (102°–104°F) malaise, headache, irritability, drowsiness, and vomiting, lasting 2–3 days. Diarrhea is usually absent	Specific serology with IgM or fourfold rise in IgG titers. Isolation of IgM in CSF fluid is most specific	Fever and somnolence are the only universal characteristics. Some cases may present with only a sudden convulsion
6–11 days	Half of patients progress to focal or generalized seizures or disorientation. Other patients gradually improve		10% of cases develop status epilepticus
10–15 days	Resolution of disease without sequelae in most patients		Patients who develop encephalopathy or coma require more time for recovery, typically at least 2 weeks

CSF, cerebrospinal fluid; IgG, IgM, immunoglobulin G, M.

Table 18–2. Differential Diagnoses of California/La Crosse Encephalitis

Herpes simplex virus (HSV) encephalitis: HSV encephalitis should be excluded because of its severe outcome and response to antiviral therapy. Rapid testing for HSV is commonly employed. A hemorrhagic, necrotizing encephalitis of the temporal lobes is typical, but it may appear as meningitis or encephalitis with seizures and coma

Enteroviral aseptic meningitis: Patients have fever, headache and nuchal rigidity. CSF studies show lymphocytic predominance with elevated protein. Enteroviral meningoencephalitis will be clinically indistinguishable from other viral CNS diseases. Serology, viral isolation or, where available, nucleic amplification testing will prove the etiology

Bacterial meningitis: A history of fever, nuchal rigidity, and headache with Kernig's and Brudzinski's signs are expected. Leukocytic predominance in the CFS with low glucose and high protein are expected as are positive bacterial cultures, gram stain, or antigen tests. Diagnosis is based on laboratory analysis of CFS

Tuberculous meningitis: Usually an insidious process associated with a miliary chest radiograph or tuberculous osteomyelitis

Cerebral malaria: Patients have periodic paroxysms of fever along with constitutional and gastrointestinal symptoms. Splenomegaly, pallor and jaundice are common. *Plasmodium falciparum* in a non-immune host may lead to cerebral malaria, blackwater fever, hepatic failure, and respiratory failure

Dengue virus with encephalopathy: Dengue is suggested by world-wide travel in the tropics and mosquito exposure; children predominantly affected with a capillary leak syndrome resulting in hemorrhage with shock

Intracranial hemorrhage/Stroke: Intracerebral hemorrhage is associated with adults; smoking or hypertension, and a variety of neurological deficits but without fever

Heat stroke: A history of insufficient fluid intake for the circumstances precedes extreme temperature elevation and seizures. Lacking is the specific geography and vector exposures, specific rash, or hepatic dysfunction

Lead encephalopathy: Exposure to automobile or battery destruction or repair, smelter activities, or lead based paint aid in diagnosis. Patient is usually a child with encephalopathy with anemia but normal white blood count

Brain abscess: Fever, signs of increased intracranial pressure, focal seizures, focal EEG, abnormal imaging (nuclear scan, CT scan, MRI), and bulging fontanelle or spread sutures are seen

Brain tumor: Afebrile, signs of increased intracranial pressure, progressive neurologic deficits, abnormal imaging (nuclear scan, CT scan, MRI), and bulging fontanelle or spread sutures are seen

Post-infectious encephalitis: Guillain-Barré presents as afebrile loss of reflexes with ascending weakness; it may progress to respiratory depression. Acute cerebellar ataxia follows varicella and shows only ataxia that appears suddenly and resolves without residual deficits

Metabolic encephalopathy: Coma or altered mental status occur with elevated ammonia or BUN, depressed glucose, or history consistent with inborn error of metabolism. Absent fever and absent focal findings typify this group of conditions

Status epilepticus (SE): A prior history of a seizure disorder, sudden onset of unresponsiveness, perhaps with stereotypic behavior and abnormal EEG, SE may resolve with antiepilepsy drugs administered acutely

Acute confusional or basilar migraine: Altered mental status or coma appear suddenly, perhaps following an aura. Episodes are quite similar. Though not postictal, somnolence may follow each attack. Fever and seizures are absent

Reye's syndrome: Depressed mental status following varicella or influenza treated with aspirin is associated with hypoglycemia, bleeding disorder, elevated ammonia, and altered liver function tests

Other arboviral encephalitides:
  Japanese encephalitis is suggested by severe encephalopathy in children in Asia in the monsoon reason
  Eastern equine encephalitis
  Western equine encephalitis
  Venezuelan equine encephalitis
  West Nile fever
  St. Louis encephalitis — See Table 15–2
  Tick-borne encephalitis
  Powassan encephalitis
  Rocky Mountain spotted fever
  Rift Valley fever
  Kyasanur Forest disease — See Table 17–2
  Colorado tick fever

BUN, blood urea nitrogen; CNS, central nervous system; CSF, cerebrospinal fluid; CT, computed tomography; EEG, electroencephalogy; MRT, magnetic resonance imaging.

from background rates in the general population [13,14]. Table 18–2 lists possible differential diagnoses.

Laboratory Findings

A peripheral leukocytosis with a left shift is frequent. The cerebrospinal fluid (CSF) shows a moderate mononuclear pleocytosis with mildly elevated protein (in one third of cases) and normal glucose. Computed tomography (CT) scans may show focal abnormalities as do brain scans. However, most CT scans appear normal [16]. Electroencephalographic findings are frequent, usually consisting of generalized symmetrical slow waves.

Pathology

Cerebral edema, perivascular cuffing, glial nodules, and neuronal degeneration are evident. All are common findings in other arboviral CNS disease.

Diagnosis

Recovery of virus from brain tissue has been reported, but viral isolation from cerebrospinal fluid (CSF) has never been successfully performed [17,18]. Detection of viral antigens also is problematic. Therefore, serology remains the cornerstone of diagnosis. Serological diagnosis requires a fourfold titer rise in hemagglutination inhibition (HI), neutralization (N), or complement fixation (CF) antibodies. Immunoglobulin M (IgM) by enzyme-linked immunosorbent assay (ELISA) is sensitive early in the disease [19], but IgM remains elevated in the serum for at least 9 months in more than 50% of patients. Thus, demonstration of IgM in CSF is the most sensitive and specific diagnostic method for patients living in endemic areas.

Treatment and Prevention

Mild cases are the most common and require only symptomatic treatment. Encephalitis cases must be supported with therapy available for sudden seizure development or acute neurological deterioration (Table 18–3). Ribavirin has been shown to have in vitro efficacy against La Crosse virus [20], but no clinical trials have yet been completed to confirm an in vivo benefit. The control of the mosquito vector requires eradication of the principal breeding sites by cementing holes of trees and removing discarded containers. Aggressive mosquito control programs in a county in Wisconsin reduced the number of cases in that area. Mosquito repellents and insecticides prevent the risk of infection by minimizing exposure to the mosquito vector.

Conclusion

La Crosse and related viruses employ a variety of mosquitoes and natural hosts endemic to the biotype, or climate. Asymptomatic infection and mild disease predominate. Clinical encephalitis has a favorable outcome in most cases, and sequelae are uncommon.

Table 18–3. Treatment of La Crosse Encephalitis

Symptom	Treatment
General	Close monitoring for changes in consciousness. If the child is disoriented, admission to an intensive care unit is necessary
Fever	Antipyretics
Headaches	Analgesics
Altered consciousness	Institute measures to limit the cerebral metabolic rate, such a fever control and seizure management. Prevention of cerebral edema is important, with maintenance of serum osmolality, avoiding hypotonic IV fluids, and monitoring for hyponatremia. Other methods include sedation, elevation of the head of the bed, hyperventilation, and osmotic agents
Seizures	Control with anticonvulsants. If this treatment is required, at least one major anticonvulsant should be continued for 1 year to reduce the risk of post-encephalitis epilepsy
Choreoathetosis	Haloperidol therapy
Irritability and confusion	Lorazepam and haloperidol

Hantaviruses

Definition

Hantaviral diseases consist of hemorrhagic fevers with renal syndrome (HFRS) in Eurasia and hantavirus pulmonary syndrome (HPS) in the Americas. These rodent-borne infections are due to a number of different hantaviruses, each with a specific rodent reservoir [23]. Four distinct viruses cause the HFRS. Hantaan virus, the prototype of this genus, is endemic in Asia and causes the most severe disease. Dobrava/Belgrade virus causes a severe infection in the Balkans. Seoul virus has a wider endemic area, and causes less severe disease. Puumala virus is the etiologic agent of a mild form of HFRS, known as nephropathia epidermica. This virus is present in Scandinavia, Russian, and western Europe. Several hantaviruses cause HPS in North and South America. Sin Nombre virus caused the first recognized epidemic in the southwestern United States in 1993. Black Creek Canal and Bayou viruses also cause HPS in the Americas (Fig. 18–4).

GEOGRAPHICAL INCIDENCE

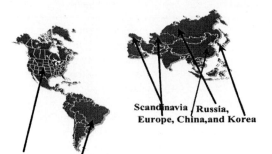

Scandinavia / Russia,
Europe, China, and Korea

North and South America

TRANSMISSION

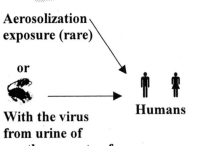

Aerosolization
exposure (rare)

or

With the virus
from urine of
or other excreta of
infected rodents.

Humans

ZOONOTIC IMPLICATIONS

Rodents } Each hantavirus has a specific
rodent reservoir:

Hantaan virus: Manchurian striped
field mouse (*Apodemus agrarius*)

Dobrava virus: Yellow-necked field
mouse (*Apdomus flavicollis*)

Seoul virus: Black rat (*Rattus rattus*) and
Norway rat (*Rattus norvegicus*)

Puumala virus: European bank vole
(*Clethrionomys glareolus*)

Sin Nombre virus: Deer mouse
(*Peromyscus maniculatus*) and white-
footed mouse (*Peromyscus leucopus*)

Black Creek Canal virus: Cotton rat
(*Sigmodon hispidus*)

Bayou virus: Rice rat (*Oryzomys*)

Figure 18–4.   Incidence and transmission of Hantaviruses.

History

The clinical syndromes associated with hantavirus infection were described as early as 960 A.D. in China [24]. Reports of the HFRS date back to 1913 in Russia [25], and sporadic epidemics have been described in Manchuria, Siberia, and Lapland during the 1930s and 1940s [26–28]. In 1940, Japanese researchers first inoculated humans and monkeys with bacteria-free serum from patients with HFRS. The serum recipients then developed the same syndrome, proving the etiology to be infectious and viral [24]. This syndrome first received worldwide attention when more than 3000 United Nations troops stationed in Korea during 1951 to 1954 (Korean War) became infected. The illness was characterized by hemorrhage, shock, and renal failure with a mortality rate of 5 to 15% and was initially known as epidemic hemorrhagic fever [29,30]. Convalescent sera from hundreds of patients were collected and stored, and approximately 20 years later, hantavirus was determined to the etiological agent by serology and viral isolation [31]. In 1993, a cluster of unexplained respiratory illnesses leading to death was found in the four corners region of the southwestern United States [32–34]. This ''new'' hemorrhagic fever was quickly demonstrated to be due to a hantavirus that is related to, but distinct from, those causing HFRS. This syndrome, known as HPS, is also rodent-borne and is associated with a high case fatality rate [35].

Incidence

The hantavirus group is distributed worldwide in rodents [36]. HFRS occurs in early summer and late fall in a band-like distribution from Scandinavia across Europe and Russia to China and Korea [37]. Hantaviruses continue to cause a considerable number of infections in certain countries, such as China, Korea, and eastern Russia, with over 100,000 known cases in China each year [38]. Milder disease characterizes the European condition, while the Asian variety is quite severe (Korean hemorrhagic fever). After the first recognized epidemic of HPS in 1993, additional cases have been recognized in almost half of the states in the continental United States, particularly in areas west of the Mississippi. As of March 1999, 211 cases of HPS have been confirmed by the CDCP, with a case fatality rate of 34% and an overall fatality of 43%. Occasional cases of HPS have also been seen in Canada and South American countries, such as Argentina, Bolivia, and Chile [39–44]. Particularly heavy snowfall preceded the United States cases, whereas excessive rainfall was noted prior to the South American cases.

Pathogenesis

Rodent hantavirus infection is chronic with lifelong excretion of virus. Adult males who hunt rodents are at greater

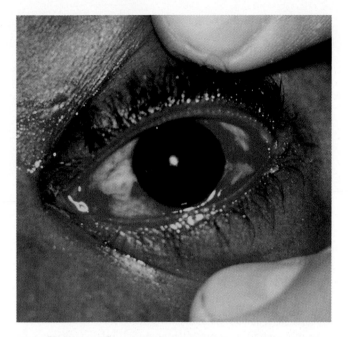

Figure 18–5. Hemorrhagic conjunctivitis secondary to infection with Hantavirus (Korean hemorrhagic fever). (Photograph courtesy of Drs. Monica McCrary and Jack Lesher, Medical College of Georgia, Augusta, GA.)

risk of acquiring infection [23]. Laboratory workers also may become infected by handling infected rodents. Human-to-human spread has not been demonstrated [45,46]. The virus presumably enters the human body via the respiratory mucosa. It can be detected in plasma during the first 7 days of clinical illness [47]. The underlying pathology of both HFRS and HPS is damage to the capillary endothelium. This is likely a consequence of viral replication and immune complex deposition [48,49]. The damage to the endothelium results in vasodilation and leakage of fluid and blood cells into tissues [47]. For unknown reasons, the viruses that cause HFRS are more tropic for the kidney, whereas those causing HPS have a predilection for lung tissue [50]. HPS demonstrates immunological mechanisms; inflammatory mediators are directed against pulmonary tissue infected with virus. Gamma interferon and tumor necrosis factor have been suspected. T-cells act on pulmonary endothelium [49]. HPS and HFRS have prominent capillary leak syndrome and cardiac depression with cardiogenic shock. HFRS has acute tubular necrosis as the principal renal insult.

Clinical Manifestations

Hemorrhagic Fever with Renal Syndrome. Prototypic HFRS involves fever, hemorrhage, and renal failure [49] (Fig. 18–5). Severe HFRS presents with headache, abdom-

Table 18–4. Clinical Manifestations of Hantavirus Hemorrhagic Fever with Renal Syndrome (HFRS)

Time after exposure	Clinical manifestations	Other notes
4–21 days	Abrupt onset of influenza-like prodrome, with high fever, chills, headache, dizziness, myalgias, abdominal pain, backache, and anorexia	
18–28 days	Abrupt defervescence of the febrile stage, followed by hypotensive stage, lasting 2 h to 3 days. Patients have nausea, vomiting, and typically develop severe clinical shock	One third of deaths due to HFRS occur during the hypotensive stage
18–31 days	Recovery from hypotension coincides with the development of the oliguric stage, lasting 3–7 days. Patients have varying degrees of renal failure, with pulmonary edema, pneumonitis, transient hypertension, and mucosal bleeding. More extensive hemorrhage may occur, with ecchymoses, hemoptysis, hematemesis, hematuria, melena, and central nervous system hemorrhage (rare)	Two thirds of the deaths due to HFRS occur during the oliguric stage, particularly due to pulmonary edema and cerebrovascular accidents (likely due to coagulopathy)
21–38 days	The polyuric stage begins in survivors of the illness and may last for weeks to months during recovery. Renal function is spontaneously restored and urine output of 3 to 6 L/day may occur. Massive fluid and electrolyte shifts may result with the diuresis	Patients who survive generally make a complete recovery, except those who develop central nervous system hemorrhages

inal pain, lumbar pain, proteinuria, and hemorrhagic manifestations with shock and renal insufficiency. Thirty to forty percent of these cases consist of minimal illness, and only 20% to 30% of patients have moderate to severe disease [51–53]. Table 18–4 summarizes the clinical manifestations.

Initially, there is a febrile phase, followed by hypotension, then by oliguria. Diuresis follows, leading into prolonged convalescence. Survival is usually associated with complete recovery, but chronic renal insufficiency may ensue. During the febrile stage, ciliary muscle involvement may cause blurred vision. With this, there is photophobia, pain of extraocular muscles, and retro-orbital pain. The face, neck, and back are flushed, and pharyngeal and conjunctival suffusion is noted. Petechiae are seen in the conjunctivae, axillae, and at points of pressure. Costovertebral angle pain reflects retroperitoneal edema. Proteinuria, disseminated intravascular coagulation (DIC), and an active urinary sediment become evident.

During the hypotensive period, a rising hematocrit corresponds with the capillary leak syndrome. There is isosthenuria along with massive proteinuria and oliguria. The presence of atypical lymphocytes and activation of kinins gives evidence for immunological activity in this stage.

The oliguric phase is associated with severe hemorrhagic phenomena and the majority of deaths. Less severe cases of HFRS (Seoul virus) develop fever with gastrointestinal symptoms followed by brief oliguria, then hypos-

---

Table 18–5. Differential Diagnoses of Hantavirus Hemorrhagic Fever

Leptospirosis: A biphasic febrile illness with myalgia precedes central nervous system manifestations. Jaundice and exposure to animals are epidemiological clues. The rash is a trunchal, erythematous, maculopapular rash. It may be urticarial, petechial, purpuric, or desquamative

Acute renal failure: A variety of etiologies leads to hematuria, proteinuria, azotemia, and/or hypertension. These include toxins/drugs, systemic lupus, HSP, malaria, and severe dehydration and shock

Murine typhus: Fever, headache, and a trunchal rash that spreads peripherally are typical. The condition is mild. Exposure to rat flea environment is necessary

Scrub typhus: Travel to the southwest Pacific, eschar from a mite bite, lymphadenopathy, hepatosplenomegaly, a rash, and pneumonia are suggestive of scrub typhus

Meningococcemia: Fever, petechiae and purpura; altered mental status; and leukocytosis precedes shock

Pyelonephritis: Fever, pyuria, bacteriuria, and costovertebral angle tenderness precede sepsis and endotoxic shock

Hemolytic uremic syndrome: A hemolytic anemia, thrombocytopenia, and azotemia follow gastroenteritis. A Shiga-like toxin has been implicated

Scarlet fever: Exudative pharyngitis, cervical adenitis, and a fine maculopapular rash with coarse, sand paper texture are characteristic. Group A β- hemolytic streptococcus on throat culture is diagnostic. This infection may lead to sepsis or necrotizing fasciitis

Acute abdomen (e.g., appendicitis): Diffuse pain migrates to the right lower quadrant, with fever and leukocytosis lead to peritoneal signs and abscess or septic shock

Heatstroke: A history of insufficient fluid intake for the circumstances precedes extreme temperature elevations and seizures. Lacking is the specific geography and vector exposures, specific rash, or hepatic dysfunction

Goodpasture's disease: Azotemia, hematuria, and proteinuria are seen with pulmonary insufficiency

Anaphylactoid purpura (Henoch-Schönlein purpura [HSP]): A purpuric rash of dependent areas (hands, feet, buttocks) is seen with hematuria of renal insufficiency, arthritis, gastrointestinal pain or bleeding, and/or intussusception

Rocky Mountain spotted fever
Other arboviral infections:
  ONN
  Sindbis
  Mayaro   } See Table 15–2
  Oropouche
  Sandfly fever
    Hantavirus pulmonary syndrome
Other hemorrhagic fevers:
  Rift Valley fever
  Kyasanur Forest disease
  Omsk hemorrhagic fever
  Colorado tick fever   } See Table 17–2
  Crimean-Congo hemorrhagic fever
  Lassa fever and the South American
    hemorrhagic fevers
  Chikungunya fever

Dengue: Suggested by world-wide travel in the tropics and mosquito exposure. Children predominantly affected with a capillary leak syndrome resulting in hemorrhage with shock

Ebola and Marburg hemorrhagic fevers: Suggested by laboratory (Europe) or wild (Africa) exposure to monkeys, patients' tissue, or secretions; by pharyngitis; conjunctival injection; toxic appearance; dehydration; basilar rales; edema; and hemorrhage

thenuria. The clinical course with mild disease is of shorter duration. Differential diagnoses are presented in Table 18–5.

Nephropathia epidemica is a milder variant of HFRS, usually caused by the Puumala virus. While 90% of these infections are asymptomatic, less than 10% are associated with hemorrhage and less than 1% are fatal [54,55].

Haantavirus Pulmonary Syndrome. HPS displays a febrile, respiratory failure pattern with prominent capillary leak syndrome. Hypotension and hemorrhagic manifestations are frequent. Tachycardia, tachypnea, and hypotension herald hypoxemia and pulmonary edema. Cutaneous and conjunctival manifestations that are seen in other hemorrhagic fevers are absent with HPS. If frank shock with severe hypoxemia and respiratory failure appear promptly, there are severe manifestations of abnormal capillary permeability, with high mortality rates despite good medical care. The case fatality rate is up to 10 times that seen in HFRS [54]. Table 18–6 depicts a timeline for hantavirus pulmonary syndrome.

Pathology

In HFRS, capillary dilation and red cell diapedesis are present, along with retroperitoneal and other interstitial edemas. Hemorrhage occurs in the skin, mucous membranes, and various organs. Kidneys are edematous and hemorrhagic, and hemorrhage can also develop in the pituitary gland and right atrium [56].

HPS pathology involves pulmonary endothelial and reticuloendothelial findings. The lungs are dense and rubbery in a serous pleural fluid. Intraalveolar edema and interstitial mononuclear infiltrate are seen. The endothelium shows generalized capillary dilitation and edema. Viral inclusions are seen on electron microscopy, with viral antigen at high levels. Cardiac endothelium is affected and may result in the myocardial depression seen clinically. Lymphoid tissues show immunoblasts in the spleen and lymph nodes.

Laboratory Findings

Neutrophilia, circulating atypical lymphocytes, hemoconcentration, and thrombocytopenia are frequent with both

Table 18–6. Clinical Manifestations of Hantavirus Pulmonary Syndrome

Time after symptom onset	Clinical manifestations	Laboratory analyses	Other notes
7–4 days	Sudden onset of prodromal symptoms, with fever, headache, myalgia, and cough, progressing to hypoxia. Over half of patients have gastrointestinal symptoms, with nausea, vomiting, abdominal pain or diarrhea, mainly mild. Some patients may also complain of malaise, dyspnea, and dizziness	Serology, with IgM acutely or fourfold rise of IgG in paired sera. Detection of viral antigens in infected tissue by PCR	
9–7 days	Rapid development of bilateral interstitial pulmonary infiltrates develop along with adult respiratory distress syndrome (ARDS). With this, the pulmonary capillary wedge pressures are <10 mm Hg. Hypotension, rhabdomyolysis, and thrombocytopenia also develop. In some patients, myocardial depression and hypovolemia develop, although systemic vascular resistance is high		The degree of hypoxia generally progresses to require mechanical ventilation. The rapidity of cardiopulmonary decompensation is the hallmark of HPS
10–18 days	Hospitalization is usually required with 3–4 days of symptom onset		
12–21 days	Maximal hemodynamic compromise peaks, with severe hypotension and pulmonary edema. Renal failure may occur in some cases but is uncommon. Survivors typically develop diuresis and recover without sequelae		Most deaths occur within 2 days of hospitalization

IgG, IgM, immunoglobulin G, M; PCR, polymerase chain reaction; HPS, hantavirus pulmonary syndrome.

syndromes. HFRS has proteinuria, azotemia, oliguria with electrolyte abnormalities, and evidence of renal insufficiency, then polyuria. There may be evidence of DIC and platelet dysfunction, possibly due to uremia. HPS shows varying degrees of hypoxia and respiratory insufficiency, progressing to respiratory failure with hypoxia, hypercapnea, and acidosis.

Diagnosis

HFRS and HPS can be confirmed serologically by a four-fold IgG antibody rise in paired sera or by IgM antibody acutely [36]. These antibodies may be detected from the initial presentation of patients with both HFRS and HPS [38]. Sin Nombre IgG ELISA is useful for epidemiological screening due to IgG persistence with clinical exposure. Reverse transcriptase-polymerase chain reaction (RT-PCR) detects hantavirus RNA in human tissue, such as blood clots, buffy coat, or fresh-frozen lung tissue [57]. Detection of viral antigens is not as effective from serum samples. Isolation of virus is difficult and not generally available for diagnostic purposes. Table 18–7 presents differential diagnoses.

Treatment and Prevention

The high case fatality rates, particularly for HPS, attest to the difficulty of treatment. Ribavirin appears to be effective if used within the first 7 days for HFRS [36]. Studies have not shown ribavirin to be of benefit in the treatment of HPS thus far, although further studies are underway. Supportive care continues to be the mainstay of treatment (Table 18–8).

Laboratory worker exposure is minimized by the use of suitable precautions while handling rodents. Household hygienic precautions to reduce vector populations are useful. The avoidance of hunting rodents for food limits disease, but protein malnutrition in economically disadvantaged areas is a risk of this strategy. A formalin-inactivated Hantaan virus vaccine is commercially available at this time, but efficacy data do not exist.

Conclusion

Hantaviral syndromes, HFRS and HPS, have an intimate relationship with rodent hosts. HPS is quite severe, and Asian HFRS more severe than the European variety. Antiviral therapy has a role early is disease, but immunological mechanisms cause the most severe manifestations. Therapy is supportive and recovery is usually complete for those who survive.

Table 18–7. Differential Diagnoses of Hantavirus Pulmonary Syndrome

Pneumonia with sepsis: Sudden onset of fever, cough, respiratory insufficiency, possibly empyema, progressing to shock and multiple organ failure, and adult respiratory distress syndrome (ARDS)

Fungal pneumonias: Coccidioidomycosis occurs in desert habitat, more often in males, and may have erythema nodosum. Usually is self-limited except to immune compromised hosts. Histoplasmosis occurs in moist areas with aerosolization of excreta of birds. In blastomycosis, pulmonary involvement results from inhalation of the agent, leading to fever malaise, cough, and chest pain. Consolidation results in chronic respiratory compromise

Plague (*Yersinia pestis*): Travel to endemic area is key with high index of suspicion when seeing chills, fever, lymphadenopathy, headache, pneumonia, DIC, purpuric skin lesions, or meningitis

Tularemia: Also may be associated with a tick bite, but the site of inoculation becomes painful and ulcerated, often with associated lymphadenopathy

Relapsing fever: Recurrent fevers, exposure to lice or ticks, headache, photophobia, nausea, vomiting, myalgia, arthralgia, and hemorrhage from skin, gastrointestinal, or GU track occur. A diffuse macular rash may appear. Hepatitis and encephalitis may occur

Brucellosis: Occurs world wide with exposure to domestic animals or unpasteurized dairy products. Triad of fever, arthralgia/arthritis, and hepatosplenomegaly is classic

Legionella: Progressive respiratory insufficiency with atypical pneumonia, chills, abdominal pain, myalgia, headache, fatigue; low or absent fever; in spite of routine antibiotic treatment progresses to respiratory failure. A variety of species and serotypes in the genus *Legionella* is etiologic

Psittacosis: An exotic avian exposure, abrupt onset of fever, chills, sweats, headache, nonproductive cough, rales, abnormal chest xray, pleural effusion, mild leukocytosis, and abnormal liver function tests characterize infection with chlamydia psittaci

Rocky Mountain spotted fever	
Leptospirosis	} See Table 15–2
Murine typhus	
Scrub typhus	
Heatstroke	
Goodpasture's disease	} See Table 18–5
Meningococcemia	
Pyelonephritis	
Pulmonary hemorrhage with Henoch-Schönlein purpura	

DIC, disseminated intravascular coagulation; GU, genitourinary.

Table 18–8. Treatment of Hemorrhagic Fever with Renal Syndrome (HFRS) and Hantavirus Pulmonary Syndrome (HPS)

Symptom	Treatment
General	Intravenous ribavirin therapy for severe cases of HFRS. Bed rest
Fever	Antipyretics. Acetaminophen is preferred over aspirin and other nonsteroid anti-inflammatories, since thrombocytopenia is already present with these syndromes
Capillary leak and hypotension	Cautious repletion with intravenous fluid and colloids. Overhydration should be avoided to prevent exacerbation of pulmonary edema
Cardiac depression	Vasopressor and inotropic agents may be beneficial
Renal insufficiency	Careful fluid and electrolyte maintenance
Renal failure	Peritoneal dialysis or hemodialysis
Respiratory insufficiency	Oxygen therapy, or if necessary, mechanical ventilation. Pulmonary artery catheterization with wedge pressure tracings is necessary in most cases

GEOGRAPHICAL INCIDENCES

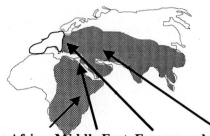

Africa, Middle East, Europe, and Asia

TRANSMISSION

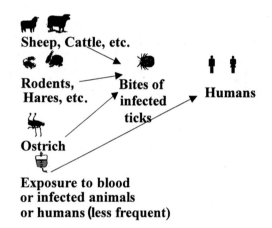

ZOONOTIC IMPLICATIONS

The details of animal reservoirs are not completely clear.

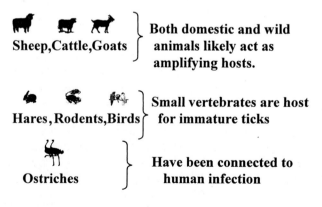

Figure 18–6. Incidence and transmission of Crimean-Congo hemorrhagic fever.

Crimean–Congo Hemorrhagic Fever

Definition

The Crimean-Congo hemorrhagic fever virus is in the genus Nairovirus. A related Nairovirus causes Nairobi sheep disease. It causes severe disease, whether tick-borne or nosocomial, and occurs across a wide area of the eastern hemisphere (Fig. 18–6).

History

From 1944 to 1945, over 200 agricultural workers in the Crimea developed a new syndrome of high fever, prostration, and occasional hemorrhagic disease with a 10% mortality. Ixodid (hard) ticks were implicated in the transmission [58], and the virus was isolated early in the disease. Antibodies to the virus were demonstrated in several of the patients. In the 1960, a new virus was isolated from patients with severe febrile illness in what is now the Republic of Congo in Africa [59]. These two viruses were later found to be identical, and the disease was termed

Crimean-Congo hemorrhagic fever (CCHF) after both locations [60,61].

Incidence

CCHF occurs in eastern Europe, the Middle East, Africa, and Asia, where *Hyalomma* species are the predominant ticks. Most patients are animal husbandry workers or medical personnel. The severity of the disease described in Europe is not generally seen in Africa. Countries with reported disease include China, India, Pakistan, Afghanistan, Iran, Iraq, United Arab Emirates, Syria, Bulgaria, Hungary, Yugoslavia, South Africa, Zimbabwe, and countries of East and West Africa [62–68]. The virus or antibody also has been found in Egypt, France, and Greece [69].

Pathogenesis

Ticks demonstrate complex natural cycles that some arboviruses exploit. Three cycles occur: one involves generations of ticks; a second, large animals and adult ticks; and a third, small animals and immature ticks. A natural cycle limited to ticks occurs with transtadial and transovarial transmission [66]. Larval ticks feed on small mammals and become infected. As these infected larval ticks feed on noninfected animals, the cycle is completed as the virus is transmitted. In maturity, these ticks are infective for large animals, which serve as amplifying hosts. This mature tick–large animal cycle permits uninfected mature ticks and large animals to acquire and transmit the virus. Large ticks transmit the virus transovarially to offspring, constituting a third natural cycle.

Infected adult *Hyalomma marginatum* or *H. anatolicum* ticks transmit the virus to large animals and to humans. *Boophilus* ticks and other *Hyalomma* species are involved in some cases. Infected birds offer the opportunity for wider virus distribution beyond the boundaries of any particular enzootic or epizootic area. Human disease occurs from tick feedings, from exposure to infected large animals or their milk or blood, or from exposure to infected humans.

Humans are accidental dead-end hosts of the virus and appear to be the only species that develops severe disease from infection. After inoculation, the virus is hematogenously spread throughout the body, resulting in a short incubation period. The exact pathogenesis of Crimean-Congo hemorrhagic fever is not well understood. The virus is known to preferentially invade the capillary endothelial cells and reticuloendothelial cells [69]. During the acute disease process and viremia, thrombocytopenia and lymphopenia occur. Although the virus involves the liver, Cri-

Table 18–9. Clinical Manifestations of Crimean-Congo Hemorrhagic Fever

Time after exposure	Clinical manifestations	Laboratory analyses	Other notes
3–6 days	Abrupt onset of influenza-like symptoms lasting 7–10 days, with fever, incapacitating chills, and severe headache. Severe myalgia, particularly of the limbs and lumbar area, nausea, vomiting, abdominal pain, diarrhea, and anorexia are also common. Conjunctival injection, pharyngeal hyperemia, flushing and edema of the face and neck, and palatal petechiae are often visible	Viral isolation Serology, with IgM or rise in IgG Detection of antigen in cells	Hepatosplenomegaly occurs in 50% of patients The mouth is dry and the breath has a foul odor. Patients appear depressed and somnolent Bradycardia is typically present, unless shock develops
6–10 days	Hemorrhagic manifestations appear in most patients, with a diffuse fine petechiae rash, ecchymoses, bruising, melena, hematemesis, epistaxis, bleeding gums, and jaundice. The petechiae typically begin on the back and spread to the entire body. Purpura and large hematomas may also develop on the skin		Hematuria, proteinuria, and azotemia are associated with severe infection and indicate a poor prognosis
11–16 days	Recovery begins, with slow improvement over 2 to 6 wk		

IgG, IgM, immunoglobulin G, M.

mean-Congo hemorrhagic fever is not primarily hepatic. Hemorrhage develops in many organs and resulting blood loss may lead to death.

The mechanism of hemorrhage is associated with DIC, and hepatic necrosis with lymphocyte depletion and necrosis in the spleen is evident. White blood cell counts over 10,000/mm³, platelets below 50,000/mm³, transaminase values over 150 mg/dL, and coagulopathy within 5 days of onset predict a case fatality rate approaching 100% [70].

Clinical Manifestations

Inapparent, subclinical infections with Crimean-Congo hemorrhagic fever must be common as some endemic areas have significant serological evidence of viral exposure [71,72]. The clinical manifestations of acute illness are outlined in Table 18–9. The fever associated with this infection is usually continuous but may sometimes be remittent or biphasic. Most cases of disease have signs of hepatitis, with hepatomegaly, jaundice, and elevated transaminases. Bleeding may occur from multiple organs and, in decreasing order of frequency, may affect the nose, gums, buccal mucosa, stomach, uterus, intestines, and lungs. CNS involvement, with nuchal rigidity, agitation, meningeal symptoms, or coma, occurs in 10 to 25% of cases and is typically associated with a poor prognosis. Capillary leakage may lead to pulmonary edema, while significant blood loss results in hypovolemic shock. These findings also signify a poor prognosis. Mortality rates vary from 10 to 50%, and death usually occurs during the second week due to severe hemorrhage, hypovolemic shock, pulmonary edema, and renal failure [71]. Potential differential diagnoses are shown in Table 18–10.

Pathology

Petechiae, ecchymoses, and bruising are seen as manifestations of the bleeding diathesis (Fig. 18–7). No specific skin lesions are described in CCHF. Hepatic and splenic necrosis is evident as is lymphocyte depletion [70].

Laboratory Findings

Profound thrombocytopenia (as low as 20,000), leukopenia, elevated liver enzymes (transaminases), and abnormalities of hemostasis are expected. Leukocytosis with thrombocytopenia and hepatic dysfunction occur in patients with the poorest outcomes [70].

Diagnosis

The virus can be isolated from blood onto cell culture or suckling mice during the first weeks of the illness. Serological diagnosis by ELISA, HI, immunofluorescence assay (IFA), immunodiffusion or plaque reduction neutralization test of paired sera is useful as is IgM antibody ELISA. In

Table 18–10. Differential Diagnoses of Crimean-Congo Hemorrhagic Fever

Gastric ulcer: Epigastric pain, relieved by food, possibly transmitted to the back. Anemia, hematochezia, and the absence of fever characterize this *Helicobacter pylori* infection or anti-inflammatory medication reaction.

Appendicitis: Diffuse pain migrates to the right lower quadrant with fever and leukocytosis leading to peritoneal signs and abscess or septic shock

Stevens-Johnson syndrome: Various skin lesions with mucous membrane involvement (conjuctivitis, stomatitis, urethritis, proctitis) result from drug reactions

Yellow fever
Rift Valley fever
Other hemorrhagic fevers:
  Dengue
  Kyasanur Forest disease
  Omsk hemorrhagic fever
  Colorado tick fever
  Crimean-Congo hemorrhagic fever   See Table 17–2
  Hantavirus hemorrhagic fever
  Lassa fever and the South American hemorrhagic fevers
  Chikungunya fever
Other arboviral infections:
  Hantavirus pulmonary syndrome
  ONN
  Sindbis
  Mayaro   See Table 15–2
  Oropouche
  Sandfly fever
Ebola/Marburg hemorrhagic fevers
Leptospirosis   See Table 18–5

nonfatal cases, IgG and IgM antibodies become demonstrable 7 to 10 days after symptoms begin [73]. Antigen can also be detected in inoculated cells. This is best performed with immunofluorescent antibody techniques.

Treatment and Prevention

The treatment of CCHF generally involves supportive therapy. Intravenous ribavirin and high titer immune convalescent plasma may have a role in the treatment of CCHF [74]. The efficacy of these treatments depends on the rapid institution of therapy early in the course of disease. For prevention of disease, tick protection is beneficial and low cost. Use of universal precautions for exposure to bodily fluids limits nosocomial spread. A vaccine, prepared from inactivated mouse-brain culture, has been used in Bulgaria and Russia [75]. However, no data on the efficacy of this

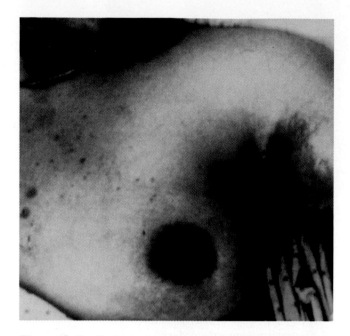

Figure 18–7. Ecchymoses and petechiae secondary to infection with Crimean-Congo hemorrhagic fever virus. (Reprinted from Samlaska CP. Viral Hemorrhagic Fevers. In: James WD ed. Military Dermatology. In: Textbook of Military Medicine. Washington, D.C., Dept. of the Army, Office of the Surgeon General, Borden Institute, 1997:201, 197–212. Photograph courtesy of David I.H. Simpson, Department of Microbiology and Immunology, The Queen's University of Belfast.)

Table 18–11. Treatment of Crimean-Congo Hemorrhagic Fever

Symptom	Treatment
General	Immediate hospitalization and strict bed rest
	Ribavirin may be useful, and is given orally as a 2 g loading dose, followed by 1 g every 6 hr for 4 days, then 0.5 g every 6 hr for 6 days
	High titer immune convalescent plasma may also be of benefit
Fever	Antipyretics: Acetaminophen is a better choice than nonsteroidal anti-inflammatory drugs, since patients often have profound thrombocytopenia and hemorrhage
Shock	Intravenous infusions of crystalloid and colloid. Avoid overhydrating the patient since this illness may be associated with a leaky capillary syndrome. Pulmonary edema may also result from fluid overload
Anemia and acute blood loss	Transfusion of red blood cells or whole blood
DIC	Fresh frozen plasma infusion
Renal failure	Fluid restriction, diuretic therapy, electrolyte management, and dialysis, if necessary

DIC, disseminated intravascular coagulation.

vaccine are available. Symptomatic treatment is shown in Table 18–11.

Conclusion

CCHF is occasionally a severe infection with the potential for a major occupational and nosocomial risk, if not a major risk for travelers. Clinical hemorrhagic fever is complicated by extensive hepatic damage, similar to yellow fever and Rift Valley fever. Though the tick exposure mechanism suggests a rural habitat, nosocomial infection may be more suburban.

Rift Valley Fever

Definition

Rift Valley fever (RVF) virus is in the genus *Phlebovirus* of the Sand fly fever group. RVF virus causes epizootic disease in sub-Saharan Africa in the wettest of rainy seasons (Fig. 18–8). It affects domestic animals, sheep most severely, but also cattle and goats. Among humans, slaughter-house workers, ranchers, and other domestic animal handlers are most commonly affected [76,77].

History

Rift Valley fever was first isolated in 1930 during investigation of an epidemic among ewes and lambs on a farm in the Rift Valley in Africa [77]. Humans in the endemic area were found to have a mild influenza-like febrile illness, with 1 to 2% having hemorrhagic disease. Other patients developed encephalitis or retinitis. By protecting parts of herds from mosquitoes while other parts were not protected, the role of mosquito vectors was first demonstrated. In 1944, the virus was isolated from wild-caught mosquitoes found in Uganda. While mild human disease was mainly recognized in the 1970s, the first cases of fatal infections were reported in South Africa in 1975 [78]. While most cases occur in sub-Saharan Africa, epidemics of the disease have been reported twice in Egypt as well as in Madagascar [79–82].

GEOGRAPHICAL INCIDENCE

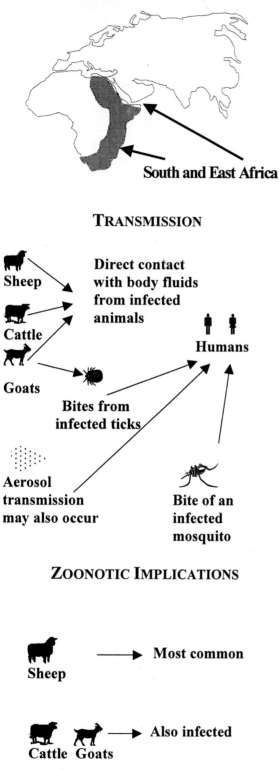

South and East Africa

TRANSMISSION

Sheep
Cattle
Goats

Direct contact
with body fluids
from infected
animals

Humans

Bites from
infected ticks

Aerosol
transmission
may also occur

Bite of an
infected
mosquito

ZOONOTIC IMPLICATIONS

Sheep ⟶ **Most common**

Cattle Goats ⟶ **Also infected**

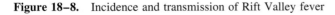

Figure 18–8. Incidence and transmission of Rift Valley fever

Incidence

Epizootic disease occurs in sub-Saharan Africa during periods of excessive rainfall and affects sheep, cattle, and goats, in descending order. Young animals die, pregnancies are aborted, and ewes are lost perinatally. During an epidemic, animal infections occur first, followed by disease in humans. The economic impact of this agent is significant. In the Kenyan epidemic of 1997, 70% of animals died, though not necessarily all from RVF. Several hundred human deaths occurred in an estimated 18,000 infections in Egypt in 1977. The case fatality rate in hospitalized Egyptian patients was 14% [79]. During the 1997 to 1998 RVF epidemic in East Africa, approximately 89,000 cases and 200 deaths were reported.

Pathogenesis

Epizootic diseases are associated with a variety of mosquitoes and, therefore, with a variety of habitats. Excessive rainfall is a constant feature of outbreaks [79]. The most common vectors include *Culex pipiens* in Egypt, *Culex theileri* in South Africa, and *Aedes* species in East Africa [83–85]. In laboratory experiments, malaria parasites present in the mosquito enhance the transmission of RVF [86]. Mosquito viral transmission may be more complex than originally thought. This phenomenon may apply to other mosquito vectors and arboviral diseases in malaria endemic areas.

Close contact with the infected animals increases risk for human infection. This suggests that the mosquito vector is less important than animal contact [76,77]. After dermal injection of the virus during feeding, local nodes are infected first and then the liver. The virus replicates in the endoplasmic reticulum of the hepatocytes. Hepatic necrosis occurs and virions are released. Encephalitis or retinitis occurs after an interval of time, which suggests an immunologic role in pathogenesis.

Clinical Manifestations

Inapparent or mild disease is frequent, and most clinical cases are uncomplicated. This clinical pattern is similar to phlebotomus fever and other arboviral fevers (Table 18–12). Bradycardia is often evident on physical examination. Many patients become delirious, sometimes with hallucinations. Hemorrhagic fever, similar to yellow fever, develops in 1 to 2% of patients with a case fatality rate of 15 to 50%. Most deaths occur during the second week, due to hemorrhagic complications with hepatic involvement. DIC seems central to the hemorrhage, compounded by hepatic disease [87]. Deaths may be due to hepatic failure from necrosis of the liver. Less than 1% of patients develop encephalitis, though much later in the course of the infection. This complication is clinically similar to Japanese

Table 18–12. Clinical Manifestations of Rift Valley Fever

Time after exposure	Clinical manifestations	Laboratory analyses	Other notes
3–6 days	Sudden onset of biphasic fever, chills, myalgias, arthralgias, and headache. Some patients may have nausea or vomiting, abdominal discomfort, photophobia, and retro-orbital pain. The face is flushed, the tongue is furred, and the conjunctivae are injected. The liver may be enlarged and tender. Jaundice may be evident in skin and conjunctiva	Viral isolation Serology (IgM or increase in IgG) Detection of viral RNA in tissue or acute sera	Viremia lasts during the acute clinical illness Less than 5% of cases are serious or fatal, with possible complications of hemorrhage and liver necrosis, retinitis and visual impairment, or meningoencephalitis Hemorrhagic manifestations of mucous membranes and skin include petechiae, ecchymoses, and bruising
7–11 days	Full resolution of symptoms in most patients		

IgG, IgM, immunoglobulin G, M.

encephalitis or other viral encephalitis, and patients typically develop intense headache, confusion, and stupor. Few patients die from the encephalitis, and most patients recover completely without permanent sequelae. A retinal vasculitis may occur quite late in the disease, in less than 1% of patients. This complication usually develops 1 to 3 weeks after the onset of the fever. Retinal edema, hemorrhage, and infarction may lead to permanent visual impairment. However, most patients gradually regain normal vision.

Pathology

Limited pathological studies have been performed on humans. Hepatocellular necrosis is evident, since the virus is cytocidal. Hemorrhage, interstitial pneumonitis, and myocardial fiber degeneration may also be present. The CNS and ophthalmologic manifestations are inflammatory, suggesting an immunological mechanism or an immunological failure [88].

Laboratory Findings

Leukopenia, thrombocytopenia, abnormal liver function tests, and indicators of DIC are seen in cases with hemorrhagic fever. If meningoencephalitis develops, the CSF findings resemble other viral encephalitides, with pleocytosis (particularly lymphocytes), a normal glucose, and a slightly increased protein level.

The mild cases can be confused with a variety of viral agents (Table 18–13). Hemorrhagic manifestations can simulate other hemorrhagic fevers, but the hepatic injury is uncommon except in yellow fever and Crimean-Congo hemorrhagic fever. Ebola, Lassa, and Marburg viruses are considerations. Other infectious encephalitides can mimic

Table 18–13. Differential Diagnoses of Rift Valley Fever

Yellow fever **Crimean-Congo hemorrhagic fever** **Lassa fever**	See Table 17–2
Other encephalitides: **Colorado tick fever** **Eastern equine encephalitis** **Western equine encephalitis** **Venezuelan equine encephalitis** **West Nile fever** **California encephalitis** **Japanese encephalitis** **St. Louis encephalitis** **Tick-borne encephalitis** **Powassan encephalitis**	See Table 15–2
Other hemorrhagic fevers: **Kyanasur Forest disease** **OMSK** **Hantavirus hemorrhagic fevers** **Chikungunya fever**	See Table 17–2
Ebola and Marburg hemorrhagic fevers **Dengue**	See Table 18–5

the encephalitis, for example, herpes simplex. The retinitis is uncommon and, in the habitat of RVF epizootic disease, should be suspected and identified. If the travel history is incomplete or includes multiple geographic regions, there may be failure to recognize the importance of coexisting RVF epizootic disease or excessive rainfall in a sub-Saharan rainy season biotype.

Diagnosis

Specific viral diagnosis may be difficult in the nonspecific phase. Virus isolation is more useful for vector surveillance than for disease detection. Serological methods (HI, CF, IgM ELISA) document human and animal disease and viral exposure. Either acute sera for IgM or paired sera (acute and convalescent) for IgG, showing a fourfold increase, can be used. IgM antibodies can also be detected in the spinal fluid in patients with encephalitis. Polymerase chain reaction (PCR) is available for detection of viral RNA in acute sera or tissue. Differential diagnoses are shown in Table 18–13.

Treatment and Prevention

The treatment for Rift Valley fever centers on palliative care (Table 18–14). Supportive therapy for DIC and circulatory integrity is pivotal (see Dengue, Table 20–4). In animal studies, treatment with interferon [89], ribavirin, and passive antibodies have demonstrated efficacy, but these agents have yet to be tested in humans. Complications, such as retinitis and encephalitis, occur after antibody development, so antiviral therapy or immune sera would not be advantageous.

Prophylaxis for Rift Valley fever includes protective gear, such as gloves and masks, in high-risk individuals to prevent contact with infected animal tissue. Unfortunately, in many poor areas of Africa, animals are kept in close proximity to family quarters, and sick or dying animals are often killed to salvage the meat for food. Animal immunization is available with live-attenuated and killed virus vaccines. For humans with high-risk of exposure, a formalin-inactivated vaccine produced in cell cultures has been developed [90]. However, this vaccine has not been licensed and is not commercially available.

Related Viruses

Sandfly fevers are self-limited, acute febrile illnesses transmitted by nocturnal biting midges, small (2–3 mm) female flies. The diseases appear in north Africa and southern Europe, southwest Asia, and India; Panamanian sandflies harbor other viral agents in the sandfly group.

Conclusion

While Rift Valley fever primarily affects sheep and cattle in endemic areas of Africa, sporadic epidemics in humans can occur. Effective animal vaccines are available and offer the potential for control. Human vaccines for animal handlers would limit disease in known high-risk personnel, but not to travelers or out-of-area animal handlers who might handle infected imported animals. Laboratory workers are protected by appropriate precautions and vaccination [79].

Arenaviridae Lassa Fever and South American Hemorrhagic Fevers

Definition

The viruses causing Lassa fever (LF, Lassa virus), Argentine hemorrhagic fever (AHF, Junin virus), Bolivian hemorrhagic fever (BHF, Machupo virus), and Venezuelan hemorrhagic fever (VHF, Guanarito virus) are rodent-borne members of the family Arenaviridae [91]. Lassa virus is found predominantly in specific rodents of Sierra Leone. This rodent is common in secondary rain forest biotypes near human habitations. Machupo virus is transmitted by a rodent whose usual habitat is the forest and grasslands of Bolivia, Paraguay, and Brazil. Junin virus is hosted by a specific rodent found in grasslands and farming areas of Argentina. The rodent reservoir for Guanarito virus is found in Central Venezuela. Disease is frequently mild with these viruses, but may be quite severe and fatal, with significant fetal wastage and maternal mortality in late pregnancy [91] (Fig. 18–9).

History

Lassa fever was described in the 1950s. However, it did not receive attention until 1969 when the disease developed

Table 18–14. Treatment of Rift Valley Fever

Symptom	Treatment
Fever	Antipyretics. Avoid nonsteroidal anti-inflammatory drugs, which may impair platelet function since thrombocytopenia is already present with this disease
Arthralgias and myalgias	Analgesics such as acetaminophen
Hemorrhagic diathesis	Transfusion of fresh frozen plasma and platelets. Avoid hepatotoxic drugs that could potentiate the condition

GEOGRAPHICAL INCIDENCE

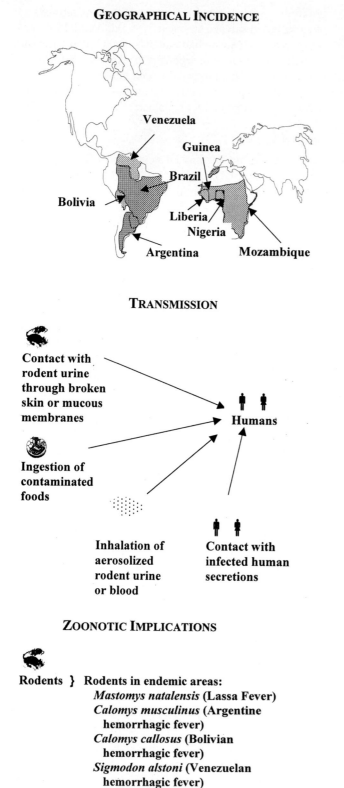

TRANSMISSION

**Contact with
rodent urine
through broken
skin or mucous
membranes**

**Ingestion of
contaminated
foods**

Humans

**Inhalation of
aerosolized
rodent urine
or blood**

**Contact with
infected human
secretions**

ZOONOTIC IMPLICATIONS

Rodents } **Rodents in endemic areas:**
Mastomys natalensis **(Lassa Fever)**
Calomys musculinus **(Argentine
hemorrhagic fever)**
Calomys callosus **(Bolivian
hemorrhagic fever)**
Sigmodon alstoni **(Venezuelan
hemorrhagic fever)**

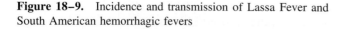

Figure 18–9. Incidence and transmission of Lassa Fever and South American hemorrhagic fevers

in missionary nurses working in a hospital in Lassa, Nigeria [92]. The virus was isolated and found to be an arenavirus closely related to lymphocytic choriomeningitis virus [93]. Epidemics have since occurred in Sierra Leone and other countries of West Africa.

Four other related arenaviruses have been found to cause hemorrhagic fever, although they are endemic in South America rather than Africa. Argentine hemorrhagic fever was clinically described in 1955, followed by isolation of the etiologic Junin virus in 1958 [94]. A similar illness was recognized in eastern Bolivia in 1959, and the causative virus isolated in 1963 was found to be similar but distinct [95]. A major epidemic of BHF occurred in 1962 to 1964 in San Joaquin, Bolivia, as the rodent vector population soared and inhabited the village housing [56]. More recently, a separate hemorrhagic disease was identified in Venezuela in 1991. The causative virus, known as Guanarito, was later isolated [96].

Incidence

Lassa fever estimates are 100,000 to 300,000 cases annually with 5,000 deaths. Because the specific rodent reservoir is restricted to endemic bush areas, this infection only arises in persons who live or have traveled to such areas or have had exposure to infected individuals. LF and BHF are generally contracted in or close to homesteads, and they affect both sexes and all ages. However, VHF is typically acquired in gardens nearby homes and, typically, affects only adults. AHF is normally contracted during the harvest of maize, and it is the only virus of this group that generally affects only adult male agricultural workers [97].

The mortality rates for these arenavirus hemorrhagic infections is similar, ranging from 15 to 20% in the absence of specific therapy. Case fatality ratios for hospitalized patients with Lassa fever approximate 16%. In endemic areas of Sierra Leone, 10 to 16% of hospitalized patients have Lassa fever [98]. The seroprevalence rates for the population in endemic areas ranges from 35 to 50% [99,100]. Lassa fever occurs throughout the year, but most hospitalizations occur during the dry season from February to May. AHF occurs in the harvest season from April to June. The frequency of BHF corresponds to the end of the rainy season from March to July in a tropical savannah biotype [56].

Pathogenesis

The viruses cause chronic infection in the rodent host. Immune tolerance probably plays a role in prolonged viral shedding. Human infection occurs when: (1) rodent urine comes in contact with broken skin or is aerosolized and inhaled; (2) rodent blood is aerosolized by farm machinery;

or (3) broken skin or mucous membranes come in contact with rodent body fluids. These events often happen when workers are hunting rodents or preparing them for food. Lassa fever is also occasionally transmitted from person-to-person through close contact. Nosocomial infection occurs through human secretions from patients in or out of hospitals [56,101]. Transmission through sexual intercourse or nursing an infant has also been described. In contrast, the South American hemorrhagic fevers are rarely transmitted from person to person.

Following viral exposure, there is an incubation period of 8 to 14 days. At the onset of symptoms, a viremia is evident. Shock and encephalopathy may ensue, probably resulting from physiological derangements instead of direct viral invasion of specific organ systems. Endothelial and platelet dysfunction develop during infection. The latter is due to a protein in serum, otherwise undefined. B-cell responses are brisk, but do not clear the viremia. T-cell responses are implicated in the above dysfunction but probably are also central in viremic clearance.

There is no DIC nor hepatic injury to explain the bleeding. It probably results from the capillary dysfunction as the capillary leaks [56]. The neurological manifestations result, not from inflammatory encephalopathy but from edema due to metabolic or circulatory changes [91].

Clinical Manifestations

Lassa fever virus infection usually has mild or nonspecific symptoms or is asymptomatic. Serologic evidence of prior infection is common in endemic areas. Patients hospitalized with other diagnoses frequently prove to have Lassa fever [98]. Conversely, infection with the South American viruses generally results in symptomatic illness. Unlike most hemorrhagic fevers, the onset of Lassa fever is insidious with a progressive course. The clinical manifestations are outlined in Table 18–15. The fever produces moist skin until shock ensues. Pulse and respiratory rates are elevated with fever, but blood pressure is low. Patients appear anxious and acutely ill. The abdomen is tender, but with active

Table 18–15. Clinical Manifestations of Lassa Fever

Time after exposure	Clinical manifestations	Laboratory analyses	Other notes
8–14 days	Insidious onset of progressive fever, weakness, and malaise	Viral isolation Serology, with IgM or paired sera for IgG Detection of viral antigens	
Slow development over the next several days	Development of generalized myalgias, arthralgias, lower back pain, and a nonproductive cough. Many patients complain of a headache, usually frontal, sore throat, retrosternal chest pain, vomiting, diarrhea, and abdominal pain		Hyperesthesia of the skin is common with AHF and BHF
12–18 days	In some patients, petechiae develop on the skin (rare in LF) and mild hemorrhage occurs from the gums, gastrointestinal tract and vagina. These signs herald the onset of hypovolemic shock. Capillary leak syndrome leads to facial edema and effusions. Neurological manifestations may occur in some patients		Hemorrhagic and neurological manifestations are more common in AHF and BHF
15–26 days	Some patients develop rapid clinical deterioration, with possible death due to hypovolemic shock or neurological sequelae. The majority of patients improve and recover completely		Patients who survive severe disease often have a slow recovery and may have significant generalized muscle wasting and limb contractures

AHF, Argentine hemorrhagic fever; BHF, Bolivian hemorrhagic fever; LF, Lassa fever.

bowel sounds and no localizing signs [56]. There is no rash, but pharyngitis and conjunctivitis are evident in some patients. More than two thirds of patients have pharyngitis, sometimes with pharyngeal and tonsillar exudates, edema, swelling, and diffuse inflammation. Conjunctival hemorrhage is less common and is a poor prognostic sign. The pharyngeal pain may lead to expectorated saliva due to dysphagia. Other respiratory symptoms are not prominent.

Hemorrhage is not frequent with Lassa fever (15–20% of cases), and develops only in the most severe cases. It usually occurs from the gums or nose, gastrointestinal (GI) or genitourinary (GU) tracts. While hemorrhage is minor and does not typically cause complications, capillary leak syndrome may become severe and lead to hypovolemic shock. Capillary leak syndrome is the hallmark of Lassa fever and the South American hemorrhagic fevers. It may lead to facial and nuchal edema without peripheral edema as well as pleural and pericardial rubs and effusions later in the course of disease. Very young children may develop a ''swollen baby syndrome,'' which consists of widespread edema (anasarca), abdominal distention, and spontaneous bleeding [102].

Deafness with tinnitus, confusion, tremors, seizures, and encephalopathy are common neurologic findings and are seen in the most severe cases with the worst outcome. Tremors precede death in fatal cases. Complications and sequelae include neurosensory hearing loss, uveitis, orchitis, effusions of pleura or pericardia, and ascites.

AHF and BHF have a similar insidious onset, but hemorrhage is more common, particularly of the skin. Petechiae are common; there is hyperemia of the face and trunk and a macular enanthem (Fig. 18–10). Neurologic findings are similar to those of Lassa fever, but are more commonly observed. A rising hematocrit and proteinuria precede and predict clinical crises; these may be lethal without appropriate supportive care. Fatal outcomes occur in patients with high levels of circulating virus or with conjunctival hemorrhage, hemorrhage with pharyngitis, or an elevated serum aspartate transaminase. Pregnancy carries a 20% fatality rate and an 80% late abortion rate. Pregnancy termination improves maternal outcome. Potential differential diagnoses are shown in Table 18–16.

Pathology

The clinical severity is strikingly out of proportion to the pathology. Focal hepatic necrosis is mild to moderate in severe Lassa fever. Otherwise, Lassa fever and the South American hemorrhagic fevers do not cause parenchymal histological damage. CNS pathology lacks inflammation, showing only edema. Interstitial edema reflects the capillary leak. Minor hemorrhagic manifestations are evident,

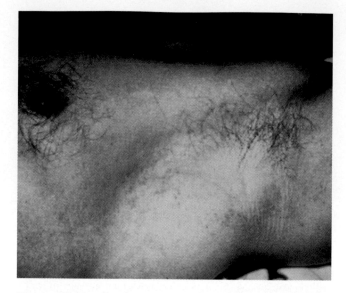

Figure 18–10. Molecular eruption in a patient with Argentine hemorrhagic fever (Junin virus). (Reprinted from Samlaska CP. Viral Hemorrhagic Fevers. In: James WD, ed. Military Dermatology. In: Textbook of Military Medicine. Washington, D.C., Dept. of the Army, Office of the Surgeon General, Borden Institute, 1997:201, 197–212. Photograph courtesy of David I.H. Simpson, Department of Microbiology and Immunology, The Queen's University of Belfast.)

Table 18–16. Differential Diagnoses of Lassa Fever and the South American Hemorrhagic Fevers

Influenza: The coryza, cough, myalgia, and fever without rash, jaundice, frequent hemorrhagic complications or encephalitis lead to the suspicion of influenza. Secondary bacterial complications pneumonia and meningitis, compound the differential diagnosis and require specific antibiotic therapy.

Rocky Mountain spotted fever	} See Table 18–2
Typhoid fever	
Malaria	
Rift Valley fever	
Other hemorrhagic fevers:	
Kyasanur Forest disease	See Table 17–2
Omsk hemorrhagic fever	
Colorado tick fever	
Crimean-Congo hemorrhagic fever	
Hantavirus hemorrhagic fever	
Chikungunya fever	
Hemolytic uremic syndrome	
Leptospirosis	See Table 18–5
Dengue	
Ebola/Marburg hemorrhagic fevers	
West Nile fever	} See Table 15–2

but these are less striking than that seen in other arboviral hemorrhagic fevers [56].

Laboratory Findings

The normal white blood cell count in Lassa fever shows a relative lymphopenia, and thrombocytopenia is evident. Neutrophilia appears late in severe cases. The hematocrit is elevated with intravascular volume depletion from capillary leakage. Blood urea nitrogen rises with dehydration and may be moderately elevated. Proteinuria is common and occurs in two thirds of patients.

The South American hemorrhagic fevers typically have leukopenia ($<4000/mm^3$) and thrombocytopenia ($<100,000/mm^3$). As in Lassa fever, proteinuria is common. Microscopic hematuria may also be present.

Diagnosis

The wide spectrum of manifestations and the insidious onset of these infections make the diagnosis difficult. Pharyngitis, proteinuria, and retrosternal chest pain in endemic areas are a specific triad for these arenaviral infections. Although this triad is present in 80% of patients with Lassa fever in endemic areas, it may only detect about 51% of cases [98]. IgM determinations or paired sera for IgG document the immunological response for diagnosis. These are best detected by indirect fluorescent antibody (IFA). Usually, an IgM titer of at least 4 or an IgG titer of at least 16 are considered diagnostic for Lassa fever. Half of all patients have measurable antibodies by day 5 of the illness, and most patients have antibodies by day 14. Conversely, antibodies with the South American hemorrhagic fevers do not appear until the third week of illness, which is 1 to 2 weeks later than that for Lassa fever. The level of neutralizing antibody rises with the declining viremia, but viremia in Lassa persists for some time after the appearance of specific antibody (up to 3–4 weeks with severe disease). With South American hemorrhagic fevers, virus can be isolated from 2 to 14 days after the onset of symptoms. PCR or viral culture are usual techniques for the demonstration of specific viral etiology. PCR detection of viral antigens in tissue is a rapid and accurate diagnostic method. Other antigen detection techniques include immunofluorescent antibody assay and ELISA.

Treatment

Ribavirin begun in the first 6 days of Lassa fever symptoms (for patients with AST greater than or equal to 150 IU/L) decreased mortality from 55 to 5% [103]. If begun 7 or more days after the onset of fever, the drug is not as effective. Limited studies have shown that ribavirin may also be effective in AHF and BHF, but further clinical trials are needed.

Administration of human convalescent plasma reduces

Table 18–17. Treatment of Lassa Fever and South American Hemorrhagic Fevers

Symptom	Treatment
General	Ribavirin administered intravenously as a 2 g loading dose, followed by 1 g every 6 hr for 4 days, then 0.5 g every 8 hr for 6 days
	Human convalescent plasma in some cases (see text)
Fever	Analgesics. Avoid aspirin and nonsteroidal anti-inflammatory drugs, which can interfere with platelet function since thrombocytopenia is already present with these infections
Dehydration	Adequate fluid replacement and management of electrolyte and acid-base balances
Hypotension and shock	Intravenous fluid replacement. Renal function, pulmonary status, and blood pressure should be monitored closely to avoid overhydration, since excess fluids may exacerbate laryngeal or pulmonary edema, and capillary leak syndrome may already be present
Neurologic deterioration	Attention to cerebral edema and seizure control without compromising cerebral perfusion and ventilation
Concurrent pregnancy	Elective termination of pregnancy by uterine evacuation, particularly in the third trimester, substantially improves maternal survival

the mortality of AHF from 16% to less than 1% if initiated within the first 7 days of clinical illness [104]. This treatment is associated with an unusual late neurological syndrome in 10% of survivors, although usually benign. Convalescent plasma has been used for the treatment of BHF as well, although studies have not proven its efficacy. Plasma therapy for LF has had equivocal results, likely due to the comparatively lower quantity of virus-neutralizing antibodies in convalescent patients with LF [105].

While ribavirin and human plasma therapy are available options for the treatment of these infections, supportive care of symptoms and complications is critical (Table 18–17). During the care of these patients, barrier nursing methods should be strictly practiced to prevent nosocomial spread of the viruses. For the prevention of disease, a live-attenuated Junin virus vaccine has been effective in decreasing the incidence of AHF. Lack of available funds has stymied promising vaccine development for LF [106].

Conclusion

These arenavirus hemorrhagic infections range from minimally or mildly symptomatic to severe and lethal. The epidemiology is defined by complex interactions with the rodent hosts during pest control of crops, encroachment into the rodent habitat, or securing food. The triad of pharyngitis, proteinuria, and retrosternal pain is useful in identification of severe disease, but it does not identify all cases. The less frequent but more severe manifestations result in morbidity and mortality in endemic areas, particularly in late pregnancy. Rodent control and vaccines would provide potential solutions, except for the rural nature of arenaviral hemorrhagic disease.

REFERENCES

1. WM Hammon, WC Reeves. California encephalitis virus, a newly described agent. I. Evidence of natural infection in man and other animals. Calif Med 77:303–309, 1952.
2. Centers for Disease Control and Prevention. Arboviral infections of the central nervous system—United States, 1984. MMWR Morbid Mortal Widely Rep 34:283–294, 1986.
3. PR Grimstad, RL Barrett, RL Humphrey, MJ Sinsko. Serologic evidence for widespread infection with La Crosse and St. Louis encephalitis viruses in the Indiana human population. Am J Epidemiol 119:913–930, 1984.
4. AA Kindle, JE McJunkin, JR Meek, MM Tomsho, DL Holbrook, DL Smith, BA Crowder, DM Rosenber, JA Burke, DC Newell, SL Sebert, JH Wright, JW Brough, LE Haddy, RC Baron. La Crosse encephalitis in West Virginia. MMWR 37:79–82, 1988.
5. TF Jones, AS Craig, RS Nasci, LE Patterson, PC Erwin, RR Gerhardt, XT Ussery, W Schaffner. Newly recognized focus of La Crosse encephalitis in Tennessee. Clin Infect Dis 28:93–97, 1999.
6. TF Tsai. Arboviral infections in the United States. Infect Dis Clin North Am 5:73–102, 1991.
7. JEM McJunkin, LL Minnich, TF Tsai. California/La-Crosse encephalitis. In: RD Feigin and JD Cherry, eds. Textbook of Pediatric Infectious Diseases, 4th ed, Philadelphia: Saunders, 1998, pp 2150–2158.
8. TM Yuill. The role of mammals in the maintenance are dissemination of LaCross virus. In: WH Thompson, CH Calister, eds. California Serogroup Viruses. New York: Alan R. Liss, 1983, pp 77–87.
9. KD Kappus, TP Monath, RM Kaminski, et al. Reported encephalitis associated with California serogroup virus infections in the United States, 1963–1981. In: CH Calisher, WH Thompson, eds. California Serogroup Viruses. New York: Alan R Liss, 1983, pp 31–41.
10. KP Johnson, RT Johnson. California encephalitis: II. Studies of experimental infection in the mouse. J Neuropathol Exp Neurol 27:390–400, 1968.
11. R Janssen, F Gonzalez-Scarano, N Nathanson. Mechanisms of bunyavirus virulence. Comparative pathogenesis of a virulent strain of La Crosse and an avirulent strain of Tahyna virus. Lab Invest 50:447–455, 1984.
12. RS Rust, WH Thompson, CG Matthews, BJ Beaty, RW Chun. La Crosse and other forms of California encephalitis. J Child Neurol 14:1–14, 1999.
13. HH Balfour Jr, RA Siem, H Bauer, PG Quie. California arbovirus (La Crosse) infections. I. Clinical and laboratory findings in 66 children with meningoencephalitis. Pediatrics 52:680–691, 1973.
14. JD Grabow, CG Matthews, RW Chun, WH Thompson. The electroencephalogram and clinical sequelae of California arbovirus encephalitis. Neurology 19:394–404, 1969.
15. HG Cramblett, H Stegmiller, C Spencer. California encephalitis virus infections in children. Clinical and laboratory studies. JAMA 198:128–132, 1966.
16. JE McJunkin, RR Khan, TF Tsai. California-La Crosse encephalitis. Infect Dis Clin North Am 12:83–93, 1998.
17. JE McJunkin, R Khan, EC de los Reyes, DL Parsons, LL Minnich, RG Ashley, TF Tsai. Treatment of severe La Crosse encephalitis with intravenous ribavirin following diagnosis by brain biopsy. Pediatrics 99:261–267, 1997.
18. WH Thompson, B Kalfayan, RO Anslow. Isolation of California encephalitis group virus from a fatal human illness. Am J Epidemiol 81:245–263, 1965.
19. CH Calisher, RE Bailey. Serodiagnosis of La Crosse virus infections in humans. J Clin Microbiol 13:344–350, 1981.
20. LF Cassidy, JL Patterson. Mechanism of La Crosse virus inhibition by ribavirin. Antimicrob Agents Chemother 33:2009–2011, 1989.
21. JD Granbow, CG Matthews, RW Chun, WH Thompson. The electroencephalogram and clinical sequelae of California arbovirus encephalitis. Neurology 19:394–404, 1969.
22. B Hjelle, SA Jenison, DE Goade, WB Green, RM Feddersen, AA Scott. Hantaviruses: clinical, microbiologic, and epidemiologic aspects. Crit Rev Clin Lab Sci 32:469–508, 1995.
23. BS Niklasson. Haemorrhagic fever with renal syndrome: virological and epidemiological aspects. Pediatr Nephrol 6:201–204, 1992.
24. KT McKee, JW LeDuc, CJ Peters. Hantaviruses. In: RB Belshe, ed. Textbook of Human Virology. 2nd ed. St. Louis: Mosby–Year Book, 1991, pp 615–632.
25. J Casals, BE Henderson, H Hoogstraal, KM Johnson, A Shelokov. A review of Soviet viral hemorrhagic fever, 1969. J Infect Dis 122:437–453, 1970.
26. DC Gajdusek. Hemorrhagic fevers in Asia: a problem in medical ecology. Geogr Rev 41:20, 1956.
27. CF Mayer. Epidemic hemorrhagic fever of the Far East, or endemic hemorrhagic nephrosonephritis, a short outline

of the disease, with supplemental data on the results of experimental inoculation of human volunteers. Milit Surg 110:276, 1952.

28. H Hortling. En epidemi av falteben in finska Lappland. Nord Med 30:1001, 1946.

29. JA Sheedy, HF Froeb, HA Batson, CC Conley, JP Murphy, RB Hunter, DW Cugell, RB Giles, SC Bershadsky, JW Vester, RH Yoe. Symposium on epidemic hemorrhagic fever. The clinical course of epidemic hemorrhagic fever. Am J Med 16:619–628, 1954.

30. JH McNinch. Far East command conference on epidemic hemorrhagic fever: introduction. Ann Intern Med 38:53–60, 1953.

31. JW LeDuc, TG Ksiazek, CA Rossi, JM Dalrymple. A retrospective analysis of sera collected by the Hemorrhagic Fever Commission during the Korean Conflict. J Infect Dis 162:1182–1184, 1990.

32. Centers for Disease Control and Prevention. Outbreak of acute illness—southwestern United States, 1993. MMWR Morbid Mortal Wkly Rep 42:421–424, 1993.

33. B Hjelle, S Jenison, G Mertz, F Koster, K Foucar. Emergence of hantaviral disease in the southwestern United States. West J Med 161:467–473, 1994.

34. JS Duchin, FT Koster, CJ Peters, GL Simpson, B Tempest, SR Zaki, TG Ksiazek, PE Rollin, S Nichol, ET Umland, et al. Hantavirus pulmonary syndrome: a clinical description of 17 patients with a newly recognized disease. The Hantavirus Study Group. N Engl J Med 330:949–955, 1994.

35. Centers for Disease Control and Prevention. Update: hantavirus pulmonary syndrome—United States, 1993. Morbid Mortal Wkly Rep 42:816–820, 1993.

36. HW Lee, G van der Groen. Hemorrhagic fever with renal syndrome. Prog Med Virol 36:62–102, 1989.

37. JB McCormick. Diseases caused by hantaviruses, In: Strickland GT, ed. Hunter's Tropical Medicine. 7th ed. Philadelphia: WB Saunders, 1991, pp 251–254.

38. CJ Peters, GL Simpson, H Levy. Spectrum of hantavirus infection: hemorrhagic fever with renal syndrome and hantavirus pulmonary syndrome. Annu Rev Med 50:531–545, 1999.

39. Centers for Disease Control and Prevention. Hantavirus pulmonary syndrome—Chile 1997. Morbid Mortal Wkly Rep 46:949–951, 1997.

40. B Hjelle, N Torrez-Martinez, FT Koster. Hantavirus pulmonary syndrome-related virus from Bolivia [letter]. Lancet 347:57, 1996.

41. N Lopez, P Padula, C Rossi, ME Lazaro, MT Franze-Fernandez. Genetic identification of a new hantavirus causing severe pulmonary syndrome in Argentina. Virology 220:223–226, 1996.

42. MD Nieves Parisi, DA Enria, NC Pini, MS Sabattini. Retrospective detection of clinical infection caused by hantavirus in Argentina [Spanish]. Medicina 56:1–13, 1996.

43. C Steven, M Johnson, A Bell. First reported cases of hantavirus pulmonary syndrome in Canada. Can Commun Dis Rep 20:121–125, 1994.

44. RJ Williams, RT Bryan, JN Mills, RE Palma, I Vera, F De Velasquez, E Baez, WE Schmidt, RE Figueroa, CJ Peters, SR Zaki, AS Khan, TG Ksiazek. An outbreak of hantavirus pulmonary syndrome in western Paraguay. Am J Trop Med Hyg 57:274–282, 1997.

45. CR Vitek, RF Breiman, TG Ksiazek, PE Rollin, JC McLaughlin, ET Umland, KB Nolte, A Loera, CM Sewell, CJ Peters. Evidence against person-to-person transmission of hantavirus to health care workers. Clin Infect Dis 22:824–826, 1996.

46. FR Nunes-Arauo, SD Nishioka, IB Ferreira, A Suzuki, RF Bonito, MS Ferreira. Absence of interhuman transmission of hantavirus pulmonary syndrome in Minas Gerais, Brazil: evidence from a serological survey. Clin Infect Dis 29:1588–1589, 1999.

47. CA Hart, M Bennett. Hantavirus: an increasing problem? Ann Trop Med Parasitol 88:347–358, 1994.

48. R Yanagihara, DJ Silverman. Experimental infection of human vascular endothelial cells by pathogenic and non-pathogenic hantaviruses. Arch Virol 111:281–286, 1990.

49. TM Cosgriff. Mechanisms of diseases in hantavirus infection: pathophysiology of hemorrhagic fever with renal syndrome. Rev Infect Dis 13:97–107, 1991.

50. H Levy, S Simpson. Hantaviral pulmonary syndrome. Am J Respir Crit Care Med 149:1710–1713, 1994.

51. HW Lee. Korean hemorrhagic fever. Prog Med Virol 28:96–113, 1982.

52. A Antoniadis, JW Le Duc, S Daniel-Alexiou. Clinical and epidemiological aspects of hemorrhagic fever with renal syndrome (HFRS) in Greece. Eur J Epidemiol 3:295–301, 1987.

53. A Gligic, N Dimkovic, SY Xiao, GJ Buckle, D Jovanovic, D Velimirovic, R Stojanovic, M Obradovic, G Diglisic, J Micic, et al. Belgrade virus: a new hantavirus causing severe hemorrhagic fever with renal syndrome in Yugoslavia. J Infect Dis 166:113–120, 1992.

54. GS Warner. Hantavirus illness in humans: review and update. South Med J 89:264–271, 1996.

55. RL Moolenaar, C Dalton, HB Lipman, ET Umland, M Gallaher, JS Duchin, L Chapman, SR Zaki, TG Ksiazek, PE Rollin, et al. Clinical features that differentiate hantavirus pulmonary syndrome from three other acute respiratory illnesses. Clin Infect Dis 21:643–649, 1995.

56. JB McCormick, S Fisher-Hock. Viral hemorrhagic fevers. In: KS Warren, AA Mahmoud, eds. Tropical and Geographic Medicine. New York: McGraw Hill, 1990, pp 700–728.

57. All About Hantavirus. CDC, Special Pathogens. March, 1999.

58. M Chumakov. Study of viral hemorrhagic fevers. J Hyg Epidemiol 7:125–140, 1963.

59. D Simpson, EM Knight, G Courtois, MC Williams, MP Weinbren, JW Kibukamusoke. Congo virus: a hitherto undescribed virus occurring in Africa. I. Human isolations—clinical notes. East Afr Med J 44:87–92, 1967.

60. J Casals. Antigenic similarity between the virus causing

Crimean hemorrhagic fever and Congo virus. Proc Soc Exp Biol Med 131:233–236, 1969.

61. M Chumakov, SE Smirnova, EA Thachenko. Relationship between strains of Crimean hemorrhagic fever and Congo viruses. Acta Virol 14:82–85, 1970.

62. SK Al-Tikriti, F Al-Ani, FJ Jurji, H Tantawi, M Al-Moslih, N Al-Janabi, MI Mahmud, A Al-Bana, H Habib, H Al-Munthri, S Al-Janabi, K AL-Jawahry, M Yonan, F Hassan, DI Simpson. Congo/Crimean hemorrhagic fever in Iraq. Bull World Health Organ 59:85–90, 1981.

63. S Al-Tikriti, FK Hassan, IM Moslih, FH Jurji, MIA Mahmud, HH Tantawi. Crimean-Congo hemorrhagic fever in Iraq: a seroepidemiologic survey. J Trop Med Hyg 84: 117–120, 1981.

64. A Antoniadis, J Casals. Serological evidence of human infection with Congo-Crimean hemorrhagic fever in Greece. Am J Trop Med Hyg 31:1066–1067, 1982.

65. M Burney. Ghafoor A, Saleen M, Webb PA, Casals J. Nosocomial outbreak of viral hemorrhagic fever caused by Crimean hemorrhagic fever-Congo virus in Pakistan, January 1976. Am J Trop Med Hyg 29:941–947, 1980.

66. H Hoogstraal. The epidemiology of tick-borne Crimean-Congo hemorrhagic fever in Asia, Europe, and Africa. J Med Entomol 15:307–417, 1979.

67. YC Yen, LX Kong, L Lee, YQ Zhang, F Li, BJ Cai, SY Gao. Characteristics of Crimean-Congo hemorrhagic fever virus (Xinjiang strain) in China. Am J Trop Med Hyg 34: 1179–1182, 1985.

68. R Swanepoel, JK Struthers, AJ Shepherd, GM McGillivray, MJ Nel, PH Jupp. Crimean-Congo hemorrhagic fever in South Africa. Am J Trop Med Hyg 32:1407–1415, 1983.

69. World Health Organization. Viral haemorrhagic fevers. World Health Org Tech Rep Ser 721:5–126, 1985.

70. R Swanepoel, DE Gill, AJ Shephard, PA Leman, JH Mynhardt, S Harvey. The clinical pathology of Crimean-Congo hemorrhagic fever. Rev Infect Dis 11(Suppl 4): 794S–800S, 1989.

71. R Swanepoel, AJ Shepherd, PA Leman, SP Shepherd, GM McGillivray, MJ Erasmus, LA Searle, DE Gill. Epidemiologic and clinical features of Crimean-Congo hemorrhagic fever in southern Africa. Am J Trop Med Hyg 36:120–132, 1987.

72. A Shepherd, R Swanepoel, SP Shepherd, GM McGillivray, LA Searle. Antibody to Crimean-Congo hemorrhagic fever virus in wild mammals from Southern Africa. Am J Trop Med Hyg 36:133–142, 1987.

73. AJ Shepherd, R Swanepoel, PA Leman. Antibody response in Crimean-Congo hemorrhagic fever. Rev Infect Dis 11(Suppl 4):S801–S806, 1989.

74. SP Fisher-Hoch, JA Khan, S Rehman, S Mirza, M Khurshid, JB McCormick. Crimean-Congo haemorrhagic fever treated with oral ribavirin. Lancet 346:472–475, 1995.

75. DM Watts, TG Ksiazek, KJ Linthicum, et al. Crimean-Congo hemorrhagic fever. In: TP Monath, ed. The Arboviruses: Epidemiology and Ecology, Vol 2. Boca Raton: CRC Press; 1989, pp 177–222.

76. J Meegan, RE Shope. Emerging concepts on Rift Valley fever. In: M Pollard, ed. Perspectives in Virology XI. New York: Alan R. Liss, 1981, pp 267–282.

77. R Daubney, JR Hudson. Enzootic hepatitis or Rift Valley fever: an undescribed virus disease of sheep, cattle, and man from east Africa. J Pathol 34:545–557, 1931.

78. J Gear. Hemorrhagic fevers in South Africa: an account of two recent outbreaks. J S Afr Vet Assoc 48:5–8, 1977.

79. World Health Organization. An outbreak of Rift Valley Fever, eastern Africa, 1997–1998. Wkly Epidemiol Rec 73:105–109, 1998.

80. RR Aruther, MS el-Sharkawy, SE Cope, BA Botros, S Oun, JC Morrill, RE Shope, RG Hibbs, MA Darwish, IZ Imam. Recurrence of Rift Valley fever in Egypt. Lancet 342:1149–1150, 1993.

81. JM Meegan. Rift Valley fever in Egypt: an overview of the epizootics in 1977 and 1978. Contrib Epidemiol Biostat 3:100–113, 1981.

82. J Morvan, PE Rollin, S Laventure, I Rakotoarivony, J Roux. Rift Valley fever epizootic in the central highlands of Madagascar. Res Virol 143:407–415, 1992.

83. F Davies, KJ Linthicum, AD James. Rainfall and epizootic Rift Valley fever. Bull World Health Organ 63:941–943, 1985.

84. J Meegan, GM Khalil, H Hoogstraal, FK Adham. Experimental transmission and field isolation studies implicating Culex pipiens as a vector of Rift Valley fever virus in Egypt. Am J Trop Med Hyg 29:1405–1410, 1980.

85. K Smithburn, AJ Haddown, JD Gillett. Rift Valley fever: isolation of the virus from wild mosquitos. Br J Exp Pathol 30:1–16, 1948.

86. JA Vaughan, MJ Turell. Facilitation of Rift Valley fever virus transmission by Plasmodium bergheisporozoites in Anopheles stephensi mosquitoes. Am J Trop Med Hyg 55: 407–409, 1996.

87. JH Gear, TP Monath, GS Bowen, GE Kemp. Arboviruses in Africa. In: Feigen RD, ed. Textbook of Pediatric Infectious Diseases. Philadelphia: WB Sanders, 1987 pp 1468–1489.

88. C Peters, GW Anderson Jr. Pathogenesis of Rift Valley fever. Contrib Epidemiol Biostat 3:21–41, 1981.

89. J Morrill, GB Jennings, TM Cosgriff, PH Gibbs, CJ Peters. Prevention of Rift Valley fever in rhesus monkeys with interferon-alpha. Rev Infect Dis 11(Suppl 4):S815–S825, 1989.

90. R Randall, CJ Gibbs, CG Anlisio, LN Binn, VR Harrison. The development of a formalin-killed Rift Valley fever vaccine for use in man. J Immunol 89:660–671, 1962.

91. D Cummins. Arenaviral haemorrhagic fevers. Blood Rev 5:129–137, 1991.

92. JD Frame, JM Baldwin, DJ Gocke, JM Troup. Lassa fever, a new virus disease in man from West Africa. I. Clinical description and pathological findings. Am J Trop Med Hyg 19:670–676, 1970.

93. SM Buckley, J Casals. Lassa fever, a new virus of man from West Africa. III. Isolation and characterization of the virus. Am J Trop Med Hyg 19:680–691, 1970.

94. NE Mettler. Argentine hemorrhagic fever: current knowledge. Sci. Publ. No. 183. Washington, D.C., Pan American Health Organization, 1969.

95. KM Johnson, NH Wiebenga, RB Mackenzie, et al. Virus isolations from human cases of hemorrhagic fever in Bolivia. Proc Soc Exp Biol Med 118:113–118, 1965.

96. R Salas, N de Manzione, RB Tesh, et al. Venezuelan haemorrhagic fever. Lancet 338:1033–1036, 1991.

97. JI Maiztegui. Clinical and epidemiological patterns of Argentine haemorrhagic fever. Bull World Health Organ 52: 567–576, 1975.

98. JB McCormick, IJ King, PA Webb, KM Johnson, R O'Sullivan, ES Smith, S Trippel, TC Tong. A case-control study of the clinical diagnosis and course of Lassa fever. J Infect Dis 155:445–455, 1987.

99. J Ter Meulen, I Lukashevich, K Sidibe, et al. Hunting of peridomestic rodents and consumption of their meat as possible risk factors for rodent-to-human transmission of Lassa virus in the Republic of Guinea. Am J Trop Med Hyg 55:661–666, 1996.

100. D Cummins. Lassa fever. Br J Hosp Med 43:186–192, 1990.

101. MD Bajani, O Tomori, PE Rollin, et al. A survey for antibodies to Lassa virus among health workers in Nigeria. Trans R Soc Trop Med Hyg 91:379–381, 1997.

102. MH Monson, AK Cole, JD Frame, JR Serwint, S Alexander, PB Jahrling. Pediatric Lassa fever: a review of 33 Liberian cases. Am J Trop Med Hyg 36:408–415, 1987.

103. JB McCormick, IJ King, PA Webb, CL Scribner, RB Craven, KM Johnson, LH Elliott, R Belmont-Williams. Lassa fever. Effective therapy with ribavirin. N Engl J Med 314: 20–26, 1986.

104. JI Maiztegui, NJ Fernandez, AJ de Damilozno. Efficacy of immune plasma in treatment of Argentine hemorrhagic fever and association between treatment and a late neurological syndrome. Lancet 2:1216–1217, 1979.

105. PB Jahrling, CJ Peters. Passive antibody therapy of Lassa fever in cynomolgus monkeys: importance of neutralizing antibody and Lassa virus strain. Infect Immun 44: 528–533, 1984.

106. SP Fisher-Hoch, JB McCormick, D Auperin, BG Brown, M Castor, G Perez, S Ruo, A Conaty, L Brammer, S Bauer. Protection of rhesus monkeys from fatal Lassa fever by vaccination with a recombinant vaccinia virus containing the Lassa virus glycoprotein gene. Proc Natl Acad Sci U S A 86:317–321, 1989.

107. ME Price, SP Fisher-Hoch, RB Craven, JB McCormick. A prospective study of maternal and fetal outcome in acute Lassa fever infection during pregnancy. BMJ 297: 584–587, 1988.

Cutaneous Manifestations of Enterovirus Infections

Wesley King Galen

Tulane University, New Orleans, Louisiana, USA
and Louisiana State University School of Medicine, New Orleans, Louisiana, USA

The study of enteroviral rashes may be somewhat perplexing, even to the most experienced clinician. Gone is the elegance of one virus for one rash, as seen in varicella in which the particular virus more or less creates the same clinical picture, albeit of varying severity, in all hosts. Instead, the clinician is confronted with one clinical syndrome that may be caused by several different enteroviral infections, or alternately, multiple widely differing clinical rashes and patterns of illness being traced to a single enteroviral cause. Recognizing this enteroviral potpourri of rashes is worthy for purposes of diagnosis and epidemiology, but it is made all the more important because it may predict associated viral involvement of other organ systems, which may be serious and life-threatening.

Enteroviruses belong to the viral family of Picornaviridae (pico = small; rna = ribonucleic acid). They contain a single strand of RNA in their central core that is covered by an icosahededral protein capsid and measure from 24 to 30 nm in size with electron microscopy. The genus *Enterovirus* is a distinctive collection of viruses that replicate in the human gastrointestinal tract [1,2]. This genus consists of four major groups of viruses: 3 polioviruses, 23 group A coxsackieviruses, 6 group B coxsackieviruses, and 32 echoviruses. These are further separated into 68 recognized serotypes by means of type-specific neutralization antisera [3]. More recent analysis by genetic sequencing may result in reorganization of these categories. For the purposes of this chapter, the standard classification is used. Newly discovered serotypes are now designated enteroviruses and numbered 68 through 71. This new terminology

acknowledges that these newer isolates did not conform to the rigid specificities with regard to effects on animals and tissue cultures applied historically to separate out coxsackie strains from echo strains. Although poliovirus infections were of great historical and clinical importance worldwide, they do not cause exanthems. Consequently, this chapter focuses on exanthematic illnesses caused by nonpolio enteroviruses (Fig. 19–1).

HISTORY

Some of the clinical diseases due to enteroviruses have been recognized since ancient times. The first documentation of poliovirus comes from an Egyptian stele dating back to 1500 B.C. that pictures a man with an atrophied, shortened, paralytic leg [4]. A London pediatrician named Underwood gave the first scientific description of poliomyelitis in 1789 [5], and the first report of a poliomyelitis outbreak in 1834 is attributed to Badham [6]. Numerous outbreaks were later documented in the 19th and 20th centuries, during which the disease process and epidemiology were elucidated. Transmission of the etiological virus from a paralytic patient to monkeys was first accomplished in 1908 [7], and propagation of the virus in human tissue was not possible until 1949 [8].

The persistent search for the viral etiology of poliomyelitis led to the serendipitous discovery of several related viruses, now known as coxsackieviruses A and B and the echoviruses. Coxsackieviruses were first isolated in 1947

TAXONOMY
Picornaviridae family
Enterovirus genus

WORLDWIDE GEOGRAPHICAL INCIDENCE

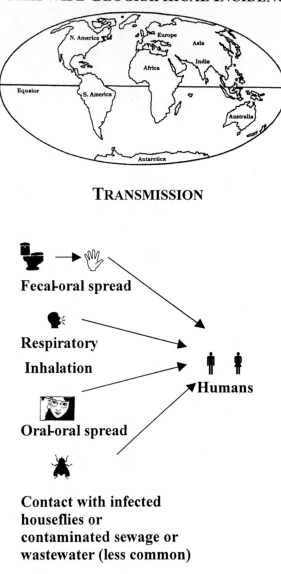

TRANSMISSION

Fecal-oral spread

Respiratory

Inhalation

Oral-oral spread

Humans

Contact with infected houseflies or contaminated sewage or wastewater (less common)

ZOONOTIC IMPLICATIONS

None

Figure 19–1.   Incidence and transmission of Enteroviruses.

by Dalldorf and Sickles [9]. Recognition of numerous strains of this virus rapidly followed, but almost 5 years passed before their association with human disease was proved [10]. The earliest recognition of an epidemic illness due to coxsackievirus A16 occurred in 1957 in Toronto, Canada [11]. This epidemic affected 60 individuals with a febrile illness associated with oropharyngeal and cutaneous lesions. The term *hand-foot-and-mouth syndrome* was first coined by Alsop and coworkers to describe a similar epidemic of coxsackievirus A16 that occurred in Birmingham, England, in 1960 [12]. Sporadic reports followed for a few years, but since the mid-1960s, the illness has been generally recognized worldwide [13–17]. Subsequently, similar clinical epidemics have been proved to be associated with other coxsackievirus strains including type A10 [18], type A5, type B1, type B3 [19], and enterovirus 71.

Several other viruses were newly discovered from tissue culture, but were not yet linked to any human diseases. These orphan viruses were grouped together and classified as *e*nteric *c*ytopathogenic *h*uman *o*rphan viruses, or *echo*viruses, for short. Within many years, numerous clinical syndromes were found to be associated with these viruses.

EPIDEMIOLOGY

Enteroviruses are distributed worldwide. Although reportedly recovered from varied animals including dogs, swine, a calf, and a fox as well as oysters, mussels, and even raw sewage, it is generally believed that the only natural hosts of enteroviral infections are humans [1]. Infections attack both sexes and all racial groups equally, but favor younger, presumably nonimmune cohorts, although not exclusively. Virus transmission is predominantly person-to-person, most often by the fecal-oral route but also by respiratory or oral-to-oral routes. Swimming pools may promote transmission in the summer as warm weather appears to increase the frequency of infections in temperate climates. Contaminated foods may be another possible source of infection [20]. Yearround outbreaks are common in tropical and subtropical climates. Epidemics or small outbreaks due to various agents occur episodically, reflecting presumably the acquisition of various sizes of nonimmune populations, especially children.

Although data are obtained from symptomatic patients (most with neurological illness), it is noted that unrecognized or presumably mildly symptomatic or asymptomatic infections occur in certain epidemics in equivalent or greater number than symptomatic infections [1]. In a survey of enteroviral isolations in the United States from 1961 through 1990, the most prevalent infections were due to echovirus types 9, 6, and 11, followed by coxsackievirus B2 and B4. Echovirus type 11 has been the most common circulating viral type reported since 1986 [1]. Survey of enteroviral epidemics reveals most clinical disease is due to a dozen serotypes, primarily Echovirus types 4, 6, 9, 11, and 30, coxsackievirus A9 and A16, coxsackievirus B2, B3, B4, and B5, and enteroviruses 70 and 71 [3]. Recently, a possible role of enteroviruses in the pathogenesis of diabetes mellitus has been postulated [1].

PATHOGENESIS

Many factors are thought to affect the clinical severity of the enteroviral illness, including the concentration of the viral innoculum, its route of inoculation, the virulence and tropism of the particular strain of virus, and the immunocompetence of the host. The age of the patient significantly affects the outcome as well, with neonatal or fetal exposure resulting in a more severe disease expression.

After the particular enterovirus is acquired, implantation occurs in both the pharynx and the lower gastrointestinal tract. Implantation proceeds to regional lymph nodes, such as the tonsils or cervical lymph nodes or Peyer's patches and mesenteric lymph nodes, within 24 hours, where the virus multiplies. By 72 hours, a mild viremia occurs with spread of the virus to many secondary locations. If a pregnant woman becomes infected and suffers a viremia, the fetus is transplacentally infected during this time. Multiplication of the virus continues at these secondary sites, such as the skin and mucous membrane, the respiratory tract, liver, heart, and/or central nervous system (CNS). This results in onset of clinical illness, which can vary from extremely minor to fatal depending on the many factors previously mentioned.

This period of viral multiplication in secondary organs usually lasts for 3 to 7 days and is often associated with a major viremia. On occasion, spread to the CNS is delayed until this period, suggesting that spread to the CNS may follow the major or secondary viremia and not only the primary viremia. The viremia and the viral infection of secondary sites usually begin to diminish about the seventh day of illness, which correlates with the increasing appearance of serum antibody. The lower gastrointestinal tract remains infected and may continue to spill virus for days, weeks, or even months, resulting in the potential spread to other nonimmune hosts [1,20]. Unfortunately, neonates and children with hypogammaglobulinemia may evidence severe and chronic enteroviral infections. Some limited success in treating these especially vulnerable patients has been accomplished using intravenous immunoglobulin (IVIG) [21].

It should be noted that, although the illnesses produced by the nonpolio enteroviruses are generally not severe, fatalities have occurred owing to myocarditis or meningoencephalitis, most often following infections with coxsackievirus B. Rare fatalities have been reported in three infants and one adult from whom coxsackievirus A1 was recovered. The adult suffered an organized pneumonitis and diffuse pancarditis associated with an exanthem, consistent with hand-foot-and-mouth disease [22]. Rare infant fatalities associated with massive hepatic necrosis have followed infections with several echovirus types including 3, 6, 7, 9, 11, 14, 19, and 21 [1]. Other echovirus-associated infant fatalities have followed adrenal and renal hemorrhage [1,23,24] and another two fatalities had extensive pneumonia.

A 1998 epidemic of enterovirus 71 infection in Taiwan was reported with mucocutaneous presentations, such as hand-foot-and-mouth disease (64–75%) and herpangina (6–11%). This epidemic resulted in severe disease in 405

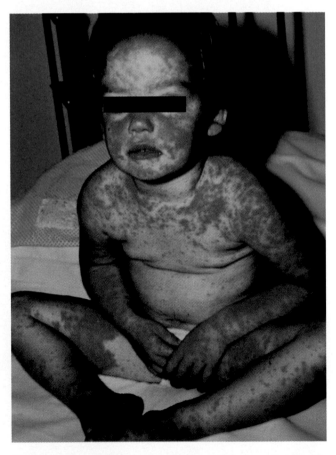

Figure 19–2. Papular, erythrodermic eruption associated with echovirus infection.

patients and 78 deaths predominantly in children younger than 5 years old. Complications included encephalitis, asceptic meningitis, pulmonary edema and hemorrhage, poliomyelitis-like acute flacid paralysis, and myocarditis [25,26].

CLINICAL PRESENTATION

Infections with enteroviruses are extremely common, and the rashes produced are protean. The most common exanthems are macular or maculopapular eruptions. In certain cases, these may coalesce into a morbilliform pattern. Such

rashes have been associated with numerous enteroviral types such as coxsackievirus A6, A9, A16, and B5 [27], but it is important to know that some of these patients also exhibited vesicles [22], petechiae, purpura, urticaria, and/or maculopapules while suffering their particular enteroviral infection (Figs. 19–2 to 19–10). Vesiculobullous eruptions mimicking herpes zoster have been described with echovirus 6 (see Fig. 5-38) [28], and petechial eruptions simulating meningococcemia have been described with echovirus 9 [29]. Acute hemangioma-like lesions have been associated with echovirus 25 infection (Fig. 19–11).

The confusion arising from these presentations is partially clarified by the two charts organized by Dr. James

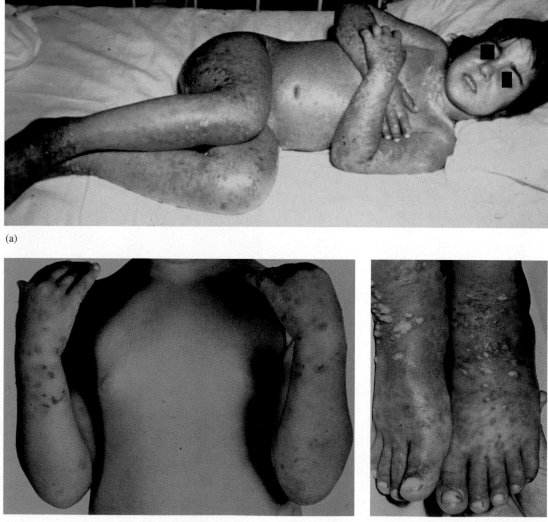

(a)

(b)   (c)

Figure 19–3.   (a–c) Pustular eruption associated with echovirus 6.

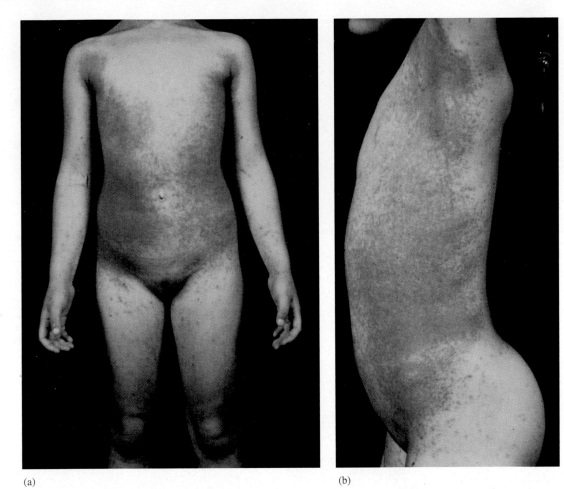

(a) (b)

Figure 19–4. (a,b) Purpuric rash due to coxsackievirus B6.

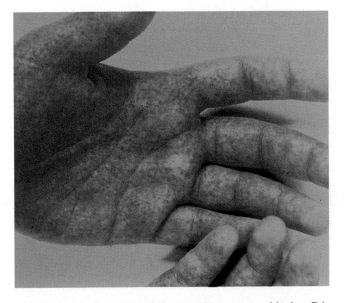

Figure 19–5. Purpuric lesions secondary to coxsackievirus B4.

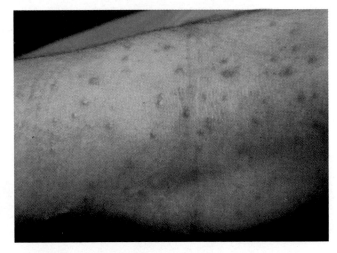

Figure 19–6. Papular lesions resulting from coxsackievirus B4.

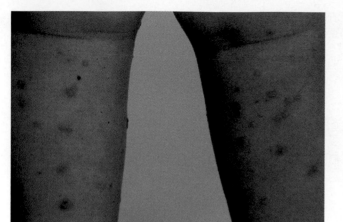

Figure 19–7. Acral pustular eruption due to enterovirus infection.

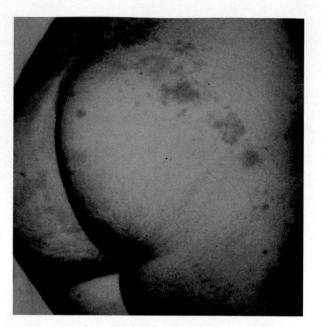

Figure 19–9. Linear distribution of papules due to coxsackievirus B5 in a patient with asceptic meningitis. (Photograph courtesy of Ronald Hansen, M.D., Department of Dermatology, University of Arizona School of Medicine, Tucson, AZ.)

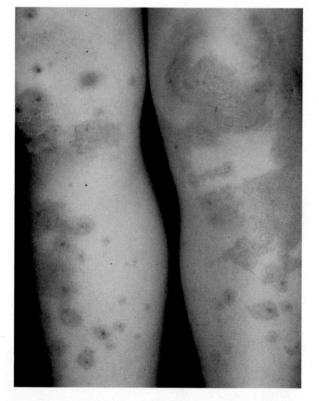

Figure 19–8. Erythema multiforme–like rash associated with coxsackievirus infection.

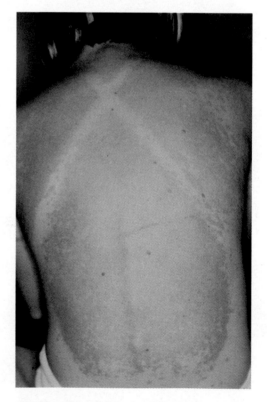

Figure 19–10. Photodistribution of macules associated with coxsackievirus infection.

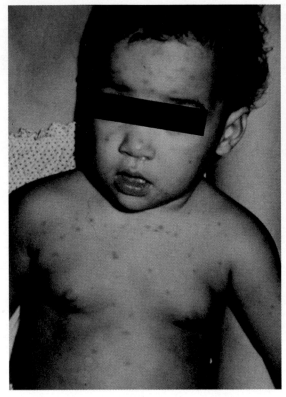

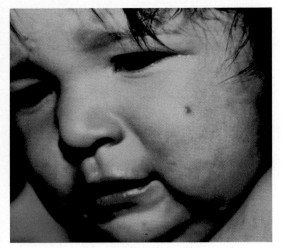

(b)

(a)

Figure 19–11. (a,b) Acute hemangioma-like lesions associated with echovirus 25 infection. (Photographs courtesy of Ronald Hansen, M.D., Department of Dermatology, University of Arizona School of Medicine, Tucson, AZ.)

D. Cherry [1]. Table 19–1 indicates the morphology of the rash and the common, occasional, and rare enteroviral illnesses producing these specified lesions. Table 19–2 indicates certain of the most prevalent enteroviral types, the age group of most affected patients, the frequency of the rash, its most common morphological features, and the associated clinical manifestations of the outbreak. This table summarizes and clarifies information from hundreds of outbreaks and will be an aid to every interested clinician.

From these tables, it is possible to deduce that certain patterns of illness, such as hand-foot-and-mouth disease, herpangina, and roseola-like illnesses, are fairly frequent enteroviral presentations. These manifestations are discussed more fully, but the clinician should consider the diagnosis of enteroviral illness every time a child or adult presents with any combination of fever, gastrointestinal symptoms, headache, meningismus, meningitis, rashes, and/or mucous membrane lesions. Table 19–3 summarizes some of the clinical rashes reported with enteroviral illnesses.

HAND-FOOT-AND-MOUTH DISEASE

In general, the illness associated with hand-foot-and-mouth disease is a mild one [17]. It predominantly affects children

between the ages of 2 and 10 years, but adults, particularly parents, are not entirely spared. Cherry [1] reports attack rates among exposed individuals of 100% in young children, 38% in school children, and 11% in adults. This illness most commonly appears in late spring, summer, or fall. Coxsackievirus A16, A5, A10, A7, A9, B1, B3, and B5 and enterovirus 71 are the etiological factors.

The syndrome of hand-foot-and-mouth disease may be complete, with both oral and cutaneous involvement, or may involve only one manifestation. The oral lesions of this disease most often involve the tongue, buccal mucosa, and gingivolabial groove. Oral discomfort and anorexia may on rare occasion lead to dehydration. In 20% of affected children, submandibular lymphadenopathy may develop [30].

The cutaneous findings of this disease begin as papular lesions and progress to papulovesicular and then vesicular lesions (Figs. 19–12 to 19–19). Most vesicles are asymptomatic but may be tender, especially when present on the palms and soles. Other exanthems noted with hand-foot-and-mouth disease include red maculopapular lesions, which are most often distributed on the buttocks and limbs of patients younger than 5 years old [11]. Hand-foot-and-mouth disease usually abates in a week, although patients may rarely exhibit a more serious, relapsing, or prolonged

Table 19–1. Clinical Exanthematous Manifestations of Coxsackieviruses and Echoviruses

Clinical feature	Associated virus subgroup	Common	Occasional	Rare
Macular rash	Coxsackievirus A			
	Coxsackievirus B		1, 2, 5	
	Echovirus and enterovirus		2, 4, 5, 13, 14, 17, 19, 30	18, 71
Maculopapular rash	Coxsackievirus A	9	2, 4, 5, 10, 16	6, 7
	Coxsackievirus B		1–5	
	Echovirus and enterovirus	4, 9	2, 5–7, 11, 16–19, 25, 30, 71	1, 3, 13, 14, 22, 27, 33
Vesicular rash	Coxsackievirus A	5, 16	8–10	4, 7
	Coxsackievirus B			1–3, 5
	Echovirus and enterovirus		11, 71	6, 9, 17
Petechial or purpuric rash	Coxsackievirus A	9	4	
	Coxsackievirus B		2–5	
	Echovirus		4, 7	3
Urticarial rash	Coxsackievirus A	9	16	
	Coxsackievirus B		4, 5	
	Echovirus		11	
Erythema multiforme or Stevens-Johnson syndrome	Coxsackievirus A		9	10, 16
	Coxsackievirus B			4, 5
	Echovirus			6, 11
Exanthem and meningitis	Coxsackievirus A		2, 9	7
	Coxsackievirus B		1, 2, 4, 5	
	Echovirus and enterovirus	4, 9	6, 11, 17, 18, 25, 30	3, 14, 33, 71
Exanthem and pneumonia	Coxsackievirus A		9	7
	Coxsackievirus B		6	1
	Echovirus			9, 11
Hand-foot-and-mouth syndrome	Coxsackievirus A	16	5, 10	7, 9
	Coxsackievirus B			1, 3, 5
	Echovirus and enterovirus		71	
Hemangioma-like lesions	Coxsackievirus A			
	Coxsackievirus B			25, 32
	Echovirus			
Herpangina and exanthem	Coxsackievirus A		4	9
	Coxsackievirus B			2
	Echovirus		16, 17	
Roseola-like illness	Coxsackievirus A			6, 9
	Coxsackievirus B		5	1, 2, 4
	Echovirus		16, 25	9, 11, 27, 30
Anaphylactoid purpura	Coxsackievirus A			4
	Coxsackievirus B			
	Echovirus			9, 18
Zoster-like rash	Coxsackievirus A			
	Coxsackievirus B			
	Echovirus			5, 6
Chronic or recurrent rash	Coxsackievirus A	16		
	Coxsackievirus B			
	Echovirus			11

Source: JD Cherry. Enteroviruses: coxsackieviruses, echoviruses, and polioviruses. In: RD Feigin, JD Cherry, eds. Textbook of Pediatric Infectious Disease, 4th edition, Philadelphia: WB Saunders, 1998, p. 1811, modified with permission.

Table 19–2. Frequency of Exanthem in Outbreaks of Illness Due to Coxsackieviruses and Echoviruses

Virus type		Age group	Occurrence of rash	Characteristic of rash	Associated manifestations
Coxsackievirus	A2	Children	Rare	Maculopapular	Fever
	A4	Children	Rare	Maculopapular, vesicular	Fever, herpangina, hepatitis
	A5	Mainly children	Occasional	Hand-foot-and-mouth syndrome	Fever
	A7	Children and adults	Rare	Morbilliform, hand-foot-and-mouth syndrome	Meningitis, pneumonia, pancarditis
	A9	Mainly children	4%	Maculopapular, vesicular, urticarial, petechial, hand-foot-and-mouth syndrome	Fever, meningitis, pneumonia
	A10	Mainly children	Occasional	Hand-foot-and-mouth syndrome	Fever
	A16	Children and adults	88%, <5 yr old 38%, 5–12 yr old 11%, adults	Hand-foot-and-mouth syndrome	Fever
	B1	Children	Occasional	Maculopapular, vesicular, (roseola-like illness)	Fever, meningitis
	B2	Children	Rare	Maculopapular, vesicular, petechial	Fever, herpangina, meningitis
	B3	Mainly children	Occasional	Maculopapular, vesicular, petechial	Fever, hepatosplenomegaly
	B4	Mainly children	Occasional	Maculopapular, vesicular, urticarial	Fever, respiratory symptoms
	B5	Mainly children	10%	Maculopapular, petechial, urticarial, roseola-like	Fever, meningitis
Echovirus	B6	Children and adults	20%	Morbilliform	Pneumonia
	1	Children	Rare	Maculopapular	Conjunctivitis
	2	Children	Rare	Macular, maculopapular	Fever, pharyngitis
	3	Children	Rare	Petechial	Fever, meningitis
	4	Mainly children	10–20%	Macular, maculopapular, petechial	Fever, meningitis
	5	Infants and adults	Occasional	Macular	Fever
	6	Mainly children	Rare	Maculopapular, macular, papulopustular, vesicular	Fever, meningitis
	7	Children	Occasional	Maculopapular	Fever, meningitis
	9	Children and adults	57%, <5 yr old 41%, 5–9 yr old 6%, >10 yr old	Maculopapular, petechial, vesicular	Fever, meningitis
	11	Mainly children	Occasional	Maculopapular, vesicular, urticarial, roseola-like	Fever, meningitis
	13	Children	Rare	Maculopapular	
	14	Mainly children	Rare	Maculopapular, scarlatiniform	Fever, meningitis
	16	Children	Occasional	Roseola-like	Fever, herpangina
	17	Children	Occasional	Macular, maculopapular, papulovesicular	Fever, diarrhea, herpangina, meningitis
	18	Children and adults	Occasional, 1 epidemic	Rubelliform	Fever, meningitis
	19	Children and adults	Occasional	Maculopapular	Fever, meningitis, upper respiratory symptoms
	22	Infants	Rare	Morbilliform	Respiratory symptoms
	25	Children	Occasional	Maculopapular, hemangioma-like	Fever, pharyngitis

(continued)

Table 19–2. *(continued)*

Virus type		Age group	Occurrence of rash	Characteristic of rash	Associated manifestations
	30	Children and adults	Occasional	Macular, maculopapular	Fever, meningitis
	32	Children	Rare	Hemangioma-like	Fever
	33	—	Rare	—	Meningitis
Enterovirus	71	Children and adults	Occasional Four epidemics	Macular, maculopapular, vesicular, hand-foot-and-mouth syndrome	Mild-to-severe illness with: fever, meningitis, herpangina, encephalitis, paralytic disease, pulmonary edema and hemorrhage, myocarditis, facial paralysis, death especially with children less than 5 yr old

Source: JD Cherry. *Enteroviruses:* coxsackieviruses, echoviruses, and polioviruses. In: RD Feigin, JD Cherry, eds. Textbook of Pediatric Infectious Diseases, 3rd ed. Philadelphia: WB Saunders, (1992), Table 157–11, p. 1718, and 4th ed. (1998). Table 170–16, p. 1813, modified with permission.

Table 19–3. Common Presentations of Enteroviruses

Approximately 30 enteroviruses cause rashes, but one virus may cause a variety of rashes

One clinical syndrome (e.g., hand-foot-and-mouth syndrome) may be caused by several enteroviruses

Common Presentations

Morbilliform	Coxsackievirus A9, B3, B5, Echovirus 2, 4, 9, 11, 19, 25 (acral)
Vesicular	Coxsackievirus A5, A16, B3, Echovirus 17, Echovirus 25 (herpangina), Coxsackievirus A1, A6, A8, A10, A16, A22, Enterovirus 71
Roseola-like	Coxsackievirus B1, B5, Echovirus 11, Echovirus 16 (Boston exanthem), Echovirus 25 persists 2–5 days, may stall on face, chest
Other presentations	Scarlatiniform, zosteriform: Echovirus 6, Coxsackievirus B5 Urticarial: Coxsackievirus B5, Echovirus 25 Petechial and pupuric: Coxsackievirus A9, A4, Echovirus 9, Coxsackievirus B3, B5 Cherry spots: Echovirus 25, 32 Gianotti-Crosti or acral papular dermatitis: Coxsackievirus A16, polio vaccine

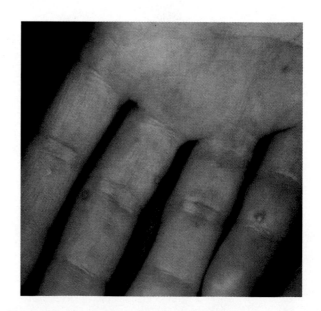

Figure 19–12. Palmar vesicles of hand-foot-and-mouth disease.

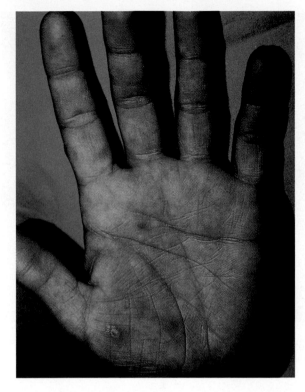

Figure 19–13. Palmar vesicles of hand-foot-and-mouth disease.

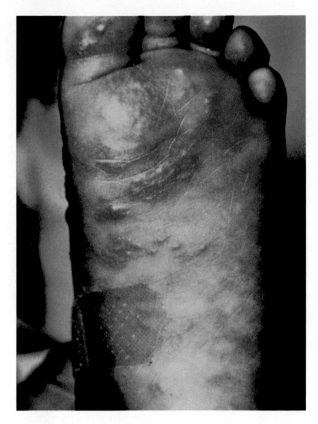

Figure 19–15. Vesicles of the feet in hand-foot-and-mouth disease. (Photograph courtesy of Ronald Hansen, M.D., Department of Dermatology, University of Arizona School of Medicine, Tucson, AZ.)

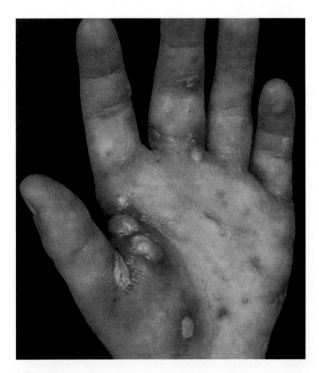

Figure 19–14. Palmar vesicles of hand-foot-and-mouth disease in a child with leukemia.

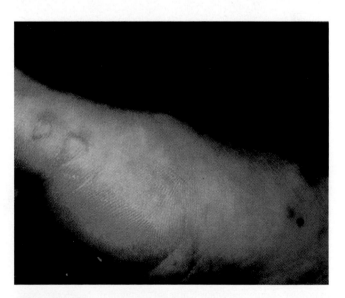

Figure 19–16. Vesicles of the feet in hand-foot-and-mouth disease.

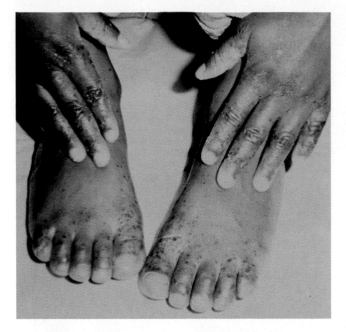

Figure 19–17. Resolving lesions of the hands and feet in hand-foot-and-mouth disease.

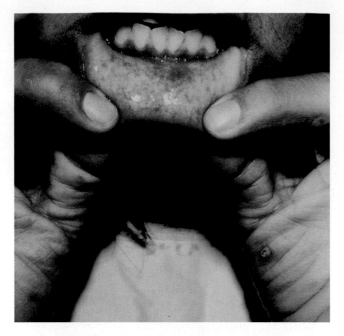

Figure 19–19. Oral and palmar vesicles of hand-foot-and-mouth disease.

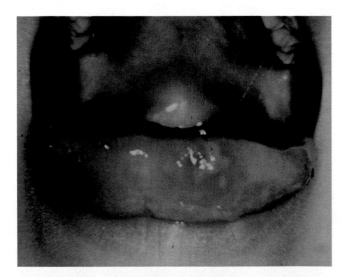

Figure 19–18. Oral vesicles of hand-foot-and-mouth disease. (Photograph courtesy of Lee Nesbitt, M.D., Department of Dermatology, Louisiana State University School of Medicine, New Orleans, LA.)

course. One chronic case in an elderly woman persisted 2½ years [31]. Rare cases have been reported with serious organ involvement, such as myocarditis, pneumonia, aseptic meningitis, or paralytic disease, with even fatal outcomes in association with hand-foot-and-mouth disease [21]. In general, however, the prognosis of hand-foot-and-mouth disease is quite good. Table 19–4 summarizes the clinical manifestations for this disease. Table 19–5 lists differential diagnoses.

ENTEROVIRUS 71

Special mention should be made of the epidemic of enterovirus 71 in Taiwan that occurred in 1998. This epidemic of hand-foot-and-mouth disease (75%) or herpangina (11%) was documented to affect 129,106 patients by 850 sentinel physicians (8.7% of MDs). Thus, some estimate these patients represented approximately 10% of the cases seen that year, implying that this epidemic may have affected over 1,300,000 from a total population of 21,178,000. The vast majority of these patients had self-limited infections and required little or no medical treatment.

There were 405 severe cases of this infection that required hospitalization. These were patients who evidenced high fever (≤38°C), tachypnea, vomiting, cardiopulmonary, or neurological complications. Seventy-eight of these patients died. Most (91%) were younger than 5 years old. Complications associated with fatal outcomes included encephalitis, encephalitis with pulmonary edema or hemorrhage, aseptic meningitis and pulmonary edema or hemor-

Table 19–4. Clinical Manifestations of Hand-Foot-and-Mouth Syndrome

Time after exposure	Clinical manifestations	Laboratory analyses	Other notes
3–6 days	Prodrome lasting 1–2 days, with sore mouth (67%), malaise (61%), anorexia (52%), low-grade fever (42%), lymphadenopathy (22%), coryza (11%), cough (11%), diarrhea (10%) and abdominal pain ↓	Leukocyte counts may be low, normal, or high, sometimes with atypical lymphocytosis	
4–7 days	90% of patients develop tiny vesicles and erosions on the tongue or oral mucosa. These lesions begin as red maculopapules that become vesicles and then rapidly break down to form shallow erosions of 4–8-mm size ↓	Viral isolation from vesicular fluid, blood, pharyngeal swabs, or less reliably, fecal specimens	Usually 1–8 oral lesions are present
4–8 days	60–70% of patients develop oval superficial vesicles (3–7 mm) with an erythematous halo. These lesions are located on the dorsum of hands, feet, palms, and soles, but may occasionally become scattered on the face, limbs, or buttocks ↓	Detection of virus-specific IgM during acute disease	Lesions may number from a few to over a hundred, and tend to cluster in areas of pressure and trauma or align along skin creases. Lesions are not typically pruritic. Occasional associated findings include high fever, malaise, diarrhea, joint pains, and lymphadenopathy (22%)
8–18 days	Crusting or resorption of vesicles, with residual red or pink spots lasting for a short time. Illness resolves in most patients		Rare but documented cases include myocarditis, pneumonia, pulmonary edema or hemorrhage, encephalitis, meningoencephalitis, aseptic meningitis, and acute flaccid paralysis

rhage, myocarditis, myocarditis with encephalitis, encephalitis with acute flaccid paralysis, or acute flaccid paralysis alone.

The large scope of this epidemic and the number of fatalities it created, especially in infants and young children, are an unpleasant reminder of the potential pathogenic virulence of enterovirus 71 and other enteroviruses [25,26].

ROSEOLA INFANTUM

True roseola infantum, also known as exanthem subitum, is now generally acknowledged to be due in major part to human herpesvirus 6, which was more recently isolated from affected infants by Yamanishi and associates [32]. The constellation of symptoms that make up this illness,

however, appears to have more than one cause; and roseola-like illnesses abound in medical offices and in the literature. Prominent among the causes of these roseola-like illnesses, particularly those outbreaks occurring in summer and fall, are enteroviruses. Several enteroviruses have been implicated, including most often coxsackievirus B5, A6, and A9. Less often reported causes of roseola-like illnesses include coxsackievirus B1, B2, B4 and echovirus 16 (the cause of Boston exanthem), 25, 9, 11, 27, and 30 [33].

Roseola and roseola-like illnesses primarily affect infants younger than 3 years old, although occasional reports of patients as old as 14 years exist. During the febrile phase, an injected pharynx may be present in 10 to 30% of patients, and suboccipital lymph nodes are frequently palpable. Some patients develop a mild cough and coryza, particular in winter months. Subtle or clear-cut signs of

Table 19–5. Differential Diagnoses of Hand-Foot-and-Mouth Syndrome

Drug eruptions: Early maculopapules of hand-foot-and mouth-disease may appear similar, but drug eruptions are typically more extensive and pruritic, rather than painful

Rubella: Early maculopapules of hand-foot-and-mouth disease may appear similar, but the rubella rash is typically more extensive

Varicella: The varicella rash is usually more extensive than that of hand-foot-and-mouth disease, and individual lesions of varicella are at different stages of development (i.e., macules, papules, vesicles, and crusts)

Erythema multiforme: This illness usually has target lesions and a greater number of oral ulcerations present when compared with hand-foot-and-mouth disease

Herpangina: Hand-foot-and-mouth disease with oral involvement only may be difficult to differentiate. The oral lesions of hand-foot-and-mouth disease most frequently involve the tongue, gingiva, and buccal mucosa, whereas herpangina lesions are usually located on the soft palate, tonsillar pillars, and anterior fauces

Herpetic stomatitis: Oral herpes infection may sometimes cause fever, but lesions usually involve the perioral area. Tzanck smear can demonstrate the characteristic cytopathic changes associated with herpes simplex virus

Aphthous stomatitis: These lesions are rarely associated with fever, Only one or a few lesions are usually present at a time

Other enterovirus exanthems: These related viral exanthems do not tend to localize to the oral mucosa and distal extremities as does hand-foot-and-mouth disease

meningismus, with or without seizures, may rarely be noted as well. Febrile seizures occur in approximately 6% of children with roseola infantum or roseola-like illnesses and are the most common cause of hospitalization of affected children. In most cases, however, the child appears alert, playful, and nontoxic in spite of the presence of fever [27]. Table 19–6 summarizes the major clinical features of roseola and roseola-like illnesses. Table 19–7 highlights differential diagnoses.

The roseola-like illness recognized as the Boston exanthem is due to echovirus 16 and was first reported in 1951 by Neva and colleagues [34–36], making it the first enteroviral exanthematous illness described. Epidemics of this illness have appeared only sporadically since then, but shared major features with roseola owing to the appearance of the described rashes at or near the resolution of the chief complaint of high fevers [1]. Hall and associates [37] described 10 affected individuals between the ages of 1 week and 7 to 16 years. All were seen during summer and early fall of 1974 in Rochester, New York. Five of these patients were neonates of 1 to 4 weeks in age and presented with fever, lethargy, irritability, vomiting, and abdominal distention requiring hospitalization, work-up, and treatment for sepsis. One 3-year-old required hospitalization for cerebellar ataxia; another had chest and leg pain suggestive of pleurodynia. Seven of the 10 children had a maculopapular rash involving the trunk, extremities, and face, which occurred during late stages of the fever in 2 patients and following its defervescence in 4. In one 3-year-old child, the rash was the only sign of illness [37]. Additionally, an increased incidence of reported cases of roseola occurred in the same and nearly adjacent communities si-

Table 19–6. Clinical Manifestations of Roseola and Roseola-like Illness

Time after exposure	Clinical manifestations	Laboratory analyses	Other notes
5–15 days	High fever suddenly develops, lasting 3–5 days, sometimes associated with lethargy, restlessness, vomiting, diarrhea, anorexia, or abdominal distention and tenderness Periorbital and palpebral edema are common	Concurrent leukopenia may be present	The fever may be intermittent or constant, and is between 38.9°C and 40.6°C. The child typically looks well
8–20 days	Fever quickly subsides and the characteristic rash rapidly appears, lasting 1–2 days Discrete, rose-pink 2–3-mm blanchable macules/papules appear on the trunk and spread to neck, arms, and legs ↓		Rash may be evanescent and is not pruritic.
9–22 days	Rash fades without desquamation or any residual effects		The disease course is generally mild with only rare complications

Table 19–7.   Differential Diagnoses of Roseola and Roseola-like Illness

Drug eruptions: Early maculopapules of roseola and roseola-like illness may appear similar, but drug eruptions are typically more extensive and pruritic rather than painful

Rubella: Early maculopapules of roseola and roseola-like illness may appear similar, but the rubella rash is typically more extensive

Varicella: The varicella rash is usually more extensive than that of roseola and roseola-like illness, and individual lesions of varicella are at different stages of development

Erythema multiforme: This illness usually has target lesions and a greater number of oral ulcerations present when compared with roseola and roseola-like illness

Scarlet fever: Exudative pharyngitis, cervical adenitis, and a fine maculopapular rash with a coarse, sandpaper texture are characteristic of scarlet fever. Group A beta-hemolytic streptococcus or *Staphylococcus aureus* on a throat culture is diagnostic. These infections may lead to sepsis or necrotizing cellulitis

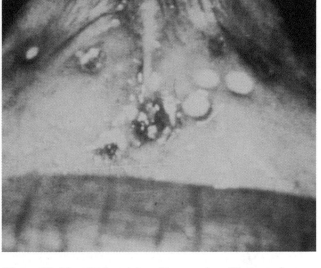

Figure 19–20.   Oral vesicles of herpangina. (Photograph courtesy of Ronald Hansen, M.D., Department of Dermatology, University of Arizona School of Medicine, Tucson, AZ.)

multaneously with these documented illnesses, implying a general appreciation of the roseola-like character of the Boston exanthem. Observation of other sporadic cases has revealed concurrent herpangina-like lesions with ulcers of the tonsillar pillars and soft palate in certain patients with the echovirus 16 exanthem [1].

HERPANGINA

Herpangina refers to an acute febrile illness most often diagnosed in summer and fall in temperate climates. It is defined by the presence of vesicular or discrete erosive lesions on the posterior buccal mucosa, soft palate, tonsillar pillars, tonsils, and pharynx (Fig. 19–20). It occurs in both epidemic and sporadic cases and is caused by several types of enterovirus. Epidemics have been traced to coxsackievirus A types 1, 2, 3, 4, 5, 6, 8, 10, 22, and B1 as well as echovirus types 16 and 25, and enterovirus 71. Sporadic cases have been cultured and documented to follow infections with coxsackievirus A types 7, 9, 16, and 22, coxsackievirus B types 1, 2, 3, 4, and 5, echovirus types 6, 9, 11, 16, 17, and 22 [38–43], and enterovirus 71 [25,26].

Herpangina, as in the majority of enteroviral infections, begins with the sudden onset of fever (from 37°C to 41.5°C) [44–48]. Young children may have a few prodromal symptoms including listlessness, anorexia, and irritability for a few hours prior to the fever's onset, but there is no pro-

drome typical for this disorder. The clinical features characteristic of herpangina are summarized on Table 19–8. Associated symptoms may include drooling (100%), sore throat (50%), coryza (45%), vomiting (25%) or diarrhea or both (36%), and headache (18%) [35,46]. Cases associated with maculopapular, petechial, vesicular, and roseola-like exanthems as well as rare reports of myocarditis, aseptic meningitis, and encephalitis have been documented [49]. See Table 19–9 for differential diagnoses.

HISTOPATHOLOGY

Specific dermatopathological findings of herpangina lesions have not been documented, because biopsies are rarely performed.

LABORATORY FINDINGS

Patients with hand-foot-and-mouth disease typically may have leukocyte counts ranging from 4000 to 16,000/mm^3, sometimes with atypical lymphocytes. Laboratory findings for herpangina are nonspecific.

Table 19–8. Clinical Manifestations of Herpangina

Time after exposure	Clinical manifestations	Laboratory analyses	Other notes
2–9 days	Sudden onset of fever, anorexia, dysphagia, and sore throat $\downarrow$	No routine testing readily available	Some patients may complain of vomiting, abdominal pain, backache, or headache
2–10 days	Shortly thereafter, the characteristic oropharyngeal lesions arise as tiny 1–2-mm papules surrounded by a red halo. These evolve into vesicles and quickly erode to become ulcerations that may slowly enlarge in size over a 2–3-day period to 3–4 mm in size $\downarrow$		Oropharyngeal lesions are most commonly seen on the anterior tonsillar pillars and may also arise on the soft palate, uvula, tonsils, pharyngeal wall, posterior buccal mucosa, and rarely, tongue
5–16 days	Abatement of all symptoms without sequelae		Complications such as myocarditis, encephalitis, acute flaccid paralysis, aseptic meningitis, pulmonary edema, or hemorrhage are rare

DIAGNOSIS

The diagnosis of most exanthemous enteroviral infections is based on clinical findings. Historically, documentation of enteroviral infections has relied on viral cultures of cerebrospinal fluid of tissue samples and subsequent neutralization with specific antisera. Both time consuming and costly, these studies are necessary for understanding the epidemiology and the study of particular viruses but have little immediate clinical benefit. These techniques are rarely used for ambulatory or recovering patients but are most often needed for those with complicated or more serious courses.

Recently, polymerase chain reaction (PCR) assays for enteroviral RNA detection in clinical material have been developed [50,51]. The Aplicor Enterovirus Test was recently reported to successfully detect enterovirus in cerebrospinal fluid. Although costly and sparsely available at present, this methodology holds great promise for the future and may become more widely applicable and available over time [3,52].

TREATMENT AND PROPHYLAXIS

Careful handwashing remains one of the most effective prophylactic measures available to prevent the spreading of these infections. Supportive treatment of symptoms (Table 19–10) and reassurance are the mainstay of therapy for most "healthy" patients with enteroviral disease.

Immunodeficient patients, especially neonates and patients with hypogammaglobulinemia, may be benefited by IVIG. This benefit is proposed to result from the presence of neutralizing antibody in the IVIG.

More recently an active broad-spectrum capsid inhibitor antipicornaviral agent with activity against enterovirus and rhinovirus has been developed. Named pleconaril, it is currently undergoing clinical evaluation for treatment of viral meningitis and viral respiratory infections. It is reported to

Table 19–9. Differential Diagnoses of Herpangina

Herpetic stomatitis: Ulcerations are usually more anterior in the oropharynx and persist longer. Fever is not a common feature with this condition

Aphthous stomatitis: These lesions are rarely associated with fever. Only one or a few lesions are usually present at a time

Hand-foot-and-mouth syndrome: Hand-foot-and-mouth syndrome with oral involvement only may frequently involve the tongue, gingiva, and buccal mucosa, whereas herpangina lesions are usually located on the soft palate, tonsillar pillars, and anterior fauces

Lymphonodular pharyngitis: Similar to herpangina, but does not result in mucosal ulcerations. The lesions associated with this illness consist of elevated white or yellow small papules on the pharynx, with an erythematous base

Table 19–10. Treatment of Enteroviral
Exanthematous Illnesses

Symptom	Treatment
General	Encourage fluids to prevent dehydration; limitation of physical activity, if needed
Fever and/or pain	Acetaminophen
Oral ulcerations	Antihistamine mouth rinses or topical application of viscous lidocaine
Nausea or vomiting	Trimethobenzamide HCI, promethazine suppositories
Diarrhea	Loperamide or diphenoxylate HCI with atropine sulfate
Dehydration	Intravenous fluids
Severe illness	Intravenous immunoglobulin; future antivirals, such as pleconaril, when available

have broad activity against 96% of the most commonly isolated serotoxic enteroviruses and an admirable safety profile thus far [52]. The development of this drug and perhaps others in its class gives rise to great hope for useful therapy especially for high-risk and seriously ill patients in the future [3,52].

CONCLUSION

Overall, enterovirus infections associated with cutaneous and mucosal manifestations have a benign clinical course with rare complications or serious sequelae. Given the vast spectrum of manifestations and overlap of symptoms commonly seen with this group of viruses, diagnosis of specific infections may sometimes present a challenge. Although no specific antiviral medications are yet available, the prognosis is good in the majority of these cases with symptomatic treatment alone. Fortunately, new antiviral agents are on the horizon for the treatment of those more seriously infected.

REFERENCES

1. JD Cherry. Enteroviruses: coxsackieviruses, echoviruses, and polioviruses. In: RD Feigen, JD Cherry, eds. Textbook of Pediatric Infectious Disease, 4th ed. Philadelphia: WB Saunders, 1998, pp. 1787–1839.
2. JL Melnick, VI Agol, HL Bachnach, F Brown, PD Cooper, W Fiers, S Gard, JH Gear, Y Ghendon, L Kasza, M LaPlaca, B Mandel, S McGregor, SB Mohanty, G Plummer, RR Rueckert, FL Schaffer, I Tagaya, DA Tyrrell, M Voroshilova, HA Wenner. Picornaviridae. Intervirology 4:303–316, 1974.
3. LI Yaresh, RW Steele. Diagnosis and prospective treatment of enteroviral infections in children. Clin Pediatr 39: 209–211, 2000.
4. DM Horstmann. The poliomyelitis story: a scientific hegira. Yale J Biol Med 58:79–90, 1985.
5. M Underwood. A Treatise on the Diseases of Children, 2nd ed. London: J Mathews, 1789.
6. J Badham. Paralysis in childhood: four remarkable cases of suddenly induced paralysis in the extremities, occurring in children, without any apparent cerebral or cerebro-spinal lesion. London Med Gazette 15:215–218, 1834.
7. K Landsteiner, E Popper. Übertragung der Poliomyelitis acuta auf Affen. Z Immun Forsch 2:377–390, 1909.
8. JR Enders, TH Weller, FC Robbins. Cultivation of the Lansing strain of poliomyelitis virus in cultures of various human embryonic tissues. Science 109:85–87, 1949.
9. G Dalldorf, GM Sickles. An unidentified, filterable agent isolated from the feces of children with paralysis. Science 108:61–62, 1948.
10. AJ Rhodes, AJ Beale. Aseptic meningitis: evidence for the etiologic role of coxsackie B "orphan" viruses. Ann N Y Acad Sci 67:212–222, 1957.
11. CR Robinson, FW Doane, AJ Rhodes. Report of an outbreak of febrile illness with pharyngeal lesions and exanthem, Toronto, Summer 1957—isolation of group A Coxsackie virus. Can Med Assoc J 79:615–621, 1958.
12. J Alsop, TH Flewett, JR Foster. "Hand, foot, and mouth disease" in Birmingham in 1959. BMJ 2:1708–1711, 1960.
13. JM Brown, JA Wright, WS Ogden. Hand, foot, and mouth disease [letter]. BMJ 1:58, 1964.
14. SR Meadow. Hand, foot, and mouth diseases. Arch Dis Child 40:560–564, 1965.
15. HB Richardson, A Leibovitz. "Hand, foot, and mouth disease" in children: an epidemic associated with Coxsackie virus A-16. J Pediatr 67:6–12, 1965.
16. GD Miller, JP Tindall. Hand, foot, and mouth disease. JAMA 203:827–830, 1968.
17. JP Tindall, GD Miller. Hand, foot, and mouth disease. Cutis 9:457–473, 1972.
18. SK Clarke, T Morley, RP Warin. Hand, foot, and mouth disease [letter]. BM J 1:58, 1964.
19. TH Flewett, RP Waren, SK Clarke. Hand, foot, and mouth disease associated with Coxsackie A5 virus. J Clin Pathol 16:53–55, 1963.
20. JD Cherry. Enteroviruses. In: JS Remington, JO Klein, eds. Infectious Diseases of the Fetus and Newborn Infant, 4th ed. Philadelphia: WB Saunders, 1995, pp. 404–446.
21. MJ Abzug, MI Keyserling, MI Lee, MJ Levin, HA Rotbart. Neonatal enterovirus infection: virology, serology, and effects of intravenous globulin. Clin Infect Dis 20: 1201–1206, 1995.
22. DA Baker, CA Phillips. Fatal hand-foot-and-mouth disease in an infant or adult caused by coxsackievirus A. JAMA 242:1065–1068, 1979.

23. JD Cherry. Enteroviruses: poliovirus (poliomyelitis), coxsackievirus, echoviruses, and enteroviruses. In: RD Feigen, JD Cherry, eds. Textbook of Pediatric Infectious Diseases, 2nd ed. Philadelphia: WB Saunders, 1987, pp 1729–1790.

24. MT Boyd, SW Jordan, LE Davis. Fatal pneumonitis from congenital echovirus type 6 infection. Pediatr Infect Dis 6: 1138–1139, 1987.

25. M Ho, ER Chin, KH Hsu, SJ Twu, KT Chen, SF Tsai, JR Wang, SR Shih. An epidemic of enterovirus 71 infection in Taiwan. Taiwan Enterovirus Epidemic Working Group. N Engl J Med 341:929–935, 1999.

26. CC Huang, CC Liu, YC Chang, CY Chen, ST Wang, TF Yeh. Neurologic complications in children with enterovirus 71 infections. N Engl J Med 341:936–942, 1999.

27. S Hurwitz. The exanthematous diseases of childhood. In: S Hurwitz, ed. Clinical Pediatric Dermatology; A Textbook of Skin Disorders of Childhood and Adolescence. Philadelphia: WB Saunders, 1981, pp. 258–276.

28. RH Meade 3rd, TW Chang. Zoster-like eruption due to Echovirus 6. Am J Dis Child 133:283–284, 1979.

29. TE Frothingham. Echovirus type 9 associated with three cases simulating meningococcemia. N Engl J Med 259: 484–485, 1958.

30. R Caputto, AB Ackerman, ED Sison-Torres. Hand-foot-and-mouth disease. In: Pediatric Dermatology and Dermatopathology, vol II. Philadelphia: Lea & Febiger, 1993, pp. 437–441.

31. AD Evans, E Waddington. Hand, foot, and mouth disease in south Wales, 1964. Br J Dermatol 79:309–317, 1967.

32. K Yamanishi, T Okuno, K Shiraki, M Takahashi, T Kondo, Y Asano, T Kurata. Identification of human herpesvirus-6 as a causal agent for exanthem subitum. Lancet 1: 1065–1067, 1988.

33. JD Cherry. Roseola infantum (exanthem subitum). In: RD Feigen, JD Cherry, eds. Textbook of Pediatric Infectious Disease, 3rd ed. Philadelphia: WB Saunders, 1992, pp. 1789–1792.

34. FA Neva, RF Feemster, IJ Gorbach. Clinical and epidemiological features of an unusual epidemic exanthem. JAMA 155:544–548, 1954.

35. FA Neva, JF Enders. Cytopathogenic agents isolated from patients during an unusual epidemic exanthem. J Immunol 72:307–314, 1954.

36. FA Neva. A second outbreak of the Boston exanthem disease in Pittsburgh during 1954. N Engl J Med 254:838–842, 1956.

37. CB Hall, JD Cherry, MH Hatch, DB Nelson, HS Winter. The return of Boston exanthem. Echovirus 16 infections in 1974. Am J Dis Child 131:323–326, 1977.

38. JD Cherry. Herpangina. In: RD Feigen, JD Cherry, eds. Textbook of Pediatric Infectious Diseases, 3rd ed. Philadelphia: WB Saunders, 1992, pp. 230–232.

39. JD Cherry, CL Jahn. Herpangina: the etiologic spectrum. Pediatrics 36:632–634, 1965.

40. TF Scott. Clinical syndromes associated with enterovirus and reovirus infection. Adv Virus Res 8:165–197, 1962.

41. S Kibrick. Current status of coxsackie and ECHO viruses in human disease. Prog Med Virol 6:27–70, 1964.

42. HA Wenner. The enteroviruses. Am J Clin Pathol 57: 751–761, 1972.

43. HA Wenner. Virus diseases associated with cutaneous eruptions. Prog Med Virol 16:269–336, 1973.

44. BB Breese Jr. Aphthous pharyngitis. Am J Dis Child 61: 669–674, 1941.

45. J Zahorsky. Herpetic sore throat. South Med J 13:871–872, 1920.

46. J Zahorsky. Herpangina (a specific infectious disease). Arch Pediatr 41:181–184, 1924.

47. RJ Huebner, RM Cole, EA Beeman, JA Bell, JH Peers. Herpangina. Etiological studies of a specific infectious disease. JAMA 145:628–633, 1951.

48. RH Parrott, S Ross, FG Burke, EC Rice. Herpangina. Clinical studies of a specific infectious disease. N Engl J Med 245:275–280, 1951.

49. ML Forman, JD Cherry. Enanthems associated with uncommon viral syndromes. Pediatrics 41:873–882, 1968.

50. HA Rotbart, MH Sawyer, S Fast, C Lewinski, N Murphy, EF Keyser, J Spadoro, SY Kao, M Loeffelholz. Diagnosis of enteroviral meningitis by using PCR with a colorimetric microwell detection assay. J Clin Microbiol 32:2590–2592, 1994.

51. MJ Abzug, M Loeffelholz, HA Rotbart. Diagnosis of neonatal enterovirus infection by polymerase reaction. J Pediatr 126:447–450, 1995.

52. DC Pevear, TM Tull, ME Seipel, JM Groarke. Activity of pleconaril against enteroviruses. Antimicrob Agents Chemother 43:2109–2115, 1999.

20

Flaviviridae

Michael R. Weir
Scott and White Clinic and Memorial Hospital, Temple, Texas, USA

Tracey E. Weir
Brackenridge Hospital, Austin, Texas, USA

The Flaviviridae family consists of almost 60 different viruses, several of which are pathogenic to humans. These viral infections are primarily mosquito- or tick-borne, and the clinical diseases associated with them range from asymptomatic infection to severe encephalitis or hemorrhagic fever. With the major morbidity and/or mortality that is associated with dengue fever, yellow fever, and Japanese encephalitis (JE), among others, this family of pathogenic viruses deserves a significant amount of medical interest (Fig. 20–1). West Nile virus, a member of the Flaviviridae family, will be discussed in Chapter 21. Hepatitis C viruses, also members of the Flaviviridae family, will be discussed in Chapter 23.

DENGUE FEVER

Definition

Dengue comes from the Swahili word *Ki-dinga,* also called breakbone fever, dandy fever, and dengue fever, and is the most common mosquito-borne viral illness worldwide [1]. It causes asymptomatic, mild (classic), severe, and fatal disease, that is, dengue hemorrhagic fever (DHF) and dengue shock syndrome (DSS). DHF is a leading cause of hospitalization and death among children in Southeast Asia [2].

Dengue viruses are single-stranded, enveloped RNA viruses. The four dengue serotypes are dengue-1 (DEN-1), dengue-2 (DEN-2), dengue-3 (DEN-3), and dengue-4 (DEN-4). All four serotypes can cause DHF, depending on the immune status and age of the host. DHF occurs predominantly under the of age 15 years.

The principal mosquito vector of dengue virus is *Aedes (Ae.) aegypti,* present in most tropical and subtropical countries. *Ae. polynesiensis* [3] and *Ae. scutellaris* are vectors in the South and Central Pacific. *Ae. albopictus,* recently introduced into the United States from Asia, is an excellent arbovirus vector.

History

In 1779, dengue-like epidemics were first described in Jakarta and Egypt, although these infections may have been caused in part by chikungunya virus [4]. Since that time, recognized outbreaks were reported in the Americas, Australia, southern Europe, North Africa, the Middle East, Asia, and islands in the Indian Ocean, South and Central Pacific Ocean, and the Caribbean [5]. For instance, the 1922 Galveston, Texas, epidemic was estimated to have 30,000 cases [6]. Although hemorrhagic manifestations were described in some of the previous infections, the 1953 to 1954 Manila outbreak documented the first DHF epidemic [7]. In 1905, Bancroft identified the *Ae. aegypti* mosquito as the vector for dengue virus [8]. DEN-1 and DEN-2 were isolated in 1944 by Sabin [9,10] and DEN-3 and DEN-4 in 1956 by Hammon and colleagues [7].

Taxonomy

Flaviviridae family
    Flavivirus genus
    Dengue fever
    Japanese encephalitis
    Omsk
    Kyasanur Forest disease
    St. Louis encephalitis
    Tick-borne encephalitis
    Yellow fever

GEOGRAPHICAL WORLDWIDE INCIDENCE

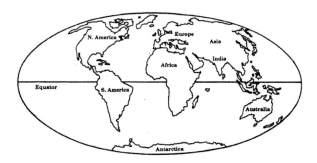

TRANSMISSION

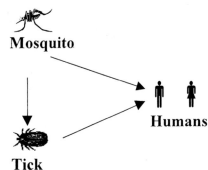

Figure 20–1. Incidence and transmission of Flaviviridae.

Incidence

An estimated 100 million cases of dengue occur worldwide each year [1]. Prior to the 1950s, major epidemics occurred at 10- to 40-year intervals. Because the virus and the mosquito vector relied on maritime transport, outbreaks occurred in port cities with spread to neighboring inland cities. Epidemics of mild, nonspecific illness rarely caused death. Urbanization and travel spread the viruses after World War II. Multiple simultaneously circulating viral serotypes led to more frequent epidemic dengue with DHF [11]. A Cuban epidemic of 10,000 cases of hemorrhagic disease resulted in 158 deaths.

During the 1980s, DHF appeared in the Americas and the Pacific, where formerly only classic dengue had been reported. Since 1984, dengue epidemics with associated cases of DHF have occurred in Aruba, Brazil, Columbia, El Salvador, French Guinea, Honduras, Mexico, Nicaragua, Puerto Rico, Santa Lucia, Surinam, and Venezuela (Fig. 20–2).

GEOGRAPHICAL INCIDENCE

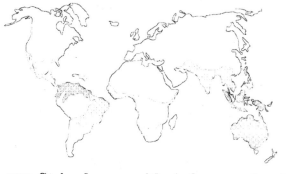

Striped areas with *Aedes aegypti* and dengue epidemics

TRANSMISSION

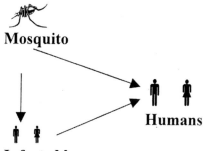

ZOONOTIC IMPLICATIONS

Mosquitoes are the only vector

Figure 20–2. Incidence and transmission of dengue fever.

Pathogenesis

Ae. aegypti and *Ae. albopictus* are excellent arboviral vectors. *Ae. aegypti* is a small, black mosquito with a silver-white, lyre-shaped figure on the upper thorax with white bands on the hind tarsi and abdomen. It is prevalent in the southern United States, whereas colder climates limit its northward spread. It thrives in wet and dry climates and bites during morning or late afternoon. This mosquito readily enters houses and prefers human blood meals, biting principally around the ankles or the back of the neck. It is usually present in peridomestic settings in dark areas, such as closets, bathrooms, behind curtains, and under beds, and is cosmotropical in distribution, breeding in manmade containers and flower vases around dwellings. Its flight range is limited (100 m).

The female *Ae. aegypti* acquires virus by feeding on viremic humans or animals, transmits virus during every feeding, and remains a vector for life. The vector can also transmit the virus immediately by a change of host when feeding is interrupted.

Ae. albopictus, the "Asian Tiger Mosquito," has a black body and silver-white markings, and a single, silver-white stripe down the center of the dorsum of the thorax. Called the "Tiger" because of the white markings on body and legs, this aggressive, daytime-biting mosquito is a competent vector for yellow fever and dengue viruses worldwide. The Asian Tiger is widely distributed in Asia, the Hawaiian Islands, and parts of the southeastern United States. It breeds in small, temporary pools of water such as tree holes or puddles in tires. The introduction of *Ae. albopictus* into the United States in 1986 is of special concern, because the species is an exceptionally efficient host for dengue viruses and is capable of transmitting both horizontally (human to human) and vertically (from infected female to her offspring), that is, transovarially. During the 1980s, Japan imported used tire casings from Asian countries for retreading in the United States. Breeding sites were found in those tires, and larvae of this and other mosquito species were found in shipments of tires from Japan and Hawaii. The patchy, discontinuous distribution of the mosquito in the United States suggested interstate transport in tire casings.

Individuals who have been immunologically sensitized to one dengue serotype develop non-neutralizing antibodies that may enhance the entry of different serotypes into mononuclear phagocytes, resulting in complement and kinin activation and release of mediators of vascular permeability [12]. Therefore, DHF occurs in persons with antibodies from a previous dengue infection, not during the initial dengue infection. DHF and DSS may also occur in infants with passive antibodies from dengue-immune mothers [13].

The virus infects mononuclear phagocytes that become the target of an immune elimination mechanism, triggering the production of mediators with the activation of complement and the clotting cascade and eventually DHF [12].

Clinical Manifestations

Dengue virus infection may range from asymptomatic disease to fatal shock. Dengue fever is defined by a spectrum of nonspecific or specific symptoms without hemorrhage. Hemorrhage defines DHF, whereas shock defines DSS.

The clinical pattern of classic dengue is outlined in Table 20–1. The fever typically lasts 3 to 7 days and may be biphasic, with a decline in temperature followed by resurgence of fever in 1 to 3 days. Physical examination also reveals relative bradycardia (despite fever), generalized lymphadenopathy, and hepatomegaly. Jaundice is rare. Some patients may complain of a metallic taste or unpleasant skin sensations. Cutaneous eruptions are present in 50% of patients hospitalized with dengue fever [14] (Figs. 20–3 to 20–9). The first rash seen with dengue fever is characterized by dilatation of capillary venules, transudation of fluid and protein into interstitial spaces, and diapedesis of red blood cells. The second rash results from an immunological response to dengue virus–infected phagocytes. Severe itching, particularly of the hands and feet, may accompany the eruption. The rash usually desquamates in recovery. Convalescence after classic dengue may last several weeks and be associated with neurological symptoms, such as weakness, depression, meningoencephalitis, and polyneuritis, as well as occasional cardiac symptoms, such as myocarditis, palpitations, extrasystole, and bradycardia.

DHF predominantly affects children and young adolescents. In patients who develop DHF, the viral prodrome is similar to that seen in classic dengue. The critical stage of DHF is usually the period from 24 hours before to 2 hours after the temperature falls to normal or below, when circulatory failure occurs. This period typically occurs on the fourth to fifth day of illness, and is characterized by sudden clinical deterioration. Signs of decreased peripheral perfusion and loss of intravascular volume, such as cool clammy skin, rapid pulse, and narrow pulse pressure, are followed by overt shock [15]. Activation of the complement and coagulation systems and increased vascular permeability occur at a time when the patient with classic dengue fever is in recovery. Whereas hemorrhagic manifestations are required for a diagnosis of DHF, the morbidity associated with the illness is primarily due to intravascular volume depletion. DHF patients demonstrate hypovolemia and thrombocytopenia, and those with DSS have hypotension or a narrow pulse pressure [12]. DSS is typically a progression of DHF, but some patients may develop shock early

Table 20–1. Clinical Manifestations of Dengue Fever

Time after exposure	Clinical manifestations	Laboratory analyses	Other notes
4–7 days	Sudden onset of high fever, chills, headache (commonly retro-orbital), eye pain, joint pain, and severe myalgia (termed *breakbone fever*). A transient, generalized erythematous flush-like rash of the face, neck, and chest, and sparing the palms and soles may be present during the first 24–48 hr of fever. Other symptoms include anorexia, nausea, vomiting, taste alteration, nonspecific respiratory symptoms, marked lassitude, cutaneous hyperesthesia, and conjunctival suffusion ↓	Serology, with acute demonstration of immunoglobulin M (IgM), or a fourfold rise in IgG titers between paired sera Viral isolation	Onset of dengue hemorrhagic fever (DHF) and dengue shock syndrome (DSS) is similar
7–12 days	In some patients, the fever and symptoms completely remit at this time and the patient recovers completely. In others, a second rash may appear as the fever subsides. This eruption can be scarlatiniform, maculopapular, petechial, or purpuric and typically begins on the trunk and spreads to the face and extremities. The rash typically desquamates after 1–3 days, leading to recovery. The hemorrhagic manifestations of DHF appear at this stage, often with petechiae and bleeding diathesis. Signs of circulatory insufficiency may appear in some patients, which may progress to DSS ↓		Patients with DHF will be restless and sweaty with cold extremities. Pleural effusion and abdominal ascites may be present. With treatment, this period lasts 24–48 hr in DHF. DSS will have these symptoms as well as rapid pulse, hypotension, generalized vasculitis, and disseminated intravascular coagulation (DIC)
11–17 days	Patients with dengue fever have complete recovery. Time to recovery varies in DHF and DSS, but is not as rapid as that in classic dengue fever		

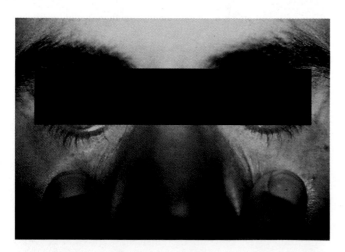

Figure 20–3. Conjunctival hemorrhages in dengue hemorrhagic fever (DHF). (Photograph courtesy of Anna Cardenas, M.D., Walter Reed Army Medical Center, Washington, D.C.)

in the course of disease [16]. The four characteristics of impending shock are intense and sustained abdominal pain, persistent vomiting, restlessness or lethargy, and a sudden change from fever to hypothermia along with sweating and prostration [17]. Once DSS has developed, the mortality rate increases dramatically in patients. Thus, admission to the hospital is critical if warning signs of shock arise.

Laboratory Findings

Plasma leak manifestations include a sudden rise in hematocrit, pleural effusion and ascites, hypoproteinemia, and reduced plasma volume. Disorders in hemostasis involve thrombocytopenia and coagulopathy as evidenced by a positive tourniquet test (Fig. 20–10). Laboratory tests confirm thrombocytopenia, disseminated intravascular coagulation (DIC), and hemoconcentration (20% or greater increase in hematocrit level). In DHF and DSS, a finding of

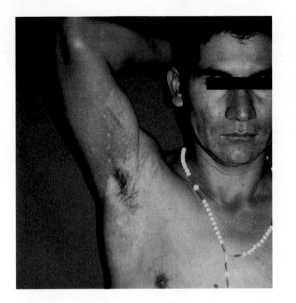

Figure 20–4. Scarlatiniform eruption of dengue fever. The "white islands within a sea of red" is a classic description for the cutaneous findings of dengue fever. (Photograph courtesy of Anna Cardenas, M.D., Walter Reed Army Medical Center, Washington, D.C.)

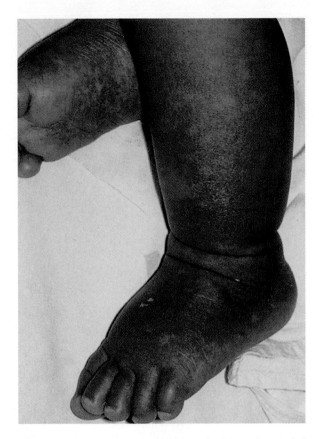

diagnostic and prognostic value is a decrease in platelet count preceding the rise in hematocrit level [18].

The mechanism of thrombocytopenia is direct action of the virus on megakaryocytes in the bone marrow. The marked destruction of cells in the marrow, followed by

Figure 20–6. Macules and petechiae of primary dengue infection in a Thai infant. (Photograph courtesy of Dr. Douglas Walsh, Armed Forces Institute Medical Sciences, Bangkok, Thailand.)

active cellular proliferation, may account for the bone pain (break-bone fever). Neutropenia and lymphopenia may also occur. The neutropenia is typically less than 5,000/ mm^3 and usually lasts at least a week [19]. A hematocrit level elevated by 20% or more is evidence of increased

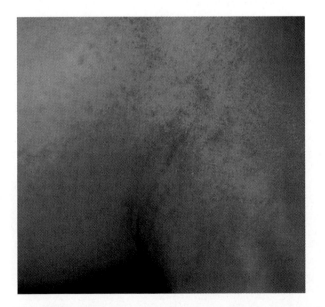

Figure 20–5. Neck petechiae in DHF. (Photograph courtesy of Dr. Siripen Kalayanarooj, Chiang Mai, Thailand.)

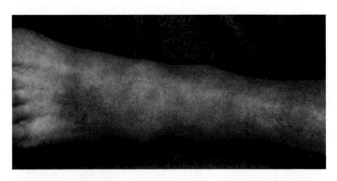

Figure 20–7. Macules and petechiae of DHF. (Photograph courtesy of Dr. James Brien, Scott and White Hospital, Temple, TX.)

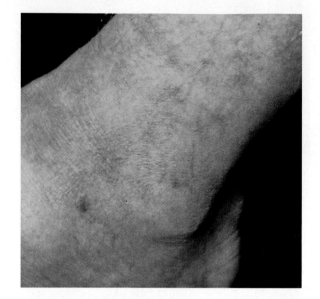

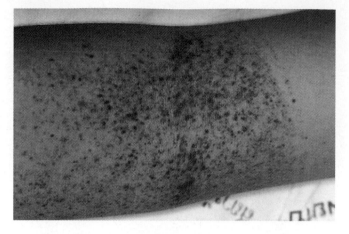

Figure 20–10. Strongly positive tourniquet test in DHF. (Courtesy of Dr. Siripen Kalayanarooj, Chiang Mai, Thailand.)

Figure 20–8. Macules and petechiae of DHF. (Photograph courtesy of Dr. J. Brien, Scott and White Hospital, Temple, TX.)

vascular permeability. Hyponatremia and reduced plasma osmolarity are commonly found in DHF and may result in convulsions. Metabolic acidosis, hypoproteinemia, hypoalbuminemia, and mildly elevated liver function tests may be present. Urinalysis is usually normal, but hematuria, albuminuria, and urinary casts may occur along with elevated blood urea nitrogen (BUN) and low complement (C′3). Chest radiographs often reveal pleural effusion, usually on the right (Fig. 20–11). The extent of pleural effusion is correlated with disease severity.

Pathology

On autopsy examination, patients with dengue fever and its associated syndromes have gross and microscopic hemorrhage in a variety of organs. Evidence of capillary leakage is also present with effusions in the serosal cavities, as well as perivascular edema microscopically demonstrable in soft tissues [20]. Biopsy specimens of skin affected by dengue show perivascular edema of the terminal capillaries, along with a monocytic infiltration [21]. Differential diagnoses are shown in Table 20–2. The diagnostic criteria for DHF and DSS have been defined by the World Health Organization (WHO) and this is shown in Table 20–3.

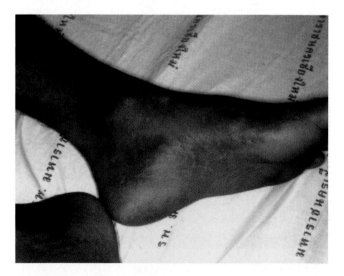

Figure 20–9. Macules and petechiae of DHF. (Courtesy of Dr. Siri Chiewchanvit, Chiang Mai, Thailand.)

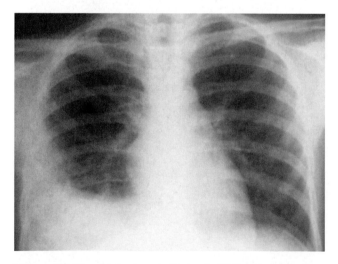

Figure 20–11. Right pleural effusion in DHF. (Courtesy of Dr. Chaicharn Phothirat, Chiang Mai, Thailand.)

Table 20–2. Differential Diagnoses of DHF

Roseola infantum (exanthem subitum): Caused by human herpesvirus 6, roseola displays fever for 3 days, then a fine maculopapular rash appears as the fever vanishes

Scarlet fever: Exudative pharyngitis, cervical adenitis, and a fine maculopapular rash with a coarse, sandpaper texture characteristic of scarlet fever. Group A beta hemolytic streptococcus on throat culture is diagnostic. This infection may lead to sepsis or necrotizing faciitis

Rocky Mountain spotted fever	} See Table 15–2
Influenza	
Typhoid fever	
Malaria	
Other hemorrhagic fevers:	
Rift Valley fever	
Chikungunya fever	
Kyasanur Forest disease (KFD)	
Omsk hemorrhagic fever (OHF)	See Table 17–2
Colorado tick fever	
Ebola and Marburg hemorrhagic fevers	
Crimean-Congo hemorrhagic fever	
Hantavirus hemorrhagic fever	
Lassa fever and the South American hemorrhagic fevers	
Meningococcemia	} See Table 18–5

Diagnosis

Virological diagnosis of dengue infection requires viral isolation during the first febrile phase (the first 5 days of illness), before the severest symptoms develop. Serological diagnosis employs paired sera for immunoglobulin G (IgG) antibody titer rise or the presence of antidengue IgM [15].

Table 20–3. World Health Organization Diagnostic Criteria for DHF and DSS

DHF
Fever
   Hemorrhagic manifestations, with either minor or major bleeding phenomena or a positive tourniquet test (except in shock cases)
   Thrombocytopenia, with platelet count $\leq 100,000/mm^3$
   Evidence of increased capillary permeability, such as hemoconcentration (hematocrit increased by $\geq 20\%$ or pleural effusions (on radiographs or other imaging study)

DSS
   All of the above, plus hypotension or narrow pulse pressure ≤ 20 mm Hg)

When a secondary dengue infection is likely, serological diagnosis depends on a fourfold or greater increase in antibody titer by the hemagglutination inhibition (HI), complement fixation (CF), enzyme-linked immunosorbent assay (ELISA), fluorescent antibody (FA), or neutralizing (N) antibody determinations. Most serological screening for dengue infection is done with IgM ELISA. IgM is detectable by the 5th day in 80% of patients, and by the 10th day in 99% [22]. This antibody persists in the serum for 2 to 3 months after acute infection. The pattern of HI response has been used to classify dengue infections as primary or secondary, based on the concept that initial or primary dengue infections tend to elicit lower HI titers than do secondary infections. Determination of IgM:IgG ratio by ELISA is an alternative method of distinguishing primary from secondary infections [23]. It is important to note that if a patient has evidence of prior dengue infection, such as presence of IgG in acute sera, there may be an increased risk for the development of DHF [22]. Diagnosis of dengue infection can also be confirmed by detection of viral RNA by reverse transcription polymerase chain reaction (PCR). Although this method is both sensitive and specific, it is available only in a research setting.

Treatment and Prevention

Treatment for dengue fever relies on palliative care (Table 20–4). Patients should be monitored for hemorrhage, signs of impending shock, or altered mental status. Isolation is unnecessary, but further mosquito contact should be avoided through the use of netting or screens.

Patients with significant hemorrhage, hemoconcentration, effusions, edema, hypoalbuminemia, or abnormal electrolyte levels should be hospitalized, possibly in an intensive care unit. The value of antiviral medications has not been established. Also, treatment with corticosteroids is not beneficial [24]. Prognosis depends on the early recognition and treatment of shock, which develops in one third of patients [18]. The case fatality rate in severe DHF with DSS is as high as 50% in patients not hospitalized, monitored, and treated promptly. However, less than 5% of patients succumb with good medical management. To avoid fluid overload, intravenous fluids should be interrupted when the hematocrit drops to approximately 40% and when urinary output and clinical signs of DHF and DSS improve (usually after 24 to 72 hours) [3]. Transfusion is contraindicated in cases with severe plasma loss in the absence of bleeding. A drop in the hematocrit level by 10%, with no clinical improvement despite adequate fluid administration, may indicate significant internal hemorrhage [18].

WHO criteria for discharging patients hospitalized with

Table 20–4. Treatment of Dengue Fever

Symptom	Treatment
General	Bed rest (during the febrile period) and adequate oral fluids. Intravenous fluid therapy is the mainstay of treatment for patients with DHF
Fever and pain	Antipyretics and analgesics. Aspirin and nonsteroidal anti-inflammatory drugs are contraindicated, because they may potentiate the hemorrhagic diathesis
Shock	Intravenous fluid therapy, with Ringer's lactate, normal saline, or a plasma expander. Close monitoring with frequent vital signs and central venous pressure measurements is recommended. The urinary output should be followed. Serial hematocrits should be performed to follow the patient's hemoconcentration. Acid-base and electrolyte disturbances should be corrected. Oxygen therapy should be given.
Hemorrhage	Fresh whole blood or red blood cell transfusions are required for uncontrollable, massive bleeding
DIC	Fresh frozen plasma or platelet transfusions. Heparin infusions may be helpful

dengue/DHF are: (1) absence of fever for 24 hours without the use of antipyretics; (2) a return of appetite; (3) visible improvement in clinical picture; (4) stable hematocrit 3 days after recovery from shock; (5) platelet count greater than 50,000/mm^3; and (6) no respiratory distress from pleural effusion/ascites [2].

A quadrivalent vaccine offers potential for future disease prevention [3]. The use of personal insect repellent, mosquito barriers, and protective clothing reduces mosquito contact. Elimination of breeding sites and the use of larvicides may help prevent outbreaks by reducing vector mosquito populations. Quarantine is not required for the patient with DHF, but suspected DHF patients should be in mosquito-proof rooms.

Conclusion

Millions of dengue cases occur worldwide each year. Dengue is usually a nonspecific febrile illness, but the clinical spectrum ranges from asymptomatic to severe hemorrhage and sudden fatal shock. The discovery that *Ae. albopictus* strains have adapted to temperate conditions could lead to increased mosquito-borne diseases. Control of dengue currently requires control of the principal vector mosquitoes. Vaccine development, the use of repellents and mosquito barriers, and habitat controls have the potential to limit dengue outbreaks. Lifesaving intervention and management of a patient with complications depend on a high level of suspicion and a complete history of travel. Once a person is infected, the key to survival is early diagnosis and appropriate treatment for life-threatening complications such as DHF and DSS.

JAPANESE ENCEPHALITIS

Definition

JE is an acute infection of the central nervous system (CNS). This flavivirus causes the greatest number of cases of childhood viral encephalitis in Asia with significant mortality and morbidity. The virus is a member of the St. Louis complex related to St. Louis, Murray Valley, West Nile, Ilheus, and Rocio encephalitis viruses. There are two immunotypes, the Nakayama strain and the JaGAr01 (Beijing-1) strain. There are also four geographically distinct genotypes: type I in Japan, China, Taiwan, Vietnam, Nepal, India, and Sri Lanka; type II in northern Thailand and Cambodia; type III in Indonesia, Malaysia, and southern Thailand; and type IV in eastern Indonesia. Types I and II occur in an epidemic pattern, and types III and IV occur as endemics [25].

History

As early as 1871, JE was recognized as a disease. In 1924, a severe epidemic occurred in Japan, with 6125 documented cases. However, it was not until 1935 when the etiological agent was serologically established as the prototypic (Nakayama) strain. The virus was isolated from *Culex tritaeniorhynchus* in 1938 [26]. Scherer and associates [27] showed that the host cycle involved pigs and birds, with transmission by *C. tritaeniorhynchus* to humans (Fig. 20–12).

Incidence

The disease occurs throughout Asia in the following countries: Japan, China, Cambodia, Indonesia, Malaysia, Korea, Philippines, India, Lao People's Democratic Republic, Myanmar, Thailand, Vietnam, and southeastern Russia [25,28] (Fig. 20–12). An estimated 1 in 300 JE infections presents

GEOGRAPHICAL INCIDENCE

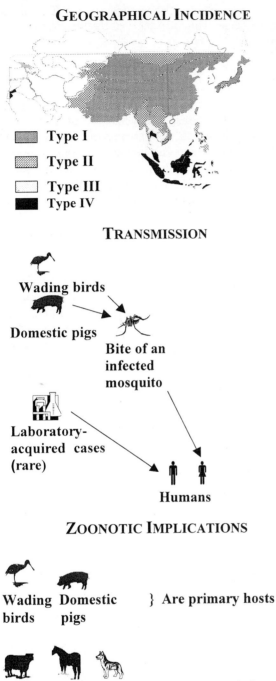

- Type I
- Type II
- Type III
- Type IV

TRANSMISSION

Wading birds

Domestic pigs

Bite of an infected mosquito

Laboratory-acquired cases (rare)

Humans

ZOONOTIC IMPLICATIONS

Wading birds Domestic pigs } Are primary hosts

Cattle Horses Dogs } Can become infected but do not have sufficiently long viremia

Figure 20–12. Incidence and transmission of Japanese encephalitis (JE).

as symptomatic illness [28,29]. The reported annual incidence of clinical infections in endemic regions is 50,000 cases, with 10,000 of these being fatal [28]. An increase in epidemics has been seen in India, Nepal, and northern Southeast Asia in the past 25 years. China and Taiwan have seen a decrease in epidemics, owing to vaccination programs, improved socioeconomics, and agricultural conditions [28].

The majority of people in endemic regions are infected by the age of 15 years, and children are most commonly clinically infected. In nonendemic regions, epidemics have a bimodal distribution affecting the elderly as well [25].

Temperate climates maintain transmission during the monsoon season of April or May through October, with incidence being highest in rural areas and in young males. Tropical areas have endemic disease with few epidemics.

Pathogenesis

The JE vector is the *Culex* mosquito, particularly *C. tritaeniorhynchus.* Other species involved in transmission occur geographically: *C. vishnui* in India; *C. gelidus* and *C. fuscocephus* in India, Malaysia, and Thailand; *C. annulus* in Taiwan; and *C. annulirostris* in Guam. The mosquito breeds in flooded rice fields and water pools. The vector rate of infection is 1 to 3% [28]. JE virus has also been isolated from *Aedes* and *Anopheles* mosquitoes. Humans and equines are not considered to be reservoirs but are "dead-end hosts" because of the short viremic period. Transmission of the virus has been shown to occur both vertically (transovarially) and sexually (venereally) in mosquitoes (Fig. 20–13). Other suggested methods of overwinter maintenance include alternate vectors (ticks or mites), vertebrate infections, reintroduction by migrating birds, and survival in hibernating mosquitoes [25].

After an infected mosquito feeds on a human, the virus

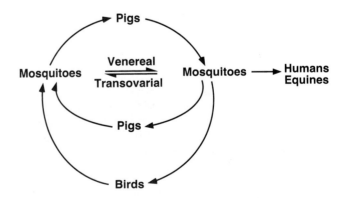

Figure 20–13. Japanese encephalitis. Relationship among pigs, birds, and mosquitoes that affects infection.

replicates in local and regional lymph nodes. This leads to viremia, with infection of various organs including the brain. Access to the CNS is thought to occur through invasion of the endothelial cells of the cerebral capillaries [30].

Clinical Manifestations

The spectrum of clinical disease with JE ranges from a febrile headache syndrome to aseptic meningitis or encephalitis. The manifestations of JE are outlined in Table 20–5. During the acute phase of illness, the most frequent complications include secondary infections (particularly pneumonia) and hyponatremia due to inappropriate ADH (antidiuretic hormone) secretion. The case-fatality rate with this disease is 5 to 40%, and may be as high as 70% in epidemics. Children and the elderly are at highest risk for mortality. A high percentage (45 to 70%) of survivors have permanent neurological and psychiatric sequelae, particularly in children younger than 10 years old [31]. These complications include seizure disorders, paralysis, mental retardation, and Parkinsonism.

There is evidence for latent and congenital human infections. A high rate of miscarriage occurs in women infected during the first and second trimester of pregnancy, but not in the third trimester [32]. Concurrent infection with JE and herpes simplex virus (HSV) suggests that JE invasion of the CNS occurs with disruption of the blood-brain barrier [33].

Pathology

CNS involvement acutely includes cerebral edema, congestion, and hemorrhage. Gray matter degeneration and necrosis, neuronophagia, perivascular inflammation, and microglial proliferation occur. Infection appears to be specific to neurons [34], with the thalamus and brainstem being most commonly involved [25]. Myocarditis, Kupffer cell involvement, pulmonary alveolar inflammation, and renal hemorrhages may be seen [25].

Laboratory Findings

A mild leukocytosis occurs. When urinary symptoms occur, the urinalysis reveals sterile pyuria, microscopic hematuria, and albuminuria. The cerebrospinal fluid (CSF) may have a high opening pressure, with leukocytes generally 10 to 500/mm^3 but rarely up to 1000/mm^3 (predominantly neutrophils initially followed by lymphocytes), and protein mildly elevated at 50 to 100 mg/dl. The electroencephalogram (EEG) shows decreased activity, generalized

Table 20–5. Clinical Manifestations of Japanese Encephalitis (JE)

Time after exposure	Clinical manifestations	Laboratory analyses	Other notes
4–14 days	Sudden onset of prodromal symptoms lasting 2–4 days, with headache, fever, chills, malaise, anorexia, nausea, and vomiting. Abdominal pain and diarrhea may be quite prominent in children. During this time, lethargy increases and behavioral changes may develop ↓	Serology, with demonstration of IgM or a fourfold rise in IgG Viral isolation (uncommon)	
7–18 days	The encephalitic phase consists of central nervous system (CNS) signs, with mental status changes (typically coma or stupor), pathological reflexes, lower motor neuron deficits, incoordination, rigidity, paresis, tremors, and cranial nerve palsies ↓		Convulsions frequently occur in children, but develop in less than 10% of adults. Meningismus occurs more frequently in adults. Death, when it occurs, typically comes on the 5th–9th day of clinical illness (days 9–23).
12–23 days	Fever begins to defervesce and neurological function slowly improves ↓		During recovery from coma and paralysis, common complications include pneumonia, bacteremia, stasis ulcers, and urinary tract infections. These may sometimes
22–33 days	Convalescent phase begins, with gradual improvement in neurological function over weeks, months, or sometimes years		be secondary causes of death.

slowing, and dysrhythmia. Brain computerized tomograms reveal abnormalities in the thalamus and basal ganglia. Magnetic resonance imaging (MRI) of survivors with sequelae generally shows abnormalities of the thalamus, globus pallidus, hippocampus, and substantia nigra [25].

Diagnosis

Serological testing with IgM-capture ELISA of the CSF or blood is specific within 4 to 7 days of disease onset [28]. Dot blot or immunoprecipitation IgM assays may also be used. A four fold rise in titer of paired sera with HI, CF, or N tests is diagnostic, although there may be a cross-reaction with other viruses [25]. Virus isolation from blood is uncommon, but may be successful if performed in the early stages of disease (during the first 6 to 7 days of symptoms); virus may be isolated from the CSF in some cases, and is generally associated with a poor prognosis [25] (Table 20–6).

Table 20–6. Differential Diagnoses of JE

Herpes simplex virus (HSV) encephalitis	
Enteroviral aseptic meningitis	
Bacterial meningitis	
Tuberculous meningitis	
Cerebral malaria	
Dengue virus with encephalopathy	
Intracranial hemorrhage/stroke	
Heat stroke	
Lead encephalopathy	See Table 18–2
Toxic encephalopathy	
Brain abscess	
Brain tumor	
Postinfectious encephalitis	
Metabolic encephalopathy	
Status epilepticus	
Acute confusional or basilar migraine	
Reye's syndrome	
Rocky Mountain spotted fever	
Other arboviral encephalitides:	
Eastern equine encephalitis	
Western equine encephalitis	
Venezuelan equine encephalitis	
West Nile fever	See Table 15–2
California encephalitis	
St. Louis encephalitis (SLE)	
Tick-borne encephalitis (TBE)	
Powassan encephalitis	
Rift Valley fever	
KFD	See Table 17–2
Colorado tick fever	

Table 20–7. Treatment of JE

Symptom	Treatment
Fever	Antipyretics
Increased intracranial pressure	Mannitol infusions, hyperventilation, elevation of head of bed
Convulsions	Anticonvulsant therapy
Altered mental status	Supportive care, with respiratory support as needed, control of fluid balance, and prevention of secondary infections
Extrapyramidal symptoms	Trihexphenidyl

Treatment and Prevention

There is no specific treatment for JE. Supportive care is essential, especially for hyperthermia, seizures, and acute neurological deterioration (Table 20–7). No specific antiviral agents are known to have efficacy against this disease. In addition, corticosteroid therapy was not shown to be beneficial [35]. Appropriate antibiotics and antiviral agents should be considered early in the course of disease until bacterial CNS disease or herpetic encephalitis can be excluded.

There are three types of JE vaccines in use. The first is a mouse brain–derived inactivated vaccine, the only one commercially available internationally. Because of a relatively high cost, large-scale immunization is less likely in poorer countries. Initial injections are given at an interval of 1 to 2 weeks, but the booster dosing intervals are poorly defined and have regional variation. A second vaccine is a cell culture–derived inactivated vaccine manufactured in China. It is inexpensive but is being replaced by a third vaccine, a cell culture–derived live attenuated vaccine. This vaccine is also manufactured in China and is inexpensive.

Side effects of immunization include local reactions in 20% of patients, and systemic effects in 20%, such as headache, fever, myalgia, and gastrointestinal symptoms. Acute encephalitis has been associated with immunization, and two fatal cases have occurred [28]. Hypersensitivity reactions may also develop, including urticaria, angioedema, respiratory distress, erythema nodosum, erythema multiforme, and rarely, anaphylaxis, with two reported fatalities [28,29]. The only contraindication to vaccination is hypersensitivity to previous vaccination. In endemic areas, JE immunization is recommended after the first birthday.

Vector control with pesticides, improvement of agricultural practices, and personal protective measures remain important methods of decreasing JE. Mosquito repellents and protective clothing are recommended during outdoor exposure in endemic areas as well as the use of bednets for sleep.

Conclusion

The frequency and severity of JE make it the most important arboviral infection. Vector control affects the frequency of disease, but vaccination constitutes the ultimate solution to human disease. Methods of interrupting the natural cycle of disease will be problematic.

KYASANUR FOREST DISEASE

Definition

Kyasanur Forest disease (KFD) is one of the tick-borne viruses that occurs in an endemic area of India. Other antigenically related flaviviruses include those that cause Omsk hemorrhagic fever (OHF) and Far Eastern tick-borne encephalitis (TBE). There is early fever and myalgia with occasional hemorrhagic symptoms. A later phase with encephalitis is seen. The maintenance of virus in the environment involves a tick-tick cycle and two tick-vertebrate cycles, with wild monkey epizootics and human disease (Fig. 20–14).

History

First isolated in 1957 in India from a monkey, thousands of human cases have since been reported. During the first documented epidemic in 1958, the virus was isolated from infected humans [36,37]. Further research showed that the human epidemic followed disease in monkeys [38]. Local villagers had already named this illness ''monkey disease'' because of the known association with dead monkeys. In 1968, Boshell and coworkers isolated the virus from ixodid ticks [39]. The disease had been limited to an area of 77 square miles of the Kyasanur Forest, which is in the state of Karnataka (formerly Mysore) in southern India. However, infection has been progressively spreading, as evidenced by more recent epidemics that encompassed larger areas of the region [40].

Incidence

Annual epidemics occur in India during the premonsoon season mid-November to mid-April. Between 400 and 500 proven cases occur annually, predominantly in persons with exposure to forested areas of the endemic region. Out-

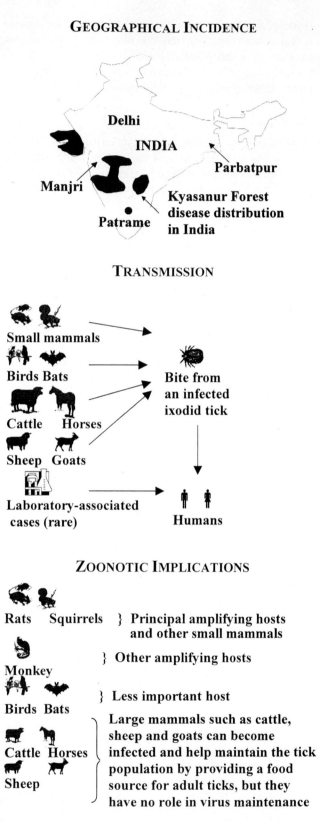

Figure 20–14. Incidence and transmission of Kyasanur Forest disease.

breaks often develop as a result of increased human activity in the endemic forest area, such as from deforestation, commercial lumbering, and cattle ranching. The density of the tick vector correlates with frequency of human disease.

Pathogenesis

A variety of ixodid tick species are implicated in the transmission of KFD virus. Nymphal *Haemaphysalis spinigera* is the vector for human disease in over 90% of cases (Fig. 20–14). Epizootics occur in wild monkeys, and monkey deaths provide a sentinel for viral activity.

In human infection, viremia is present between the 2nd and the 12th days of clinical illness. During this period, the virus is widely disseminated and can be demonstrated in various organs, such as heart, lung, kidneys, liver, spleen, and skeletal muscle. The virus can occasionally be isolated from the CSF in severe cases. The neurological symptoms that develop late in the course of disease are due to delayed infection of the CNS rather than a postinfectious phenomenon.

Clinical Manifestations

The clinical manifestations of KFD are outlined in Table 20–8.. Table 20–9 lists the most common signs and symptoms of KFD. During the acute phase of illness, lymphadenopathy (particularly axillary and cervical lymph nodes) and bronchiolar involvement are common, and bradycardia is expected [41]. No skin discoloration or cutaneous eruption are observed with most cases of this illness [41], although petechiae have been reported in patients. Death is unusual, but usually results from coma or pneumonia [42]. Most patients recover completely. Differential diagnoses are shown in Table 20–10.

Pathology

Degeneration of hepatic and renal parenchyma, hemorrhagic pneumonia, an increase in the hepatic and splenic reticuloendothelial tissues, and erythrophagocytosis characterize the pathology [43]. Skin lesions relate to mucus membrane and cutaneous hemorrhagic phenomenon, probably due to DIC.

Table 20–8.   Clinical Manifestations of KFD

Time after exposure	Clinical manifestations	Laboratory analyses	Other notes
3–8 days	Sudden onset of fever and severe headache. Back pain, myalgias, listlessness, and prostration follow. Cough, sore throat, diarrhea, or vomiting may or may not be present. Conjunctival and pharyngeal suffusion appear, with papulovesicular palatine lesions ↓	Viral isolation during the first 12 days of clinical disease Serology with acute IgM or fourfold rise in IgG	
7–15 days	In over half of patients, the illness progresses to involve hemorrhage, neurological signs indicative of brain involvement, or pulmonary findings of dyspnea and cyanosis ↓		Hemorrhagic signs include hematemesis, melena, hemoptysis, and gingival bleeding Hepatosplenomegaly or splenomegaly may occasionally develop
17–22 days	The acute phase of illness resolves, with recovery for some patients at this time. In 15% of cases, an afebrile period of 1–3 wk occurs, followed by recurrence of fever and prodromal symptoms along with hemorrhage and mild meningoencephalitis ↓		Signs of CNS involvement include severe headache, neck stiffness, coarse tremors, abnormal reflexes mental disturbance, and giddiness. Generalized convulsions indicate a poor prognosis. Death may sometimes occur in this second phase of illness
19–34 days	Recovery begins in the remaining patients. Convalescence in survivors is prolonged and may last up to 4 wk.		

Table 20–9. Signs and Symtoms of KFD

Signs	Percent of cases	Symptoms	Percent of cases
Fever	99	Fever	99
Hypotension	61	Weakness	90
Conjunctival congestion	54	Headache	69
Hemorrhage	54	Vomiting	55
Facial flushing	50	Hemorrhage	54
Hepatomegaly	50	Severe myalgia	53
Gingival hyperplasia	46	Altered sensorium	45
Neurological signs	45	Diarrhea	22
Pulmonary signs	45	Convulsions	22
Second phase of fever	14	Cough	13
Petechiae	13	Arthralgia	13
Stomatitis	11	Sore throat	6
Anemia	7		
Splenomegaly	3		

Table 20–10. Differential Diagnoses of KFD

TBE	
HSV encephalitis	
Bacterial meningitis	See Table 20–6
Influenza-like illnesses	
Leptospirosis	
Other hemorrhagic fevers:	
Dengue	See Table 18–2
Ebola and Marburg hemorrhagic	
fevers	
Other arboviral encephalitides:	
Eastern equine encephalitis	
Western equine encephalitis	
Venezuelan equine encephalitis	
West Nile fever	See Table 15–2
California encephalitis	
JE	
SLE	
Powassan encephalitis	
Other hemorrhagic fevers:	
Rift Valley fever	
OHF	
Colorado tick fever	
Crimean-Congo hemorrhagic fever	See Table 17–2
Hantavirus hemorrhagic fever	
Lassa fever and the South American	
hemorrhagic fevers	

Laboratory Findings

Leukopenia and elevated serum aspartate transaminase (AST) are frequently seen. The presence of atypical lymphocytes is a consistent feature [41]. Thrombocytopenia of varying degree and anemia may also be present. Albuminuria occurs in most cases during the acute febrile period, and granular casts may occasionally be observed. In the presence of hemorrhage, laboratory documentation of DIC is expected. Patients with meningeal signs later in the course of disease may have abnormalities in the CSF, with a mild mononuclear pleocytosis and an increase in protein.

Diagnosis

Viremia occurs on days 2 to 12, during the nonspecific phase, earlier than the more severe and more specific findings. The virus can be isolated during this acute phase of disease. Standard serological testing (IgM ELISA or paired sera for CF, HI, or N testing) can also give the diagnosis, but cross reaction from previous flavivirus infections may complicate results.

Treatment and Prophylaxis

The treatment for KFD is supportive, particularly for shock, DIC, and acute neurological deterioration (Table 20–11). No specific antiviral therapy is available. A formalin-inactivated vaccine made in chick embryo fibroblasts is effective and available to high-risk groups and during epidemics in India.

Table 20–11. Treatment of KFD

Symptom	Treatment
Fever and myalgias	Antipyretics and analgesics. Aspirin and nonsteroidal anti-inflammatory drugs should be avoided because thrombocytopenia and hemorrhage can occur with this infection.
Hypotension and shock	Intravenous fluids
Convulsions	Anticonvulsants
Hemorrhage	Blood transfusions for severe bleeding
DIC	Fresh frozen plasma or platelet transfusions, as needed

Conclusion

KFD virus is a significant problem in its endemic area. The variety of tick vectors, the tick–small animal perpetual cycle, the use of large animals by the tick population, and the tick-tick transmission are potent transmission strategies for the virus. The increase in worldwide travel and commerce has the potential to further disperse this already spreading virus.

OMSK HEMORRHAGIC FEVER

Definition

OHF is caused by a flavivirus of the TBE complex. It occurs in a remote part of northwestern Siberia. It is closely related virologically and clinically to KFD.

History

The OHF was first isolated during the 1945 to 1949 epidemic in western Siberia. Travel to this area was restricted, and experience was limited to Soviet physicians. An evolving Russian tourist industry may change the Western medical experience, although the disease frequency has diminished in recent years.

Incidence

Few cases are now seen in rural residents of the forest-steppe Omsk region of western Siberia. Almost 1500 cases were reported in the endemic area between 1945 and 1958 [44]. Seroprevalence rates in some areas of the endemic

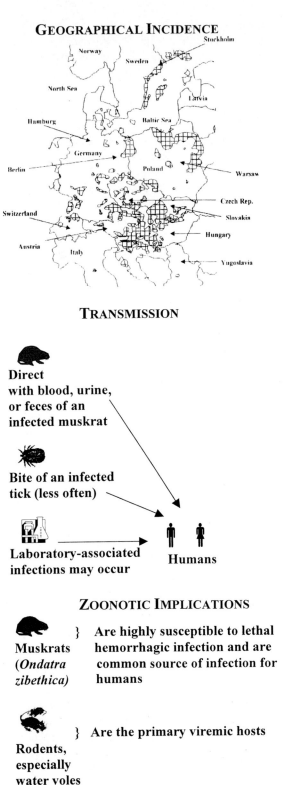

Figure 20–15. Incidence and transmission of Omsk hemorrhagic fever.

region are higher than 30%. There is a spring-summer-fall distribution coinciding with *Dermacentor pictus* activity and a more common winter disease distribution related to muskrat hunting. The mortality rate with this disease is less than 5%.

Pathogenesis

The vector for OHF is an ixodid tick, *D. pictus,* possibly *D. reticularus* or *D. marginatus* (Fig. 20–15). A maintenance cycle is thought to involve another tick, *Ixodes apronophorus* [25]. The host animals excrete virus in urine and feces, which plays a role in horizontal infection [45]. Infection of humans generally occurs in muskrat hunters with direct contact while skinning the animals. Family members of hunters account for 28% of infection [45], likely owing to exposure of the infected animal's tissue or fluids. Individuals prone to tick-borne disease are agricultural workers of the area and gatherers of mushrooms and wild berries. No direct human-human transmission of the virus has been documented [40].

Clinical Manifestations

Clinical illness with OHF closely resembles that of KFD, except that hemorrhagic manifestations have an earlier

onset. In addition, OHF more commonly has sequelae of psychomotor retardation, hearing loss, hair loss, and depression [25,45]. Table 20–12 outlines the clinical course of OHF. Table 20–13 lists differential diagnoses.

Pathology

Autopsies show scattered hemorrhages, endothelial damage, interstitial pneumonia, normal lymphoid tissues, and focal necrosis of brain tissue. The pathology is not specific to OHF and is common with other hemorrhagic fevers.

Laboratory Findings

Leukopenia, thrombocytopenia, and plasmacytosis are common. Transaminases may be elevated. Hemoconcentration, albuminuria, and hematuria are evident in the most severely ill.

Diagnosis

Diagnosis is made by isolation of the virus during the acute phase of illness or by serological testing with ELISA, N,

Table 20–12. Clinical Manifestations of OHF

Time after exposure	Clinical manifestations	Laboratory analyses	Other notes
3–7 days	Sudden onset of fever and chills, followed by headache, myalgias, and prostration. Conjunctivitis, cervical adenopathy, and gastrointestinal symptoms often occur ↓	Isolation of virus during acute disease Fourfold rise in IgG or seroconversion in paired sera	
10–17 days	Uncomplicated cases resolve after 7–10 days of symptoms. 30–50% of cases have remission of symptoms, with an afebrile period lasting 1–2 wk followed by recurrence of fever ↓		
17–31 days	Development of second phase of fever, with headache, vomiting meningismus, or other CNS symptoms. Hemorrhage may occur, with epistaxis, gastrointestinal bleeding, metrorrhagia, and hemorrhagic pneumonitis. A papulovesicular eruption may also occur on the soft palate. Hyperemia of the face, upper body, and mucous membranes often occurs ↓		The second febrile phase is typically more severe than the first Hemorrhage tends to be less severe than that of KFD. Bleeding predominately occurs from the nasal, enteric, lung, and uterine tissues Complications include bronchopneumonia, meningoencephalitis, shock, and rarely, death
Days to weeks	Most patients recover completely, but sequelae may occur (see text). Convalescence may be prolonged with weeks of persistent weakness		

Table 20–13. Differential Diagnoses of OHF

Enteroviral aseptic meningitis	} See Table 18–2
HSV encephalitis	
Leptospirosis	
Other hemorrhagic fevers:	
Dengue	See Table 18–5
Ebola and Marburg hemorrhagic	
fevers	
Congo-Crimean hemorrhagic fever	
Hantavirus hemorrhagic fever	
Lassa fever and the South	
American hemorrhagic fevers	
Chikungunya fever	See Table 17–2
Other encephalitides:	
Rift Valley fever	
KFD	
Colorado tick fever	
Eastern equine encephalitis	
Western equine encephalitis	
Venezuelan equine encephalitis	
West Nile fever	See Table 15–2
California encephalitis	
JE	
SLE	
Powassan encephalitis	
TBE	} See Table 20–6

HI, and CF antibodies [45,46]. Paired serum in infected individuals will show seroconversion or a fourfold rise in IgG titers.

Treatment and Prevention

Treatment remains supportive, aimed at controlling hemorrhage and replacing blood loss. Refer to Table 20–11 for the treatment of KFD. The mainstay of prevention is limiting exposure to the tick vector and careful handling of muskrat hosts in endemic areas, as well as laboratory safety measures. A vaccine was reported to be available in the former Soviet Union [46]. TBE vaccine may provide cross-protective immunity and is used in high-risk populations [25].

Conclusion

OHF occurred in an isolated part of the world, and there is limited medical experience with this disease. As the former Soviet Union is increasingly open to industry and travel, more cases may be seen. Alternately, the virus may eradi-

cate the non-native muskrat population, which would lead to eradication of the disease.

ST. LOUIS ENCEPHALITIS

Definition

St. Louis encephalitis (SLE) disease is defined by the CNS manifestations caused by the SLE virus. Wild birds and mosquitoes constitute the natural cycle of the virus, which has the potential to cause massive epidemics in the United States. The large epidemic in St. Louis and Kansas City in 1933 gave rise to the name.

History

The first recognized epidemic occurred in Paris, Illinois, in 1932, and was followed by the St. Louis epidemic. The etiological virus was isolated from the brain of a fatal case in 1933, and the disease was later proved to be mosquito-borne [47]. Outbreaks have subsequently occurred in the Pacific coast states, other Western states, Texas, Florida, and the Ohio-Mississippi river valley. During these various outbreaks, different vectors were identified for each region [25]. Figure 20–16 illustrates incidence, transmission, and zoonosis.

Incidence

In the United States, SLE is the most common pathogen transmitted by mosquitoes [48]. It occurs in epidemics in the Midwest and Southeast, but the virus can be found throughout the continental 48 states. A single outbreak of disease was reported in northern Mexico [49]. Although natural disasters such as floods and hurricanes increase the vector density, there is no evidence of increased transmission to humans [50]. Most cases of SLE occur in late summer or early autumn, during the period of increased mosquito activity.

Pathogenesis

Culex mosquitoes transmit SLE among wild birds. Humans are incidental dead-end hosts and are not involved in the transmission cycle [48]. The vectors involved in the Ohio-Mississippi basin and eastern Texas are *C. pipiens* and *C. quinquefasciatus*. *C. nigripalpus* is the vector in Florida, whereas the western states have *C. tarsalis* as the vector species. SLE may occur in conjunction with Western equine encephalitis (WEE), because *C. tarsalis* is the vector for WEE as well. Various amplification mechanisms

GEOGRAPHICAL INCIDENCE

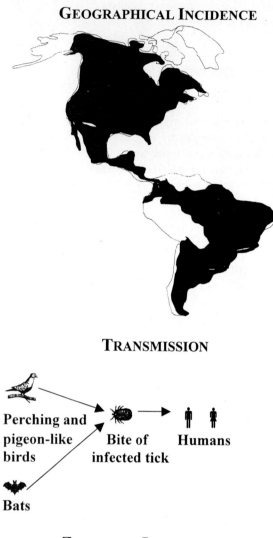

TRANSMISSION

Perching and
pigeon-like
birds

Bite of
infected tick

Humans

Bats

ZOONOTIC IMPLICATIONS

Perching
(passerine)
and pigeon-
like birds
(columbiforme)

} Act as amplifying hosts for
the virus

Bats

} May provide overwintering
maintenance

Figure 20–16. Incidence and transmission of St. Louis encephalitis.

exist, including vertical transmission and possibly over-winter maintenance by bats [25].

After inoculation from an infective mosquito, the virus replicates in local tissue and regional lymph nodes. This leads to viral dissemination in the blood, with replication at secondary sites, such as lymphoreticulum, endocrine, muscle, and other tissues. Access to the CNS most likely occurs through involvement of the vascular endothelial cells [30]. The most affected regions of the brain are the substantia nigra, thalamus, and hypothalamus, and the virus spreads from cell to cell [51].

Clinical Manifestations

Less than 1% of cases of SLE are clinically apparent [48]. Although approximately 75% of symptomatic cases involve encephalitis, other clinical illness may include aseptic meningitis or a febrile illness with associated headache [52]. The disease is typically more severe in the elderly. Significant comorbidity such as diabetes, hypertension, and alcoholism are also associated with increased severity and poor outcome.

The clinical course of SLE is outlined in Table 20–14. With CNS involvement, physical examination may reveal an altered level of consciousness, nystagmus, tremor, ataxia, meningeal signs, myoclonus, abnormal reflexes, and cranial nerve abnormalities (most commonly cranial nerve VII) [25]. Urinary frequency, urgency, and dysuria occur in 25% of cases [53]. Possible complications of illness include bacterial infection such as pneumonia, thrombophlebitis and pulmonary embolus, stroke, and gastrointestinal hemorrhage. Permanent neurological sequelae may occur, particularly psychomotor retardation in infants. Differential diagnoses are described in Table 20–15.

Pathology

During autopsy, histopathological examination of the brain reveals perivascular and parenchymal inflammation. Pathological changes are widely dispersed throughout the brain and spinal cord, but the midbrain, thalamus, brain stem, cerebral cortex, and cerebellum have more pronounced involvement.

Laboratory Findings

Leukocytosis, elevated transaminases, and increased BUN and creatinine phosphokinase may be seen. Urinalysis may show hematuria, proteinuria, and pyuria. In patients with CNS involvement, the CSF has pleocytosis and increased protein. Hyponatremia and hypo-osmolarity can be seen with the syndrome of inappropriate ADH. Radionuclide

Table 20–14. Clinical Manifestations of SLE

Time after exposure	Clinical manifestations	Laboratory analyses	Other notes
4–21 days	Insidious onset of malaise, myalgia, headache, fever, nausea, cough, and anorexia ↓	Serology, with IgM in the acute phase or fourfold rise in IgG titers in paired sera	In elderly patients, illness may first present with delirium, seizures, coma, or a focal neurological deficit
5–25 days	Progressive CNS involvement, with a stiff neck, disorientation, altered consciousness, vomiting, and photophobia. Clumsiness, tremor, dysarthria, or ataxia may occur. 10% of patients have seizures ↓	Viral isolation (rarely successful)	Seizure is a poor prognostic sign. The overall mortality rate is 7%, although up to 22% of cases in the elderly result in death.
Over several days	The fever resolves and neurological improvement begins in survivors. A prolonged convalescence is typical, often with emotional disturbance, forgetfulness, headache, tremor, unsteadiness, and dizziness. These symptoms may persist for months to years after acute illness, particularly in the elderly		Convalescent patients may also have gait or speech disturbances and sensorimotor impairment.

brain scans are normal, and computerized tomographic scans of the head are either normal or reveal mild, generalized edema. The EEG shows generalized diffuse slowing and delta waves.

Diagnosis

Diagnosis can be made with serology of paired sera, demonstrating a fourfold rise in antibody titers. HI may be used after the first week. Cross-reactions may occur with dengue. CF antibodies are present from the second week up to a year. Neutralization tests may be used in the first week and for years after infection. IgM-capture ELISA is useful from 3 to 5 days up to 60 days. IgM antibodies may persist in some individuals for up to a year, making this diagnostic modality less specific of acute infection. The demonstration of IgM in the CSF is a more accurate and rapid means of diagnosis. Other diagnostic tests are indirect fluorescent antibody test and use of monoclonal antibodies [48,50]. The virus has rarely been successfully isolated from blood or CSF in infected patients.

Treatment and Prevention

The treatment of SLE remains supportive (Table 20–16), and includes treatment of complications such as septice-

mia, bacterial pneumonia, pulmonary embolism, and gastrointestinal bleed. No vaccine is available against SLE. The mainstay of prevention continues to be personal protective measures such as limiting vector exposure times, proper clothing, and mosquito repellent. Public insecticide spraying is also an important factor, particularly during epidemics.

Conclusion

SLE continues to be a significant cause of viral encephalitis in the United States. During epidemic periods, this virus is the most common cause of viral encephalitis in this country. Lacking specific therapy and a vaccine, prevention rests on protective measures, vector control, and surveillance of sentinel avians.

TICK-BORNE ENCEPHALITIS

Definition

The TBE viruses consist of 14 antigenically related viruses, 8 of which cause human disease. The most common infections include Far Eastern TBE (Russian spring-summer encephalitis, RSSE) and Central European TBE (CEE). A

Table 20–15. Differential Diagnoses of SLE

HSV encephalitis
Enteroviral aseptic meningitis
Bacterial meningitis
Tuberculous meningitis
Cerebral malaria
Dengue virus with encephalopathy
Intracranial hemorrhage/stroke
Heat stroke
Lead encephalopathy
Toxic encephalopathy   } See Table 18–2
Brain abscess
Brain tumor
Postinfectious encephalitis
Metabolic encephalopathy
Status epilepticus
Acute confusional or basilar migraine
Reye's syndrome
Other arboviral encephalitides:
  Japanese encephalitis
  Eastern equine encephalitis
  Western equine encephalitis
  Venezuelan equine encephalitis
  West Nile fever   } See Table 15–2
  California encephalitis
  Powassan encephalitis
  Rocky Mountain spotted fever
  TBE   } See Table 20–6
  Rift Valley fever
  KFD   } See Table 17–2
  Colorado tick fever

unique feature of these viruses is the relative resistance to low pH, such as gastric secretions. This characteristic has favored the oral transmission of these viruses in infected milk, causing a condition previously known as biphasic milk fever. Figure 20–17 highlights the incidence, types of transmission, and zoonotic implications.

Table 20–16. Treatment of SLE

Symptom	Treatment
General	Maintenance of fluid and electrolyte balance
Fever and myalgia	Antipyretics and analgesics
Seizures	Anticonvulsants
SIADH (syndrome of inappropriate antidiuretic hormone)	Water restriction

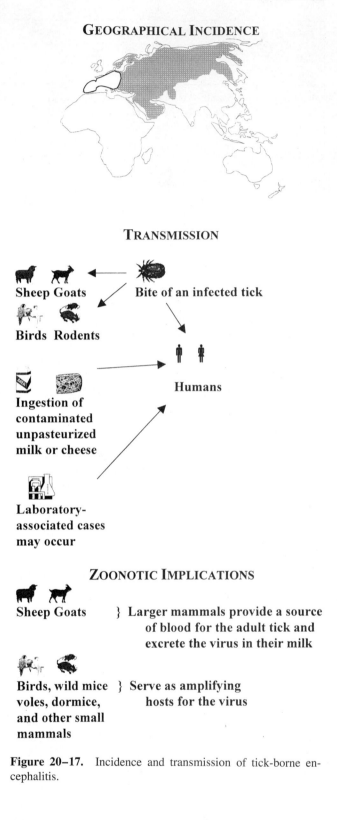

GEOGRAPHICAL INCIDENCE

TRANSMISSION

Sheep Goats

Birds Rodents

Bite of an infected tick

Humans

Ingestion of contaminated unpasteurized milk or cheese

Laboratory-associated cases may occur

ZOONOTIC IMPLICATIONS

Sheep Goats   } Larger mammals provide a source of blood for the adult tick and excrete the virus in their milk

Birds, wild mice voles, dormice, and other small mammals   } Serve as amplifying hosts for the virus

Figure 20–17. Incidence and transmission of tick-borne encephalitis.

History

RSSE was first described in 1934 in Siberia, with virus isolation and tick transmission shown in 1937 [54,55]. CEE was first seen in a 1948 epidemic in Czechoslovakia, an area of high disease frequency. Milk-borne transmission of these viruses was first recognized during an outbreak in 1951 to 1952. The disease has been recognized in all central and eastern European countries, with Scandinavia, Italy, Greece, Albania, and France reporting cases frequently.

Incidence

Two thousand cases a year are observed for these European outbreaks. Asymptomatic and mild infections are much more common, over 30 times as frequent as apparent clinical disease. In outbreaks, infection rates have ranged from 5 to 20 cases per 100,000 persons [56]. The tick-borne virus has two peaks of activity in Europe—May to June and September to October—corresponding to adult tick activity. A single late summer peak occurs in Scandinavia. The 10 days following excessively heavy rainfall is a period of greatest disease activity [57]. Outbreaks occur in families as a result of ingestion of unpasteurized milk or cheese, usually from goats [58]. Laboratory infections can occur if suitable precautions are not implemented [59]. RSSE has a case fatality rate of 20% with 30 to 60% having sequelae. The CEE case fatality rate is 1 to 5% with infrequent sequelae [60].

Pathogenesis

Ixodes ricinus and *Ix. persulcatus* are vectors in Europe and Russia, respectively. The virus cycles between ticks and vertebrates, usually small animals (Fig. 20–18). Transmission occurs transovarially to offspring and transtadially as the tick matures. Transmission of the virus from an infective tick to another unaffected tick has been shown. Viremia in the host is not involved, shown by transmission

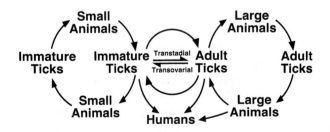

Figure 20–18. Tick-borne Arbovirus infections. Transmission occurs transovarially to offspring and transtadially as the tick matures.

in immune animals. The mechanism has to do with local virus replication at the feeding site and migration of infected cells to other feeding sites [61].

After inoculation, infection of the local dermal cells leads to seeding of the regional lymph nodes, where further replication takes place. This results in viral dissemination in the blood, with generalized infection, particularly involving the reticuloendothelial cells. A second period of viremia leads to neuroinvasion, which occurs through infection of mononuclear cells and vascular endothelial cells. Failure to establish an early CSF IgM response has been associated with clinical encephalitis [62]. Viral infection of macrophages alters the cellular ability to manufacture nitric oxide, important in antiviral defense [63].

Clinical Manifestations

The clinical course of TBE is outlined in Table 20–17. With CEE, children are less severely affected than adults. With neurological involvement, physical examination may reveal signs of meningeal irritation, photophobia, and irritability. Seizures, altered level of consciousness, and focal neurological signs are less frequent in children. Overall, there is a case fatality rate of 1 to 2%. Ten to 20% of individuals with severe disease develop long-term or permanent neuropsychiatric sequelae, although generally mild.

In contrast to the biphasic course of CEE, RSSE has a monophasic course, with fatalities after a week of symptoms. Children are more severely affected than adults. The variety of neurological disturbances that may occur with this disease include paralysis, paresis, sensory loss, and seizures. Neurological sequelae are frequent (30 to 60%) [60], particularly flaccid paralysis of the upper extremities consistent with the anterior horn cell pathology. The virus has a propensity to develop persistent infection in immune-impaired animals and by implication in humans. The Central European disease has lower mortality and neurological sequelae. Differential diagnoses are shown in Table 20–18.

Laboratory Findings

Thrombocytopenia, leukopenia, and occasional abnormal liver function define the hematological and chemistry abnormalities [64]. The CSF pleocytosis is initially neutrophilic, but becomes lymphocytic [65].

Pathology

Gross CNS changes include edema and petechiae. Histologically, there is perivascular and meningeal inflammation, neuronal necrosis and neuronophagia, and glial nod-

Table 20–17. Clinical Manifestations of TBE

Time after exposure	Clinical manifestations	Laboratory analyses	Other notes
3–7 days	Onset of fever, headache, myalgia, and malaise, mimicking influenza. ↓	Serology, with acute IgM or fourfold rise in IgG titers in paired sera	Central European tick-borne encephalitis (CEE) is milder than Russian spring-summer encephalitis (RSSE) and usually has a biphasic course. The onset of RSSE illness is normally gradual, rather than acute
10–14 days	Symptoms remit for 1 wk, other than fatigue. Most patients have no further symptoms and recover completely ↓	Alternatively, antibodies can be detected in the cerebrospinal fluid	
17–21 days	In some patients (up to 33%) a second phase abruptly begins, with high fever, headache, and emesis. CNS involvement develops in this phase, with aseptic meningitis, myelitis, encephalitis, or radiculitis ↓	Viral isolation is possible, but is less successful	RSSE has a longer prodromal phase, with fever, headache, anorexia, nausea, vomiting, and photophobia, but it has a shorter course overall. These symptoms are followed by nuchal rigidity, visual disturbances, neurological dysfunction, or sensorial changes.
20–25 days	In uncomplicated cases, the fever remits and convalescence begins. Most patients recover completely. In patients with encephalitis, the fever may persist for up to 1 wk		

ule formation. These pathological changes predominantly involve the anterior horn cells, but also affect the cerebral and cerebellar cortices, basal ganglia, and brain stem [66].

Diagnosis

Diagnosis is most commonly made by serology, especially with demonstration of IgM antibodies by ELISA [67,68]. However, with sensitive methods, IgM may be detected for up to 9 to 10 months after acute disease [69]. A fourfold rise in IgG titers between paired sera can also make the diagnosis. Antibodies to IgG or IgM can be detected in the CSF by ELISA [70]. Virus can be isolated from blood early in the disease or from brain in fatal cases. This method uses infant mice, embryonated eggs, or chick embryo cell cultures, but is usually unrewarding, being positive in only 10% of patients [25].

Treatment and Prophylaxis

Treatment is symptomatic and supportive (Table 20–19). No specific antiviral therapy is currently available. Passive protection with specific TBE globulin is preventive if given within 96 hours of tick exposure, but is not therapeutic. This treatment could have detrimental effects if administered to a patient with current disease [71,72]. A vaccine is used for persons with high risk of exposure, such as forest workers, military, and laboratory workers. Repellents and protective clothing are recommended, but are of little utility for those with constant or repeated exposure. Avoiding habitat and unpasteurized milk is beneficial.

Related Viruses

Louping ill is a disease of sheep in Scotland, England, Ireland, and Wales. It occurs infrequently in humans, usually in laboratory workers or in abattoir workers, butchers, and veterinarians directly exposed to sick animals. The disease in humans is biphasic with fever lasting 2 to 10 days, then remission for 5 days followed by fever and meningoencephalitis for 4 to 10 days. Abortive influenza-like disease occurs, as does asymptomatic disease [73,74]. *Ix. ricinus* is the agent for humans, sheep, and grouse. A killed vaccine for Louping ill has been used. TBE vaccine may provide protection due to cross-reaction of TBE antibody with the Louping ill virus. A similar virus has been recovered in Norway from sheep [75]. A distinct virus causes Turkish sheep encephalitis [76].

Rocio encephalitis appeared in epidemics in 1975 to 1976 in Sao Paulo State, Brazil, and then vanished. It caused a disease similar to SLE, although it is more closely related to JE antigenically. The specific vector was probably a mosquito. Wild birds may have completed the natural cycle.

Powassan virus encephalitis occurs in Russia, Canada,

Table 20–18. Differential Diagnoses of TBE

HSV encephalitis	
Enteroviral aseptic meningitis	
Bacterial meningitis	
Tuberculous meningitis	
Cerebral malaria	
Dengue virus with encephalopathy	
Intracranial hemorrhage/stroke	
Heat stroke	
Lead encephalopathy	
Toxic encephalopathy	See Table 18–2
Brain abscess	
Brain tumor	
Postinfectious encephalitis	
Metabolic encephalopathy	
Status epilepticus	
Acute confusional or basilar migraine	
Reye's syndrome	
Rocky Mountain spotted fever	
Other arboviral encephalitides:	
Japanese encephalitis	
Eastern equine encephalitis	
Western equine encephalitis	
Venezuelan equine encephalitis	
West Nile fever	
California encephalitis	See Table 15–2
SLE	
Powassan encephalitis	
Rift Valley fever	
KFD	

and the United States. Small mammals and Ixodid ticks appear to be the natural cycle. Virus has also been isolated from ticks and mosquitoes, but mosquito transmission is unproved. Cases have been more common and more severe in the young, usually boys, probably due to outdoor activi-

Table 20–19. Treatment of TBE

Symptom	Treatment
General	Bed rest
Fever and myalgias	Antipyretics and analgesics. Acetaminophen is preferred, owing to the thrombocytopenia associated with this disease
Convulsions	Anticonvulsants. Chronic anticonvulsive therapy is rarely indicated
Increased intracranial pressure	Hyperventilation, elevation of head of bed, and mannitol infusions, if needed

ties. Disease is severe, and sequelae are common [25]. The virus is more widely distributed than reported cases, a situation suggesting that many cases are mild and unrecognized. The increasing distribution of *Ix. dammini* portends greater disease frequency in the future. These two factors predict more recognized clinical disease in the northern United States and Canada in the future.

Modoc is a virus isolated from the white-footed deer mouse in California, Oregon, Montana, and Ontario. A single proven case of human disease presented as aseptic meningitis [25].

Negishi was isolated from two fatal cases and a febrile laboratory infection. Human cases occur in China, but the frequency is unknown. The agent is a member of the TBE virus complex but is similar to the JE agent [25].

Conclusion

TBE viruses constitute a group of several agents that cause human disease. Tick-bite history is incomplete, usually only in half of the cases. Transmission occurs between infected and noninfected ticks feeding on the same nonviremic animal. Personal protection from tick exposure, particularly after heavy rainfall periods, is recommended. Laboratory workers handling the virus and persons in contact with sick animals are at substantial risk and are vaccine candidates.

YELLOW FEVER

Definition

The yellow fever virus is the prototypic virus of the family Flaviviridae. The name for this virus resulted from the jaundice that occurs in severe cases. This mosquito-borne hemorrhagic fever that causes severe hepatic injury was one of the great scourges of the world. The clinical course of this infection involves two distinct phases that are separated by a transient remission. The first phase has viremia, and the second involves multiorgan dysfunction and hemorrhage of varying degree. In spite of an effective vaccine, yellow fever remains a major public health problem in Africa and the Americas. See Figure 20–19 for additional details.

History

Yellow fever was initially recognized in the Yucatan in 1648. Although this illness was first recognized in the New World, yellow fever probably originated in Africa and was spread to the Americas through the slave trade. The tropical areas of the Americas experienced large outbreaks from

GEOGRAPHICAL INCIDENCE

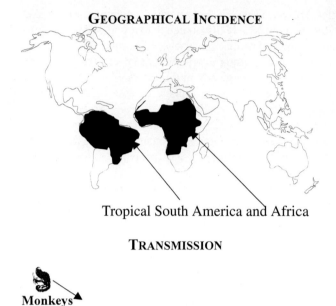

Tropical South America and Africa

TRANSMISSION

Monkeys

Bite of an
infected mosquito

Humans

ZOONOTIC IMPLICATIONS

} Cercopithecid and celobid monkeys of Africa
and howler, spider, owl, capuchin, and
wooly monkeys of tropical South America
are primary vertebrate hosts

Figure 20–19. Incidence and transmission of yellow fever.

the 17th to the 20th centuries. Nott first suggested that mosquitoes were the vector. Walter Reed demonstrated the agent and transmission by the *Ae. aegypti* mosquito in 1900. Soper initially proposed the concept of jungle yellow fever, and later it was shown that this cycle involved wild monkeys and sylvanic mosquito species [77]. The virus was isolated in 1927 by Mahaffy and Bauer [78].

Incidence

Yellow fever is a serious public health concern in tropical South America and sub-Saharan Africa. WHO estimates 200,000 cases annually with 30,000 deaths, although significant underreporting and misidentification occur. Prior

to the 1900s, there were also outbreaks in Europe, the Caribbean, and Central and North America. Yellow fever has never been reported in Asia, although WHO considers the area to be at risk, because the appropriate vectors and primates exist there. Nine South American countries have endemic yellow fever, with Bolivia, Brazil, Ecuador, Columbia, and Peru considered the highest risk [79]. Incidence in South America occurs via sylvanic transmission, primarily in young adult males from January to March due to peak rain and humidity during forest-clearing activities. Incidence in Africa occurs during the late rainy season, with background immunity the primary factor in determining age distribution. African countries in which yellow fever is endemic include Angola, Benin, Cameroon, Congo, Gabon, Gambia, Ghana, Guinea, Liberia, Nigeria, Sierra Leone, and Sudan [25].

Pathogenesis

There are four topotypes (geographic genetic types): two in Africa (one occurring in the eastern countries and the other occurring in the western countries), and two in South America (only one of which has been identified as causing outbreaks) [79,80]. The virus primarily affects humans and primates. Transmission can be horizontal by the biting mosquito as the vector between one animal and another, or vertically (transovarial). The mosquito vectors include the *Aedes* species or, in South America, *Haemagogus* species. There are three cycles of yellow fever: sylvatic, urban, and intermediate. In sylvatic yellow fever, an infected monkey is bitten by a wild mosquito, which then is able to transmit the virus to uninfected monkeys. Sporadic human cases occur when infective mosquitoes enjoy a human blood meal from an itinerant worker or traveler. This occurs primarily in tropical rainforests. Urban yellow fever is transmitted directly from human to human via an infective domestic mosquito. Details of transmission are shown in Figure 20–20. There is no monkey involvement, and large epidemics occur. Intermediate yellow fever involves trans-

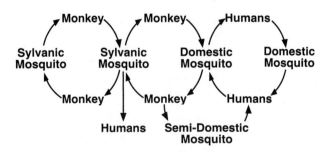

Figure 20–20. Yellow fever transmission.

mission from a semidomestic mosquito to both monkeys and humans. This mode occurs in the "zone of emergence" in the African savannah, which borders equatorial forests and has high concentrations of vector and monkey [81]. Intermediate yellow fever results in small-scale epidemics.

After inoculation, the virus replicates in regional lymph nodes, followed by dissemination through the bloodstream to other tissues, such as bone marrow, myocardium, liver, and spleen. In the liver, the virus infects Kupffer cells and then certain hepatocytes, leading to coagulative necrosis of these cells. The bleeding diathesis that occurs with yellow fever is a result of depletion of hepatic clotting factors, platelet dysfunction, and intravascular coagulation.

Clinical Manifestations

The spectrum of disease with yellow fever ranges from a nonspecific febrile illness to a fulminating, sometimes fatal illness. The clinical course of yellow fever is outlined in Table 20–20. The characteristic course of disease progresses through three phases, known as the periods of infection, remission, and intoxication. Patients with yellow fever infection may demonstrate the Faget sign, which is a paradoxically slow pulse with high fever, a common feature of arboviral disease. The most significant dermatological manifestations other than icterus are the petechiae and ecchymosis associated with the bleeding diathesis. This is likely due not only to decreased synthesis of vitamin K dependent factors but also to increased vascular permeability, altered platelet function, and ultimately, disseminated intravascular coagulopathy. The eyes may become jaundiced (Fig. 20–21).

During the phase of intoxication, renal manifestations may include albuminuria and oliguria or frank renal failure and anuria. CNS involvement can be seen as delerium, seizures, and coma. The jaundice associated with yellow fever may not be significant and may be undetectable until after death. Signs that often precede death include worsening jaundice, hemorrhage, hypotension, oliguria, azotemia, and rising pulse. Poor prognostic indicators include hypothermia, intractable hiccups, agitation, delerium, hypogly-

Table 20–20. Clinical Manifestations of Yellow Fever

Time after exposure	Clinical manifestations	Laboratory analyses	Other notes
3–6 days	Abrupt onset of fever, chills, headache, significant lumbosacral pain, myalgia, anorexia, nausea, vomiting, and possibly, mild epistaxis or gingival bleeding. This "period of infection" typically lasts 3 days ↓	Serology, with acute IgM or fourfold rise in IgG titers	During this phase, the patient has a high viral titer and is infective to the mosquito
6–9 days	The "period of remission" begins, with defervescence. Most patients begin to recover without further symptoms ↓	Viral isolation during the acute phase of illness	
7–10 days	In severe cases, the disease progresses. The "period of intoxication" consists of a recurrence of fever and other symptoms, which progress to worsened vomiting, epigastric pain, prostration, altered consciousness, and jaundice. Hemorrhage occurs from multiple sites, with coffee-ground emesis ("vomito negro"), melena, petechiae, ecchymosis, metrorrhagia, oozing from mucous membranes, and DIC. Renal and CNS involvement may occur ↓		During this period, viremia is absent and antibodies are present. Dehydration results from vomiting and increased insensible losses. Death occurs in 20–50% of cases, typically 7–10 days after disease onset
14–28 days	Survivors begin to recover, typically without sequelae. Convalescence involves significant weakness for 1–2 wk		

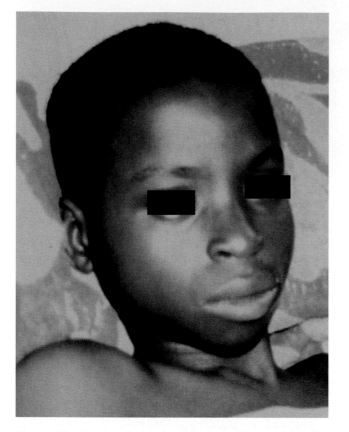

Figure 20–21. Jaundice and scleral icterus in a patient with yellow fever. (Reprinted from Samlaska CP. Viral Hemorrhagic Fevers. In: James WD, ed., Military Dermatology. In: Textbook of Military Medicine. Washington, D.C. Department of the Army, Office of the Surgeon General. Borden Institute, 1997, vol. 201, pp. 197–212.) (Courtesy of Thomas P. Monath, M.D., formerly Walter Reed Army Institute of Research, Washington, D.C.)

Table 20–21. Differential Diagnoses of Yellow Fever

Q fever: Is a self-limited febrile illness with pneumonitis and granulomatous hepatitis, headache and myalgia. Leukopenia and thrombocytopenia may occur. Chronic endocarditis with negative blood cultures occurs. Diagnosis is serological

Viral hepatitis: A prodrome of malaise is followed by hepatic tenderness, possibly jaundice and markedly elevated transaminases. Specific antigen or antibody identifies the actual viral etiology. Risk factors may be identified, e.g., travel, intravenous drug use, sexual, household, or daycare contact with known hepatitis or high-risk patients. Anicteric disease occurs. Coagulopathy, cutaneous or gastrointestinal bleeding, and progression to hepatic failure are uncommon

Drug-induced hepatitis: A variety of natural products, herbal treatments, and medications results in hepatic injury. Fever, rash, and arthralgia are seen clinically, with hepatic enzyme elevation and chemical and clinical evidence of hepatic dysfunction in the most severe injuries

West Nile fever } See Table 15–2

Malaria
Typhoid } See Table 17–2

Murine typhus
Scrub typhus
Leptospirosis
Other hemorrhagic fevers: } See Table 18–5
  Ebola and Marburg hemorrhagic fevers

Dengue
Rift Valley fever
KFD } See Table 17–2
OHF

cemia, stupor, and coma. Rarely, late death during convalescence occurs owing to cardiac or renal involvement. Table 20–21 lists possible differential diagnoses.

Laboratory

Findings are nonspecific and include leukopenia, elevated bilirubin and transaminases, albuminuria, thrombocytopenia, and prolonged prothrombin and bleeding time. Transaminases remain elevated for at least 2 months. An electrocardiogram may show nonspecific ST changes.

Pathology

Numerous changes occur in the liver. Initially, there is swelling of the hepatocytes, followed by coagulation necrosis. This mainly occurs in the midzone of the lobule and spares the cells bordering the central vein. Eosinophilic degeneration of hepatocytes produces Councilman bodies. When these degenerate, as occurs with delayed death, they are known as Villela bodies. Torres bodies are hepatocytes with intranuclear eosinophilic granular inclusions. Fatty changes occur, and there is minimal inflammatory response. In recovered cases, there is complete healing. Renal manifestations include acute tubular necrosis and fatty changes. Glomerular changes are insignificant. The glomerular basement membrane undergoes Schiff-positive transformation, possibly causing altered permeability and albuminuria. Myocardial fibers degenerate with fatty infiltration and edema. The CNS can be affected by edema, and petechial hemorrhage can occur in the brain. The reticuloendothelial system may show depletion of lymphocytic elements in the spleen and lymph nodes, as well as accumulation of monocytes and histiocytic cells in the spleen [80].

Diagnosis

Isolation of the virus is usually best during the first 4 days of disease, but serum up to 14 days after disease onset and from the liver at death can also be used. Antibodies can be detected by HI, CF, and N tests, indirect immunofluorescence, ELISA, and RIA. Clinical suspicion must be high in patients from endemic or epidemic areas or with recent travel history. Specific IgM or a rise in antibody titer in paired serum samples is diagnostic. Serological cross-reaction does occur with other flaviviruses [82].

Treatment and Prevention

The mainstay of treatment continues to be supportive care (Table 20–22). Antiviral therapies are not effective against this virus, and no specific therapy is available.

The most important factor for prevention is immunization. This is recommended 7 to 10 days prior to travel to endemic areas. Seroconversion occurs in 95% of recipients within 1 week. Although the vaccine is recommended every 10 years, immunity may be lifelong. Serious side effects from the vaccine are rare. The vaccine is not recommended for children under 6 months of age, pregnant women (except during an emergency vaccination campaign), persons with allergy to egg, and persons with immunodeficiency or taking immunosuppressive medications [79].

The Pan American Health Organization had vector control programs in the 1950s and 1960s that virtually eliminated *Ae. aegypti* in most countries. However, the programs were not continued, and reinfestation has occurred in all Latin American countries except Chile and Uruguay [83]. Mosquito control programs against sylvanic infections are not cost-effective. For the urban cycle, elimination of mosquito breeding sites, treatment of potable water, and organophosphate spraying are beneficial but must be continuously supported. The United States has *Ae. aegypti* vector present in the southeastern region, and is therefore a potential area of epidemic in the future.

Conclusion

Vigilant surveillance is necessary for early recognition of yellow fever, with control of epidemics through emergency vaccination campaigns. Urban areas where yellow fever has been eradicated, such as the southeastern United States, may face potential future outbreaks owing to lapsing vaccine use in current endemic areas and inattention to vector control.

Table 20–22. Treatment of Yellow Fever

Symptom	Treatment
General	Bed rest, maintenance of fluid and electrolyte balance, and close monitoring of vital organ function. Supplemental oxygen may be helpful in some cases
Fever	Analgesics. Aspirin and nonsteroidal anti-inflammatory agents that impair platelet function should be avoided because of the associated hemorrhage and thrombocytopenia
Dehydration	Oral fluid replacement, or if necessary, intravenous fluid infusions
Hemorrhage	Transfusion of fresh whole blood or packed red blood cells is useful for severe bleeding
DIC	Transfusion of fresh frozen plasma is indicated. Heparin therapy is controversial, but may be helpful in certain situations that have a predominant fibrinolytic process
Renal insufficiency	Close monitoring of fluid balance and electrolytes. Hemodialysis may become necessary for severe renal impairment

REFERENCES

1. I Kautner, MJ Robinson, U Kuhnle. Dengue virus infection: epidemiology, pathogenesis, clinical presentation, diagnosis, and prevention. J Pediatr 131:516–524, 1997.
2. World Health Organization. Dengue Hemorrhagic Fever: Diagnosis, Treatment and Control. Geneva: World Health Organization, 1986.
3. DW Vaughn, S Green. Dengue and dengue hemorrhagic fever. In: GT Strickland, ed. Hunter's Tropical Medicine, 8th ed. Philadelphia: WB Saunders, 1991, pp. 240–245.
4. DE Carey. Chikungunya and dengue: a case of mistaken identity. J Hist Med Allied Sci 26:243–262, 1971.
5. NJ Ehrenkranz, AK Ventura, RR Cuadrado, WL Pond, JE Porter. Pandemic dengue in Caribbean countries and the southern United States: past, present and potential problems. N Engl J Med 285:1460–1469, 1971.
6. L Rice. Dengue fever: a clinical report of the Galveston epidemic of 1922. Am J Trop Med Hyg 3:73–90, 1923.
7. WM Hammon, A Rudnik, GE Sather. Viruses associated with epidemic hemorrhagic fevers of the Philippines and Thailand. Science 131:1102–1103, 1960.
8. GF Lumley, FH Taylor. Dengue. School of Public Health and Tropical Medicine Service Publication Number 3.

Glebe: Australasian Medical Publishing Company, 1943, p. 74.

9. AB Sabin. The dengue group of viruses and its family relationships. Bacteriol Rev 14:225–232, 1950.

10. AB Sabin. Research on dengue during World War II. Am J Trop Med Hyg 1:30–49, 1952.

11. DJ Gubler, DW Trent. Emergence of the epidemic dengue/ dengue hemorrhagic fever as a public health problem in the Americas. Infect Agents Dis 2:383–393, 1994.

12. SB Halstead. The pathogenesis of dengue. Am J Epidemiol 114:632–648, 1981.

13. SB Halstead. Observations related to pathogenesis of dengue hemorrhagic fever. VI. Hypothesis and discussion. Yale J Biol Med 42:350–362, 1970.

14. CG Hayes, TF O'Rourke, V Fogelman, DD Leavengood, G Crow, MM Albersmeyer. Dengue fever in American military personnel in the Phillippines: clinical observations on hospitalized patients during a 1984 epidemic. Southeast Asian J Trop Med Public Health 20:1–8, 1989.

15. EB Hayes, DJ Gubler. Dengue and dengue hemorrhagic fever. Pediatr Infect Dis J 11:311–317, 1992.

16. SK Lam. Dengue and dengue hemorrhagic fever. Southeast Asian J Trop Med Public Health 21:520–521, 1990.

17. JG Rigau-Pérez, GG Clark, DJ Gubler, P Reiter, EJ Sanders, AV Vorndam. Dengue and dengue haemorrhagic fever. Lancet 352:971–977, 1998.

18. DJ Gubler. Question and Answers About DHF. Atlanta: Centers for Disease Control and Prevention, August 1995, pp. 1–9.

19. ER Nelson. Dengue fever: a thrombocytopenic disease? JAMA 190:99–103, 1964.

20. N Bhamarapravati, P Toochinda, V Boonyapaknavik. Pathology of Thailand hemorrhagic fever: a study of 100 autopsy cases. Ann Trop Med Parasitol 61:500–510, 1967.

21. RM de Andino, MV Botet, DJ Gubler, C Garcia, E Laboy, F Espada, SH Waterman. The absence of dengue virus in the skin lesions of dengue fever. Int J Dermatol 24:48–51, 1985.

22. JH McBride. Dengue fever: an Australian perspective. Aust Fam Physician 28:319–323, 1999.

23. BL Innis, A Nisalak, S Nimmanitya, S Kusalerdchariya, V Chongswasdi, S Suntayakorn, P Puttisri, CH Hoke. An enzyme-linked immunosorbent assay to characterize dengue infections where dengue and Japanese encephalitis cocirculate. Am J Trop Med Hyg 40:418–427, 1989.

24. S Tassniyom, S Vasanawathana, A Chirawatkul, S Rojanasuphot. Failure of high-dose methylprednisolone in established dengue shock syndrome: a placebo-controlled, double-blind study. Pediatrics 92:111–115, 1993.

25. TP Monath, FX Heinz. Flaviviruses. In: FN Fields, DM Knipe, PM Howley, et al., eds. Fields Virology, 3rd ed. Philadelphia: Lippincott-Raven, 1996, pp. 961–1034.

26. R Inada. Compute rendu des recherches sur l'encephalite epidemique au Japon. Offic Internat d'Hyg Pub Bull Mens 29:1389–1401, 1937.

27. WF Scherer, EL Buescher. Ecologic studies of Japanese encephalitis in Japan. Parts I–IX. Am J Trop Med Hyg 8: 644–722, 1959.

28. World Health Organization. Japanese Encephalitis Vaccines, position paper. Geneva: World Health Organization, updated Jan 18, 1999.

29. MW Benenson, FJ Top Jr, W Gresso, CW Ames, LB Altstatt. The virulence to man of Japanese encephalitis virus in Thailand. Am J Trop Med Hyg 24:974–980, 1975.

30. B Dropulic, CL Masters. Entry of neurotropic arboviruses into the central nervous system: an in vitro study using brain endothelium. J Infect Dis 161:685–691, 1990.

31. R Kumar, A Mathur, KB Singh, P Sitholey, M Prasad, R Shukla, SP Agarwal, J Arockiasamy. Clinical sequelae of Japanese encephalitis in children. Indian J Med Res 97: 9–13, 1993.

32. TF Tsai. Japanese encephalitis vaccines. In: S Plotkin, ed. Vaccines, 2nd ed. Philadelphia: WB Saunders, 1994, pp. 671–713.

33. K Hayashi, T Arita. Experimental double infection of Japanese encephalitis virus and herpes simplex in mouse brain. Jpn J Exp Med 47:9–13, 1977.

34. RT Johnson, DS Burke, M Elwell, CJ Leake, A Nisalak, CH Hoke, W Lorsomrudee. Japanese encephalitis: immunocytochemical studies of viral antigen and inflammatory cells in fatal cases. Ann Neurol 18:567–573, 1985.

35. CH Hoke Jr, DW Vaughn, A Nisalak, P Intralawan, S Poolsuppasit, V Jongsawas, U Titsyakorn, RT Johnson. Effect of high-dose dexamethasone on the outcome of acute encephalitis due to Japanese encephalitis virus. J Infect Dis 165: 631–637, 1992.

36. TH Work. Russian spring-summer virus in India. Kyasanur Forest disease. Prog Med Virol 1:248–279, 1958.

37. PN Bhatt, TH Work, MG Varma, H Trapido, DP Murthy, FM Rodrigues. Kyasanur forest diseases. IV. Isolation of Kyasanur forest disease virus from infected humans and monkeys of Shimogadistrict, Mysore state. Indian J Med Sci 20:316–320, 1966.

38. TH Work, FR Rodriquez, PN Bhatt. Kyasanur forest disease: virological epidemiology of the 1958 epidemic. Am J Public Health 49:869–874, 1959.

39. MJ Boshell, Rajagopalan PK, Patil AP, Pavri KM. Isolation of Kyasanur Forest disease virus from ixodid ticks: 1961–1964. Indian J Med Res 56:541–568, 1968.

40. World Health Organization. Viral haemorrhagic fevers. World Health Org Tech Rep Ser 721:5–126, 1985.

41. K Pavri. Clinical, clinicopathologic, and hematologic features of Kyasanur Forest disease Rev Infect Dis 11(suppl 4):S854–S859, 1989.

42. MR Prabha, MG Prabhu, CV Raghuveer, M Bai, MA Mala. Clinical study of 100 cases of Kyasanur Forest disease with clinicopathological correlation. Indian J Med Sci 47: 124–130, 1993.

43. CG Iyer, RR Laxmana, TH Work, DP Narasimha Murthy. Kyasanur forest disease VI. Pathologic findings in 3 fatal human cases of Kyasanur Forest Disease. Indian J Med Sci 13:1011–1022, 1959.

44. NN Kharitonova, YA Leonov. Omsk Hemorrhagic Fever. Ecology of the Agent and Epizootiology. New Delhi: Amerind Publishing Company, 1985.

45. BD Schoub, NK Blackburn. Flaviviruses. In: AJ Zuckerman, JE Banatvala, JR Pattison, eds. Principles and Practice of Clinical Virology, 3rd ed. Chichester: John Wiley & Sons, 1994, pp. 512–513.

46. AS Benenson, ed. Control of Communicable Diseases Manual: An Official Report of the American Public Health Association, 16th ed. Washington, DC. The Association, 1995, pp. 25–54.

47. TF Tsai. Arboviral infections in the United States. Infect Dis Clin North Am 5:73–102, 1991.

48. National Center for Infectious Diseases. Information on Arboviral Encephalitides. Atlanta: Centers for Disease Control and Prevention. Available at: http://www.cdc.gov/ncidod/dvbid/arbor/arbdet.htm. Accessed Feb 13, 2000.

49. A Gonzalez Cortes, ML Zarate Aquino, JG Bahena Guzman, J Miro Abella, G Cano Avila, M Aguilera Arrayo. St. Louis encephalomyelitis in Hermosillo, Sonora, Mexico. Pan Am Health Org Bull 9:306–316, 1975.

50. RS Nasci, CG Moore. Vector-borne disease surveillance and natural disasters. Emerg Infect Dis 4:333–334, 1998.

51. A Desai, SK Shankar, V Revi, A Chandramuki, M Gourie-Devi. Japanese encephalitis virus antigen in the human brain and its topographic distribution. Acta Neuropathol 89:368–373, 1995.

52. RM Zwighaft, C Rasmussen, D Brolnitsky, JC Lashof. St. Louis encephalitis: the Chicago experience. Am J Trop Med Hyg 28:114–118, 1979.

53. DT Quick, JM Thompson, JO Bond. The 1962 epidemic of St. Louis encephalitis in Florida. IV. Clinical features of cases in the Tampa Bay area. Am J Epidemiol 81:415–427, 1965.

54. RJ Whitley. Arthropod-borne encephalitides. In: WM Scheld, RJ Whitley, DT Durack, eds. Infections of the Central Nervous System, 2nd ed. Philadelphia: Lippincott-Raven, 1997, pp. 147–168.

55. AA Smorodintsev. Tick-borne spring-summer encephalitis. Prog Med Virol 1:210–248, 1958.

56. D Blaskovic, G Pucekova, L Kubinyi. An epidemiological study of tick-borne encephalitis in the Tribec region: 1956–1963. Bull World Health Organ 36:89–94, 1967.

57. V Danielova, C Benes. Possible role of rainfall in the epidemiology of tick-borne encephalitis. Cent Eur J Public Health 5:151–154, 1997.

58. DH Clarke, J Casals. Arboviruses group B. In: FL Horsfall, I Tanner, eds. Viral and Rickettsial Infection of Man. Philadelphia: JB Lippincott, 1965, pp. 606–658.

59. WF Scherer, GA Eddy, TP Monath, et al. Laboratory safety for arboviruses and certain other viruses of vertebrates. The Subcommittee on Arbovirus Laboratory Safety of the American Committee on Arthropod-Borne Viruses. Am J Trop Med Hyg 29:1359–1381, 1980.

60. IB Galant. Certain features of the course of contemporary Far Eastern tick-borne encephalitis. Prob Virol 4:66–68, 1959.

61. M Labuda, JM Austyn, E Zuffova, O Kozuch, N Fuchsberger, J Lysy, PA Nuttall. Importance of localized skin infection in tick-borne encephalitis virus transmission. Virology 219:357–366, 1996.

62. G Gunther, M Hahlund, L Lindquist, B Skoldenberg, M Forsgren. Intrathecal IgM, IgA and IgG antibody response in tick-borne encephalitis. Long-term follow-up related to clinical course and outcome. Clin Diagn Virol 8:17–29, 1997.

63. TR Kreil, MM Eibl. Viral infection of macrophages profoundly alters requirements for induction of nitric oxide synthesis. Virology 212:174–178, 1995.

64. S Lotric-Furlan, F Strle. Thrombocytopenia, leukopenia and abnormal liver function tests in the initial phase of tick-borne encephalitis. Zentralbl Bakteriol 282:275–278, 1995.

65. T Jeren, A Vince. Cytologic and immunoenzymatic findings in CSF from patients with tick-borne encephalitis. Acta Cytol 42:330–334, 1998.

66. LA Zilber, VD Soloviev. Far Eastern tick-borne spring-summer encephalitis. Annu Rev Med Spec 5(suppl):1–75, 1946.

67. H Hofmann, C Kunz, FX Heinz. Laboratory diagnosis of tick-borne encephalitis. Arch Virol 1(suppl):153–159, 1990.

68. M Roggendorf, F Heinz, F Deinhardt, C Kunz. Serological diagnosis of acute tick-borne encephalitis by demonstration of antibodies of the IgM class. J Med Virol 7:41–50, 1981.

69. H Hofmann, C Kunz, FX Heinz, H Dippe. Detectability of IgM antibodies against TBE virus after natural infection and after vaccination. Infection 11:164–166, 1983.

70. FX Heinz, M Roggendorf, H Hofmann, C Kunz, F Dienhardt. Comparison of two different enzyme immunoassays for detection of immunoglobulin M antibodies against tick-borne encephalitis virus in serum and cerebrospinal fluid. J Clin Microbiol 14:141–146, 1981.

71. G Kluger, A Schottler, K Waldvogel, D Nadal, W Hinrichs, GF Wundisch, MC Laub. Tickborne encephalitis despite specific immunoglobulin prophylaxis [letter]. Lancet 346:1502, 1995.

72. C Kunz. Tick-borne encephalitis in Europe. Acta Leidensia 60:1–14, 1992.

73. HE Webb, JH Connolly, FF Kane, KJ O'Reilly, DI Simpson. Laboratory infections with louping ill with associated encephalitis. Lancet 2:255–258, 1968.

74. JH Lawson, WG Mauderson, EW Hurst. Louping ill meningoencephalitis. A further case and a serologic survey. Lancet 2:696–699, 1949.

75. HW Reid. Louping ill. In: Monath, ed. The Arboviruses: Epidemiology and Ecology, vol III. Boca Raton: RC Press, 1988, pp. 118–135.

76. GF Gao, MH Hussain, HW Reid, EA Gould. Classification of a new member of the TBE flavivirus subgroup by its immunological, pathogenetic and molecular characteristics: identification of subgroup-specific pentapeptides. Virus Res 30:129–144, 1993.

77. FL Soper. Jungle yellow fever: new epidemiological entity in South America. Rev Hyg Saude Publica 10:107–144, 1936.

78. World Health Organization. Prevention and Control of Yellow Fever in Africa. Geneva: World Health Organization, 1986.

79. National Center for Infectious Diseases. Summary of Health Information for International Travel (The Blue Sheet). Atlanta: Centers for Disease Control and Prevention. Available at: http://www.cdc.gov/travel/bluesheet.htm. Accessed Feb 13, 2000.

80. M Germain, M Cornet, J Mouchet, JP Herve, V Robert, JL Camicas, R Cordellier, JP Hervy, JP Digoutte, TP Monath, JJ Salaun, V Deubel, Y Robin, J Coz, R Taufflieb, JF Saluzzo, JP Gonzalez. [Sylvatic yellow fever in Africa recent advances and present approach (author's transl)]. Med Trop (Mars) 41:31–43, 1981.

81. AS Benenson, ed. Control of Communicable Disease Manual: An Official Report of the American Public Health Association, 16th ed. Washington D.C.: The Association, 1995, pp. 519–524.

82. D Brandling-Bennett, F Pinheiro. Infectious diseases in Latin America and the Caribbean: are they really emerging and increasing? Emerg Infect Dis 2:59–61, 1996.

83. JM McFarland, LM Baddour, JE Nelson, SK Elkins, RB Craven, BC Cropp, GJ Chang, AD Grindstaff, AS Craig, RJ Smith. Imported yellow fever in a United States citizen. Clin Infect Dis 25:1143–1147, 1997.

21

Togaviridae

Michael R. Weir
Scott and White Clinic and Memorial Hospital, Temple, Texas, USA

Tracey E. Weir
Brackenridge Hospital, Austin, Texas, USA

The *Alphavirus* genus is one of four groups of the Togaviridae family. This genus consists of mosquito-borne viruses that have a natural worldwide distribution in birds or mammals. For the most part, humans are incidental hosts of the transmission cycle. In humans, these viruses cause either encephalitis or a syndrome of fever, polyarthritis, and rash. Three groups of importance to humans are described: eastern equine encephalitis (EEE), western equine encephalitis (WEE), and Venezuelan equine encephalitis (VEE). Chikungunya fever and other alphaviruses are less well known but may be equally important if they spread to more densely populated areas (Fig. 21–1). Rubella, also a member of the Togaviridae family, will be discussed in Chapter 22.

EASTERN EQUINE ENCEPHALITIS

Definition

EEE is an alphavirus centered in North America. There are two closely related alphaviruses, one centered in the Amazon basin and one seen in Panama, Trinidad, Ecuador, Guyana, and Argentina [1]. This arthropod-borne virus infects humans, horses, and other vertebrates, primarily in coastal locations (Fig. 21–2).

History

Epidemics were noted as early as 1931 and appeared to be related to salt marsh habitats. This suggested a mosquito cycle with avian reservoirs and led to demonstration of a virus distinct from WEE [2]. Isolation of the virus from human tissue occurred in 1938 [3]. EEE has become recognized as a severe and sometimes fatal cause of encephalitis.

Incidence

Infections occur along the Atlantic and Gulf coasts, and to a lesser extent in the interior. The natural cycle involves *Culex melanura,* the mosquito, and numerous birds, which function as amplifying hosts. Other mosquitoes, such as *Aedes* and *Coquillettidia sp.,* feed on birds and become infected. This creates a secondary natural cycle with birds and small mammals. Humans, horses, and pheasants sustain clinical disease, but these are considered dead-end hosts with little opportunity for viral transmission because of the short period of viremia. Whereas equine cases occur year round, human cases develop sporadically from early spring until autumn [4]. Few cases of EEE occur each year, with an average of three reported infections annually in the United States [5]. The infection rate in epidemics is about 2% [6,7]. Mild, febrile disease is 20 times more frequent than that of encephalitis. However, encephalitis caused by EEE frequently results in neurological sequelae among the survivors.

Pathogenesis

Culex melanura mosquitoes acquire the virus by feeding on viremic birds. The virus must spread from the mosquito

TAXONOMY

Togaviridae family
Alphavirus genus
- Eastern equine encephalitis (EEE)
- Western equine encephalitis
- Venezuelan equine encephalitis (VEE)
- Chikungunya fever (CHIK)
- O'nyong-nyong (ONN)
- Sindbis (Ockelbo)
- Ross River virus (RRV)
- Barmah forest vırus

WORLDWIDE GEOGRAPHICAL INCIDENCE

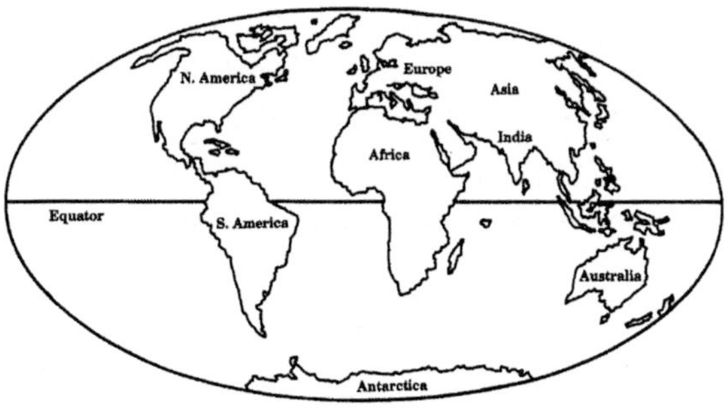

Figure 21–1. Taxonomy and incidence of Togaviridae.

gut through the hemolymph to the salivary system before transmission can occur [8]. The virus damages the mosquito intestine, which is contradictory to the usual assumption that the vector is uninjured [9]. There is not sufficient evidence to suggest transtadial or transovarial transmission. The off-season reservoir is probably the migratory bird population. Because *C. melanura* does not feed on humans, other vectors must acquire the virus from the birds and then transmit it to horses, humans, and pheasants.

Viremia occurs shortly after inoculation and may be accompanied by a febrile prodromal period. The virus is disseminated through the blood to visceral organs. Infection in the brain occurs after viremia and visceral spread, which suggests access to the central nervous system through hematogenous spread.

Clinical Manifestations

EEE is a severe encephalitis with death or disability as a frequent outcome. Death occurs more often in children and the elderly, with severe sequelae in many survivors [10]. Sequelae include spastic paralysis, personality change, seizures, and intellectual impairment or developmental delay, particularly in infant survivors. The clinical course of EEE is outlined in Table 21–1. Table 21–2 includes possible differential diagnoses.

GEOGRAPHICAL INCIDENCE OF EASTERN EQUINE ENCEPHALITIS

TRANSMISSION

ZOONOTIC IMPLICATIONS

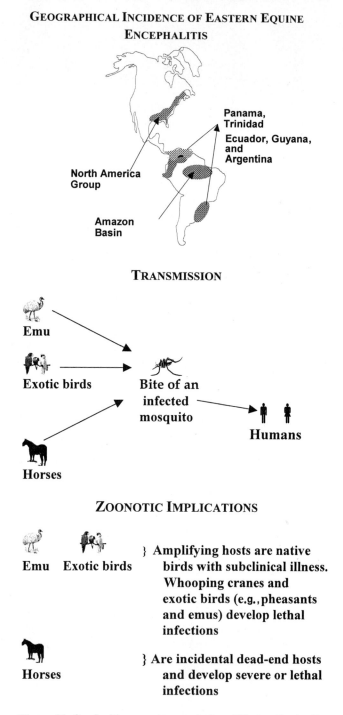

Figure 21–2. Incidence and transmission of Eastern Equine Encephalitis.

Table 21–1. Clinical Manifestations of Eastern Equine Encephalitis

Time after exposure	Clinical manifestations	Laboratory analyses	Other notes
3–10 days	Prodrome of fever, chills, headache, photophobia, and myalgia, often with nausea and vomiting ↓	Serological tests, with detection of IgM or IgG in any sera Viral isolation early in the course of disease	The clinical course progresses more rapidly in infants, with high fever, irritability, vomiting, and diarrhea, which rapidly progresses to somnolence or intermittent seizures. This may lead to coma within 24 to 48 hours of symptom onset
6–17 days	Symptoms suddenly progress, with severe headache, dizziness, nuchal rigidity, lethargy, decreased level of consciousness, and focal neurological signs. Seizures may occur ↓	Viremia disappear prior to the onset of most dramatic symptoms	
Several days later	Many patients progressively worsen and die within the first several days of hospitalization. Survivors frequently have permanent sequelae	Detection of viral antigens by immunohisto-chemical staining of tissue in fatal cases	With improved intensive care techniques, the overall case fatality rate is 30%. However, 67–78% of elderly cases result in death, while 20–62% of childhood illness results in death

Pathology

Neuronal necrosis and thrombosis of small vessels occur in the central nervous system. Cellular infiltration by neutrophils is early, and lymphocytic infiltration occurs later. Scattered lesions are more common in the basal ganglia and thalamus and less so in the cortex, hippocampus, and pons. Even less involvement occurs in the cerebellum and spinal cord [12].

Laboratory Findings

Polymorphonuclear leukocytosis occurs in blood and cerebrospinal fluid (CSF) and is associated with a normal or decreased CSF level of glucose and a mildly elevated level of protein. Polymorphonuclear cells predominate in the early phase of the disease but are replaced by mononuclear cells later in the course of infection [5]. Viremia occurs in the first few days but is usually not detected because it disappears prior to the most dramatic symptoms. Antibody is present by days 3 to 5, although the disease continues to progress, with virus detected in the brain as neuronal damage occurs. Computed tomographic scans of the brain may be normal or reveal only diffuse cerebral edema. Electroencephalogram patterns typically reveal focal or generalized slowing. Other patterns, such as burst suppression patterns, disorganized background activity, or high voltage delta wave slowing, are associated with a poor prognosis [13].

Diagnosis

Severe febrile central nervous system disease and deaths of horses and pheasants occurring in hot, wet summers near salt marsh biotypes in endemic areas suggest EEE. The virus can be isolated early during the initial febrile phase before the central nervous system manifestations are evident [14]. The encephalopathy and neurological symptoms occur when antibody production has displaced the viremia. In fatal cases, diagnosis can also be documented by detection of viral antigens in brain tissue by immunohistochemical stains.

Serological tests are the usual means of diagnosis. Hemagglutination inhibition or neutralization tests on paired sera or IgM antibodies detected by enzyme-linked immunosorbent assay confirm the diagnosis [15]. Because seroprevalence rates are low, even in endemic areas, the presence of EEE-specific antibody in acute serum indicates a high probability of current infection [5].

Treatment and Prophylaxis

Supportive care for encephalitis is indicated (Table 21–3). No specific antiviral therapy for this illness is available. Intensive care of encephalitis involves frequent reassessment of neurological progression or resolution, as with using the Glasgow Coma Scale [16]. Imaging and testing for compromise of circulatory function, ventilation suffi-

Table 21–2. Differential Diagnoses of Eastern Equine Encephalitis

Herpes simplex virus encephalitis Enteroviral aseptic meningitis Bacterial meningitis Tuberculous meningitis Cerebral malaria Dengue virus with encephalopathy Intracranial hemorrhage/stroke Heat stroke Lead encephalopathy Toxic encephalopathy Brain abscess Brain tumor Postinfectious encephalitis Metabolic encephalopathy Status epilepticus Acute confusional or basilar migraine Reye's syndrome	See Table 18–2

Other arboviral encephalitides:
  Japanese encephalitis
  Western equine encephalitis
  Venezuelan equine encephalitis
  West Nile fever
  California encephalitis
  St. Louis encephalitis
	See Table 15–2

Powassan encephalitis Rift Valley fever Kyasanur Forest disease Colorado tick fever Tick-borne encephalitis Rocky Mountain spotted fever	See Table 17–2

Table 21–3. Treatment of Eastern Equine Encephalitis

Symptom	Treatment
Fever and headache	Antipyretics and analgesics
Seizures	Anticonvulsants—observe for changes in neurological and ventilation status
Elevated intracranial pressure	Hyperventilation, sedation, elevation of head of bed, and fluid restriction to 30–50% of maintenance, with diuretics and osmotic agents (mannitol infusion). These methods help to limit the impact of associated cerebral edema
Decreased level of consciousness	Airway protection and frequent monitoring

Conclusion

EEE is the most severe of the arboviral encephalitides. It results in small, annual outbreaks and occasional larger epidemics. Current therapy is supportive. Vaccination has limited utility. Currently, avoiding endemic swamps in hot damp months reduces exposure. The vector winters as larvae in a dark, organic-rich habitat; a floating root mat is ideal. The complicated requirements for epidemics, which include dense vector population and infected birds in a salt marsh biotype, limit spread. The significant public health threat of EEE requires a solution to the natural cycle. However, no such solution is at hand.

ciency, and cerebral perfusion are central measures of progression. Ventilatory support is adjusted to maintain oxygenation and to maximize cerebral perfusion. Medical treatment of agitation or seizures may obscure neurological status and worsen ventilation.

Recent human and animal exposures to EEE can be treated prophylactically with immune sera. However, the evidence for an immunological mechanism for the central nervous system manifestations would limit such therapy for encephalitis. An equine vaccine is available for the infrequent epidemics. The human vaccine from the Center for Disease Control (CDC) or the US Army Medical Research Institute for Infectious Disease (Fort Detrick, MD) is indicated for potential laboratory exposure. The human vaccine is also effective in whooping cranes in which EEE is lethal [8]. Vaccination does not affect the natural cycle in native birds and mosquitoes. Climate vector and habitat control may influence annual outbreaks.

WESTERN EQUINE ENCEPHALITIS

Definition

The WEE virus is an alphavirus that is mosquito-transmitted in a natural cycle in birds. The virus is a recombinant virus, deriving the glycoprotein structural genes from Sindbis virus (SIN), the prototype alphavirus, and capsid and nonstructural genes from EEE [17]. WEE is less neuroinvasive and neurovirulent than EEE [18]. The disease is less severe than other arbovirus encephalitis cases in humans, although the veterinary impact is grave (Fig. 21–3).

History

WEE was first isolated in 1930 from the brain of an infected horse during a California equine epizootic [19]. In 1938, the virus was then isolated from the brain of a child who had succumbed to the disease [20]. WEE was later

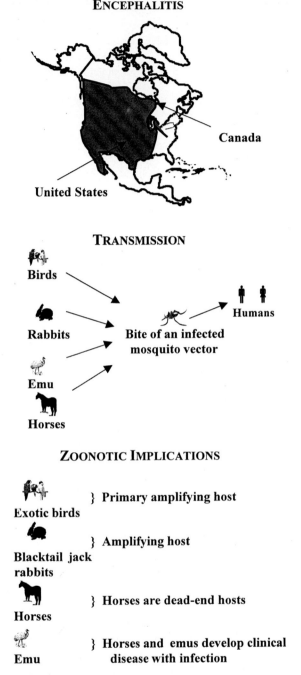

GEOGRAPHICAL INCIDENCE OF WESTERN EQUINE ENCEPHALITIS

Canada

United States

TRANSMISSION

Birds

Rabbits

Emu

Horses

Bite of an infected mosquito vector

Humans

ZOONOTIC IMPLICATIONS

Exotic birds } Primary amplifying host

Blacktail jack rabbits } Amplifying host

Horses } Horses are dead-end hosts

Emu } Horses and emus develop clinical disease with infection

Figure 21–3. Incidence and transmission of Western Equine Encephalitis.

isolated from *Culex tarsalis,* and mosquito transmission was implicated in the disease [18]. The use of the equine vaccine and declining wild horse populations led to decreased occurrence of the illness.

Incidence

WEE occurs predominantly in June and July in the western United States and Canada. The 1941 epidemic in the United States and Canada resulted in an attack rate of 23 to 172 per 100,000 and a case fatality rate of 8 to 15%. The 1952 California epidemic attack rate was 50 per 100,000 [21]. In recent years, the number of cases has dramatically decreased, with the last known case reported in 1994. Investigations of epidemics reveal an increased risk of infection on rural farms, with significantly less risk in towns and urban dwellings in the same endemic areas [5]. Increased risks of infection, morbidity, and mortality occur at the extremes of age, in infants, and in the elderly.

Pathogenesis

Culex tarsalis is the mosquito vector, with birds as the natural amplifying hosts. An additional natural cycle involves the blacktail jack rabbit and *Aedes melanimon* [22]. Horses and humans are accidental dead-end hosts in the avian-mosquito amplification cycle, with no real opportunity for viral spread. No human-to-human transmission has been observed.

In animal studies, inoculation of WEE leads to virus replication in extraneural sites, such as viscera, muscle, and probably vascular endothelial cells. The viral replication results in viremia, followed by central nervous system involvement. Infection in the central nervous system in humans results from hematogenous dissemination [23].

Clinical Manifestations

Infection with WEE may range from subclinical disease, a mild, undifferentiated febrile syndrome, to severe fatal encephalitis. Aseptic meningitis and febrile disease are more common than encephalitis. WEE has no typical features that distinguish it from other causes of viral encephalitis or aseptic meningitis. The typical clinical course of this infection is outlined in Table 21–4. Once neurological involvement occurs, physical examination reveals an altered mental status, weakness and tremulousness, and pathological reflexes. A small percentage of patients (<5%) develop motor weakness, spasticity, convulsions, or a cranial nerve palsy. Children more commonly show paralysis, involuntary movements, and rigidity. Infants commonly develop generalized convulsions and spastic paresis. The anterior fontanelle may be tense or bulging in this age group. No associated cutaneous manifestations have been described. Deaths occur early in the course of disease, but uncommonly (3–4%) and more often in the elderly. Significant neurological sequelae occur in 13% of all cases and

Table 21–4. Clinical Manifestations of Western Equine Encephalitis

Time after exposure	Clinical manifestations	Laboratory analyses	Other notes
5–10 days	Sudden onset of fever, malaise, headache, nausea, vomiting, vertigo, photophobia, sore throat, abdominal pain, and myalgia. The headache worsens with time ↓	Serological tests, with IgM or fourfold rise in IgG titers in paired sera	Some patients may have upper respiratory symptoms during the prodromal period
Progression over several days	Restlessness, drowsiness, stupor, and coma may evolve. Neck stiffness is present in 50%. Neurological abnormalities may develop (see text) ↓	Viral isolation from the blood or CSF is rarely successful in live patients	Seizures may occur in children, particularly infants (up to 80%)
15–20 days	Resolution of fever, followed by gradual improvement in symptoms and convalescence. After encephalitis, convalescence may last for 2 months	Antigen detection in brain tissue can be performed in fatal cases	Major neurological sequelae include quadriplegia, hemiplegia, spasticity, epilepsy, and developmental delay

are most common in infants less than 1 year of age (30% of cases) [24].

Pathology

A histopathological examination of the brain shows perivascular cuffing, meningeal inflammation, endothelial cell swelling with infarction, and foci of necrosis without cellular infiltrate in the striatum, globus pallidus, cerebral cortex, thalamus, and pons [25,26]. Infiltration with polymorphonuclear leukocytes is evident in areas of necrosis [27].

Laboratory Findings

The peripheral blood typically shows either a polymorphonuclear leukocytosis or leukopenia. Analysis of the CSF reveals a moderate pleocytosis with normal glucose and slightly elevated protein levels.

Diagnosis

WEE should be suspected in febrile central nervous system disease in endemic areas, particularly if equine deaths have occurred. Virus isolation from the CSF, brain, or throat is sometimes accomplished using suckling mice or embryonated egg models [8]. In fatal cases, viral antigens can be demonstrated in brain tissue with immunohistochemical stains. The most common and direct method of diagnosis is

serologic testing. Complement fixation, hemagglutination inhibition, or neutralization testing on paired sera or IgM antibodies can be utilized [28]. Differential diagnoses are shown in Table 21–5.

Treatment and Prophylaxis

Care is supportive and symptomatic (Table 21–6). No specific antiviral therapy exists. An equine vaccine exists and a human vaccine benefits laboratory workers and high-risk personnel, but it is not for general use. In the summer in endemic areas, mosquito protection (e.g., screened windows and air conditioning) of infants constitutes important prevention.

Conclusion

Although WEE has been a detrimental infection in equine populations, its incidence and severity are of less consequence in humans when compared with other arboviral encephalitides. It is hoped that the current trend of reducing infection will continue, as equine vaccination, personal protection, and mosquito control are maintained.

VENEZUELAN EQUINE ENCEPHALITIS
Definition

Considered the most important arboviral disease in tropical America, Venezuelan equine encephalitis (VEE) is the pro-

Table 21–5. Differential Diagnoses of Western Equine Encephalitis

Herpes simplex virus
  encephalitis
Enteroviral aseptic meningitis
Bacterial meningitis
Tuberculous meningitis
Cerebral malaria
Dengue virus with
  encephalopathy
Intracranial hemorrhage/stroke
Heat stroke   See Table 18–2
Lead encephalopathy
Toxic encephalopathy
Brain abscess
Brain tumor
Postinfectious encephalitis
Metabolic encephalopathy
Status epilepticus
Acute confusional or basilar
  migraine
Reye's syndrome
Other arboviral encephalitides:
  Japanese encephalitis
  Eastern equine encephalitis
  Venezuelan equine encephalitis
  West Nile fever
  California encephalitis   See Table 15–2
  St. Louis encephalitis
  Tick-borne encephalitis
  Powassan encephalitis
  Rocky Mountain spotted fever
  Rift Valley fever
  Kyasanur Forest disease   See Table 17–2
  Colorado tick fever

Table 21–6. Treatment of Western Equine Encephalitis

Symptom	Treatment
General	Bed rest and maintenance of fluid and electrolyte balance
Fever	Antipyretics
Increased intracranial pressure	Hyperventilation, elevation of head of bed, and mannitol infusions, as needed
Decreased level of consciousness	Close monitoring of neurological function and appropriate airway protection
Seizures	Anticonvulsants

totype virus for a group of related alphaviruses. The VEE virus has six subtypes; subtype I is divided into variants A through F. Variants A and B are now considered identical. IABC variants are pathogenic for horses and exist in epizootics (animal epidemics) in Peru, Colombia, Venezuela, and Ecuador in tropical dry or tropical thorn forests during rainy seasons with particularly heavy rainfall. Equine cases precede human cases. The elevated and prolonged equine viremia is central to the amplification cycle. Possible transmission from human to human by *Aedes aegypti* has been implicated but is not central to the genesis of epizootic and epidemic disease [31]. The reservoir for the interepizootic periods is problematic. Genetic similarities between epizootic and prior enzootic virus suggest a dynamic relationship between the two, as though the enzootic strains drift during conditions that favor epizootics [32]. Variants IDEF and subtypes II–VI occur in enzootics in American subtropical or tropical swamps or forests [8] (Fig. 21–4).

History

VEE is a significant cause of severe disease in northern South America. Epidemics involving up to tens of thousands of human and equine infections occurred over the past 10 years. Local inhabitants referred to *peste loca,* but VEE was not documented in equine epizootics until 1938. As is common in the viral etiology for EEE and WEE, VEE variants (IABC) are present in brains of dead horses [33,34]. The first documented human epidemic occurred in Colombia in 1952 [35]. Related VEE strains (IDEF) lack significant equine disease but cycle in rodents and *Culex* mosquitoes, which causes human disease outside the natural cycle (Fig. 21–5). A third group (II–VI) proved similar to the latter strains (IDEF) a member of this group occurred in the Florida Everglades. Recently, IAB disease has diminished, and these variants may be extinct. Recent epizootics were related to virus strain ID; this provides evidence of the potential for change in this arbovirus group [32].

Incidence

Seroconversion rates vary. In epizootic disease, attack rates of 10–60% are seen in humans. Horses are universally infected, developing immunity or succumbing to disease [8]. In enzootic disease, a high seroprevalence rate is reported [8]. Because horses also serve as amplifying hosts, equine epidemics usually precede those of humans by 1–2 weeks. A peak in VEE transmission coincides with periods of heavy rainfall, particularly in areas that have a distinct rainy season. Epizootics occur primarily in Colombia, Venezuela, Peru, and Ecuador. From 1969–1982, a single outbreak extended from Guatemala through the Central Amer-

GEOGRAPHICAL INCIDENCE OF VENEZUELAN EQUINE ENCEPHALITIS

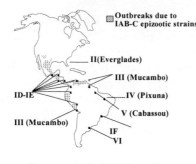

Outbreaks due to
IAB-C epizootic strains

II(Everglades)

III (Mucambo)

ID-IE

IV (Pixuna)

III (Mucambo)

V (Cabassou)

IF
VI

Shown are sylvatic viral subtypes of
Venezuelan equine encephalitis

TRANSMISSION

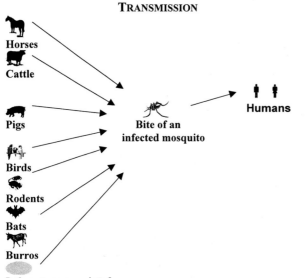

Horses

Cattle

Pigs

Birds

Rodents

Bats

Burros

Bite of an
infected mosquito

Humans

Laboratory-associated
cases may occur through
aerosol spread of the virus

ZOONOTIC IMPLICATIONS

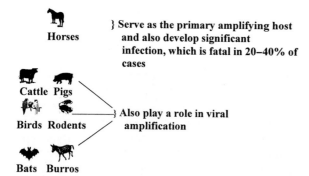

Horses } Serve as the primary amplifying host
and also develop significant
infection, which is fatal in 20–40% of
cases

Cattle Pigs

Birds Rodents } Also play a role in viral
amplification

Bats Burros

Figure 21–4. Incidence and transmission of Venezuelan Equine Encephalitis.

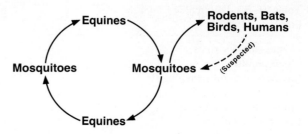

Equines

Rodents, Bats,
Birds, Humans

Mosquitoes

Mosquitoes

(Suspected)

Equines

Figure 21–5. Vectors and hosts in transmission of Venezuelan Equine Encephalitis.

ican countries and into Mexico and Texas [36]. Asymptomatic or mild cases probably predominate, but only a few patients become ill enough for hospitalization or potential fatality.

Pathogenesis

In enzootic disease, the vector is *Culex tarsalis,* a twilight feeder with a short feeding range. In epizootic disease, a variety of vectors may be involved. No single mosquito species predominates [8]. Following a mosquito bite, viremia occurs with central nervous system involvement. Invasion of the central nervous system may be through the endothelium but more likely involves the olfactory bulbs. Following injection of the virus into animals, the virus is evident first in the olfactory bulbs, then in the proximal neuroepithelium. Thus, an olfactory mode of entry into the central nervous system appears to be early and central to pathogenesis [37]. Other methods of central nervous system entry have been demonstrated following olfactory entry [38]. Antibodies appear as the viremia clears. The humoral response to infection has a role in viremia clearance, but inflammation of the central nervous system may be aggravated by the antibody response.

Clinical Manifestations

The vast majority of individuals infected with VEE develop clinical illness. Most patients have an undifferentiated febrile disease, or more commonly an influenza-like illness. Fortunately, neurological involvement occurs in only a small percentage of cases. The clinical course of typical VEE is outlined in Table 21–7. On physical examination, injection of the conjunctivae and pharynx is evident, as well as flushed facies and muscular tenderness. The mortal-

Table 21–7. Clinical Manifestations of Venezuelan Equine Encephalitis

Time after exposure	Clinical manifestation	Laboratory analyses	Other notes
2–5 days	Sudden onset of malaise, high fever, chills, headache, sore throat, and myalgia. Some patients have prostration, vomiting, and photophobia	Viral isolation from blood or throat swabs during the first 3 days of symptoms Serological tests, with IgM or fourfold rise in IgG	
	↓		
Over several days	Some patients (5–10%) may progress to have neurological involvement, with nuchal rigidity, confusion, agitation, and mild alteration of consciousness. Fever patients (<5%) have severe symptoms, with motor weakness, paralysis, seizures, cranial nerve palsy, or coma		Only 4% of patients with clinical infection develop frank encephalitis, with children more often than adults
	↓		
7–12 days	Complete recovery without sequelae in the majority of cases. Convalescence is usually prolonged, with asthenia, headaches, and memory difficulties for up to 1–2 months		Patients rarely develop persistent sequelae, such as sensory or motor abnormalities

ity rate with VEE is 0.5%; but of those who develop encephalitis, 10–25% of infections lead to death [39].

Pathology

The pathological changes with VEE are similar to, but less striking than, those of EEE [41]. Because the virus is both lymphotropic and neurotropic [36], pathological changes occur in the brain, gastrointestinal lymphoid tissue, lymph nodes, spleen, liver, and lungs. Some fatalities show lymphoid depletion with little central nervous system pathology. Punctate hemorrhages may be seen. Histologically, there is perivascular cuffing with lymphocytic infiltration.

Laboratory Findings

The peripheral blood typically reveals a modest thrombocytopenia and leukopenia with an early lymphopenia, which later changes to a neutropenia. Elevation of aspartate aminotransferase and lactate dehydrogenase levels may also occur. The CSF shows a pleocytosis that may be composed of polymorphonuclear cells early in disease but later becomes lymphocytic. The CSF also has a normal or slightly decreased glucose and a moderately elevated protein level.

Diagnosis

If residents are from an area with rising equine deaths (or travelers have just been there), symptomatic WEE should be suspected. The virus can be isolated from sera and the nasopharynx in the first 2 to 3 days of symptoms until as late as day 6 [42]. Viral culture is best accomplished in Vero cell or suckling mice models. The virus can also be isolated from horses in affected herds but not in those severely affected or at necropsy.

For diagnosis later in the course of disease, serologic tests are more useful. Hemagglutination inhibition and neutralizing antibodies appear with disappearance of the viremia. IgM can be obtained from both blood and CSF specimens, and a single positive specimen confirms the diagnosis of VEE. Paired sera that document a rise in IgG titers can also be used for diagnosis. Table 21–8 lists differential diagnosis.

Treatment and Prophylaxis

Medical treatment of mild disease is routine and symptomatic (Table 21–9). No specific antiviral treatment for VEE is available. Monitoring of intracranial and central venous pressures augments oxygenation and respiratory measures to improve cerebral blood flow. Cerebral blood flow is

Table 21–8. Differential Diagnosis of Venezuelan Equine Encephalitis

Herpes simplex virus encephalitis	
Enteroviral aseptic meningitis	
Bacterial meningitis	
Tuberculous meningitis	
Cerebral malaria	
Dengue virus with encephalopathy	
Intracranial hemorrhage/stroke	
Heat stroke	See Table 18–2
Lead encephalopathy	
Toxic encephalopathy	
Brain abscess	
Brain tumor	
Postinfectious encephalitis	
Metabolic encephalopathy	
Status epilepticus	
Acute confusional or basilar migraine	
Reye's syndrome	
Other arboviral encephalitides:	
Japanese encephalitis	
Eastern equine encephalitis	
Western equine encephalitis	
West Nile fever	
California encephalitis	See Table 15–2
St. Louis encephalitis	
Powassan encephalitis	
Rocky Mountain spotted fever	
Colorado tick fever	
Rift Valley fever	See Table 17–2
Kyasanur Forest disease	
Tick-borne encephalitis	See Table 20–6

Table 21–9. Treatment of Venezuelan Equine Encephalitis

Symptom	Treatment
General	Bed rest and maintenance of fluid and electrolyte balance
Fever and headache	Antipyretics and analgesics Acetaminophen is preferred because of the thrombocytopenia that may occur with this illness
Seizures	Anticonvulsants
Neurological deterioration	Frequent monitoring of neurological function and control of increased intracranial pressure

a balance of intracranial pressure and volume restriction. Patients should be protected from further mosquito exposure until they are afebrile. Blood and bodily fluid protection is indicated.

Because VEE is highly infectious by aerosol, laboratory workers must maintain a strict protective technique. Live attenuated and formalin inactivated vaccines are available, but both have side effects of fever and myalgia. A biodegradable microencapsulated vaccine is under development [43]. Personal protection from the vector for the traveler or inhabitant consists of insect repellants, protective clothing, and habitat avoidance. The *Culex* vector is a crepuscular feeder and does not venture far from its habitat [8]. Epizo-

otic disease can be controlled by equine vaccine that interrupts the equine role in vertebrate viral amplification.

Related Viruses

''Everglades'' virus is VEE subtype II, an enzootic strain, which causes encephalitis in Florida. Mosquitoes are the vector. Tonate mosquito fever is an enzootic strain of VEE subtype III in South America. Mucambo virus causes fever in South America. It is a mosquito-transmitted enzootic strain of VEE subtype III. VEE subtypes IV–VI have also been isolated from mosquitoes. These strains include Pixuna and Cabassous.

Semliki Forest virus is a significant alphavirus, as it is used as a serological marker in African studies and as a model laboratory virus. The Central African Republic epidemic occurred when green monkeys were infected by *Aedes Africans*. The virus spilled into the human population and into urban *Aedes aegypti*. Infected patients developed fever, pronounced headache, myalgia, and arthralgia. Abdominal pain, diarrhea, and conjunctivitis also were evident in some cases [44].

Conclusion

Epizootic disease occurs when vector populations explode in very wet, tropical habitats and interface with a population of nonimmune equine hosts for virus amplification. Viral antigens or virulence have been demonstrated to change as well. For VEE, appropriate vaccination of horses should dampen or completely thwart both equine and human outbreaks.

CHIKUNGUNYA FEVER

Definition

The chikungunya (CHIK) virus, several species in the genus *Alphavirus,* causes a febrile arthralgia syndrome with occasional hemorrhagic disease. CHIK is in the Semliki Forest antigenic group. This virus was originally a forest virus of primates of Africa, transmitted by sylvatic *Aedes* species. However, CHIK has become a major public health problem in urban centers with *Aedes aegypti* as the vector. Sylvatic cycles probably involve primates and *Aedes* species (Fig. 21–6).

History

The term chikungunya comes from a Tanzanian tribal word meaning ''that which contorts or bends up.'' Local inhabitants described the characteristic posture assumed by afflicted individuals with severe joint pains. The virus was first isolated during an epidemic in Tanzania in 1952 [45]. However, historical evidence cited by Carey [46] strongly suggests that sporadic outbreaks of the disease have occurred in India and Southeast Asia for over 200 years.

Incidence

Disease occurs in the rainy season as humans impinge upon the primate-*Aedes* cycle. There are also urban epidemics of mosquito-human cycles. During outbreaks, CHIK typically appears suddenly and infects a substantial portion of the susceptible population, then disappears [46]. In the urban areas of sub-Saharan Africa, India, Southeast Asia, and the Philippines, regular epidemics occur among the susceptible population, especially the young, whose symptoms may be atypical and less dramatic. Epidemics of hemorrhagic fever in Bangkok show CHIK titer rises in 8% of cases, with most of the remainder caused by dengue fever [47]. Although it is not usually considered a hemorrhagic fever, CHIK causes a significant amount of clinical Thai hemorrhagic fever.

Pathogenesis

With alphavirus infection, the bite of an infected mosquito results in a viremia with target organ involvement. High levels of viremia are present during the first 2 days of symptoms, with resolution of the viremia within 5 days of disease onset. Manifestations result from direct viral infection or an immunological (i.e., lymphocytic) reaction. The presence of specific antibody heralds resolution of the fever and of other early systemic manifestations. The later symptoms appear to result from an immunological reaction to the virus rather than from the infection itself [8].

Clinical Manifestations

Fever and arthralgia characterize CHIK infections. The sequence of clinical manifestations of CHIK are shown in Table 21–10. Because of the severe arthralgias, patients

Table 21–10. Clinical Manifestations of Chikungunya Fever

Time after exposure	Clinical manifestations	Laboratory analyses	Other notes
2–6 days	Sudden onset of high fever, significant arthralgia, muscle pains, and headache (frontal or orbital). Patients may often have photophobia, nausea, vomiting, and diarrhea. A flushed face often develops early in the disease and lasts 24 hours ↓	Viral isolation during the first 2 to 4 days of illness Serological tests, with acute IgM or fourfold rise in IgG among paired sera	Small children may have seizures and fever only. Arthritic manifestations are less common in children The fever is often biphasic, with an afebrile period that develops after 1–4 days and lasts 1–2 days before return of fever The rash may recur with repetitive waves of viremia
5–11 days	A generalized, fine and discrete maculopapular exanthem develops along with lymphadenopathy. The rash involves the trunk and limbs as well as the palms and soles. The rash either fades or desquamates after 1–5 days ↓		
10–13 days	Resolution of symptoms, with persistence of myalgia and arthralgia from 1 week to more than a year at times		Middle-aged adults experience more prolonged joint manifestations than younger patients

typically prefer to lie in flexion positions and complain of pain when moved. The arthralgia affects small joints more than large ones and may aggravate previous arthritic conditions. Associated central nervous system disease and myocarditis have been described but are quite rare. However, children may have febrile convulsions. A maculopapular rash involves the trunk, limbs, palms and soles. Manifestations suggesting hemorrhagic fever affect few patients, but CHIK infections are so common that CHIK hemorrhagic disease is not unusual. Petechiae may occur along with gingival bleeding, but severe hemorrhage is rare. A significant portion (8–10%) of presumed dengue hemorrhagic fever patients prove to have serological evidence of CHIK.

Pathology

Biopsies of skin lesions show lymphocytic perivascular cuffing with erythrocytic extravasation [49]. Otherwise, little is known about the associated pathology of this disease.

Laboratory Findings

Significant laboratory abnormalities are uncommon. Most frequently, patients have an elevated erythrocyte sedimentation rate and high C-reactive protein level. In one fourth of patients, rheumatoid factor is present in low titers [48]. A leukopenia with a lymphocytosis and a low platelet count may sometimes occur.

Diagnosis

The suddenness and severity of the fever, the startling joint pain, and the rash should suggest the diagnosis in endemic or epidemic settings or in a patient who has recently traveled in these areas. Virus can be isolated from blood samples in the first 2 to 4 days of clinical illness. Later, hemagglutination inhibition (HI) and neutralizing antibodies appear when the viremia declines (after the first 5 days of symptoms) [8]. A fourfold rise in IgG titers of paired (acute and convalescent) sera establishes the diagnosis. Specific CHIK-IgM can be shown by capture enzyme-linked immunosorbent assay [50]. Possible differential diagnoses are shown in Table 21–11.

Treatment and Prophylaxis

The arthralgia is improved by mild exercise with symptomatic and supportive care (Table 21–12). Severe exercise is contraindicated because of worsening of arthritic symptoms. Prevention is by mosquito protection directed at *Aedes aegypti*. Both a formalin-inactivated vaccine and a

Table 21–11. Differential Diagnoses of Chikungunya Fever

Dengue fever
Hantavirus pulmonary syndrome
Other arbovirus infections: } See Table 17–2
O'nyong-nyong
Sindbis
Mayaro
Oropouche } See Table 15–2
Sandfly fever
Lyme disease

Parvovirus B19: Parvovirus B19 causes erythema infectiosum or Fifth disease in infants. In adults, arthritis or anthralgia is common. Fever is not prominent, and other manifestations are lacking except for aplastic crisis in patients with hemolytic anemia

Rheumatic fever: Fever, arthritis, carditis, chorea, and subcutaneous nodules in combination typify the condition

Reiter's syndrome: Fever, arthritis, urethritis, and conjunctivitis are typical of this condition

Coxsackievirus: This virus usually causes minor disease but may cause carditis and viral sepsis with multisystem failure

Mumps: The clinical spectrum spans mild, self-limited febrile illness with parotitis or orchitis to encephalomyelitis, nephritis, pancreatitis, or diabetes

Rubella: Associated with fever, posterior cervical adenopathy, and maculopapular exanthem. Adults frequently have anthralgia, but frank arthritis is uncommon. The disease is self-limited except in the fetus. The embryopathy is significant, with cardiac and central nervous system involvement the most significant

Disseminated gonococcal infection: Fever and a petechial rash that is gram positive along with positive cervical culture are diagnostic

Hepatitis B prodrome: The prodrome is associated with malaise and anorexia. Anthralgia and arthritis may occur, along with glomerulonephritis and a variety of skin lesions (Gianotti-Crosti is classic). Jaundice and abnormal liver function tests are seen

Henoch-Schönlein purpura } See Table 18–5

Rheumatological conditions: Fever, arthritis, carditis, chorea, and subcutaneous nodules in combination typify the conditions

Autoimmune disease: Most patients have gradual onset of fever and joint symptoms. Conditions persist well beyond the time course of CHIK

live attenuated vaccine have been developed. Although the development of neutralizing antibodies has been demonstrated, the efficacy of these vaccines has not been evaluated [51].

Table 21–12. Treatment of Chikungunya Fever

Symptom	Treatment
Fever	Antipyretics. Because of the hemorrhagic potential for CHIK, aspirin and any medicines that inhibit platelet function should be avoided. Bed rest is indicated during the febrile period
Arthralgia	Analgesics and, if needed, mild sedation
Nausea or vomiting	Oral rehydration for fluid losses
Seizures	Anticonvulsants

Related Viruses

O'nyong-nyong (ONN) first appeared in the Acholi province of Uganda. The name derives from an Acholi word meaning "weakening of the joints." The epidemic has affected 2 million people in Africa, usually with an attack rate of over 50% [52]. The mosquito vectors include *Anopheles (An.) funestus* and *An. gambiae*. Fever, arthritis, and a morbilliform rash occur. ONN causes less fever than CHIK but manifests startling lymphadenopathy. The locale is sub-Saharan Africa. Diagnosis is by virus isolation in mice or chick embryo cell culture. Once isolated, identification is by mouse antisera for CHIK and ONN. Hemagglutination inhibition, complement fixation, and neutralization assays document seroconversion.

Sindbis (ockelbo) is the prototype alphavirus and causes predominantly mild or asymptomatic disease. The classic clinical pattern is fever, rash, and arthritis. The virus has been used as a model laboratory virus for studies of viral biology. It is found in Europe, Asia, Africa, and Australia and is transmitted in a natural cycle involving *Culex* mosquitoes and birds that develop viremia but not disease.

Mayaro virus disease manifests with fever, chills, headache, myalgia, arthralgia, and a CHIK-like maculopapular rash as the fever fades. Diagnosis is by virus isolation in Vero cells or paired sera. *Haemagogus* species are the vectors for the disease in Trinidad and Brazil (Fig. 21-7).

For Ross River virus (RRV), the mosquito is the agent for epidemic polyarthritis seen in military personnel and civilians in rural Australia. Clinically, there is sudden onset of joint symptoms, predominantly migratory and polyarticular. Later, there is a rash, usually macular, papular, or both, occasionally with vesiculation of the papules or petechiae. Skin biopsies show mononuclear infiltration and perivascular edema, with extravasation of red blood cells.

Joints show mononuclear cells and highly vacuolated macrophages [8].

Barmah Forest disease occurs in Australia and produces fever, arthritis, and rash. Specific virus identification is necessary to distinguish this virus from RRV; *Culex annulirostris* and *Aedes vigilax* are the mosquito vectors. Treatment is symptomatic and supportive.

Conclusion

The exact time of onset of fever and the severe, incapacitating arthralgia with rash can be noted and recalled in typical CHIK disease. The joint symptoms are striking and may persist for months. Despite the significant joint symptoms, disease tends to be mild and does not appear to be life-threatening [53]. The presence of *Aedes aegypti* and *Aedes albopictus* in the United States raises the risk of future epidemics in warm, wet southern climates. Care is supportive, while prevention is based on vector control and on personal protection from the vector.

OTHER ARBOVIRAL FEVERS

West Nile fever is a mosquito-borne flavivirus found in rural Africa, southern Europe, central and south Asia and has recently been reported in the northeastern United States. A variety of avian and mammalian hosts are involved. *Culex* species are the vector, and birds are amplifying hosts. Following a 3- to 6-day incubation period, small children have a nonspecific febrile illness. Adults have a dengue-like condition with fever, headache, backache, myalgia, lymphadenopathy, and leukopenia. The rash is nonpruritic, maculopapular mainly on the trunk, and resolves without desquamation. Sore throat and gastrointestinal symptoms may occur. Meningeal signs occur infrequently but are more common in the elderly, for whom the disease may prove fatal. Generally, the disease is brief, 3 to 6 days, and self-limited. The diagnosis can be proved by viral isolation during the acute phase. Paired sera can be attempted, but cross-reactions with related flaviviruses limit the usefulness. Weakness and fatigue may persist after the acute phase for 1 to 2 weeks.

Oropouche virus is of the Simbu serogroup of the family Bunyaviridae, genus *Bunyavirus*. It is transmitted by *Culicoides paraensis* midges in Trinidad or northern South America. It causes Oropouche fever, a febrile illness with a good outcome. The symptoms are fever, chills, myalgia, arthralgia, anorexia, headache, dizziness, and photophobia. There is no rash and no hepatosplenomegaly or lymphadenopathy. Leukopenia is common. Diagnosis is by viral isolation or by serological evidence.

GEOGRAPHICAL INCIDENCE

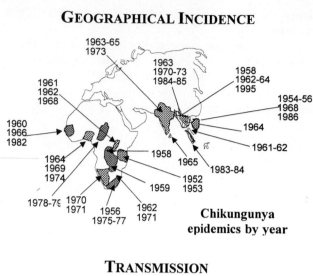

Chikungunya
epidemics by year

TRANSMISSION

**Wild primates
appear to be principal
reservoir for disease**

Humans

**Bite of an
infected mosquito**

**Laboratory-associated
infections can occur
through aerosolization
of the virus**

ZOONOTIC IMPLICATIONS

**Wild primates
(e.g., baboons,
chimpanzees,
monkeys)**

} **Appear to be principal
reservoir for disease**

Aedes sp.

} **Principal vector of disease**

Figure 21–6. Incidence and transmission of Chikungunya fever.

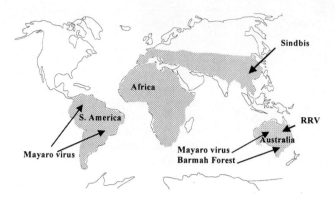

Figure 21–7. Geographical distribution of Mayaro virus.

Phlebotomus (sandfly) fever refers to a group of Bunya viruses that produce similar diseases. Classic disease involves sudden onset of fever, headache, myalgia, photophobia, retroorbital pain, and conjunctival injection. There is an erythematous flush to the skin but not a frank rash. Marked leukopenia with an initial lymphopenia and a protracted neutropenia is seen. The acute phase lasts 2 to 4 days, followed by prolonged weakness and depression. No deaths occur, and sequelae are not described. Diagnosis is presumptive, based on epidemiology in travel, because the viremia is brief. Serological testing is useful to exclude influenza and other arboviral disease.

These conditions occur in Africa, southern Europe, central Asia, and the Americas. These flies are small (2 to 3 mm) midges with limited flight range. They breed in organic debris and leaf litter. The virus is maintained by transovarial mechanisms, permitting survival in adverse climates. The disease is seasonal and occurs primarily in the summer when the female flies are active and biting, principally at night. Prevention involves habitat disinfection, insecticides, and sleeping under fine mesh netting.

Conclusion

These less common conditions are principally identified by classic symptoms, exposure to vectors, and geographic locale.

REFERENCES

1. SC Weaver, A Hagenbaugh, LA Bellow, L Gousset, V Mallampalli, JJ Holland, TW Scott. Evolution of alphaviruses in the eastern equine encephalomyelitis complex. J Virol 68:158–169, 1994.
2. C TenBroeck, EW Hurst, E Traub. Epidemiology of eastern equine encephalomyelitis in the eastern United States. J Exp Med 62:677–685, 1935.

3. LD Fothergill, JH Dingle, S Faber, ML Connerley. Human encephalitis caused by a virus of the eastern variety of equine encephalomyelitis. N Engl J Med 219:411, 1938.

4. Tsai TF. Arboviral infections in the United States. Infect Dis Clin North Am 5:73–102, 1991.

5. LP Levitt, FG Lovejoy, JB Daniels. Eastern equine encephalitis in Massachusetts: first human case in 14 years. N Engl J Med 284:540, 1971.

6. RF Feemster. Outbreak of encephalitis in man due to the eastern virus of equine encephalomyelitis. Am J Public Health 28:1403–1410, 1938.

7. RF Feemster, RE Wheeler, JB Daniels, HD Rose, M Schaeffer, RE Kissling, RO Hayes, ER Alexander, WA Murray. Field and laboratory studies on equine encephalitis. N Engl J Med 259:107–113, 1958.

8. RE Johnston, CJ Peters. Alphaviruses. In: BN Fields, ed. Fields Virology, 3rd ed. Philadelphia: Lippincott-Raven, 1996, pp 843–898.

9. SC Weaver, TW Scott, LH Lorenz, K Lerdthusnee, WS Romoser. Togavirus-associated pathologic changes in the mid gut of a natural mosquito vector. J Virol 62:2083–2090, 1988.

10. DH Clarke. Two nonfatal human infections with the virus of eastern encephalitis. Am J Trop Med Hyg 10:67–70, 1961.

11. MM Przelomski, E O'Rourke, GF Grady, VP Berardi, HG Markley. Eastern equine encephalitis in Massachusetts: a report of 16 cases 1970–1984. Neurology 38:736–739, 1988.

12. FO Bastion, RD Wend, DB Singer, RS Zeller. Eastern equine encephalitis. Histopathologic and ultrastructural changes with isolation of the virus in a human case. Am J Clin Pathol 64:10–13, 1975.

13. TW Scott, SC Weaver. Eastern equine encephalomyelitis virus; epidemiology and evolution of mosquito transmission. Adv Virus Res 37:277–328, 1989.

14. RF Feemster. Equine encephalitis. Public Health 28:1403–1410, 1938.

15. M Goldfild, BF Taylor, JN Welsh. The 1959 outbreak of equine encephalitis in New Jersey. 6. The frequency of prior infection. Am J Epidemiol 87:39–49, 1968.

16. G Teasdale, B Jennett. Assessment of coma and impaired consciousness. A practical scale. Lancet 2:81–84, 1974.

17. CS Hahn, S Lustig, EG Strauss, JH Strauss, RO Hayes. Western equine encephalitis virus is a recombinant virus. Proc Natl Acad Sci USA 85:5997–6001, 1988.

18. RO Hayes. Eastern and western encephalitis. In: GW Beran, ed. Viral Zoonoses. Boca Raton: CRC Press, 1981, pp 29–57.

19. KF Meyer, CM Haring, B Howitt. The etiology of epizootic encephalomyelitis of horses in the San Joaquin Valley. Science 74:227–228, 1931.

20. BF Howitt. Recovery of the virus of equine encephalomyelitis from the brain of a child. Science 88:455–456, 1938.

21. WC Reeves, WM Hammon. Epidemiology of the arthropod-borne viral encephalitides in Kern County California, 1943–1952. Univ Calif Pub Public Health 4:257, 1962.

22. JL Hardy. The ecology of WEE virus in the central valley of California, 1945–1985. Am J Trop Med Hyg 37(suppl): 18S–32S, 1987.

23. TP Monath, CB Cropp, AK Harrison. Mode of entry of a neurotropic arbovirus into the central nervous system. Reinvestigation of an old controversy. Lab Invest 48:399–410, 1983.

24. CDC. Western equine encephalitis—United States and Canada, 1987. MMWR 36:655–659, 1987.

25. KH Finley. Postencephalitis manifestations of viral encephalitides. In: NS Fields, RJ Blattner, eds. Viral Encephalitis. Springfield, IL: Charles C Thomas, 1959, pp 69–91.

26. H Herzon, JT Shelton, HB Bruyn. Sequelae of western equine and other arthropod-borne encephalitides. Neurology 7:535–548, 1957.

27. MP Earnest, HA Goolishian, JR Calverley, RO Hayes, HR Hill. Neurologic, intellectual, and psychologic sequelae following western encephalitis. Neurology 21:969–974, 1971.

28. CH Calisher, AO eL-Kafrawi, MI Al-Deen Mahmud, AP Travassos da Rosa, CR Bartz, M Brummer-Korvenkontio, S Haksohusodo, W Suharyono. Complex-specific immunoglobulin M antibody patterns in humans infected with alphaviruses. J Clin Microbiol 23:155–159, 1986.

29. H Koprowski, HR Cox. Human laboratory infection with Venezuelan equine encephalomyelitis virus. N Engl J Med 236:647–654, 1947.

30. AK Shubladze, SY Gaidmovich, VI Gavrilov. A virological study of laboratory infections with Venezuelan equine encephalomyelitis [Russian]. Vopr Virusol 3:305, 1959.

31. OM Suarez, GH Bergold. Investigations of an outbreak of Venezuelan equine encephalitis in towns of eastern Venezuela. Am J Trop Med Hyg 17:877–880, 1968.

32. AM Powers, MS Oberste, AC Brault, R Rico-Hesse, SM Schmura, JF Smith, W Kang, WP Sweeney, SC Weaver. Repeated emergence of epidemic/epizootic Venezuelan equine encephalitis from a single genotype of enzootic subtype ID virus. J Virol 71:6697–6705, 1997.

33. CE Beck, RW Wyckoff. Venezuelan equine encephalomyelitis. Science 88:530, 1938.

34. V Kubes, FA Rios. The causative agent of infectious equine encephalomyelitis in Venezuela. Science 90:20–21, 1939.

35. C Sanmartin-Barberi, H Groot, E Osborno-Mesa. Human epidemic in Colombia caused by the Venezuelan equine encephalomyelitis virus. Am J Trop Med Hyg 3:283–293, 1954.

36. S de la Monte, F Castro, NJ Bonilla, A Gaskin de Urdaneta, GM Hutchins. The systemic pathology of Venezuelan equine encephalitis virus infection in humans. Am J Trop Med Hyg 34:194–202, 1985.

37. AB Ryzhikov, EI Ryabchikova, AN Sergeev. Spread of Venezuelan equine encephalitis virus in mice olfactory tract. Arch Virol 140:2243–2254, 1995.

38. PC Charles, E Walters, F Margolis, RE Johnston. Mechanism of neuroinvasion of Venezuelan equine encephalitis virus in the mouse. Virology 208:662–671, 1995.

39. AL Rossi. Rural epidemic encephalitis in Venezuela caused

by a group A arbovirus (VEE). Prog Med Virol 9:176–203, 1967.

40. GS Bowen, TR Fashinell, PB Dean, MB Gregg. Clinical aspects of human Venezuelan equine encephalitis in Texas. Bull Pan Am Health Org 10:46–57, 1976.

41. KM Johnson, A Shelokov, PH Peralta, GJ Dammin, NA Young. Recovery of Venezuelan equine encephalomyelitis virus in Panama. A fatal case in man. Am J Trop Med Hyg 17:432–440, 1968.

42. GS Bowen, CH Calisher. Virological and serological studies in Venezuelan equine encephalomyelitis in humans. J Clin Microbiol 4:22–27, 1986.

43. TE Greenway, JH Eldridge, G Ludwig, JK Staas, JF Smith, RM Gilley, SM Michalek. Enhancement of protective immune responses to Venezuelan equine encephalitis (VEE) virus with microencapsulated vaccine. Vaccine 13: 1411–1420, 1995.

44. CC Mathiot, G Grimaud, P Garry, JC Bouquety, A Mada, AM Daguisy, AJ Georges. An outbreak of human Semliki Forest virus infection in Central African Republic. Am J Trop Med Hyg 42:386–393, 1990.

45. MC Robinson. An epidemic of virus disease in Southern Province, Tanganyika Territory, in 1952–1953. Trans R Soc Trop Med Hyg 49:28–32, 1955.

46. DE Carey. Chikungunya and dengue: a case of mistaken identity? J Hist Med 26:243–262, 1971.

47. S Nimmannitya, SB Halstead, SN Cohen, MR Margiotta. Dengue and chikungunya virus infection in man in Thailand, 1962–1964. I. Observations on hospitalized patients with hemorrhagic fevers. Am J Trop Med Hyg 18:954–971, 1969.

48. JG Morrison. Chikungunya fever. Int J Dermatol 18: 628–629, 1979.

49. ED Fourie, JGL Morrison. Rheumatoid arthritis syndrome after chikungunya fever. S Afr Med J 56:130–132, 1979.

50. R Tan, J Meegan, J LeDuc, C Bartz. Enzyme-linked immunosorbent assay for diagnosis of chikungunya disease. Presented at the 34th Annual Meeting of the American Society of Tropical Medicine and Hygiene. Miami, FL, Nov 3–7, 1985.

51. NH Levitt, HH Ramsburg, SE Hasty, PM Repik, FE Cole Jr, HW Lupton. Development of an attenuated strain of chikungunya virus for use in vaccine production. Vaccine 4:157–162, 1986.

52. MC Williams, JP Woodall, JD Gillett. O'nyong-nyong fever: an epidemic virus disease in East Africa. VII. Virus isolations from man and serological studies up to July 1961. Trans R Soc Trop Med Hyg 59:186–197, 1962.

53. JJ Deller, PK Russell. Chikungunya disease. Am J Trop Med Hyg 17:107–111, 1968.

22

Rubella (German Measles)

Lourdes Tamayo
Instituto Nacional de Pediatría, Mexico City, Mexico

Edith Garcia-Gonzalez
Instituto Nacional de Perinatología, Mexico City, Mexico

Tricia J. Brown
University of Oklahoma Health Sciences Center, Oklahoma City, Oklahoma, USA

Rubella, also known as German measles or 3-day measles, is typically a subclinical or inconsequential viral exanthem of childhood. However, the serious potential for teratogenic effects with congenital rubella syndrome makes this infection of great importance to public health.

HISTORY

It is known that early Arabian physicians recognized a rash that presumably was rubella. They considered it to be a variant of measles and referred to it as *al-hamikah*. In 1752 and 1758, Bergen and Orlow, respectively, described rubella as a separate entity from measles. German physicians in the early 1800s called it Rötheln [1]. Warner, in 1829, distinguished this infection from measles and scarlet fever. In 1866, the Scottish physician Henry Veale described 30 cases of this disease and proposed the current name "rubella" [2]. The commonly known name, German measles, was used in several European countries because of the continued interest that Germans had in this disease during the 18th and 19th centuries [3].

In 1938, Hiro and Tasaka, inoculated humans and monkeys with filtered nasal secretions taken from infected individuals and demonstrated the viral etiology of rubella. This infection was considered to be a benign disease until 1941, when Sir Norman McAlister Gregg first linked rubella to congenital cataracts and malformations [4]. This observation was quickly confirmed by others. In 1942, Habel was able to reproduce the disease in monkeys, and in 1953 Krugman isolated the rubella virus from blood. In 1962, two different groups first isolated the virus in tissue cultures. Soon thereafter, the worldwide pandemic of rubella began. In the United States, this resulted in 12 million cases of rubella infection, with 30,000 stillbirths and 20,000 deformed infants caused by congenital rubella. These devastating figures prompted the rapid development of the rubella vaccine, which would soon turn the tables in the fight against this viral disease (Fig. 22–1).

INCIDENCE

This worldwide infection most frequently occurs in the spring months. Epidemics occur every 5 to 7 years. Both sexes are equally affected, although most infections are subclinical. The ratio of subclinical to overt disease is 2:1 [5]. Infection is more frequent in schoolchildren, adolescents, and young adults, but prior to widespread immunization younger children were more often affected [5].

PATHOGENESIS

The rubella virus is transmitted from person to person via inhalation of infected droplets from respiratory secretions.

519

TAXONOMY
Togaviridae family
Rubivirus genus

WORLDWIDE GEOGRAPHICAL DISTRIBUTION

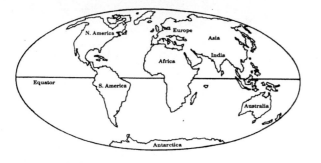

TRANSMISSION

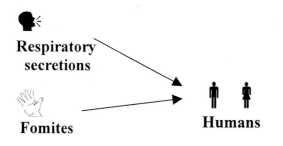

ZOONOTIC IMPLICATIONS

None

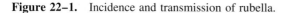

Figure 22–1.   Incidence and transmission of rubella.

Transmission of the secretions by contact and fomites is also possible [3]. Rubella is a moderately communicable infection. In the family setting, less than 50 to 60% of susceptible family members acquire rubella from the infected person [5].

The portal of entry for the rubella virus is primarily the nasopharynx. Viral replication begins in the respiratory

epithelium and then spreads via the lymphatics to regional lymph nodes. Seven to nine days after exposure, viremia develops, and the virus spreads to multiple sites of the body. The extent of viremia peaks immediately before the development of the exanthem, then disappears quickly thereafter. Viral excretion from the nasopharynx persists for 6 days after onset of the exanthem and may continue for up to 13 days after the onset of rash (Fig. 22–2) [6].

CLINICAL MANIFESTATIONS

Rubella produces a mild exanthematous macular rash (Figs. 22–3 to 22–5) except when it is transmitted in utero (7). Subclinical infections represent 50 to 80% of the infections [8]. When eruption is present, it starts on the face and neck with mild pink erythematous macules and papules that spread, fade quickly, and leave no desquamation (Fig. 22–6) [9]. The clinical manifestations of postnatal rubella infection are outlined in Table 22–1. Up to 25 to 40% of rubella patients do not develop a rash [10], and 50 to 80% of infections are clinically inapparent [8]. Lymphadenopathy with prominent enlargement and tenderness, particularly involving the suboccipital and preauricular nodes, is the main prodromal characteristic of rubella infection [11–13]. Forschheimer's sign is also present in 20% of cases; this is an exanthem consisting of dull red petechiae on the soft palate. This manifestation generally appears during the prodromal period or during the first day of the rash [10]. In younger children there is usually no prodrome; in older individuals there is fever, malaise, sore throat, nausea, lymphadenopathy and painful eye movement. Cutaneous petechiae and purpura may develop infrequently with rubella infection [12]. Thrombocytopenic purpura develops in 1 out of 1500 to 3000 cases and more commonly affects children [14,15]. This complication may persist for weeks or even months but typically resolves completely.

Polyarticular arthritis or arthralgias are common complications of infection, more frequently involving adolescent girls and women. These sequelae affect 30% of females and 5% of males [16] and typically begin 1–6 days after the appearance of the rash. Articular symptoms may include pain, swelling, effusions, warmth, erythema, arthritis, and decreased movement of the joint. Joint manifestations may persist for one month up to several months and only rarely lead to chronic arthritis. Rubella virus has been isolated from peripheral blood lymphocytes in women with rubella-associated arthritis [17] and from synovial cells of patients with juvenile rheumatoid arthritis [18].

Complications involving the central nervous system, such as encephalitis, develop in 1 out of 6000 cases and more commonly affect adults [14]. Neurological symp-

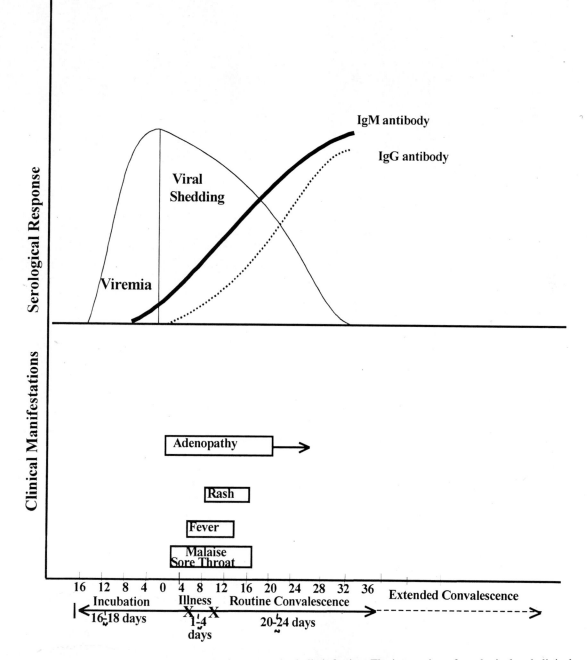

Figure 22–2. Pathogenesis and acquired immunity in postnatal rubella infection. The interaction of serological and clinical manifestations are shown over time. Although IgM antibody expression occurs most rapidly, most of the antibody disappears in less than a year. IgG levels, however, develop more slowly but are associated with lifetime immunity.

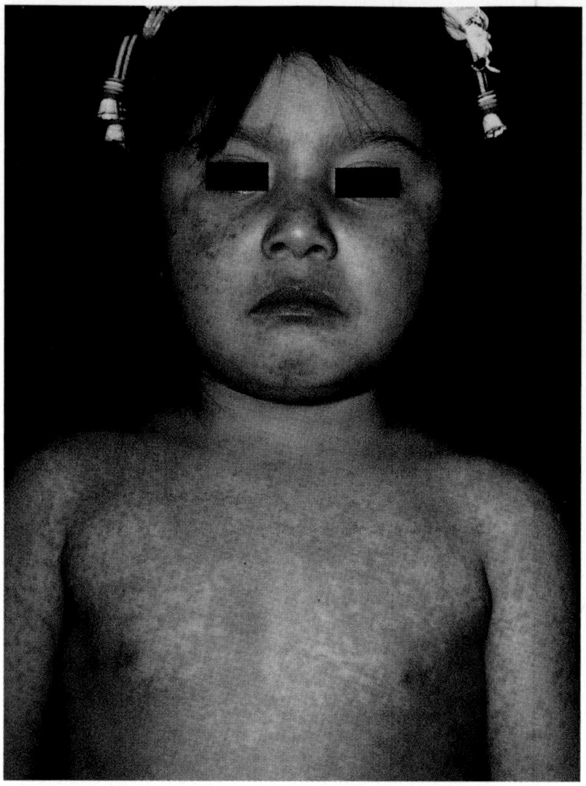

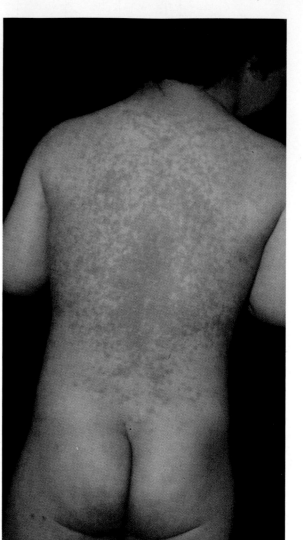

Figure 22–3. Erythematous macules of acute rubella. The exanthem starts on the face and neck. In young children, there is no prodromal syndrome. The lesions are mild, pink, erythematosus macules and papules that spread and fade in 2 or 3 days with no desquamation.

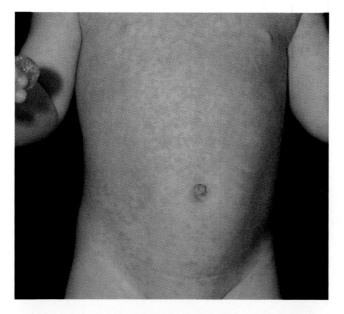

Figure 22–5. Erythematous macules of acute rubella.

Figure 22–4. Erythematous macules of acute rubella.

toms, which may include headache, vomiting, nuchal rigidity, lethargy and seizures, suddenly appear 2 to 6 days after the rash onset in most cases. Encephalitis resulting from rubella is clinically similar to that of measles, although less severe [3]. Examination of the cerebrospinal fluid commonly reveals a mild increase in white blood cells (20 to 100 cells/mm^3), predominantly composed of lymphocytes. The protein concentration may be normal or slightly increased, and the glucose concentration is normal [3]. Rare neurological complications reported in rubella infection include panencephalitis (19,20), optic neuritis (21), peripheral neuritis (22,23), Guillain-Barré syndrome (24), and polyradiculoneuritis associated with encephalitis (25). Potential differential diagnoses are shown in Table 22–2.

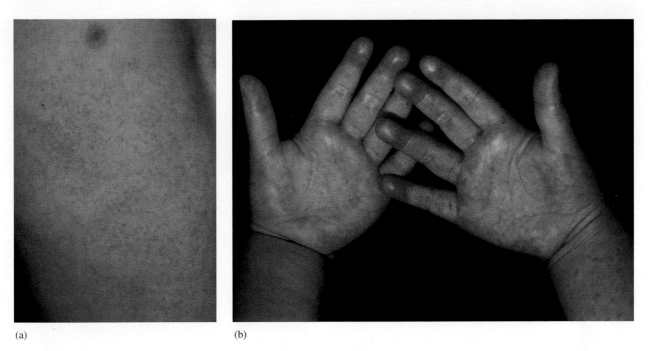

(a)   (b)

Figure 22–6. (a, b) The macular erythematous rash spreads to the trunk and goes to the lower extremities in 24 to 48 hours, as seen here.

Table 22–1. Clinical Manifestations of Rubella (German Measles)

Time after exposure	Clinical manifestations	Laboratory analysis	Other notes
13–15 days	Viral prodrome of low-grade fever and the following symptoms lasting 1–3 days: headache, conjunctivitis, sore throat, rhinitis, malaise, cough, and diffuse lymphadenopathy. Petechiae may be seen on the soft palate at the end of the viral prodrome. ↓	Serological tests, with rubella-specific IgM or a fourfold rise in IgG. Isolation of the virus by nasal or throat swabs	Prodromal period is not always apparent in children Extremely elevated temperature is rare, and patients are not generally ill to a significant degree Tender lymph nodes resolve rapidly, but lymphadenopathy may remain for weeks The rash is not exceptionally distinctive and may look similar to an enteroviral or heat rash
16–18 days	Pink-red maculopapules appear. The rash initially begins on the forehead and spreads down to the face, trunk, and extremities during the first day. Lesions on the trunk may become confluent. The viral prodrome remits quickly after appearance of the rash. ↓		
17–19 days	The facial rash begins to fade. ↓		
18–21 days	The viral exanthem completely disappears after 2 to 3 days. Mild scaling may occur.		

Table 22–2. Differential Diagnoses of Rubella
(German Measles)

Measles: Koplik's spots in the oral cavity, and the viral exanthem lasts 3–5 days. Rubella does not include photophobia, fever is slight or absent, and the rash persists for
no more than 3 days. Lymph node enlargement strongly
supports the diagnosis of rubella

Scarlet fever: Puncate, pinhead-sized yellow-red lesions on
erythematous skin. There is a sandpaper-like quality to
the skin rash. Scarlet fever typically has a significant
postexanthem desquamation, particularly on the hands
and feet

Infectious mononucleosis: Similar to rubella, this disease
may have a diffuse rash and lymph node enlargement but
is distinguished by the characteristic hematological findings

Exanthem subitum (roseola infantum): Rash appears after resolution of the febrile prodromal stage rather than at
the peak of these symptoms

Enteroviral infections: These viral infections may also
cause a diffuse rash but can typically be differentiated by
respiratory and/or gastrointestinal manifestations and the
absence of retroauricular adenopathy

Drug rash: Exanthem may appear similar, but lymphadenopathy is lacking

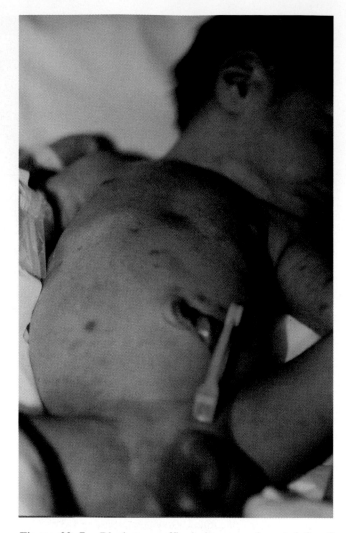

Figure 22–7. Blueberry-muffin lesions are characteristic of
congenital rubella infection (20–50% of affected children), although congenital cytomegalovirus infection can also produce
these lesions. They are areas of extramedullary hematopoiesis
that can be associated with petechiae and purpura.

CONGENITAL RUBELLA SYNDROME

Rubella infection of the embryo or fetus occurs equally
in all races and is most commonly the result of infection
acquired during the first trimester of pregnancy. After Sir
Normal Gregg first linked congenital rubella infection to
cataract formation, the many effects of this syndrome were
recognized during the large rubella pandemic of 1962 to
1965.

Not all infants exposed in utero become infected. In
addition, not all infected infants have signs of disease during the neonatal period. Of all infected neonates, approximately 30% have clinical signs of rubella at birth whereas
nearly 70% have subclinical infections [26].

There is a risk of 65% for congenital rubella if the infection occurs in the first 16 weeks of pregnancy [24]. The skin
manifestations in the immediate neonatal period include
multiple "blueberry-muffin spots" (Fig. 22–7), which are
areas of extramedullary hematopoiesis. These sequelae develop in 20 to 50% of cases [28]. The lesions appear at birth
or during the first 48 hours after birth. They can be macular
or papular and are dark blue, dark red, or blue-grey in
color. These lesions are frequently diffuse but often have
a predilection for the trunk, scalp, and neck [26]. Thrombo-

cytopenia commonly occurs in infants with congenital rubella syndrome, although actual petechiae and purpura are
uncommon [26]. The hair, nails, and mucous membranes
are spared in congenital rubella syndrome, but necrosis of
the inner enamel of the teeth has been described [29].

Visceral abnormalities can be present in up to 75% of
patients with congenital rubella syndrome. The manifestations of congenital rubella syndrome are listed in Table
22–3. The classic triad of congenital rubella syndrome includes cataracts (Fig. 22–8), deafness, and heart defects
(e.g., patent ductus arteriosus). If the mother is infected
with rubella virus before becoming pregnant, the virus is
not transmitted across the placenta. The greatest impact of

Table 22–3. Manifestations of Congenital Rubella Syndrome

Transient Sequelae
Extramedullary hematopoiesis (blueberry-muffin rash)
Diffuse lymphadenopathy
Thrombocytopenia (+/− petechiae, purpura)
Hepatosplenomegaly
Hepatitis
Hyperbilirubinemia and jaundice
Interstitial pneumonitis
Myocarditis
Myositis
Meningoencephalitis
Nephritis
Bony radiolucencies
Hemolytic anemia
Growth retardation (intrauterine and postnatal)

Permanent Sequelae
Ocular defects: cataracts, retinopathy, glaucoma, microphthalmia
Sensorineural hearing loss
Heart defects: patent ductus arteriosus, pulmonary artery stenosis, pulmonary valvular stenosis, ventricular septal defects
Mental retardation, psychomotor retardation, behavior disorders

viral transmission is during the first trimester. If the virus is transmitted after the first trimester, the impact of viral transmission declines until it nearly disappears at 20 weeks of gestation. The interval of viral transmission from the onset of rash in the mother is about 10 days to the placental

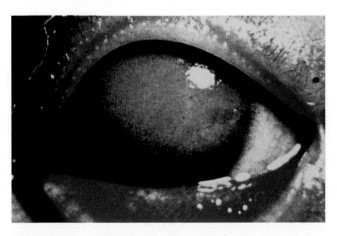

Figure 22–8. Glaucoma and cataracts are seen with the congenital rubella syndrome.

villi and 20–30 days to the fetus. A phylogenetic tree of 61 virus isolates suggested no difference in virulence or teratogenicity among the virus isolates [30]. If infection occurs before the 20th week of gestation, the fetal damage and clinical findings are more severe. These neonates frequently have multiple congenital defects, particularly those of the classic triad, and often are of low birth weight and mentally retarded. Infection acquired after the 20th week of gestation rarely leads to congenital defects [14]. These neonates who are infected in utero after complete organ development often have a different array of manifestations, which may include myocarditis, hepatitis, encephalitis, pneumonitis, or other sequelae. In infants with congenital rubella, the virus can be isolated from peripheral leukocytes, stool, and urine for months to years after birth [12]. These infants are considered infectious for the first 6 to 12 months of life [26]. Sequelae of rubella virus infection include three distinct neurological syndromes: a postinfectious encephalitis following acute infection, a spectrum of neurological manifestations following congenital infections, and progressive rubella panencephalitis (PRP). PRP is an extremely rare neurodegenerative disorder that may follow either congenital or postnatal infection. The pathogenesis of the three neurological syndromes is not understood. There may be an autoimmune reaction triggered by molecular mimicry between viral and host epitopes, as there is an apparent lack of virus in the brain except in cases of PRP [27].

Dermatopathology

There are no specific well-known histopathological findings in rubella infection. Some examined cases have shown a sparse superficial perivascular infiltrate of atypical lymphocytes (Türk's cells) with mild spongiosis [31].

Laboratory Findings

Leukopenia may be present early and may be followed by an increase in plasma cells or atypical lymphocytes. Little is known about the cellular immune response to rubella virus structural proteins, although both helper T-lymphocyte proliferation and cytotoxic T-lymphocyte responses occur during viral infections [32]. Most rubella virus infections produce lifelong immunity mediated by circulating antibodies and specific T lymphocytes [33].

Diagnosis

The most definitive form of diagnosis is made by isolation of the rubella virus in sensitive tissue culture. Throat or nasal swabs can readily isolate the virus for 6 days before or after the onset of the viral exanthem [34]. In infants with congenital rubella syndrome, virus can be isolated from the nasopharynx, conjunctivae, urine, feces, blood buffy coat, and cerebrospinal fluid.

Despite the accuracy of viral isolation, most cases of rubella are diagnosed by serological testing. A fourfold rise of rubella-specific IgG in sequential serum samples taken during the acute and convalescent phases (at least 1–2 weeks apart) is diagnostic of rubella infection. Some experts recommend drawing the convalescent phase serum at least 28 days after exposure [14]. For those patients who do not present sufficiently early in the course of disease, the presence of rubella-specific IgM is diagnostic of recent infection. Rubella-specific IgM becomes detectable quickly after the rash onset, and testing for this antibody can be done as early as 1–2 days after the appearance of the rash [14]. The rubella-specific antibodies can be identified by complement fixation, hemagglutination-inhibition, immunofluorescence, enzyme-linked immunosorbent assay, or platelet aggregation [35–39]. Hemagglutination-inhibition testing has been the predominant screening method for rubella antibodies in the past, but enzyme-linked immunosorbent assay and other newer methods are now more commonly employed [14]. The presence of IgM and the persistence of IgG antibody in neonates are both indicative of congenital infection [10]. If exposure to rubella is suspected in a pregnant woman with uncertain rubella immunity, serological testing should be performed close to the time of exposure. If the woman already has antibodies to rubella, she is considered immune. If no rubella antibody is detected on serological examination, the test should be repeated in 3–4 weeks. Seroconversion at that time would confirm exposure to rubella, and information regarding the risks and alternative approaches for congenital rubella syndrome should be discussed with the mother [40].

Treatment and Prophylaxis

Antiviral agents such as amantadine and interferon have been tried in some cases of rubella infection with equivocal results at best. The mainstay of treatment for this condition continues to be supportive therapy (Table 22–24). Infected individuals should refrain from exposure to others for 7 days after the onset of the rash because of infectivity.

Because no antiviral treatment is available for rubella, widespread vaccination has been a priority. The World Health Organization set the goal to eliminate indigenous measles and congenital rubella in Europe by the end of the year 2000; however, some outbreaks have continued to occur. The immunization of children and susceptible

Table 22–4. Treatment of Rubella Infection

Symptom	Treatment
Pruritus	Starch baths or antipruritics
Arthritis in adults	Aspirin or nonsteroidal antiinflammatory drugs and bed rest, if needed
Encephalopathy or encephalitis	Maintenance of fluids and electrolytes and other supportive care

women of child-bearing age is now a standard public health measure.

Several live-attenuated rubella vaccines have been used since 1966. The rubella vaccine is typically given as part of the combined MMR (measles, mumps, rubella) vaccine in childhood. One vaccine dose, usually given between 12–15 months of age, generally confers durable immunity against rubella. However, most experts recommend giving a second dose at 4–6 years of age [14]. Immunity after two vaccine doses is considered to be long-lasting, and waning immunity with increased susceptibility to rubella has not been observed in long-term surveillance [41]. Infants with colds or upper respiratory infections at the time of immunization have a significant seroconversion failure rate [42]. Interferon induced by a concomitant viral illness may be responsible for the vaccine failure. However, it is currently recommended that immunization be postponed for persons with severe illnesses only and not for those with minor illnesses [14].

Rubella vaccination is contraindicated in the following situations: pregnancy; persons on systemic corticosteroids for more than 2 weeks; leukemic or immunosuppressed patients; recipients of immune globulin treatment other than anti-Rho(D) therapy during the previous 3 months or in the following 2 weeks; and those with a history of anaphylactic reaction to neomycin [14].

Conclusion

Although widespread rubella immunization has significantly diminished the frequency of occurrence of this disease, many developing countries continue to have epidemics and high rates of infection because of the lack of vaccine availability. Although most cases of rubella are subclinical or insignificant, the possibility of fetal involvement with congenital rubella syndrome demands accurate diagnosis and monitoring of all potential infections.

REFERENCES

1. JA Forbes. Rubella: historical aspects. Am J Dis Child 118: 5–11, 1969.

2. C Wesselhoeft. Rubella (German measles). N Engl J Med 236:943–950; 978–988, 1947.

3. JD Cherry. Rubella virus. In: RD Feigin, JD Cherry, eds. Textbook of Pediatric Infectious Diseases, 4th ed. Philadelphia: WB Saunders, 1998, pp 1922–1949.

4. NM Gregg. Congenital cataract following German measles in the mother. Trans Ophthalmol Soc Aust 3:35–46, 1941.

5. CF Phillips. Viral infections and those presumed to be caused by virus. In: RE Behrman, RM Kliegman, WE Nelson, VC Vaughan III, eds. Nelson Textbook of Pediatrics, 14th ed. Philadelphia: Saunders, 1992, pp 795–796.

6. RH Green, MR Balsamo, JP Giles, S Krugman, GS Mirick. Studies of the natural history and prevention of rubella. Am J Dis Child 110:348–365, 1965.

7. IJ Friedman, NS Penneys. Viral infections. In: Schachner LA, Hausen RC, eds. Pediatric Dermatology, 2nd ed. New York: Churchill Livingstone, 1995, pp 1371–1413.

8. DM Horstmann. Rubella. In: AS Evans, ed. Viral infections of Humans. Epidemiology and Control. New York: Plenum, 1976, p 409.

9. BR Krafchik. Viral exanthems. In: J Harper, A Oranje, N Prose, eds. Textbook of Pediatric Dermatology. London: Blackwell Science Ltd, 2000, pp 329–351.

10. JC Sterling, JB Kurtz. Viral infections. In: RH Champion, JL Burton, DA Burns, SM Breathnach, eds. Textbook of Dermatology, 6th ed. Malden, MS: Blackwell Science, 1998, pp 995–1095.

11. SE Gellis. Rubella (German measles). In: TB Fitzpatrick, AZ Eisen, K Wolff, IM Freedberg, KF Austen, eds. Dermatology in General Medicine, 4th ed. New York, NY: McGraw-Hill Inc, 1993, pp 2513–2515.

12. Viral infections. In: WL Weston, AT Lane, JG Morelli, eds. Color Textbook of Pediatric Dermatology, 2nd ed. St. Louis: Mosby Year Book, 1996, pp 97–130.

13. EH Tschen, HC Burgdoff. Diseases due to viruses. In: P Ruiz-Maldonado, LC Parish, JM Beare, eds. Textbook of Pediatric Dermatology. Philadelphia: Grune & Stratton, 1989, pp 441–457.

14. Centers for Disease Control and Prevention. Measles, mumps, and rubella—vaccine use and strategies for elimination of measles, rubella, and congenital rubella syndrome and control of mumps: recommendations of the Advisory Committee on Immunization Practices (ACIP). MMWR 47(No. RR-8):4–8, 1998.

15. K Ueda, F Sasaki, K Tokugawa, K Segawa, H Fujii. The 1976–1977 rubella epidemic in Fukuoka city in southern Japan: epidemiology and incidences of complications among 80,000 persons who were school children at 28 primary schools and their family members. Biken J 27: 161–168, 1984.

16. J Fry, JB Dillane, L Fry. Rubella. BMJ 2:833–834, 1962.

17. JK Chantler, DK Ford, AJ Tingle. Persistent rubella infection and rubella-associated arthritis. Lancet 1:1323–1325, 1982.

18. JR Fraser, AL Cunningham, K Hayes, R Leach, B Lunt. Rubella arthritis in adults. Isolation of virus, cytology and other aspects of synovial reaction. Clin Exp Rheumatol 1: 287–293, 1983.

19. JS Wolinsky. Rubella virus and its effect on the developing nervous system. In: RT Johnson, G Lyon, eds. Virus Infections and the Developing Nervous System. Boston, MA: Kluwer Academic Publishers, 1988, pp 125–142.

20. JS Wolinsky, PC Dau, E Buimovici-Klein, J Mednick, BO Berg, PB Lang, LZ Cooper. Progressive rubella panencephalitis: immunovirological studies and results of Isoprinosine therapy. Clin Exp Immunol 35:397–404, 1979.

21. JH Connolly, WM Hitchinson, IV Allen, JA Lyttle, MW Swallow, E Dermott, D Thomsom. Carotid artery thrombosis, encephalitis, myelitis, and optic neuritis associated with rubella virus infections. Brain 98:583–594, 1975.

22. EW Witney. Neuritis following rubella (Letter). BMJ 1: 831, 1940.

23. GM Hodges. Neuritis following rubella (Letter). BMJ 1: 830–831, 1940.

24. AA Saeed, LS Lange. Guillain-Barré syndrome after rubella. Postgrad Med J 54:333–334, 1978.

25. DI Chang, JH Park, KC Chung. Encephalitis and polyradiculoneuritis following rubella virus infection—a case report. J Korean Med Sci. 12:168–170, 1997.

26. AM Wagner, RC Hansen. Neonatal skin and skin disorders. In: LA Schachner, RC Hausen, eds. Pediatric Dermatology, 2nd ed. New York: Churchill Livingstone, 1995, pp 263–346.

27. TK Frey. Neurological aspect of rubella virus infection. Intervirology 40:167–175, 1997.

28. ED McIntosh, MA Menser. A fifty-year follow-up of congenital rubella. Lancet 340:414–415, 1992.

29. G Tondury, DW Smith. Fetal rubella pathology. J Pediatr 68:867–879, 1966.

30. S Katow. Rubella virus genome diagnosis during pregnancy and mechanism of congenital rubella. Intervirology 41: 163–169, 1998.

31. ZM Khan, CJ Cockerell. Cutaneous viral infections. In: RL Barnhill, ed. Textbook of Dermatopathology. New York, NY: McGraw-Hill, 1998, pp 439–456.

32. D Ou, P Chong, O Tripet, S Gillam. Analysis of T- and B-cell epitopes of capsid protein of rubella virus by using synthetic peptides. J Virol 66:1674–1681, 1992.

33. T Zhang, CO Mauracher, LA Mitchell, AJ Tingle. Detection of rubella virus-specific immunoglobulin G (IgG), IgM and IgA antibodies by immunoblot assays. J Clin Microbiol 30: 824–830, 1992.

34. WJ Davis, HE Larson, JP Simarian, PD Parkman, HM Meyer Jr. A study of rubella immunity and resistance to infection. JAMA 215:600–608, 1971.

35. JL Sever, RJ Huebner, A Fabiyi, GR Monif, GA Castellano, CL Cusumano, RG Traub, AC Ley, MR Gilkeson, JM Roberts. Antibody responses in acute and chronic rubella. Proc Soc Exp Biol Med 122:513–516, 1966.

36. GL Stewart, PD Parkman, HE Hopps, RD Douglas, JP Hamilton, HM Meyer Jr. Rubella-virus hemagglutination-inhibition test. N Engl J Med 276:554–557, 1967.

37. A Vaheri, T Vesikari. Small size rubella virus antigens and soluble immune complexes: analysis by the platelet aggregation technique. Arch Gesamte Virusforsch 35:10–24, 1971.

38. GC Brown, HF Maassab, JA Veronelli, TJ Francis Jr. Rubella antibodies in human serum. Detection by the indirect fluorescent-antibody technic. Science 145:943–945, 1964.

39. M Vejtorp, E Fanoe, J Leerhoy. Diagnosis of postnatal rubella by the enzyme-linked immunosorbent assay for rubella IgM and IgG antibodies. Acta Pathol Microbiol Scand 87: 155–160, 1979.

40. American Academy of Pediatrics. Rubella. In: G Peter, ed. 1994 Red Book: Report of the Committee on Infectious Diseases, 23rd ed. Elk Grove Village, IL: American Academy of Pediatrics, 1994, p 406.

41. CE Johnson, ML Kumar, J Whitwell, BO Staehle, LP Rome, C Dinakar, W Hurni, DR Nalin. Antibody persistence after primary measles-mumps-rubella vaccine and response to a second dose given at four to six vs. eleven to thirteen years. Pediatr Infect Dis J 15:687–692, 1996.

42. MS Krober, CE Stracener, JW Bass. Decreased measles antibody response after measles-mumps-rubella vaccine in infants with colds. JAMA 265:2095–2096, 1991.

23

Hepatitis Viruses

A. Michele Hill
Kansas University School of Medicine, Kansas City, Kansas, USA

Catherine C. Newman and Sharon S. Raimer
University of Texas Medical Branch, Galveston, Texas, USA

Tricia J. Brown
University of Oklahoma Health Sciences Center, Oklahoma City, Oklahoma, USA

Viral hepatitis is a worldwide health problem of immense proportions caused by several distinct DNA and RNA viruses, with the incidence of disease varying significantly among different populations (Fig. 23–1). This condition is most commonly caused by one of three viruses: hepatitis A virus (HAV), hepatitis B virus (HBV), or hepatitis C virus (HCV). Hepatitis D (HDV) and hepatitis E (HEV) occur less frequently and, to date, are not associated with any specific cutaneous findings. Hepatitis G virus (HGV) has been discovered more recently, but its role in hepatitis is not well established [1]. Other viruses that are known to cause hepatitis rarely include herpes simplex virus, cytomegalovirus, Epstein-Barr virus, varicella-zoster virus, and yellow fever virus.

This chapter focuses primarily on hepatitis viruses B and C, since the predominant cutaneous manifestations occur in these diseases. Hepatitis A virus infection may occasionally (less than 14% of cases) produce a transient, discrete, maculopapular, urticarial, or petechial rash that develops in the prodromal period [2,3]. Papular acrodermatitis of childhood has been described in association with HAV in at least one case [4]. On rare occasions, persistent cholestatic hepatitis A infection may develop as cryoglobulinemia with cutaneous vasculitis [5–7]. A similar vasculitis during the acute phase of an HAV infection has been reported in a 2-year-old child [8]. HDV may coinfect individuals (along with HBV) or superinfect carriers of hepatitis B surface antigen (HBsAg). Because HDV infection requires concurrent involvement with HBV, dermatological manifestations with this infection are similar to those for HBV infection [9]. HEV infection has a high rate of associated disseminated intravascular coagulation, and cutaneous signs of this disorder may be evident [10]. Although HGV has been found in a large proportion of HCV-infected individuals, several different studies have determined that this virus plays no role in the pathogenesis of mixed cryoglobulinemia [11,12], vasculitis [13], or other extrahepatic manifestations [14].

HEPATITIS B VIRUS (HBV)

Definition

HBV is caused by an antigenically complex deoxyribonucleic acid (DNA) virus, which is transmitted mainly percutaneously or sexually in Western countries but primarily by the perinatal route in the Far East and in Africa (Fig. 23–2). The intact virion of HBV, known as the Dane particle, is composed of double-stranded DNA that contains the core antigen (HBcAg). The "e" antigen (HBeAg) is

GEOGRAPHICAL INCIDENCE

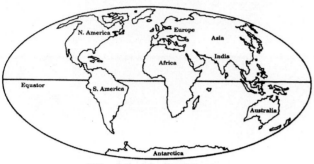

Worldwide Incidence

TAXONOMY
Picornaviridae family (hepatitis A virus)
Hepadnaviridae family (hepatitis B virus)
Flaviviridae family
　　Hepacivirus genus (hepatitis C virus)
Deltaviridae family (hepatitis D virus)
Caliciviridae family (hepatitis E virus)
Flaviviridae family (hepatitis G virus)

Figure 23–1.　Incidence and taxonomy of viral hepatitis.

closely associated with hepatitis B infectivity, whereas the surface antigen (HBsAg) consists of various antigens, which allows for subtyping.

History

Hepatitis with associated jaundice has been a recognized clinical entity since antiquity, although the differentiation of the various causes is a more recent event. Lürman, in 1885, first suggested that parenteral inoculation and icterus were associated with hepatitis [15]. He noted that almost 200 shipyard workers in Germany developed jaundice between 2 and 8 months after they received smallpox vaccination prepared from a human lymph node. Through the years, several other outbreaks of hepatitis were found to be associated with inoculation of products derived from human sources or containing human blood [16–22]. These cases were eventually grouped together and termed homologous serum jaundice [23]. The nature of HBV was serendipitously discovered in 1965, while researchers were investigating serum protein polymorphisms in multiply transfused hemophiliacs from around the world [24]. Blumberg and colleagues [24] found a unique antigen, initially termed the Australia antigen, which is now known

GEOGRAPHICAL INCIDENCE

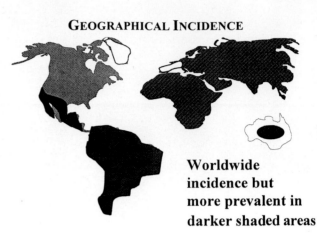

Worldwide incidence but more prevalent in darker shaded areas

TRANSMISSION

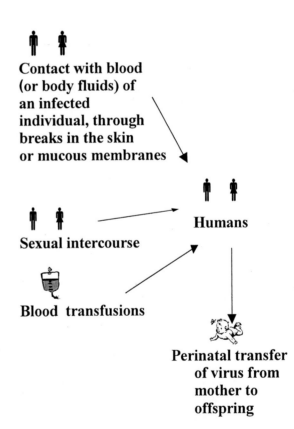

Contact with blood (or body fluids) of an infected individual, through breaks in the skin or mucous membranes

Sexual intercourse

Blood transfusions

Humans

Perinatal transfer of virus from mother to offspring

ZOONOTIC IMPLICATIONS

None

Figure 23–2.　Incidence and transmission of hepatitis B virus.

as the hepatitis B surface antigen (HBsAg). This antigen was later found to be associated with hepatitis, particularly post-transfusion cases [25–27]. Subsequent studies begun in the 1950s at the Willowbrook State School in New York have further broadened our knowledge and understanding of HBV [28–32].

Incidence

The World Health Organization estimates that there are approximately 350 million carriers of HBV worldwide, with over 1 million deaths each year caused by hepatocellular carcinoma or HBV-associated cirrhosis. Five to fifteen percent of the world's population shows evidence of exposure to HBV. However, the seroprevalence of HBV varies markedly throughout the world [33]. The majority of cases occur in China, sub-Saharan Africa, and other developing countries. Prevalence in the United States has remained at 5% since the 1970s [34]. Approximately 140,000 to 320,000 infections occur each year in the United States; of these infections, 70,000 to 160,000 are symptomatic. Of all HBV infections in the United States, 8000 to 32,000 chronic infections occur each year and 5000 to 6000 deaths occur each year from chronic liver disease, including primary liver cancer. Infections with HBV cost an estimated $700 million each year. In most countries, lower socioeconomic status correlates with higher HBV seroprevalence.

Pathogenesis

The predominant mode of HBV transmission varies with location. In Asia, approximately half of infections are acquired perinatally. However, in Africa and other developing countries, the virus is more often acquired during the first decade of life, with exposure to infected family members or other children. HBV is commonly transmitted through sexual intercourse as well. In industrialized nations, such as the countries of Europe and the United States, HBV is usually acquired through sexual exposure or intravenous drug use. Prior to universal screening of blood, transfusions were a prominent source of infection. Transmission of the virus may occur from infected persons to health care workers, tattoo recipients, barbers, and others if appropriate preventive and protective measures are not employed [35]. It is estimated that 30% of percutaneous exposures to HBV in nonimmunized people lead to seroconversion [36]. In addition to its presence in blood, HBsAg has been found in various body fluids, including semen, saliva, tears, urine, and in impetiginous skin lesions [37]. However, HBV infection only rarely develops after exposure to these other body fluids.

Liver injury with HBV infection varies from minimal hepatocellular injury and subclinical illness to extensive parenchymal involvement with subsequent liver failure. HBV does not appear to be directly cytopathic to hepatocytes [38]. On the contrary, evidence suggests that the clinical manifestations are determined by the immunological responses of the host. After ingestion or inoculation, the virus reaches the liver and enters an incubation period, during which extensive virus replication occurs within the hepatocytes.

During infection, hepatitis B virions are present in highest concentrations in the blood and liver. Rather than exerting a direct cytopathic effect on infected hepatocytes, HBV alters the antigenic structure of the membrane of infected cells. Minute quantities of HBsAg, HBcAg, and HBeAg combine with HLA class I antigens on the cell surface of infected cells and act as a target. This results in an immune response against the HBV-infected cells, which involves both B and T lymphocytes. It is primarily the sensitized cytotoxic T lymphocytes and other components of the cell-mediated immune system that are considered responsible for destruction and necrosis of infected cells.

The extent of the necrosis may vary with the degree of immune response and may also vary depending on the particular subtype of virus with which a person is infected. Chronic hepatitis develops when there is failure of the T lymphocytes to respond adequately to infected hepatocytes and HBsAg is not cleared. The presence of neutralizing antibody to HBsAg strongly correlates with the development of immunity to HBV.

Clinical Manifestations

Acute HBV may be symptomatic or asymptomatic. Asymptomatic infection is common in neonates and young children. Adults and adolescents usually develop symptoms. Only 25% develop jaundice. The remainder display milder and less prolonged symptoms. When symptomatic, acute HBV infection consists of five phases: (1) incubation, (2) prodrome, (3) icteric, (4) convalescent, and (5) a possible chronic disease phase. The clinical course of HBV is outlined in Table 23–1. The majority of asymptomatic carriers have mild infection, although the risk of cirrhosis is significant in those with evidence of active viral replication. During the icteric phase, the physical examination may reveal hepatomegaly with a tender liver edge and splenomegaly. In less than 1% of adults, fulminant hepatitis occurs and manifests as hepatic encephalopathy with marked prolongation of the prothrombin time. Chronic hepatitis occurs when liver enzyme elevation and serological evidence of viral hepatitis persist 6 months following the acute infection. Overall, the risk of chronic infection in immunocompetent adults is less than 5% [39]. Approxi-

Table 23–1.   Clinical Manifestations of Hepatitis B

Time after exposure	Clinical manifestations	Laboratory analyses	Other notes
4 months (ranges from 2–6 months)	Insidious onset of prodromal period, with nonspecific symptoms of anorexia, nausea and vomiting, right upper quadrant abdominal pain, fever, headache, malaise, fatigue, myalgia, coryza, and/or perversions of taste or smell. 10% of patients may have a serum-sickness like illness, with fever, malaise, urticaria, and symmetrical small joint arthritis	Serological assays, with detection of HBsAg, HBcAg, and others. Detection of HBV DNA in serum (although this method is not widely available)	Minimal symptoms may be present during the prodrome. Fewer then 50% of patients experience a prodromal period
	↓		
4 months and 10 days	Progression to the jaundice phase, with subsidence of prodromal symptoms shortly thereafter. A yellowish discoloration of the skin, sclera, conjunctiva, and mucous membranes becomes evident. The stools turn pale, and urine becomes dark		Approximately 50% of patients remain anicteric. Less than 0.5% of cases develop fulminant hepatitis, with encephalopathy, coagulopathy, and fluid electrolyte imbalance, which has a high rate of mortality
	↓		
4 months and 2–3 weeks	Jaundice and symptoms begin to fade, and convalescence begins. Increased fatigue may persist for months		
	↓		
5 months	The majority of cases are completely resolved		Some patients have persistent antigenemia and elevated liver enzymes, with or without associated symptoms

mately 30% of children under the age of 6 develop chronic infection, while up to 90% of neonates have chronic HBV. Males and/or patients with impaired immunity, such as organ transplant recipients or human immunodeficiency virus/(HIV)-infected persons, also have a greater risk of chronic infection. In 15 to 20% of persons with evidence of active viral replication, cirrhosis develops within 5 years [40–42]. Patients with chronic HBV infection, particularly with cirrhosis, have a 100- to 200-fold increased risk for the development of hepatocellular carcinoma. Approximately 2.5% of patients with chronic HBV infection develop these slow-growing tumors each year.

Cutaneous Findings in Acute HBV Infection

The majority of the skin findings in early hepatitis other than those of papular acrodermatitis of childhood appear to be caused by the development of immune complexes involving HBsAg. It is known that a state of antigen excess produces soluble antigen-antibody complexes that are pathogenic for tissue. Antigen (HBsAg) appears prior to the onset of symptoms. As the individual begins to develop antibodies, symptoms begin to appear. As the titer of antibody rises, the immune complexes formed become less soluble and are cleared rapidly from the circulation. This is paralleled by a decrease in symptoms and clinical findings.

Serum Sickness-like Syndrome

The most common skin eruption associated with HBV infection has been described as a serum sickness-like illness that generally occurs in the prodromal period of the disease [43,44]. It occurs in 20 to 30% of patients infected with HBV and may be the sole manifestation of the disease. This syndrome consists most commonly of urticaria, angioedema, arthropathy, lymphadenopathy, and proteinuria or hematuria. The onset is usually 1 to 6 weeks prior to the commencement of jaundice and it frequently improves or clears when jaundice appears. The articular involvement generally manifests as arthralgia or arthritis involving the small joints of the hands, the shoulders, knees, and ankles [45]. The duration of joint symptoms usually lasts 20 days. The dermatological manifestations are varied but urticaria is the most common, although its appearance may be somewhat atypical. Angioedema occurs in approximately 4% of patients. Renal involvement is less frequent than the articular and dermatological manifestations and is commonly mild with complete resolution. The serum sickness–like syndrome is attributable to the deposition of circulating immune complexes involving HBsAg on endothelial surfaces. The clinical manifestations are produced by the subsequent activation of complement and the induction of an inflammatory response.

Gianotti-Crosti Syndrome

Papular acrodermatitis of childhood (Gianotti-Crosti syndrome) is another skin eruption frequently associated with HBV infection in areas of the world with a relatively high incidence of hepatitis B, such as Europe and Japan. This eruption is seen most frequently in young children between the ages of 1 and 6 years and rarely after the age of 10, although its occurrence has been recorded in young adults. In this disease the papules, usually 2–5 mm in diameter, frequently erupt first on the buttocks and thighs, and then generally extend to involve the arms, legs, face, and ears, with relative sparing of the trunk (Fig. 23–3). Koebnerization of the papules frequently occurs. The eruption tends to be relatively persistent but generally clears by the 11th week. Papular acrodermatitis of childhood is not a specific skin finding for hepatitis B infection, although in southern

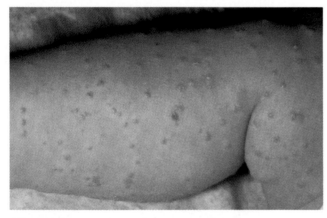

(a)

Figure 23–3. (a) Skin eruption of papular acrodermatitis of childhood (Gianotti-Crosti syndrome) on the legs of infants. Note that some of the papules appear to be slightly umbilicated, which is a frequent finding in this eruption. (b) The papules have coalesced above the knee. (c) This close-up view shows the papules on the dorsal hand.

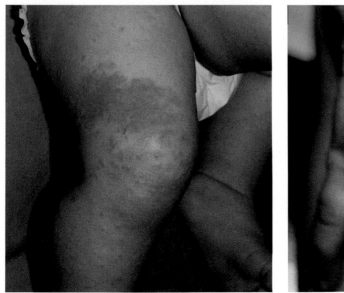

(b)

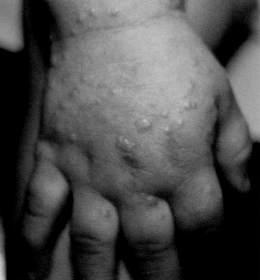

(c)

Europe, the majority of cases appear to be associated with hepatitis B, subtype ayw. The eruption is seen most frequently with an anicteric form of the disease. In the United States, this eruption has more commonly been associated with viral infections other than hepatitis [46].

Others

In addition to the serum sickness–like manifestations, nonspecific macular and maculopapular eruptions, a scarlatiniform rash, petechiae, palpable purpura and Henoch-Schönlein type purpura, erythema multiforme, erythema nodosum, and a lichenoid dermatitis have all been described in the acute phase of HBV infection [47–49]. There have also been two reported cases of localized angioedema of the tongue, which for 6 months was the sole manifestation of the infection [50].

Cutaneous Findings in Chronic HBV Infection

About 5% of patients with hepatitis B fail to clear HBsAg from the blood and become chronic carriers. Patients with defects in their cell-mediated immunity appear to be at greater risk for chronic hepatitis. The most common skin lesions associated with chronic hepatitis are those seen with mixed cryoglobulinemia and polyarteritis nodosa (PAN).

Mixed Cryoglobulinemia

Mixed cryoglobulinemia, which recent evidence suggests is more often associated with HCV than with HBV [50], is thought to be caused by immune complexes that have the physical characteristics of precipitating at temperatures below 37°C. The cryoglobulin precipitates have a mixed pattern, with almost equal amounts of IgG and IgM [51]. Symptoms of cryoglobulinemia associated with hepatitis include purpuric skin lesions (95%), arthropathy (45%), and renal disease (48%) [43]. Patients without nephritis generally have a protracted but benign course, whereas those with renal involvement may have a rapidly deteriorating course. Palpable purpura or small vessel vasculitis is the most common dermatological finding and usually begins on the lower extremities. The condition initially appears as erythematous palpable papules and plaques that do not completely blanch when pressure is applied. Lesions may develop vesicles or bullae. Over the next 1–3 days, plaques without bullae flatten and become purplish in color. Bullae, when present, generally rupture and result in ulcerations. Lesions frequently appear in crops, so that lesions of different ages may be present in the same patient. Other findings may include Raynaud's phenomenon, urticaria, livedo reticularis, and acrocyanosis [52]. An acquired

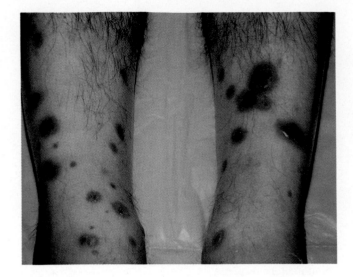

Figure 23–4. Small vessel vasculitis (palpable purpura) on the legs of a 37-year-old man with HBV infection.

form of cold-induced urticaria has been reported in association with hepatitis B and cryoglobulins [53]. Cold sensitivity, however, is clinically apparent in fewer than half of the patients with cryoglobulinemia. Small-vessel vasculitis manifesting as palpable purpura may also be associated with hepatitis in the absence of demonstrable cryoglobulinemia (Fig. 23–4).

Polyarteritis Nodosa (PAN)

It has been estimated that 1 in 200 to 1 in 500 HBV infections result in PAN. In a 1991 report, PAN appeared to be caused by HBV in 30 to 50% of cases, when the standard polyclonal radioimmunoassay for HBsAg was used for antigen detection. When the more sensitive monoclonal radioimmunoassay was used, along with studies to detect HBV DNA sequences, the percentage of PAN cases associated with HBV infection seemed to be much higher [54]. However, since the development of an HBV vaccine, there has been a dramatic decrease in the number of new cases. A 1995 report indicated that HBV-related PAN represented only 7–8% of PAN vasculitidies [55].

PAN is a systemic vasculitis that develops less than 6 months after infection with HBV, and it may be the initial manifestation of the infection. The vasculitis is not an antineutrophil cytoplasmic antibody (ANCA)–related disease, as is classic PAN. However, it appears to be an immune complex-mediated event and may be caused by decreased clearance of immune complexes by the reticuloendothelial system [55]. PAN affects both medium and small arteries in various organs of the body, including the kidneys, central

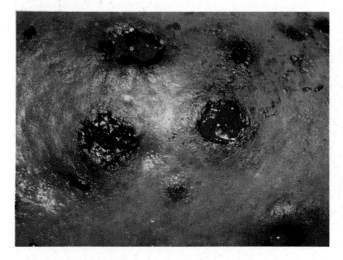

Figure 23–5. Cutaneous lesions of polyarteritis nodosa on the calf of the leg. Lesions began as tender nodules that progressed to painful ulcerations.

nervous system, and skin. This form of PAN is characterized by fever, polyarthralgia, calf pain, and systemic complaints related to involved organ systems. Dermatological manifestations in PAN occur in about 10–15% of cases [56]. The most common skin finding is tender subcutaneous nodules approximately 1–2 cm in diameter on the lower extremities. These nodules may progress to painful ulcerations (Fig. 23–5). Livedo may be present, and occasionally urticarial lesions and angioedema are seen. With end artery involvement, acral gangrene is a common finding.

A cutaneous form of PAN without apparent systemic involvement has been described in association with HBV [57]. This entity probably represents part of the spectrum of PAN rather than a separate disease, because cutaneous PAN may sometimes progress to systemic disease many years after the initial more limited involvement.

In addition, several nonspecific skin manifestations may be seen with acute fulminant hepatitis or from extensive liver damage from chronic hepatitis. These include findings such as jaundice, pruritus, spider nevi, palmar erythema, and purpura.

Dermatopathology

There are few reports in the literature of histopathological studies on skin eruptions accompanying early hepatitis infection. Specimens from one series of patients demonstrated a primarily lymphocytic venulitis with focal necrosis in patients with urticarial and maculopapular eruptions [47]. Histologically, the lesions of the serum sickness–like

prodrome may show a neutrophilic vasculitis of small vessels with immune complexes involving HBsAg, IgG, IgM, and C3 when studied by direct immunofluorescence. Histopathological studies of papular acrodermatitis of childhood (PAC) reveal a superficial perivascular lymphocytic infiltrate with some mild endothelial swelling (Fig. 23–6). Direct immunofluorescence of skin lesions of PAC is negative, and there is no evidence of vasculitis [58]. Skin lesions of palpable purpura associated with mixed cryoglobulinemia show a leukocytoclastic vasculitis of small vessels that has positive immunofluorescence for IgM, IgG, and complement.

PAN is a necrotizing vasculitis of small and medium-sized muscular arteries. Histologically, the lumina of vessels are often partially or completely thrombosed and the vessel wall is thickened, variably necrotic, and infiltrated with neutrophils. Eosinophils and extravasated red blood cells are frequently present in the adjacent dermis. The presence of nuclear dust is variable. The vascular lesions of PAN are characteristically focal and segmental. Multiple histological sections may have to be obtained to demonstrate the characteristic vascular changes. HBsAg, IgM, and complement are characteristically detected in endothelial membranes by immunofluorescence and electron microscopy.

Laboratory Findings

Patients with HBV infection typically have elevated serum alanine aminotransferase (ALT) and serum aspartate aminotransferase (AST) levels. ALT is usually more elevated than AST. These enzymes begin to increase 2–4 weeks before the onset of clinical symptoms and persist through-

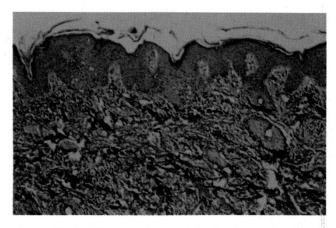

Figure 23–6. Histological examination of the papules of Gianotti-Crosti syndrome reveals a superficial perivascular lymphocytic infiltrate with mild endothelial swelling.

out the period of jaundice. Bilirubin levels may be modestly elevated as well. The white blood cell count is often low, with a relative lymphocytosis. A decreased complement level may be present when active vasculitis is associated with hepatitis. In the presence of renal involvement with vasculitis or PAN, elevated blood urea nitrogen or serum creatinine levels may be evident.

Diagnosis

The diagnosis of hepatitis is usually made by obtaining appropriate serological tests. Hepatitis B infection must be differentiated from a number of other viral and nonviral causes of hepatitis (Table 23–2). The diagnosis of associated skin diseases is made by clinical findings and, when appropriate, histological examination of skin lesions and confirming laboratory tests. A patient with a typical case of hepatitis B infection has a predictable serological response. HBsAg is detectable in the serum 2–8 weeks before the onset of clinical illness and may persist into the convalescence period. Antibody to hepatitis B core antigen (anti-HBc) generally is detectable with the onset of clinical illness. Following clinical illness, the titer of HBsAg declines and eventually is undetectable. Antihepatitis B surface antibody (anti-HBs) appears after the HBsAg disappears. Occasionally, there is a lag period between the disappearance of HBsAg and the appearance of anti-HBs, which is referred to as a serological "window phase." Diagnosis of acute HBV infection at this time is made by finding a positive anti-HBc. A positive anti-HBc result alone may indicate either active HBV infection in the "window phase" or a healthy asymptomatic chronic carrier and may also be found in patients previously infected with HBV in whom the titer of anti-HBs is undetectable.

The association of HBeAg with HBsAg indicates the presence of infectious virus and correlates with high infectivity and prolonged duration of disease. Concomitant HBsAg and anti-HBs are sometimes found and are particularly common in patients with renal failure on hemodialysis. Failure to clear the HBsAg and develop anti-HBs 6 months after infection constitutes serological evidence of a chronic carrier state for hepatitis B. Patients who have received a series of hepatitis B vaccinations have anti-HBs only in their serum.

HBV DNA can be detected in serum with polymerase chain reaction or direct hybridization techniques. The presence of HBV DNA correlates with viral replication and infectivity. These viral antigens are detectable early in the acute phase of disease and persist with chronic infection. However, this diagnostic modality is primarily limited to research environments at this time.

Treatment

Current therapies for chronic hepatitis B infection either inhibit viral replication or modulate immunity (Table 23–3). Recombinant alpha interferon has been used in the treatment of chronic hepatitis B and may result in patient improvement during the time of treatment; however, long-term benefits are questionable. Lamivudine (Epivir HBV) is a more recently approved antiviral agent that results in significant improvement or complete suppression of HBV DNA. Upon discontinuation of therapy, however, most patients return to pretreatment levels.

The treatments of the skin eruptions associated with hepatitis are the same as for skin eruptions from other etiologies (Table 23–4). The serum sickness–like syndrome occurs during acute HBV infection, which is typically benign and self-limited. No specific therapy is usually indicated. The urticaria and angioedema are most commonly treated with antihistamines, as is pruritus when associated with maculopapular eruptions. Mild palpable purpura and mixed cryoglobulinemia without systemic involvement do not require specific treatment, but when causing ulceration or when associated with systemic involvement, these conditions may require systemic corticosteroids. Other drugs,

---

Table 23–2.   Differential Diagnosis

Other viral hepatitides	
Hemochromatosis	
Wilson's disease	
Alpha$_1$-antitrypsin deficiency	Clinical differentiation can be difficult and laboratory analysis is required
Primary biliary cirrhosis	
Primary sclerosing cholangitis	
Autoimmune hepatitis	
Alcoholic cirrhosis	

Table 23–3.   Antiviral Therapy of HBV Infection

FDA-Approved Treatments
Interferon alpha (Intron A)
Lamivudine (Epivir)

Therapies Under Investigation
Famciclovir (Famvir)
Interferon alpha plus lamivudine
Interferon alpha plus famciclovir
Adefovir dipivoxil

Table 23–4. Treatment of HBV-Related Skin Disorders

Symptom	Treatment
Serum sickness–like syndrome	Antihistamines for urticaria, angioedema, or pruritus of the maculopapular eruption
Mixed cryoglobulinemia with palpable purpura	Systemic corticosteroids, dapsone, or colchicine may be required for severe involvement or ulceration
Gianotti-Crosti syndrome	No therapy is indicated
Polyarteritis nodosa	Short course (1–2 weeks) of corticosteroids followed by antiviral agents (e.g., lamivudine or interferon alpha) and plasma exchange
	Lamivudine plus interferon alpha
	Interferon alpha and plasma exchange
	Interferon alpha and famciclovir (famciclovir is not currently approved for HBV therapy)
	Interferon alpha alone

such as dapsone or colchicine, should be considered as alternatives to systemic corticosteroids if long-term treatment becomes necessary or if the use of systemic corticosteroids is contraindicated. Dapsone and colchicine require monitoring of blood counts and liver function. Occasionally, chemotherapeutic agents are required to control the symptoms of the disease.

Gianotti-Crosti syndrome is a benign and self-limited disease that does not require specific therapy. Affected children with chronic hepatitis B infection should typically receive therapy for the underlying viral disorder.

Conventional treatment of PAN has included the use of corticosteroids, immunosuppressive drugs, and plasma exchange. However, the use of steroids and immunosuppressive drugs in HBV-associated PAN has recently been shown to facilitate viral replication and the development of a chronic HBV infection [55]. The most effective treatment regimen is a short (1 to 2 week) course of corticosteroid therapy followed by an antiviral agent (e.g., lamivudine or alpha interferon) and plasma exchange [59–62]. Other reports of successful treatment include lamivudine plus interferon alpha [63], interferon alpha and plasma exchange [64], interferon alpha and famciclovir [65], interferon alpha alone [66,67], and corticosteroids and cyclophosphamide [68].

One mutant form of HBV incapable of synthesizing HBeAg, the precore mutant HBV, tends to produce a more severe liver disease and to progress more rapidly to cirrhosis. This precore mutant HBV-associated PAN responds poorly to the above treatment guidelines compared with the wild-type virus. It should be considered an individual entity, and no clear treatment approach has been defined [69].

Prevention

Prophylaxis is extremely important in preventing a disease that is widespread in distribution and for which there is no completely effective treatment. Active immunization is recommended using vaccines of human-derived or recombinant surface antigen for people at risk of infection with hepatitis B, such as health-care workers, hemodialysis patients, and intravenous drug abusers. Hepatitis B vaccine is now also recommended as a routine childhood vaccination in the United States and other countries. Passive immunization with high-titer anti-HBs human immunoglobulin in conjunction with vaccine is recommended for newborn babies of hepatitis B carrier mothers or for adults following accidental exposures, such as a needlestick injury [70]. Immunoglobulin should be given within 48 hours of exposure in order to be of maximum benefit and should be followed by a full immunization protocol.

The first hepatitis B vaccine, made available in 1982, was Hevac B (Pasteur Vaccines). This is a formalin-inactivated suspension containing noninfectious HBsAg purified from plasma of healthy HBsAg carriers. The majority of reactions to this vaccine have consisted of mild local redness and tenderness; however, urticaria, lichen planus, and a case of generalized dermatitis have been reported [71,72]. Recombinant DNA techniques have permitted the development of vaccines to hepatitis B that are prepared by cloning and expressing the HBsAg gene in yeast cells. In 1987 Recombivax-HB (Merck) and Engerix-B (SmithKline Beecham) became available in the United States. Gen Hevac B (Pasteur Institute) is a recombinant vaccine produced from mammalian cells that is available only in France. Recently a combination vaccine for the prevention of HAV and HBV was approved. This vaccine (Twinrix) contains the antigenic components of Havrix (HAV vaccine) and Engerix-β (HBV vaccine).

There are two pathogenic mechanisms involved in the cutaneous reactions associated with the recombinant vaccines. The immediate reactions, including reported cases of anaphylaxis, urticaria, and angioedema, are mediated by an immediate hypersensitivity reaction involving histamine release. This is probably triggered by the minute quantities of yeast lipid, the aluminum hydroxide, or the thimerosal

[73,74]. There are several reports of more delayed reactions to the recombinant vaccines. These include lichenoid eruptions, lichen planus, erythema nodosum, erythema multiforme, Stevens-Johnson syndrome, cutaneous vasculitis, serum sickness–like illness, and systemic lupus erythematosus [72,75–79]. These reactions are thought to be caused by the simultaneous presence of relatively large amounts of HBsAg and small amounts of anti-HBs in the serum that is induced following administration of the vaccine. This antigen excess is the same as that seen in the prodromal phase of the HBV infection, and it induces the same antigen-antibody complexes that result in clinical disease. Scalp hair loss resembling telogen effluvium has also been reported following vaccine administration [79]. In conclusion, cutaneous manifestations of HBV infection may also occur following hepatitis B vaccination, although most of these conditions do not occur at a higher rate than in the unvaccinated population. Once a serious, life-threatening adverse event occurs, a patient should not undergo further vaccination.

Conclusion

Viral hepatitis is a worldwide health problem resulting in notable morbidity in many infected individuals as well as significant mortality from acute fulminant disease or from the sequelae of chronic infection. Hepatitis B infection may produce myriad dermatological manifestations and syndromes. Even though these conditions are not specific for HBV disease, this diagnosis should be considered as a possible etiology in patients with the appropriate skin findings.

HEPATITIS C VIRUS (HCV)

Definition

HCV is a worldwide health problem (Fig. 23–7). The predominant cutaneous manifestations of hepatitis viruses are associated with HCV [1,2]. The majority of cases of non-A, non-B type hepatitis appear to be caused by HCV [80]. Hepatitis C is a single-stranded RNA virus composed of at least three structural proteins. It has been the most common cause of post-transfusion hepatitis, although appropriate screening measures have now significantly decreased this risk. Prior to widespread blood screening, an estimated 40% of cases of HCV were acquired by routes other than blood transfusion (Fig. 23-7) [81]. Today these routes (e.g., needle sticks, intravenous drug use, tatoos, sexual transmission) are responsible for over 90% of new cases of HCV.

History

After the discovery and increased understanding of HBV infection, several new cases were encountered of post-

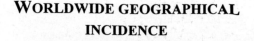

WORLDWIDE GEOGRAPHICAL INCIDENCE

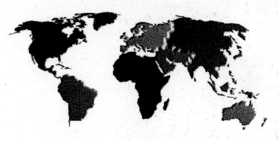

TRANSMISSION

Percutaneous exposure to blood, such as needle sticks or intravenous drug use

Transfusion of blood products in areas without appropiate screening measures

Humans

Sexual transmission (uncommon)

Perinatal transmission

ZOONOTIC IMPLICATIONS

None

Figure 23–7. Incidence and transmission of hepatitis C virus.

transfusion hepatitis with no evidence of HBV involvement. In 1974, Prince and his colleagues analyzed a group of post-transplantation hepatitis patients with no serological evidence for HBV or cytomegalovirus infection and with incubation periods longer than that expected for HBV

[82]. Through their investigations, it was first recognized that a virus other than HBV could be involved in transfusion-associated hepatitis. In 1988, the genome of HCV was first isolated and cloned from the liver and plasma of an experimentally infected chimpanzee [83,84]. This virus was later found to be the primary cause of parenterally acquired non-A, non-B hepatitis across the world [85,86].

Incidence

HCV has a prevalence of 1–2% in most countries [87]. However, some areas such as particular regions of Egypt and Japan have significantly higher rates, with 20 to 40% of the population infected (Fig. 23–7). Overall, the World Health Organization estimates that 3% of the worldwide population has had HCV infection and that over 170 million individuals are chronic carriers of the virus. Prior to proper blood screening, HCV was responsible for 80 to 90% of the cases of post-transfusion hepatitis as well as 12 to 15% of sporadic hepatitis cases. Since the implementation of HCV screening of blood donors, the incidence of transfusion-associated hepatitis has decreased to less than 1% [88,89].

Although it is not as efficiently transmitted as HIV or HBV, HCV may be sexually transmitted in up to 20% of cases. Injection drug use is the predominant risk factor for HCV transmission in low endemic countries. Transmission from mother to infant is less than 5%. Nosocomial transmission of HCV has also been reported [90]. In a 1992 study of 175 intravenous drug users in the United States, 83% were positive for HCV [91]. This virus is the primary cause of chronic liver disease in many countries, such as the United States, Japan, and Egypt. It is estimated that 4 million Americans are infected with hepatitis C virus. About 70% of infected patients go on to develop chronic liver disease. It is the cause of 40 to 60% of chronic liver disease in the United States and is the leading indication for adult liver transplant. Although survival for liver transplantation for HBV infection has greatly increased during the past 10 years, outcomes for transplantation for HCV remain poor because HCV reinfection is universal. Yearly, 8000 to 10,000 deaths in the United States are caused by HCV. Current medical costs are estimated to be more than $600 million annually.

Pathogenesis

The risk of transmission of HCV by needlestick is 4–10%, demonstrating less infectivity than HBV [36]. Once inoculation occurs, the primary site of HCV infection and viral replication is the liver. The incubation period for HCV is typically 6 to 7 weeks, but viremia has been detected within 2 weeks of exposure. Although HCV is not considered to be directly cytopathic to hepatocytes, infection results in hepatic cell injury and necrosis during the acute phase. Contrary to HBV, hepatitis C is an extremely rare cause of acute fulminant hepatic necrosis [92,93]. However, this virus more commonly results in chronic disease, cirrhosis, and liver cancer than HBV. Factors known to increase the probability of HCV disease progression include male sex, older age at infection, alcohol abuse, and concurrent viral infection, particularly with HBV or human immunodeficiency virus (HIV) or both. The prevalence of HCV/HIV coinfection ranges from 30% to over 50%. Patients who are coinfected with HIV and HCV tend to progress faster to cirrhosis and experience higher rates of morbidity and mortality. The leading risk factor for coinfection is intravenous drug use, but a history of alcohol use is also common. In a study of 4000 HIV patients, it was determined that having a positive HCV serological response was associated with a 50% higher risk of dying as compared with HCV-seronegative patients [94]. One factor contributing to the increased mortality rate is that coinfected patients often must discontinue highly active antiretroviral therapy (HAART) secondary to hepatic toxicity.

Clinical Manifestations

Most acute HCV infections are subclinical and unrecognized. The clinical course of HCV infection is reviewed

Table 23-5.   Clinical Manifestations of HCV

Time after exposure	Clinical manifestations	Laboratory analyses	Other notes
6–7 weeks (varies from 2 weeks to 6 months)	Symptoms begin, with a clinical course that is indistinguishable from that of HBV and other hepatitis viruses. Refer to Table 23–1	Serological tests, with selection of anti-HCV in serum Detection of HCV RNA in serum by polymerase chain reaction	At least two thirds of cases are anicteric and mild or completely asymptomatic

in Tables 23–1 and 23–5. Clinical illness occurs less frequently in children compared with adults. From 70–85% of infected persons develop chronic hepatitis, sometimes progressing to cirrhosis or hepatocellular carcinoma. HCV can cause persistent infection, accompanied by elevations of ALT, even without evidence of chronic liver disease [95]. The physical examination should include the following markers of liver damage: jaundice, hepatomegaly, splenomegaly, ascites, encephalopathy, palmar erythema, spider angiomas, telangiectasias, and purpura.

Cutaneous Findings in HCV Infection

Urticaria [96,97], erythema multiforme–like reactions [98], erythema nodosum [99], mixed cryoglobulinemia with leukocytoclastic vasculitis [100–114], urticarial vasculitis [115], Henoch-Schönlein purpura [116], necrolytic acral erythema [117], porphyria cutanea tarda [118–126], lichen planus [127–133], prurigo [134], and polyarteritis nodosa all have been associated with hepatitis C infections. Hepatitis C appears to be a much less frequent cause of polyarteritis nodosa than hepatitis B [135].

Mixed Cryoglobulinemia

HCV appears to be a frequent cause of mixed cryoglobulinemia (MC). Cryoglobulins are anti-immunoglobulin immunoglobulins, which precipitate at temperatures less than 37°C. There are three types of cryoglobulins, as defined by

Brouet et al. in 1974 [106]. Type I consists of monoclonal immunoglobulins without rheumatoid factors and is generally paraneoplastic. Type II consists of polyclonal IgG and monoclonal IgM rheumatoid factors. In type III, both IgG and IgM are polyclonal. MC is considered "essential" (i.e., idiopathic) if not associated with any disease other than Sjögren's syndrome. Secondary MC occurs in association with chronic liver disease, infections, autoimmune disease, and as a paraneoplastic phenomenon. It has been estimated that 80% of MC, which would have been considered essential prior to 1998, is secondary to HCV infection [107].

MC typically results in mild to severe vasculitis that may manifest with a classic triad of purpura, weakness, and arthralgias and may result in glomerulonephritis and peripheral neuropathy. The pathogenesis of cutaneous vasculitis in HCV infection is still unknown, but it is widely accepted that the disease is mediated by deposition of immune complexes and activation of complement [105,107]. This theory is supported by finding anti-HCV antibody and HCV RNA concentrated in the cryoprecipitate [112] and by the clinical manifestations of the decrease of vasculitis with the concentration of these circulating immune complexes [108]. The cutaneous lesions reported with this condition include palpable purpura, petechiae, urticaria, vascular occlusions, and ulcerative lesions with and without necrosis (Fig. 23–8). Raynaud's phenomenon and Sjögren's syndrome may also be present.

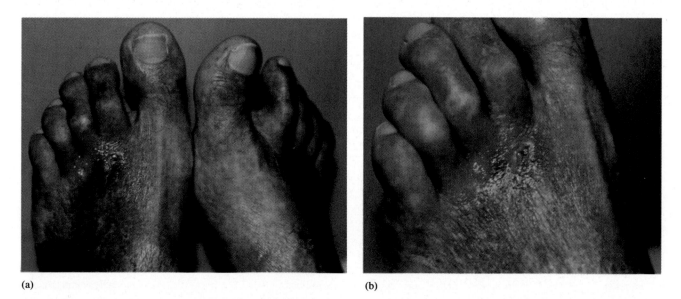

(a)   (b)

Figure 23–8. (a, b) Leukocytoclastic vasculitis in a hepatitis C patient with mixed cryoglobulinemia manifested as palpable purpura and ulcerations.

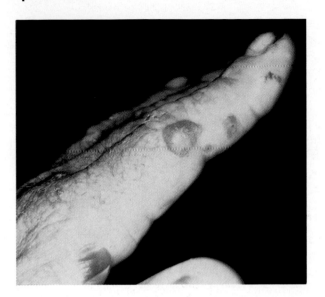

Figure 23–9. Slightly hemorrhagic bullae of porphyria cutanea tarda.

Porphyria Cutanea Tarda

Recent reports have documented the increased incidence of porphyria cutanea tarda (PCT) in patients with HCV infection (Figs. 23–9 and 23–10) [118–120,126,136,137]. HCV tends to induce PCT in predisposed individuals. The reported prevalence of antibodies to HCV in PCT varies from 8 to 79%, with a higher prevalence in southern Eu-

rope, the United States, and Japan [118–120]. The mechanism of this relationship is poorly understood, but in theory it is thought to begin with viral-induced liver damage that decompartmentalizes hepatic iron stores. This results in increased free iron and the formation of free radicals, which alter cytochrome P450. This leads to the reduction in uroporphyrinogen decarboxylase activity, an enzyme active in the metabolism of uroporphyrins, and a subsequent buildup of uroporphyrins [123]. PCT is often the first sign of hepatocyte injury provoked by HCV and manifests as subepidermal bullae, superficial erosions, hypertrichosis, and hyperpigmentation in sun-exposed skin. The skin lesions are a result of photosensitization by porphyrins, which accumulate in the disease [119].

Lichen Planus

There is a probable association of chronic HCV infection with lichen planus [138,139], particularly with the erosive type of chronic oral lichen planus (Figs. 23–11, 23–12) [87,127–132]. This association, as in the association between HCV infection and PCT [129,130], tends to be strongest in populations at greatest risk of exposure to HCV [135,136]. Reports have indicated a 20% prevalence of lichen planus in patients with chronic HCV infection compared with a less than 1% prevalence of lichen planus in the general population [127]. Skin involvement typically consists of flat-topped violaceous papules, most commonly on the dorsal hands and wrist. HCV RNA has been detected by polymerase chain reaction in the tissue of oral lichen planus, suggesting a pathological role of HCV in this disease [131].

Although several other cutaneous conditions have been linked to chronic HCV infection, as mentioned earlier,

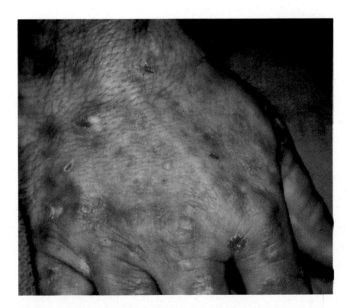

Figure 23–10. Healing erosions and scarring lesions of porphyria cutanea tarda on the dorsal hand.

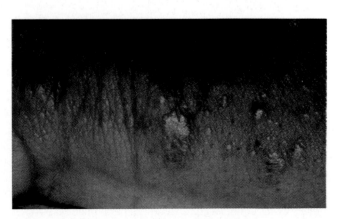

Figure 23–11. Violaceous flat-topped papules and plaques typical of lichen planus. Lesions are located near the wrist.

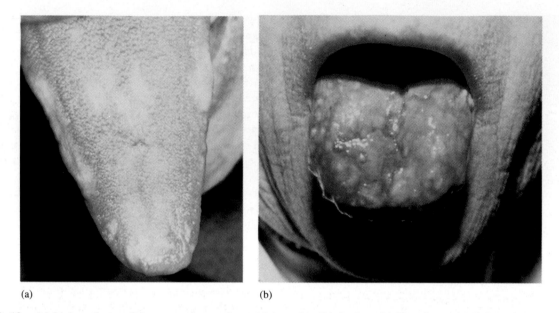

(a)   (b)

Figure 23–12. (a) Lichen planus of the tongue in a patient with hepatitis C infection. (b) Chronic erosive lichen planus on the tongue of a 60-year-old woman. Not infrequently, such lesions appear to be associated with HCV infection.

these associations are not definitive. As with hepatitis B, serious liver damage from chronic hepatitis C may result in jaundice, pruritus, spider nevi, palmar erythema, and purpura.

Pathology

Histopathological features of chronic HCV infection include lymphocytic infiltration with lymphoid cell aggregation and bile duct damage [140,141]. Microvesicular fatty changes and acidophilic changes in the hepatocytes may also be evident. Severe lobular necrosis and inflammation are less frequently seen.

Skin biopsy samples in essential MC reveal evidence of a vasculitis, with destruction of dermal blood vessels and infiltration of neutrophils in and around the vessel wall [142]. Histologically, lichen planus lesions show degeneration of keratinocytes and dense infiltration of lymphocytes in the upper dermis, which are hugging the border of the epidermis [143].

Laboratory Findings

The laboratory findings in HCV infection may vary. Basic laboratory tests for detecting HCV should include a complete blood count with differential and platelets, ALT, AST, albumin, globulin, and glucose determinations, renal function tests, prothrombin time, partial thromboplastin time, viral load, and genotype. Ancillary tests may include

HAV antibody, HBV antibody, thyroid profile, alpha-fetoprotein (AFP) (in cirrhotics), cryoglobulins, and rheumatoid factor. The most characteristic feature is a fluctuating pattern of serum ALT elevations [144]. In general, serum bilirubin and transaminase levels are lower in acute HCV infection when compared to those in HAV or HBV.

Diagnosis

Hepatitis caused by HCV, like that due to HBV, must be differentiated from hepatitides of other etiologies (Table 23–2). The viral RNA of HCV can be detected by polymerase chain reaction in the serum shortly after infection. This diagnostic modality can begin to detect HCV RNA 1 to 2 weeks after exposure, which is long before symptoms or liver enzyme abnormalities develop. Detection of HCV RNA indicates current infection and transmissibility of HCV.

Specific antibodies to HCV are not usually detected earlier than 3 to 4 months after initial exposure [145]. Therefore, testing should be repeated in patients suspected of having HCV infection who have negative serological findings. A new second-generation enzyme-linked immunosorbent assay test for anti-HCV adds two new antigens—HC31 and HC34—to the single antigen C100-3 found in the first-generation test, thus increasing its sensitivity. Unfortunately, no diagnostic modalities are able to differentiate acute disease from chronic involvement with HCV. The diagnosis of chronic infection is usually based on the persistence of elevated ALT enzyme levels for at least 6 months.

Treatment

Current indications for HCV therapy include patients older than 18 years with HCV-RNA in the serum, elevated enzyme levels, a liver biopsy showing fibrosis or moderate-to-severe necrosis and inflammation, and no contraindications to treatment. The standard treatment for chronic HCV infection has been alpha interferon [146] (Table 23–6). However, the more recent combination of alpha interferon and ribavirin, a nucleoside analogue shown to inhibit the replication of DNA and RNA viruses, has shown more promising results. Clinical studies have demonstrated significantly improved response rates with this combination when compared with the response to alpha interferon alone [147–149]. Two large, randomized, controlled trials published in 1998 compared interferon alone with combination therapy (interferon alpha plus ribavirin) [150,151]. Combined data showed that only 29% of patients treated with interferon monotherapy became polymerase chain reaction–negative, whether they were treated for 6 or 12 months. Combination therapy, however, showed better results, with 50 to 55% of patients being polymerase chain reaction–negative at the end of therapy.

When combination therapy was stopped, there was a higher sustained response rate of 33 to 41%; extended therapy resulted in yet a higher sustained response rate and a lower relapse rate.

Genotype was the main predictive factor in sustained virological response, with types 2 and 3 having a two- to threefold higher response rate than genotype 1. Unfortunately, in the United States the predominant genotype is type 1, which ranges from 70 to 90% of all HCV patients. In addition, younger patients, patients with lower fibrosis scores, and women were more likely to have a sustained virological response. Studies suggest that interferon mono-

therapy should be reserved only for those patients who have contraindications to ribavirin.

Longer-lasting forms of interferon 40kDa, branched peginterferon alpha-2a and alpha-2b may be more effective than standard interferon therapy for patients with HCV and cirrhosis [152]. In a study of patients treated for 48 weeks with interferon alpha-2a (3 million IU injected three times weekly) or 40kDa, branched peginterferon alpha-2a (either 90 µg or 180 µg injected once weekly), 6% of patients on sustained interferon alpha-2a maintained sustained viral loss after 6 months. Twenty-nine percent of patients on 40kDa, branched peginterferon alpha-2a maintained sustained viral loss after the same time period. Again, response varied according to genotype. In those patients with a non-1 genotype, there was a 53% sustained viral loss, but for those patients with genotype 1, the sustained viral loss was only 10%. Viral load also contributed to the difference, with those with low viral loads having a 35% sustained response, compared with 23% for patients with a high viral load. In 2001, the Food and Drug Administration approved peginterferon alpha-2b as once weekly therapy for HCV infection in patients 18 years and older who had not previously been treated with interferon alpha and who had compensated liver disease. A pilot study looking at ribavirin in combination with 40kDa, branched peginterferon alpha-2a, found that the combination works better than standard interferon alpha-2a. At week 48 in the pilot study, which included 16 patients with genotype 1 virus and four with genotype 2, 70% of patients had undetectable levels of HCV in their blood. Combination therapy with once weekly peginterferon alpha-2b plus daily ribavirin achieved a 61% rate of sustained virological response overall in previously untreated adults with chronic HCV. The response range was 48% for genotype 1 and 88% for genotypes 2 and 3 [153]. This combination is now approved therapy.

Recently, there have been many reports of the successful treatment of mixed cryoglobulinemia secondary to HCV infection with subcutaneous alpha interferon [104,108,111, 113,114] (Table 23–7). This indicates the importance of screening all patients with vasculitis for HCV infection, as it would be more beneficial to these patients to treat them with antiviral therapy rather than systemic corticosteroids or cytotoxic drugs. Although alpha interferon attenuates mixed cryoglobulinemia in most of these cases, relapse is frequent after discontinuation of the drug [154]. Cytotoxic agents (i.e., cyclophosphamide and azathioprine) used in the conventional treatment of MC should generally be avoided in the treatment of HCV-associated mixed cryoglobulinemia [58]. These agents, however, may sometimes be necessary for treatment of the most severe forms of the disease. The same principle stands for steroid therapy,

---

Table 23–6.   Antiviral Therapy of HCV Infection

FDA Approved Treatments
Inteferon alpha (Intron A)
Peginterferon alpha-2b (pegylated interferon) (PEG-Intron)
Alpha interferon plus ribavirin (Rebetol)
Pegylated interferon plus ribavirin

Therapies Under Investigation
Protease inhibitors
Helicase inhibitors
Antisense oligoribonucleotides

Table 23–7. Treatment of HCV-Related Cutaneous Disorders

Symptom	Treatment
Mixed cryoglobulinemia	Interferon alpha,* 3–6 million U given subcutaneously three times/week for 6–12 months. Increased doses and longer duration of treatment are frequently used
	Steroid therapy, in severe cases only
	Plasma exchange therapy, typically combined with alpha interferon or low-dose steroids
	Cytotoxic agents, only in the most severe cases
Porphyria cutanea tarda	Interferon alfa,* 3 million U given subcutaneously three times/week for 6–12 months
Lichen planus	Topical corticosteroids
	Interferon alpha therapy*
	Systemic corticosteroids should be reserved for severe cases only

* Or interferon alpha plus ribavirin

which may be necessary in cases not responsive to alpha interferon alone. If HCV-associated mixed cryoglobulinemia is refractory to all medications, plasma exchange, which removes immune complexes and rheumatoid factors from circulation, may be effective [58,109]. Relapse often occurs after withdrawal of this therapy.

The treatment of porphyria cutanea tarda (Table 23–7) in patients with HCV infection has not been as thoroughly evaluated. Several reports have described the complete resolution of this condition after treatment with interferon alpha [155–159]. However, one case of ineffective interferon treatment has also been reported [160]. Interferon alpha should probably be considered for primary therapy in these patients.

Lichen planus is most commonly treated with topical steroids (Table 23–7), however, systemic corticosteroids are occasionally used in extensive, symptomatic cases. Numerous reports have indicated the beneficial effect of alpha interferon in the treatment of lichen planus associated with HCV infection [128,161,162]. However, there have also been reports of worsening or induction of lichen planus lesions with the use of this drug [129,163–168]. The efficacy of alpha interferon therapy is difficult to appreciate in cases of lichen planus because its evolution is unpredict-

able, with occasional remissions occurring even in the absence of any treatment. To date, insufficient data are available to define the exact role of interferon in the treatment of lichen planus associated with HCV infection. However, certain authors recommend that interferon alpha therapy should be attempted in patients with HCV and LP, with the knowledge that some patients may improve, others will deteriorate, and some may remain unchanged [143].

Prevention

Immunoglobulin has been shown to be ineffective in preventing hepatitis C. A prototype vaccine that induces antibodies to HCV envelope protein is being studied but is currently not available. The major difficulty in vaccine development is that HCV is a heterogenous virus with a high mutation rate. The six major genotypes are represented by major variants with up to 30% sequence differences. Not only do multiple subtypes exist within each genotype, but minor sequence variations, on the order of 1 to 2% are common. Despite recent screening for hepatitis C antibody in blood donors, hepatitis C remains the most common (although rare) cause of transfusion-related hepatitis, most probably because of the 3- or 4-month period between the time of infection and the development of circulating antibodies that allow detection of the infection. In a recent study in which high-risk blood donors were tested for viremia by polymerase chain reaction, antibodies detected by the most sensitive of the serological assays were present in only 68% of the positive serum samples. Although blood transfusion becomes safer as testing improves, it will never be risk-free, and transfusions should be avoided unless the benefits to be derived clearly offset the risks. Whenever possible, autologous transfusions should be considered.

Conclusion

Hepatitis C virus infection continues to be a significant cause of chronic hepatitis around the world. Because the majority of acute HCV infections go unrecognized, the development of particular cutaneous manifestations should warrant further investigation into possible chronic infection. While this virus was only recently discovered and our current knowledge of HCV is incomplete, it is hoped that future research and investigation will provide us with effective methods of treatment and prevention.

REFERENCES

1. K Kiyosawa, E Tanaka. GB virus C/hepatitis G virus. Intervirology 42:185–195, 1999.
2. JA Routenberg, JL Dienstag, WO Harrison, ME Kil-

patrick, RR Hooper, FV Chisari, RH Purcell, MF Fornes. Foodborne outbreak of hepatitis A: clinical and laboratory features of acute and protracted illness. Am J Med Sci 278:123–137, 1979.

3. S Dollberg, Y Berkun, E Gross-Kielselstein. Urticaria in patients with hepatitis A virus infection. Pediatr Infect Dis J 10:702–703, 1991.

4. EF Sagi, N Linden, D Shonval. Papular acrodermatitis of childhood associated with hepatitis A virus infection. Pediatr Dermatol 3:31–33, 1985.

5. Y Ilan, M Hillman, R Oren, A Zlotogorski, D Shouval. Vasculitis and cryoglobulinemia associated with persisting cholestatic hepatitis A virus infection. Am J Gastroenterol 85:586–587, 1990.

6. M Dan, R Yaniv. Cholestatic hepatitis, cutaneous vasculitis, and vascular deposits of immunoglobulin M and complement associated with hepatitis A virus infection. Am J Med 89:103–104, 1990.

7. RD Inman, M Hodge, ME Johnston, J Wright, J Heathcote. Arthritis, vasculitis, and cryoglobulinemia associated with relapsing hepatitis A virus infection. Ann Intern Med 105: 700–703, 1986.

8. J Press, S Maslovitz, I Avinoach. Cutaneous necrotizing vasculitis associated with hepatitis A virus infection. J Rheumatol 24:965–967, 1997.

9. ME Parsons, GG Russo, LE Millikan. Dermatologic disorders associated with viral hepatitis infections. Int J Dermatol 35:77–81, 1996.

10. K Krawczynski. Hepatitis E. Hepatology 17:932–941, 1993.

11. M Crovatto, C Mazzaro, S Mishiro, G Santini, S Baracetti, F Zorat, G Pozzato. GBV-C/HGV and HCV infection in mixed cryoglobulinemia. Br J Haematol 106:510–514, 1999.

12. M Casan, D Lilli, D Rivanera, FG De Rosa, B Laganá, C Mancini. HCV/HGV coinfection in mixed cryoglobulinemia. J Hepatol 28:355–356, 1998.

13. A Servant, M Bogard, C Delaugerre, P Cohen, P Dény, L Guillevin. GB virus C in systemic medium- and small-vessel necrotizing vasculitides. Br J Rheumatol 37: 1292–1294, 1998.

14. A Grasso, G Menardo, N Campo, A Picciotto. Hepatitis G virus and HCV related extrahepatic disease. Am J Gastroenterol 94:1120–1121, 1999.

15. A Lürman. Eine Icterusepidemic. Berlin Klin Wochenschr 22:20–23, 1885.

16. GM Findlay, PO MacCallum. Note on acute hepatitis and yellow fever immunization. Trans R Soc Trop Med Hyg 31:297–308, 1937.

17. WA Sawyer, KF Meyer, MD Eaton. Jaundice in army personnel in the western region of the United States and its relation to vaccination against yellow fever. Am J Hyg 39: 337–430, 1944.

18. SA Propert. Hepatitis after prophylactic serum. Br Med J 2:677–678, 1938.

19. PB Beeson, G Chesney, AM McFarlan. Hepatitis following injection of mumps convalescent plasma. I. Use of plasma in the mumps epidemic. Lancet 1:814–815, 1944.

20. AM McFarlan, G Chesney. Hepatitis following injection of mumps convalescent plasma. II. Epidemiology of the hepatitis. Lancet 1:816–821, 1944.

21. PB Beeson. Jaundice occurring one to four months after transfusion of blood or plasma. JAMA 121:1332–1334, 1943.

22. HV Morgan, DA Williamson. Jaundice following administration of human blood products. Br Med J 1:750–753, 1943.

23. Memorandum prepared by Medical Officers of the Ministry of Health. Homologous serum jaundice. Lancet 1: 83–88, 1943.

24. BS Blumberg, BJ Gerstley, DA Hungerford, WT London, AI Sutnick. A serum antigen (Australia antigen) in Down's syndrome, leukemia and hepatitis. Ann Intern Med 66: 924–931, 1967.

25. WT London, AI Sutnick, BS Blumberg. Australia antigen and acute viral hepatitis. Ann Intern Med 70:55–59, 1969.

26. AM Prince. An antigen detected in the blood during the incubation period of serum hepatitis. Proc Natl Acad Sci USA 60:814–821, 1968.

27. AM Prince, RL Hargrove, W Szmuness, CE Cherubin, VJ Fontana, GH Jeffries. Immunologic distinction between infectious and serum hepatitis. N Engl J Med 282: 987–991, 1970.

28. R Ward, S Krugman, JP Giles, AM Jacobs, O Bodansky. Infectious hepatitis. Studies of its natural history and prevention. N Engl J Med 258:407–416, 1958.

29. S Krugman, R Ward, JP Giles. The natural history of infectious hepatitis. Am J Med 32:717–728, 1962.

30. S Krugman, JP Giles, J Hammonds. Infectious hepatitis. Evidence for two distinctive clinical, epidemiological and immunological types of infection. JAMA 200:365–373, 1967.

31. S Krugman, JP Giles. Viral hepatitis. New light on an old disease. JAMA 212:1019–1029, 1970.

32. S Krugman, JP Giles, J Hammond. Hepatitis virus: effect of heat on the infectivity and antigenicity of the MS-1 and MS-2 strain. J Infect Dis 122:432–436, 1970.

33. F Deinhardt, ID Gust. Viral hepatitis. Bull World Health Org 60:661–691, 1982.

34. PJ Coleman, GM McQuillan, LA Moyer, SB Lambert, HS Margolis. Estimated incidence of hepatitis B virus infections in the United States. Abstract. International Conference on Emerging Infectious Diseases, Atlanta, GA, March 8–12, 1998.

35. HS Margolis, MJ Alter, SC Hadler. Hepatitis B: evolving epidemiology and implications for control. Semin Liver Dis 11:84–92, 1991.

36. K Kiene, B Hsu, D Rowe, A Carruthers. Hepatitis, HIV, and the dermatologist: a risk review. J Am Acad Dermatol 30:108–115, 1994.

37. RJ Gerity. Hepatitis B transmission between dental and medical workers and patients. Ann Intern Med 95: 229–231, 1981.

38. SC Hadler, HS Margolis. Viral hepatitis. In: AS Evans, ed. Viral Infections of Humans: Epidemiology and Control, 3rd ed. New York: Plenum, 1989, pp 351–391.

39. KC Hyams. Risks of chronicity following acute hepatitis B virus infection: a review. Clin Infect Dis 20:992–1000, 1995.

40. YF Liaw, DI Tai, CM Chu, TJ Chem. The development of cirrhosis in patients with chronic type B hepatitis; a prospective study. Hepatology 8:493–496, 1988.

41. FE de Jongh, HL Janssen, RA de Man, WC Hop, SW Schalm, M van Blankenstein. Survival and prognostic indicators in hepatitis B surface antigen-positive cirrhosis of the liver. Gastroenterology 103:1630–1635, 1992.

42. G Fattovich, L Brollo, G Giustina, F Noventa, P Pontisso, A Alberti, G Realdi, A Ruol. Natural history and prognostic factors for chronic hepatitis type B. Gut 32:294–298, 1991.

43. PB Gregory, CM Knauer, RL Kempson, R Miller. Steroid therapy in severe viral hepatitis. A double-blind, randomized trial of methylprednisolone versus placebo. N Engl J Med 294:681–687, 1976.

44. C Newman, JS Newman. Acute viral hepatitis. In: DJ Demis, ed. Clinical Dermatology. Philadelphia: JB Lippincott, 1995, vol 3, pp 1–11.

45. R Fernandez, DJ McCarty. The arthritis of viral hepatitis. Ann Intern Med 74:207–211, 1971.

46. ZK Draelos, RC Hansen, WD James. Gianotti-Crosti syndrome associated with infections other than hepatitis B. JAMA 256:2386–2388, 1986.

47. JW Popp Jr, TJ Harrist, JL Dienstag, AK Bhan, JR Wands, JT LaMont, MC Mihm Jr. Cutaneous vasculitis associated with acute and chronic hepatitis. Arch Intern Med 141:623–629, 1981.

48. AE Prestia, YL Lynfield. Scarlatiniform eruption in viral hepatitis. Arch Dermatol 101:352–355, 1970.

49. G Maggiore, S Grifeo, MD Marzani. Erythema nodosum and hepatitis B virus (HBV) infection. J Am Acad Dermatol 9:602–603, 1983.

50. M Geller. Association of chronic localized angioedema of the tongue with hepatitis B. Ann Allergy Asthma Immunol 81:96, 1998.

51. C Ferri, LA La Civita, G Longombardo, F Greco, S Bombardieri. Hepatitis C virus and mixed cryoglobulinaemia. Eur J Clin Invest 23:399–405, 1993.

52. NA Lockshir, H Hurley. Urticaria as a sign of viral hepatitis. Arch Derm 105:570–571, 1972.

53. P Barranco Sanz, C Lopez Serrano. Cold urticaria associated with serological markers of hepatitis B and cryoglobulinemia [Spanish]. Allergol Immunopathol (Madr) 15:167–169, 1987.

54. P Marcellin, Y Calmus, H Takahashi, AL Zignego, Chatenoud, L LP Galanaud, M Leibowitch, JF Bach, JP Benhamou, P Tiollais, et al. Latent hepatitis B virus (HBV) infection in systemic necrotizing vasculitis. Clin Exp Rheumatol 9:23–28, 1991.

55. L Guillevin, F Lhote, P Cohen, F Sauvaget, B Jarrousse, O Lortholary, LH Noel, C Trepo. Polyarteritis nodosa related to hepatitis B virus. A prospective study with long-term observation of 41 patients. Medicine (Baltimore) 74:238–253, 1995.

56. PS McElgunn. Dermatologic manifestations of hepatitis B virus infection. J Am Acad Dermatol 8:539–548, 1983.

57. SJ Whittaker, JS Dover, MW Greaves. Cutaneous polyarteritis nodosa associated with hepatitis B surface antigen. J Am Acad Dermatol 15:1142–1145, 1986.

58. F Gianotti. Papular acrodermatitis of childhood and other papulo-vesicular acro-located syndromes. Br J Dermatol 100:49–59, 1979.

59. L Guillevin, F Lhote, R Ghérardi. The spectrum and treatment of virus-associated vasculitides. Curr Opin Rheumatol 9:31–36, 1997.

60. L Guillevin, F Lhote, B Jarrousse, P Bironne, J Barrier, P Deny, C Trepo, MF Kahn, P Godeau. Polyarteritis nodosa related to hepatitis B virus. A retrospective study of 66 patients. Ann Med Interne (Paris) 143(suppl 1):63–74, 1992.

61. L Guillevin, F Lhote, A Leon, F Fauvelle, L Vivitski, C Trepo. Treatment of polyarteritis nodosa related to hepatitis B virus with short term steroid therapy associated with antiviral agents and plasma exchanges. A prospective trial in 33 patients. J Rheumatol 20:289–298, 1993.

62. WC Maddrey. Chronic hepatitis. Dis Mon 39:53–126, 1994.

63. JW Olivier, G Pizzolato, F Sarasin, L Guillevin, JM Dayer, C Chizzoline. Successful treatment of polyarteritis nodosa related to hepatitis B virus with a combination of lamivudine and interferon alpha [letter]. Rheumatology (Oxford) 38:183–185, 1999.

64. L Guillevin, F Lhote, F Sauvaget, P Deblois, F Rossi, D Levallois, J Pourrat, B Christoforov, C Trepo. Treatment of polyarteritis nodosa related to hepatitis B virus with interferon-alpha and plasma exchanges. Ann Rheum Dis 53:334–337, 1994.

65. M Krüger, KH Böker, H Zeidler, MP Manns. Treatment of hepatitis B-related polyarteritis nodosa with famciclovir and interferon alfa-2b. J Hepatol 26:935–939, 1997.

66. E Avsar, B Savas, N Tözün, NB Ulusoy, C Kalayci. Successful treatment of polyarteritis nodosa related to hepatitis B virus with interferon alpha as first-line therapy. J Hepatol 28:525–526, 1998.

67. H Simsek, H Telatar. Successful treatment of hepatitis B virus-associated polyarteritis nodosa by interferon alpha alone. J Clin Gastroenterol 20:263–265, 1995.

68. BJ McMahon, WL Heyward, W Templin, D Clement, AP Lanier. Hepatitis B-associated polyarteritis nodosa in Alaskan Eskimos; clinical and epidemiologic features and long-term follow-up. Hepatology 9:97–101, 1989.

69. M Miguelez, J Bueno, P Laynez. Polyarteritis nodosa associated with precore mutant hepatitis B virus infection [letter]. Ann Rheum Dis 57:173, 1998.

70. Centers for Disease Control and Prevention. Immune globulins for protection against viral hepatitis. Recommenda-

tions of the Immunization Practices Advisory Committee (IPAC). MMWR 30:423–428, 433–435, 1981.

71. RL Rietschel, RM Adams. Reactions to thimerosal in hepatitis B vaccines. Dermatol Clin 8:161–164, 1990.

72. CA Saywell, RA Wittal, S Kossard. Lichenoid reaction to hepatitis B vaccination. Australas J Dermatol 38:152–154, 1997.

73. I Grotto, Y Mandel, M Ephros, I Ashkenazi, J Shemer. Major adverse reactions to yeast-derived hepatitis B vaccines—a review. Vaccine 16:329–334, 1998.

74. TJ Hudson, M Newkirk, F Gervais, J Suster. Adverse reactions to the recombinant hepatitis B vaccine. J Allergy Clin Immunol 88:821–822, 1991.

75. Havrix, SmithKline Beecham. Physicians' Desk Reference, 52nd ed. Montvale, NJ: Medical Economics Data Production Co, 1998, p 2827.

76. HB Recombivax, Merck. Physicians' Desk Reference, 52nd ed. Montvale, NJ: Medical Economics Data Production Co, 1998, p 1741.

77. B Engerix, SmithKline Beecham. Physicians' Desk Reference, 52nd ed. Montvale, NJ: Medical Economics Data Production Co, 1998, p 2820.

78. MF Ferrando, MS Doutre, M Beylot-Barry, I Durand, C Beylot. Lichen planus following hepatitis B vaccination [letter]. Br J Dermatol 139:350, 1998.

79. M Vanoli, D Gambini, R Scorza. A case of Churg-Strauss vasculitis after hepatitis B vaccination [letter]. Ann Rheum Dis 57:256–257, 1998.

80. K Hosoda, M Omata, O Yolosuka, N Kato, M Ohto. Non-A, non-B chronic hepatitis is chronic hepatitis C: a sensitive assay for detection of hepatitis C virus RNA in the liver. Hepatology 15:777–781, 1992.

81. MJ Alter, RE Sampliner. Hepatitis C: and miles to go before we sleep. N Engl J Med 321:1538–1540, 1989.

82. AM Prince, B Brotman, GF Grady, WJ Kuhns, C Hazzi, RW Levine, SJ Millian. Long-incubation post-transfusion hepatitis without serological evidence of exposure to hepatitis B virus. Lancet 2:241–246, 1974.

83. G Kuo, QL Choo, HJ Alter, GL Gitnick, AG Redeker, RH Purcell, T Miyamura, JL Dienstag, MJ Alter, CE Stevens, et al. An assay for circulating antibodies to a major etiologic virus of human non-A, non-B hepatitis. Science 244:362–364, 1989.

84. QL Choo, G Kuo, AJ Weiner, LR Overby, DW Bradley, M Houghton. Isolation of a cDNA clone derived from a blood-borne non-A, non-B viral hepatitis genome. Science 244:359–362, 1989.

85. S Kleinman, H Alter, M Busch, P Holland, G Tegtmeier, M Nelles, S Lee, E Page, J Wilber, A Polito. Increased detection of hepatitis C virus (HCV)-infected blood donors by a multiple-antigen HCV enzyme immunoassay. Transfusion 32:805–813, 1992.

86. Centers for Disease Control and Prevention. Public Health Service inter-agency guidelines for screening donors of blood, plasma, organs, tissues, and semen for evidence of hepatitis B and hepatitis C. MMWR 40(RR-4):1–17, 1991.

87. C Jubert, JM Pawlotsky, F Pouget, C Andre, L DeForges, S Bretagne, JP Mavier, J Duval, J Revuz, D Dhumeaux, et al. Lichen planus and hepatitis C virus-related chronic active hepatitis. Arch Dermatol 130:73–76, 1994.

88. HJ Alter. Transfusion transmitted hepatitis C and non-A, non-B, non-C. Vox Sang 67(suppl 3):19–24, 1994.

89. Japanese Red Cross Non-A, Non-B Hepatitis Research Group. Effect of screening for hepatitis C virus antibody and hepatitis B virus core antibody on incidence of post-transfusion hepatitis. Lancet 338:1040–1041, 1991.

90. G Krause, S Whisenhunt, M Trepka, et al. Patient to patient transmission of hepatitis C virus associated with use of multidose saline vials in a hospital. 4th Decennial International Conference on Nosocomial and Healthcare-Associated Infections. March 5–9, 2000, Atlanta, GA.

91. GD Kelen, GB Green, RH Purcell, DW Chan, BF Qaqish, KT Sivertson, TC Quinn. Hepatitis B and hepatitis C in emergency department patients. N Engl J Med 326:1399–1404, 1992.

92. TL Wright. Etiology of fulminant hepatic failure: is another virus involved? Gastroenterology 104:640–643, 1993.

93. TJ Liang, L Jeffers, RK Reddy, MO Silva, H Cheinquer, A Findor, M De Medina, PO Yarbough, GR Reyes, ER Schiff. Fulminant or subfulminant non-A, non-B viral hepatitis: the role of hepatitis C and E viruses. Gastroenterology 104:556–562, 1993.

94. BH McGovern. Morbidity and mortality in patients with HIV and HCV coinfection. Presented at Issues and Controversies in Hepatitis C and HIV/HCV Coinfection. Sept. 7, 2000, New Orleans, LA.

95. MJ Alter, HS Margolis, K Krawczynski, FN Judson, A Mares, WJ Alexander, PY Hu, JK Miller, MA Gerber, RE Sampliner, et al. The natural history of community-acquired hepatitis C in the United States. N Engl J Med 327:1899–1905, 1992.

96. M Reichel, TM Mauro. Urticaria and hepatitis C. Lancet 336:822–823, 1990.

97. K Kanazawa, H Yaoita, F Tsuda, H Olamoto. Hepatitis C virus infection in patients with urticaria. J Am Acad Dermatol 35:195–198, 1996.

98. S Antinori, R Esposito, C Aliprandi, G Tadini. Erythema multiforme and hepatitis C [letter]. Lancet 337:428, 1991.

99. P Domingo, J Ris, E Martinez, F Casas. Erythema nodosum and hepatitis C [letter]. Lancet 336:1377, 1990.

100. JM Durand, P Lefevre, JR Harle, J Boucrat, L Vitviski, J Soubeyrand. Cutaneous vasculitis and cryoglobulinemia type II associated with hepatitis C virus infection [letter]. Lancet 337:499–500, 1991.

101. M Pascual, L Perrin, E Giostra, JA Schifferli. Hepatitis C virus in patients with cryoglobulinemia type II [letter]. J Infect Dis 162:569–570, 1990.

102. M Hearth-Holmes, S Zahrodka, BA Baethge, RE Wolf. Leukocytoclastic vasculitis associated with hepatitis C. Am J Med 90:765–766, 1991.

103. AS Pakula, JM Garden, SI Roth. Cryoglobulinemia and

cutaneous leukocytoclastic vasculitis associated with hepatitis C virus infection. J Am Acad Dermatol 28:850–853, 1993.

104. V Agnello, G Abel. Localization of hepatitis C virus in cutaneous vasculitic lesions in patients with type II cryoglobulinemia. Arthritis Rheum 40:2007–2015, 1997.

105. Y Abe, Y Tanaka, M Takenaka, H Yoshida, H Yatsuhashi, M Yano. Leukocytoclastic vasculitis associated with mixed cryoglobulinemia and hepatitis C virus infection. Br J Dermatol 136:272–274, 1997.

106. JC Brouet, JP Clauvel, F Danon, M Klein, M Seligmann. Biologic and clinical significance of cryoglobulins. A report of 86 cases. Am J Med 57:775–788, 1974.

107. V Agnello. The etiology and pathophysiology of mixed cryoglobulinemia secondary to hepatitis C virus infection. Springer Semin Immunopathol 19:111–129, 1997.

108. S Nityanand, G Holm, AK Lefvert. Immune complex mediated vasculitis in hepatitis B and C infection and the effect of antiviral therapy. Clin Immunol Immunopathol 82:250–257, 1997.

109. G von Kobyletzki, M Stucker, K Hoffman, D Pohlau, V Hoffmann, P Altmeyer. Severe therapy-resistant necrotizing vasculitis associated with hepatitis C virus infection: successful treatment of the vasculitis with extracorporeal immunoadsorption [letter]. Br J Dermatol 138:926–927, 1998.

110. PL Karlsberg, WM Lee, DL Casey, CJ Cockerell, PD Cruz Jr. Cutaneous vasculitis and rheumatoid factor positivity as presenting signs of hepatitis C virus-induced mixed cryoglobulinemia. Arch Dermatol 131:1119–1123, 1995.

111. MS Daoad, RA el-Azhary, LE Gibson, ME Lutz, S Daoud. Chronic hepatitis C, cryoglobulinemia, and cutaneous necrotizing vasculitis. Clinical, pathologic, and immunopathologic study of twelve patients. J Am Acad Dermatol 34: 219–223, 1996.

112. GF Buezo, M Garcia-Buey, L Rios-Buceta, MJ Borque, M Aragues, E Dauden. Cryoglobulinemia and cutaneous leukocytoclastic vasculitis with hepatitis C virus infection. Int J Dermatol 35:112–115, 1996.

113. RW McMurray. Hepatitis C-associated autoimmune disorders. Rheum Dis Clin North Am 24:353–374, 1998.

114. JC Mertens, HK Ronday, AA Masclee, FC Breedveld. Rheumatic manifestations of hepatitis C virus infection. Neth J Med 51:225–227, 1997.

115. CM Shearer, JM Jackson, JP Callen. Symmetric polyarthritis with livedo reticularis: a newly recognized manifestation of hepatitis C virus infection. J Am Acad Dermatol 37:659–662, 1997.

116. B Frankum, CH Katelaris. Hepatitis C infection and Henoch-Schönlein purpura [letter]. Aust N Z J Med 25:176, 1995.

117. M el Darouti, M Abu el Ela. Necrotizing acral erythema: a cutaneous marker of viral hepatitis C. Int J Dermatol 35: 252–256, 1996.

118. N Tsukazaki, M Watamabe, H Irifune. Porphyria cutanea tarda and hepatitis C virus infection. Br J Dermatol 138: 1015–1017, 1998.

119. GH Elder. Porphyria cutanea tarda. Semin Liver Dis 18: 67–75, 1998.

120. E Dabrowska, I Jablonska-Kaszewska, B Falkiewicz. High prevalence of hepatitis C virus infection in patients with porphyria cutanea tarda in Poland. Clin Exp Dermatol 23: 95–96, 1998.

121. A Piperno, R D'Alba, L Roffi, M Pozzi, A Farina, L Vecchi, G Fiorelli Hepatitis C virus infection in patients with idiopathic hemochromatosis (IH) and porphyria cutanea tarda (PCT). Arch Virol 4(suppl):215–216, 1992.

122. B Cribier, D Rey, G Uhl, C Le Coz, C Hirth, E Libbrecht, D Vetter, JM Lang, F Stoll-Keller, E Grosshans. Abnormal urinary coproporphyrin levels in patients infected by hepatitis C virus with or without human immunodeficiency virus. A study of 177 patients. Arch Dermatol 132: 1448–1452, 1996.

123. H Gomi, K Hatanaka, T Miura, I Matsuo. Type of impaired porphyrin metabolism caused by hepatitis C virus is not porphyria cutanea tarda but chronic hepatic porphyria [letter]. Arch Dermatol 133:1170–1171, 1997.

124. KA Stuart, F Busfield, EC Jazwinska, P Gibson, LA Butterworth, WG Cooksley, LW Powell, DH Crawford. The C282Y mutation in the haemochromatosis gene (HFE) and hepatitis C virus infection are independent cofactors for porphyria cutanea tarda in Australian patients. J Hepatol 28:404–409, 1998.

125. MY Sheikh, RA Wright, JB Burrus. Dramatic resolution of skin lesions associated with porphyria cutanea tarda after interferon alpha therapy in a case of chronic hepatitis C. Dig Dis Sci 43:529–533, 1998.

126. S Fargion, A Piperno, MD Cappellini, M Sampietro, AL Fracanzani, R Romano, R Caldarelli, R Marcelli, L Vecchi, G Fiorelli. Hepatitis C virus and porphyria cutanea tarda: evidence of a strong association. Hepatology 16: 1322–1326, 1992.

127. J Sanchez-Perez, MD Castro, GF Buezo. Lichen planus and hepatitis C virus: prevalence and clinical presentation of patients with lichen planus and hepatitis C virus infection. Br J Dermatol 134:715–719, 1996.

128. M Lapidoth, N Arber, D Ben-Amitai, J Hagler. Successful interferon treatment for lichen planus associated with chronic active hepatitis due to hepatitis C virus infection [letter]. Acta Derm Venereol 77k1–172, 1997.

129. JV Bagan, C Ramon, L Gonzales, M Diago, MA Milian, R Cors, E Lloria, F Cardona, Y Jimenez. Preliminary investigation of the association of oral lichen planus and hepatitis C. Oral Surg Oral Med Oral pathol Oral Radiol Endod 85:532–536, 1998.

130. N Dupin, O Chosidow, F Luncl, C Fretz, H Szpirglas, C Frances. Oral lichen planus and hepatitis C virus infection: a fortuitous association? [letter]. Arch Dermatol 133: 1052–1053, 1997.

131. Y Nagao, T Kameyama, M Sata. Hepatitis C virus RNA detection in oral lichen planus tissue [letter]. Am J Gastroenterol 95:850, 1998.

132. AS Boyd, LB Nanney, LE King Jr. Immunoperoxidase

evaluation of lichen planus biopsies for hepatitis C virus. Int J Dermatol 37:260–262, 1998.

133. R Tanei, Y Ohta, K Katsuoka. Lichen planus and Sjögren-type sicca syndrome in a patient with chronic hepatitis C. J Dermatol 24:20–27, 1997.

134. K Kanazawa, H Yaoita, F Tsuda, K Murata, H Okamoto. Association of prurigo with hepatitis C virus infection [letter]. Arch Dermatol 131:852–853, 1995.

135. L Theilmann, B Gmelin, B Kallinowski, B Kommerell, J Koderisch, K Andrassy. Prevalence of antibodies to hepatitis C virus in sera from patients with systemic necrotizing vasculitis [letter]. Nephron 57:482, 1991.

136. J Lacour, I Bodokh, J Castanet, S Bekri, JP Ortonne. Porphyria cutanea tarda and antibodies to hepatitis C virus. Br J Dermatol 128:121–123, 1993.

137. C Herrero, A Vicente, M Bruguera, MG Ercilla, JM Barrera, J Vidal, J Teres, JM Mascaro, J Rodes. Is hepatitis C virus infection a trigger of porphyria cutanea tarda? Lancet 341:788–789, 1993.

138. M Mokni, M Rybojad, D Puppin Jr, S Catala, F Venezia, R Djian, P Morel. Lichen planus and hepatitis C virus. J Am Acad Dermatol 24:792, 1991.

139. TY Chaung, L Stitle, R Brashear, C Lewis. Hepatitis C virus and lichen planus: a case-control study of 340 patients. J Am Acad Dermatol 41:787–789, 1999.

140. PJ Scheuer, P Ashrafzadeh, S Sherlock, D Brown, GM Dusheiko. The pathology of hepatitis C. Hepatology 15:567–571, 1992.

141. MA Gerber, K Krawczynski, MJ Alter, RE Sampliner, HS Margolis. Histopathology of community acquired chronic hepatitis C. Mod Pathol 5:483–486, 1992.

142. JM Levey, B Bjornsson, B Banner, M Kuhns, R Malhotra, N Whitman, PL Romain, TG Cropley, HL Bonkovsky. Mixed cryoglobulinemia in chronic hepatitis C infection. A clinicopathologic analysis of 10 cases and review of recent literature. Medicine (Baltimore) 73:53–67, 1994.

143. SJ Hadziyannis. Nonhepatic manifestations and combined diseases in HCV infection. Dig Dis Sci 41 (suppl): 63S–74S, 1996.

144. Centers for Disease Control and Prevention. Recommendations for prevention and control of hepatitis C virus (HCV) infection and HCV-related chronic disease. MMWR 47(No. RR-19):1–39, 1998.

145. M Roggendorf, V Schlopkoter. Hepatitis C virus [German]. Bietr Infusionsther 28:13–21, 1991.

146. L Viladomiu, J Genesca, JI Esteban, H Allende, A Gonzalez, JC Lopez-Talavera, R Esteban, J Guardia. Interferon-alpha in acute posttransfusion hepatitis C: a randomized, controlled trial. Hepatology 15:767–769, 1992.

147. J Pawlotsky, D Dhumeaux, M Bagot. Hepatitis C virus in dermatology. A review. Arch Dermatol 131:1185–1193, 1995.

148. SW Schalm, BE Hansen, L Chemello, A Bellobuono, JT Brouwer, O Weiland, L Cavalletto, R Schvarcz, G Ideo, A Alberti. Ribavirin enhances the efficacy but not the adverse effects of interferon in chronic hepatitis C. Meta-analysis

of the individual patient data from European centers. J Hepatol 26:961–966, 1997.

149. R Schvarcz, ZB Yun, A Sonnerborg, O Weiland. Combined treatment with interferon alpha-2b and ribavirin for chronic hepatitis C in patients with a previous non-response or non-sustained response to interferon alone. J Med Virol 46:43–47, 1995.

150. GL Davis, R Esteban-Mur, V Rustgi, J Hoefs, SC Gordon, C Trepo, ML Shiffman, S Zeuzem, A Craxi, MH Ling, J Albrecht. Interferon alfa-2b alone or in combination with ribavirin for the treatment of relapse of chronic hepatitis C. N Engl J Med 339:1493–1499, 1998.

151. O Reichard, G Norkrans, A Fryden, JH Braconier, A Sonnerborg, O Weiland. Randomized double-blind, placebo-controlled trial of interferon a-2b with and without ribavirin for chronic hepatitis C. Lancet 351:83–87, 1998.

152. J Hoofnagle. Antiviral therapy of hepatitis C. Plenary session VI. Presented at the 10th International Symposium on Viral Hepatitis and Liver Disease. April 9–13, 2000, Atlanta, GA.

153. MP Manns, JG McHutchison, S Gordon, et al. Peg-interferon alfa 2-b plus ribavirin compared to interferon alfa-2b plus ribavirin for the treatment of chronic hepatitis C. Presented at the 51st Annual Meeting of the American Association for the Study of Liver Diseases. October 27–31, 2000, Dallas, TX.

154. P Cohen, QT Nguyen, P Deny, F Ferriére, D Roulot, O Lortholary, B Jarrousse, F Danon, JH Barrier, J Ceccaldi, J Constans, B Crickx, JN Fiessinger, E Hachulla, A Jaccard, M Seligmann, M Kazatchkine, L Laroche, JF Subra, P Turlure, L Guillevin. Treatment of mixed cryoglobulinemia with recombinant interferon alpha and adjuvant therapies. A prospective study on 20 patients. Ann Med Interne (Paris) 147:81–86, 1996.

155. C Ferri, AL Zignego, G Longombardo, M Monti, L La Civita, F Lombardini, F Greco, A Mazzoni, G Pasero, P Gentilini, et al. Effect of alpha-interferon on hepatitis C virus chronic infection in mixed cryoglobulinemia patients. Infection 21:93–97, 1993.

156. LB Siegel, BB Eber. Porphyria cutanea tarda remission [letter]. Ann Intern Med 121:304–309, 1994.

157. H Takikawa, R Yamazaki, S Shoji, K Miyake, M Yamanaka. Normalization of urinary porphyrin level and disappearance of skin lesions after successful interferon therapy in a case of chronic hepatitis C complicated with porphyria cutanea tarda. J Hepatol 22:249–250, 1995.

158. D Grasset, J Nougue, C Seigneuric, M Landreaud, JJ Voigt. Porphyria cutanea tarda and chronic hepatitis C. Course after interferon therapy [letter]. Gastroenterol Clin Biol 18:1148–1149, 1994.

159. J Okano, Y Horie, H Kawasaki, M Kondo. Interferon treatment of porphyria cutanea tarda associated with chronic hepatitis type C. Hepatogastroenterology 44:525–528, 1997.

160. M Fureta, M Kaito, E Gabazza, N Fujita, S Ishida, S Tamaki, R Ikeda, S Wakisawa, H Hayashi, S Watanabe, Y

Adachi. Ineffective interferon treatment of chronic hepatitis C-associated porphyria cutanea tarda, but with a transient decrease in HCV RNA levels. J Gastroenterol 35: 60–62, 2000.

161. MS Doutre, C Beylot, P Couzigou, P Long, P Royer, J Beylot. Lichen planus and virus C hepatitis: disappearance of the lichen under interferon alpha therapy [letter]. Dermatology 184:229, 1992.

162. MS Daoud, LE Gibson, S Daoud, RA el-Azhary. Chronic hepatitis C and skin diseases: a review. Mayo Clin Proc 70:559–564, 1995.

163. T Barreca, G Corsini, R Franceschini, C Gambini, A Garibaldi, E Rolandi. Lichen planus induced by interferon-alpha-2a therapy for chronic active hepatitis C. Eur J Gastroenterol Hepatol 7:367–368, 1995.

164. Nagao, M Sata, T Ide, H Suzuki, K Tanikawa, K Itoh, T Kameyama. Development and exacerbation of oral lichen planus during and after interferon therapy for hepatitis C. Eur J Clin Invest 26:1171–1174, 1996.

165. L Jauregui, V Garcia-Patos, R Pedragosa, J Vidal, A Castells. Liquen plano asociado a hepatopatia por virus de la hepatitis C. Gastroenterol Hepatol 19:507–510, 1996.

166. R Strumia, D Venturini, S Boccia, S Gamberini, S Gullini. UVA and interferon-alfa therapy in a patient with lichen planus and chronic hepatitis C [letter]. Int J Dermatol 32: 386, 1993.

167. S Boccia, S Gamberini, M Dalla Libera, R Strumia, D Venturini. Lichen planus and interferon therapy for hepatitis C [letter]. Gastroenterology 105:1921–1922, 1993.

168. U Protzer, FR Ochsendorf, A Leopolder-Ochsendorf, KH Holtermüller. Exacerbation of lichen planus during interferon alfa-2a therapy for chronic active hepatitis C. Gastroenterology 104:903–905, 1993.

Index

Acquired immunodeficiency syndrome (AIDS)
  human immunodeficiency virus (HIV) and, 307–395
Adhesion molecules
  E-selectin, 32
  ELAM-1, 32
  ICAM-1, 32
  ICAM-2, 32
  P-selectin, 32
  VCAM, 32, 34
Aedes, 444, 473, 481, 496, 499
  Ae. aegypti, 473, 475, 496, 499
  Ae. albopictus, 475
  Ae. polynesiensis, 473
  Ae. scutellaris, 473
  Ae. triseriatus, 431
Adenoviruses, 4
Angiocentric cutaneous lymphoma, 157
Anopheles, 481
Antivariola sera, 8
Antivaccinia sera, 8
Arenaviridae, 446–450
  Lassa fever, 430, 446–450
  South American hemorrhagic fever viruses, 430, 446–450
  taxonomy, 430

B virus (herpesvirus simiae), 15, 235
Bacillary angiomatosis, 228, 229
Barmah Forest disease, 515
Biological warfare
  anthrax, 55, 58
  smallpox, 42, 44
Buschke-Lowenstein tumor, 273, 274
Bunyaviridae, 429–446

California/La Crosse encephalitis, 429–433
  related viruses, 429, 434, 439, 443, 446
Crimean-Congo hemorrhagic fever, 439–443
hantaviruses, 434–439
Rift Valley fever, 443–446
taxonomy, 430

Cabassous, 512
California/La Crosse encephalitis, 429–433
  clinical manifestations, 431, 433
  definition, 429
  diagnosis, 433
  differential diagnoses, 432
  history, 429, 430
  incidence, 430
  laboratory findings, 433
  pathogenesis, 431
  pathology, 433
  related viruses, 429, 434, 439, 443, 446
  transmission, 430–431
  treatment and prevention, 433
    ribavirin, 433
  zoonotic implications, 430
CD1, 27
cdc2-kinase, 30
Cell mediated immunity (CMI), 27, 32
Cell structure
  asymmetrical periflexural exanthem
  cellular pathology (CMV), 177
  of childhood (APEC), 1
  CMV-induced cytopathic effect, 183
  CMV-specific macromolecular, 179
  Cowdry type A

[Cell structure]
    intranuclear inclusion, 90, 91
    nuclear inclusion and CMV, 183
  cowpox, 51
  cytomegaly and CMV, 183
  EBV encoded RNA transcript (EBER-1), 157
  EBV lymphocytes, 151
  EBV Reed-Sternberg cells of Hodgkin's disease, 157
  EBV Kikuchi's disease, 160
  eczema vaccinatum, 46
  endothelial cells, 32–34
  HIV and HSV, 313
  HPV
    condyloma acuminatum, 279
    HeLa cells, 257
    HPV capsid antigens, 281
    SiHa cells, 257
    squamous cell carcinoma, 267–270
    verruca vulgaris, 279
    verrucous carcinoma, 280
  HSV and cytopathology, 91–94
  keratinocytes, 28–31
  Langerhans' cells, 25–28
  measles
    microtubules of paramyxovirus, 414
    multinucleated giant cells, 404, 413
    spindle cell transformation, 404, 413
    syncytial-type multinucleated giant cells, 413
    Warthin-Finkelday giant cells, 413
  molluscum contagiosum, 60–61
  mononucleosis (CMV), 180
  monkeypox, 49–50
  morphological changes (CMV), 178
  Owl's eyes (CMV), 188, 186
  SALT, 25
  smallpox, 42
  T cells, 31, 32
  unilateral laterothoracic exanthem (ULE), 1
  vaccinations and, 9, 10
Centers for Disease Control and Prevention (CDCP)
    (formerly CDC)
  equine vaccine, 506
  measles, 404–405, 410
    eradication of, 404
    estimate of cases, 404
  monkey pox, 48
  smallpox, 43
Chikungunga fever (CHIK), 513–515
  clinical manifestations, 513, 514
  definition, 513
  diagnosis, 514
  differential diagnoses, 514
  history, 513
  incidence, 513, 516
  laboratory findings, 514
  mosquito vector
    Aedes aegypti, 513

[Chikungunga fever]
  pathogenesis, 513
  pathology, 514
  related viruses and vectors:
    Mayaro, 515
    O'nyong-nyong (ONN), 515
    Ross River virus, 515
    Sindbis (Ockelbo), 515
    Barmah Forest, 515
  transmission, 516
  treatment/prophylaxis, 514, 515
  zoonotic implications, 516
Children
  asymmetrical periflexural exanthem of childhood (APEC),
    1
  classic exanthems, 14
  cowpox, 51
  coxsackieviruses
    associated manifestations, 463
    characteristics of rash, 463
  cytomegalovirus (CMV)
    ''blueberry muffin'' syndrome, 184
    clinical manifestations, 180
    complications, 180
    congenital infection in neonates, 176, 177, 180, 181, 192
    cutaneous vasculitis, 185
    effect on fetus, 177
    infection with, 175–177
    mononucleosis, 180
    pathogenesis, 174–178, 180
    vaccine, 192
  eczema vaccinatum, 46
  molluscum contagiosum (MC), 60–61
  monkeypox, 49–50
  smallpox, 42
  dengue fever, 475
  Echovirus
    associated manifestations, 463–464
    characteristics of rash, 463–464
    occurrence of rash, 463–464
  enteroviruses, 455–472
  Epstein-Barr virus (EBV), 14
    clinical manifestations, 148
    diagnosis of, 152
    Gianotti-Crosti syndrome, 14, 149
  Hemophilus influenza and measles, 411
  hepatitis B, 535
    perivascular lymphocytic infiltrate, 535
    vaccine, 537
  hepatitis C, 539, 543, 544
  herpes labialis, 74, 75
  Heck's disease, 272
  HSV and infants, 79, 96
  HSV and neonates, 87–90, 96
  human herpesvirus 6 (HHV-6), 14, 15, 198, 199
    exanthem subitum (roseola infantum), 14, 198
  human herpesvirus 8 (HHV-8)

[Children]
    horizontal transmission, 220
    lymphadenopathy, 225
    mother to child transmission, 220
  HPV, infection with, 248, 250, 262, 270, 272
  keratoconjunctivitis, 84
  measles
    and rubella vaccine (MR), 415
    measles, mumps, rubella vaccine (MMR), 415
    modified measles in infants, 409
    respiratory complications, 411
    vaccine, 415
  Neisseria meningitides and measles, 411
  neonatal HSV infections, 87–90
  parvovirus (B19) infection, 296
    clinical manifestations, 295–297
    fifth disease, 295, 296
    "slapped cheek" syndrome, 295, 297
  rubella
    congenital rubella, 524
    pregnancy, 524, 525
    vaccine contraindications, 526
    vaccination, 526
    WHO, 526
  Streptococcus pyogenes and measles, 411
  unilateral laterothoracic exanthem (ULE), 1
  varicella-zoster virus (VZV), 119
    chickenpox, 119, 122
    fetal complications, 123
    treatment for, 133
    varicella, 119
    yellow fever vaccine and, 499
    zoster, 125, 126, 128
Clinical manifestations
  acute exanthem, 309
  B virus, 238
  Chikungunya fever (CHIK), 513
  CMV-induced mononucleosis, 181
  Colorado tick fever, 398
  cowpox, 51
  Crimean-Congo hemorrhagic fever, 441
  dengue fever, 476
  eastern equine encephalitis (EEE), 505
  erythema infectiosum, 298
  exanthem subitum, 201, 215
  hand-foot-and-mouth syndrome, 467
  hantavirus hemorrhagic fever:
    with renal syndrome (HFRS), 436
  hantavirus pulmonary syndrome, 438
  hepatitis B virus (HBV), 532
  hepatitis C virus (HCV), 539
  herpangina, 470
  herpes genitalis, 76
  herpes labialis, 74
  herpes zoster, 130
  HPV, 258
  infectious mononucleosis, 150

[Clinical manifestations]
  Japanese encephalitis (JE), 482
  Kaposi's sarcoma, 223
  Kikuchi's disease, 159
  Kyasanur Forest disease (KFD), 485
  La Crosse infection, 431
  Lassa fever, 448
  Marburg and Ebola hemorrhagic diseases, 425
  measles, 407
  molluscum contagiosum (MCV), 61
  monkeypox, 49
  Omsk hemorrhagic fever (OHF), 488
  oral hairy leukoplakia, 162
  orf, 55
  papular-purpuric gloves-and-socks syndrome (PPGSS), 301
  pseudocowpox/paravaccinia, 57
  Rift Valley fever, 444
  roseola and roseola-like illness, 468
  rubella (German measles), 523
  St. Louis encephalitis (SLE), 291
  smallpox, 43
  tanapox, 59
  tick-borne encephalitis (TBE), 491
  vaccinia, 45
  varicella, 123
  Venezuelan equine encephalitis (VEE), 511
  western equine encephalitis (WEE), 508
  yellow fever, 497
Colorado tick fever, 397–401
  clinical manifestations, 398
  definition, 397
  diagnosis, 400
  differential diagnoses, 399
  history, 397
  incidence, 397
  laboratory findings, 400
  pathogenesis, 397, 398
  prevention, 400
  taxonomy, 398
  transmission, 398
  treatment, 400
  vectors, 398
    Dermacentor andersoni, 398
  zoonotic implications, 398
Cowpox, 50–51
  clinical manifestations, 50–51
  definition, 50
  dermatopathology, 51
  diagnosis, 50–51
  differential diagnoses, 52
  history, 50
  incidence, 50
  pathogenesis, 50
  transmission, 50
  treatment/prophylaxis, 51
  zoonotic implications, 50
Coxsackieviruses, 3, 5

Crimean-Congo hemorrhagic fever, 439–443
    clinical manifestations, 441
    definition, 439
    diagnosis, 442
    differential diagnoses, 442
    history, 439
    incidence, 440
    laboratory findings, 440
    pathogenesis, 440
    pathology, 441
    transmission, 440
    treatment and prevention of, 442, 443
    zoonotic implications, 440
Culex, 481
    annulirostris, 481
    annulus, 481
    fuscocephus, 481
    gleidus, 481
    nigripalpus, 489
    pipiens, 444, 489
    quinquefasciatus, 489
    tarsalis, 489
    theileri, 444
    tritaeniorhynchus, 480–481
    vishnui, 481
Cutaneous lymphocyte-associated antigen (CLA), 31
Cutaneous virology
    classic childhood exanthems, 14
    clinical manifestations, 1
    diagnosis, 3
    differential diagnoses, 5
    DNA viruses, 3–17
        hepatitis B and D, 20
        herpesviruses, 12–16
        parvoviruses, 16–17
        papillomaviruses, 8–12
        poxviruses, 5–8
    FDA-approved
        anti-HPV agents, 12
        anti-herpesvirus agents, 16
        anti-retroviral agents, 20
        anti-hepatitis agents, 21
        anti-influenza agents, 21
    human disease, 4
    immunoglobulins (IG), 10
    miscellaneous viruses, 20
        hemorrhagic fever viruses, 20
    pathophysiology, 3
    RNA viruses, 6
        enteroviruses, 17
        hepatitis C, 20
        paramyxoviruses, 17–18
        retroviruses, 18–19
        togaviruses, 18
    taxonomy, 6
    viral exanthems, 3

[Cutaneous virology]
    virus vaccines
        administration, 9–10
        timeline, 8
Cytokines, 26–27, 30, 31
    colony-stimulating factor-1, 28
    granulocyte-macrophage colony-stimulating factor (GMC-SF), 28, 30
    IFN-α, 33
    IFN-β, 30, 32, 33
    IFN-γ, 32, 33
    IL-1, 30
    IL-1α, 28
    IL-1β, 26, 32, 33
    IL-2, 28, 30, 32
    IL-2 receptor, 28
    IL-4, 32
    IL-5, 32
    IL-6, 32, 33
    IL-10, 32
    IL-12, 32
    IL-15, 32
    IL-18, 32
    TGF-β1, 30, 31
    tumor necrosis factor-α (TNF-α), 26, 30, 31, 32, 33
Cytomegalovirus (CMV), 2, 4, 14, 32–33, 173–195
    cell structure
        cellular pathology, 177
        Cowdry type nuclear inclusion and CMV, 183
        cytomegaly and CMV, 183
        induced cytopathic effect, 183
        macromolecules, 179
        mononucleosis, 180
        morphological changes, 178
        owl's eyes, 188, 186
    cellular pathology, 177–180
        effect of HIV on replication, 177
        morphological changes, 178
        replication of, 177
        reservoirs of virus, 178
    children
        ''blueberry muffin'' syndrome, 14, 184
        clinical manifestations, 180
        complications, 180
        congenital infection in neonates, 176, 177, 180, 181, 192
        cutaneous vasculitis, 185
        effect on fetus, 177
        infection with, 175–177
        mononucleosis, 180
        vaccine, 192
    Chlamydia trachomatis and CMV, 182
    clinical manifestations, 180–184
        CMV-induced mononucleosis, 181
        congenital infections, 180–181
        HIV and mononucleosis syndrome, 180
        immunocompromised, 182–184

[Cytomegalovirus]
    perinatal infections, 181–182
    related diseases, 180
  control of CMV infection, 189
  cutaneous manifestations, 184–186
    herpes simplex virus coinfection, 185
    immunocompromised, 185, 186
    Staphylococcus coinfection, 185
  definition, 173
  diagnosis, 188–189
    complement fixation, 188
    enzyme-linked immunosorbent assay (ELISA), 188
    hemagglutination, 188
    immunofluoresence, 188
    latex agglutination, 188
    neutralization tests, 188
    viral isolation, 188
  differential diagnoses, 181
  dermatopathology, 186
    cutaneous ulcerations, 186, 187
    owl's eye, 186, 188
    viral isolation, 186
  history, 173
  immunocompromised:
    clinical syndromes with, 182
    cutaneous manifestations, 186
    cutaneous ulcerations, 186, 187
    gastrointestinal involvement, 176
    HIV effect on replication and, 177
    lungs, 176
    mononucleosis syndrome, 180
    mortality rate, 186
    prevention/therapy, 190
    renal transplants, 176
    synergy with HIV, 182–184
  incidence, 174
  Kaposi's sarcoma and CMV, 176, 185
  ocular
    CMV retinitis in HIV patients, 182, 183
  pathogenesis, 174
    congenital CMV, 177
    early childhood, 174–178, 180
    early infection, 175, 176
    immunosuppression, 177
    mononucleosis syndrome, 176
  Pneumocystis carinii and CMV, 185
  prophylaxis, 189, 190
  Staphylococcus aureus and CMV, 185
  taxonomy, 174
  transmission, 174
  treatment, 189–190
    CMV-induced mononucleosis, 189
    CMV infection, 190
  vaccine, 192
  viral genome structure, 173–174
  zoonotic implications, 174
Cytotoxic T lymphocytes, 27, 31, 32

Dengue fever, 473–480
  clinical manifestations, 475–477
    children and young adolescents, 475
  definition, 473
  diagnosis, 478, 479
  history, 473
  incidence, 474
  laboratory findings, 477–478
  pathogenesis, 475
  pathology, 478
  treatment and prevention, 479, 480
DC-SIGN, 26
Delayed type hypersensitivity (DTH), 32
Dendritic cells, 29, 29, 31
Dermacentor
  ard, 347
  pictus, 483
Differential diagnoses
  B virus, 241
  California/La Crosse encephalitis, 432
    in other diagnoses, 399, 445, 483, 486, 489, 492, 495, 506, 509, 512
  Chikungunya fever (CHIK), 514
    in other diagnoses, 425, 437, 442, 445, 449, 479, 489
  Colorado tick fever, 399
    in other diagnoses, 425, 432, 437, 442, 445, 449, 479, 483, 486, 489, 492, 506, 509, 512
  cowpox, 52
    in other diagnoses, 55
  Crimean-Congo hemorrhagic fever, 442
    in other diagnoses, 425, 437, 442, 445, 449, 479, 486, 489
  cytomegalovirus (CMV), 181
  dengue hemorrhagic fever (DHF), 473
    in other diagnoses, 425, 437, 442, 445, 449, 486, 489, 498, 514
  eastern equine encephalitis (EEE), 506
    in other diagnoses, 399, 432, 445, 483, 486, 489, 492, 495, 509, 512
  erythema infectiosum, 299
    in other diagnoses, 204, 216, 409
  exanthem subitum, 216
    in other diagnoses, 409, 479, 524
  hand-foot-and-mouth syndrome, 468
    in other diagnoses, 123, 302, 470
  hantavirus hemorrhagic fever, 437
    in other diagnoses, 425, 442, 445, 449, 479, 486, 489, 514
  hantavirus pulmonary syndrome, 439
  hepatitis B, 536
  herpangina, 470
    in other diagnoses, 76, 468
  herpes genitalis, 78
  herpes labialis, 76
  herpes zoster, 130
    in other diagnoses, 241

[Differential diagnoses]
human papillomavirus (HPV), 281
human herpesvirus 6, 204
in other diagnoses, 151
infectious mononucleosis, 151
in other diagnoses, 76, 181, 204, 216, 409, 524
Japanese encephalitis (JE), 483
in other diagnoses, 399, 432, 445, 483, 486, 489, 492, 495, 506, 509, 512
Kaposi's sarcoma, 226
Kikuchi's disease, 159
Kyasanur Forest disease (KFD), 486
in other diagnoses, 425, 432, 437, 442, 445, 449, 479, 483, 489, 498, 506, 509, 512
Lassa fever and the South American hemorrhagic fever viruses, 449
in other diagnoses, 425, 437, 442, 445, 479, 486, 489
hemorrhagic fevers, 449
Marburg and Ebola hemorrhagic diseases, 425
in other diagnoses, 432, 437, 445, 449, 479, 486, 489, 498
measles, 409
in other diagnoses, 204, 216, 299, 524
molluscum contagiosum (MCV), 62
in other diagnoses, 55, 281
monkeypox, 50
in other diagnoses, 43, 59
Omsk hemorrhagic fever (OHF), 489
in other diagnoses, 425, 437, 442, 445, 449, 479, 486, 498
oral hairy leukoplakia, 162
orf, 55
in other diagnoses, 58
other entries
anthrax, 55, 58
enteroviruses, 204, 216, 399, 409, 524
herpes simplex virus (HSV), 62, 123, 130, 241, 483
Kawasaki's disease, 159, 204, 216, 302
keratoacanthomas, 55, 62, 281
leptospirosis, 437, 439, 432, 449, 486
malaria, 425, 449, 479, 498
Mayaro, 399, 432, 437, 514
O'nyong nyong virus (ONN), 399, 437, 432, 514
oropuche, 399, 432, 437, 514
Powassan encephalitis, 399, 432, 483, 486, 489, 492, 495, 506, 509, 512
Rocky Mountain spotted fever, 204, 216, 302, 399, 432, 437, 439, 449, 479, 483, 492, 495, 506, 509, 512
sandfly fever, 399, 432, 437, 514
scarlet fever, 204, 216, 299, 409, 437, 469, 479, 524
Sindbis, 399, 432, 437, 514
syphilis, 43, 162
typhoid fever, 425, 449, 479, 498
West Nile fever, 399, 425, 432, 445, 449, 483, 486, 489, 492, 495, 498, 506, 509, 512
pseudocowpox, 57

[Differential diagnoses]
Rift Valley fever, 445
in other diagnoses, 425, 432, 442, 437, 442, 445, 449, 479, 483, 486, 489, 492, 495, 498, 506, 509, 512
roseola and roseola-like illness, 469
rubella (German measles), 524
in other diagnoses, 151, 204, 216, 299, 409, 468, 469, 514
St. Louis encephalitis (SLE), 492
in other diagnoses, 399, 432, 445, 483, 486, 489, 495, 506, 509, 512
smallpox, 43
in other diagnoses, 50, 123
tanapox, 59
tick-borne encephalitis (TBE), 495
in other diagnoses, 399, 432, 445, 483, 486, 489, 492, 509, 512
vaccinia, 46
varicella, 123
in other diagnoses, 43, 50, 468, 469
Venezuelan equine encephalitis (VEE), 512
in other diagnoses, 399, 432, 445, 483, 486, 489, 492, 495, 506, 509
western equine encephalitis (WEE), 509
in other diagnoses, 399, 432, 445, 483, 486, 489, 492, 495, 506, 512
yellow fever (YE), 498
in other diagnoses, 425, 442, 445
DNA viruses
hepatitis B and D, 529–550
herpesviruses, 69–245
papillomaviruses, 247–294
parvovirus B19, 295–306
poxviruses, 39–68

Eastern equine encephalitis (EEE), 503–506
clinical manifestations, 504, 505
definition, 503
diagnosis, 505
differential diagnoses, 506
history, 503
incidence, 503, 504
laboratory findings, 505
mosquito vectors:
Culex melanura, 503
Aedes sp, 503
Coquillettidia sp., 503
pathogenesis, 503, 504
pathology, 505
taxonomy, 504
transmission, 504
treatment and prophylaxis, 505, 506
immune sera, 506
zoonotic implications, 504
Ebola, 421–426
clinical manifestations, 422, 423

[Ebola]
definition, 421
diagnosis, 425, 426
differential diagnoses, 425
history, 421
incidence, 421, 422
laboratory findings, 424
pathogenesis, 422
pathology, 425
treatment/prevention, 426
Echovirus, 463
Elderly
arboviral fevers, 515
vaccinia, 45–46
virus vaccines, 9, 10
VZV, 120
shingles, 120
herpes zoster, 120
postherpetic neuralgia, 129
Endothelial cells, 32–34
Endothelium, 31
E-selectin, 31
Eta-1, 32
Enterovirus infections, 455–471
clinical manifestations, 458–461
enterovirus 71, 17, 457, 466–467
hand-foot-and-mouth disease, 461–466
clinical manifestations, 467
differential diagnoses, 468
herpangina, 462, 469–471
clinical manifestations, 470
differential diagnoses, 470
history, 455
incidence, 456–457
pathogenesis, 457–458
related diseases, 464
roseola infantum, 467–469
clinical manifestations, 468
differential diagnoses, 469
taxonomy, 456
transmission, 456
treatment, 471
virus type, 462–464
coxsackievirus, 462–464
echovirus, 462–464
enterovirus, 462–464
zoonotic implications, 456
Enzyme-linked immunosorbent-assay (ELISA)
acute HIV exanthem, 310
California/La Crosse encephalitis, 433
CMV infections, 188
Crimean-Congo hemorrhagic fever, 442
dengue fever, 479
diagnosis of hepatitis B, 542
fifth disease, 302–303
HSV infection and, 92

[Enzyme-linked immunosorbent-assay (ELISA)]
Japanese encephalitis, 483
Kyasanur Forest disease, 486
Marburg and Ebola hemorrhagic diseases, 426
measles, 415
Omsk hemorrhagic fever (OHF), 488
orf, 55
Rift Valley fever, 445
St. Louis encephalitis, 491
tick-borne encephalitis, 494
yellow fever, 499
Epidermodysplasia verruciformis, 249, 253
clinical manifestations, 258
progression of, 276–278
treatment of, 286
Epstein-Barr virus (EBV), 3, 5, 14, 145–171
angiocentric cutaneous lymphoma, 157
cellular
encoded RNA transcript (EBER-1), 157
Kikuchi's disease, 160
lymphocytes, 151
Reed-Sternberg cells of Hodgkin's disease, 157
children
clinical manifestations, 148
diagnosis of, 152
Gianotti-Crosti syndrome, 149
dermatological manifestations, 149–151
asymptomatic primary EBV infection, 149
infectious mononucleosis, 145–173
antibody response in infectious mononucleosis, 152, 153
associated diseases and syndromes, 146
clinical manifestations, 148–151
definition, 145
dermatopathology, 151
diagnosis, 151
differential diagnoses, 151
epidemiology, 2, 146, 147
Gianotti-Crosti syndrome, 149
Guillain-Barré, 148
history, 145
incidence, 146, 147
pathogenesis, 147
Reye's syndrome, 148
taxonomy, 146
zoonotic implications, 146
immunocompromised:
B cell lymphoma, 155, 156
Kikuchi's histiocytic necrotizing lymphadenitis, 158
lymphoproliferative disease, 153, 154
T cell lymphoma, 155, 156
treatment, 158
Kikuchi's histiocytic necrotizing lymphadenitis:
clinical manifestations, 158, 159
dermatopathology, 159
diagnosis, 160
differential diagnoses, 159

[Epstein-Barr virus]
  epidemiology, 158
  pathogenesis, 158
  treatment, 161
  laboratory findings, 151
  lymphoproliferative disease/malignancy, 153
    clinical and dermatological manifestations, 154, 155
    dermatopathology, 156, 157
    diagnosis, 157
    epidemiology, 153
    histiocytoid lymphoma, 157
    laboratory findings, 156
    pathogenesis, 154
    treatment, 158
  oral hairy leukoplakia (OHL), 161–166
    clinical manifestations, 161, 162
    dermatopathology, 162–164
    diagnosis, 164, 165
    differential diagnoses, 162
    epidemiology, 161
    laboratory findings, 161, 162
    pathogenesis, 161
    treatment, 165–166
  Reed-Sternberg cells (EBV), 157
  subcutaneous lymphoma, 157
  Toxoplasma gondii and EBV, 158
  transmission, 146
  treatment, 152, 153
  vesiculopapular eruptions and EBV, 157
  Yersinia enterocolitica and EBV, 158
Erythema infectiosum (*see also* parvovirus B19), 14, 295–303
Everglades virus, 512
Exanthem subitum, 14, 198
Exanthems, viral, 3

Flaviviridae family, 473–499
  dengue fever, 473–480
  incidence, 474
  Japanese encephalitis, 480–484
  Kyasanur Forest disease, 484–487
  Omsk hemorrhagic fever, 487–489
  St. Louis encephalitis, 489–491
  taxonomic families, 474
  transmission, 474
  yellow fever, 489–491
Fibroblast growth factor-beta (β-FGF), 34
Filatov-Dukes (Fourth disease), 14
Filoviridae family
  Marburg and Ebola, 421–426
    clinical manifestations, 422, 423
    definition, 421
    diagnosis, 425, 426
    differential diagnoses, 425
    history, 421

[Filoviridae family]
  incidence, 421, 422
  laboratory findings, 424
  pathogenesis, 422
  pathology, 425
  prevention, 426
  transmission, 422
  treatment/prevention, 426
  zoonotic implications, 422
Food and Drug Administration (FDA), 14, 100, 101, 102, 134, 387

Gianotti-Crosti syndrome
  EBV and, 149
  hepatitis B and, 533–535
Guillain-Barré syndrome
  EBV and, 148
  VZV and, 122

Hand-foot-and-mouth disease, 17, 470, 461–466
  clinical manifestations, 467
  differential diagnoses, 468
Hantaviruses, 434–439
  clinical manifestations, 435, 436
    hemorrhagic fever with renal syndrome (HFRS), 435
    hantavirus pulmonary syndrome (HPS), 436, 438
  definition, 434
  diagnosis, 437
  differential diagnoses, 434
  history, 434
  incidence, 435
  laboratory findings, 436
  pathogenesis, 435
  pathology, 434
  related viruses, 429, 434, 439, 443
  rodent vectors and
    Apodemus agrarius, 434
    Apodemus flavicollis, 434
    Clethrionomys glareolus, 434
    Oryzomys, 434
    Peromyscus maniculatus, 434
    Rattus rattus, 434
    Sigmodon hispidus, 434
  transmission, 434
  treatment and prevention of, 429, 439
    ribavirin, 438
  zoonotic implications, 434
Hantavirus pulmonary syndrome (HPS), 436–439
  clinical manifestations, 438
  diagnosis, 438
  differential diagnoses, 439
  laboratory findings, 438, 439
  pathology, 436
  treatment and prevention of, 438–439
    ribavirin, 438
Heck's disease, 272

Hemorrhagic fever viruses, 3, 436–439
  clinical manifestations, 436
  diagnosis, 438
  differential diagnoses, 437
  laboratory findings, 438, 439
  pathology, 436
  treatment and prevention, 438–439
Henoch-Schönlein purpura
  parvovirus B-19 and, 297
  VZV and, 123
Hepatitis
  Caliciviridae family, 530
  Deltaviridae family, 530
  Flaviviridae family, 530
  Hepacivirus genus, 530
  Hepadnaviridae family, 530
  hepatitis B, 529–537
  hepatitis C, 538–544
  Picornaviridae family, 530
Hepatitis A virus
  Engerix-b, 9
  Havrix, 9
  Twinrix, 9
Hepatitis B virus, 3, 20–21, 529–537
  antiviral therapy, 536
  chronic hepatitis B, cutaneous manifestations, 534
    mixed cryoglobulinemia, 534
    polyarteritis nodosa (PAN), 534–535
  clinical manifestations, 531–534
    acute hepatitis B infection, 532
    Gianotti-Crosti syndrome, 533–535
    other manifestations, 534
    serum sickness-like infection, 532–533
  definition, 529–530
  dermatopathology
    papular acrodermatitis of childhood (PAC), 535
  diagnosis, 536
    serological window phase, 536
  differential diagnoses, 536
  history, 531, 532
  incidence, 530–532
  laboratory findings, 535–536
    serum alanine aminotransferase (ALT), 535
    serum aspartate aminotransferase (AST), 535
  pathogenesis, 531
    Africa and developing nations, 531
    antigens, 531
    Asia, 531
    liver injury, 531
    necrosis, 531
    US and Europe, 531
  prevention, 537
  transmission, 531
  taxonomy, 530
  treatment, 536, 537
    adefovir dipiroxil, 536
    Epivir HBV, 536

[Hepatitis B virus]
    famciclovir, 536
    immunity modulation, 536
    interferon alpha, 536
    interferon alpha + famciclovir, 536
    interferon alpha + lamivudine, 536
    Intron A, 536
    lamivudine, 536
  vaccines
    Comvax, 9
    Engerix-b, 9
    recombivax HB, 9
  viral replication inhibition, 536
  zoonotic implications, 530
Heptatitis C virus, 3, 20–21, 538–544
  antiviral therapy, 543
  clinical manifestations, 539, 540
  cutaneous findings, 540
    mixed cryoglobulinema, 540
    porphyria cutanea tarda (PCT), 540, 541
    lichen planus, 541, 542
  definition, 538
  diagnosis, 542
    antibody detection, 542
    enzyme-linked immunosorbent assay (ELISA), 542
  history, 538
  incidence, 538, 539
  laboratory findings, 542
  pathogenesis
    cirrhosis, 539
    liver cancer, 539
    risk factors, 539
  pathology, 542
  prevention, 544
  transmission, 538, 539
    sexual transmission, 539
  treatment, 543, 544
    alpha interferon, 543
    alpha interferon + ribavirin (Rebetol), 543
    antisense oligoribonucleotide, 543
    helicase inhibitors, 543
    peginterferon alfa-2b-pegylated (interferon) (PEG-intron), 543
    pegylated interferon + ribavirin, 543
    protease inhibitors, 543
  zoonotic implications, 538
Herpangina, 17, 469–471
  clinical manifestations, 470
  diagnosis, 470
  differential diagnoses, 470
  laboratory findings, 17, 469–470
  pathology, 17
  treatment and prevention, 470–471
Herpes B virus, 4, 5, 15, 16, 235–245
  clinical manifestations, 237–240
    aerosol inhalation, 239
    asymptomatic infection, 239
    recurrent vesicular eruption, 239

[Herpes B virus]
    control and prevention, 241
        laboratory technique, 242
        monkey, screens, 242
        passive immunization, 241
        vaccine, 241
    definition, 235
    dermatopathology, 240–241
    diagnosis, 241
    differential diagnoses, 241
    epidemiology, 235
    history, 235
    pathogenesis, 237
        direct inoculation of, 237
        nervous system involvement in, 237
        viral replication of, 237
    taxonomy, 236
    transmission, 236
    treatment, 242–243
        acyclovir, 242
        ganciclovir, 242
        wound cleansing, 242
    zoonotic implications, 236
Herpes simplex viruses (HSV), 2, 12, 13, 69–117
    clinical manifestations
        herpes genitalis, 75, 76
        herpes labialis, 74, 75
    diagnosis, 91–93
        polymerase chain reaction (PCR), 92
        serologic assays, 92, 93
    differential diagnoses
        herpes labialis, 76
        herpes genitalis, 78
    eczema herpeticum, 80
    encephalitis
        Cowdry type A inclusion, 91
        progression of, 91
        symptoms, 91
    erythema multiforme, 80
    eye, involvement of, 84
    history, 69–71
    incidence, 70–72
    immunocompromised, 85–87
    keratoconjunctivitis, 84, 85, 96
        cornea, involvement of, 84
        treatment of, 96
        uveitis, 84, 85
    mimics of, 104
    non-viral "herpes", 105
    pathology
        symptoms, 93
    pathogenesis, 72–74
    prevention, 102, 103
        barrier protection, 102
        viral vaccines, 103
    risk during pregnancy, 77, 79, 87, 88
    severity of, 77

[Herpes simplex viruses]
    taxonomy, 70
    transmission, 70
    treatment, 94–102
        experimental therapy, 102
        viral resistance, 102
    Whitlow, herpetic, 80, 81
    zoonotic implications, 70
Herpes simplex encephalitis, 90–105
    diagnosis, 91–93
    pathology, 93–94
    treatment, 94–102
HSV-2 gD protein, 31–32
Herpes simplex keratoconjunctivitis, 84–85
Highly active antiretroviral therapy (HAART), 20
    AIDS-associated Kaposi's sarcoma and, 227
    HIV infections and, 307–308, 313, 318, 325, 331, 337,
        344, 362, 379, 384, 387–389
Histiocytoid lymphoma, 157
HIV, 19, 33
    acanthamebiasis, 331–333
    AIDS and, 26–28, 34, 307–395
    bacillary angiomatosis, 320, 321, 323–325
        Bartonella and, 320, 321
    bacterial infections and, 320–325
        Haemophilus, 320, 323, 325
        Mycobacterium, 320, 325, 326, 327, 328
        Neisseria, 320
        Pseudomonas, 320, 323
        Staphylococcus, 320, 321
        Streptococcus, 320, 321
    botryomycosis
        S. aureus and, 321, 322
    clinical manifestations, 309
    cutaneous drug eruptions and, 363–366
    cutaneous manifestations, 309
    diagnosis, 309–310
    gingivitis, 370, 371
    hair abnormalities, 366–367
        alopecia, 366
        trichomegaly, 366
    highly active antiretroviral therapy (HAART), 378–389
        nucleoside reverse transcriptase inhibitors (NRTIs), 379,
            380
        non-nucleoside reverse transcriptase inhibitors
            (NNRTIs), 381
        nucleotide reverse transcriptase inhibitors, 381
        protease inhibitors, 382, 383
        treatment with, 313
    HPV and, 316–318
    hyperpigmentation, 370, 371
    Kaposi's sarcoma and, 307, 338, 370, 373, 376–378
        effect of Th2 cytokines, 307
        mimics of, 338, 370
        neoplastic disorders, 376–378
        treatment, 373
    Kawasaki's disease, 369–370

[HIV]

kwashiorkor, 370
Langerhans' cells, 25–28
lymphadenitis
    Streptococcus and, 321, 323
malignant melanoma, 378
measles and, 319
metabolic and nutrition disorders and, 367–370
mononucleosis, 313
nail disorders and, 367
    Beau's lines, 367
    caused by *Candida*, 367
    Muehrcke's nails, 367
    Terry's nails, 368
neoplastic disorders, 370, 372–379
    Hodgkin's and non-Hodgkin's lymphoma, 373–375
    Kaposi's sarcoma, 370, 376–378
    malignant melanoma, 378
    multiple dysplastic nevi, 378–379
parvovirus B19 (fifth disease) and, 319
pellagra, 370
psoriasis and, 344–351
    Candida, 344
    Staphylococcus, 344
    Streptococcus, 344
poxviruses and, 61, 63–65, 318, 319
Reiter's syndrome:
    Campylobacter fetus, 344
    Shigella flexneri, 344
    Ureaplasma urealyticum, 344
    HLA-B27, 344, 351
seborrheic dermatitis, 347–351
    Pityrosporum ovale, 343
septicemia:
    Pseudomonas aeruginosa or *P. cepacia* and, 323
treatment
    abacavir, 20, 379, 381, 384
    abacavir + lamivudine + zidovudine, 20, 379, 384
    ABC, 379, 381
    adefovir, 388
    Agenerase, 20, 379, 383, 387
    amikacin, 331
    amphotericin B, 339, 343
    amprenavir, 20, 379, 383, 387
    azithromycin, 321
    AZT, 379–380
    bacitracin, 321
    bleomycin, 375
    ceftriaxone, 321
    cephalexin, 321
    ciprofloxacin, 321, 331
    clarithromycin, 321
    clofazimine, 321
    Combivir, 20, 379, 381, 384
    Crixivan, 20, 379, 382, 387
    cyclophosphamide, 375
    ddC, 379, 380

[HIV]

ddI, 379, 380, 384
D4T, 379, 380, 384
delaviridine, 20, 379, 385
dicloxacillin, 321
didanosine, 20, 379, 380, 384
doxorubicin, 375
doxycycline, 321
efavirenz, 20, 379, 381, 385
Epivir, 20, 379, 380, 384
erythromycin, 321
Fortovase, 20, 382
Hivid, 20
indinavir, 20, 382
Invirase, 20, 379, 382, 386
interferon-α, 16, 382
itraconzaole, 343
Kaletra, 20, 379, 383, 387
ketoconazole, 343
lamivudine, 20, 379, 380, 384, 388
lamivudine + zidovudine, 20, 379, 384
lopinavir + ritonavir, 20, 379, 383, 387
methotrexate, 375
minocycline, 321
mupirocin ointment, 321
nelfinavir, 20, 379, 382, 387–388
nevirapine, 20, 379, 381, 385
norfloxacin, 321
Norvir, 20, 379, 381, 386
olfloxacin, 331
penicillin G benzathine, 321
polymyxin B sulfate, 321
potassium iodide, 343
prednisone, 375
Preveon, 388
pyrazinamide, 331
Rescriptor, 20, 379, 381, 385
Retrovir, 20, 379, 380, 382, 386
rifampin, 321
ritonavir, 20, 379, 381
saquinavir, 20, 379, 382, 386
spectinomycin, 321
stavudine, 20, 379, 380, 384
Sustiva, 20, 379, 381, 385
tenofovir, 20, 379, 381, 385
3TC, 379, 380, 384
trimethoprim-sulfamethoxazole, 321
Trizivir, 20, 379, 381, 384
Videx, 20, 379, 380, 384
vincristine, 375
Viracept, 20, 379, 382, 387
Viramune, 20, 379, 381, 385
Viread, 20, 379, 381, 385
zalcitibine, 20, 379, 380, 384
Zerit, 20, 379, 380, 384
Ziagen, 20, 379, 380, 384
zidovudine, 20, 379, 380, 388

[HIV]
  treatment of bacterial infections
    Bartonella, 320
    Corynebacterium, 323
    Nocardia, 323
    Rhodococcus, 323
    Streptomyces, 323
  ectoparasites
    Demodex folliculorum, 331
    Sarcoptes scabiei, 331
  fungal infections, 342–344
    Aspergillus, 342
    Cladosporium cladosporioides, 344
    Curvularia, 344
    Microsporum canis, 342
    Penicillium marneffei, 345
    Pityrosporum orbiculare, 343
    Pityrosporum ovale, 343
    Pseudallescheria boydii, 342
    Scedosporium inflatum, 342
    Tinea corporis, 343
    Trichosporon beigelii, 343, 344
    Zygomycosis, 343
  hair abnormalities, 366–367
    alopecia, 366
    trichomegaly, 366
  internal parasites, 332–335
    Leishmania donovani, 333, 335
    Pneumocystis carinii, 332
    Strongyloides stercoralis, 332
    Toxoplasma gondii, 332
  nail disorders, 367
    Beau's lines, 367
    caused by *Candida*, 367
    caused by *Hendersonula toruloidea*, 367
    Muehrcke's nails, 367
    Terry's nails, 368
  noninfectious papular pruritic disorders, 353–356
  noninfectious skin disorders, 344–347
    seborrheic dermatitis, 344
    psoriasis, 344
    Reiter's syndrome, 344
  other papulosquamous disorders, 351–353
    exfoliative erythroderma, 352
    pityriasis rubra pilaris, 351
  parasitic infestations:
    acanthamebiasis, 331–333
    demodicidosis, 331–333
    ectoparasites, 331–333
    scabies, 330–333
  photoinduced and photoaggravated conditions, 360–363
  systemic fungal infections and, 335
    B. dermatitidis, 337
    Histoplasma capsulatum, 328, 341
    Paracoccidioides brasiliensis, 328
  vascular and vascular-related abnormalities, 356–360
  venereal disease and, 325–329

[HIV]
  chancroid, 325
  gonorrhea, 325
  lymphogranuloma venereum, 325
  syphilis, 325, 328, 329
  vitamin A deficiency, 370
  vitamin C deficiency, 370
HIV-derived transactivator (tat) protein, 30, 34
HIV infection, 307–395
  acute exanthem of, 308–310
  human herpes infections and, 310–313, 315
  bacterial infections and, 320–325
  CMV and (*see also* Chapter 7), 313, 315, 316
  Epstein-Barr virus and, 313, 316
  incidence, 308
  OHL and, 313, 316
  parvovirus B19 (fifth disease) and, 302
  pathogenesis, 307–309
  transmission, 308
  VZV and (*see also* chapter 5), 313–314
HIV patients
  molluscum contagiosum (MCV), 61–65
  vaccinia, 46
HLA-B7, 31, 32
HLA-DR+, 29–31
HLA-DQ+, 29–31
Hodgkin's and non-Hodgkin's lymphoma, 373–375
Human herpesviruses (HHV)
  HHV-1 (Herpes simplex 1), 2–5, 12–13, 31, 32, 69–117
  HHV-2 (Herpes simplex 2), 2–5, 12–13, 31, 32, 69–117
  HHV-3 (VZV), 2–5, 12–13, 119–144
  HHV-4 (Epstein-Barr virus), 3, 145–171
  HHV-5 (CMV), 2, 4, 173–195
  HHV-6, 1, 2, 3, 5, 12, 14, 15, 197–211
  HHV-7, 12, 15, 213–218
  HHV-8, 12, 15, 34, 219–234
Human herpesvirus 6 (HHV-6), 1, 2, 5, 14–15, 197–211
  children
    exanthem subitum (roseola infantum), 198
  clinical manifestations, 200–202
    exanthem subitum, 200–202
    clinical features, 200
  definition, 197
  dermatopathology, 202–204
  diagnosis, 204–205
  rashes, 205
  serologic assays, 205
  differential diagnoses, 204
  history, 197
  incidence, 198
    exanthem subitum, 198
    roseola infantum, 198
  laboratory findings, 202
  pathogenesis
    infants and children, 199
    latent infection, 199
    related disorders, 199

[Human herpesvirus 6]
  pregnancy, 199
  Rosai-Dorfman syndrome, 203
  taxonomy, 198
  transmission, 198
  treatment/prophylaxis, 205
    foscarnet, 205
    ganciclovir, 205
  zoonotic implications, 198
Human herpesvirus 7 (HHV-7), 14, 213–218
  clinical manifestations, 215
    exanthem subitum and HHV-6, 214
  definition, 213
  diagnosis, 215
    polymerase chain reaction, 215
    serology, 215
  different diagnoses, 216
  history, 213
  incidence, 213, 214
  immunocompromised, 214
  pathogenesis, 213–215
    latency, 214
    relationship with HHV-6, 214
  taxonomy, 214
  transmission, 214
  treatment, 216, 217
    acyclovir, 216
    cidofovir, 216
    ganciclovir, 216
    foscarnet, 216
    lobucavir, 216
  zoonotic implications, 214
Human herpesvirus 8 (HHV-8), 3, 14, 34, 219–234
  children
    horizontal transmission, 220
    infant concerns, 79, 96
    lymphadenopathy, 225
    mother to child transmission, 220
    neonatal, 87–90, 96
  classic KS, 226
  clinical manifestations, 222–225
    AIDS and, 222
    oral lesions, 222
    classic Kaposi's sarcoma, 222
  definition (Kaposi's sarcoma), 219
    African endemic, 219
    classic Mediterranean, 219
    HIV-associated, 219
    immunosuppressed (organ transplant), 219
  dermatopathology, 225
    cytology, 226
    histopathology, 225, 226
  diagnosis, 226
  differential diagnoses, 226
  history, 219
  incidence, 219, 220
  immunosuppressed

[Human herpesvirus 8]
    gastrointestinal involvement, 222
    genital mucosa, 222
    HAART, 227
    HIV and, 221–224
    organ transplantation and, 221
    oral mucosa, 222
  pathogenesis, 220–222
    genome evolution, 220
    immunosuppressed patients, 221
    JAK1/STAT 1/3 pathways, 221
  transmission, 220
  treatment/prevention, 226–229
    Alitretinoin, 227
    cidofovir, 228
    foscarnet, 227, 228
    ganciclovir, 227, 228
    highly active antiretroviral therapy (HAART), 227
    interferon α, 226
  zoonotic implications, 220
Human immunodeficiency virus (HIV), 3, 19, 20, 307–395
  laboratory findings, 20
  pathology, 19, 20
Human papillomaviruses (HPV), 1, 3, 8, 32, 247–294
  clinical manifestations, 258
    Bowenoid papulosis, 258, 264, 266, 279
    cervical cancer, 267
    condyloma acuminata, 11, 273
    epidermodysplasia verruciformis, 11, 258
    oral papillomas, 258
    respiratory papillomatosis, 258
    squamous cell carcinoma, 267–270
    verrucous carcinoma, 258
    warts, 11, 258
  definition, 247
  diagnosis, 280–282
    polymerase chain reaction (PCR), 282
  differential diagnoses, 281
    Bowenoid papulosis, 281
    condyloma acuminata, 281
    epidermodysplasia verruciformis, 281
    flat warts, 281
    oral papillomatosis, 281
    paronychial warts, 281
    plantar warts, 281
    verruca vulgaris, 281
  epidermodysplasia verruciformis, 249, 253, 258, 275–278
    progression of, 276–278
  histopathology, 277–280
  history, 247
  HIV infection and, 270
  HPV and, 32
  incidence, 248, 250
    in adults, 248, 250, 251
    in children, 248, 250
  pathogenesis, 251–253
    development of lesions, 251

[Human papillomaviruses]
    immune response, 252, 253
    viral replication, 252
  taxonomy, 248
  transmission, 248
  treatment, 282–288
    cidofovir, 283, 286
    destructive therapies, 283–284, 286
    epidermodysplasia verruciformis, 286–288
    imiquimed, 283–285
    interferon, 283–285
    topical therapies, 282–283
  vaccines, 286–288
    prophylactic, 287–288
    therapeutic, 286
  viral oncogenesis, 253–259
    cervical cancer, 253, 267
    dysplasia, 254
    E6,E7 oncoproteins, 254–257
    epidermodysplasia verruciformis (EV), 249, 253, 258, 275–277
    HeLa cells, 257
    non-melanoma skin cancers, 253
    p53, mechanisms of, 254, 255
    SiHa cells, 257
    squamous cell carcinoma, 267–270
    tumor necrosis factor, 257
  virology, 247–250
    genotypes, lesions, 249
    proteins, 250
    structure, 247–249
  zoonotic implications, 248
Human rabies
  Bayrab, 10
  Imogam-rabies, 10
  Hyperab, 10
Humoral, 27, 32
Hutchinson's sign and VZV, 127

Imiquimed, 283–285
Immunocompromised
  acquired immunodeficiency syndrome (AIDS) (*see also* HIV)
  EBV
    B cell lymphoma, 155, 156
    Kikuchi's histiocytic necrotizing lymphadenitis, 158
    lymphoproliferative disease, 153, 154
    T cell lymphoma, 155, 156
    treatment, 158
  HHV-6
    HIV-infected, 200
    transplants, 199, 200
  HHV-7, 214
  HHV-8
    gastrointestinal involvement, 222
    genital mucosa, 222
    HAART, 227
    HIV and, 221–224

[Immunocompromised]
    organ transplantation and, 221
  HIV and, 307–395
  HPV infection and, 270
  HSV and, 85–87
  measles
    HIV+, 414
    respiratory complications, 412
    ribavirin treatment, 416
    subacute sclerosing panencephalitis complications, 412
  parvovirus B19
    transient aplastic crisis, 300
  rubella
    vaccine contraindications, 526
  transplants, increased risk with HSV, 85–87
    gastrointestinal, 85
    HIV, 87
    renal, cardiac, 85
    respiratory tract, esophagus, 85
  varicella zoster virus (VZV), 5, 120–137
    bone marrow transplant, 120
    gabapentin for PHN, 137
    Hodgkin's disease, 120
    sign of HIV, 121
    treatment of postherpetic neuralgia, 136–137
    treatment of varicella, 134
    treatment of zoster, 135
    varicella complications, 125
    zoster complications, 129, 132
Immunoglobulins (IG)
  cytomegalovirus, 10
  hepatitis B IG, 10
  human rabies IG, 10
  intramuscular IG, 10
  respiratory syncytial virus IG, 10
  varicella zoster IG, 10
Influenza vaccines
  Fluogen, 9
  Flushield, 9
  Fluvirin, 9
  Fluzone, 9
Influenza A, 21
Influenza B, 21
Integrin
  alpha v beta, 33
Intercellular adhesion molecule (ICAM-1), 30, 31
Ixodes, 488
  apronophorus, 488
  dammini, 495
  ricinus, 493
  persuleatus, 493

Janus Kinus, 1, 33
Japanese encephalitis (JE), 480–484
  clinical manifestations, 482
  definition, 480
  diagnosis, 483
  differential diagnoses, 483

[Japanese encephalitis]
history, 480
incidence, 480, 481
laboratory findings, 482
pathogenesis, 481
pathology, 482
transmission, 481
treatment and prevention, 483
JE-VAX, 10
zoonotic implications, 481
JAK 1/STAT 1/3 pathway, 221
in HHV-8, 221

Kaposi's sarcoma, 3, 15, 34, 219–229, 307, 338, 370, 373,
376, 378
effect of TH2 cytokines, 307
histopathology, 226
mimic of, 338, 370
neoplastic disorder, 376–378
treatment, 373
Keratinocytes, 28–31
Kikuchi's histiocytic necrotizing lymphadenitis
clinical manifestations, 158, 159
dermatopathology, 159
diagnosis, 160
differential diagnoses, 159
epidemiology, 158
pathogenesis, 158
treatment, 161
Kyasanur Forest disease (KFD), 484–487
clinical manifestations, 485, 486
definition, 484
diagnosis, 486
differential diagnoses, 486
history, 484
incidence, 484, 485
laboratory findings, 486
pathogenesis, 485
pathology, 485
symptoms, 486
transmission, 484
treatment and prevention, 486, 487
zoonotic implications, 484

Langerhans' cells, 25–28, 29, 30, 32, 33
Lassa fever and South American hemorrhagic fevers,
446–450
clinical manifestations, 447–449
definition, 446
diagnosis, 449, 450
differential diagnoses, 449
history, 446
incidence, 446, 447
laboratory findings, 449
pathogenesis, 447
pathology, 449
transmission, 447

[Lassa fever and South American hemorrhagic fevers]
treatment and prevention, 450
ribavirin, 450
zoonotic implications, 447
Latency-associated nuclear antigen (LANA), 221
Lymph nodes, 27
Lymphoma cells, 34
Lymphocytes
T cells
CD4+, 26, 28, 30, 31, 32, 33
CD8+, 30, 31, 32
CD14+, 27
CD16+, 28
CD34+, 27
CD54+, 31
CD58+, 31
Lymphocyte function-associated antigen-1 (LFA-1), 29, 30,
34
Lymphoproliferative disorders
EBV and, 157

Major histocompatibility complex (MHC) class I, 28, 30, 31,
32, 33
Major histocompatibility complex (MHC) class II, 28, 30, 31,
32, 33
Marburg (*see also* Ebola), 421–426
clinical manifestations, 422, 423
definition, 421
diagnosis, 425, 426
differential diagnoses, 425
history, 421
incidence, 421, 422
laboratory findings, 424
pathogenesis, 422
pathology, 425
treatment/prevention, 426
Mayaro, 515, 516
mosquito vector, 515
Haemagogus sp., 515
Melanoma, malignant, 378
Measles, 4, 14, 17, 403–420
atypical measles, 410–411
killed virus vaccine and, 410
mimics, 410
symptoms, 410
children
modified measles in infants, 409
respiratory complications, 411
vaccine, 415
clinical manifestations, 406
erythematous macules, 406, 407
erythematous papules, 406, 407
Koplik's spots, 407, 408
complications, 411
black measles, 412
encephalitis, 412
hepatitis, 412

[Measles]
    pregnancy, 413
    respiratory manifestations, 411
    subacute sclerosing panencephalitis, 412
    transitory hypocalcemia, 413
    ulcerations, 413
  definition, 403
  diagnosis
    ELISA, 415
  differential diagnoses, 409
  epidemiology, 404–405
    clinical diagnosis, 405
    unpreventable cases, 405
  incidence, 404
  history, 403
  laboratory findings, 414
    leukopenia, 414
    lymphocytosis, 414
  modified measles, 409
  pathogenesis, 405
    viral multiplication, 405
    viremia, 405
  pathology, 413–414
    multinucleated giant cells, 413
    syncytial-type multinucleated giant cells, 413
    Warthin-Finkleday giant cells, 413
  prevention
    immunity, 415
    measles and rubella (MR) vaccine, 415
    measles, mumps, rubella (MMR), 9, 18, 415
    measles vaccines, 415
  taxonomy, 404
  transmission, 404
  treatment, 415–416
    ribavirin, 416
    vitamin supplements, 416
  virology, 403–404
    multinucleated giant cells, 404
    spindle cell transformation, 404
    temperature and humidity effects, 404
  zoonotic implications, 404
MMR (measles, mumps, rubella), 9
  Attenuvax, 9
  Biavax II, 9
  Meruvax, 9
  Mrvax II, 9
  Mumpsvax, 9
Medications
  abacavir, 20, 379, 381, 384
  abacavir + lamivudine + zidovudine, 9, 20, 379, 384
  ABC, 379, 381
  Abreva, 16
  acyclovir, 16, 102, 216
    treatment for varicella, 134, 135
    treatment for herpes B virus, 242
    treatment for HSV, 94–96
    treatment for EBV, 157–158

[Medications]
  adefovir, 16, 388
  adefovir dipicoxil, 536
  Agenerase, 20, 379, 383, 387
  Aldara, 12
  Alferon, 12
  Alitretinon, 227
  amantadine, 21
  amikacin, 331
  amphotericin B, 339, 343
  ampicillin, 14
  amprenavir, 20, 379, 383, 387
  Attenuvax, 9
  azithromycin, 321
  AZT, 379, 380
  bacitracin, 321
  BAYGAM, 10
  BAYRAB, 10
  BAYHEPB, 10
  BIAVAX, 9
  bleomycin, 375
  bupivacaine, 137
  capsaicin, 137
  ceftriaxone, 321
  cephalexin, 321
  chlorprothixene, 137
  cidofovir, 16, 96, 102, 190, 191, 216, 228, 283, 286
  ciprofloxacin, 321, 331
  clarithromycin, 321
  clofazimine, 321
  Combivir, 20, 379, 381, 384
  Comvax, 9
  cryoanalgesia, 137
  Crixivan, 20, 379, 381, 387
  cyclophosphamide, 375
  cytarabine, 190
  Cytogam, 10
  cytomegalovirus immune globulin, 191
  Cytovene, 16
  ddC, 379, 380
  ddI, 379, 380, 384
  D4T, 379, 380, 384
  Delaviridine, 20, 379, 385
  Denavir, 16
  dicloxacillin, 321
  didanosine, 20, 379, 380, 384
  docosanol, 102
  doxorubicin, 375
  doxycycline hydrochloride, 321
  efavirenz, 20, 379, 381, 385
  EMLA, 137
  Epivir, 20, 379, 380, 384
  Epivir-HBV, 21, 536
  erythromycin, 321
  famciclovir, 16, 96, 536
    treatment for varicella, 134, 135
    treatment of HSV, 96–101, 536

[Medications]

Famvir, 16
floxuridine, 190
fluconazole, 343
flucytosine, 343
Flumadine, 21
Fluogen, 9
fluphenazine, 137
Fluvirin, 9
Flushield, 9
Fluzone, 9
fomivirsen, 16, 190, 191
Fortovase, 20, 379, 381, 386
foscarnet, 16, 96, 102, 190, 191, 205, 216, 227, 228
foscavir, 16
ganciclovir, 16, 190, 205, 216, 227, 228, 242
gentamicin, 321
gabapentin
  pain treatment for post-herpetic neuralgia, 137
HAART (highly active antiretroviral therapy), 227
haloperidol, 137
Hivid, 20, 379, 380, 384
Hyper Hep, 10
HYPERAB, 10, 210
idoxuridine, 190
imidazoles, 339, 343
imiquimod, 12, 283, 285
Imovax, 9
Imovax-rabies, 9
indinavir, 20, 379, 381, 387, 388
Infergen, 21
interferons, 190
interferon α, 12, 16, 21, 536, 543
  Alferon, 12
  HPV treatment, 283–285
  Intron A, 12, 16, 21, 536, 543
  Roferon A, 12, 16
interferon alpha + lamivudine, 536
interferon alpha + famciclovir, 536
interferon alpha + ribavirin, 21
Intron A, 12, 16, 21, 536, 543
Invirase, 20, 379, 381, 386
IPOL, 10
itraconazole, 343
JE-VAX, 10
Kaletra, 20, 379, 383, 387
ketoconazole, 343
lamivudine, 20, 21, 379, 380, 384, 388, 536
lamivudine + zidovudine, 21, 379, 384
lidocaine, 137
lobucavir, 216
lopinavir + ritonavir, 20, 379, 383, 387
mannitol, 483
methotrexate, 375
methylprednisolone with lidocaine, 137
minocycline, 321
MERUVAX, 9
MRVAX II, 9

[Medications]

MUMPSVAX, 9
mupirocin ointment, 321
n-docosanol, 16
nelfinavir, 20, 379, 381, 387, 388
nevirapine, 20, 379, 381, 385
norfloxacin, 321
Norvir, 20, 379, 381, 386
olfloxacin, 331
oseltamivir, 21
peginterferon alpha-2b + ribavirin, 21
Peg Intron + rebetol, 21
penciclovir, 16
penicillin, 14
penicillin G benzathine, 321
Poliovax, 10
polymyxin B sulfate, 321
potassium iodide, 343
prednisone, 375
Preveon, 388
pyrazinamide, 331
RABIE-VAX, 9
Ramantadine, 21
Rebetron, 21
Recombivax HB, 9
Relenza, 21
Rescriptor, 20, 379, 385
resiquimod, 102
Retrovir, 20, 379, 380, 386
ribavirin, 190, 416
rifampin, 321
ritonavir, 20, 379, 381
Roferon-A, 12, 16, 21, 134
Rotashield, 9
saquinavir, 20, 379, 382, 386
spectinomycin, 321
stavudine, 20, 379, 380, 384
Sustiva, 20, 379, 385
Symmetrel, 21
Tamiflu, 21
tenofovir, 20, 379, 381, 385
thiosemicarbezone, 8
3TC, 379, 380, 384
trifluridine, 16, 96, 190
trihexphenidyl, 483
trimethoprim-sulfamethoxazole, 321
trizivir, 20, 379, 381, 384
valacyclovir, 16, 96, 134, 135, 190
Valcyte, 16
valganciclovir, 16
Valtrex, 16
vidarabine, 16, 102, 134, 190
Videx, 20, 379, 380, 384
vincristine, 375
Vira A, 16
Viracept, 20, 379, 381, 387
Viramune, 20, 379, 381, 385
Viread, 20, 379, 385

[Medications]
  Viroptic, 16
  Vistide, 16
  Vitrasene, 16
  Vitrasert, 16
  VZIG, 134
  zalcitibine, 20, 379, 380
  zanamivir, 21
  Zerit, 20, 379, 380, 384
  Ziagen, 20, 379, 380, 384
  zidovudine, 20, 379, 380, 388
  zidovudine + lamivudine, 20
  Zovirax, 16
Milker's nodules, 3, 5, 8, 55–57
  clinical manifestations, 53–55
  dermatopathology, 54–55
  diagnosis, 55
  differential diagnoses, 55
  history, 53
  incidence, 53
  laboratory findings, 54–55
  transmission, 53
  treatment, 55
Mixed cryoglobulinemia
  Hepatitis B, 534
    arthropathy, 534
    dermatological findings, 534
    purpuric skin lesions, 534
    renal disease, 534
  Hepatitis C, 540
    Type I, 540
    Type II, 540
    Type III, 540
Monocytes, 33
Molluscum contagiosum (MCV), 3–5, 59–65
  clinical manifestations, 60–62
  dermatopathology, 62
  description, 59
  diagnosis, 64, 65
  differential diagnoses, 62
  history, 59–60
  incidence, 60
  in HIV patients, 61–65
  laboratory findings, 62, 64
  pathogenesis, 60
  transmission, 60
  treatment/prophylaxis, 64, 65
  zoonotic implications, 60
Monkeypox, 48–50
  clinical manifestations, 49
  definition, 48
  differential diagnoses, 50
  effects of smallpox vaccine on, 48
  history, 48
  pathogenesis/epidemiology, 48–50
  transmission, 49
  zoonotic implications, 49

Mononucleosis, 14, 153
  CMV-induced
    clinical manifestations, 181
  Epstein-Barr virus induced
    differential diagnoses, 181
Mucambo virus, 512
Multiple dysplastic nevi, 378–379
Mosquito vectors
  Anopheles, 481
  Aedes, 444, 473, 481, 496, 499
    aegypti, 499, 473, 475, 496
    albopictus, 475
    polynesiensis, 473
    scutellaris, 473
    triseriatus, 431
  Culex
    annulirostis, 481
    annulus, 481
    fuscocephus, 481
    gleidus, 481
    nigripalpus, 489
    pipiens, 444, 489
    quinquefasciatus, 489
    tarsalis, 489
    theileri, 444
    tritaeniorhynchus, 480–481
    vishnui, 481
  Haemagogus, 496
Mycobacterium
  avium- intracellulare, 325
  bovis, 325
  chelonae, 325
  haemophilum, 325
  leprae, 325
  marinum, 325
  thermoresistible, 325

Neonatal HSV infection, 87–90

Ocular
  conjunctival warts and HPV, 265
  CMV retinitis in HIV patients, 182, 183
  keratoconjunctivitis and HSV, 84, 85, 96
  retinal necrosis and VZV, 132
  conjunctivitis (measles), 405
Omsk hemorrhagic fever, 487–491
  clinical manifestations, 488
  definition, 487
  diagnosis, 488, 489
  differential diagnoses, 489
  history, 487
  incidence, 487, 488
  laboratory findings, 488
  pathogenesis, 488
  pathology, 488
  transmission, 487
  treatment and prevention, 489
  zoonotic implications, 487

Oncogenes
 c-*myc*, 30
O'nyong-nyong (ONN)
 mosquito vector
  Anopheles funestus, 515
  Anopheles gambiae, 515
Oral hairy leukoplakia (OHL), 161–166
 clinical manifestations, 161
 diagnosis, 164, 165
 differential diagnoses, 162
 epidemiology, 161
 laboratory findings, 161, 162
 pathogenesis, 161
 treatment, 165–166
Orf, 8, 51–55
 clinical manifestations, 53, 55
 definition, 51–52
 dermatopathology, 54
 diagnosis, 56
 differential diagnoses, 55
 history, 53
 incidence, 53
 laboratory findings, 54, 55
 milker's nodules, 55
 pathogenesis, 53
 transmission, 53
 treatment, 55
 zoonotic implications, 53
Oropouche
 midge vector
  Culicoides paragensis, 515
 symptoms, 515
Osteopontin, 32
Owl's eyes, 188, 186

p48, 33
Papular acrodermatitis of childhood (PAC):
 perivascular lymphocyte infiltrate:
  children, 535
  endothelial swelling, 535
Paramyxoviruses (*see measles*), 17, 18
Parapoxvirus, 40, 51–65
 molluscum contagiosum, 59–65
 orf, 51
 paravaccinia, 56
 pseudocowpox, 56
 tanapox, 57
Parvovirus B19, 3, 16, 295–306
 clinical manifestations, 296–300
  children, 296
  fifth disease, 296
  juvenile rheumatoid arthritis, 297
  Henoch-Schönlein, 297
 definition
  fifth disease, 295, 296
 dermatopathology, 302
 diagnosis, 302, 303

[Parvovirus B19]
 differential diagnoses, 299
 history, 295
 incidence, 295, 296
 laboratory findings, 302
 papular-purpuric gloves-and-socks syndrome, 300
  clinical manifestations, 301
  complications, 300, 302
  differential diagnoses, 302
 parvovirus infection in adults, 287
  arthropathy, 299
  mimics of, 299
  rash, 300
 pathogenesis, 296
 taxonomy, 296
 transient aplastic crisis, 295, 300
 transmission, 296
 treatment/prophylaxis, 303
 zoonotic implications, 296
Phlebotomus fever (*see* sandfly fever)
Polymorphonuclear (PMN) cells, 33
Polyarteritis nodosa (PAN), 534
 dermatological manifestations, 535
 systemic vasculitis, 534
Post-herpetic neuralgia, 129
 clinical manifestations, 125–130
 complications of herpes zoster, 129
 treatment of pain:
  gabapentin, 137
  topical, 137
  tricyclic antidepressants, 136
Poxviridae, 5, 39–68
 cell structure, 39
 hosts and portal of entry, 40
 orthopoxviruses, 39–51
  cowpox, 50
  monkeypox, 47–50
  smallpox, 39–44
  vaccinia, 44–47
 parapoxvirus, 40, 51–65
  molluscum contagiosum, 59–65
  orf, 51
  paravaccinia (see pseudocowpox), 56
  pseudocowpox, 56
  tanapox, 57
 taxonomy, 40
Pregnancy
 hepatitis B, 537
  vaccines, 537
 HHV-6, 199
 measles complications, 413
 parvovirus B19
  chronic anemia, 301
  intrauterine infection, 302
 yellow fever vaccine and, 499
Pseudocowpox
 clinical manifestations, 56–57

[Pseudocowpox]
  definition, 56
  dermatopathology, 56
  differential diagnoses, 58
  history, 56
  incidence, 56
  laboratory findings, 56
  milker's nodules, 56–58
  pathogenesis, 56
  transmission, 56
  treatment, 56
  zoonotic implications, 56
Psoriasis
  HIV infection and, 351

Rabies, 2, 9
  Imovax, 9
  RabAvert, 9
  RABIE-VAX, 9
Retroviruses, 6, 18
Reyes syndrome
  EBV complications of, 148
  VZV and, 122
Ribavirin, treatment for, 21, 433
  California/La Crosse encephalitis, 429–433
  hantavirus pulmonary syndrome (HPS), 438
  Lassa fever, 450
  South American hemorrhagic fevers, 450
Rift Valley fever, 1, 443–446
  clinical manifestations, 444, 445
  definition, 443
  diagnosis, 445
  differential diagnoses, 445
  history, 444
  incidence, 443, 444
  laboratory findings, 445
  pathogenesis, 444
  pathology, 445
  related viruses, 446
  transmission, 443
  treatment and prevention, 445, 446
  zoonotic implications, 443
RNA viruses, 17–20
  bunyaviridae and arenaviridae, 429–454
  enteroviruses, 455–472
  flaviviridae, 473–502
  hepatitis A,C,E,G, 529–550
  HIV infections, 307–395
  Marburg and Ebola hemorrhagic fevers, 421–427
  measles, 403–420
  rubella, 519–528
  togaviridae, 503–518
Rosai-Dorfman syndrome and HHV-6, 203
Roseola infantum, 198, 467–469
  clinical manifestations, 468
  differential diagnoses, 469

Ross River virus, 515
Rotavirus, 6
Rubella (German measles), 3, 5, 14, 18, 469, 519–526
  clinical manifestations, 520–523
    encephalitis, 520
    polyarticular arthritis, 520
    rashes, 520
  congenital rubella syndrome, 3, 524
    "blueberry muffin" lesions, 3, 524
    glaucoma and cataracts, 525
    manifestations, 525
  definition, 519
  dermatopathology, 525
  diagnosis, 525, 526
  differential diagnoses, 524
  history, 519
  incidence, 519, 520
  laboratory findings, 525
  pathogenesis, 519–521
    immunity, 521
    nasopharynx, 520
    viral replication, 520–523
  taxonomy, 520
  transmission, 520
  treatment/prophylaxis, 526
  zoonotic implications, 520
Rubeola (measles), 3, 403–420

St. Louis encephalitis, 489–491
  clinical manifestations, 490, 491
  definition, 489
  diagnosis, 491, 492
  differential diagnoses, 492
  history, 489
  incidence, 489, 490
  laboratory findings, 490, 491
  pathogenesis, 489–490
  pathology, 490
  transmission, 490
  treatment and prevention, 491, 492
  zoonotic implications, 490
Sandfly fever, 516
  symptoms, 516
  vector, 516
Scarlet fever, 14, 469
Seborrheic dermatitis:
  HIV infection and, 351
Selectin ligand, 31
Semliki Forest virus, 512
Shingles, 120
Smallpox, 5, 39–43
  Centers for Disease Control (CDC), 43
  clinical manifestations, 42–43
  definition, 39
  dermatopathology, 43
  destruction of, 44

[Smallpox]
  differential diagnoses, 43
  history, 39–41
  incidence, 41–42
  laboratory findings, 43
  pathogenesis/epidemiology, 42
  symptomatic treatment, 44
  transmission, 41
  taxonomy, 40
  treatment/prophylaxis, 43–44
  variola major, 43
  variola minor, 43
  zoonotic implications, 41
South American hemorrhagic fevers and Lassa fever,
      446–450
  clinical manifestations, 448–450
  diagnosis, 449, 450
  differential diagnoses, 449
  history, 446
  incidence, 446, 447
  laboratory findings, 449
  pathogenesis, 447
  pathology, 449
  transmission, 447
  treatment and prevention, 450
    ribavirin, 450
  zoonotic implications, 447
Subcutaneous lymphoma, 157
Syphilis, 162

Tanapox, 57–59
  clinical manifestations, 59
  definition, 57–58
  differential diagnoses, 59
  history, 57–58
  incidence, 59
  pathogenesis, 58–59
  transmission, 58
    effects of smallpox vaccines, 59
  treatment/prophylaxis, 59
  zoonotic implications, 58
T cells, 28, 29, 31–32
TH1, 32
TH2, 32
Tick-borne encephalitis, 491–495
  clinical manifestations, 493, 494
  definition, 491
  diagnosis, 494, 495
  differential diagnoses, 495
  history, 493
  incidence, 493
  laboratory findings, 493
  pathogenesis, 493
  pathology, 493, 494
  related viruses, 491, 492, 494
    louping ill, 494

[Tick-borne encephalitis]
    Modoc, 495
    Negishi, 495
    Powassan virus, 494–495
    Rocio encephalitis, 494
  transmission, 492, 493
  treatment and prophylaxis, 494, 495
  zoonotic implications, 492
Tick vectors, 485
  Haemaphysalis spinigera, 485
  Hyalomma sp., 440
    anatolicum, 440
    marginatum, 440
  Boophilus, 440
T lymphocytes, 33
Togaviridae, 18, 503–518
  Chikungunya (CHIK), 513–515
  eastern equine encephalitis (EEE), 503–506
  other arboviral fevers, 515
    oropouche, 515
    phlebotomus (Sandfly fever), 516
  Venezuelan equine encephalitis (VEE), 508–512
  western equine encephalitis (WEE), 506–508
Toxoplasma gondii, 158
Transendothelial migration, 34
Treatment
  bacterial infections, 321
  B virus infections, 243
  Chikungunya fever (CHIK), 515
  Colorado tick fever, 400
  cowpox, 51
  Crimean-Congo hemorrhagic fever, 443
  dengue fever, 480
  eastern equine encephalitis (EEE), 506
  enteroviral exanthematous illnesses, 471
  exanthem subitum, 217
  Hantavirus pulmonary syndrome, 439
  hemorrhagic fever renal syndrome, 439
  hepatitis B virus (HBV)-related skin disorders, 537
  hepatitis C virus (HCV)-related cutaneous disorders, 544
  herpesvirus infections
    acyclovir-resistant HSV infection, 96
    herpes genitalis, 96
    herpes labialis, 96
    herpes simplex encephalitis, 96
    herpes simplex keratoconjunctivitis, 96
    mucocutaneous HSV, 96
    other cutaneous HSV infections, 96
    neonatal herpes simplex infection, 96
    neonatal HSV, 96
    recurrent orolabial or genital HSV infections, 96
  infectious mononucleosis, 153
  Japanese encephalitis (JE), 483
  Kaposi's sarcoma, 227
  Kikuchi's disease, 161
  Kyasanur Forest disease (KFD), 487
  La Crosse encephalitis, 433

[Treatment]
    Lassa fever and South American hemorrhagic fevers, 450
    Marburg and Ebola hemorrhagic diseases, 426
    measles, 415
    molluscum contagiosum, 64
    neoplastic disorders, 373
    noninfectious papular pruritic disorders, 357
    oral hairy leukoplakia, 166
    orf, 55
    parasitic infestations, 333
    parvovirus B19 infection, 303
    photoinduced and photoaggravated conditions, 362
    postherpetic neuralgia, 136
    psoriasis, 351
    rubella infection, 526
    seborrheic dermatitis, 351
    St. Louis encephalitis (SLE), 492
    smallpox, 43
    systemic fungal infections, 343
    tanapox, 59
    tick-borne encephalitis (TBE), 495
    varicella, 134
    vasculitis and vascular-related abnormalities, 360
    Venezuelan equine encephalitis (VEE), 512
    warts, 283
    western equine encephalitis (WEE), 509
    yellow fever, 499
    zoster, 135
Tumor suppressor genes
    p53, 30
    pRb, 30

Vaccine adverse event reporting system, 21
Vaccines/vaccinations
    adenovirus types 4 and 7, 10
    in AIDS patients
        vaccinia, 46
    CMV humoral immune response, 192
    hepatitis B
        childhood vaccinations, 537
        pathogenic mechanisms, 537
    hepatitis C
        development of, 544
    herpes B virus vaccine, 241, 242
    HSV vaccine, 102, 103
    HPV prophylactic vaccines, 287
    HPV therapeutic vaccines, 286
    Japanese encephalitis
        JE-VAX, 10
    Measles vaccine, 415
    Measles and rubella (MR) vaccine, 415, 526
    Measles, mumps, rubella vaccine (MMR), 415, 526
    monkeypox, 50
    papillomavirus vaccine, 286
    poliomyelitis
        Poliovax, 10

[Vaccines/vaccinations]
    IPOL, 10
        Orimune, 10
    rubella vaccination, 526, 415
    smallpox, 44, 48, 49
    varicella zoster vaccine, 134
    Yellow fever, 499
        YF-VAX, 10
Vaccinia, 4, 5, 44
    clinical manifestations, 45
    definition, 44
    differential diagnoses, 43
    elderly, 45–46
    future of, 47–48
    history, 45
    incidence, 44–45
    pathogenesis, 45
    transmission, 44
    vaccination complications, 45
    zoonotic implications, 44
Varicella, 3–4
Varicella-zoster virus (VZV), 13, 14, 119–144
    children
        chickenpox, 119, 122
        fetal complications, 123
        treatment for, 133
        varicella, 119
        zoster, 125, 126, 128
    clinical manifestations, 121–132
        varicella, 121–123
        zoster, 125–130
    complications of herpes zoster infection, 129–132
        elderly, 129
        immunocompromised, 132
        postherpetic neuralgia, 129
        pregnancy, 129
    complications of primary varicella infection, 122–124
        pregnancy, 123, 124
    definition, 119
    dermatopathology, 133
    differential diagnoses of herpes zoster, 130
    differential diagnoses of varicella, 123
    elderly, 45–46
    future of, 47–48
    Henoch-Schönlein and VZV, 123
    history, 45, 119
    Hutchinson's sign and VZV, 127
    incidence, 44–45, 119–120
    immunocompromised:
        bone marrow transplant, 120
        Hodgkin's disease, 120
        HIV, 121
    laboratory findings, 133
    ocular, 124
    pathogenesis, 45, 120, 121
    retinal necrosis, 132

[Varicella-zoster virus]
Reyes syndrome and VZV, 122
Streptococcus and VZV, 123
taxonomy, 120
transmission, 120
treatment of postherpetic neuralgia, 136–137
gabapentin, 137
topical, 137
tricyclic antidepressants, 136
treatment of varicella, 133, 134
antiviral, 134
treatment of zoster, 135–136
acyclovir, 135
famciclovir, 135
valacyclovir, 135
prevention of postherpetic neuralgia, 137
prevention of varicella, 134, 135
VZIG, 134–136
VZV vaccine (Oka), 134, 135
zoonotic implications, 120
Variola (smallpox), 4, 39–48
Venezuelan equine encephalitis (VEE), 508–512
clinical manifestations, 510, 511
definition, 508, 509
diagnosis, 511
differential diagnoses, 512
history, 509
incidence, 509, 510
laboratory findings, 511
mosquito vectors
Culex tarsalis, 509, 510
Aedes africans, 512
Aedes aegypti, 512
pathogenesis, 510
pathology, 511
related viruses, 512
Everglades virus, 512
Tonate mosquito fever, 512
Mucambo, 512
Pixuna, 512
Cabassous, 512
Semliki Forest, 512
transmission, 510
treatment/prophylaxis, 511, 512
zoonotic implications, 510
Viral exanthems, 3
Viral inclusion bodies, 4
Virology, cutaneous
clinical manifestations, 1–3
diagnosis, 3
microscopic examination, 3, 4
serology, 3, 4
viral antigen detection, 3, 4
viral cultures, 3
viral DNA or RNA detection, 3, 4
differential diagnoses, 5

[Virology]
DNA viruses (ds), 5, 6, 55
adenoviruses, 6
herpesviruses 1–8, 6, 12–16
papillomaviruses, 6, 8, 11, 12
parvoviruses, 6, 16–17
poxviruses, 5
DNA viruses (ss)
parvoviruses, 6
DNA/RNA reverse transcribing viruses, 6
hepatitis B, 6
HIV, 6, 19–20
RNA (ds), 6
coltivirus, 6
RNA (ss, negative), 6
Crimean-Congo, 7
Ebola, 7
Hantaan virus, 7
La Crosse, 7
measles, 6
mumps, 6
Rift Valley, 7
RNA (ss, positive)
enteroviruses, 7, 17
equine encephalitis, 7
flavivirus, 7
rubella, 7, 19
Varicella-zoster immune globulin (VZIG), 10, 134, 135
Varicella-zoster (VZV) vaccine (Oka), 134, 135

Warts
HPV infection and, 258
anogenital, 258, 262–264
Butcher's, 258
common, 258, 259, 260
condyloma acuminata, 11, 258, 262–264
destructive procedures, 284
flat, 258, 261, 278
filiform, 258, 260, 278
palmar, plantar, 11, 258, 261, 278
paronychial, 258, 259
Western equine encephalitis (WEE), 506–508
clinical manifestations, 507, 508
definition, 506
diagnosis, 508
differential diagnoses, 509
history, 506–507
incidence, 507
laboratory findings, 508
mosquito vectors:
Culex tarsalis, 507
Aedes melanimon, 507
pathogenesis, 507
pathology, 508
transmission, 507
treatment/prophylaxis, 508, 509
zoonotic implications, 507

West Nile fever virus, 1, 515
  symptoms, 515
  vectors, 515
World Health Organization (WHO)
  diagnostic criteria
    dengue fever (DHF), 479
    dengue shock syndrome (DSS), 479
  diagnostic criteria for DHF and DSS, 479
  eradication of rubella, 526
  HBV, 531
  measles, 404, 416
    eradication of, 404
    estimates of cases, 404
  monkeypox, 48
  smallpox, 41, 43, 44
  yellow fever, 496

Yellow fever, 495–499
  clinical manifestations, 497, 498
  definition, 495
  diagnosis, 499
  differential diagnoses, 498
  history, 496
  incidence, 496
  laboratory findings, 498
  pathogenesis, 496, 497
  pathology, 498
  transmission, 496
  treatment and prevention, 499
    YF-VAX, 10
  zoonotic implications, 496
Yersinia enterocolitica
  EBV and, 158

Zoonotic implications
  California/La Crosse encephalitis, 430
  Chikungunya fever (CHIK), 516
  cowpox, 50
  Crimean-Congo hemorrhagic fever, 440

[Zoonotic implications]
  cytomegalovirus (CMV), 174
  dengue fever, 474
  eastern equine encephalitis (EEE), 504
  Ebola virus, 422
  enteroviruses, 456
  Epstein-Barr virus (EBV; HHV-4), 146
  flaviviridae, 474
  hantaviruses, 434
  hepatitis B virus, 530
  hepatitis C virus, 538
  herpes B, 236
  herpes simplex viruses (HSV), 70
  human herpesvirus 6 (HHV-6), 198
  human herpesvirus 7 (HHV-7), 214
  human herpesvirus 8 (HHV-8), 220
  human papillomaviruses (HPV), 248
  Japanese encephalitis (JE), 481
  Kyasanur Forest disease (KFD), 484
  Lassa fever, 447
  Marburg virus, 422
  measles, 404
  molluscum contagiosum (MC), 60
  monkeypox, 49
  Omsk hemorrhagic fever, 487
  orf, 53
  parvovirus B19, 296
  pseudocowpox, 56
  Rift Valley fever, 443
  rubella, 520
  St. Louis encephalitis (SLE), 490
  smallpox, 41
  South American hemorrhagic fever, 447
  tanapox, 58
  tick-borne encephalitis (TBE), 492
  vaccinia, 44
  varicella-zoster virus (VZV), 120
  Venezuelan equine encephalitis (VEE), 510
  western equine encephalitis (WEE), 507
  yellow fever, 496